Geriatric Gastroenterology

C. S. Pitchumoni • T. S. Dharmarajan

Editors

Geriatric Gastroenterology

Second Edition

Volume 2

With 662 Figures and 499 Tables

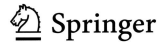

Springer

Editors
C. S. Pitchumoni
Department of Medicine
Robert Wood Johnson School
of Medicine
Rutgers University
New Brunswick, NJ, USA

Department of Medicine
New York Medical College
Valhalla, NY, USA

Division of Gastroenterology
Hepatology and Clinical Nutrition
Saint Peters University Hospital
New Brunswick, NJ, USA

T. S. Dharmarajan
Department of Medicine
Division of Geriatrics, Montefiore
Medical Center
Wakefield Campus
Bronx, NY, USA

Department of Medicine
Albert Einstein College of Medicine
Bronx, NY, USA

Department of Medicine
New York Medical College
Valhalla, NY, USA

ISBN 978-3-030-30191-0   ISBN 978-3-030-30192-7 (eBook)
ISBN 978-3-030-30193-4 (print and electronic bundle)
https://doi.org/10.1007/978-3-030-30192-7

This Springer imprint is published by the registered company Springer Nature Switzerland AG.
The registered company address is: Gewerbestrasse 11, 6330 Cham, Switzerland

Dedicated to my parents,
My wife Prema
And children Sheila, Shoba, and Suresh, and
Grandchildren Shreya, Salena, Tara, Ajay, and Aneel
For all their love and support

CSP

Dedicated to my mother,
My wife Lekshmi,
And Kumar, Kavita, Iyla, and Jaiya,
With much love and gratitude!

TSD

Foreword

I'll never forget the first time I met Professor C.S. Pitchumoni. It was 1997 and I was a fourth-year medical student still contemplating how to focus my career. I wanted to become a surgeon, but wasn't sure I could awaken before dawn for the rest of my working life. I liked psychiatry, but wasn't sure I could pursue a non-procedural specialty. I had not thought of gastroenterology as a career at that point, not for a nanosecond. Professor Pitchumoni changed all of that.

I attended one of Dr. Pitchumoni's lectures on irritable bowel syndrome where I came to realize that gastroenterology is, in fact, a curious hybrid between surgery and psychiatry. Here was this ebullient, articulate, engaging master clinician who held me spellbound with patient stories. He described the "brain-gut axis," explained that many people with IBS have concurrent psychosocial distress, yet also emphasized that some patients need a colonoscopy to rule out underlying organic disease. Gastroenterology, it seemed, required a deep and abiding knowledge about mind *and* body. I realized this was a field like no other, and I was being taught by a professor like no other.

There was something magical about this man. Something about how he entranced his audience, how he brought a topic like IBS to life, how he exuded expertise in biopsychosocial medicine, and how people could laugh hysterically at his unique humor while maintaining a serious focus on the material. To this day, Dr. Pitchumoni is the most effective teacher I have ever witnessed. I am here, writing this foreword, because he inspired me to become a gastroenterologist. Early in his academic career, Dr. Pitchumoni focused his research on pancreatic disorders, but his clinical interests always spanned across the entire spectrum of gastroenterology. In over five decades of his academic career, he has authored over 200 peer-reviewed papers and over 100 chapters in textbooks, in addition to editing 7 books.

If it weren't for C.S. Pitchumoni, I probably would be doing an appendectomy right now or rounding at 5:00 AM in the SICU. Instead, I am writing about a truly special man who has now co-authored a truly special second edition of his masterwork, *Geriatric Gastroenterology*.

Dr. Pitchumoni is joined by another master educator and co-author T.S. Dharmarajan, Professor of Medicine, Vice Chair of Medicine, and

Clinical Director of Geriatrics at Montefiore Medical Center (Wakefield Campus), Albert Einstein College of Medicine, Bronx, New York. Dr. Dharmarajan leads one of the largest hospital-based geriatric programs and geriatric medicine fellowships and has an extensive track record of exceptional scholarship in his burgeoning field. He has published over 200 papers, presented over 400 scientific abstracts, and has been a principal investigator for a wide range of impactful studies in geriatric medicine. Together with Dr. Pitchumoni, Dr. Dharmarajan has teamed up to publish a number of previous studies and textbooks, most notably the very successful first edition of the current text. Now, after their book became a best seller, this dynamic duo returns with their second edition to expand and further strengthen an extraordinary text.

One glance at the table of contents reveals an expansive treatment of geriatric gastroenterology. The text is organized into 15 parts and detailed in over one hundred authoritative chapters written by key opinion leaders. The book begins with a thoughtful overview of perspectives and trends, including views from both the geriatrician and gastroenterologist about the importance of understanding how age affects the digestive system. Next comes a detailed review of the relevant basic science and physiology of aging, with special reference to the alimentary canal, together with key facts and figures regarding the epidemiology of GI diseases. A comprehensive part on pharmacology follows, including a discussion about the pharmacology of aging, GI toxicities of special interest to the geriatric population, and drug-nutrient interactions – an area often underappreciated in traditional GI educational programs. The part on nutrition is of special interest given the expanding evidence that what we eat truly matters to GI health. Chapters in this part cover geriatric nutritional assessment, tube feeding and enteral nutrition, and peri-operative nutrition in geriatric populations; this part also contains a series of chapters on individual vitamin and mineral deficiencies, often prevalent yet underdiagnosed in senior populations. The book continues with careful treatments about the role of endoscopy in older adults, GI radiology considerations in the geriatric population, common motility disorders, and clinical approaches to prevalent symptoms, including abdominal pain, gas and bloating, constipation, and diarrhea, among others. Later parts offer deep discussions about hepatobiliary and pancreatic issues among seniors; common luminal disorders like peptic ulcer disease, intestinal ischemia, diverticular disease, and intestinal infections; and an expansive part on neoplasms. Appropriate for this volume, the book also includes a thoughtful part about palliative care considerations for the gastroenterologist.

This is a master work edited by two master clinicians who have dedicated their respective careers to educating the next generations (note the plural) of gastroenterologists and geriatricians. I count myself as one of the lucky students to have been inspired by these authors, who have supported and crafted many careers far beyond my own. I hope you enjoy reading this comprehensive and insightful book as much as I have enjoyed writing about it, and I thank the authors for giving me the opportunity of writing the foreword to their magisterial work.

American Journal of   Brennan Spiegel, MD, MSHS, FACG, AGAF
Gastroenterology   Co-Editor-in-Chief
Professor of Medicine
and Public Health
Cedars-Sinai Medical Center
Assistant Dean of Clinical and
Translational Research
David Geffen School of
Medicine at UCLA
Los Angeles, California
September 2020

Preface to Second Edition

We are pleased to present *Geriatric Gastroenterology*, the second edition and a Major Reference Work, a Springer publication. Although initially reluctant to take on what appeared to be an intimidating, massive venture, the considerable success of the first edition of *Geriatric Gastroenterology* published in 2012 has made a difference in encouraging us on. The first edition was a best seller in the Springer category of books, with over 150,000 chapter downloads, providing us the stimulus to move forward with this work. The entire work has been completed in about 3 years. Importantly, the final year of work was done amidst the COVID-19 pandemic. The final product far exceeded the initial plans of the editors in terms of content and scope of work.

Trends in global aging have focused attention on the manner in which we care for older adults, and we must be prepared to meet the demands of health-related disorders and societal concerns in our aging population. Most specialties, gastroenterology included, have increasingly promoted the blending of medical subspecialty training with expertise in the care of the older adult. The American Gastroenterology Association Future Trends Committee Report highlighted several years ago the areas for improvement in healthcare delivery, including the need to identify "best evidence-based care" for the older adult, to develop guidelines for care of specific gastrointestinal issues in geriatrics, to modify current practices to meet the complex needs of older individuals, and to adapt the healthcare workforce to meet the demands of specialized treatments in gastroenterology for older people.

As editors, specialized in gastroenterology and geriatric medicine, we believe in the concept of editing and writing material for textbooks to address the physiology, pathology, evaluation, and management of digestive disorders in older people. Too often, most clinical complaints are attributed to "old age" by patients and providers alike. Physicians must be better trained to discern physiological and pathological processes and distinguish healthy aging from the disease. Providers of care must understand the impact of polypharmacy and adverse drug events, which often mimic gastrointestinal disorders, and increase healthcare burden and costs. They need to be aware that the average older adult presenting with digestive disorders will likely manifest multiple comorbid diseases, some obvious and some hardly recognizable. And physicians must be focused and sensitive to ethical aspects of care the old. Effort has been made to limit (but not exclude) the term "elderly" and briefly address the controversies associated with the use of terms such as "elderly, older, and geriatric" individuals. We have preferentially used the term "older adults" in conformity with the current trends. This book attempts to clarify several challenging and controversial aspects related to the diagnosis and care of the geriatric individual.

The standard format adopted for the first edition has been retained. Most chapters begin with an introduction, followed by discussion, and conclude with key points. The concept of key points at the end of each chapter is retained as in the first edition. Numerous tables and figures present succinct accounts to emphasize content. Certain chapters are mostly pictorial and abundant on pictures focusing on endoscopy, radiography, dermatological disorders, and pathology relevant to gastroenterology. The book offers value to residents, fellows, nutritionists, and practicing physicians alike.

The current work differs in many ways from the first edition. As a major reference work, it has 50% more chapters, for a total of 105 and a page content well in excess of 2000, over three times the content of the first version. The parts have been altered and many chapters substantially enlarged in information. The parts of nutrition and pharmacology, both most relevant in the care of older adults, have been substantially broadened to include several relevant and new topics. The topic of medical ethics has been given due importance and also obesity in older adults, including bariatric surgery. Imaging and dermatology chapters are studded with illustrations that are succinctly explained. There is a marked increase in tables and figures, with many illustrations in color. Each chapter is preceded by an abstract which briefly describes its content. We did not hesitate to add a chapter on COVID-19, the hottest topic in medicine today, under the current circumstances. The popular "key points" that present bulleted themes regarding the entire text at the end of each chapter have been improved upon, based on the feedback received from readers of the first edition, who remarked that "if one is too busy to read the book, the least that an individual can do is to review the key points at the end of each chapter."

Although a major reference work, it is by no means all inclusive, yet offers a comprehensive range of chapters in the field of geriatric gastroenterology. Credit is due to two pioneers who wrote books on the field: *Gastrointestinal Disorders of the Elderly* by Lawrence J. Brandt, MD, and *Aging and the Gastrointestinal Tract* by Peter R. Holt, MD. The two provided the initial motivation for our efforts. We salute the numerous giants in the field of geriatrics: William R. Hazzard, Christine K. Cassel, Joseph G. Ouslander, Mary E. Tinetti, Laurence Z. Rubenstein, John E. Morley, and others; and in the field of Gastroenterology: Howard M. Spiro, Henry L. Bockus, Sir Francis Avery Jones, Dame Sheila Sherlock, Marvin H. Sleisenger, John S. Fordtran, Edward J. Berk, Lawrence R. Schiller, and others. These scholars blazed the trail for us to follow.

Special thanks are due to Dr. Brennan Spiegel who graciously agreed to write the foreword to the book. We are indebted to the numerous physicians and surgeons who contributed to the work and gave their precious time, which added tremendous value to the work. Their efforts during the COVID-19 pandemic have been remarkable, in that they responded favorably to our calls almost invariably.

Springer was supportive all along and instrumental in helping us formulate the concepts and implement the process to produce a major reference work. The staff was most helpful in the submission, e-proofing, and publication of each chapter throughout the editing process; their patience with the editors is highly appreciated. The Meteor system introduced by Springer was new to us and it took a while to comprehend its benefits. Both the editors had earlier written a series of articles on the theme of geriatric gastroenterology, and Springer was largely instrumental in bringing to fruition the concept of our initial textbook of geriatric gastroenterology in 2012. Springer followed by helping our dream of creating a major reference work for the current second edition come true to life.

We appreciate the tremendous support from members of our families, as always, throughout, for which we remain eternally grateful. Our families were a source of encouragement and inspiration; their patience, understanding, and sacrifices during the period are commendable.

As teachers and mentors, we acknowledge our students, residents, fellows, and professional colleagues in providing the stimulus to enrich our knowledge and clinical skills. But above all, we pay tribute to our older patients in community, hospital, and nursing home settings, from whom we have learnt so much and without whom we do not matter!

In this work, we have emphasized the importance of function, quality of life, and ethical aspects (besides the disease) in caring for the old. It is important to care, even if one cannot cure. We quote Abraham Lincoln: "And in the end, it's not the years in your life that count. It's the life in your years," and Jeanne Louise Calment (1875–1997), the oldest documented individual: "I had to wait 110 years to become famous; I wanted to enjoy it as long as possible."

C. S. Pitchumoni, MD
T. S. Dharmarajan, MD

Preface to the First Edition

Over the past several decades, trends in global aging have focused attention on the manner in which we care for older adults. How can we be best prepared to meet the demands of medical illness in our aging population? Many of the medical societies have increasingly promoted the blending of medical sub-specialty training with expertise in the care of the older adult. In this regard, the American Gastroenterologic Association Future Trends Committee Report recently highlighted several areas for improvement in health care delivery, including the need to identify 'best evidence-based care' for the older adult; to develop guidelines for care of specific gastrointestinal issues in geriatrics; to modify current practices in order to meet the complex needs of older individuals; and to adapt the healthcare workforce to meet the demands of specialized treatments in gastroenterology for older people. Until there are sufficient trained personnel in both geriatrics and gastroenterology, providers must handle the daunting task with knowledge gained in other ways.

As editors specialized in gastroenterology and geriatric medicine, we see the need for a textbook to address the physiology, pathology, evaluation and management of digestive disorders in the elderly. Too often, clinical complaints are attributed to 'old age' by patient and provider alike. Physicians must be better trained to discern physiological from pathological processes and normal aging from disease. Disorders such as constipation and diverticular disease are common in the old, but are they pathological, or the result of aging? As age is associated with immune dysfunction, the role of the gut in the elderly has become a subject of increasing importance. How should the age-related decline in homeostatic mechanisms, known as homeostenosis, alter medical care in the elderly? Added to the complex situation is the impact of polypharmacy and adverse drug events which often mimic gastrointestinal disorders, with increasing health care costs. How can we learn to be more focused and sensitive to these issues? This book attempts to clarity these challenging and controversial issues in the diagnosis and care of the geriatric individual.

A standard format has been adopted for this text, whereby most chapters conclude with key summary points. Numerous tables and figures are included to emphasize content. There are abundant pictures focusing on endoscopy, radiography and pathology. Several relevant gastrointestinal topics unique to the older person are included. We anticipate the book will be a valuable resource for residents, fellows, and practicing physicians alike. A section providing Questions with multiple choice Answers and brief discussions relating to the chapters is hosted in an electronic platform (Springer Extras); this may be an additional benefit particularly to residents and fellows in training.

This work is by no means all-inclusive, but does offer solid grounding in geriatric gastroenterology. It is also not the first text on the subject: the first comprehensive book was written in 1984 by Lawrence J. Brandt MD, Emeritus Chairman of Gastroenterology at Albert Einstein College of Medicine, entitled "Gastrointestinal Disorders of the Elderly." Tremendous credit is due to Peter R. Holt MD of Saint Luke's Hospital of New York-Presbyterian Medical Center for pioneering the concept of 'Aging and the Gastrointestinal Tract'. These two provided the initial motivation for our efforts. We salute as well many pioneers in the field of Geriatrics: William R. Hazzard, Christine K. Cassel, Joseph G. Ouslander, Mary E. Tinetti, Laurence Z. Rubenstein, John E. Morley, and others; and the field of Gastroenterology: Howard M. Spiro, Henry L. Bockus, Sir Francis Avery Jones, Dame Sheila Sherlock, Marvin H. Sleisenger, John S. Fordtran, Edward J. Berk, and others. All of these scholar-mentors in medicine paved the path for us to follow.

Special thanks are due to Martin H. Floch MD of Yale University, who has graciously provided the Foreword for the book. We are grateful to the many contributors who responded to our call and gave generously of their time to provide chapters for the book. Springer has been supportive from the start of this venture and throughout the editing process. Both of us wrote a series of articles over the past 15 years on the theme of geriatric gastroenterology, and Springer has been instrumental in bringing to fruition our dream of a textbook of geriatric gastroenterology.

Support and encouragement from our family was ever present, and for this we are eternally grateful. Our families were a source of strength and inspiration; their patience, understanding and sacrifices commendable. As teachers and mentors, we acknowledge our students, residents, fellows and professional colleagues for providing the opportunity to enrich our knowledge and clinical skills. And above all, we pay tribute to our older adult patients in community, hospital and nursing home settings, from whom we have learned so much.

It is our hope that this textbook serves as a resource towards fulfillment of a goal so aptly stated by Abraham Lincoln: "And in the end, it's not the years in your life that count. It's the life in your years."

C. S. Pitchumoni, MD
T. S. Dharmarajan, MD

Acknowledgments

The editors remain forever grateful and
acknowledge

All Authors for contributing
the many valuable chapters to this work

And

Vasowati Shome, Consultant, Major Reference Works,
Mohanapriya Caliamourthy, Project Manager,
Alexa Steele, Editor, Major Reference Work,
And all others at Springer
Who helped make this work happen!

Contents

About the Editors

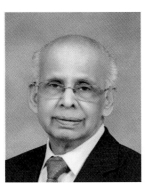

C. S. Pitchumoni MD, MPH, MACP, MACG, FRCPC, FRCPE, AGAF
Clinical Professor of Medicine, Robert Wood Johnson School of Medicine
Rutgers University, New Brunswick, NJ, USA
Adjunct Professor, New York Medical College, Valhalla, New York, USA
Emeritus Chief of the Division of Gastroenterology, Hepatology and Clinical Nutrition
Saint Peters University Hospital, New Brunswick, NJ, USA

Professor C.S. Pitchumoni is an acclaimed author, a dedicated teacher, a well-published researcher, and an editor of several popular books and prestigious journals in the field of clinical gastroenterology. For his many academic contributions spanning more than five decades at New York Medical College, Robert Wood Johnson School of Medicine, and Drexel University, Dr. Pitchumoni has the rare distinction of being recognized as a master of two leading professional organizations, the American College of Physicians as well as the American College of Gastroenterology. Medical students and residents in internal medicine and fellows in gastroenterology look up to Dr. Pitchumoni, or "Pitch," as they affectionately call him, fondly remember his guidance during the period of training and beyond for many decades. His mentors in gastroenterology at Yale and New York Medical College, Dr. Howard Spiro, Dr. Martin H Floch, and Dr. Gerzy B Glass, inculcated in him the value of hard work and readiness to share knowledge. Following his role models, he has no desire to retire from teaching and writing. True to his learning, Dr. Pitchumoni shares his knowledge and experience and continues to teach and help many students worldwide despite the COVID-19 pandemic restrictions.

Dr. Pitchumoni's publication of over 250 articles in major peer-reviewed journals and more than 100 chapters in the reputable textbooks are in addition to 7 edited books. A long period of six decades in academic medicine, Dr. Pitchumoni considers, is a boon to satisfy his desire to learn and teach. The return is his vast knowledge of internal medicine and gastroenterology.

Dr. Pitchumoni has received various awards and recognitions. The one award that he takes pride in is the recognition by students of Drexel University with the covetable Blockley-Osler award for excellence in teaching clinical medicine at bed side in the tradition of Sir William Osler. The Royal Colleges of Physicians of Ottawa, Canada, and the Royal College of Physicians of Edinburgh have honored Dr. Pichumoni as a fellow of the respective colleges.

Dr. Pitchumoni is board certified in internal medicine, gastroenterology, and clinical nutrition. The MPH qualification from New York Medical College substantially expands his broad knowledge in clinical medicine, clinical epidemiology, and research methods. With his professional experience at senior levels in teaching and administration for over 50 years, he is currently the emeritus chief of gastroenterology, hepatology, and clinical nutrition at Saint Peters University Hospital, Robert Wood Johnson School of Medicine; emeritus chairman of medicine at Our Lady of Mercy Medical Center of New York Medical College; adjunct Professor of medicine at New York Medical College; and clinical Professor of medicine at Rutgers University.

The initial publications that brought him to the academic forefront were focused on pancreatology; his pioneering work in the field is well quoted in the literature.

However, his passion was to be a general gastroenterologist, he expanded his interests to cover nutrition and geriatrics. The desire to emphasize the older adults' unique needs encouraged Dr. Pitchumoni to work closely with Professor Dharmarajan, a longtime professional colleague with a similar background and professional achievements. Both the editors, one with tremendous experience in the science of geriatrics and the other an experienced clinical gastroenterologist, perceived the need for a comprehensive book in geriatric gastroenterology. The success of the first edition of *Geriatric Gastroenterology* by Springer, which was released in 2012, prompted the authors to expand the book with many more chapters in the second edition. The editors expect the same enthusiastic reception for the second edition.

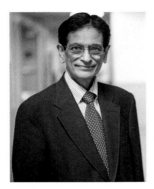

T. S. Dharmarajan MD, MACP, AGSF, FRCPE
Vice Chairman, Department of Medicine
Clinical Director, Division of Geriatrics
Program Director, Geriatric Medicine Fellowship Program
Montefiore Medical Center, Wakefield Campus, Bronx, NY, USA
Professor of Medicine, Albert Einstein College of Medicine, Bronx, NY, USA
Adjunct Professor of Medicine, New York Medical College, Valhalla, NY, USA

T. S. Dharmarajan, MD, is vice chairman, Department of Medicine; clinical director, Division of Geriatrics; and program director of the geriatric medicine fellowship program at Montefiore Medical Center (Wakefield Campus) Bronx, a University Hospital of Albert Einstein College of Medicine (AECOM), Bronx, New York. He is a Professor of medicine, AECOM, and adjunct Professor of medicine at New York Medical College. He was formerly Professor of medicine and Associate Dean of New York Medical College, Valhalla, New York, and chairman of the Department of Medicine at Our Lady of Mercy Medical Center, until its transition to Montefiore Medical Center.

Dr. Dharmarajan is certified by the American Boards in Internal Medicine, Nephrology and Geriatric Medicine. He is a fellow of the American Geriatrics Society (AGSF), Master of the American College of Physicians (MACP), and fellow of Royal College of Physicians, Edinburgh (FRCPE).

Dr. Dharmarajan was instrumental in developing a reputable inpatient geriatric medicine program at Our Lady of Mercy Medical Center in the Bronx (currently Montefiore Medical Center), with clinical, academic, and research components, including a fully accredited fellowship program (for 10 fellows) in geriatrics.

Dr. Dharmarajan co-edited the textbook *Clinical Geriatrics* (CRC Press/Parthenon Publishing) released in 2003. His second textbook, *Geriatric Gastroenterology* (Springer), co-edited with CS Pitchumoni, was released in July 2012. Dr. Dharmarajan authored several chapters in the two books. The latter was a best seller in the Springer category of textbooks. Based on its success, he co-edited *Geriatric Gastroenterology*, a Major Reference Work (Springer), a far more comprehensive work. His publications in peer-reviewed journals and textbooks number around 200. He has over 500 scientific presentations (abstracts) in county, state, national, and international conferences. He has been a principal investigator for several research projects, including national multicenter studies for the AMDA Foundation. He won the Howard Gutterman Award for best research project in the National Annual AMDA (2006) meeting; several of his abstracts were winners in county, state, or national society meetings. At Montefiore, he received the first prize for best clinical science paper published in 2016 and the second prize in 2019. He received a Lifetime Achievement Award at New York City in April 2019 and in the same year received Recognition for Leadership and Community Services from Montefiore at the tenth anniversary celebrations.

Dr. Dharmarajan is a regular speaker at local, national, and international conferences. Some of his many recognitions in medicine include: Teacher of the Year; Peer to Peer recognition by the Bronx County Society; Dedication as Teacher and Mentor to young Physicians in the Bronx (from American Assn. of Physicians of Indian origin); and Unparalleled Leadership in the Medical Community for medicine and research (from the Bronx County Society). In 2013, he was featured on the cover of *AgingWell* magazine, as one of five noteworthy geriatricians.

Dr. Dharmarajan was the president of the Montefiore Physician Council, Wakefield Campus, for 5 years until 2015; he was a member of the board of trustees at Our Lady of Mercy Medical Center.

For much of his professional career, Dr. Dharmarajan has been fortunate to be associated with a renowned colleague and master teacher, Professor CS Pitchumoni. During the period that spanned decades, the two initially published a series of articles in the field of geriatric gastroenterology, which caught Springer's attention, and became the foundation for the first edition of *Geriatric Gastroenterology*. The huge success of the first edition laid the platform for the more comprehensive second edition of *Geriatric Gastroenterology*, the current Major Reference Work.

Contributors

Hamzah Abu-Sbeih Department of Gastroenterology, Hepatology and Nutrition, The University of Texas MD Anderson Cancer Center, Houston, TX, USA

Ritu Agarwal Division of Liver Diseases, The Mount Sinai Hospital, Icahn School of Medicine, New York, NY, USA

Nanakram Agarwal New York Medical College, Valhalla, NY, USA
Montefiore Medical Center, Bronx, NY, USA

Gaurav Aggarwal GA Bellevue Medical Center, Bellevue, WA, USA
Division of Epidemiology, Mayo Clinic, Rochester, MN, USA

Joseph J. Alukal Mercy Medical Center, Institute of Digestive Health and Liver Diseases, Baltimore, MD, USA

Judith K. Amorosa Robert Wood Johnson School of Medicine, Rutgers University, New Brunswick, NJ, USA
Faculty Development and Academic Affairs, Department of Radiology, RUTGERS Robert Wood Johnson Medical School, Rutgers University, New Brunswick, NJ, USA
University Radiology Group, East Brunswick, NJ, USA

Allen Andrade Brookdale Department of Geriatrics and Palliative Care, Icahn School of Medicine at Mount Sinai, New York, NY, USA

Krishna P. Aparanji Department of Critical Care Medicine, Springfield Clinic, Springfield, IL, USA
Southern Illinois University School of Medicine, Springfield, IL, USA

Kellie Arita Lauren Cornell Nutrition, Inc., Los Angeles, CA, USA

Harry R. Aslanian Yale University School of Medicine, New Haven, CT, USA

Nilesh N. Balar New York Medical College, Valhalla, NY, USA
Department of Surgery, St. Michael's Medical Center, Newark, NJ, USA

Lorraine Bonkowski Adult Liver Transplant/Hepatology Clinic, Michigan Medicine, Ann Arbor, MI, USA

Arkady Broder Division of Gastroenterology and Hepatology, Saint Peter's University Hospital – Rutgers Robert Wood Johnson School of Medicine, New Brunswick, NJ, USA

Marco A. Bustamante Bernal Department of Internal Medicine, Texas Tech University Health Science Center, El Paso, TX, USA

Department of Internal Medicine, Division of Gastroenterology, Texas Tech University Health Science Center, El Paso, TX, USA

Naga P. Chalasani Division of Gastroenterology and Hepatology, Indiana University School of Medicine, Indianapolis, IN, USA

Suresh T. Chari Department of Gastroenterology, Hepatology and Nutrition, Division of Internal Medicine, The University of Texas MD Anderson Cancer Center, Houston, TX, USA

Abhijeet Chaubal Department of Anatomic Pathology, Saint Peters University Hospital, New Brunswick, NJ, USA

Rahul Chaudhari University of Pennsylvania Health System, Philadelphia, PA, USA

Luis O. Chavez Department of Internal Medicine, Texas Tech University Health Science Center, El Paso, TX, USA

Mario Cherubino Department of Biotechnology and Life Sciences, University of Insubria, Varese, Italy

Jennifer Chuy Department of Medical Oncology, Montefiore Medical Center, Bronx, NY, USA

Steven R. Cohen Department of Medicine, Division of Dermatology, Albert Einstein College of Medicine and Montefiore Medical Center, Bronx, NY, USA

Elise Marie Collins Chakra Tonics Inc., San Francisco, CA, USA

Eugene C. Corbett Jr Division of General Medicine, Geriatrics and Palliative Care, University of Virginia Health Science Center, Charlottesville, VA, USA

Lauren Cornell Lauren Cornell Nutrition, Inc., Los Angeles, CA, USA

Nicholas J. Costable Department of Internal Medicine, Icahn School of Medicine at Mount Sinai, New York, NY, USA

Jaime de la Fuente Division of Gastroenterology and Hepatology, Mayo Clinic College of Medicine and Sciences, Rochester, MN, USA

Gopal Desai Department of Radiation Oncology, Saint Peters University Hospital, New Brunswick, NJ, USA

Mitesh A. Desai Centers for Disease Control and Prevention, Atlanta, GA, USA

Alana Deutsch Department of Medicine, Division of Dermatology, Albert Einstein College of Medicine and Montefiore Medical Center, Bronx, NY, USA

Jill K. Deutsch Section of Digestive Diseases – Department of Internal Medicine, Yale University School of Medicine – Yale New Haven Hospital, New Haven, CT, USA

Kumar Dharmarajan Clover Health, Jersey City, NJ, USA

Yale School of Medicine, New Haven, CT, USA

T. S. Dharmarajan Department of Medicine, Division of Geriatrics, Montefiore Medical Center, Wakefield Campus, Bronx, NY, USA

Department of Medicine, Albert Einstein College of Medicine, Bronx, NY, USA

Department of Medicine, New York Medical College, Valhalla, NY, USA

Nicolle Dickey Boise State University, Boise, ID, USA

Pietro G. di Summa Department of Surgery, Centre Hospitalier Universitaire Vaudois (CHUV), Lausanne, Switzerland

Bethany Doerfler Northwestern Medicine, Division of Gastroenterology and Hepatology, Digestive Health Center, Chicago, IL, USA

Lindsay Dowhan Hoag Cleveland Clinic, Center for Gut Rehabilitation and Transplantation, Cleveland, OH, USA

Douglas A. Drossman Division of Gastroenterology and Hepatology, University of North Carolina, Center for Education and Practice of Biopsychosocial Care and Drossman Gastroenterology PLLC, Chapel Hill, NC, USA

Anwar Dudekula Division of Gastroenterology and Hepatology, Department of Internal Medicine, Saint Peter's University Hospital/Rutgers-RWJ Medical School, New Brunswick, NJ, USA

Geoffrey P. Dunn Depaertment of Surgery, UPMC Hamot, Erie, PA, USA

Lucia C. Fry Department of Gastroenterology, Helios Frankenwaldklinik, Kronach, Germany

Department of Geriatrics, Helios Frankenwaldklinik, Kronach, Germany

Chiranjeevi Gadiparthi Division of Gastroenterology and Hepatology, Saint Peter's University Hospital, New Brunswick, NJ, USA

Salvatore Giordano Department of Surgery, Vaasa Central Hospital, and University of Turku, Turku, Finland

---

Geoffrey P. Dunn has retired.

Roy J. Goldberg Division of Geriatrics, Albert Einstein College of Medicine, Bronx, NY, USA

Kings Harbor Multicare Center, Bronx, NY, USA

Debra R. Goldstein Department of Gastroenterology, Saint Peters University Hospital, New Brunswick, NJ, USA

Rutgers University School of Medicine, New Brunswick, NJ, USA

Maria Fernanda Gomez Department of Psychiatry and Behavioral Sciences, Montefiore Medical Center, Albert Einstein College of Medicine, Bronx, NY, USA

Rafael Gonzalez Alonso Department of Psychiatry and Behavioral Sciences, Montefiore Medical Center, Albert Einstein College of Medicine, Bronx, NY, USA

Rebecca Goodrich DaVita Kidney Care, Santa Monica, CA, USA

Pavel Goriacko Center for Pharmacotherapy Research and Quality, Department of Pharmacy, Montefiore Medical Center, Bronx, NY, USA

David Y. Graham Department of Medicine, Michael E. DeBakey Veterans Affairs Medical Center, and Baylor College of Medicine, Houston, TX, USA

David A. Greenwald Department of Internal Medicine, Division of Gastroenterology, Icahn School of Medicine at Mount Sinai, New York, NY, USA

Julia B. Greer Division of Gastroenterology, Hepatology and Nutrition, Department of Medicine, University of Pittsburgh School of Medicine, Pittsburgh, PA, USA

Rasim Gucalp Department of Medical Oncology, Montefiore Medical Center, Bronx, NY, USA

Vineet Gudsoorkar Lynda K and David M Underwood Center for Digestive Disorders, Division of Gastroenterology and Hepatology, Houston Methodist Hospital, Houston, TX, USA

Srinivas Guptha Gunturu Advanced Endoscopy, Gastroenterology, Phoebe-Putney Memorial Health System, Albany, GA, USA

Emily Haller Division of Gastroenterology and Hepatology, Michigan Medicine, Ann Arbor, MI, USA

Elizabeth Hames Kiran Patel College of Osteopathic Medicine, Nova Southeastern University, Fort Lauderdale, FL, USA

Barbara Hammaker Department of Dental Hygiene, Broward College, Davie, FL, USA

Noam Harpaz Department of Pathology, Molecular and Cell-Based Medicine, Icahn School of Medicine at Mount Sinai, New York, NY, USA

Mary S. Haumschild St. Petersburg College, St. Petersburg, Florida, USA
Bachelors Health Services Administration, State College of Florida, Bradenton, FL, USA

R. Ann Hays Division of Gastroenterology, University of Virginia, Charlottesville, VA, USA

Hilary Hertan Montefiore Medical Center-Wakefield Campus, The Bronx, NY, USA

T. Patrick Hill Edward J. Bloustein School of Planning and Public Policy, Rutgers University, New Brunswick, NJ, USA

David Hirschl Albert Einstein College of Medicine, Montefiore Medical Center, Bronx, NY, USA

Andrew Ho Division of Gastroenterology and Hepatology, Stanford University School of Medicine, Stanford, CA, USA
Division of Gastroenterology and Hepatology, Santa Clara Valley Medical Center, San Jose, CA, USA

Lisa C. Hutchison College of Pharmacy and College of Medicine, University of Arkansas for Medical Sciences, Little Rock, AR, USA

Kelly Issokson Cedars-Sinai, Digestive Diseases Center, Los Angeles, CA, USA

Prasad G. Iyer Division of Gastroenterology and Hepatology, Mayo Clinic, Rochester, MN, USA

Vishal Jain Coastal Gastroenterology Associates, Brick, NJ, USA

Mahesh Jhurani Kings Harbor Multicare Center, Bronx, NY, USA

Charles J. Kahi Roudebush VA Medical Center, Indiana University School of Medicine, Indianapolis, IN, USA

Holly Kanavy Department of Medicine, Division of Dermatology, Albert Einstein College of Medicine and Montefiore Medical Center, Bronx, NY, USA

Seymour Katz Department of Medicine Gastroenterology Division, New York University School of Medicine, New York, NY, USA

Natalia Khalaf Department of Medicine, Michael E. DeBakey Veterans Affairs Medical Center, and Baylor College of Medicine, Houston, TX, USA

Abraham Khan Division of Gastroenterology. Department of Medicine, NYU Langone Health, NYU School of Medicine, New York, NY, USA

Rita M. Knotts Division of Gastroenterology. Department of Medicine, NYU Langone Health, NYU School of Medicine, New York, NY, USA

Maanit Kohli Division of Hospital Medicine, Department of Medicine, Icahn School of Medicine at Mount Sinai, New York, NY, USA

Andrew Korman Division of Gastroenterology and Hepatology, Saint Peter's University Hospital, New Brunswick, NJ, USA

Noah Kornblum Department of Medical Oncology, Montefiore Medical Center, Bronx, NY, USA

Steven Krawitz VA New Jersey Health Care System, East Orange VA Medical Center, East Orange, NJ, USA

Jessica Lebovits Irving Medical Center, Columbia University, New York, NY, USA

Yingheng Liu Department of Medicine, Division of Gastroenterology and Hepatology, Mount Sinai Beth Israel, New York, NY, USA

D. Lourdusamy Geriatrics, Montefiore Medical Center, Bronx, NY, USA

Jorge D. Machicado Division of Gastroenterology and Hepatology, Mayo Clinic Health System, Eau Claire, WI, USA

Shounak Majumder Division of Gastroenterology and Hepatology, Mayo Clinic College of Medicine and Sciences, Rochester, MN, USA

Ashish Malhotra Department of Gastroenterology and Hepatology, Seton Hall University of Health and Medical Sciences, Paterson, NJ, USA

Mohandas K. Mallath Department of Digestive Diseases, Tata Medical Center, Kolkata, India

Fernanda Samara Mazzariol Radiology, New York Presbyterian Hospital/ Weill Cornell Medicine, New York, NY, USA

Richard W. McCallum Department of Internal Medicine, Texas Tech University Health Science Center, El Paso, TX, USA

Department of Internal Medicine, Division of Gastroenterology, Texas Tech University Health Science Center, El Paso, TX, USA

Ethan D. Miller Department of Gastroenterology, Hepatology and Nutrition, The University of Texas MD Anderson Cancer Center, Houston, TX, USA

Sidharth P. Mishra Department of Internal Medicine- Molecular Medicine, Wake Forest School of Medicine, Winston-Salem, NC, USA

Sonmoon Mohapatra Division of Gastroenterology and Hepatology, Saint Peter's University Hospital – Rutgers Robert Wood Johnson School of Medicine, New Brunswick, NJ, USA

Klaus Mönkemüller Department of Gastroenterology, Helios Frankenwaldklinik, Kronach, Germany

Otto-von-Guericke University, Magdeburg, Germany

University of Belgrade, Belgrade, Serbia

Melanie Moses Albert Einstein College of Medicine, Montefiore Medical Center, Bronx, NY, USA

Thiruvengadam Muniraj Yale University School of Medicine, New Haven, CT, USA

Mandakolathur R. Murali Division of Rheumatology, Allergy and Clinical Immunology, Department of Medicine, Massachusetts General Hospital and Harvard Medical School, Boston, MA, USA

Sajan Nagpal University of Chicago, Chicago, IL, USA

Murali D. Nair Suzanne Dworak-Peck School of Social work, University of Southern California, Los Angeles, CA, USA

Satheesh Nair Medical Director of Liver Transplantation, Endowed Chair of Excellence in Transplant Medicine, University of Tennessee Health Science Center, Memphis, TN, USA

Shreya Narayanan Morsani College of Medicine, University of South Florida, Tampa, FL, USA

Carolyn Newberry Innovative Center for Health and Nutrition in Gastroenterology, Weill Cornell Medical Center, New York, NY, USA

Tam H. Nguyen Larkin Community Hospital, Miami, FL, USA

Mumtaz Niazi Department of Medicine, Division of Gastroenterology and Hepatology, Rutgers University, New Jersey Medical School, Newark, NJ, USA

Michael J. Nissenblatt Regional Cancer Care Associates, East Brunswick, NJ, USA

Robert A. Norman Center for Geriatric Dermatology, Integrative Dermatology and Neuro-Dermatology, Nova Southeastern University, Tampa, FL, USA

Custon Nyabanga Department of Medicine, NYU Langone Health, NYU School of Medicine, New York, NY, USA

Mary Alice O'Dowd Department of Psychiatry and Behavioral Sciences, Montefiore Medical Center, Albert Einstein College of Medicine, Bronx, NY, USA

Juan J. Omana Adventhealth, Kissimmee, FL, USA

Carlo M. Oranges Department of Surgery, Geneva University Hospital, Geneva, Switzerland

Rona Orentlicher Albert Einstein College of Medicine, Montefiore Medical Center, Bronx, NY, USA

Sangeetha Pabolu Saint Peters University Hospital, New Brunswick, NJ, USA

Jennifer Pan Division of Gastroenterology and Hepatology, Stanford University School of Medicine, Stanford, CA, USA

Division of Gastroenterology and Hepatology, Veterans Affairs Palo Alto Medical Center, Palo Alto, CA, USA

Naushira Pandya Kiran Patel College of Osteopathic Medicine, Nova Southeastern University, Fort Lauderdale, FL, USA

Sanjiv K. Patankar Colon and Rectal Surgery, Colon and Rectal Surgeons of Central New Jersey, East Brunswick, NJ, USA

Trupal Patel American University of Antigua COM MSIV University of Florida, B.S. Biology, Gainesville, FL, USA

Carlos A. Pelaez Iowa Methodist Medical Center, Des Moines, IA, USA

Carver College of Medicine, University of Iowa, Iowa City, IA, USA

Frederick B. Peng Department of Medicine, Baylor College of Medicine, Houston, TX, USA

Gloria Petersen Department of Health Sciences Research, Mayo Clinic, Rochester, MN, USA

Octavia Pickett-Blakely GI Nutrition, Obesity and Celiac Disease Program, University of Pennsylvania Perelman School of Medicine, Perelman Center for Advanced Medicine, Philadelphia, PA, USA

Rodolfo Pigalarga GastroHealth, Miami, FL, USA

Ileana Pino School of Health Sciences, Miami Dade College Medical Campus, Miami, FL, USA

C. S. Pitchumoni Department of Medicine, Robert Wood Johnson School of Medicine, Rutgers University, New Brunswick, NJ, USA

Department of Medicine, New York Medical College, Valhalla, NY, USA

Division of Gastroenterology, Hepatology and Clinical Nutrition, Saint Peters University Hospital, New Brunswick, NJ, USA

Amanda J. Podolski Department of Medical Oncology, Montefiore Medical Center, Bronx, NY, USA

Nikolaos Pyrsopoulos Department of Medicine, Division of Gastroenterology and Hepatology, Physiology, Pharmacology and Neuroscience, Medical Director Liver Transplantation, Rutgers – New Jersey Medical School, University Hospital, Newark, NJ, USA

Eamonn M. M. Quigley Lynda K and David M Underwood Center for Digestive Disorders, Division of Gastroenterology and Hepatology, Houston Methodist Hospital, Houston, TX, USA

Waqar Qureshi Section of Gastroenterology and Hepatology, Department of Medicine, Baylor College of Medicine, Houston, TX, USA

Mohammad Raoufi Department of Pathology and Laboratory Medicine, Henry Ford Health System, Detroit, MI, USA

Adharsh Ravindran Department of Internal Medicine, University at Buffalo, Buffalo, NY, USA

Nishal Ravindran Robert Wood Johnson School of Medicine, Rutgers University, New Brunswick, NJ, USA
Saint Peters University Hospital, New Brunswick, NJ, USA

Eduardo Redondo-Cerezo Endoscopy Unit. Gastroenterology Department, 'Virgen de las Nieves' University Hospital, Granada, Spain

Douglas K. Rex Indiana University School of Medicine, Indianapolis, IN, USA

Marnie E. Rosenthal Department of Medicine, St. Peter's University Hospital and Rutgers Robert Wood Johnson Medical School, New Brunswick, NJ, USA

Abbas Rupawala Alpert Medical School of Brown University, Providence, RI, USA

Negar M. Salehomoum Department of Surgery, John Muir Medical Center, Walnut Creek, CA, USA

Avishkar Sbharwal Hackensack University Medical Center, Hackensack, NJ, USA

Kate Scarlata For a Digestive Peace of Mind, LLC., Medway, MA, USA

Lawrence R. Schiller Baylor University Medical Center, Dallas, TX, USA
Texas A&M College of Medicine, Dallas Campus, Dallas, TX, USA

Courtney Schuchmann Section of Gastroenterology, Hepatology and Nutrition, University of Chicago Medicine, Chicago, IL, USA

Samir A. Shah Alpert Medical School of Brown University, Providence, RI, USA
Gastroenterology Associates Inc, The Miriam Hospital, Providence, RI, USA

Edward Sheen Division of Gastroenterology and Hepatology, Stanford University School of Medicine, Stanford, CA, USA

Pratik A. Shukla Department of Radiology, Division of Interventional Radiology, Rutgers University, New Jersey Medical School, Newark, NJ, USA

Dhruv P. Singh Department of Gastroenterology, Mayo Clinic, Rochester, MN, USA

Amit Sohagia Twin River Gastroenterology Center, Easton, PA, USA

Christina Surawicz Division of Gastroenterology, University of Washington, Seattle, WA, USA

Paul J. Thuluvath Mercy Medical Center, Institute of Digestive Health and Liver Diseases, Baltimore, MD, USA

Department of Medicine, University of Maryland School of Medicine, Baltimore, MD, USA

George Triadafilopoulos Division of Gastroenterology and Hepatology, Stanford University School of Medicine, Stanford, CA, USA

Chung Sang Tse Alpert Medical School of Brown University, Providence, RI, USA

Keith T. Veltri Touro College of Pharmacy, New York, NY, USA

Montefiore Medical Center, Bronx, NY, USA

Rajanshu Verma Division of Transplant Hepatology, University of Tennessee Health Science Center, Memphis, TN, USA

Cynthia L. Vuittonet Director of Addiction Medicine, Jewish Renaissance Medical Center, Perth Amboy, NJ, USA

Jonathan B. Wallach Department of Radiation Oncology, Saint Peter's University Hospital, New Brunswick, NJ, USA

David Widjaja Bogor Senior Hospital, Bogor, Indonesia

Katherine Woods St. Petersburg College, Pinellas Park, FL, USA

Dhiraj Yadav Division of Gastroenterology, Hepatology and Nutrition, Department of Medicine, University of Pittsburgh School of Medicine, Pittsburgh, PA, USA

Hariom Yadav Department of Internal Medicine- Molecular Medicine, Wake Forest School of Medicine, Winston-Salem, NC, USA

Osman Yilmaz Alpert Medical School of Brown University, Providence, RI, USA

Hongfa Zhu Hackensack Pathology Associates, Hackensack University Medical Center, Hackensack, NJ, USA

Gastrointestinal Endoscopy: Considerations

37

Klaus Mönkemüller and Lucia C. Fry

Contents

K. Mönkemüller (✉)
Department of Gastroenterology, Helios
Frankenwaldklinik, Kronach, Germany

Otto-von-Guericke University, Magdeburg, Germany

University of Belgrade, Belgrade, Serbia
e-mail: moenkemueller@yahoo.com

L. C. Fry
Department of Gastroenterology, Helios
Frankenwaldklinik, Kronach, Germany

Department of Geriatrics, Helios Frankenwaldklinik,
Kronach, Germany

© Springer Nature Switzerland AG 2021
C. S. Pitchumoni, T. S. Dharmarajan (eds.), *Geriatric Gastroenterology*,
https://doi.org/10.1007/978-3-030-30192-7_31

Abstract

Despite the increasing percentage of the older population, there is still little literature on gastrointestinal endoscopy in this patient group. Importantly, because of population demographics, the use of endoscopy is expected to rise in this section of the population worldwide. Older adults represent a special group, as aging results in changes in pathophysiology of the gastrointestinal tract. A substantial significant percentage of geriatric patients suffer from comorbid diseases. The spectrum of gastrointestinal disorders differs from that in younger patients and the elderly are, in general, more susceptible to complications from therapeutic endoscopic interventions. Indeed, due to the decreased physiologic reserve and associated diseases, complications in this age group tend to be more severe than in subjects younger than 65 years. Moreover, ethical considerations play a special role in frail patients with a potential poor prognosis, where the indication for endoscopy may be correct, but conducting endoscopy may not lead to a better prognosis. Thus, the endoscopist needs to pay special attention to the geriatric patient, indication and potential benefit when considering or performing endoscopy.

In this chapter, we review the role of endoscopy in the geriatric patient, with emphasis on the perioperative period, including pre-endoscopic assessment, management of anticoagulants, sedation, endoscopic procedures, and post-endoscopic care.

Keywords

Endoscopy · Older adults · Elderly · Extreme elderly · Octogenarians · Anticoagulation · Sedation · Endoscopic retrograde cholangiopancreatography · Colonoscopy · Esophagogastroduodenoscopy · Gastrointestinal · Enteroscopy

Introduction

The use of diagnostic and therapeutic gastrointestinal endoscopy in geriatric patients is increasing (ASGE Standards of Practice Committee et al. 2013; Lippert et al. 2015; Mönkemüller et al. 2009; Jafri et al. 2010; Cangemi et al. 2015). The increase is the result of safer techniques, advances in equipment, and more importantly, a change in population demographics (https://data.worldbank.org/indicator/sp.pop.65up.to.zs). Indeed, in countries such as Germany and Japan, the percentage of population over 65 years is over 20% and those over 85 comprise 3–5% (https://data.worldbank.org/indicator/sp.pop.65up.to.zs; https://www.census.gov/prod/cen2010/briefs/c2010br-09.pdf). In the USA in the year 2010, 40.3 million people (13% of the total population) were 65 years of age and older, and 5.5 million were aged 85 years and older (https://data.worldbank.org/indicator/sp.pop.65up.to.zs; https://www.census.gov/prod/cen2010/briefs/c2010br-09.pdf). By the year 2030, the percentage of individuals 65 years and older is expected to increase to more than 20% of the total US population (https://data.worldbank.org/indicator/sp.pop.65up.to.zs; https://www.census.gov/prod/cen2010/briefs/c2010br-09.pdf).

Essentially, any type of gastrointestinal endoscopy can be performed in geriatric patients (ASGE Standards of Practice Committee et al. 2013; Lippert et al. 2015; Mönkemüller et al. 2009; Jafri et al. 2010; Cangemi et al. 2015; Qumseya et al. 2014; Cha et al. 2016; Obana et al. 2010).

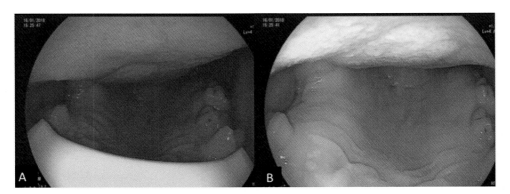

Fig. 1 Poor dentition is a common problem in elderly patients. Both images show lack of teeth (**a, b**)

Paradoxically, some complex procedures such as endoscopic retrograde cholangiopancreatography (ERCP) are associated with fewer complications in the older age group compared to those younger (Obana et al. 2010). Nevertheless, elderly patients are more prone to complications related to sedation and most interventional endoscopies (Ukkonen et al. 2016; Finkelmeier et al. 2015; Gómez et al. 2014; Warren et al. 2009; Katsinelos et al. 2006). Furthermore, as geriatric patients often have multiple comorbidities and changes in physiologic status, most complications intend to be more catastrophic. Thus, the clinician considering an endoscopic intervention and the endoscopist performing it must pay close attention to the indication and carefully consider the pros and cons of any invasive procedure in this group of patients. Indeed, the "ethical, clinical and therapeutic consequence" of any given intervention is the key factor determining the need for gastrointestinal endoscopy in the elderly (Lieberman et al. 2012; DeLegge et al. 2005).

Thus, it is evident that gastrointestinal endoscopy in older adults is a part of gastroenterology and gerontology that requires the clinician to pay closer attention to detail and focus on the pros and cons of the investigation with careful judgment.

Gastrointestinal Tract in the Elderly

Before embarking on the spectrum of gastrointestinal endoscopic procedures, it is important to briefly review key pathophysiologic aspects of the gastrointestinal tract in aging patients (Durazzo et al. 2017; Thomson 2009; Azzolino et al. 2019).

Oropharynx

The use of dental prosthesis is much more prevalent; additionally, poor dentition remains a problem. This leads to chewing, maldigestive, and nutritional problems. These patients often develop vitamin deficiencies, such as folate- and B12-deficiency-related megaloblastic anemia, which in turn cause glossitis and mouth pain, thus decreasing alimentary intake. Poor dentition is a common problem in these patients (Fig. 1).

Esophagus

The elderly are more prone to suffer from dysmotility disorders of the esophagus, such as achalasia (Grande et al. 1999; Schechter et al. 2011) (Fig. 2). In addition, due to decreased immune system response and the presence of comorbidities that affect the immune system such as diabetes mellitus, vasculitis, and rheumatoid disorders requiring immunomodulating agents, patients often present with candida esophagitis (Weerasuriya and Snape 2008) (Fig. 3). Furthermore, neurodegenerative disorders such as Parkinson's disease and dementia often lead to oropharyngeal dysphagia and esophageal dysmotility (Sung et al. 2010; Wirth et al. 2016).

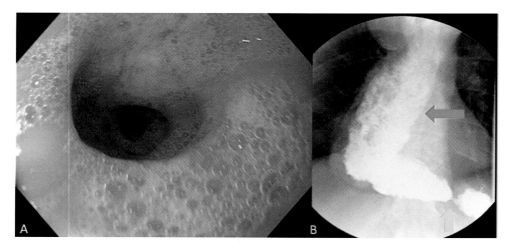

Fig. 2 Achalasia is more commonly found in elderly patients. Panel (**a**) shows the typical findings of hyper-contracted esophagus with lots of saliva in the lumen, which does not advance to the stomach due to hypocontractility (**a**). Panel **b** shows a massively dilated esophagus (red arrow) with the bird-beak appearance of the distal esophagus (yellow arrow)

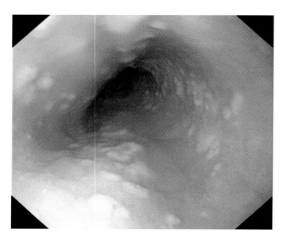

Fig. 3 Candida esophagitis with typical cottage cheese-like deposits on the mucosa

In these cases, the indication for endoscopy (i.e., dysphagia) may be correct, but conducting an endoscopy may not be indicated at all, as the oropharyngeal dysphagia should be evaluated first using other noninvasive means.

Because of decreased chewing capability and the presence of dental prosthesis, older patients sometimes present with acute foreign body dysphagia or accidentally swallowed prosthesis or tooth-bridges (Fig. 4).

Other esophageal diseases that are much more common include Zenker's diverticulum and huge hiatal hernias with upside-down stomachs (Al-Kadi et al. 2010; Treskatsch et al. 2013; Gryglewski et al. 2016) (Figs. 5 and 6). It is not uncommon for these stomachs located inside of the thoracic cavity to compress on the heart and lead to arrhythmias and chest pains. Lastly, esophageal cancer is seen more frequently in patients over the age of 65 years. Indeed, for different types of esophageal cancer, the risk increases with age, with a mean age at diagnosis of 67 years (Drahos et al. 2016) (Fig. 7).

Stomach

Table 1 shows various changes occurring in the stomach, including reduced acid production, gastric atrophy, and disturbed motility. Chronic infection with *H. pylori* leads to chronic atrophic gastritis (Watari et al. 2014). Autoimmune gastritis and pernicious anemia are much more common (Fig. 8) (Murphy et al. 2015; Kuipers 2015; Carmel 1996). Due to mucosal and immunomodulation changes, the stomach of patients older than 65 years of age is more prone to suffer damage from nonsteroidal anti-inflammatory

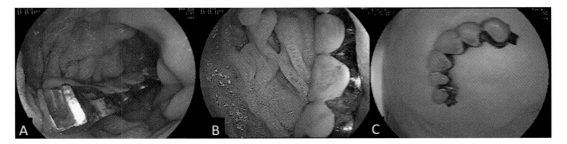

Fig. 4 Accidentally swallow endoprosthesis or tooth-bridges. (**a**) Prothesis in the jejunum. (**b**) The patient received intravenous glucagon to decrease small bowel motility, while the endoscopist utilized a snare to catch the dentures. (**c**) Dentures successfully removed

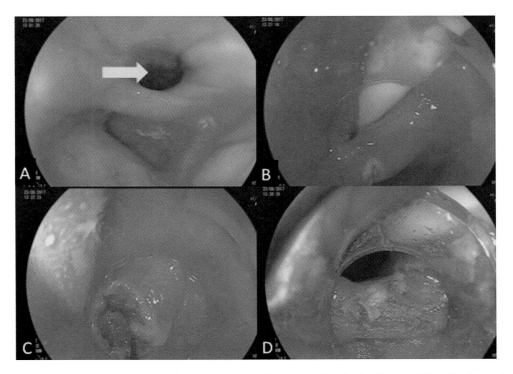

Fig. 5 This image shows the typical endoscopic appearance of a Zenker's diverticulum. (**a**) The yellow arrow shows the esophageal lumen, the diverticulum is in the back. (**b**) Endoscopic resection of the diverticulum. (**c**) The septum is incised with a special needle. We prefer to use a hook knife needle. (**d**) Complete transection of the septum

agents, including peptic ulcer related hemorrhage (Higuchi et al. 2014; Lanza et al. 2009) (Fig. 9). Large hiatal hernias with Cameron lesions are also more common in this age group (Fig. 10). The reason for the higher prevalence of large para-esophageal hiatal hernias with erosions leading to occult blood loss and anemia in the old remain unknown. Neoplasia of the stomach such as adenocarcinomas, lymphomas, and neuroendocrine tumors are also more common in the geriatric population (Kuipers 2015; Cui et al. 2017; Modlin et al. 2003) (Fig. 11).

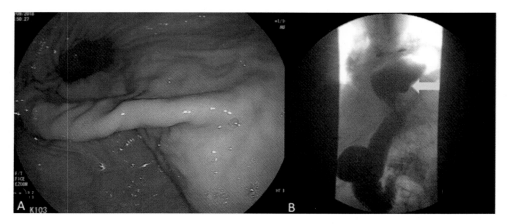

Fig. 6 Huge hiatal hernia with upside-down stomach. (**a**) Endoscopic view. (**b**) Radiologic view showing the upside-down stomach. The arrow shows the antrum inside the chest

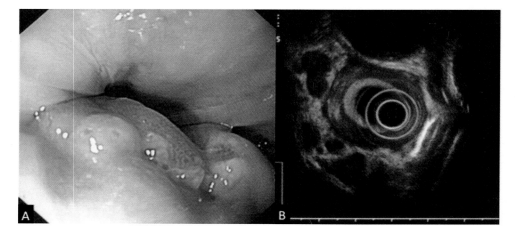

Fig. 7 Esophageal cancer. (**a**) Endoscopic view. (**b**). Endosonographic appearance

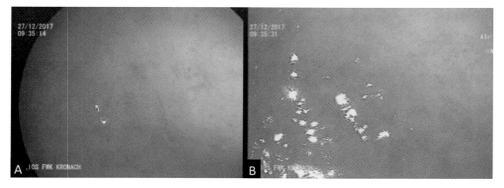

Fig. 8 Autoimmune gastritis with pernicious anemia. Panel **a** shows the atrophic gastritis. (**b**) Massive light reflections (shiny reflections) are typical of the atrophic mucosa

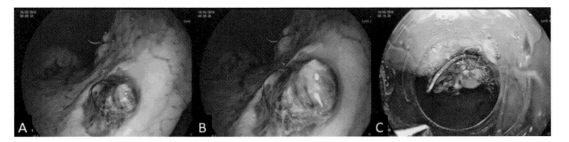

Fig. 9 Peptic ulcer hemorrhage. (**a**) Bleeding ulcer at the incisura angularis of the stomach. (**b**) Close-up showing a large vessel covered with blood clot. (**c**) This lesion was successfully treated endoscopically with an over-the-scope clip

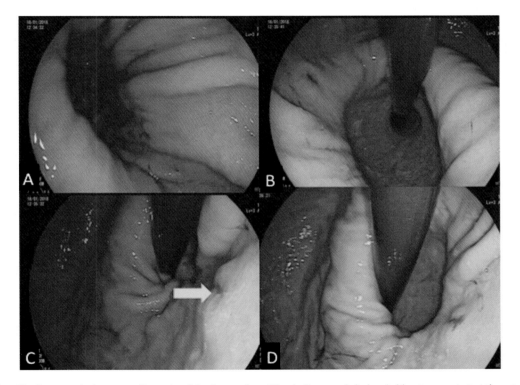

Fig. 10 Cameron lesions are often missed by inexperienced endoscopists. (**a**) The yellow arrow shows the bleeding erosion at the level of the diaphragmatic pinch. (**b**) Classic Cameron's lesion (without arrow, to test the astute eye of the reader)

Small Bowel

Few studies evaluating the changes of small bowel in geriatric patients have been conducted. Most data show that with ageing, there is decreased mesenteric blood flow, diminished absorption surface, and decreased absorption and uptake of proteins and vitamins (Durazzo et al. 2017; Lawson 2018). While the increase in breath hydrogen in elderly individuals compared to controls may be due to malabsorption of carbohydrates, it may be also due to bacterial overgrowth in the small intestine (Durazzo et al. 2017). Small bowel bacterial overgrowth may be associated with gastric hypochlorhydria, altered intestinal motor function, or reduced secretion of

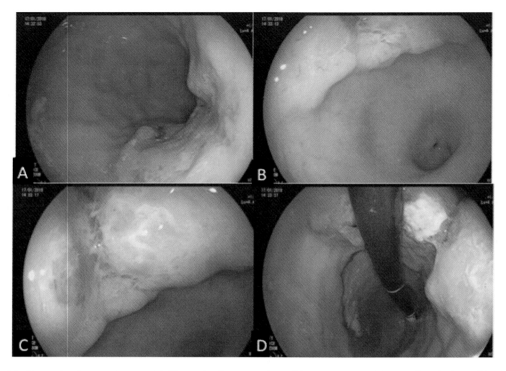

Fig. 11 Stomach adenocarcinoma. (**a**) The entire lesser curvature is involved by an ulcerated and exophytic tumor. (**b**) The tumor extends towards the antrum. (**c**) Close-up view of the tumor mass. (**d**) Retroflexed view of the large adenocarcinoma

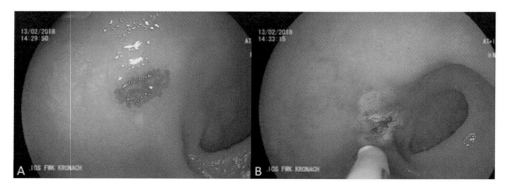

Fig. 12 Small bowel angiodysplasias. (**a**) Typical angiodysplasias. (**b**) Ablation using argon plasma coagulation

luminal IgA (Durazzo et al. 2017; Thomson 2009). Elderly patients are also more prone to suffer from acute and chronic mesenteric ischemia (Lawson 2018; Stone and Wilkins 2015; Kolkman and Geelkerken 2017). Mesenteric ischemia not only leads to abdominal pain, a common indication for EGD and colonoscopy, but also to blood loss and anemia. Therefore, the endoscopist evaluating these patients with abdominal pain should be alert to vascular insufficiency (Kolkman and Geelkerken 2017). Occult bleeding from small bowel is more common in the old, usually due to angiodysplasias (Fig. 12).

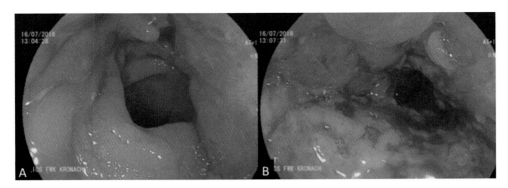

Fig. 13 Colon cancer. (**a**) Stenosing sigmoid adenocarcinoma. (**b**) The proximal part of the tumor is severely stenosed impeding the passage of the colonoscope

Colon

The most important physiologic change of the colon in geriatric patients is slower colonic transit time leading to constipation (Durazzo et al. 2017; Wiskur and Greenwood-Van Meerveld 2010). The use of multiple medications including anti-cholinergics and opiates worsens this problem substantially (Chokhavatia et al. 2016). Despite decreasing incidence likely due to effective screening strategies, colon cancer remains one of the three most common neoplasms in men and women, especially in the geriatric population (Maratt and Calderwood 2019) (Fig. 13). Of course, the incidence of adenomas, the precursors of colon cancer, increases with age (Fig. 14). Other disorders that occur more commonly in geriatric patients are diverticular disease, chronic diarrhea, angiodysplasias of the colon, nonsteroidal associated colitis and ischemic colitis (Dumic et al. 2019) (Figs. 15, 16, 17, and 18].

Biliary Tract

Astonishingly, there are almost no studies published evaluating changes of the pancreatobiliary tract in the elderly. In one Iranian study, a retrospective chart review of 371 cholecystectomy materials was performed (Yaylak et al. 2016). In our experience, geriatric patients tend to have larger diameter bile ducts, higher incidence of choledocal cysts, recalcitrant fibrotic distal bile duct strictures, and complex bile duct stones and, of course, higher incidence of cholangiocellular carcinoma (CCA) (Figs. 19, 20, and 21). Whereas the data on CCA has been clearly demonstrated in epidemiological studies, the anatomic appearance of bile ducts and its function in elderly remains to be studied.

Indications for Endoscopy

Although the indications for endoscopy in the old are essentially the same as for other patients, careful attention must be paid to several exceptions. Geriatric patients tend to suffer more often from nutritional anemia and weight loss versus younger patients. Before embarking on endoscopy, clinical and laboratory testing is mandatory. However, in elderly patients, the clinical presentation of various diseases such as cholangitis, cholecystitis, and peptic ulcer may be atypical. This, the astute endoscopist should be alert to these atypical presentations. Screening colonoscopy is not usually offered to patients older than 75 years of age (van Hees et al. 2015). Furthermore, surveillance after polyp resection is usually stopped once the patient reaches 80 years of age (US Preventive Services Task Force et al. 2016). Table 1 details some suggestions for quality perioperative endoscopic care in older adults.

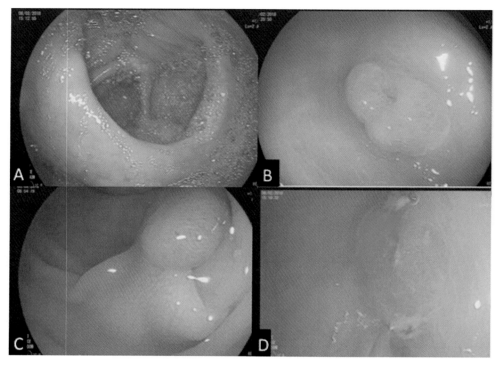

Fig. 14 Colonic polyps. (**a**) The cecum is still filled with liquid stool and bubbles, impeding an adequate inspection. All remaining liquid stool and bubbles should be cleansed endoscopically to perform adequate inspection and decrease the chances of missing a flat polyp (**b**). (**c**) Typical pedunculated adenoma. (**d**) Serrated adenomas tend to secrete mucus and retain stool on their surface and are thus more difficult to find for the inexperienced endoscopist

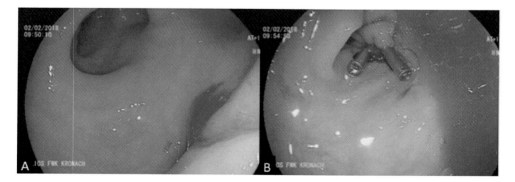

Fig. 15 Colonic diverticular bleeding. (**a**) Bleeding diverticulum. (**b**). Successful hemostasis with clips

Patient Preparation

The patient should undergo a detailed pre-operative history and physical examination and be informed by the physician about the benefits and risks of endoscopy. The informed consent should not only include information about the endoscopic risks but also those risks associated with sedation. In elderly patients, routine pre-operative laboratory blood testing is indicated before most endoscopic procedures, especially if there is clinical evidence or suspicion

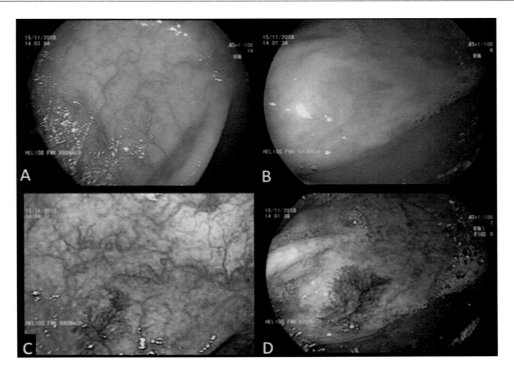

Fig. 16 Angiodysplasias of the colon. (**a**). Occasionally the angiodysplasias may be missed in the spider-like submucosal circulation. (**b**) Typical angiodysplasias. Using virtual chromoendoscopy methods such as computerized imaging these lesions become more evident as seen in panels **c** and **d**

of a blood dyscrasia or patients are being treated with coumarin oral anticoagulants or heparin and its derivatives. Table 1 shows essential steps recommended by us for appropriate perioperative care of elderly patients.

In addition, the physician needs to indicate clearly to the patient which medications he or she can take on the day of the procedure. Specifically, insulin and antidiabetic medications should be adjusted appropriately, especially during the bowel preparation period. On the day of endoscopy, the patient should receive his hypoglycemic medications based on the glucose levels (Lieberman et al. 2012; DeLegge et al. 2005). Insulin may best be withheld until procedure is over.

Both routine and emergency preparation for endoscopy in geriatric patients is somewhat different from that in younger patients. Although it is logical to approach endoscopy methodically in all patient groups, assessing elderly patients should follow a strict pattern of standards and checklists in order to reduce potential complications. The physiologic reserve of geriatric patients is lower than that of younger patients and lack of attention to any of the pre-operative, intra-operative, and postoperative standards is more likely to result in negative outcomes (Mönkemüller et al. 2009; Jafri et al. 2010; Lieberman et al. 2012; DeLegge et al. 2005; Travis et al. 2012). International experts in gerontology have intensively been searching for appropriate tools to predict morbidity, mortality, and outcomes in geriatric patients undergoing invasive procedures including gastrointestinal endoscopy. Unfortunately, no tool exists so far to risk-stratify and orient the care of older patients presenting with gastrointestinal disease Therefore, we strongly recommend using mental and written checklists to ensure a smooth pre-, intra-, and post-endoscopic period.

In our hospital, we also have three safety levels that include checklists to ensure smooth and safe endoscopy. First, the procedure is ordered and entered into a digital system, to include indication,

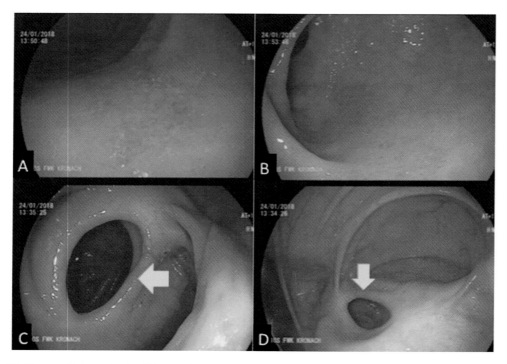

Fig. 17 Nonsteroidal associated colitis. Usually this colitis presents as "patchy colitis" (Panels **a** and **b**). Rarely, stenosis and ring-like stricture can be seen, especially in the cecum (**c**). The yellow arrow shows the fibrotic rings (**c, d**)

brief clinical history, coagulation parameters such as INR, platelet count, and partial prothrombin time. In addition, information is transmitted on the isolation or contagious status of the patient and whether the procedure is considered routine, urgent, or emergent. A contact phone number of the physician must be provided (Lieberman et al. 2012; DeLegge et al. 2005). The order is then worked-up by both endoscopist and endoscopy nurse, including NPO status, verifying the presence of consent, securing an intravenous access, and coordinating the transportation of the patient to the endoscopy unit. Patients undergoing colonoscopy undergo bowel preparation using specific protocols. In order to ensure a clean preparation, floor nurses have been instructed on how to best conduct them, including feedback from the patient and inspecting the progress of preparation. If the results of the bowel preparation appear inadequate, further contact is established with the GI endoscopy team to include additional preparation.

Preoperative bowel preparation is best accomplished with polyethylene glycol solutions. Laxatives containing phosphates and magnesium should not be used in geriatric patients as these lead to electrolyte disturbances including hypernatremia, hyperphosphatemia, hypokalemia, and worsening kidney function (Lieberman et al. 2012; DeLegge et al. 2005; Martens and Bisschops 2014). These changes have been reported to lead to death in the old, including those without preexisting kidney disease. Therefore, we focus on dietary measures, including a clear-liquid diet for 24 h before the procedure. In addition, seeds and fresh vegetables are eliminated from the diet for at least 72 h. Of course, during emergency colon preparation, these dietary instructions cannot be followed. We want to emphasize that geriatric patients often have poorer bowel preparations as compared to the young, but we circumvent this problem by a personalized bowel preparation, assisting the

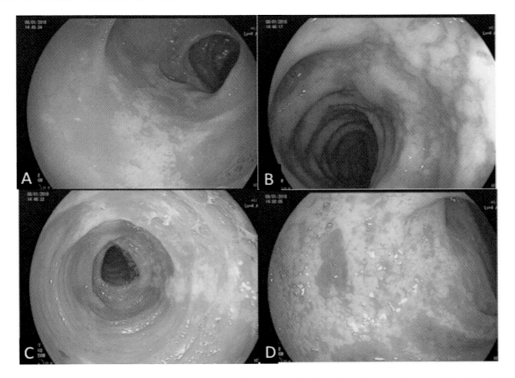

Fig. 18 Left-sided ischemic colitis is more common in elderly patients. Panel **a** shows a linear ulcerative lesion. Panel **b** shows circumferential ulcers and erosions. In Panel c, another lengthy ulcer can be seen. Panel **d** depicts a moderate ischemic colitis with exudates over the sigmoid mucosa

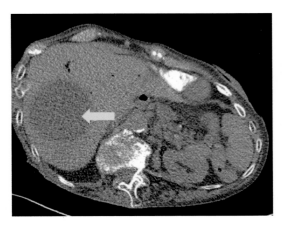

Fig. 19 Computer tomography of the abdomen showing a liver abscess in a patient with choledocal cyst and choledocholithiasis with cholangitis

patient during the bowel prep and checking its progress. In addition, although there are no data, we prefer to do a split preparation, which entails administering half the solution the previous evening and half on the morning of procedure.

Management of Anticoagulants and Antiplatelet Agents

The elderly are more likely to be taking oral anticoagulants, antiplatelet agents, and many other medications (Veitch et al. 2016). Since national and international geriatric and neurologic societies recommend the use of oral anticoagulants for stroke prophylaxis in patients with atrial fibrillation, physicians are confronted every day with the management of this therapy before invasive procedures, especially in those presenting with acute gastrointestinal hemorrhage (Bo et al. 2016). Other important indications, such as prosthetic metal heart valve, require continuous anticoagulation (Sanaani et al. 2018). Revascularizations with the use of percutaneous coronary

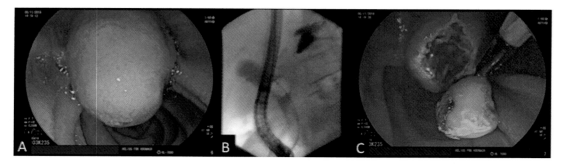

Fig. 20 Common bile duct stone. (**a**) Impacted stone in the papilla of Vater. (**b**) Cholangiography showing the dilated bile duct and stone. (**c**) Endoscopic extraction of the large bile duct stone after endoscopic sphincterotomy

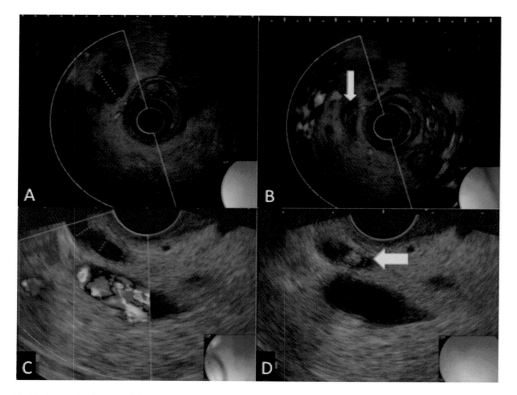

Fig. 21 Endoscopic ultrasound (EUS) is the most sensitive method to detect bile duct stones. (**a**) Radial EUS showing a dilated choledocus. (**b**) The yellow arrow shows the stone inside of the choledocus. (**c**) Linear EUS showing a dilated bile duct. (**d**) The arrow shows the stone inside the bile duct

intervention are now also performed very often, and such individuals need dual antiplatelet therapy for up to 12 months depending of the type of stent placement (Stähli and Landmesser 2018).

Management of anticoagulation should be based on the underlying condition. Table 2 provides information about pre-endoscopic management of anticoagulants (Veitch et al. 2016; Bo et al. 2016; Kirchhof et al. 2016; Sanaani et al. 2018; Stähli and Landmesser 2018; Gralnek et al. 2015; Shah et al. 2019; Gressenberger 2019). Table 3 provides information about new direct

Table 1 Suggestions for quality perioperative endoscopic care in older adults

1. Obtain a thorough history and physical examination
2. In patients with significant comorbidities (ASA 3 or higher), consult an anesthesiologist to assist with conscious sedation or provide general anesthesia
3. Always have a surgical back-up when performing advanced endoscopy
4. Review all medications, including anticoagulants
5. Ensure proper instructions for bowel preparation
6. Obtain informed consent using accepted written documentation forms. Use adequate chart documentation
7. Check whether prophylactic antibiotics are needed peri-procedurally
8. Create a pre-, intra-, and postoperative checklist for all endoscopies
9. Verify that all endoscopic equipment and accessories needed and potentially required for a given procedure are working, utilizable, and readily available
10. Give clear post-procedure orders, communicating with the geriatric team and inform of the results and plan after the endoscopy

Table 2 Pre-endoscopic management of patients taking oral anticoagulation (ASGE Standards of Practice Committee et al. 2013; Veitch et al. 2016; Sanaani et al. 2018; Gralnek et al. 2015)

Pre-endoscopic management		
Patients taking vitamin K antagonists (VKAs): withhold VKA In patients with hemodynamic instability, consider administration of vitamin K, prothrombin complex concentrate (PCC) or fresh frozen plasma (FFP) if PCC is unavailable Cardiologist consultation In case of hemodynamic stability: international normalized ratio (INR) value <2.5 should be reached before performing endoscopy **Patients taking DOAC**: withheld DOAC Considered PCC for patients with severe or life-threatening bleeding Vitamin K or FFP are not useful as reversal agents Hemodialysis may be used for dabigatran		
Endoscopic findings		

High-risk endoscopic stigmata identified (FIa, FIb, FIIa, FIIb)	APA used for primary prophylaxis
	    Withhold low-dose acetylsalicylic acid (ASA)
	    Reevaluate risks and benefits of ongoing low dose ASA use
	    Resume low-dose ASA after ulcer healing or earlier if clinically indicated
		APA used for secondary prophylaxis
		1. Patients on low-dose ASA alone
		    Resume low-dose ASA by day 3 following index endoscopy
		    Second-look endoscopy may be considered
		2. Patients on dual antiplatelet therapy (DAPT)
		    Continue low-dose ASA
		    Cardiology consultation regarding management of second APA
		    Second-look endoscopy may be considered

Low-risk endoscopic stigmata identified (FIIc, FIII)	APA used for primary prophylaxis
	    Withhold low-dose ASA
	    If clinically indicated, resume low-dose ASA at discharge
		APA used for secondary prophylaxis (known cardiovascular disease)
		1. Patients on low-dose ASA alone
		    Continue low-dose ASA without interruption
		2. Patients on dual antiplatelet therapy (DAPT)
		    Continue DAPT without interruption

Resume anticoagulation after 7 days
High-risk patients (see Table 3): resume anticoagulation within the first week following an acute bleeding event
Bridging therapy using unfractionated or low-molecular-weight heparin may be considered

anticoagulants (Veitch et al. 2016; Bo et al. 2016; Kirchhof et al. 2016; Sanaani et al. 2018; Stähli and Landmesser 2018; Gralnek et al. 2015; Shah et al. 2019; Gressenberger 2019). Table 4 provides information about management of anticoagulants during elective endoscopic procedures (Veitch et al. 2016; Bo et al. 2016; Kirchhof et al. 2016; Sanaani et al. 2018; Stähli and Landmesser 2018; Gralnek et al. 2015; Shah et al. 2019; Gressenberger 2019).

Although the limited data available do not demonstrate any increased risk of bleeding after therapeutic endoscopic procedures in patients taking NSAIDs, aspirin or clopidogrel, in those taking these medications for cardiovascular purposes, we do stop either aspirin or clopidogrel (not both) 1 week before the procedure (Veitch et al. 2016).

Emergency Gastrointestinal Endoscopy for Patients with Acute Gastrointestinal Bleeding on Oral Anticoagulants

In patients who present with acute gastrointestinal bleeding, it is important to assess the hemodynamic situation. In case of hemodynamic instability, it is advisable to delay the EGD for a few hours in order to improve the hemodynamic and coagulation status (Gralnek et al. 2015). Whereas emergency endoscopy may be performed with abnormal coagulation parameters, hemodynamic instability almost always precludes endoscopic intervention, as resuscitating the patient and ensuring appropriate organ perfusion and oxygenation have priority (Mönkemüller et al. 2009; Jafri et al. 2010).

In most cases, it suffices to stop the anticoagulant; in case of vitamin K antagonists, it is necessary to check the international normalized ratio (INR) status. Ideally, an INR value <2.5 before performing endoscopy is advisable. Measures to correct vitamin K antagonist-induced coagulopathy include administration of vitamin K, intravenous prothrombin complex concentrate or fresh frozen plasma if prothrombin complex concentrate is unavailable. Patient's cardiovascular risk should be considered and a consultation with a cardiologist is highly recommended.

In those under therapy with the new direct oral anticoagulants (DOACs), temporarily withholding the DOACs is recommended. In most, loss of anticoagulation effect will take place within 12–24 h if hepatic and/or renal function are normal (Table 3). There are no routine laboratory tests available to measure anticoagulant activity in patients taking DOACs. Both vitamin K and FFP have no effect as reversal therapy against the DOACs. However, prothrombin complex concentrates (activated PCC) may be considered in those with severe or life-threatening bleeding. Furthermore, hemodialysis can be used to reduce the blood concentration of dabigatran; it will not reduce rivaroxaban and apixaban levels, which are more tightly bound to plasma proteins (Veitch et al. 2016; Bo et al. 2016; Kirchhof et al. 2016; Sanaani et al. 2018; Stähli and Landmesser 2018; Gralnek et al. 2015; Shah et al. 2019; Gressenberger 2019).

For dabigatran, a specific reversal agent for emergency use was developed (Shah et al. 2019; Gressenberger 2019). Idarucizumab is a humanized monoclonal antibody fragment that specifically binds to dabigatran to reverse its anticoagulant effects with a dosage-dependent inhibition that has 300-times more affinity to dabigatran than thrombin (Shah et al. 2019; Gressenberger 2019). Recently, andexanet alfa was developed as a specific antidote for the anti-Xa inhibitors apixaban and rivaroxaban (Shah et al. 2019; Gressenberger 2019). Furthermore, a universal reversal agent for all DOACs and low-molecular-weight heparin, ciraparantag is under investigation (Gressenberger 2019). Despite its promising results, we have not yet used any of these antagonists, and current practice focuses on discontinuation of DOACs followed by endoscopy as soon as the patient is stable hemodynamically.

Acute Gastrointedstinal Bleeding While on Antiplatelet Agents

Antiplatelet activity remains for at least 5–7 days after holding the medication. The timing to perform the EGD depends on hemodynamic instability and comorbidities. The timing to resume the

Table 3 Characteristics of direct oral anticoagulation drugs (Shah et al. 2019; Gressenberger 2019)

	Dabigatran	Apixaban	Rivaroxaban	Edoxaban
Renal elimination (%)	85	27	66	50
Half life (hours)	9–13	12	9–13	10–14
Antidote	Idarucizumab	Andexanet alfa	Andexanet alfa	

Table 4 Management of oral anticoagulation in patients who undergo elective endoscopic procedures (Veitch et al. 2016)

Low-risk procedure	Antiplatelet therapy	Continue therapy

Diagnostic procedures with biopsy: EGD, colonoscopy, enteroscopy, EUS, ERCP with stenting	Oral anticoagulants	Vitamin K antagonists
		  INR can be in therapeutic range
		DOAC
		  Omit the day of the procedure

High-risk procedure
  ERCP with sphincterotomy
  Ampullectomy
  Polypectomy/ESD/EMR
  EUS with FNA
  PEG
  Variceal therapy
  Dilation of strictures
  Esophageal, enteral, or colonic stenting
	Low-risk condition (APA)
	  Ischemic heart disease without stent
	  Cerebrovascular disease
	  Peripheral vascular disease
		Continue AAS
		  P2Y12 receptor antagonist: withhold 5 days before procedure

	High-risk condition (APA)
	  Coronary artery stents
		Cardiologist consultation
		Consider stop P2Y12 receptor antagonist
		  Drug-eluting stents >12 months
		  Bare metal stents >1 month after insertion

	Low-risk condition (oral anticoagulants)
	  AF without valvular disease
	  Prosthetic metal heart valve in aortic position
	  Xenograft heart valve
	  Thrombophilia syndromes
		Vitamin K antagonist
		  Stop 5 days before endoscopy
		  INR should be <1,5 before procedure
		  Restart warfarin same day of procedure

	High-risk condition (oral anticoagulation)
	  Prosthetic metal hearth valve in mitral position
	  Prosthetic metal hearth valve and AF
	  Mitral stenosis and AF
	  Less than 3 months after thromboembolic ereignis
		Vitamin K antagonist
		  Stop 5 days before endoscopy
		  Stop heparin at least 24 h before procedure
		  Restart warfarin same day of procedure and continue heparin until INR in therapeutic range

	DOAC	Stop DOAC at least 48 h before procedure In case of dabigatran: if eGFR is between 30 ml/min and 50 ml/min, this drug should be stopped 72 h before procedure

antiplatelet agent therapy after the index endoscopy will depend on the endoscopic findings and risk of rebleeding as well as the indication for the antiplatelet agent therapy. We use the Forrest classification to determine the risk of rebleeding and to determine timing of resuming antiplatelet therapy. In patients taking aspirin as a primary prophylaxis, there are two options. One, aspirin is discontinued, or two, long-term gastric acid inhibition with proton pump inhibitors is instituted (Veitch et al. 2016; Bo et al. 2016; Kirchhof et al. 2016; Sanaani et al. 2018; Stähli and Landmesser 2018; Gralnek et al. 2015). When antiplatelet therapy is used for secondary prophylaxis because of known cardiovascular disease, ASA (if used as only therapy) should be resumed by day 3 following index endoscopy, if the ulcers were clean based (Forrest III and IIc). A second-look endoscopy should be performed in patients with high-risk Forrest lesions (Ia, Ib, IIa). In these cases, patients on dual antiplatelet therapy for coronary artery disease should continue the low dose ASA therapy without interruption. An early cardiology consultation regarding continuation or pause of the second APT is mandatory. Again, a second-look endoscopy at the discretion of the endoscopist may be considered. In all cases, high dose PPI is mandatory (Gralnek et al. 2015). The substitution of dual APT with low-molecular-weight heparins or unfractionated heparin is ineffective and should be discouraged (Veitch et al. 2016).

Elective Endoscopy

Patients who undergo elective endoscopic procedures and are receiving antiplatelet or anticoagulant therapy need to be thoroughly evaluated. The first point is to classify the endoscopies as low- or high-risk procedures (ASGE Standards of Practice Committee et al. 2013; Mönkemüller et al. 2009; Jafri et al. 2010; Travis et al. 2012). Low-risk procedures are diagnostic endoscopy with or without biopsies, including EGD, colonoscopies, EUS, and enteroscopies (Veitch et al. 2016). High-risk procedures include polypectomies, endoscopic mucosal resection,

endoscopic submucosal dissection, ERCP with sphincterotomy, ampullectomy, variceal ligation, dilation of strictures, percutaneous endoscopic gastrostomy, endoscopic ultrasound with fine-needle aspiration or puncture, and esophageal, colonic, or enteral stenting. For low-risk procedures, antiplatelet agents could be continued (Veitch et al. 2016). In case of DOAC, they should be held the day of the procedure. Importantly, there is no need for bridging with heparins in patients taking DOACs. Patients treated with warfarin can undergo low-risk endoscopy if INR is in therapeutic range.

Patients who need to undergo high-risk endoscopic procedures need to be individually evaluated. Those at high thrombotic risk should be evaluated by a cardiologist pre-procedure. Withholding the clopidogrel 5 days before the endoscopy should be considered; ASA can be continued. In patients on vitamin K antagonists and low-risk conditions, endoscopies could be performed if the INR <1.5; vitamin K antagonists can be given the day of the procedure. Patients with a high-risk condition should stop warfarin 5 days before procedure and INR needs to be <1.5 prior to the procedure; bridging therapy with heparin is needed but should be withheld 24 h before the endoscopic procedure. Otherwise the risk of bleeding from the therapeutic intervention is too high. Warfarin can be started the evening after procedure; heparin restarted 6–24 h after the procedure, depending on the intervention carried out and continued until therapeutic INR is reached. In patients undergoing high-risk therapeutic endoscopy, DOACs should be withheld at least 48 h before procedure. However, in patients with chronic kidney disease (i.e., glomerular filtration rate of 30–50 ml/min) and on dabigatran, this drug should be stopped 72 h before the procedure.

Pacemakers and Internal Defibrillators

The management and handling of cardiac defibrillators and pacemakers before endoscopy is not standardized. Most devices can be safely continued (Li et al. 2015). However, patients who are pacemaker dependent or mostly in a paced rhythm should be switched to automated pacing (Parekh et al. 2013). This is accomplished by placing a ring magnet on the skin whenever monopolar electrosurgical currents are used (Li et al. 2015; Parekh et al. 2013). Monopolar currents are used for snare resection of polyps, sphincterotomy, hot biopsy forceps, and argon plasma coagulation (Li et al. 2015; Parekh et al. 2013; Borgaonkar et al. 2016). However, when using electrosurgical currents, intracardiac defibrillators should be inactivated.

Sedation

Most GI endoscopy is performed with light to moderate sedation. However, there are significant variations from country to country. Physician or qualified nurse anesthetist controlled propofol sedation is the standard of care. Data is needed to standardize effective and safe sedation in this population. Of course, it is well known that geriatric patients are more prone to develop hypotension, hypoxia, and arrhythmias (Lippert et al. 2015; Mönkemüller et al. 2009; Jafri et al. 2010; Finkelmeier et al. 2015; Katsinelos et al. 2006; de Wit et al. 2016; Hong et al. 2015). These changes occur because of the increased residual pulmonary volumes, the increased tissue elasticity, and the decreased vital capacity, among others (de Wit et al. 2016; Hong et al. 2015; Lin 2017; Leslie et al. 2017). In addition, the patient's central nervous system response to hypercapnia and hypoxia is altered. Thus, sedatives such as midazolam or diazepam and narcotics such as meperidine or morphine can deeply affect their cardiorespiratory function. On the other side, propofol may also lead to rapid drop in blood pressure and decreased cardiac output, especially if the heart function is compromised (ASGE Standards of Practice Committee et al. 2013; Mönkemüller et al. 2009; Jafri et al. 2010; Travis et al. 2012).

The age-related increase in body lipid fraction provides an expanded distribution volume for pharmacologic agents that are highly lipid soluble, including benzodiazepines, leading to prolonged post-endoscopic recovery periods (Lin 2017; Miyanaga et al. 2018). Because the body composition of geriatric patients is different, with decreased muscle mass and altered function of the kidneys and liver, these patients are more prone to develop hypothermia during prolonged procedures (de Wit et al. 2016; Hong et al. 2015; Lin 2017; Leslie et al. 2017; Miyanaga et al. 2018). Thus, careful attention to appropriate clothing and covers should be paid. Finally, most elderly patients have multiple medical problems including renal dysfunction, chronic obstructive pulmonary disease, and coronary heart disease, which make them additionally more susceptible to complications from the use of sedatives and narcotics. Hence, it is mandatory to always use monitoring of vital signs and oxygen saturation. In addition, routine oxygen administration to keep the saturation above 90% reduces risk of desaturation during and after the procedure.

Sedation with the short-acting anesthetic agent propofol has shown several advantages, particularly in interventional endoscopy and thus has become popular. Currently, nurse-assisted propofol sedation (NAPS) or physician-controlled propofol sedation (PCPS) is an accepted alternative to standard sedation with benzodiazepine and opiates (Riphaus et al. 2005, 2013; Friedrich et al. 2012). Nevertheless, there are only few studies specifically evaluating NAPS in the elderly (Riphaus et al. 2005, 2013; Friedrich et al. 2012).

Riphaus et al. showed that propofol is as safe as standard sedation for routine ERCP in high-risk octogenarians (Riphaus et al. 2005). Propofol sedation requires the presence of a nurse or physician to administer the drug and monitor the patient. This implies that the endoscopist concentrates on the endoscopy and a technician or nurse assists the endoscopist during the procedure. Thus, propofol implies the availability of three subjects in the endoscopy suite.

Esophagogastroduodenoscopy (EGD)

Because of risks of aspiration with blunting of airway protective reflexes, patients undergoing sedation should be asked to fast for a specific time period (ASGE Standards of Practice Committee et al. 2013). There are no data to support a direct relationship between duration of fasting and the risk of pulmonary aspiration, and the literature contains varying recommendations for oral intake before procedural sedation (ASGE Standards of Practice Committee et al. 2013). There is no practice standard for pre-procedural fasting that has been universally accepted. The ASA guidelines indicate that patients should not drink fluids or eat solid foods for a sufficient period of time to allow for gastric emptying before the procedure. Specifically, these guidelines state that patients should fast a minimum of 2 h after ingestion of clear liquids and 6 h after ingestion of light meals before sedation is administered (ASGE Standards of Practice Committee et al. 2013). In situations where gastric emptying is impaired or in emergent situations, the potential for pulmonary aspiration of gastric contents is increased (ASGE Standards of Practice Committee et al. 2013).

Similar to the young, older patients should have fasted at least 6 h before undergoing an EGD. Expert guidelines suggest waiting 8 h if solids were ingested and 4 h if the previous meal was liquid (ASGE Standards of Practice Committee et al. 2013). The only exception includes an acute episode of upper GI bleeding, in which case the necessity of the endoscopy is mandated by the severity of the bleeding. The routine use of EGD in elderly patients is not associated with more complications as compared to younger patients (Cangemi et al. 2015). However, the endoscopist needs to always remember that conditions such as Zenker's diverticula are more common in the old requiring more attention to the intubation process of the scope (Wirth et al. 2016; Al-Kadi et al. 2010). From the endoscopist's perspective, it is crucial to always examine the oral cavity. The presence of dentures mandates their removal before any esophagogastroduodenoscopy. In addition, attention should be paid to the presence of loose or absent teeth (Fig. 1). Patients may be partly or completely edentulous; endoscopy may accidentally cause injury to gums or remaining. Any endoscopy unit treating geriatric patients should have various types of bite blocks, as occasionally

normal sized bite blocks cannot be placed in the mouth of these patients. In those cases, smaller or pediatric type bite blocks are essential.

In a retrospective study of 3147 older adults undergoing EGD, Buri et al. found significant findings in almost 50% of patients (Buri et al. 2013). The yield of finding a disease process was in relation to the indication for EGD, being highest for GI hemorrhage (74%), reflux symptoms (53%), weight loss (53%), dysphagia 50%), and anemia (49%) (Buri et al. 2013). The prevalence of peptic ulcer disease or malignancy was threefold in patients older than 85 years compared to those 65–69 years of age (Buri et al. 2013). In a multivariate analysis, the following risk factors were associated with positive findings: male sex, weight loss, bleeding, and symptoms of GERD (Buri et al. 2013). In a study of outcomes following therapeutic EGD, Lee et al. found that success and outcomes did not differ between geriatric and younger patients, with similar rates of successful therapy, mortality, and hospitalization (Lee et al. 2007). Exceptions to this are percutaneous endoscopic gastrostomies (PEG). Age is a predictor of post-PEG death, with geriatric patients having 30-day mortality up to 24% (Callahan et al. 2000; Grant et al. 1998). Although most deaths occurred due to underlying comorbidities and were not related to the procedure itself, these data clearly show that a more conservative approach is warranted before implanting a needless PEG in these patients with poor prognosis (Callahan et al. 2000; Grant et al. 1998).

One retrospective study evaluated the etiology, clinical outcomes, and factors related to mortality of acute upper gastrointestinal bleeding in the elderly and very elderly patients during a 2-year period (Theocharis et al. 2008). The patients were divided into two groups: Group A (65–80 years old) with 269 patients and Group B (>80 years) with 147 patients. Comorbidity was more common in Group B, octogenarians, over 80 years ($P = 0.04$). The main cause of bleeding was peptic ulcer in both groups. Incidences of rebleeding and emergency surgery were uncommon in octogenarians and were similar in both groups. But, in-hospital complications and mortality were more common in octogenarians (Theocharis et al. 2008). The major determinant of poor outcome of elderly patients in this study was the presence of multiple comorbidities in the old.

In the recent past, an increasing variety of therapeutic interventions have become available. These include advanced endoscopic resection methods such as endoscopic mucosal resection and endoscopic submucosal dissection (Qumseya et al. 2014; Yamaguchi et al. 2019; Yang et al. 2015; Toya et al. 2018; Son et al. 2019) (Fig. 22). In a retrospective study form the USA, Qumseya et al. identified 136 patients who underwent esophageal endoscopic mucosal resection (Qumseya et al. 2014). Of those, 40% ($n = 55$) were aged ≥ 75 years (elderly group) and 60% ($n = 81$) were aged <75 years (younger group). There was no difference in rate of stricture formation, early or delayed bleeding when we compared the elderly to younger patients. None of the patients had esophageal perforation following the procedure (Qumseya et al. 2014). In a Japanese study in geriatric patients undergoing endoscopic submucosal dissection for early gastric cancer, the authors found that mortality due to endoscopy and gastric cancer was very low, and

the main reason for death at 3- and 5-years follow-up were the presence of comorbidities as reflected by the Charlson comorbidity index (Toya et al. 2018). Son et al. from Korea also reported on excellent results of endoscopic submucosal dissection for gastric neoplasia in those older than 80 years of age (Son et al. 2019). In a study group of more than 400 patients, the authors did not find any differences in procedural and clinical outcomes among patients younger than 80 years versus those over this age (Son et al. 2019). The only significant difference was the time needed to achieve hemostasis during the operative procedure, which was longer in patients over 80 years of age (Son et al. 2019).

Colonoscopy

Despite its widespread use, there are few data evaluating the effectiveness of colonoscopy in elderly patients (Lukens et al. 2002; Karajeh et al. 2006; Virk et al. 2019; Day et al. 2011; van Hees et al. 2015). Nevertheless, more data are being generated in recent years, including

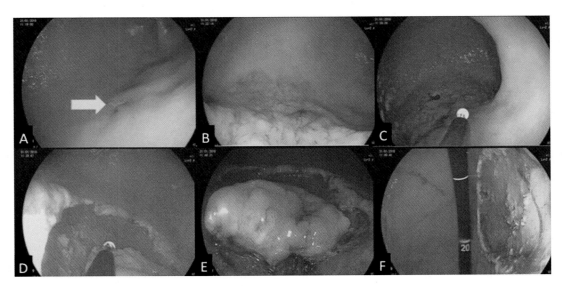

Fig. 22 Endoscopic submucosal dissection of early cancer of the stomach. (**a**) Early cancer is shown by the yellow arrow. (**b**) Using chromoendoscopy, the lesion can be better defined. (**c**) Special knives such as the ceramic tip knife are especially useful for dissection. (**d**) Circumferential incision and dissection. (**e**) The lesions have been liberated and now vertical dissection continues. (**f**). Large wound after complete resection of the cancer. The patient was cured

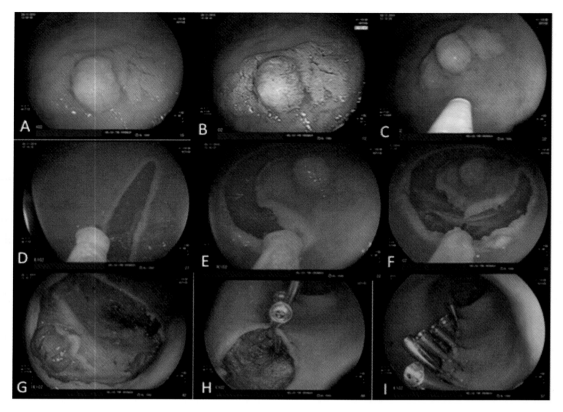

Fig. 23 Endoscopic submucosal dissection of colorectal lesions. (**a**) Laterally spreading tumor, granular type, sessile, and polypoid (LST-G polypoid). (**b**) Chromoendoscopy of the lesion. (**c**) Injection of the base of the lesion prior to incision. (**d**) Circumferential incision. (**e**) Incision and dissection. (**f**) Completed circumferential incision. (**g**) Complete vertical resection. (**h**) Closing the wound with clips to prevent bleeding and perforation. (**i**) Completed closure using seven clips

therapeutic interventions such as endoscopic submucosal dissection (Pontone et al. 2017; Tamai et al. 2012) (Fig. 23). In a prospective study involving 250 patients, including 100 octogenarians, Lukens et al. aimed to determine whether there were differences between octogenarians and non-octogenarians in adequacy of colonic preparation, success in completing colonoscopy, and complications of conscious sedation (Lukens et al. 2002). The investigators found that in octogenarians and non-octogenarians preparation tolerance (86% and 90%, respectively) was similar. Endoscopic success rate was slightly lower in octogenarians (90% vs. 99%, $p = 0.002$). However, preparation was poor in 16% of octogenarians compared with 4% of non-octogenarians ($p = 0.001$). This was independent of the type of preparation used. In addition, they found that oxygen desaturation was more common in octogenarians (27% vs. 19%, $p = 0.0007$). The authors concluded that colonic preparations were well tolerated and colonoscopic success rates were high in octogenarians and non-octogenarians. However, poor colonic preparation was four times as likely in octogenarians and was the most important impediment to adequate colonoscopy (Lukens et al. 2002). When using colon preparation in older adults, the use of phosphate containing agents is contraindicated, especially in those with heart failure and chronic kidney disease (Mönkemüller et al. 2009; Jafri et al. 2010).

In another study, Karajeh et al. prospectively evaluated the incompletion rates, diagnostic yield, complication rates, and 30-day mortality between patients aged ≥ 65 years and patients aged <65 undergoing colonoscopy in a study of 2000 patients (Karajeh et al. 2006). The median age was 75 years (51% women) for the elderly group and 54 years (59% women) for controls. The proportion of patients who received sedation was similar for both groups (59% vs. 62%, $p = 0.97$). In the elderly group, the mean dose of midazolam was lower (3.8 mg vs. 4.5 mg, $P < 0.0001$); the crude completion rate was lower (81.8% vs. 86.5%, $p = 0.004$); the overall diagnostic yield was higher (65% vs. 45%, $P < 0.0001$), with higher rates of carcinoma detected (7.1% vs. 1.3%, $P < 0.0001$). The complication rate was low (0.2% per group). This study shows us that colonoscopy in the elderly is safe and effective with a high diagnostic yield (Karajeh et al. 2006).

In a retrospective study, Cha et al. from the USA compared data from 76 extremely elderly patients (90 years or older) with data from 140 elderly patients (75–79 years old, controls), all of whom underwent diagnostic colonoscopy during a 3-year period (Cha et al. 2016). The findings were that in the extremely elderly: more colonoscopies were performed under general anesthesia, compared with controls ($P < 0.001$); lower doses of midazolam and fentanyl were given, compared with controls ($P < 0.001$); colonoscopies were completed in a lower proportion of patients (88.2% vs. 99.3% for controls, $P < 0.001$); and a higher incidence of inadequate bowel preparation (29.7% vs. 15.0% for controls, $P = 0.011$). Further, in the extremely elderly, colonoscopies were associated with cardiopulmonary events in a higher proportion of patients ($P = 0.006$) as well as overall adverse events, versus controls ($P = 0.002$); more patients were found to have advanced neoplasia (28.4% vs. 6.4% of controls, $P < 0.001$) as well as any neoplasia ($P < 0.001$ vs. controls); a greater percentage had large lesions ($P = 0.002$) and malignancies detected by histology ($P < 0.001$ vs. controls); 11 patients (14.9%) had cancer or high-grade dysplasia by colonoscopy. In summary, in those 90 years or older, diagnostic colonoscopy is associated with increased yield of finding advanced neoplasia at the expense of higher risk for incomplete procedure, inadequate bowel preparation, and adverse events (Cha et al. 2016).

In a large meta-analysis including 20 studies, Day et al. found that colonoscopy is associated with higher rates of adverse events in those over 65 years of age (Day et al. 2011). Pooled incidence rates for adverse events (per 1000 colonoscopies) were 26.0 (95% CI, 25.0–27.0) for cumulative GI adverse events, 1.0 (95% CI, 0.9–1.5) for perforation, 6.3 (95% CI, 5.7–7.0) for GI bleeding, 19.1 (95% CI, 18.0–20.3) for cardiopulmonary complications, and 1.0 (95% CI, 0.7–2.2) for mortality. Among octogenarians, adverse events (per 1000 colonoscopies) were as follows: cumulative GI adverse event rate of 34.9 (95% CI, 31.9–38.0), perforation rate of 1.5 (95% CI, 1.1–1.9), GI bleeding rate of 2.4 (95% CI, 1.1–4.6), cardiopulmonary complication rate of 28.9 (95% CI, 26.2–31.8), and mortality rate of 0.5 (95% CI, 0.06–1.9) (Warren et al. 2009). Overall, patients 80 years and older experienced higher rates of cumulative GI adverse events (incidence rate ratio 1.7; 95% CI, 1.5–1.9) and a greater risk of perforation (incidence rate ratio 1.6, 95% CI, 1.2–2.1) compared to younger patients below 80 years of age.

A multinational group has proposed to personalize colonoscopy screening in the old based on screening history, cancer risk and comorbidity (van Hees et al. 2015). Using a microsimulation model (Microsimulation Screening Analysis-Colon) calibrated to the incidence of colorectal cancer in the USA and the prevalence of adenomas reported in autopsy studies to determine the appropriate age at which to stop colonoscopy screening in 19,200 cohorts (of ten million individuals), defined by sex, race, screening history, background risk for colorectal cancer, and comorbidity status (van Hees et al. 2015). The summary was that the current approach to colorectal cancer screening in the old, where decisions are often based primarily on age, is inefficient, resulting in underuse of screening for some and overuse of screening for others. Colorectal cancer screening is more effective if individual factors for each patient are considered (van Hees et al. 2015).

Nevertheless, several studies continue to show that therapeutic interventions in selected elderly patients are safe and effective, improving patient's outcomes. In an observational, retrospective study of 90 octogenarians that underwent colon endoscopic mucosal resection ≥2 cm, Gomez et al. found that adverse events occurred in 6.4%, with 94% of patients not requiring an operation as a result of successful resection of the colonic lesion (Cangemi et al. 2015).

A study compared outcomes after colonic endoscopic mucosal resection in 50 patients younger and older than 65 years. Although 10 patients still required surgery for incomplete resection, the incidence of complications was similar for younger and geriatric patients (Pontone et al. 2017).

For larger and more complex lesions, we prefer to perform endoscopic submucosal dissection (Fig. 18). Although endoscopic submucosal dissection has become the standard of care to remove large colonic lesions in Japan, Korea, and some Western countries, there are still no outcome data available on the old. Nevertheless, outcomes and efficiency are excellent, based on Japanese data on over 16,000 patients who underwent endoscopic submucosal dissection, with almost 40% of patients being older than 65 years of age (Tamai et al. 2012).

Endoscopic Retrograde Cholangiopancreatography (ERCP)

ERCP is a procedure performed frequently in the geriatric population. This is because of the relatively high incidence of biliary tract disorders in this age group such as cholelithiasis, biliary tract tumors, and pancreatic head cancer. There are several studies on the role of ERCP in the old (Ukkonen et al. 2016; Finkelmeier et al. 2015; Gómez et al. 2014; Katsinelos et al. 2006; Lukens et al. 2010; Amornyotin et al. 2012; Fritz et al. 2006).

We will describe six studies of clinical interest in which the focus was the very elderly group of patients (Obana et al. 2010; Ukkonen et al. 2016; Katsinelos et al. 2006; Riphaus et al. 2005; Lukens et al. 2010; Fritz et al. 2006). Obana

et al. from Japan evaluated outcomes in octogenarians (Obana et al. 2010). The cannulation rates and bile duct stone clearance, as well as adverse events were similar in older versus younger patients, despite the poorer general health status of octogenarians (Obana et al. 2010). Ukkonen et al. evaluated all patients older than 65-years of age undergoing ERCP during the 5-year study period (Ukkonen et al. 2016). A total of 480 elderly patients (median age 78; range 65–97; 48% men) underwent 531 ERCPs during the study period. The most common indications were bile duct stones (56.1%) and biliary obstruction caused by malignancy (33.7%). Successful stone extraction was achieved in 72.8%. Post-ERCP complications developed in 3.4% of the patients. These included pancreatitis in 1.7%, hemorrhage in 0.6%, and duodenal perforation in 0.2% of the patients. Procedure-related mortality was zero, but overall 30-day mortality was 10%, being 24% in the patients with malignancy (Ukkonen et al. 2016). Katsinelos et al. went further and focused on patients older than 90 years of age (Katsinelos et al. 2006). The investigators compared the results of ERCP in patients >90 years ($n = 63$) and patients between 70 and 89 years of age ($n = 350$), thus focusing on two groups of elderly patients. Although all patients >90 years had concomitant diseases, as compared to 72.8% of patients 70–79 years-old, the rate of post-ERCP early complications was similar (6.3% and 8.4%, respectively). The frequency of ERCP-related mortality was 1.6% (1 patient) in patients >90 years and 0.6% in patients 70–79 years (Katsinelos et al. 2006). In a study investigating the safety of ERCP in the very elderly, Riphaus et al. compared the results of 118 consecutive patients older than 80 years with 1842 ERCPs performed in patients <80 years (Riphaus et al. 2005). Of interest, 75% of the patients > had an ASA status > III. The investigators did not find any difference in outcomes and complications between both groups of patients. Post-ERCP pancreatitis occurred in 4.2% of very elderly patients as compared to 4.1% in patients <80 years. The incidence of post-sphincterotomy bleeding was also similar in both groups (4.1% vs. 4.3%) (Riphaus et al. 2005). In a large study evaluating ERCP in octogenarians, Lukens et al. evaluated 628 patients older than 80 and compared outcomes to a younger group with mean age of 59 years (Lukens et al. 2010). The authors found that the endoscopic success rate was lower in octogenarians (96.9 vs. 98.3%, $P = 0.004$). However, the overall, complication rates between both groups was significantly less in older compared to younger patients (1.64 vs. 3.50%, $P = 0.006$). Of importance, complication and failure rates were higher as procedure complexity increased in all patients (Lukens et al. 2010). In another retrospective cohort study, Fritz et al. also compared the success, complication, and outcomes of ERCP in patients older and younger than 80 years (Fritz et al. 2006). Although the comorbidities were higher in the very elderly patient group, the success rate (88% vs. 86%) and complications (6.8% vs. 5.1%) were similar in both groups (Fritz et al. 2006). In sum, these studies show that advanced age per se should not impinge on decisions relating to its use.

Enteroscopy

Over the past decade, the advent of capsule endoscopy and balloon-assisted enteroscopy has revolutionized the approach to small intestinal diseases (Teshima and May 2012). Double-balloon enteroscopy was the first type of balloon-assisted endoscopy and is the method for which there are the most data. Single-balloon enteroscopy has since been introduced as an alternative balloon-assisted method, followed more recently by the development of spiral overtube-assisted enteroscopy (Teshima and May 2012). The most common indication for deep enteroscopy is obscure gastrointestinal bleeding, followed by investigation of ulcerative diseases, malabsorption, and polyposis syndromes (Teshima and May 2012; Cangemi et al. 2015; Mönkemüller et al. 2006; Heine et al. 2006; Di Caro et al. 2005; Rondonotti et al. 2018a; b). There is only one study specifically evaluating double-balloon enteroscopy in elderly patients. Cangemi et al. (2015) retrospectively reviewed a large database, including procedures during a 6-year period.

The authors found 215 double-balloon enteroscopies performed in 130 patients aged 80 or older. The mean age was 83.6 ± 3.03 years (range: 80–94). The most common indication for DBE was obscure gastrointestinal bleeding ($N = 204$, 94.9%). The overall diagnostic yield of double-balloon enteroscopy was 77.2% ($N = 166$). There were no immediate postprocedural complications or failed procedures. Therefore, double-balloon enteroscopy may be considered a safe and effective technique for investigation of the small bowel in octogenarians (Teshima and May 2012; Cangemi et al. 2015; Mönkemüller et al. 2006; Heine et al. 2006; Di Caro et al. 2005; Rondonotti et al. 2018a, b).

In that vein, most studies evaluating the utility of balloon-assisted enteroscopy for small bowel disorders have included a significant number of older adults (Mönkemüller et al. 2006; Heine et al. 2006; Di Caro et al. 2005). Indeed, the median age for most studies has ranged from 52 to 65 years old (Lukens et al. 2010; Amornyotin et al. 2012; Fritz et al. 2006; Teshima and May 2012; Cangemi et al. 2015; Mönkemüller et al. 2006). In most studies, the yields of balloon-assisted enteroscopy have been high and up to 70% of patients have undergone therapeutic interventions (Lukens et al. 2010; Amornyotin et al. 2012; Fritz et al. 2006; Teshima and May 2012; Cangemi et al. 2015; Mönkemüller et al. 2006). The potential complications associated with balloon enteroscopy include pancreatitis, perforation, bleeding, and intestinal necrosis (Carmel 1996).

Capsule Endoscopy (CE)

The topic has been dealt with elsewhere in the book. Similar to balloon-assisted enteroscopy, capsule endoscopy is performed for the evaluation of a large variety of small bowel diseases; it is a safe procedure with very few reported complications (Teshima and May 2012; Cangemi et al. 2015; Mönkemüller et al. 2006; Heine et al. 2006; Di Caro et al. 2005; Rondonotti et al. 2018a, b). The most important complications of CE attributed to patient age may be bronchial aspiration of the capsule, retention of a CE in a Zenker's diverticulum, stomach emptying problems, and inability to swallow the capsule (Rondonotti et al. 2018a, b; Knapp and Ladetsky 2005). Another important issue is the potential interaction of CE with cardiac defibrillators. Although there was initial concern on the use of CE in patients with automated cardiac defibrillators, two studies have not found any detrimental interaction (Barkin and O'Loughlin 2004; Leighton et al. 2004; Moneghini et al. 2016).

Key Points

- Because of population demographics, the use of endoscopy is expected to rise in the geriatric population worldwide.
- Older adults represent a special group, as aging results in changes in pathophysiology of the gastrointestinal tract.
- The endoscopic approach to this group of patients is different as a substantial significant percentage of geriatric patients suffer from comorbid diseases.
- The spectrum of gastrointestinal disorders differs between the elderly and that in younger patients.
- Elderly patients are, in general, more susceptible to complications from therapeutic endoscopic interventions.
- Due to the decreased physiologic reserve and associated diseases, complications in this age group tend to be more severe than in subjects younger than 65 years.
- Ethical considerations play a special role in frail patients with a potential poor prognosis, where the indication for endoscopy may be correct, but conducting endoscopy may not lead to a better prognosis.
- The clinician considering an endoscopic intervention and the endoscopist performing it must pay close attention to the indication and carefully consider the pros and cons of any invasive procedure in this group of patients.
- The "ethical, clinical and therapeutic consequence" of any given intervention is the key factor determining the need for gastrointestinal endoscopy in the elderly.

- In sum, the endoscopist needs to pay special attention to the geriatric patient, indication and potential benefit when considering or performing endoscopy.

References

Al-Kadi AS, Maghrabi AA, Thomson D, Gillman LM, Dhalla S. Endoscopic treatment of Zenker diverticulum: results of a 7-year experience. J Am Coll Surg. 2010;211:239–43. https://doi.org/10.1016/j.jamcollsurg.2010.04.011.

Amornyotin S, Leelakusolvong S, Chalayonnawin W, Kongphlay S. Age-dependent safety analysis of propofol-based deep sedation for ERCP and EUS procedures at an endoscopy training center in a developing country. Clin Exp Gastroenterol. 2012;5:123–8. https://doi.org/10.2147/CEG.S31275. Epub 2012 Jul 9

ASGE Standards of Practice Committee, Chandrasekhara V, Early DS, Acosta RD, Chathadi KV, Decker GA, Evans JA, Fanelli RD, Fisher DA, Foley KQ, Fonkalsrud L, Hwang JH, Jue T, Khashab MA, Lightdale JR, Muthusamy VR, Pasha SF, Saltzman JR, Sharaf R, Shergill AK, Cash BD. Modifications in endoscopic practice for the elderly. Gastrointest Endosc. 2013;78:1–7. https://doi.org/10.1016/j.gie.2013.04.161.

Azzolino D, Damanti S, Bertagnoli L, Lucchi T, Cesari M. Sarcopenia and swallowing disorders in older people. Aging Clin Exp Res. 2019. https://doi.org/10.1007/s40520-019-01128-3.

Barkin JS, O'Loughlin C. Capsule endoscopy contraindications: complications and how to avoid their occurrence. Gastrointest Endosc Clin N Am. 2004;14:61–5.

Bo M, Sciarrillo I, Li Puma F, Badinella Martini M, Falcone Y, Iacovino M, Grisoglio E, Menditto E, Fonte G, Brunetti E, Maggiani G, Isaia GC, Gaita F. Effects of oral anticoagulant therapy in medical inpatients ≥65 years with atrial fibrillation. Am J Cardiol. 2016;117(4):590–5. https://doi.org/10.1016/j.amjcard.2015.11.032.. Epub 2015 Dec 2. PubMed PMID: 26718230

Borgaonkar MR, Pace D, Lougheed M, Marcoux C, Evans B, Hickey N, O'Leary M, McGrath J. Canadian Association of Gastroenterology indicators of safety compromise following colonoscopy in clinical practice. Can J Gastroenterol Hepatol. 2016;2016:2729871. https://doi.org/10.1155/2016/2729871. Epub 2016 Jun 21. PubMed PMID: 27446832; PubMed Central PMCID: PMC4932159

Buri L, Zullo A, Hassan C, Bersani G, Anti M, Bianco MA, Cipolletta L, Giulio ED, Matteo GD, Familiari L, Ficano L, Loriga P, Morini S, Pietropaolo V, Zambelli A, Grossi E, Tessari F, Intraligi M, Buscema M, SIED Appropriateness Working Group. Upper GI endoscopy in elderly patients: predictive factors of relevant endoscopic findings. Intern Emerg

Med. 2013;8:141–6. https://doi.org/10.1007/s11739-011-0598-3.

Callahan CM, Haag KM, Weinberger M, Tierney WM, Buchanan NN, Stump TE, Nisi R. Outcomes of percutaneous endoscopic gastrostomy among older adults in a community setting. J Am Geriatr Soc. 2000;48 (9):1048–54.

Cangemi DJ, Stark ME, Cangemi JR, Lukens FJ, Gómez V. Double-balloon enteroscopy and outcomes in patients older than 80. Age Ageing. 2015;44:529–32. https://doi.org/10.1093/ageing/afv003.

Carmel R. Prevalence of undiagnosed pernicious anemia in the elderly. Arch Intern Med. 1996;156:1097–100.

Cha JM, Kozarek RA, La Selva D, Gluck M, Ross A, Chiorean M, Koch J, Lin OS. Risks and benefits of colonoscopy in patients 90 years or older, compared with younger patients. Clin Gastroenterol Hepatol. 2016;14:80–6.e1. https://doi.org/10.1016/j.cgh.2015.06.036.

Chokhavatia S, John ES, Bridgeman MB, Dixit D. Constipation in elderly patients with non-cancer pain: focus on opioid-induced constipation. Drugs Aging. 2016;33:557–74. https://doi.org/10.1007/s40266-016-0381-2.

Cui X, Zhou T, Jiang D, Liu H, Wang J, Yuan S, Li H, Yan P, Gao Y. Clinical manifestations and endoscopic presentations of gastric lymphoma: a multicenter seven year retrospective survey. Rev Esp Enferm Dig. 2017;10:566–71. https://doi.org/10.17235/reed.2017.4882/2017.

Day LW, Kwon A, Inadomi JM, Walter LC, Somsouk M. Adverse events in older patients undergoing colonoscopy: a systematic review and meta-analysis. Gastrointest Endosc. 2011;74:885–96. https://doi.org/10.1016/j.gie.2011.06.023.

de Wit F, van Vliet AL, de Wilde RB, Jansen JR, Vuyk J, Aarts LP, de Jonge E, Veelo DP, Geerts BF. The effect of propofol on haemodynamics: cardiac output, venous return, mean systemic filling pressure, and vascular resistances. Br J Anaesth. 2016;116(6):784–9. https://doi.org/10.1093/bja/aew126.

DeLegge MH, McClave SA, DiSario JA, Baskin WN, Brown RD, Fang JC, Ginsberg GG. ASGE Task Force on enteral nutrition. Ethical and medicolegal aspects of PEG-tube placement and provision of artificial nutritional therapy. Gastrointest Endosc. 2005;62:952–9.

Di Caro S, May A, Heine DG, et al. The European experience with double-balloon enteroscopy: indications, methodology, safety, and clinical impact. Gastrointest Endosc. 2005;62:545–50.

Drahos J, Xiao Q, Risch HA, Freedman ND, Abnet CC, Anderson LA, Bernstein L, Brown L, Chow WH, Gammon MD, Kamangar F, Liao LM, Murray LJ, Ward MH, Ye W, Wu AH, Vaughan TL, Whiteman DC, Cook MB. Age-specific risk factor profiles of adenocarcinomas of the esophagus: a pooled analysis from the international BEACON consortium. Int J Cancer. 2016;138:55–64. https://doi.org/10.1002/ijc.29688.

Dumic I, Nordin T, Jecmenica M, Stojkovic Lalosevic M, Milosavljevic T, Milovanovic T. Gastrointestinal tract disorders in older age. Can J Gastroenterol Hepatol. 2019;2019:6757524. https://doi.org/10.1155/2019/6757524.

Durazzo M, Campion D, Fagoonee S, Pellicano R. Gastrointestinal tract disorders in the elderly. Minerva Med. 2017;108:575–91. https://doi.org/10.23736/S0026-4806.17.05417-9.

Finkelmeier F, Tal A, Ajouaou M, Filmann N, Zeuzem S, Waidmann O, Albert J. ERCP in elderly patients: increased risk of sedation adverse events but low frequency of post-ERCP pancreatitis. Gastrointest Endosc. 2015;82:1051–9. https://doi.org/10.1016/j.gie.2015.04.032.

Friedrich K, Stremmel W, Sieg A. Endoscopist-administered propofol sedation is safe – a prospective evaluation of 10,000 patients in an outpatient practice. J Gastrointestin Liver Dis. 2012;21:259–63. PubMed PMID: 23012666

Fritz E, Kirchgatterer A, Hubner D, Aschl G, Hinterreiter M, Stadler B, Knoflach P. ERCP is safe and effective in patients 80 years of age and older compared with younger patients. Gastrointest Endosc. 2006;64:899–905.

Gómez V, Racho RG, Woodward TA, Wallace MB, Raimondo M, Bouras EP, Lukens FJ. Colonic endoscopic mucosal resection of large polyps: Is it safe in the very elderly? Dig Liver Dis. 2014;46:701–5. https://doi.org/10.1016/j.dld.2014.03.012.

Gralnek IM, Dumonceau JM, Kuipers EJ, Lanas A, Sanders DS, Kurien M, Rotondano G, Hucl T, Dinis-Ribeiro M, Marmo R, Racz I, Arezzo A, Hoffmann RT, Lesur G, de Franchis R, Aabakken L, Veitch A, Radaelli F, Salgueiro P, Cardoso R, Maia L, Zullo diagnosis and management of nonvariceal upper gastrointestinal hemorrhage: European Society of Gastrointestinal Endoscopy (ESGE) Guideline. Endoscopy. 2015; 47(10):a1–46. https://doi.org/10.1055/s-0034-1393172. Epub 2015 Sep 29.

Grande L, Lacima G, Ros E, Pera M, Ascaso C, Visa J, Pera C. Deterioration of esophageal motility with age: a manometric study of 79 healthy subjects. Am J Gastroenterol. 1999;94:1795–801.

Grant MD, Rudberg MA, Brody JA. Gastrostomy placement and mortality among hospitalized Medicare beneficiaries. JAMA. 1998;279:1973–6.

Gressenberger P. Reversal strategies in patients treated with direct oral anticoagulants. Vasa. 2019;5:1–4. https://doi.org/10.1024/0301-1526/a000777. PubMed PMID: 30719950

Gryglewski A, Kuta M, Pasternak A, Opach Z, Walocha J, Richter P. Hiatal hernia with upside-down stomach. Management of acute incarceration: case presentation and review of literature. Folia Med Cracov. 2016;56:61–6.

Heine GD, Hadithi M, Groenen MJ, et al. Double-balloon enteroscopy: indications, diagnostic yield, and complications in a series of 275 patients with suspected small-bowel disease. Endoscopy. 2006;38:42–8.

Higuchi T, Iwakiri R, Hara M, Shimoda R, Sakata Y, Nakayama A, Nio K, Yamaguchi S, Yamaguchi D, Watanabe A, Akutagawa T, Sakata H, Fujimoto K. Low-dose aspirin and comorbidities are significantly related to bleeding peptic ulcers in elderly patients compared with nonelderly patients in Japan. Intern Med. 2014;53:367–73.

Hong MJ, Sung IK, Lee SP, Cheon BK, Kang H, Kim TY. Randomized comparison of recovery time after use of remifentanil alone versus midazolam and meperidine for colonoscopy anesthesia. Dig Endosc. 2015;27:113–20. https://doi.org/10.1111/den.12383.

Jafri SM, Monkemuller K, Lukens FJ. Endoscopy in the elderly: a review of the efficacy and safety of colonoscopy, esophagogastroduodenoscopy, and endoscopic retrograde cholangiopancreatography. J Clin Gastroenterol. 2010;44:161–6. https://doi.org/10.1097/MCG.0b013e3181c64d64.

Karajeh MA, Sanders DS, Hurlstone DP. Colonoscopy in elderly people is a safe procedure with a high diagnostic yield: a prospective comparative study of 2000 patients. Endoscopy. 2006;38:226–30.

Katsinelos P, Paroutoglou G, Kountouras J, Zavos C, Beltsis A, Tzovaras G. Efficacy and safety of therapeutic ERCP in patients 90 years of age and older. Gastrointest Endosc. 2006;63:417–23.

Kirchhof P, Benussi S, Kotecha D, et al. 2016 ESC Guidelines for the management of atrial fibrillation developed in collaboration with EACTS. Eur Heart J. 2016;37(38):2893–962.

Knapp AB, Ladetsky L. Endoscopic retrieval of a small bowel enteroscopy capsule lodged in a Zenker's diverticulum. Clin Gastroenterol Hepatol. 2005;3:xxxiv.

Kolkman JJ, Geelkerken RH. Diagnosis and treatment of chronic mesenteric ischemia: an update. Best Pract Res Clin Gastroenterol. 2017;31(1):49–57. https://doi.org/10.1016/j.bpg.2017.01.003.

Kuipers EJ. Pernicious anemia, atrophic gastritis, and the risk of cancer. Clin Gastroenterol Hepatol. 2015;13:2290–2. https://doi.org/10.1016/j.cgh.2015.07.013.

Lanza FL, Chan FK, Quigley EM. Practice parameters Committee of the American College of Gastroenterology. Guidelines for prevention of NSAID-related ulcer complications. Am J Gastroenterol. 2009;104:728–38. https://doi.org/10.1038/ajg.2009.115.

Lawson RM. Mesenteric Ischemia. Crit Care Nurs Clin North Am. 2018;30:29–39. https://doi.org/10.1016/j.cnc.2017.10.003. Epub 2017 Nov 20. PMID: 29413213

Lee TC, Huang SP, Yang JY, Chang CY, Liou JM, Liu CH, Huang MS, Wang HP. Age is not a discriminating factor for outcomes of therapeutic upper gastrointestinal endoscopy. Hepato-Gastroenterology. 2007;54:1319–22.

Leighton JA, Sharma VK, Srivathsan K, et al. Safety of capsule endoscopy in patients with pacemakers. Gastrointest Endosc. 2004;59:567–9.

Leslie K, Allen ML, Hessian EC, Peyton PJ, Kasza J, Courtney A, Dhar PA, Briedis J, Lee S, Beeton AR, Sayakkarage D, Palanivel S, Taylor JK, Haughton AJ, O'Kane CX. Safety of sedation for gastrointestinal endoscopy in a group of university-affiliated hospitals: a prospective cohort study. Br J Anaesth. 2017;118:90–9. https://doi.org/10.1093/bja/aew393.

Li Y, Han Z, Sun Y, Li A, Zhang W, Li A, Liu S. Endoscopic polypectomy for pacemaker patients: is it safe? ANZ J Surg. 2015;85(11):834–7.

Lieberman DA, Rex DK, Winawer SJ, Giardiello FM, Johnson DA, Levin TR. Guidelines for colonoscopy surveillance after screening and polypectomy: a consensus update by the US Multi-Society Task Force on Colorectal Cancer. Gastroenterology. 2012;143:844–57. https://doi.org/10.1053/j.gastro.2012.06.001.

Lin OS. Sedation for routine gastrointestinal endoscopic procedures: a review on efficacy, safety, efficiency, cost and satisfaction. Intest Res. 2017;15:456–66. https://doi.org/10.5217/ir.2017.15.4.456.

Lippert E, Herfarth HH, Grunert N, Endlicher E, Klebl F. Gastrointestinal endoscopy in patients aged 75 years and older: risks, complications, and findings – a retrospective study. Int J Color Dis. 2015;30:363–6. https://doi.org/10.1007/s00384-014-2088-3.

Lukens FJ, Loeb DS, Machicao VI, Achem SR, Picco MF. Colonoscopy in octogenarians: a prospective outpatient study. Am J Gastroenterol. 2002;97:1722–5.

Lukens FJ, Howell DA, Upender S, Sheth SG, Jafri SM. ERCP in the very elderly: outcomes among patients older than eighty. Dig Dis Sci. 2010;55:847–51. https://doi.org/10.1007/s10620-009-0784-6.

Maratt JK, Calderwood AH. Colorectal cancer screening and surveillance colonoscopy in older adults. Curr Treat Options Gastroenterol. 2019. https://doi.org/10.1007/s11938-019-00230-9.

Martens P, Bisschops R. Bowel preparation for colonoscopy: efficacy, tolerability and safety. Acta Gastroenterol Belg. 2014;77:249–55.

Miyanaga R, Hosoe N, Naganuma M, Hirata K, Fukuhara S, Nakazato Y, Ojiro K, Iwasaki E, Yahagi N, Ogata H, Kanai T. Complications and outcomes of routine endoscopy in the very elderly. Endosc Int Open. 2018;6(2):E224–9. https://doi.org/10.1055/s-0043-120569.

Modlin IM, Lye KD, Kidd M. Carcinoid tumors of the stomach. Surg Oncol. 2003;12:153–72.

Moneghini D, Lipari A, Missale G, Minelli L, Cengia G, Bontempi L, Curnis A, Cestari R. Lack of interference between small bowel capsule endoscopy and implantable cardiac defibrillators: an 'in vivo' electrophysiological study. United European Gastroenterol J. 2016;4:216–20.

Mönkemüller K, Weigt J, Treiber G, et al. Diagnostic and therapeutic impact of double-balloon enteroscopy. Endoscopy. 2006;38:67–72.

Mönkemüller K, Fry LC, Malfertheiner P, Schuckardt W. Gastrointestinal endoscopy in the elderly: current issues. Best Pract Res Clin Gastroenterol. 2009;23:821–7. https://doi.org/10.1016/j.bpg.2009.10.002.

Murphy G, Dawsey SM, Engels EA, Ricker W, Parsons R, Etemadi A, Lin SW, Abnet CC, Freedman ND. Cancer risk after pernicious anemia in the US elderly population. Clin Gastroenterol Hepatol. 2015;13:2282–9. e1-4. https://doi.org/10.1016/j.cgh.2015.05.040.

Obana T, Fujita N, Noda Y, Kobayashi G, Ito K, Horaguchi J, Koshita S, Kanno Y, Yamashita Y, Kato Y, Ogawa T. Efficacy and safety of therapeutic ERCP for the elderly with choledocholithiasis: comparison with younger patients. Intern Med. 2010;49:1935–41.

Parekh PJ, Buerlein RC, Shams R, Herre J, Johnson DA. An update on the management of implanted cardiac devices during electrosurgical procedures. Gastrointest Endosc. 2013;78(6):836–41.

Pontone S, Palma R, Panetta C, Pironi D, Eberspacher C, Angelini R, Pontone P, Catania A, Filippini A, Sorrenti S. Endoscopic mucosal resection in elderly patients. Aging Clin Exp Res. 2017;29(Suppl 1):109–13. https://doi.org/10.1007/s40520-016-0661-z.

Qumseya B, David W, Woodward TA, Raimondo M, Wallace MB, Wolfsen HC, Lukens FJ. Safety of esophageal EMR in elderly patients. Gastrointest Endosc. 2014;80:586–91. https://doi.org/10.1016/j.gie.2014.02.010.

Riphaus A, Stergiou N, Wehrmann T. Sedation with propofol for routine ERCP in high-risk octogenarians: a randomized, controlled study. Am J Gastroenterol. 2005;100:1957–63.

Riphaus A, Geist F, Wehrmann T. Endoscopic sedation and monitoring practice in Germany: re-evaluation from the first nationwide survey 3 years after the implementation of an evidence and consent based national guideline. Z Gastroenterol. 2013;51:1082–8. https://doi.org/10.1055/s-0033-1335104.

Rondonotti E, Spada C, Pennazio M, de Franchis R, Cadoni S, Girelli C, Hassan C, Marmo R, Riccioni ME, Scarpulla G, Soncini M, Vecchi M, Cannizzaro R. Adherence to European Society of Gastrointestinal Endoscopy recommendations of endoscopists performing small bowel capsule endoscopy in Italy. Dig Liver Dis. 2018a. https://doi.org/10.1016/j.dld.2018.11.031. pii: S1590-8658(18)31270-2.

Rondonotti E, Spada C, Adler S, May A, Despott EJ, Koulaouzidis A, Panter S, Domagk D, Fernandez-Urien I, Rahmi G, Riccioni ME, van Hooft JE, Hassan C, Pennazio M. Small-bowel capsule endoscopy and device-assisted enteroscopy for diagnosis and treatment of small-bowel disorders: European Society of Gastrointestinal Endoscopy (ESGE) Technical Review. Endoscopy. 2018b;50:423–46. https://doi.org/10.1055/a-0576-0566.

Sanaani A, Yandrapalli S, Harburger JM. Antithrombotic management of patients with prosthetic heart valves. Cardiol Rev. 2018;26(4):177–86. https://doi.org/10.1097/CRD.0000000000000189. Review. PubMed PMID: 29608496

Schechter RB, Lemme EM, Novais P, Biccas B. Achalasia in the elderly patient: a comparative study. Arq Gastroenterol. 2011;48:19–23.

Shah SB, Pahade A, Chawla R. Novel reversal agents and laboratory evaluation for direct-acting oral anticoagulants (DOAC): An update. Indian J Anaesth. 2019;63:169–81. https://doi.org/10.4103/ija.IJA_734_18.

Son YW, Kim A, Jeon HH. Efficacy and safety of endoscopic submucosal dissection for gastric epithelial neoplasia in elderly patients aged 80 years and older. Aging Clin Exp Res. 2019. https://doi.org/10.1007/s40520-019-01133-6.

Stähli BE, Landmesser U. Dual antiplatelet therapy after percutaneous coronary intervention for stable CAD or ACS: redefining the optimal duration of treatment. Herz. 2018;43(1):11–9. https://doi.org/10.1007/s00059-017-4654-2. PubMed PMID: 29236148

Stone JR, Wilkins LR. Acute mesenteric ischemia. Tech Vasc Interv Radiol. 2015;18:24–30. https://doi.org/10.1053/j.tvir.2014.12.004.

Sung HY, Kim JS, Lee KS, Kim YI, Song IU, Chung SW, Yang DW, Cho YK, Park JM, Lee IS, Kim SW, Chung IS, Choi MG. The prevalence and patterns of pharyngoesophageal dysmotility in patients with early stage Parkinson's disease. Mov Disord. 2010;25:2361–8. https://doi.org/10.1002/mds.23290.

Tamai N, Saito Y, Sakamoto T, Nakajima T, Matsuda T, Tajiri H. Safety and efficacy of colorectal endoscopic submucosal dissection in elders: clinical and follow-up outcomes. Int J Color Dis. 2012;27:1493–9. https://doi.org/10.1007/s00384-012-1514-7.

Teshima CW, May G. Small bowel enteroscopy. Can J Gastroenterol. 2012;26(5):269–75.

Theocharis GJ, Arvaniti V, Assimakopoulos SF, Thomopoulos KC, Xourgias V, Mylonakou I, Nikolopoulou VN. Acute upper gastrointestinal bleeding in octogenarians: clinical outcome and factors related to mortality. World J Gastroenterol. 2008;14:4047–53.

Thomson AB. Small intestinal disorders in the elderly. Best Pract Res Clin Gastroenterol. 2009;23:861–74. https://doi.org/10.1016/j.bpg.2009.10.009.

Toya Y, Endo M, Nakamura S, Akasaka R, Yanai S, Kawasaki K, Koeda K, Eizuka M, Fujita Y, Uesugi N, Ishida K, Sugai T, Matsumoto T. Long-term outcomes and prognostic factors with non-curative endoscopic submucosal dissection for gastric cancer in elderly patients aged ≥ 75 years. Gastric Cancer; 2018. https://doi.org/10.1007/s10120-018-00913-9.

Travis AC, Pievsky D, Saltzman JR. Endoscopy in the elderly. Am J Gastroenterol. 2012;107:1495–501. https://doi.org/10.1038/ajg.2012.246.

Treskatsch S, Ocken M, Lembcke A, Spies C, Braun JP. Upside-down stomach as a rare cause of obstructive shock and cardiac arrest. Intensive Care Med. 2013;39:2209–10.

Ukkonen M, Siiki A, Antila A, Tyrväinen T, Sand J, Laukkarinen J. Safety and Efficacy of Acute Endoscopic Retrograde Cholangiopancreatography in the Elderly. Dig Dis Sci. 2016;61:3302–8.

US Preventive Services Task Force, Bibbins-Domingo K, Grossman DC, Curry SJ, Davidson KW, Epling JW Jr, García FAR, Gillman MW, Harper DM, Kemper AR, Krist AH, Kurth AE, Landefeld CS, Mangione CM, Owens DK, Phillips WR, Phipps MG, Pignone MP, Siu AL. Screening for colorectal cancer: US Preventive Services Task Force Recommendation Statement. JAMA. 2016;315:2564–75. https://doi.org/10.1001/jama.2016.5989.

van Hees F, Saini SD, Lansdorp-Vogelaar I, Vijan S, Meester RG, de Koning HJ, Zauber AG, van Ballegooijen M. Personalizing colonoscopy screening for elderly individuals based on screening history, cancer risk, and comorbidity status could increase cost effectiveness. Gastroenterology. 2015;149:1425–37. https://doi.org/10.1053/j.gastro.2015.07.042.

Veitch AM, Vanbiervliet G, Gershlick AH, Boustiere C, Baglin TP, Smith LA, Radaelli F, Knight E, Gralnek IM, Hassan C, Dumonceau JM. Endoscopy in patients on antiplatelet or anticoagulant therapy, including direct oral anticoagulants: British Society of Gastroenterology (BSG) and European Society of Gastrointestinal Endoscopy (ESGE) guidelines. Endoscopy. 2016;48:385.

Virk GS, Jafri M, Ashley C. Colonoscopy and colorectal cancer rates among octogenarians and nonagenarians: nationwide study of US veterans. Clin Interv Aging. 2019;14:609–14. https://doi.org/10.2147/CIA.S192497.

Warren JL, Klabunde CN, Mariotto AB, Meekins A, Topor M, Brown ML, Ransohoff DF. Adverse events after outpatient colonoscopy in the Medicare population. Ann Intern Med. 2009;150:849–57, W152

Watari J, Chen N, Amenta PS, Fukui H, Oshima T, Tomita T, Miwa H, Lim KJ, Das KM. *Helicobacter pylori* associated chronic gastritis, clinical syndromes, precancerous lesions, and pathogenesis of gastric cancer development. World J Gastroenterol. 2014;20:5461–73. https://doi.org/10.3748/wjg.v20.i18.5461.

Weerasuriya N, Snape J. Oesophageal candidiasis in elderly patients: risk factors, prevention and management. Drugs Aging. 2008;25:119–30.

Wirth R, Dziewas R, Beck AM, Clavé P, Hamdy S, Heppner HJ, Langmore S, Leischker AH, Martino R, Pluschinski P, Rösler A, Shaker R, Warnecke T, Sieber CC, Volkert D. Oropharyngeal dysphagia in older persons – from pathophysiology to adequate intervention: a review and summary of an international expert meeting. Clin Interv Aging. 2016;11:189–208. https://doi.org/10.2147/CIA.S9748.

Wiskur B, Greenwood-Van Meerveld B. The aging colon: the role of enteric neurodegeneration in constipation. Curr Gastroenterol Rep. 2010;12:507–12. https://doi.org/10.1007/s11894-010-0139-7.

Yamaguchi H, Fukuzawa M, Kawai T, Matsumoto T, Suguro M, Uchida K, Koyama Y, Madarame A, Morise T, Aoki Y, Sugimoto A, Yamauchi Y, Kono S, Tsuji Y, Yagi K, Itoi T. Impact of gastric endoscopic submucosal dissection in elderly patients: the latest single center large cohort study with a review of the literature. Medicine (Baltimore). 2019;98:e14842. https://doi.org/10.1097/MD.0000000000014842. PubMed PMID: 30882676; PubMed Central PMCID: PMC6426470

Yang TC, Hou MC, Chen PH, Hsin IF, Chen LK, Tsou MY, Lin HC, Lee FY. Clinical outcomes and complications of endoscopic submucosal dissection for superficial gastric neoplasms in the elderly. Medicine (Baltimore). 2015;94:e1964. https://doi.org/10.1097/MD.0000000000001964.

Yaylak F, Deger A, Bayhan Z, Kocak C, Zeren S, Kocak FE, Ekici MF, Algın MC. Histopathological gallbladder morphometric measurements in geriatric patients with symptomatic chronic cholecystitis. Ir J Med Sci. 2016;185:871–6.

Eduardo Redondo-Cerezo

Contents

Abstract

Gastrointestinal endoscopy has never been comfortable for patients. As it evolves, more complex, lengthy, and interventional procedures are performed, and patients prefer sedation to undergo endoscopy. Sedation needs to be adapted to the singularities of older adults, who essentially manifest a higher burden of comorbidities. They require lower doses of most usual sedatives required to reach an acceptable level of sedation while preserving safety. Endoscopy requires the whole range of the anesthetic spectrum, from superficial sedation to general anesthesia, a judicious selection of the type of sedation, the setting of the procedure, the sedation plan, and the drug utilized,

E. Redondo-Cerezo (✉)
Endoscopy Unit. Gastroenterology Department, 'Virgen de las Nieves' University Hospital, Granada, Spain
e-mail: eredondoc@gmail.com

© Springer Nature Switzerland AG 2021
C. S. Pitchumoni, T. S. Dharmarajan (eds.), *Geriatric Gastroenterology*,
https://doi.org/10.1007/978-3-030-30192-7_103

as a prerequisite for endoscopy. When performed by endoscopists, midazolam and a sedative versus propofol-based sedation are the two main options. Anesthesiologists are required in some situations, and they must actively collaborate with the endoscopy team to provide the best sedation regime for each patient. Individual characteristics as well as local expertise and regulations are the key points to choose either option. Regardless of the particularities of older patients, general principles about sedation can be applied to most individuals.

Keywords

Sedation for endoscopy · Older adults and sedation · Propofol for endoscopy · Non-anesthesiologist sedation for endoscopy · Unsedated endoscopy in the older adult · Risks for sedation · Midazolam · Propofol · ASA classification · Sedation · Moderate and deep · Fentanyl · GABA

Introduction

The evolution of gastrointestinal endoscopy has led to more complex procedures, which are time-consuming and require precision. Indeed, gastrointestinal endoscopy was never comfortable for patients, but longer interventional procedures, as well as a society that is increasingly concerned about suffering and discomfort, have raised requests for sedation and anesthesia for both diagnostic and interventional endoscopy. Thus, the vast majority of endoscopies are done with the aid of intravenous sedation, and this should be offered virtually to every patient who receives endoscopy, regardless of the type of procedure or the age and comorbidities of the patient.

Technological advances in endoscopy have allowed for faster and less painful examinations. Advances like the utilization of thinner endoscopes, variable stiffness colonoscopes, CO_2 insufflation, and water immersion techniques (in colonoscopy) allow for less painful procedures. Although helpful, these options are probably not as effective with regard to patients' comfort as intravenous sedation has shown to be, although they have been valuable auxiliary tools to improve tolerability.

Indeed, there has been a continuous evolution regarding sedation practices for endoscopy since the early 1960s, when pentobarbital use was described. Meperidine as an analgesic was an initial strategy, followed by the widespread adoption of the combination with diazepam, which led to midazolam as the staple of moderate sedation. There was an FDA warning about this drug, but it was successfully addressed by the agency and the American Society of Gastrointestinal Endoscopy (ASGE). Subsequently, propofol used by anesthesiologists and even by gastroenterologists in nurse-administered propofol sedation (NAPS) has revolutionized sedation in endoscopy, leading to deep sedation performed by trained endoscopists and nurses (Ferreira and Cravo 2015).

The physician role with regard to sedation is to minimize pain and discomfort balancing this goal with a minimization of adverse events related to the procedure (perforation, bleeding, and others) and to the sedation (hypoxemia, aspiration, and cardiac events) (Thomson et al. 2010).

As far as patients referred to endoscopy are concerned, we should consider the clear aging tendency in Western countries, as well as the increasing proportion of those patients that seek gastrointestinal healthcare, with growing numbers of gastrointestinal procedures in elderly individuals. Indeed, endoscopic procedures are now better tolerated due to technological progress and sedation.

In this chapter we will address sedation for endoscopic procedures in older individuals, focusing on the general aspects of sedation in this particular population.

Definition of Sedation

The American Association of Anesthesiologists (ASA) state that "sedation and analgesia" comprise a continuum of states ranging from minimal sedation (anxiolysis) through "general anesthesia" (American Society of Anesthesiologists

Table 1 Definition of general anesthesia and levels of sedation/analgesia

	Minimal sedation or anxiolysis	Moderate sedation or analgesia ("conscious sedation")	Deep sedation or analgesia	General anesthesia
Responsiveness	Normal response to verbal stimulation	Purposeful response to verbal or tactile stimulation	Purposeful response following repeated or painful stimulation	Unarousable even with painful stimulus
Airway	Unaffected	No intervention required	Intervention may be required	Intervention often required
Spontaneous ventilation	Unaffected	Adequate	Maybe inadequate	Frequently inadequate
Cardiovascular function	Unaffected	Usually maintained	Usually maintained	Maybe impaired

Task Force on and Analgesia by non-anesthesiologists 2002). Therefore, there are different levels of sedation, and the whole four levels (see Table 1) are used in endoscopy at different situations, depending on the procedure and patients' characteristics. In this wide range, minimal sedation, also called *anxiolysis*, is a drug-induced state during which patients respond normally to verbal commands. Although cognitive function and physical coordination may be impaired, airway reflexes and ventilatory and cardiovascular functions are normal. *Moderate sedation*, also called conscious sedation, is a drug-induced depression of consciousness during which patients respond purposefully to verbal commands, either alone or accompanied by light tactile stimulation. No interventions are required to maintain a patent airway, and spontaneous ventilation is adequate. Cardiovascular function is usually maintained. *Deep sedation* is a drug-induced depression of consciousness during which patients cannot be easily aroused but respond purposefully following repeated or painful stimulation. The ability to independently maintain ventilatory function may be impaired. Patients may require assistance in maintaining a patent airway, and spontaneous ventilation may be inadequate. Cardiovascular function is usually maintained. The last stage is *general anesthesia*, sometimes needed in interventional and complex endoscopy, as the safest and most adequate method (American Society of Anesthesiologists Task Force on and Analgesia by non-anesthesiologists 2002).

The Older Individual, Singularities, and Special Features

Biological age is the result of pathophysiologic aging processes, comorbidity, and genetic factors, and it has largely been recognized as more important than chronological age in defining the degree of fitness and performance of a given individual when facing health issues (Demongeot 2009). Geriatric population presents, with respect to the rest of the population, some clinical singularities that should be considered before performing endoscopy, such as the higher prevalence of cardiovascular, respiratory, renal, and metabolic conditions (Bettelli 2018). In accordance with the ASA (American Society of Anesthesiologists) physical status classification system, surgical risk is influenced by the patient's basal health conditions (Table 2). Indeed, relationships between comorbidities and postoperative complications are well-known. Further, functional status, which has been proven to predict mortality among older hospitalized patients, is the sum of behaviors needed to maintain daily activities, including social and cognitive functions. Comprehensive geriatric assessment (CGA) is used by anesthesiologists in the preoperative assessment of surgical risk of elderly individuals (Partridge et al. 2017).

It is essential to keep in mind that patients over 70 years suffer from at least one associated condition and in 30% of them two or even more. Multiple prescriptions are the norm, with the subsequent associated risk of drug interaction, poor adherence, and increased risks derived from drugs with effects

Table 2 ASA physical status classification system

Classification	Definition	Adult examples (including but not limited to)
ASA I	A normal healthy patient	Healthy, non-smoking, no or minimal alcohol use
ASA II	A patient with mild systemic disease	Mild diseases only without substantive functional limitations. Examples include (but not limited to) current smoker, social alcohol drinker, pregnancy, obesity (30 < BMI < 40), well-controlled DM/HTN, mild lung disease
ASA III	A patient with severe systemic disease	Substantive normal limitations; one or more moderate to severe diseases. Examples include(but not limited to) poorly controlled diabetes, HTN, COPD, morbid obesity, active hepatitis, alcohol dependence or abuse, implanted pacemaker, moderate reduction of ejection fraction, ESRD undergoing regularly scheduled dialysis, premature infant PCA <60 weeks, history (>3 months) of IM, TIA, or CAD/stents
ASA IV	A patient with severe systemic disease that is a constant threat to life	Examples include (but not limited to) recent (<3 months) MI, TIA, or CAD/stents, ongoing cardiac ischemia or severe valve dysfunction, severe reduction of ejection fraction, sepsis, DIC, ARD, or ESRD not undergoing regularly scheduled dialysis
ASA V	A moribund patient who is not expected to survive without the operation	Examples include (but not limited to) ruptured abdominal/thoracic aneurysm, massive trauma, intracranial bleed with mass effect, ischemic bowel in the faces of significant cardiac pathology or multiple organ/system dysfunction
ASA VI	A declared brain death patient whose organs are being removed for donor purposes	

From the American Society of Anaesthesiologists website (amended October 23, 2019)

on the central nervous system and thromboembolic and other complications (Bettelli 2018).

It is also well-known that essential pharmacokinetic and pharmacodynamic changes are associated with the process of aging. Regarding sedation, the brain becomes more sensitive to sedative agents, such as benzodiazepines and propofol. The measurement of specific propofol drug effects on electroencephalography (EEG) demonstrated an increased sensitivity to the propofol drug effect in the elderly (Schnider et al. 1999). Aging determines an increased half time for lipophilic drugs, as well as impaired renal and hepatic clearance, that must be considered when calculating drug dosages. Those facts can prolong the recovery of those patients after sedation.

Some factors have been recommended as a part of presurgical evaluation of geriatric patients undergoing endoscopy, which are depicted in Table 3. Although such a thorough evaluation is probably not necessary for simple diagnostic procedures, most of these issues should be taken into account before performing advanced endoscopy in this population (Bettelli 2018).

Table 3 Elements recommended as part of preoperative assessment

Cognitive function and metal capacity
Depression
Alcohol and other substance abuse
Cardiac evaluation
Respiratory evaluation
Functional status
Nutritional status
Medications
Treatment goals and patient's expectations
Availability of family support

Sedating the Older Adult: Who Should Perform Sedation?

The obvious answer to this question is that a proficient, specifically trained provider should sedate older individuals undergoing endoscopy. In light of the published evidence, gastroenterologist-guided propofol sedation has been successfully performed from the first decade of the current century in the elderly (Heuss et al.

2003), as well as in complex procedures and high-risk patients (Fatima et al. 2008; Redondo-Cerezo et al. 2012). After those initial experiences, large series have been issued, supporting the ability of gastroenterologists to perform sedation for endoscopic procedures (Heuss et al. 2012; Rex et al. 2009).

As advised by the several gastroenterology societies, the physician who performs sedation needs to be specifically trained for the procedure. In fact, this provider should be able to resuscitate or rescue a patient whose level of sedation is deeper than deep sedation. A specific training in sedation should be a requirement, teaching from minimal to moderate sedation, and rescuing techniques when the sedation process goes too far. A multi-society sedation curriculum has been developed with this purpose (ASGE Standards of Practice Committee et al. 2018; American Association for the Study of Liver et al. 2012).

Regarding the personnel involved in sedation, it seems reasonable and has been advised as a grade A recommendation, that non-anesthesiologist sedation should be controlled by a specific person, dedicated to this purpose exclusively (Dumonceau et al. 2015). Regardless of the professional level, physician or nurse, the key point is adequate training of the professional, who might be under the guidance of the physician, either an anesthesiologist or a gastroenterologist.

When it comes to legal concerns, practitioners should be aware of the legislations in their countries. Although some controversy has historically arisen with anesthesiology societies, looking at the published evidence, we must assume that gastroenterologist-directed sedation is safe (Rex 2016).

Sedating Older Patients: A Tailored Sedation Schedule

When applying intravenous sedation to an old patient, we need to consider two different aspects:

- Patient-related issues
- Procedure-related issues

Although no clear guidelines have been established, it is recommended that complex, lengthy, and risky procedures should be sedated or anesthetized by an anesthesiologist, experienced in sedation and anesthesia for endoscopic procedures (ASGE Standards of Practice Committee et al. 2018). This must be emphasized for geriatric patients, in which additional risks exist beyond the procedure complexity. Although there is a thin line, with differences in practices in different countries and even in the same country, we might state that sedation for long procedures, both upper and lower, comprises more risks (Fisher et al. 2006). Moreover, upper procedures are more reflexogenic, the airway is more exposed, and, apart from basic upper endoscopy, ERCP, EUS, or enteroscopy are complex and skill-demanding techniques. In those cases, an anesthesiologist is of help, a stress-relieving support for the endoscopist.

The other important point is to make the minimal assessment necessary to know patients' added risks. In this sense, some simple issues to address are the following (ASGE Standards of Practice Committee et al. 2018):

1. History of snoring, stridor, or sleep apnea
2. Drug allergies and current medications
3. Prior adverse reactions to sedation or anesthesia
4. Tobacco, alcohol, or other substance abuse

ASA classification has also been recognized as a risk marker, and it has been largely recognized as an essential tool for the stratification of risk in endoscopy (ASGE Standards of Practice Committee et al. 2018). Indeed, based on the CORI database (Clinical Outcomes Research Initiative), increasing ASA class was associated with a stepwise increase in the probability of serious adverse events, and ESGE recommends sedation guided by an anesthesiologist in individuals with ASA ≥ 3 (Dumonceau et al. 2015).

Body mass index (BMI) has been associated with sedation-related complications, and care should be taken in obese and overweight patients, usually associated with a wider neck circumference and obstructive sleep apnea (OSA). OSA, together with older age, higher BMI, and total dose of propofol, is an independent predictor of hypoxemia during colonoscopy under propofol sedation (Dumonceau et al. 2015). For the diagnosis of OSA, a usually underdiagnosed entity, simple questionnaires such as the STOP-BANG previous to the endoscopy provide a high negative predictive value for the diagnosis of moderate and severe OSA (Table 4) (Chung et al. 2008).

A final but unavoidable evaluation of patients' airway should be performed, with the aim to predict complications and to seek help from an airway expert such as the anesthesiologist. Mallampati classification is an easy tool that identifies potential obstructive sleep apnea and predicts difficulties with endotracheal intubation (Fig. 1) (ASGE Standards of Practice Committee et al. 2018). However, a simpler and easier test, the upper lip bite test showed the most favorable diagnostic test accuracy properties regarding the same goals (Roth et al. 2018) (Fig. 2). Other simple characters that anyone performing sedation should take into account beforehand are the following (ASGE Standards of Practice Committee et al. 2018):

1. Previous problems with anesthesia or sedation, particularly with tracheal intubation
2. A story of sleep apnea
3. Dysmorphic facial features
4. Oral abnormalities, such a small opening (<3 cm in adults), gross dental abnormalities, high-arched palate, macroglossia, tonsillar hypertrophy, or nonvisible uvula
5. Neck abnormalities, such as obesity affecting the neck or face, short neck, limited neck

Table 4 STOP-BANG questionnaire (16)

S *(snoring)*	Do you snore loudly? (Louder than talking or loud enough to be heard through closed doors)
T *(tiredness)*	Do you often feel tired, fatigued, or sleepy during daytime?
O *(observed)*	Has anyone observed you stop breathing during your sleep?
P *(blood pressure)*	Do you have or are your been treated for high blood pressure?
B *(BMI)*	>35 kg/m^2
A *(age)*	>50 year
N *(neck)*	> 40 cm
G *(gender)*	Male

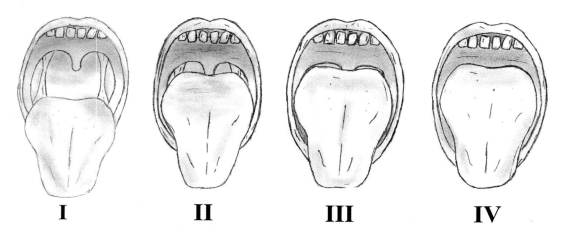

Fig. 1 Mallampati classification. (Illustrations: Mr. Eduardo Redondo-Godino)

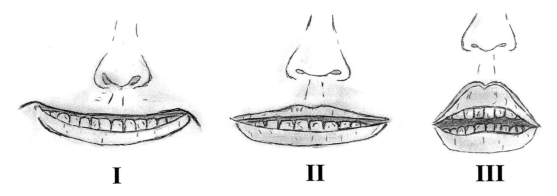

Fig. 2 Bite test. (Illustrations: Mr. Eduardo Redondo-Godino)

extension, neck masses, cervical spine disease or trauma, or diminished hyoid-mental distance (<3 cm)
6. Jaw abnormalities, such as micrognathia, retrognathia, trismus, or malocclusion

In the general population, which is also applicable to older people, the American Society of Anesthesiology recommends the assistance of an anesthesiologist in the following situations (ASGE Standards of Practice Committee et al. 2018):

• Prolonged or therapeutic endoscopic procedures
• Anticipated intolerance to standard sedatives
• Severe comorbidity (ASA class IV or V)
• Increased risk of airway obstruction related to anatomic abnormalities

Sedation Plan and Patient Monitoring During Procedure

As stated by the ASGE guideline, for both moderate and deep sedation, the level of consciousness and vital signs must be assessed and documented at different moments (ASGE Standards of Practice Committee et al. 2018):

1. Before the beginning of the procedure
2. After administration of sedative agents
3. Every 5 min during the procedure
4. During initial recovery
5. Before discharge

The sedation plan should be adapted to the characteristics of the patient, especially in older individuals who are probably more prone to adverse events. The first accepted need for monitoring is an intravenous access, preferably a catheter, until full patient's recovery (Dumonceau et al. 2015). A continuous infusion of saline has been used and recommended, in order to secure the intravenous line and to provide a quick way to infuse fluids in case of hypotension, a usual and recognized adverse event (Heuss et al. 2003; Redondo-Cerezo et al. 2012). Oxygen administered through a nasal probe has shown to reduce oxygen desaturation, and it has been recommended by every major society (ASGE Standards of Practice Committee et al. 2018; Dumonceau et al. 2015). Moreover, it has been suggested that preoxygenation for some minutes before sedation with a fraction of inspired oxygen (FiO_2) as close to one as possible may protect from hypoxemia the majority of patients that eventually progress to apnea, given the narrow therapeutic window for older individuals (Homfray et al. 2018; Redondo-Cerezo et al. 2012).

In general, when the patient is sedated, it is recommended to use continuous pulse oximetry and automated noninvasive blood pressure measurement (at baseline and then at 3–5 min intervals) throughout the sedation and the recovery period. Continuous electrocardiography is optional in selected patients with history of cardiac and/or pulmonary disease. It has also been suggested to assess baseline oxygen blood saturation, heart rate, and blood pressure (Dumonceau et al. 2015). Capnography is not really a must, because it has not proved to increase patients safety; it has been only endorsed in specific situations, including high-risk individuals, when we intend deep sedation or in long procedures (ASGE Standards of Practice Committee et al. 2018; Dumonceau et al. 2015).

It is wise to have clear goals regarding the endoscopic procedure, the complexity of the procedure itself, and the sedation plan. A short time-out before the beginning of the procedure should consist in a stop of other activities and a verification of patient identification and the general plan for the procedure, including the sedation plan, which should be clear for everyone before endoscopy is begun (ASGE Standards of Practice Committee et al. 2018). Awareness about the most usual complications related to sedation and endoscopic procedure should be clear to all staff members, as well as the needed devices and drugs for the procedures itself and for the most usual complications.

The sedation plan should take into account the patient's individual features, allergies, as well as the drugs and first infusion doses meant to be used.

Special Situations in Older Adult Sedation

- Endoscopy Post-Myocardial Infarction

  As a general rule, emergency endoscopy should not be delayed in an otherwise hemo-dynamically stable patient with a recent myo-cardial infarction. By contrast, elective endoscopy is more controversial. The American Heart Association recommends waiting 60 days for noncardiac surgery following a myocardial infarction if the patient has not undergone coronary revascularization. The recommendation is to wait 14 days after bal-loon angioplasty and 30 days after bare-metal stent implantation. If a drug-eluting stent is inserted, elective noncardiac surgery should be delayed 365 days, if possible (180 days if the risk of delay is greater than the risk of ischemia and stent thrombosis) (Fleisher et al. 2014).

- Implanted Cardiac Defibrillators

  In most situations they do not interfere with the endoscopic procedure. Pacemakers are not usually affected by electrosurgical units, but defibrillators might in some instances. Thus, it is advisable to make sure which device has been implanted in the patient, and ask a cardi-ologist to deactivate the defibrillator while the endoscopy is performed. Interferences can be avoided by placing magnets (Thomson et al. 2010).

- Other Situations

  In general, chronic use of narcotics, benzo-diazepines, alcohol, or other drugs has been associated with the need for greater dosages of the sedative agent. Obesity is always a chal-lenge, as stated before, and can be a risk factor for hypoxemia (Friedrich et al. 2012).

The Endoscopy Room, Drugs, and Emergency Equipment

The room where the sedated endoscopy is performed should be large enough to accom-modate the endoscopic equipment and monitor-ing devices, as well as to allow the easy movement of the health-care workers and a quick access to patient's airway in case compli-cations happen.

The most usual devices used in each procedure should be organized in shelves, with an easy access for the auxiliary personnel. Obviously, suc-tion and oxygen outlets are a must in those facil-ities that might be located close to operating theaters, intensive care units, and cardiac resusci-tation teams. An appropriate recovery area, with at least two boxes (with required resuscitation mate-rial) per endoscopy room, is needed in every endoscopy unit.

Appropriate resuscitation equipment should be easily accessible, with oral and nasal airways of different sizes, endotracheal tubes, laryngoscopes, laryngeal masks, Ambu bag with masks, and intravenous catheters and fluids and a wide range of drugs for life support and reversal agents, including adrenaline, atropine, steroids, naloxone, and flumazenil, among others. A defibrillator is also needed in units where sedation for endoscopy is performed (Thomson et al. 2010).

Depending on the type of procedure, the depth of the sedation required, the length and difficulty of the technique, and patient's comorbidities and characteristics, an anesthesiologist might be required. Without fixed rules in this sense, therapeutic endoscopy, such as ERCP, interventional EUS, ESD, etc., requires the presence of an anesthesiologist or a dedicated trained individual to exclusively control the sedation.

Music in the endoscopy unit has shown to reduce anxiety, heart rate, and arterial blood pressure in patients, although no differences have been found in the doses of drugs utilized. As it is simple and inexpensive, it has been recommended by major endoscopic societies (Dumonceau et al. 2015).

Currently, there is no standard sedation regimen, and the choice of the sedation agent depends on the endoscopist's preference, the procedure, the local protocols, and the legal regulation in each country. Benzodiazepines, mostly midazolam, opioids such as meperidine (not favored in the USA), fentanyl, propofol, ketamine, droperidol, and dexmedetomidine are the most widespread ones:

- Midazolam

    Probably it is the most widely used drug (Versed, as known in the USA) for sedation in everyday endoscopic work. Doses for adults undergoing endoscopy usually range from 1 to 5 mg. It is lipophilic, distributing quickly to the central nervous system, inducing hypnosis within few minutes after its intravenous administration. Its action is due to the potentiation of the neural inhibition mediated by gamma-aminobutyric acid. It has also a dose-dependent ventilatory depressive effect and causes a reduction in arterial blood pressure and an increase in heart rate. It is metabolized by cytochrome P450 enzymes and glucuronide conjugation. The duration of action is greater in older people, probably because of their reduced hepatic and renal metabolic activity, reduced muscle mass, and the associated relative increase of fat relative to body mass. Of note, a paradoxical response to midazolam, where excitement rather than sedation is induced, has been described more commonly in the elderly (Horn and Nesbit 2004; Thomson et al. 2010). The main advantage of midazolam in this population is that it can be reversed by administration of flumazenil, which competitively blocks GABA receptors.

- Propofol

    Propofol (2,6-diisopropylphenol) is a more potent sedative agent with a narrower therapeutic window than benzodiazepines. It is also lipophilic, and it is formulated with soy, benzyl alcohol, sometimes metabisulfite, and egg lecithin, so it must be avoided in patients with allergies to eggs, sulfites (usually present in red wines), or soybeans. Propofol has a high volume of distribution and moves to the central nervous system and other tissues rapidly. This allows a very quick onset of sedation, with hypnosis induced within 40 s, and a short duration of action, with a phase of elimination of around 2–3 min. The drug is mainly a hypnotic, with little analgesic effect and also an amnestic effect, although less than midazolam, as well as an antiemetic effect. Pharmacokinetics are significantly influenced by patients' individual characteristics, such as age, weight, sex, and comorbidities, particularly cardiovascular comorbidities.

    Recommended doses for sedation in endoscopy are between 0.5 and 1 mg/kg as induction, followed by repeated boluses, between 10 and 30 mg each 30–60 s, until the needed level of sedation is achieved. In lengthy procedures, continuous infusion of propofol, 2–8 mg/kg/h, can be more adequate to avoid unstable levels of sedation. In old patients, doses might be adjusted, and extra boluses are tailored to patient's level of sedation. In patients older than 70 years, a dose of 0.5 mg/kg should be enough as first infusion, and in individuals older than 90 years, a dose less than half of that administered to the average patient might provide similar levels of sedation (Dumonceau et al. 2015).

    Local pain occurs in 30% of patients during its infusion, and it can be avoided adding small quantities of lidocaine. It also can reduce systemic vascular resistance and cardiac contractility, causing hypotension. It can also decrease the cardiac output. Propofol can cause cardiorespiratory depression; slow administration of boluses or a continuous infusion is recommended to avoid cardiorespiratory complications. Of note, propofol can provoke convulsions, particularly in epileptic patients who have ceased their medication, usually while the patient is recovering from sedation. In the elderly, the dose should be reduced due to the abovementioned particularities. In these patients, impaired cardiac function might also potentiate the effects of propofol, but hepatic and renal impairment do not have any influence on these effects, nor does propofol precipitate hepatic encephalopathy (Thomson et al. 2010; Nonaka et al. 2015).

- Fentanyl

  It is an opioid with good analgesic effect and a rapid onset of action, of around 30 s, and a half-life between 30 and 120 min. Main side effects are hypoxia, bradycardia, hypotension, and nausea. It has been used in combination with other drugs, such as midazolam or propofol with an initial dose of 50 mcg and repeated boluses of 25–50 mcg. Its effects can be reverted with naloxone, and its use is preferred to meperidine for sedation in endoscopy (Moon 2014).

- Meperidine

  Meperidine is an opioid agent with a low analgesic effect and a long half-life. The initial dose should be of 50–100 mg and has to be used with caution in patients with hepatic or renal impairment. In those with renal impairment, the use is associated with seizures or neurotoxicity. It is used in combination with benzodiazepines. It causes more nausea than fentanyl (Moon 2014).

- Droperidol

  Droperidol is a butyrophenone, with antidopaminergic and antipsychotic effects similar to haloperidol, actually used for the management of psychosis/agitation, as an antiemetic, for vertigo, as an adjunct analgesic (especially in opioid-tolerant patients) and

as a treatment for benign headache. It also has sedative effects. It has been used in patients difficult to sedate in different randomized trials, but a warning of the FDA restricted its use only when first-line agents cannot be used. It is contraindicated in patients with a prolonged QTc interval and should be used with caution in patients with known risk of developing this abnormality, because they have an increased risk of ventricular tachyarrhythmias (other drugs that might prolong QT interval, congestive heart failure, bradycardia, diuretic, alcohol abuse, cardiac hypertrophy, hypomagnesemia, and elderly patients) (Yimcharoen et al. 2006). However, the drug has been widely used after the FDA warning by psychiatrists, emergency physicians, and anesthesiologists for the treatment of headache, nausea, agitation, acute pain, chronic pain, pain in the context of opioid tolerance, and refractory abdominal pain with no significant adverse events (Gaw et al. 2019).

- Diphenhydramine

  Diphenhydramine, a histamine-1 receptor antagonist, is a central nervous system depressant that has been widely used as a sedative for dental and ophthalmologic procedures. Diphenhydramine, which is available as an over-the-counter medication, is a first-generation antihistamine that is used in a variety of conditions to treat and prevent dystonia, insomnia, pruritus, urticaria, vertigo, and motion sickness. It also possesses local anesthetic properties for those patients who have allergies to other, more commonly used local anesthetics (Li et al. 2019). It has been administered to patients who are difficult to sedate with a benzodiazepine and opioid combination, or when sedation difficulties are expected. However, it has shown disappointing results in randomized clinical trials (Sachar et al. 2018).

- Dexmedetomidine (DEX)

  It is a relatively new highly selective blocker of α2 receptors present in noradrenaline neurons and induces sedation by suppressing upper neuron activity through negative feedback. It has a limited affinity for gamma-aminobutyric acid (GABA) receptors, and, therefore, there is almost no respiratory depression. Sedation by DEX has been reported as useful for upper and lower endoscopy and ESD. Moreover, it has also been reported as useful in combination with other sedatives, such as midazolam, in the older patients for complex and painful procedures such as ERCP and for reducing respiratory complications (Inatomi et al. 2018).

- Other Drugs

    Other drugs have been used as sedatives, such as ketamine, with less respiratory depression, as well as hypertension as a secondary effect, that can be of some help in patients hemodynamically unstable, such as the ones with gastrointestinal bleeding. Its main side effect is hallucinations, usually throughout the recovery period, that can be avoided by premedication with benzodiazepines such as midazolam.

    In the near future, new drugs such as the powerful sedative remifentanil, remimazolam, or fospropofol could be included among the different pharmacologic schedules used in the intravenous sedation for endoscopy in older people (Rex 2016).

    The use of pharyngeal anesthesia has been controversial in sedated endoscopy, and, although it has been widely used, actual recommendation is not to use it because it neither improves sedation nor reduces the dosage of other drugs (Dumonceau et al. 2015; Sun et al. 2018).

Dosing Drugs for Endoscopic Sedation (Table 5)

Although traditionally the use of a narcotic combined with a benzodiazepine has provided an adequate sedation for most procedures, in a wide range of patients, this approach is suboptimal. Robust evidence supports propofol administration by gastroenterologists in schedules that offer a better quality of sedation without compromising safety compared to traditional sedation practices, even improving the occurrence of delayed side

effects and giving way to outpatient programs in advanced endoscopy (Dumonceau et al. 2015; Han et al. 2017; Katsinelos et al. 2011; Wadhwa et al. 2017).

In general, there are two approaches to propofol administration:

1. "Combination" or "balanced" regimes in which a benzodiazepine or an opioid is given and, after a pause, propofol infusion is initiated. In frail patients or the elderly, the opiate should be avoided.
2. Propofol alone administered either as a continuous infusion or as incremental doses.

Minimal and moderate sedation regimens consist of a benzodiazepine to minimize anxiety and a narcotic analgesic to minimize pain and discomfort. Most endoscopists use midazolam as a benzodiazepine and fentanyl or meperidine as opiates. Fentanyl has a quicker onset of action and clearance and has lower incidence of nausea compared to meperidine. Flumazenil and naloxone should be available, and we should take into account that the effects of the reversal agents are shorter than the effects of the benzodiazepines themselves. Those regimes need longer recovery periods, and their generalized use in an endoscopy unit might require more emergency recovery boxes in the recovery area (ASGE Standards of Practice Committee et al. 2018; Triantafillidis et al. 2013). Some small trials have found alternatives to opioids in combination regimes with midazolam, with the intention to minimize the incidence of hypoxia. In this sense, dexmedetomidine has proven successful in a small trial (Inatomi et al. 2018), and, not surprisingly, propofol has also showed a reasonable level of safety when compared to opioids in a randomized study that included older individuals (Paspatis et al. 2002).

However, we agree with the ESGE statement about the preference of propofol as monotherapy when the person in charge of the sedation is not an anesthesiologist. Indeed, there are some papers that show no advantages in combination therapy (Wang et al. 2013). Adding midazolam as a premedication might be beneficial in some

Table 5 Characteristics of the pharmacological agents used to achieve a moderate level of sedation in gastrointestinal endoscopy

Drug	Onset of action (min)	Peak effect (min)	Duration of action (min)	Initial dose	Main adverse events	Antidote
Midazolam	1–2	3–4	15–80	1–3 mg	Hypoxemia Arrhythmia	Flumazenil
Diazepam	2–3	3–5	360	1–3 mg	Hypoxemia	Flumazenil
Propofol	<1	1–2	4–8	<70 years: 0.5–1 mg ≥70 years: 0.5 mg ≥90 years: 0.25 mg	Hypoxemia Apnea Hypotension Bradycardia Upper airway obstruction Pain in the site of injection	Ninguno
Meperidine	3–6	5–7	60–180	25–50 mg	Hypoxemia Cardiovascular instability Nausea	Naloxone
Fentanyl	1–2	3–5	30–60	25–50 mg	Hypoxemia Muscle hypertonia	Naloxone

circumstances, such as in patients with anxiety, long-lasting procedures in those with need of sedatives, or limited ventricular function with previous propofol-induced hypotension (Dumonceau et al. 2015).

In geriatric patients, administration of propofol must be prudent and careful, beginning with a bolus of 0.5 mg/kg in patients ASA I–II and even a lower dose (0.25–0.4 mg/kg) in patients with ASA ≥3 (Nonaka et al. 2015). After this initial dose, boluses of 10–20 mg every 30–60 s can be administered, always checking for signs of discomfort and being cautious as a general rule. We must be aware that propofol has no reversal drug or antidote and that we can always increase the dose if it is needed by clinical signs, but reversion takes some time, and excessive doses can lead to serious complications. Sedation with propofol has a similar efficacy and safety but with a shorter recovery time, even for long procedures such as ERCP (Han et al. 2017).

Although it is a controversial issue, and there are no clear rules, we should state the conditions in which an anesthesiologist might perform the sedation:

1. Patients conditions:
   (a) Patients with ASA >3
   (b) Predictors of difficult airway management: Mallampati 4, Bite test 3, mouth opening <3 cm, short neck
2. Procedure conditions:
   (a) Lengthy or complex procedures, such a ERCP, interventional EUS, enteroscopy or ESD
3. Hospital conditions:
   (a) Endoscopist lacking proper training for sedation
   (b) Legal issues that prevent endoscopists to provide sedation

Notwithstanding, it has been proved that for conventional procedure endoscopist-guided sedation is at least as safe as anesthesiologist-guided sedation, regardless of patient's age (ASGE Standards of Practice Committee et al. 2018).

Complications of Intravenous Sedation and Their Management

There are three major complications related to sedation in endoscopy: hypoxemia, bradycardia, and hypotension. Hypoxemia is defined as a decrease of SpO_2 below 90%, hypotension as a decline of systolic blood pressure to less than

90 mmHg, and bradycardia as a heart rate less than 50 bpm.

Of these three side effects, the most worrisome and usual is hypoxemia. It needs to be addressed in a stepwise routine, with most cases resolved by very simple measures. The first and most obvious one is to stop the infusion of sedating drugs. Along with this, we should increase oxygen flow through the nasal cannula and gently perform the jaw-thrust maneuver, if the two first measures are not enough to revert the situation. At this point, if hypoxemia subsides, we could even continue with the procedure. In case it persists, the endoscope should be retrieved, aspiration of upper airway secretions should be performed, a Mayo cannula should be inserted, and the patient should be ventilated with a mask, oxygen, and an Ambu. At this time it is sensible to call for an upper airway expert (anesthesiologist or critical care practitioner) to continue with patient's resuscitation (Lee and Lee 2014). Severe hypoxemia with the need for endotracheal intubation is exceptional even among high-risk patients undergoing complex procedures (Redondo-Cerezo et al. 2012).

The second most usual complication is hypotension, induced by a reduced peripheral vascular resistance caused by some drugs, such as propofol. It is normally irrelevant, and there is no need for additional measures to revert the condition. In case it is clinically relevant or persistent, crystalloids infusion is the treatment of choice, without a need for vasoactive drugs administration.

Arrhythmias, essentially bradycardia and tachycardia, are rare and usually subside spontaneously. However, in case bradycardia is persistent, it can be treated with 0.5–1 mg of atropine. Routinely, tachycardia is not a problem, and it is related to anxiety before the procedure. As a general recommendation, patients with known cardiac disease should have cardiac monitoring during the procedure and first recovery phase.

Geriatric patients have comorbidities and are on multiple medications, and the need to fast before endoscopy can be a problem. As a general recommendation, patients can take their antihypertensive and anticonvulsant medications before endoscopy with a small amount of water up to 2 h before the procedure, regardless of the type of endoscopy to be performed.

Recovery and Discharge from the Endoscopy Unit

The recovery room of an endoscopy unit should be attended by nurses. A discharge protocol must be available to warrant perfect conditions of the patient to be discharged. In this protocol, a scoring system, such as the Aldrete scoring system (Table 6) or the post-anesthetic discharge scoring system (PADSS) (Table 7), should be used for determining when the patient can be safely discharged from the recovery room (Trevisani et al. 2013).

Monitoring vital signs and conscious state after sedation is essential, because patients may progress into a deeper level of sedation after the procedure and may develop apnea and hypotension. The same resuscitation equipment available in the endoscopy room should also be accessible in the recovery room, and the same conditions regarding staff skills and possibilities of resuscitation maneuvers are a must in this area.

The recovery time is variable, depending on patient characteristics such as comorbidities, age and weight, and the sedation regime used. The main advantage of propofol-based sedation is that, compared to combination regimes or to regimes based on benzodiazepines, propofol monotherapy has the least impact on post-procedure cognitive function and, consequently, the vast majority of patients can be discharged within the first hour after the procedure (Dumonceau et al. 2015).

Information after sedated endoscopy is important. The physician should wait until the patient is awake, taking into consideration that, to some extent, the effects of the drugs will last after discharge. For this reason, written instructions should be given to patients about the inadmissibility of driving, operating machinery, engaging in legally binding decisions, or performing activities with inherent risks for the patient's own life or others. ESGE recommends those restrictions for 24 h in ASA >2 patients and for 6 h in patients ASA 1–2 who have received low-dose propofol monotherapy

Table 6 Modified Aldrete scoring system

Assessment items	Condition	Grade
Activity Able to move voluntarily or on command	4 extremities 2 extremities No	2 1 0
Breathing	Able to breathe deeply and cough freely Dyspnea, shallow or limited breathing Apnea	2 1 0
Consciousness	Fully awake Arousable on calling Unresponsible	2 1 0
Circulation Blood pressure	±20% pre-sedation level ±20–49% pre-sedation level ±50% pre-sedation level	2 1 1
SpO$_2$	Maintains SpO$_2$ >92% in ambient air Maintains SpO$_2$ >90% with O$_2$ Maintains SpO$_2$ <90% with O$_2$	2 1 0

Total score (patients' scoring ≥9 for two consecutive measurements is considered fit for discharge home)

Table 7 Modified post-anesthetic discharge scoring system

Assessment items	Condition	Grade
Vital signs Blood pressure and heart rate	± 20% of pre-endoscopy value ± 20–40% of pre-endoscopy value ± 40% of pre-endoscopy value	2 1 0
Activity	Steady gait, no dizziness, or meets pre-endoscopy level Requires assistance Unable to ambulate	2 1 0
Pain	Minimal or no pain (numerical analogue scale = 0–3) Moderate (numerical analogue scale = 4–6) Severe (numerical analogue scale = 7–10)	2 1 0
Surgical bleeding	±20% pre-sedation level ±20–49% pre-sedation level ±50% pre-sedation level	2 1 1
SpO$_2$	None or minimal (not requiring intervention) moderate (1 episode of hematemesis or rectal bleeding) Severe (≥2 episodes of hematemesis or rectal bleeding)	2 1 0

Total score (patients' scoring ≥9 for two consecutive measurements is considered fit for discharge home)

(Dumonceau et al. 2015). Furthermore, patients must also receive written information about their condition, the results of the procedure, delayed complications, future appointments, and future steps regarding the disorder that brought them to the endoscopy room. We must keep in mind that older individual's understanding of the medical procedures, risks, and complications is generally low, and an additional effort should be taken to increase patients' awareness about the procedure, prior to its performance, and about, complications, results, and future steps (Sherlock and Brownie 2014).

It is advisable to keep written structured records as a part of the quality process of sedation that should include the following (Dumonceau et al. 2015):

- Vital signs at regular intervals (oxygen saturation, heart rate, and blood pressure)
- Drugs (names and dosages), intravenous fluids, and oxygen rate administered
- Sedation-associated complications and their management
- Fulfillment of discharge criteria

Unsedated Endoscopy in the Elderly

Selected patients may be able to undergo endoscopic procedures without sedation. In this population topical pharyngeal anesthesia is generally used, as it may decrease discomfort, as well as in the ones receiving non-propofol-mediated sedation. Some technical variations, such as the use of small-diameter endoscopes for upper endoscopy or the use of water-assisted or carbon dioxide insufflation, may reduce pain during and after the endoscopy. Older patients, men, anxious patients, and the ones with a history of abdominal pain may be more willing to undergo unsedated endoscopy. Nevertheless, it is recommended to perform a standard pre-endoscopic preparation for sedation and monitoring, including intravenous line insertion, in the event that the patient does not tolerate the procedure or develops complications (ASGE Standards of Practice Committee et al. 2018). However, in contrast to the idea that unsedated endoscopy is safer, some complications such as tachycardia or hypertension are more usual, whereas hypoxemia is most common in sedated endoscopy, and this should be considered before deciding for a given option especially in old and frail patients (Zheng et al. 2018).

Hypnosis has been used to aid endoscopic procedures with little success in terms of patient discomfort or amnesia (Thomson et al. 2010).

Training Programs for Intravenous Sedation in Endoscopy

Today, sedation is an intrinsic part of any endoscopic procedure, so it must be included as another competence in gastroenterology training programs. Every member of the endoscopy unit staff should be specifically trained in sedation, with a scheduled periodical recertification as an essential tool to keep skills updated. National and international endoscopic societies have committed to provide courses and teaching resources for the education of trained endoscopists and nurses involved in sedation (Dumonceau et al. 2013; Kochhar et al. 2016).

Key Points

- The majority of endoscopic procedures are done with the aid of intravenous sedation, and this should be offered virtually to every patient who receives endoscopy, including older patients.
- Geriatric patients present some clinical singularities that should be considered before performing endoscopy, such as the higher prevalence of cardiovascular, respiratory, renal, and metabolic conditions and pharmacodynamic changes.
- In older patients the brain becomes more sensitive to sedative agents; they manifest increased half time for lipophilic drugs and impaired renal and hepatic clearance.
- The physician who performs sedation needs to be specifically trained for the procedure. An anesthesiologist is sometimes needed, especially in high-risk individuals or in complex procedures.
- An individualized sedation plan should be established, taking into account the patient's individual features, allergies, drugs, and first infusion doses meant to be used. Accurate monitoring of level of consciousness and vital signs is mandatory.
- Adequate facilities and appropriate resuscitation equipment are needed. Music can be used in the endoscopy room.
- The choice of the sedation agent depends on the endoscopist's preference, the procedure, the local protocols, and the legal regulation in each country.
- There are three major complications related to sedation in endoscopy: hypoxemia, bradycardia, and hypotension. They are usually mild and can be managed with simple measures without stopping the procedure.
- A recovery area, assisted by nurses, equipped with resuscitation equipment and with a discharge protocol is needed in every endoscopy unit.

References

American Association for the Study of Liver Diseases, American College of Gastroenterology, American Gastroenterological Association Institute, American Society for Gastrointestinal Endoscopy, Society for Gastroenterology Nurses and Associates, et al. Multisociety sedation curriculum for gastrointestinal endoscopy. Gastroenterology. 2012;143(1):e18–41. https://doi.org/10.1053/j.gastro.2012.05.001.

American Society of Anesthesiologists Task Force on Sedation & Analgesia by Non-anesthesiologists. Practice guidelines for sedation and analgesia by non-anesthesiologists. Anesthesiology. 2002;96(4):1004–17. https://doi.org/10.1097/00000542-200204000-00031.

ASGE Standards of Practice Committee, Early DS, Lightdale JR, Vargo JJ 2nd, Acosta RD, Chandrasekhara V, et al. Guidelines for sedation and anesthesia in GI endoscopy. Gastrointest Endosc. 2018;87(2):327–37. https://doi.org/10.1016/j.gie.2017.07.018.

Bettelli G. Preoperative evaluation of the elderly surgical patient and anesthesia challenges in the XXI century. Aging Clin Exp Res. 2018;30(3):229–35. https://doi.org/10.1007/s40520-018-0896-y.

Chung F, Yegneswaran B, Liao P, Chung SA, Vairavanathan S, Islam S, et al. STOP questionnaire: a tool to screen patients for obstructive sleep apnea. Anesthesiology. 2008;108(5):812–21. https://doi.org/10.1097/ALN.0b013e31816d83e4.

Demongeot J. Biological boundaries and biological age. Acta Biotheor. 2009;57(4):397–418. https://doi.org/10.1007/s10441-009-9087-8.

Dumonceau JM, Riphaus A, Beilenhoff U, Vilmann P, Hornslet P, Aparicio JR, et al. European curriculum for sedation training in gastrointestinal endoscopy: position statement of the European Society of Gastrointestinal Endoscopy (ESGE) and European Society of Gastroenterology and Endoscopy Nurses and Associates (ESGENA). Endoscopy. 2013;45(6):496–504. https://doi.org/10.1055/s-0033-1344142.

Dumonceau JM, Riphaus A, Schreiber F, Vilmann P, Beilenhoff U, Aparicio JR, et al. Non-anesthesiologist administration of propofol for gastrointestinal endoscopy: European Society of Gastrointestinal Endoscopy, European Society of Gastroenterology and Endoscopy Nurses and Associates Guideline – Updated June 2015. Endoscopy. 2015;47(12):1175–89. https://doi.org/10.1055/s-0034-1393414.

Fatima H, DeWitt J, LeBlanc J, Sherman S, McGreevy K, Imperiale TF. Nurse-administered propofol sedation for upper endoscopic ultrasonography. Am J Gastroenterol. 2008;103(7):1649–56. https://doi.org/10.1111/j.1572-0241.2008.01906.x.

Ferreira AO, Cravo M. Sedation in gastrointestinal endoscopy: where are we at in 2014? World J Gastrointest Endosc. 2015;7(2):102–9. https://doi.org/10.4253/wjge.v7.i2.102.

Fisher L, Fisher A, Thomson A. Cardiopulmonary complications of ERCP in older patients. Gastrointest Endosc. 2006;63(7):948–55. https://doi.org/10.1016/j.gie.2005.09.020.

Fleisher LA, Fleischmann KE, Auerbach AD, Barnason SA, Beckman JA, Bozkurt B, et al. 2014 ACC/AHA guideline on perioperative cardiovascular evaluation and management of patients undergoing noncardiac surgery: a report of the American College of Cardiology/American Heart Association Task Force on practice guidelines. J Am Coll Cardiol. 2014;64(22):e77–137. https://doi.org/10.1016/j.jacc.2014.07.944.

Friedrich K, Stremmel W, Sieg A. Endoscopist-administered propofol sedation is safe – a prospective evaluation of 10,000 patients in an outpatient practice. J Gastrointestin Liver Dis. 2012;21(3):259–63. https://www.ncbi.nlm.nih.gov/pubmed/23012666.

Gaw CM, Cabrera D, Bellolio F, Mattson AE, Lohse CM, Jeffery MM. Effectiveness and safety of droperidol in a United States emergency department. Am J Emerg Med. 2019. https://doi.org/10.1016/j.ajem.2019.09.007.

Han SJ, Lee TH, Park SH, Cho YS, Lee YN, Jung Y, et al. Efficacy of midazolam- versus propofol-based sedations by non-anesthesiologists during therapeutic endoscopic retrograde cholangiopancreatography in patients aged over 80 years. Dig Endosc. 2017;29(3):369–76. https://doi.org/10.1111/den.12841.

Heuss LT, Schnieper P, Drewe J, Pflimlin E, Beglinger C. Conscious sedation with propofol in elderly patients: a prospective evaluation. Aliment Pharmacol Ther. 2003;17(12):1493–501. https://doi.org/10.1046/j.1365-2036.2003.01608.x.

Heuss LT, Froehlich F, Beglinger C. Nonanesthesiologist-administered propofol sedation: from the exception to standard practice. Sedation and monitoring trends over 20 years. Endoscopy. 2012;44(5):504–11. https://doi.org/10.1055/s-0031-1291668.

Homfray G, Palmer A, Grimsmo-Powney H, Appelboam A, Lloyd G. Procedural sedation of elderly patients by emergency physicians: a safety analysis of 740 patients. Br J Anaesth. 2018;121(6):1236–41. https://doi.org/10.1016/j.bja.2018.07.038.

Horn E, Nesbit SA. Pharmacology and pharmacokinetics of sedatives and analgesics. Gastrointest Endosc Clin N Am. 2004;14(2):247–68. https://doi.org/10.1016/j.giec.2004.01.001.

Inatomi O, Imai T, Fujimoto T, Takahashi K, Yokota Y, Yamashita N, et al. Dexmedetomidine is safe and reduces the additional dose of midazolam for sedation during endoscopic retrograde cholangiopancreatography in very elderly patients. BMC Gastroenterol. 2018;18(1):166. https://doi.org/10.1186/s12876-018-0897-5.

Katsinelos P, Kountouras J, Chatzimavroudis G, Zavos C, Terzoudis S, Pilpilidis I, et al. Outpatient therapeutic endoscopic retrograde cholangiopancreatography is safe in patients aged 80 years and older. Endoscopy.

2011;43(2):128–33. https://doi.org/10.1055/s-0030-1255934.

Kochhar GS, Gill A, Vargo JJ. On the horizon: the future of procedural sedation. Gastrointest Endosc Clin N Am. 2016;26(3):577–92. https://doi.org/10.1016/j.giec.2016.03.002.

Lee TH, Lee CK. Endoscopic sedation: from training to performance. Clin Endosc. 2014;47(2):141–50. https://doi.org/10.5946/ce.2014.47.2.141.

Li YY, Zeng YS, Chen JY, Wang KF, Hsing CH, Wu WJ, et al. Prophylactic diphenhydramine attenuates postoperative catheter-related bladder discomfort in patients undergoing gynecologic laparoscopic surgery: a randomized double-blind clinical study. J Anesth. 2019. https://doi.org/10.1007/s00540-019-02724-3.

Moon SH. Sedation regimens for gastrointestinal endoscopy. Clin Endosc. 2014;47(2):135–40. https://doi.org/10.5946/ce.2014.47.2.135.

Nonaka M, Gotoda T, Kusano C, Fukuzawa M, Itoi T, Moriyasu F. Safety of gastroenterologist-guided sedation with propofol for upper gastrointestinal therapeutic endoscopy in elderly patients compared with younger patients. Gut Liver. 2015;9(1):38–42. https://doi.org/10.5009/gnl13368.

Partridge JS, Harari D, Martin FC, Peacock JL, Bell R, Mohammed A, et al. Randomized clinical trial of comprehensive geriatric assessment and optimization in vascular surgery. Br J Surg. 2017;104(6):679–87. https://doi.org/10.1002/bjs.10459.

Paspatis GA, Manolaraki M, Xirouchakis G, Papanikolaou N, Chlouverakis G, Gritzali A. Synergistic sedation with midazolam and propofol versus midazolam and pethidine in colonoscopies: a prospective, randomized study. Am J Gastroenterol. 2002;97(8):1963–7. https://doi.org/10.1111/j.1572-0241.2002.05908.x.

Redondo-Cerezo E, Sanchez-Robaina A, Martinez Cara JG, Ojeda-Hinojosa M, Matas-Cobos A, Sanchez Capilla AD, et al. Gastroenterologist-guided sedation with propofol for endoscopic ultrasonography in average-risk and high-risk patients: a prospective series. Eur J Gastroenterol Hepatol. 2012;24(5):506–12. https://doi.org/10.1097/MEG.0b013e328350fcbd.

Rex DK. Endoscopist-directed propofol. Gastrointest Endosc Clin N Am. 2016;26(3):485–92. https://doi.org/10.1016/j.giec.2016.02.010.

Rex DK, Deenadayalu VP, Eid E, Imperiale TF, Walker JA, Sandhu K, et al. Endoscopist-directed administration of propofol: a worldwide safety experience. Gastroenterology. 2009;137(4):1229–37;. quiz 1518-9. https://doi.org/10.1053/j.gastro.2009.06.042.

Roth D, Pace NL, Lee A, Hovhannisyan K, Warenits AM, Arrich J, et al. Airway physical examination tests for detection of difficult airway management in apparently normal adult patients. Cochrane Database Syst Rev. 2018;5:CD008874. https://doi.org/10.1002/14651858.CD008874.pub2.

Sachar H, Pichetshote N, Nandigam K, Vaidya K, Laine L. Continued midazolam versus diphenhydramine in difficult-to-sedate patients: a randomized double-blind trial. Gastrointest Endosc. 2018;87(5):1297–303. https://doi.org/10.1016/j.gie.20 17.01.028.

Schnider TW, Minto CF, Shafer SL, Gambus PL, Andresen C, Goodale DB, et al. The influence of age on propofol pharmacodynamics. Anesthesiology. 1999;90(6):1502–16. https://doi.org/10.1097/00000542-199906000-00003.

Sherlock A, Brownie S. Patients' recollection and understanding of informed consent: a literature review. ANZ J Surg. 2014;84(4):207–10. https://doi.org/10.1111/ans.12555.

Sun X, Xu Y, Zhang X, Li A, Zhang H, Yang T, et al. Topical pharyngeal anesthesia provides no additional benefit to propofol sedation for esophagogastroduodenoscopy: a randomized controlled double-blinded clinical trial. Sci Rep. 2018;8(1):6682. https://doi.org/10.1038/s41598-018-25164-7.

Thomson A, Andrew G, Jones DB. Optimal sedation for gastrointestinal endoscopy: review and recommendations. J Gastroenterol Hepatol. 2010;25(3):469–78. https://doi.org/10.1111/j.1440-1746.2009.06174.x.

Trevisani L, Cifala V, Gilli G, Matarese V, Zelante A, Sartori S. Post-anaesthetic discharge scoring system to assess patient recovery and discharge after colonoscopy. World J Gastrointest Endosc. 2013;5(10):502–7. https://doi.org/10.4253/wjge.v5.i10.502.

Triantafillidis JK, Merikas E, Nikolakis D, Papalois AE. Sedation in gastrointestinal endoscopy: current issues. World J Gastroenterol. 2013;19(4):463–81. https://doi.org/10.3748/wjg.v19.i4.463.

Wadhwa V, Issa D, Garg S, Lopez R, Sanaka MR, Vargo JJ. Similar risk of cardiopulmonary adverse events between propofol and traditional anesthesia for gastrointestinal endoscopy: a systematic review and meta-analysis. Clin Gastroenterol Hepatol. 2017;15(2):194–206. https://doi.org/10.1016/j.cgh.20 16.07.013.

Wang D, Wang S, Chen J, Xu Y, Chen C, Long A, et al. Propofol combined with traditional sedative agents versus propofol- alone sedation for gastrointestinal endoscopy: a meta-analysis. Scand J Gastroenterol. 2013;48(1):101–10. https://doi.org/10.3109/00365521.2012.737360.

Yimcharoen P, Fogel EL, Kovacs RJ, Rosenfeld SH, McHenry L, Watkins JL, et al. Droperidol, when used for sedation during ERCP, may prolong the QT interval. Gastrointest Endosc. 2006;63(7):979–85. https://doi.org/10.1016/j.gie.2006.01.052.

Zheng HR, Zhang XQ, Li LZ, Wang YL, Wei Y, Chen YM, et al. Multicentre prospective cohort study evaluating gastroscopy without sedation in China. Br J Anaesth. 2018;121(2):508–11. https://doi.org/10.1016/j.bja.201 8.04.027.

Gastrointestinal Luminal Stenting

39

Chiranjeevi Gadiparthi and Andrew Korman

Contents

Abstract

Gastrointestinal (GI) stenting has advanced rapidly in recent years and has emerged as an essential alternative to surgery especially in patients with malignant obstruction or strictures of the GI tract. In addition to malignancy, GI stenting is expanded to several other nonmalignant indications. Future development of stents with bigger diameter may be useful in other conditions such as achalasia. Operator expertise and a better understanding of the stent characteristics may result in optimal placement and decreased complications. As advancing age is a known risk factor for cancers in general, older adults who develop malignant obstruction and strictures in the GI tract are commonly encountered in clinical practice. In those, luminal stenting remains a valuable and minimally invasive palliative option. Patients highly desire the restoration of oral nutrition, which can be achieved by GI luminal stenting in the majority of cases, and relief of obstruction results in significant improvement in the quality of life.

Keywords

Stents · Stricture · Obstruction · Cancer · Luminal · Nutrition · Self-expandable metal

C. Gadiparthi · A. Korman (✉)
Division of Gastroenterology and Hepatology, Saint Peter's University Hospital, New Brunswick, NJ, USA
e-mail: akorman@saintpetersuh.com

© Springer Nature Switzerland AG 2021
C. S. Pitchumoni, T. S. Dharmarajan (eds.), *Geriatric Gastroenterology*,
https://doi.org/10.1007/978-3-030-30192-7_32

stents (SEMS) · Partially covered (PC) and fully covered (FC) SEMS · Boerhaave's syndrome · Tracheo-esophageal fistulae · Benign strictures · Fistulae · Gastric outlet obstruction (GOO) · Cholangiocarcinoma · Lymphoma · Metastatic disease · Achalasia · Refractory benign esophageal strictures (RBES)

Introduction

Over the past two decades, gastrointestinal (GI) luminal stenting has become widely available and is increasingly used in clinical practice. Stents are safe and effective alternatives or bridge to surgery and have shown to improve quality of life in patients with a variety of GI disorders, more so in GI malignancies. The common indications for GI luminal stenting are malignant obstruction from tumors or strictures, extrinsic compression of the GI tract, fistulae, malignant perforation, and in select cases of benign strictures that require recurrent endoscopic dilations and other interventions (Sabharwal et al. 2005; Varadarajulu et al. 2011). Malignant obstruction of the GI tract is a frequent cause of morbidity. GI stents are useful in providing excellent palliative symptom relief in patients with obstructed caused by advanced GI malignancies, mainly when they are not suitable candidates for curative surgical resection and/or chemoradiotherapy (Dormann et al. 2003).

Therefore, one of the goals of stent placement is to provide palliation by relieving the obstruction, resume oral nutrition as much as possible and by doing so, improve quality of life. The commonly used GI luminal stents based on anatomical location are esophageal, gastroduodenal, and colonic stents. A variety of GI stents of various sizes and designs are available in the market and continue to evolve over the years. In this chapter, we discuss the role of stents GI disorders, types of stents, special considerations based on the anatomical location, indications, and complications, as they relate to older adults.

Stent Types and Characteristics

Frimberger first reported expandable metal stents in 10 patients with esophageal adenocarcinoma (Frimberger 1983). These spiral stents, which were wound around the shaft of a pediatric endoscope, were then deployed across the malignant strictures. Following this report, a new era of self-expandable metal stents (SEMS) began in the management of luminal strictures which swiftly evolved with advent of several new designs and types. For a long period, rigid stents made of plastic, latex, or polyethylene were used, and these stents required aggressive dilatation of the stricture prior to placement leading to inadvertent complications and pain (Baron and Siersema 2019). The superiority of expandable stents over rigid plastic stents in the management of dysphagia caused by malignant esophageal strictures was demonstrated by a landmark study published several years later (Symonds 1887). The first set of commercially available SEMS were made of stainless steel and were uncovered. This often led to tumor ingrowth, causing recurrent obstruction. SEMS by design exert more radial than axial force on GI luminal wall and slowly expand until they reach maximum predetermined diameter.

The development of partially covered and fully covered metal stents has addressed this issue and were particularly useful in the treatment and palliation of malignant strictures and trachea-esophageal fistulas (Baron and Siersema 2019). Over the years, the use of SEMS has expanded to include refractory benign strictures, fistulas, and leaks. Newer stents are compressed and constrained within a delivery device allowing placement within tight stenosis without the need for dilation beforehand thus minimizing complications such as perforation and migration (Varadarajulu et al. 2011), but are associated with increased migration risk due to reduced anchorage compared to uncovered SEMS (Baron and Siersema 2019). But, the latest modifications such as flared ends, partial cover, and double stent design have decreased the migration rates (Sabharwal et al. 2003; Sabharwal et al. 2005). Among the several materials used in SEMS, nitinol, an alloy of titanium and nickel, has become the most widely used metal among expandable metal stents due to its inherent property of shape memory and "superelasticity" (Castaño et al. 2010).

Special Considerations Based on Anatomical Location

Esophageal Stents

In current clinical practice, although esophageal stents are utilized in a variety of esophageal disorders, palliation for malignant dysphagia due to esophageal cancer remains the most common indication. However, compared to esophageal stents, palliative brachytherapy may be a more effective treatment option for esophageal dysphagia (Homs et al. 2004). Esophageal stents are classified based on the materials used (metal, plastic, and biodegradable), type of force exerted on the esophageal wall (radial and axial), and the kind of covering around the stent mesh (Vermeulen and Siersema 2018). Although specific stent characteristics are helpful to predict the occurrence of particular symptoms or complications following stent placement, the clinical behavior of each type of stent is much more complex and cannot be attributed to these factors alone (Hirdes et al. 2013).

Furthermore, no robust randomized controlled trials are available comparing different stents and their clinical outcomes. Therefore, the selection of a stent for each particular clinical situation is largely dependent on operator preference, expertise, and local availability. In general, for malignant esophageal dysphagia, fully or partially covered SEMS are preferred and recommended in the clinical guidelines (Spaander et al. 2016).

Over the past decades, the increasing rates of curative chemoradiotherapy of esophageal cancers have led to a decrease in the usage of esophageal stents for malignant strictures in developed countries (Reijm et al. 2019). On the other hand, esophageal stents are increasingly used in dysphagia caused by refractory benign esophageal strictures (RBES), which has become a novel indication. For example, esophageal stenting can be considered if RBES was not successfully dilated to a diameter of at least 14 mm after 5 successful esophageal dilation (bougie or balloon) sessions at 2-week intervals (Kochman et al. 2005). Common causes of RBES are esophagogastric anastomotic strictures, caustic injuries, postradiation, and strictures following endoscopic therapy such as radiofrequency ablation for circumferential Barrett's and endoscopic mucosal resection for esophageal nodules or early esophageal cancer, etc. (Repici et al. 2016). Another indication for the esophageal stent is esophageal leakage. Esophageal leakage can be caused by a variety of conditions including spontaneous (Boerhaave's syndrome) or iatrogenic (endoscopic and instrumental) esophageal rupture, postsurgical (esophagectomy or gastrectomy and reconstructive surgeries) anastomotic leakage, and malignancy (esophagus-tracheal fistula). Esophageal leakage can result in severe and life-threatening complications, including mediastinitis and sepsis for which esophageal stenting can be temporizing or definitive mode of therapy.

There are of course limitations to esophageal stent placement. A relatively higher frequency of adverse events compared to other luminal stenting is a major limitation of esophageal stent placement. Stent migration is the most common complication, which can be minimized to some extent by utilizing newer stent design or anchoring the stent to the esophageal wall using a suture or hemostatic clips (Mudumbi et al. 2014; Walter et al. 2014). Covered stents have a wider diameter and therefore have a lower risk of migration. Other major and minor adverse complications include bleeding, aspiration pneumonia, perforation, retrosternal chest pain, recurrent dysphagia due to tumor ingrowth, and reflux symptoms

(Reijm et al. 2019). Despite these substantial risks, esophageal stenting remains a necessary palliative and therapeutic option in clinical practice in carefully selected patients.

Duodenal Stents

Benign and malignant etiologies cause gastric outlet obstruction (GOO). Intramural obstruction due to gastric, duodenal, ampullary cancers, and extrinsic compression by pancreatic cancers may result in GOO. Rare causes of malignant GOO include cholangiocarcinoma, lymphoma, and metastatic disease. Typical symptoms of GOO are nausea, vomiting, abdominal pain, and inability to tolerate oral nutrition. In addition to decreased life span in patients suffering from these cancers, quality of life is drastically affected due to the symptoms of GOO. Duodenal stenting alleviates such symptoms and restores the ability to drink or eat, which are essential quality of life measures to these patients. Traditionally, GOO was treated by bypass surgeries such as gastrojejunostomy; however, duodenal stenting is a less invasive, safer, and effective alternative.

Furthermore, in patients with advanced cancers with a shorter life span, Roux-en-Y gastrojejunostomy may not be feasible and comes with increased morbidity (Del Piano et al. 2005). On the other hand, duodenal stenting relieves obstruction quickly with the ability to resume oral feeding promptly. However, duodenal stenting is associated with higher rates of stent obstruction and the need for reintervention compared to surgical gastrojejunostomy (Khashab et al. 2013). Endoscopic ultrasound-guided gastroenterostomy (EUS-GE) is another novel approach that delivers sustained symptom relief and is minimally invasive as compared to surgery (Chen et al. 2017).

If endoscopic retrograde cholangiopancreatography is necessary for concomitant biliary obstruction, this should ideally be performed at the time of enteral stent placement whenever possible (Brimhall and Adler 2011). Contraindications for enteral stents in malignant GOO include life expectancy less than 2 weeks, obstruction at multiple levels caused by peritoneal carcinomatosis, and underlying motility disorders (Adler and Baron 2002; Wai et al. 2001). The technical success of enteral stent placement is 75–100%. Common causes of mechanical failure include the inability to traverse the stricture by guidewire and catheter, failure of the delivery system with the deployment, and finally, stent migration (Jeurnink et al. 2007). Minor complications such as mild pain, low-grade fever, vomiting without obstruction, and significant complications such as severe pain, peroration, development of fistula, bleeding, and stent migration are associated with enteral stent placement (Jeurnink et al. 2007).

Lumen-Apposing Metal Stents

The lumen-apposing metal stent (LAMS) has revolutionized gastrointestinal endoscopy. First reported by Binmoeller and shah in 2011 for transluminal drainage to provide anchorage across non-adherent luminal structures (Mussetto et al. 2018). They were first designed for drainage of pancreatic collections, both walled-off necrosis and pseudocysts. LAMS are unique in their design. They have a barbell shape with flanged ends and have a large luminal diameter of varying sizes. The benefit of this design allows for minimal risk of migration. Currently, there are many types LAMS available, those with or without an electrocautery-enhanced delivery system. Over time, both in-and-off label use LAMS have been proposed and are currently in practice.

As discussed, the elderly are more susceptible and at higher risk for malignancy. One special consideration is the risk of acute cholecystitis in the elderly with or without a concomitant neoplastic process. Options for those unfit for surgery are percutaneous gallbladder drainage (PTGBD) by interventional radiology and/or transpapillary drainage through ERCP with a plastic stent. Both have their own risks including catheter obstruction, infection, pain, and bleeding. In 2017, a multicenter study evaluated patients with acute cholecystitis deemed too high risk for surgery (Dollhopf et al. 2017). The technical and clinical success rates were 98.7% and 95.9%, respectively. The procedure-related and short- and long-term adverse events occurred in 10.7% of the entire cohort. The authors reported serious stent- or procedure-related adverse events in 13% of patients.

Future use of LAMS has been studied in endoscopic ultrasound-guided gastroenterostomy (EUS-GE) for patients with benign and malignant gastric outlet obstruction (GOO) as well as for benign luminal strictures, primarily from anastomotic strictures. In another small study, the use of LAMS for EUS-gastrojejunostomy in patients with benign and malignant GOO was associated with 92.3% technical success (24/26 patients) and 84.6% clinical success (22/26 patients, defined as those who were able to tolerate an oral diet) (Tyberg et al. 2016).

Colon Stents

Over the past two decades, colonic stenting has been well described and increasingly used as palliation or bridge to surgery in colonic obstruction caused by colorectal cancer (Sebastian et al. 2004; Van Hooft et al. 2014). Advanced colon cancer-causing significant bowel obstruction is seen in 8–13% (Cheynel et al. 2007; Jullumstrø et al. 2011). SEMS in these circumstances are considered a safe and alternatives to emergent surgery with many advantages. They may also be used as a bridge to surgery so that the patient may complete a bowel preparation beforehand (Ormando et al. 2019). Uncovered stents appear to be a better option in malignant bowel obstruction as they are associated with fewer complications. Colonic stenting for blockage caused by extracolonic malignancy is less characterized than luminal malignant colonic obstruction; however, it is not contraindicated. In a large retrospective single-center series of 187 patients, 75.9% of patients

achieved professional success and 54.5% achieved clinical success. However, patients with peritoneal carcinomatosis and multifocal disease have lower technical and clinical success rates (Faraz et al. 2018). In this study, the procedure-related adverse events were reported in 6.4%, and the stent occlusion rate in 14.7% after 3 months in patients who achieved clinical success.

It is important to note that prophylactic stenting is not recommended, and only patients with imaging evidence of large bowel obstruction without perforation and those with clinical symptoms should be considered for colon stenting (Van Hooft et al. 2020). Obtaining a contrast-enhanced computed tomography (CECT) scan of the abdomen and pelvis should be obtained, if possible, before colon stent placement. CTCT scan helps in identifying the obstruction in a majority of cases (96% sensitivity), defines the site (94% cases) and etiology (81% cases) of obstruction, and assists in staging of cancer (Frager et al. 1998; Frago et al. 2014). In general, colon stenting is performed for left-sided colon cancers proximal to recto-sigmoid, including sigmoid, descending colon, and splenic flexure. Most randomized control trials excluded rectal cancer (8–10 cm from the anal verge) and cancers proximal to splenic flexure. Colon stenting is usually avoided in rectal cancers due to tenesmus, pain, incontinence, and stent migration. In fact, for potentially curable left-sided cancers with malignant obstruction, colon stenting is a bridge to surgery and should be considered with shared decision-making. For better outcomes, at least a 2-week interval is suggested between stent placement and elective surgery in curable left-sided colon cancers. For proximal colon cancers, colon stenting may serve as bridge to surgery or as a palliative measure. Additionally, colon stenting should be performed by an operator who is experienced and competent in these procedures to minimize the complications and increase the clinical and technical success rates.

The primary contraindication for colon stenting is bowel perforation. Generally, colonic stenting should be avoided for benign colon strictures mimicking colon obstruction. For example, stenosis associated with the active diverticular disease is a contraindication due to the high risk of perforation. It is beneficial to obtain tissue from the obstructing lesion to confirm the diagnosis at the time of stent placement; however, this may be challenging in emergent endoscopy for colonic obstruction (Brouwer et al. 2009). Although bowel preparation is contraindicated in colonic obstruction, a partial bowel preparation with enema(s) to clean the colon distal to the obstruction may facilitate and aid in visualization of stent placement (Van Hooft et al. 2020). Prophylactic

antibiotics are not recommended during colon stent placement as the risk of bacterial translocation is very low.

Initiation of Nutrition After Stent Placement

Usually patients feel symptomatic relief immediately after successful GI stenting. Oral intake is restored by initiating a liquid diet which is advanced over a period of several days. Low-fiber diet is recommended and patients are asked to take small bites and chew thoroughly.

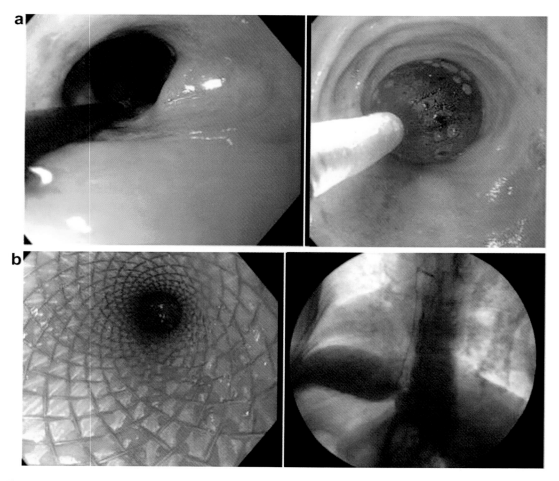

Fig. 1 (**a**) Endoscopic images showing RBES before (left) and after (right) after balloon dilation. (**b**) Endoscopic image (left) and fluoroscopic images after deployment of 18 × 100 mm fully covered SEMS

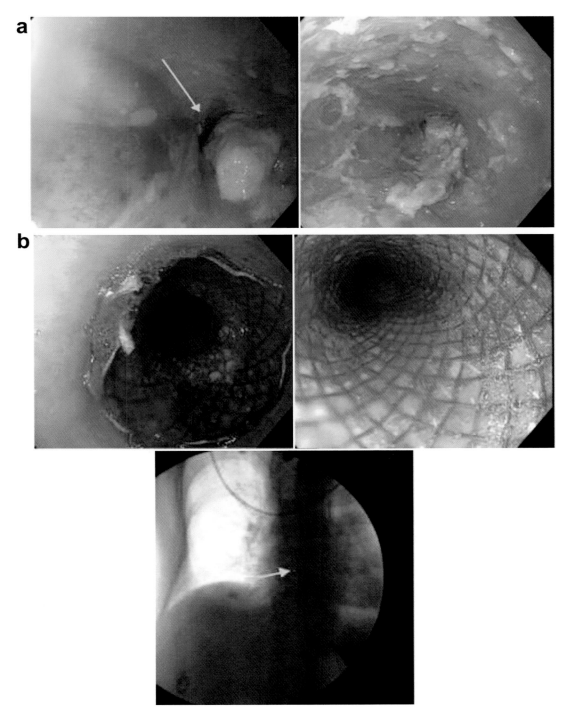

Fig. 2 (a) Endoscopic images showing severe malignant stricture in the mid-esophagus (20 cm from incisors). (b) Endoscopic (upper) and fluoroscopic (lower) images after placement 18 × 120 mm partially covered SEMS

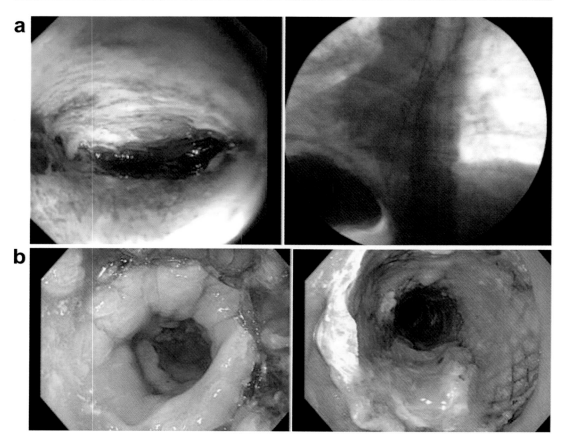

Fig. 3 (a) Endoscopic image (left) of severe malignant stricture and fluoroscopic picture (right) after stent placement (18 mm × 120 cm fully covered SEMS). (b) Proximal (left) and distal (right) ends of esophageal stent seen in follow-up endoscopy

Supervised feeding, especially in older adults, is advised. To keep adequate calorie intake, protein supplements should be considered and where possible, consultation with a certified nutritionist and/or dietician would be preferable. If there is development of recurrent symptoms, diet should be downgraded to pureed or liquids until the symptoms resolve and recurrent obstruction has been excluded.

In conclusion, GI stenting has advanced rapidly in recent years and has emerged as an important alternative to surgery especially in patients with malignant obstruction or strictures of GI tract. In addition to malignancy, GI stenting is expanded to several other nonmalignant indications. Future development of stents with bigger diameter may be useful in other conditions such as achalasia. Operator expertise and better understanding of the stent characteristics may result in optimal placement and decreased complications. As advancing age is a known risk factor for cancers in general, older adults who develop malignant obstruction and strictures in GI tract are the commonly encountered in clinical practice and in those, luminal stenting remains a valuable and minimally invasive palliative option. Restoration of oral nutrition is highly desired by patients, can be achieved by GI luminal stenting in the majority of cases, and relief of obstruction results in significant improvement in quality of life.

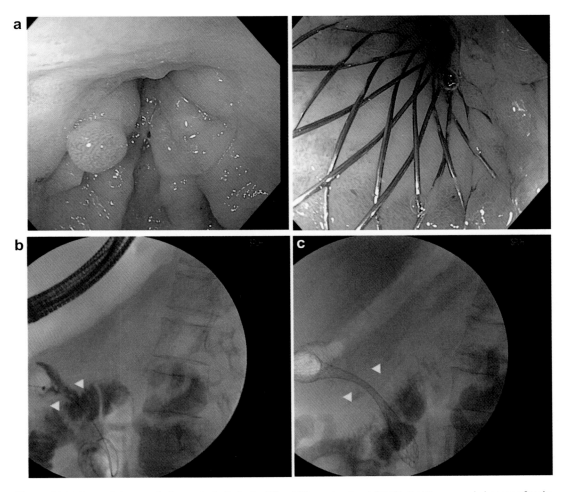

Fig. 4 (**a**) Endoscopic images (before and after) placing 22 × 120 mm duodenal SEMS. (**b**) Fluoroscopic images after the SEMS placement. (**c**) Small bowel series showing the oral contrast flowing through the stent

Key Points

1. GI stents improve quality of life in patients with a variety of GI disorders, more so in GI malignancies.
2. Stents can be temporary (bridging) or permanent.
3. Esophageal stents are primarily indicated as palliation for malignant dysphagia due to esophageal cancer. GI stents are safe and effective alternatives or bridge to surgery.
4. Esophageal stents are also increasingly used in dysphagia caused by refractory benign esophageal strictures (RBES), which has become a novel indication.
5. Duodenal stenting is associated with higher rates of stent obstruction and the need for reintervention compared to surgical gastrojejunostomy.
6. In addition to drainage of pancreatic collections, use of LAMS has been expanded to drainage of gallbladder in patients with acute cholecystitis who are unfit for surgery,

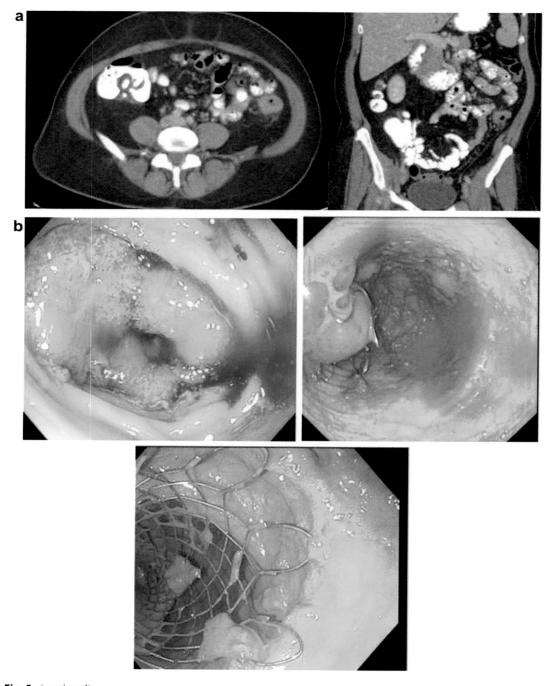

Fig. 5 (continued)

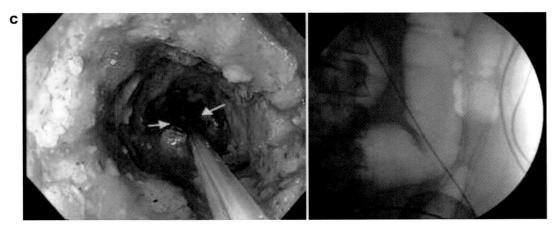

Fig. 5 (**a**) CT scan of the abdomen pelvis axial and coronal views showing descending colon mass. (**b**) Endoscopic images showing the descending colon cancer (left sided) before and after placement of 22 × 90 mm self-expandable metal stent (SEMS) under fluoroscopic and endoscopic guidance. (**c**) Guidewire and delivery system traversing the malignant colonic stricture (left) and fluoroscopic image after placement of second SEMS (25 mm × 120 cm) showing a stent inside the stent (right)

EUS-guided gastroenterostomy in benign and malignant GOO, etc.

7. Prophylactic colonic stenting is not recommended.
8. Only patients with imaging evidence of large bowel obstruction and those with clinical symptoms should be considered for colon stenting.
9. The primary contraindication for colon stenting is bowel perforation.
10. Stenosis associated with the active diverticular disease is a contraindication due to the high risk of perforation.

Patient 1: 89-year-old female with dysphagia due to refractory benign esophageal stricture (RBES) (Fig. 1).

Patient 2: 84-year-old female patient with progressive dysphagia admitted to hospital with food impaction (Fig. 2).

Patient 3: 60-year-old male patient with esophageal cancer (Fig. 3).

Patient 4: 67-year-old with complete gastric outlet obstruction (GOO) due to large tumor in second portion of duodenum (Fig. 4).

Patient 5: 70-year-old female patient with obstructing descending colon mass (left sided) (Fig. 5).

References

Adler DG, Baron TH. Endoscopic palliation of malignant gastric outlet obstruction using self-expanding metal stents: experience in 36 patients. Am J Gastroenterol. 2002;97:72–8.

Baron TH, Siersema PD. Stents for the gastrointestinal tract. Endoscopy. 2019;51:611–2.

Brimhall B, Adler DG. Enteral stents for malignant gastric outlet obstruction. Gastrointest Endosc Clin N Am. 2011;21:389–403.

Brouwer R, Macdonald A, Matthews R, Gunn J, Monson JR, Hartley JE. Brush cytology for the diagnosis of colorectal cancer. Dis Colon Rectum. 2009;52:598–601.

Castaño R, Lopes TL, Alvarez O, Calvo V, Luz LP, Artifon EL. Nitinol biliary stent versus surgery for palliation of distal malignant biliary obstruction. Surg Endosc. 2010;24:2092–8.

Chen YI, Itoi T, Baron TH, Nieto J, Haito-Chavez Y, Grimm IS, Ismail A, Ngamruengphong S, Bukhari M, Hajiyeva G, Alawad AS, Kumbhari V, Khashab MA. EUS-guided gastroenterostomy is comparable to enteral stenting with fewer re-interventions in malignant gastric outlet obstruction. Surg Endosc. 2017;31:2946–52.

Cheynel N, Cortet M, Lepage C, Benoit L, Faivre J, Bouvier AM. Trends in frequency and management of obstructing colorectal cancers in a well-defined population. Dis Colon Rectum. 2007;50:1568–75.

Del Piano M, Ballarè M, Montino F, Todesco A, Orsello M, Magnani C, Garello E. Endoscopy or surgery for malignant GI outlet obstruction? Gastrointest Endosc. 2005;61:421–6.

Dollhopf M, Larghi A, Will U, Rimbaş M, Anderloni A, Sanchez-Yague A, Teoh AYB, Kunda R. EUS-guided gallbladder drainage in patients with acute cholecystitis and high surgical risk using an electrocautery-enhanced lumen-apposing metal stent device. Gastrointest Endosc 2017;86:636–43.

Dormann AJ, Eisendrath P, Wigginghaus B, Huchzermeyer H, Devière J. Palliation of esophageal carcinoma with a new self-expanding plastic stent. Endoscopy. 2003;35:207–11.

Faraz S, Salem SB, Schattner M, Mendelsohn R, Markowitz A, Ludwig E, Zheng J, Gerdes H, Shah PM. Predictors of clinical outcome of colonic stents in patients with malignant large-bowel obstruction because of extracolonic malignancy. Gastrointest Endosc. 2018;87:1310–7.

Frager D, Rovno HD, Baer JW, Bashist B, Friedman M. Prospective evaluation of colonic obstruction with computed tomography. Abdom Imaging. 1998;23:141–6.

Frago R, Ramirez E, Millan M, Kreisler E, Del Valle E, Biondo S. Current management of acute malignant large bowel obstruction: a systematic review. Am J Surg. 2014;207:127–38.

Frimberger E. Expanding spiral–a new type of prosthesis for the palliative treatment of malignant esophageal stenoses. Endoscopy. 1983;15(Suppl 1):213–4.

Hirdes MM, Vleggaar FP, De Beule M, Siersema PD. In vitro evaluation of the radial and axial force of self-expanding esophageal stents. Endoscopy. 2013;45:997–1005.

Homs MY, Steyerberg EW, Eijkenboom WM, Tilanus HW, Stalpers LJ, Bartelsman JF, Van Lanschot JJ, Wijrdeman HK, Mulder CJ, Reinders JG, Boot H, Aleman BM, Kuipers EJ, Siersema PD. Single-dose brachytherapy versus metal stent placement for the palliation of dysphagia from oesophageal cancer: multicentre randomised trial. Lancet. 2004;364: 1497–504.

Jeurnink SM, Van Eijck CH, Steyerberg EW, Kuipers EJ, Siersema PD. Stent versus gastrojejunostomy for the palliation of gastric outlet obstruction: a systematic review. BMC Gastroenterol. 2007;7:18.

Jullumstrø E, Wibe A, Lydersen S, Edna TH. Colon cancer incidence, presentation, treatment and outcomes over 25 years. Color Dis. 2011;13:512–8.

Khashab M, Alawad AS, Shin EJ, Kim K, Bourdel N, Singh VK, Lennon AM, Hutfless S, Sharaiha RZ, Amateau S, Okolo PI, Makary MA, Wolfgang C, Canto MI, Kalloo AN. Enteral stenting versus gastrojejunostomy for palliation of malignant gastric outlet obstruction. Surg Endosc. 2013;27:2068–75.

Kochman ML, Mcclave SA, Boyce HW. The refractory and the recurrent esophageal stricture: a definition. Gastrointest Endosc. 2005;62:474–5.

Mudumbi S, Velazquez-Aviña J, Neumann H, Kyanam Kabir Baig KR, Mönkemüller K. Anchoring of self-expanding metal stents using the over-the-scope clip, and a technique for subsequent removal. Endoscopy. 2014;46:1106–9.

Mussetto A, Fugazza A, Fuccio L, Triossi O, Repici A, Anderloni A. Current uses and outcomes of lumen-apposing metal stents. Ann Gastroenterol 2018;31:535–40.

Ormando VM, Palma R, Fugazza A, Repici A. Colonic stents for malignant bowel obstruction: current status and future prospects. Expert Rev Med Devices. 2019;16:1053–61.

Reijm AN, Didden P, Schelling SJC, Siersema PD, Bruno MJ, Spaander MCW. Self-expandable metal stent placement for malignant esophageal strictures - changes in clinical outcomes over time. Endoscopy. 2019;51:18–29.

Repici A, Small AJ, Mendelson A, Jovani M, Correale L, Hassan C, Ridola L, Anderloni A, Ferrara EC, Kochman ML. Natural history and management of refractory benign esophageal strictures. Gastrointest Endosc. 2016;84:222–8.

Sabharwal T, Hamady MS, Chui S, Atkinson S, Mason R, Adam A. A randomised prospective comparison of the flamingo Wallstent and Ultraflex stent for palliation of dysphagia associated with lower third oesophageal carcinoma. Gut. 2003;52:922–6.

Sabharwal T, Morales JP, Irani FG, Adam A. Quality improvement guidelines for placement of esophageal stents. Cardiovasc Intervent Radiol. 2005;28:284–8.

Sebastian S, Johnston S, Geoghegan T, Torreggiani W, Buckley M. Pooled analysis of the efficacy and safety of self-expanding metal stenting in malignant colorectal obstruction. Am J Gastroenterol. 2004;99:2051–7.

Spaander MC, Baron TH, Siersema PD, Fuccio L, Schumacher B, Escorsell À, Garcia-Pagán JC, Dumonceau JM, Conio M, De Ceglie A, Skowronek J, Nordsmark M, Seufferlein T, Van Gossum A, Hassan C, Repici A, Bruno MJ. Esophageal stenting for benign and malignant disease: European Society of Gastrointestinal Endoscopy (ESGE) clinical guideline. Endoscopy. 2016;48:939–48.

Symonds CJ. The treatment of malignant stricture of the OEsophagus by Tubage or permanent Catheterism. Br Med J. 1887;1:870–3.

Tyberg A, Perez-Miranda M, Sanchez-Ocaña R, Peñas I, De La Serna C, Shah J, Binmoeller K, Gaidhane M, Grimm I, Baron T, Kahaleh M. Endoscopic ultrasound-guided gastrojejunostomy with a lumen-apposing metal stent: a multicenter, international experience. Endosc Int Open. 2016;4:E276–81.

Van Hooft JE, Van Halsema EE, Vanbiervliet G, Beets-Tan RG, Dewitt JM, Donnellan F, Dumonceau JM, Glynne-Jones RG, Hassan C, Jiménez-Perez J, Meisner S, Muthusamy VR, Parker MC, Regimbeau JM, Sabbagh

C, Sagar J, Tanis PJ, Vandervoort J, Webster GJ, Manes G, Barthet MA, Repici A. Self-expandable metal stents for obstructing colonic and extracolonic cancer: European Society of Gastrointestinal Endoscopy (Esge) clinical guideline. Endoscopy. 2014;46:990–1053.

Van Hooft JE, Veld JV, Arnold D, Beets-Tan RGH, Everett S, Götz M, Van Halsema EE, Hill J, Manes G, Meisner S, Rodrigues-Pinto E, Sabbagh C, Vandervoort J, Tanis PJ, Vanbiervliet G, Arezzo A. Self-expandable metal stents for obstructing colonic and extracolonic cancer: European Society of Gastrointestinal Endoscopy (ESGE) guideline - update 2020. Endoscopy. 2020;52:389–407.

Varadarajulu S, Banerjee S, Barth B, Desilets D, Kaul V, Kethu S, Pedrosa M, Pfau P, Tokar J, Wang A, Song LM, Rodriguez S. Enteral stents. Gastrointest Endosc. 2011;74:455–64.

Vermeulen BD, Siersema PD. Esophageal stenting in clinical practice: an overview. Curr Treat Options Gastroenterol. 2018;16:260–73.

Wai CT, Ho KY, Yeoh KG, Lim SG. Palliation of malignant gastric outlet obstruction caused by gastric cancer with self-expandable metal stents. Surg Laparosc Endosc Percutan Tech. 2001;11:161–4.

Walter D, Van Den Berg MW, Van Hooft JE, Boot H, Scheffer RC, Vleggaar FP, Siersema PD. A new fully covered metal stent with anti-migration features for the treatment of malignant dysphagia. Endoscopy. 2014;46:1101–5.

Role of ERCP in Older Adults

40

Sonmoon Mohapatra and Arkady Broder

Contents

S. Mohapatra · A. Broder (✉)
Division of Gastroenterology and Hepatology, Saint
Peter's University Hospital – Rutgers Robert Wood
Johnson School of Medicine, New Brunswick, NJ, USA
e-mail: sonmoon0mohapatra@gmail.com;
abroder@saintpetersuh.com

© Springer Nature Switzerland AG 2021
C. S. Pitchumoni, T. S. Dharmarajan (eds.), *Geriatric Gastroenterology*,
https://doi.org/10.1007/978-3-030-30192-7_33

Abstract

With increasing age, the incidence of pancreatic and biliary diseases rises. Endoscopic retrograde cholangiopancreatography (ERCP) is a commonly performed endoscopic procedure in older adults to diagnose and treat pancreaticobiliary disorders. However, older patients are usually associated with multiple comorbid conditions and, thus, may be more susceptible to complications during the endoscopic interventions. Additionally, complications in older patients can be more severe compared to younger individuals because of the decreased physiological reserve, presence of concomitant systemic diseases, and possible serious drug interactions. Therefore, the endoscopist should be aware of the risks and needs to pay special attention to the risk versus benefits before considering the endoscopic interventions in geriatric patients. This chapter will focus on the yield, safety, and indications of ERCP in older adults.

Keywords

Endoscopic retrograde cholangiopancreatography (ERCP) · Older adults · Choledocholithiasis · Acute cholecystitis · Benign biliary stricture · Malignant biliary obstruction

Introduction

Approximately 50 years ago, endoscopic retrograde cholangiopancreatography (ERCP) was primarily developed as a diagnostic modality, to facilitate radiographic images of the biliary system and pancreas. It was first introduced in 1968 by William McCune and his colleagues who published the first report of endoscopic cannulation of the ampulla of Vater (McCune et al. 1968). At that time, computed tomography (CT) was in its infancy. In 1969, Oi and colleagues developed the side-viewing fiber-optic duodenoscope with a channel and an elevator lever to enable manipulation of the cannula (Oi 1970). In the early 1970s, the therapeutic applications of ERCP emerged. Common bile duct stones were accurately diagnosed at the time of cholangiography, biliary sphincterotomy was performed, and the stones were left in the bile duct to pass on their own. Dr. Peter Cotton reported cannulation in 60 patients who presented with undiagnosed persistent jaundice, recurrent biliary tract symptoms, or suspected pancreatic disease in 1972 (Cotton et al. 1972). In the subsequent year, Drs. Meinhard Classen in Germany and Keiichi Kawai in Japan performed the first biliary sphincterotomy (Kawai et al. 1974). ERCP gained its popularity over the next decade and was well adopted by the endoscopists throughout the world. Pathologic interpretation of endoscopic biopsies and cytologic assessment of brushings continued to improve. During this time, the domain of bile duct stones and palliation of malignancies predominantly shifted from surgeons to the endoscopists. In the subsequent decade (1990–2000), CT and magnetic resonance imaging (MRI)/magnetic resonance cholangiopancreatography (MRCP) to image noninvasively the pancreatobiliary system was introduced, which ultimately transformed the indications for ERCP from a diagnostic/therapeutic procedure to a predominately therapeutic modality (Wallner et al. 1991).

In general, the procedure involves passing of an endoscope to the ampulla (the opening of the bile and pancreatic ducts) located in the second part of the duodenum. After visualizing the ampulla, a catheter is passed through the channel of the endoscope into the duct of interest, and a contrast medium is injected under fluoroscopic guidance to outline the ductal structures or to measure sphincter pressure. If necessary, therapeutic maneuvers can be performed by incising the sphincter muscle at the opening of the bile duct or pancreatic duct (biliary and pancreatic duct sphincterotomy, respectively). Depending on the indication, other accessories may be passed through the endoscope channel into the duct of interest to remove stones, insert stents, or ablate tissue.

ERCP is a frequent procedure performed in geriatric patients. This is because of the relatively higher incidence of pancreaticobiliary diseases in this age group such as choledocholithiasis, biliary tract malignancy, and pancreatic cancer (Harness et al. 1986). Common bile duct stones and malignancies account for more than 70% of cases of jaundice in the older population. Indeed, the most common indication for abdominal surgery in these patients is biliary tract disease. However, compared to younger patients, surgical therapy in these patients carries a higher potential risk of complication and mortality. In view of the reported increased morbidity and mortality of surgical interventions in older individuals, endoscopic alternatives may be preferred for the management of certain biliary tract disorders. In this chapter, we aim to summarize the indications, contraindications, success rates, and complication rates of diagnostic and therapeutic ERCP in the geriatric population.

Preprocedural Evaluation

Similar to that of all patients, geriatric patients require to be evaluated to determine whether they are at increased risk before undergoing an endoscopic procedure. The preprocedural assessment should include determination of the patient's ability to provide informed consent, evaluation of the patient's cardiopulmonary status, and associated comorbid conditions which may affect procedural sedation or the performance of the procedure (ASGE Standards of Practice Committee et al. 2013). It is essential to provide appropriate information before each endoscopic procedure to confirm patient comprehension, especially in the presence of possible coexisting disabilities (i.e., cognitive impairment, visual disturbances, hard of hearing, etc.). Cognitive impairment may limit the ability to actively participate in this process, especially in extremely older patients, and the endoscopist has the responsibility to obtain informed consent from the legal guardian or surrogate of the patient (Giampieri 2012).

Elderly patients are more likely to have underlying cardiovascular disease, and implanted cardiac devices, thus, special precautions, are required before performing an endoscopic procedure as discussed below. Additionally, it has been shown that elderly patients are more likely to require anticoagulation therapy at some point, either on a short- or a long-term basis. The most frequently encountered indications for anticoagulation in these patients are atrial fibrillation, with a prevalence of approximately 10% in patients over 80 years of age, and the prevention and treatment of venous thromboembolism (VTE) (Go et al. 2001). Indeed, the incidence of deep vein thrombosis and pulmonary embolism increases almost exponentially with age, and the majority of all VTE events occur in patients over 70 years of age (Naess et al. 2007). Presently, several recommendations have been published from various societies to guide the endoscopist in the management of anticoagulants in peri-endoscopic period (Chan et al. 2018; ASGE Standards of Practice Committee et al. 2016; Veitch et al. 2016).

Implanted Cardiac Pacemakers and Internal Defibrillators

Many older patients have implanted cardiac devices, such as pacemakers or pacemaker-defibrillators. These devices have the potential for electromagnetic interference during electrocautery (e.g., sphincterotomy); adverse events such as intracardiac device malfunction in this setting include pacing inhibition, pacing triggering, automatic mode switching, spurious tachyarrhythmia detection, ventricular fibrillation, electrical reset, myocardial burns, the runaway pacemaker syndrome, and irreversible loss of output have been reported (Petersen et al. 2007). Presently, there is insufficient literature regarding the safety of endoscopic electrocautery use in patients with implanted cardiac pacemakers, and thus, the handling of pacemaker before endoscopy is not standardized.

American Society of Gastrointestinal Endoscopy (ASGE) and the American Heart Association (AHA) recommend the use of continuous electrocardiographic rhythm monitoring in addition to pulse oximetry during the entire procedure (Parekh et al. 2013; Fleisher et al.

2009). In addition to this, indication for the device, type of cardiac device, the patient's underlying cardiac rhythm, and degree of pacemaker-dependence before the endoscopic procedure need to be determined. Although the routine use of electrocautery appears safe in most patients with cardiac pacemakers, reprogramming the pacemaker to an asynchronous mode via application of a magnet over the pulse generator should be considered for the patients who are pacemaker dependent or in whom prolonged electrocautery is anticipated. Preprocedural assessment of device function in collaboration with the cardiologist should be considered, especially in patients with ICDs. Intracardiac defibrillators should be turned off prior to the use of electrocautery. Use of bipolar cautery should be considered if the patient with an ICD who is pacemaker dependent and the ICD cannot be reprogrammed to an asynchronous mode, and prolonged cautery application is anticipated.

Prophylactic Antibiotics

Prophylactic antibiotics are not recommended for most of the endoscopic procedures regardless of the patient's age. For ERCP, antibiotics are recommended in patients with incomplete biliary drainage (such as with hilar carcinoma or primary sclerosing cholangitis) or those with immunosuppression (ASGE Standards of Practice Committee et al. 2015). Additionally, routine administration of antibiotics is recommended in patients with post-liver transplantation biliary strictures who plan to undergo ERCP. Recommendations regarding the use of prophylactic antibiotics for all other endoscopic procedures is beyond the scope of this chapter and have been outlined in guidelines from the ASGE (ASGE Standards of Practice Committee et al. 2015).

Sedation

Majority of the endoscopic procedures are performed using moderate sedation. Compared to the younger patients, although geriatric patients

better tolerate the upper endoscopy or colonoscopy with little or no sedation (common practice outside the USA), ERCPs are usually performed under conscious sedation (Baron and Fleischer 2002).

In older adults, one of the main risks of performing endoscopy is the sedation use during the procedure. Sedation in the geriatric patients requires awareness of their increased response to sedatives (Muravchick 2002). A variety of physiologic changes contribute to the increase in sensitivity and sedation risk in geriatric patients (Boss and Seegmiller 1981). Compared to younger patients, an increased risk of hypotension, hypoxia, arrhythmias, and aspiration occur in older patients undergoing procedural sedation (Clarke et al. 2001; Riphaus et al. 2005; Fritz et al. 2006; Katsinelos et al. 2006, 2011; Thomopoulos et al. 2007). This perhaps occurs mainly because of the increased residual pulmonary volumes, increased vascular tissue elasticity, and decreased vital capacity in the older adults.

With aging, arterial oxygenation progressively deteriorates, and cardiorespiratory stimulation in response to hypoxia or hypercarbia is blunted and delayed. The risk of arterial desaturation from the sedative medications increases with increase in the number of comorbid illness (such as coronary artery disease, chronic obstructive pulmonary disease, and renal dysfunction), especially in patients with low cardiac index and a worse functional class, according to New York Heart Association. An increased risk of respiratory depression and a higher incidence of transient apneic episodes have been reported with the use of narcotic and nonnarcotic central nervous system (CNS) depressants. In the older adults, a greater distribution of the lipid-soluble pharmacological agents (such as benzodiazepines) occurs because of the age-related increase in the lipid fraction of body mass.

Current ASGE guideline recommends choosing a drug with a short half-life, with minimally active metabolites, and limited side effects. The primary modification in sedation practices requires the administration of fewer agents at a slower rate with a lower cumulative dose, usually to start with a half the recommended standard dose. Midazolam and/or narcotics are commonly used in geriatric patients. Fentanyl has a quicker onset of action and shorter half-life and may have an advantage over meperidine in the older patients (Hayee et al. 2009). Although propofol has a narrower safety margin, it has been shown to be safe when used in older adults (Cohen et al. 2004).

Efficacy of ERCP in Older Adults

Several studies have investigated the role of ERCP in the older patients and demonstrated that the therapeutic success rates of ERCP in these patients are comparable to the success rates in younger patients (Fritz et al. 2006; Katsinelos et al. 2006; Thomopoulos et al. 2007; Koklu et al. 2005; Cariani et al. 2006; Ali et al. 2011). In fact, ERCP in the geriatric patients is a safer option with a lower rate of morbidity and mortality compared with alternative operative interventions. Studies have reported that successful cannulation of the bile duct is achieved in 88–98% with a diagnostic yield of 82% and therapeutic yield of 85–87% of the older adults (Fritz et al. 2006; Thomopoulos et al. 2007; Riphaus et al. 2008). A prospective study of 118 older patients have demonstrated that biliary obstruction was one of the leading indications for ERCP (73.7%) (Riphaus et al. 2008). Compared to younger patients, older patients ($\geq$80 years) were more likely to present with cholangitis (28.5% vs. 16.1%, P <0.001) based on the result of a retrospective study (Fritz et al. 2006). Another study who have compiled 11 cohort studies involving 1372 older patients (often octogenarians and nonagenarians), consisting of at least 1476 ERCPs demonstrated that successful stone clearance was achieved in 93% of the patients (Fritz et al. 2006; Thomopoulos et al. 2007; Koklu et al. 2005; MacMahon et al. 1993; Ashton et al. 1998; Sugiyama and Atomi 2000; Mitchell et al. 2003; Rodriguez-Gonzalez et al. 2003; Hui et al. 2004; Katsinelos et al. 2007; Chong et al.

2005). Among these, $\geq$2 procedures were required in 17% of patients and mechanical lithotripsy was performed in 22% of procedures (DiSario 2008). Adverse events occurred in 6% of procedures and included, in decreasing order of frequency, bleeding, cholangitis, pancreatitis, perforation, and cardiorespiratory problems. Procedure-related death occurred in <1% of patients. Although periampullary diverticula have been noted more frequently in older adults, this anatomic finding has not been reported to affect cannulation rates (Fritz et al. 2006; Katsinelos et al. 2006).

Adverse Events Related to ERCP in Older Adults

Overall, adverse events including pancreatitis, perforation, and bleeding from ERCP in the older patients are similar compared to the younger populations, although patients of advanced age are more prone to prolonged sedation and hypotension (Fritz et al. 2006; Katsinelos et al. 2011; Sugiyama and Atomi 2000; Freeman et al. 1996). The list of commonly recognized complications related to ERCP is shown in Box 1.

Box 1 Complications of ERCP
- Pancreatitis
- Post-sphincterotomy bleeding
- Perforation
- Infection
- Cardiopulmonary
- Stent-related complications such as migration, occlusion, perforation, acute cholecystitis, biliary or pancreatic duct injury
- Miscellaneous
  - Hepatic abscess
  - Duodenal hematoma
  - Portal venous air
  - Ileus
  - Perforation of duodenal diverticula

Post-ERCP Pancreatitis

Increasing age appears to be protective against post-ERCP pancreatitis (PEP). Compared to younger patients, patients ≥65 years of age were 70% less likely to develop PEP based on the result of a recent meta-analysis (IRR 0.3; 95% CI 0.3–0.4; $P = 0.7$ for heterogeneity) (Day et al. 2014). Several other studies support this finding (Ali et al. 2011; Lukens et al. 2010; Behlul et al. 2014; Yun et al. 2014; Maitin-Casalis et al. 2015). Possible reasons for this lower rate of pancreatitis include pancreatic atrophy, increased fibrosis of the pancreas, and reduced pancreatic enzyme secretion in the elderly (Lukens et al. 2010). Alteration of guidewire cannulation techniques (using a wire probe instead of contrast injection) and pancreatic stent placement are some of the strategies to reduce the incidence of PEP (ASGE Standards of Practice Committee et al. 2017). Recently, several meta-analyses of rectal NSAID use have demonstrated that these agents reduce the risk of moderate or severe PEP, with a number needed to treat to prevent 1 case of PEP ranging from 11 to 17 (ASGE Standards of Practice Committee et al. 2017; Sethi et al. 2014; Yang et al. 2017; Patai et al. 2017). The result of a subgroup analysis in another meta-analysis indicated that prophylactic rectal indomethacin is not suitable for all patients undergoing ERCP but is safe and effective to prevent PEP only in high-risk patients. In addition, they demonstrated that rectal indomethacin administration before ERCP is superior to its administration after ERCP for the prevention of PEP (Wan et al. 2017). However, a multicenter, single-blinded, randomized, controlled trial of 2600 patients undergoing ERCP in China who also included low-risk individuals showed a significant reduction in PEP in those who universally received rectal indomethacin (4%) before the procedure, compared with a group that received the medication after the procedure based on risk stratification (8%, RR 0.47; 95% CI 0.34–0.66; $P < 0.0001$) (Luo et al. 2016).

Bleeding After ERCP

A prospective multicentric study from the USA and Canada have shown that age solely was not a risk factor for adverse events after biliary sphincterotomy (Freeman et al. 1996). The rate of complications after a biliary sphincterotomy was largely dependent on the indication of the procedure; it was highest in patients with suspected sphincter of Oddi (21.7%) dysfunction and lowest in patients with bile duct stones removal within 30 days of laparoscopic cholecystectomy (4.9%) (Freeman et al. 1996). Post-sphincterotomy bleeding in the geriatric patients have been reported to be 1–2%, which is not different from the younger population (Freeman et al. 1996; ASGE Standards of Practice Committee et al. 2017; Masci et al. 2001). In contrast, Koklu et al. have reported bleeding as the most frequent complication in the older adults (6.2% vs. 3%) compared to the younger patients (Koklu et al. 2005). There was a significantly higher rate of procedure-related bleeding within the elderly cohort (3.3%) compared with the nonelderly cohort (0.8%; $P = 0.016$) in another large cohort of older patients with 600 ERCPs. However, most of the post-procedure bleeding episodes in that study were minor and did not require blood transfusions. In line with this, the result of a recent meta-analysis has shown that nonagenarians had twice the risk of bleeding (IRR 2.4; 95% CI 1.1–5.2; $P = 0.4$ for heterogeneity) compared to the patients with <90 years of age. This observation may be due to increased prevalence of coagulopathy, big stones requiring larger sphincterotomy, increased number of therapeutic maneuvers, and/or periampullary diverticulum in the older population (Day et al. 2014).

Cardiopulmonary Complications

Despite the overall consistency in the published studies, older patients carry an increased risk of cardiopulmonary complications (Day et al. 2014). This observation may be because of the longer procedural time and associated medical comorbidities carried by older adults rather than with age alone (Fisher et al. 2006). In general, cardiopulmonary complications secondary to ERCP are rare, occurring in 1% of cases with an associated fatality rate of 0.07% in older adults (Andriulli et al. 2007). In a study comparing patients older than 65 years of age with younger patients, standard cardiac risk factors and hemodynamic and electrocardiographic changes such as ERCP-related transient hypoxemia, tachycardia, and hypotension during the procedure were reported as more common in the group older than 65 years but were not statistically significant (Fisher et al. 2006). Eight percent (6/74) of patients older than 65 years of age had a sustained myocardial injury especially with prolonged procedures (>30 min) (Fisher et al. 2006). Nonagenarians were shown to have a fourfold increase in the cardiopulmonary adverse events compared to younger patients (Day et al. 2014). It is important to note that therapeutic ERCP appears to be relatively safe in patients who have a recent myocardial infarction or unstable angina (30 days or less) especially when the benefits outweigh procedural complications (Nojkov and Cappell 2010).

Safety of sedation is one of the most important issues when ERCP is performed in older adults with multiple comorbidities. Propofol is associated with shorter recovery times, better sedation, and higher rates of amnesia without higher rates of cardiopulmonary adverse events compared to traditional medications (Garewal et al. 2012). Sedation with propofol is considered safe in older patients, and the required dose was significantly lower in the elderly cohort compared to younger patients (Fritz et al. 2006). Advanced age and poor general condition classified as ASA class III or more in the older adults have not associated with an increased mortality rate following ERCP. In some instances, patients with advanced age are unable to tolerate endoscopic procedures because either they are critically ill or uncooperative. In these cases, ERCP can be performed safely under general anesthesia with endotracheal intubation.

Risk of Perforation

Perforation has been reported in 1% of the younger patients compared to 1.5% in the older adults and can often be treated with conservative management alone (Koklu et al. 2005). Patient-related and procedure-related risk factors for perforation during ERCP have been well described. Older patient age is one of the patient-related factors along with others such as suspected SOD, female sex, and surgical or altered anatomy (i.e., situs inversus or Billroth II gastrectomy) (ASGE Standards of Practice Committee et al. 2017). Procedure-related factors include difficult cannulation, longer duration of procedure, intramural injection of contrast material, sphincterotomy and precut papillotomy, biliary stricture dilation, procedure performed by lesser experienced operators, and endoscopic papillary large-balloon dilation. Prompt recognition of periampullary perforation and conservative treatment with biliary and duodenal drainage coupled with broad-spectrum antibiotics result in a clinical resolution in up to 86% of patients (Enns et al. 2002).

Infections and Mortality

Post-ERCP bacteremia or cholangitis and acute cholecystitis do not seem to have a statistically increased risk in the older adults compared to younger. Despite an extremely rare mortality rate of <0.5% among older adults, patients >80 years of age have a two- to fourfold increased risk of mortality compared to the younger population (Day et al. 2014; Freeman 2002a, b). A multivariate analysis has shown that older age solely is not responsible for an increased risk of mortality following ERCP and is likely related to the degree of comorbid disease (Freeman 2002a).

Indications for ERCP in the Elderly

Biliary obstruction (mainly secondary to choledocholithiasis) is the most frequent indication of ERCP in the elderly. Among the malignant causes, pancreatic cancer is the most frequent cancer in the older population, followed by cholangio-carcinoma and ampullary carcinoma (Koklu et al. 2005). A summary of the indications and contraindications of ERCP are illustrated in Boxes 2 and 3. Common indications for ERCP in the geriatric patients are described below in detail.

Box 2 Indications for ERCP
- Jaundice secondary to biliary obstruction
- Clinical, biochemical, or imaging evidence of pancreatic or biliary tract disease
- Diagnosis and treatment of ampullary carcinoma
- Recurrent pancreatitis
- Tissue sampling for pancreatic or biliary carcinoma
- Stent placement for benign or malignant strictures, postoperative bile leak, fistulae, common bile duct stones
- Pancreatic pseudocysts
- Balloon dilation of ductal strictures
- Sphincter of Oddi manometry
- Endoscopic sphincterotomy
  - Type 1 sphincter of Oddi dysfunction
  - Choledocholithiasis
  - Facilitate biliary stent placement or balloon dilation
  - Ampullary carcinoma who are poor surgical candidates
  - Choledochocele involving the major papilla

Box 3 Contraindications to ERCP
- Recent myocardial infarction
- Uncontrolled systemic infection or sepsis
- High suspicion or known perforated viscus
- Coagulopathy
- Severe pulmonary disease
- Uncooperative patient or when consent cannot be obtained

Box 3 Contraindications to ERCP (continued)
- Anatomic abnormalities (gastroduodenal disease or surgical alteration) limiting access to papilla
- Prior history of allergy to ERCP contrast medium
- Endoscopist with inadequate training in ERCP

Choledocholithiasis

Choledocholithiasis is a frequent cause of biliary obstruction in the older adults. Similarly, choledocholithiasis with concomitant cholecystitis is frequently found in older patients with a prevalence rate of 10–20% compared to 5% in the general population. Common bile duct (CBD) stones often present with biliary colic, acute cholangitis, acute pancreatitis, and rarely, hepatic abscesses because of obstruction and superimposed biliary infection.

Clinical Presentation
Clinical presentation of choledocholithiasis can be quite variable. Typical biliary pain in the older patients may be lacking on presentation. Instead, they may have a difficulty in localizing upper abdominal pain with or without any other associated symptoms. Some patients with choledocholithiasis can present with painless jaundice, often mimicking an obstructive tumor in the pancreatobiliary system. In extremely older patients (>80 years), bile duct stones can manifest as an acute confusional state especially when cholangitis ensues.

Risk Stratification and Management
Choledocholithiasis may be diagnosed in the patient either before or after cholecystectomy. Occasionally, common bile duct stones get diagnosed intraoperatively at the time of cholecystectomy. Although there is no single variable that consistently strongly predicts choledocholithiasis in patients with symptomatic cholelithiasis,

studies have showed that the probability of a CBD stone is higher in the presence of multiple abnormal prognostic signs. Based on these results, the 2010 ASGE guideline has proposed a risk stratification system to categorize patients into low (10%), intermediate (10–50%), and high (50%) probability of choledocholithiasis by using factors such as age, liver test results, and ultrasound findings (ASGE Standards of Practice Committee et al. 2010). However, since that time, the guidelines have been the subject of multiple validation studies which subsequently demonstrated that the 2010 ASGE guidelines may result in performance of diagnostic ERCP in 20–30% of cases. Therefore, the 2010 criterion was recently revised to decrease the use of diagnostic ERCP, which has significant risk but minimal benefit.

The 2019 ASGE guideline recommend the following high-risk criteria: A CBD stone visualized in the US or cross-sectional imaging, cholangitis, a combination of total bilirubin level higher than 4 mg/dL and a dilated CBD on US (ASGE Standards of Practice Committee et al. 2019). A dilated CBD is defined as >6 mm in adults who have not undergone and 8 mm in those who have undergone cholecystectomy. This criterion is no different in the older patients although a significant correlation between the CBD size and age has been reported in previous studies (Bachar et al. 2003; Daradkeh et al. 2005). Intermediate criteria were defined as abnormal liver tests, age >55 years, and dilated common bile duct on US (intermediate risk for choledocholithiasis) in patients with suspected choledocholithiasis. Given a lack of association, gallstone pancreatitis was removed as a criterion. It was proposed that patients with any of the high-risk criteria proceed to ERCP and those with intermediate-risk criterion undergo EUS, MRCP, or laparoscopic IOC or laparoscopic intraoperative US for further evaluation. In fact, patients >55 years solely meets the intermediate risk criteria for choledocholithiasis and, thus, should be evaluated with EUS or MRCP even without presence of any liver enzyme abnormalities or dilated CBD on the US. Patients without any clinical risk factors (low risk) should undergo cholecystectomy with or without IOC or intraoperative US for symptomatic cholelithiasis.

Clinicians can either follow one-step approaches (when one combined surgical procedure is used) versus a variety of two-step approaches (using surgery and a minimally invasive bile duct clearance procedure) for the management of choledocholithiasis when cholecystectomy is planned. For high-risk patients, ERCP (with either endoscopic sphincterotomy (ES) or endoscopic papillary balloon dilation (EPBD)) before cholecystectomy is a frequently used two-step approach. Another alternative two-step pathway is to perform laparoscopic cholecystectomy with intraoperative cholangiogram (IOC) and subsequent postoperative ERCP for positive CBD stone in the IOC. However, in patients with a history of cholecystectomy, ERCP is the preferred method for removing bile duct stones. A retrospective study comparing 43,338 older patients (≥60 years) with 45,295 younger patients (<60 years) from the Nationwide Inpatient Sample database suggested that ERCP followed by cholecystectomy was characterized by lowest mortality among the older patients and should be the preferred method of management for patients with complicated gallstone disease, regardless of the age (Nassar and Richter 2019). However, in this study, although mortality was found to be significantly higher in ERCP compared to ERCP followed by cholecystectomy in patients 60–79 years old, death rates were noted to be comparable between the two groups in patients more than 80 years old. Another study by Yasui et al. who compared the outcomes of patients who underwent ERCP with and without cholecystectomy among the elderly concluded that cholecystectomy after the ERCP does not provide a benefit to patients older than 80 years (Yasui et al. 2012).

Laparoscopic common bile duct exploration (LCBDE) has emerged as a recommended alternative to endoscopic retrograde cholangiopancreatography (ERCP) for the management of choledocholithiasis. Platt et al. have demonstrated that LCBDE in older patients is safe and effective and has similar outcomes compared to younger patients, despite higher frequency of comorbidities and ASA grade (Platt et al. 2018). However, the size of their study cohort was too small to identify differences in complications between the groups, particularly in subgroup analysis of patients aged ≥80.

Management of Large and Difficult Choledocholithiasis

Nearly 85–90% of biliary stones can be removed with a balloon or basket after ES or EPBD. However, in patients with large bile duct stones (≥1 cm), endoscopic sphincterotomy followed by large balloon dilation (ES-LBD) rather than ES alone is the preferred approach to facilitate the removal of large stones (Yang and Hu 2013; Dong et al. 2019). Current evidence suggest that adverse events for ESLBD were comparable with ES alone (Karsenti et al. 2017). EPBD is a safe and effective technique for the treatment of bile duct stones even in high-risk geriatric patients without an increased risk of pancreatitis and bleeding (Ito et al. 2008). Large and difficult bile duct stones particularly due to other reasons (i.e., anatomic abnormalities or impaction) may be managed either by intraductal therapy or by conventional therapy. Intraductal therapy includes cholangioscopy and fluoroscopically guided laser and electrohydraulic lithotripsy, whereas conventional therapy included mechanical lithotripsy, balloon extraction, and papillary dilation (Chen and Pleskow 2007; Moon et al. 2009).

Role of Bile Duct Stents in the Management of Choledocholithiasis

Biliary stents are an effective way for decompression of the biliary system and can be used as a temporary measure in patients with CBD stones in whom sphincterotomy may be high-risk because of certain comorbid conditions such as bleeding diathesis and/or recent myocardial infarction. Another advantage of biliary plastic stent placement over sphincterotomy and stone extraction is that stenting usually involves a shorter procedure time allowing less exposure to sedation and risk for development of cardiopulmonary complications in the setting of acutely severely ill patients. In contrary, this approach often requires a second

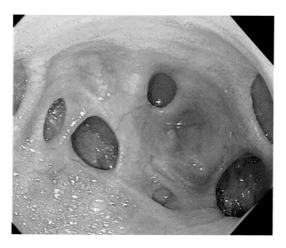

Fig. 1 Endoscopic appearance of multiple periampullary diverticula in an old male patient

procedure in the future for sphincterotomy and definitive stone extraction.

Stone disease complicated with strictures can be treated either in multiple sessions or palliated by providing long-term stent placement. Endoscopic sphincterotomy and stone extraction complications are divided into early (within 3 months after the procedure) or delayed (more than 3 months after the procedure). One of the delayed complications includes recurrent bile duct stones occurring in 4–24% of patients despite increasing experience and success with the procedure. The prevalence of periampullary diverticula increases with age and is reported to be greater than 30% in patients above age 70 undergoing ERCP (Fig. 1). Periampullary diverticula are also known to be a risk factor for recurrent CBD stones, CBD cannulation difficulty, prolonged procedure times, and procedure failure. In addition, this is perhaps one of the reasons for the higher prevalence of recurrent symptomatic CBD stones in older adults compared to the younger population.

Gallstone Pancreatitis

Cholelithiasis is determined as the main cause of acute pancreatitis (AP) among the older patients. Compared with younger patients, older patients admitted for acute biliary pancreatitis (ABP) have increased rates of severe acute pancreatitis and mortality (Koziel et al. 2019; Patel et al. 2019). In a retrospective study consisting of 184,763 ABP cases, 41% were older adults (Patel et al. 2019). Mortality was increased in the elderly versus younger patients, with an odds ratio of 2.8 (95% CI 2.2–3.5).

The consensus recommends that ERCP and ES should be restricted to patients who presents with biliary sepsis or obstructive jaundice (ASGE Standards of Practice Committee et al. 2019). Early ERCP (within 48 h) is preferred in patients who presents with concomitant cholangitis as evidence suggests that urgent ERCP is of benefit in these patients if done in the first 48 h. In the absence of biliary sepsis or obstructive jaundice, severity alone is not an indication for ERCP given the lack of benefit and potential increase risk of adverse events. In ABP patients with suspected choledocholithiasis, MRCP and EUS are useful in the diagnosis of biliary obstruction before performing ERCP. Same admission cholecystectomy is recommended for patients with mild ABP (Jee et al. 2018). However, adherence to current recommendations for the management of mild ABP has been shown to be low in older patients. Recent data suggest that over 40% of patients who did not undergo cholecystectomy would have benefited from early definitive therapy (Trust et al. 2011).

Acute Cholecystitis

Acute cholecystitis may present atypically, especially in the older adult population. The definitive treatment of acute cholecystitis is urgent cholecystectomy or cholecystostomy in patients who are unable to tolerate surgery. However, it has been shown that older patients who require emergency cholecystectomy have a poor outcome compared to younger patients. Among the older patients, the mortality rates for emergency cholecystectomy range from 6% to 15% (Glenn and Hays 1955). Therefore, a thorough clinical assessment of these patients is necessary before subjecting them to cholecystectomy. In certain clinical situations, especially in extremely older or ill patients, minimally invasive techniques such as ERCP may be a safer alternative.

In patients with acute calculous cholecystitis, stones can be dislodged by vigorously injecting contrast material into the cystic duct or by manipulating the obstructing stone with catheters and guidewires (Siegel et al. 1994). Trans-papillary stents can be placed into the affected gall bladder via the cystic duct establishing free flow of bile and purulent material to drain into the duodenum thus palliating acute cholecystitis. These ERCP-guided palliative procedures can be implemented in patients of any age who are considered unfit for surgery, but more appropriate in acutely ill, older patients who present with serious comorbid conditions (Hosking et al. 1989; Margiotta et al. 1988). Although EUS-guided gallbladder drainage is outside the scope of our discussion, it is important to note that this is a commonly accepted and highly successful intervention in the non-operable patient (Dollhopf et al. 2017).

Benign Biliary Strictures

The most common cause of benign biliary stricture is an iatrogenic injury during surgery, especially following cholecystectomy, or at the site of biliary anastomosis after hepatic resection or liver transplantation. Other causes relevant to the older population include traumatic, parasitic, inflammatory, and idiopathic biliary strictures (Laasch and Martin 2002). About 10–30% of patients with advanced chronic pancreatitis develop symptomatic biliary stenosis. Alternatively, in acute pancreatitis biliary obstruction may be caused by the compression of the bile duct by an edematous pancreatic head or a fluid collection, which may resolve spontaneously or require ERCP intervention. On the other hand, an obstruction caused by a fibrotic stricture does not resolve spontaneously and almost always needs therapeutic intervention.

Overall, differentiating between benign and malignant strictures, especially in an older patient, is of utmost importance and often can be very difficult. With the development of intraductal

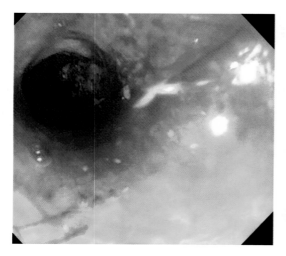

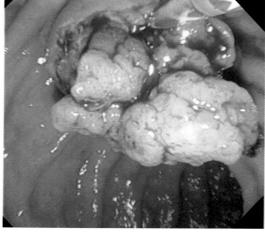

Fig. 2 Direct cholangioscopy showing a malignant biliary stricture with an infiltrative grown pattern

Fig. 3 Carcinoma of ampulla of Vater detected while performing endoscopic retrograde cholangiography

cholangioscopy, it has become easier to identify intraductal lesions for better differentiation between benign and malignant strictures. The criteria for differentiation based on direct cholangiography findings include irregular margins, asymmetric dilation of the biliary radicles, abrupt or gradual tapering of the strictures, presence or absence of a mass, and length of the stricture (Saluja et al. 2007). Malignant strictures are generally long with an infiltrative growth pattern spreading intramurally beneath the epithelial lining (Fig. 2).

ERCP should be performed if an older patient requires urgent relief of obstruction. ERCP serves as both a diagnostic and therapeutic tool when brushings/biopsies are taken, and the obstruction is relieved after balloon dilation and stent placement. In the appropriate setting, patients can be given the option of repeated endoscopic insertion of plastic stents. Alternatively, larger diameter self-expandable metal stents (SEMS) are an attractive alternative to single or multiple plastic stents. SEMS can be uncovered, partially covered, or fully covered and provide superior durability and longer-standing patency then plastic stents. Uncovered SEMS are susceptible for tissue ingrowth through the meshes of the stent which can make stent removal extremely difficult or impossible.

This can be prevented by using a covered or partially covered metal stent, but, unfortunately, these are more prone for migration. To overcome this problem, fully covered stents with anti-migration flaps have been developed. Due to the inherent properties of SEMS, their use has become preferable in the setting of chronic fibrotic strictures.

Malignant Biliary Strictures

Malignant strictures of the pancreaticobiliary system are often difficult to diagnose and treat. Majority of the patients present in more advanced stages of disease, contributing to poor prognosis and outcome. Painless jaundice is the most common presentation of malignant biliary obstruction. The different etiologies of distal malignant obstruction include carcinoma of ampulla of Vater (Fig. 3), pancreatic cancer (Fig. 4), gallbladder cancer, distal cholangiocarcinoma, and metastatic disease that involves the head of the pancreas or the common bile duct. Malignant biliary obstruction of the hilum and proximal intrahepatic ducts can occur from primary pancreatobiliary cancers (Fig. 5a), primary liver cancers, portal lymphadenopathy, or metastatic disease.

Fig. 4 Cholangiogram showing markedly dilated bile duct secondary to pancreatic cancer

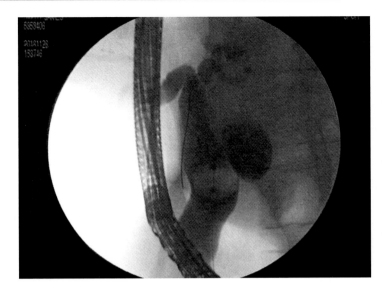

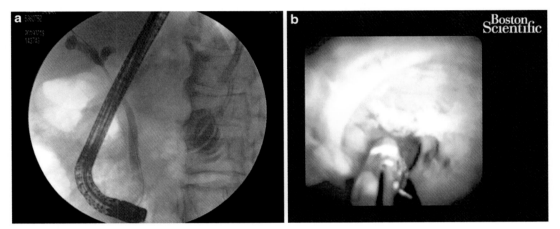

Fig. 5 (**a**) Endoscopic retrograde cholangiography in a patient with hilar cholangiocarcinoma with Bismuth-Corlette classification type I. (**b**) Intraductal biliary biopsy obtained through direct cholangiography in the same patient

Pancreatic Cancer

Pancreatic cancer, the most common cause of malignant biliary obstruction in the USA, accounts for nearly 43,920 new cases per year and ranks fourth in cancer-related death in both sexes (American Cancer Society 2012). The number of pancreatic cancer-related deaths is expected to increase in the USA, and pancreatic cancer may become the second leading cause of cancer-related deaths by 2030 (Rahib et al. 2014). Among various risk factors (such as cigarette smoking, daily alcohol consumption (30–40 g of

alcohol per day), chronic pancreatitis, obesity, family history, and certain genetic syndromes), advanced age is the most significant risk factor for pancreatic cancer. The median age at diagnosis of pancreatic cancer in the USA is 72 years. Apart from painless jaundice, advanced forms of pancreatic cancer can present with epigastric pain radiating to the back, suggesting pancreatic duct obstruction and infiltration of retroperitoneal structures, palpable gallbladder, dyspepsia, unintentional weight loss, early satiety because of gastric outlet obstruction, new-onset glucose intolerance or diabetes mellitus, and acute pancreatitis.

Cholangiocarcinoma

Cholangiocarcinoma can either be intrahepatic or extrahepatic and is the second most common primary hepatic malignancy. The peak age of presentation for cholangiocarcinoma is the seventh decade with a higher incidence in men. The incidence of cholangiocarcinoma appears to be rising in the Western world, although the data is not consistent in all studies (Bergquist and von Seth 2015). The risk factors for cholangiocarcinoma include advanced age, male gender, and underlying conditions such as primary sclerosing cholangitis (PSC), fibropolycystic liver disease, Caroli's disease, choledochal cysts, HNPCC, and bile duct adenomas. However, specific risk factors are identified only in a minority of patients and majority of cases are sporadic. Cholangiocarcinoma commonly presents with abdominal pain mostly in the right upper quadrant, jaundice, pruritus, and weight loss.

Gallbladder Cancer

Gallbladder cancer is the fifth common gastrointestinal cancer and the most common cancer involving the biliary tract in the USA. Risk factors for gallbladder cancer include advanced age, female gender, and specific geographic areas. The incidence of gallbladder cancer is higher in South American countries such as Chile, Ecuador, and Bolivia and in Asian countries such as India, Pakistan, Japan, and Korea. Other conditions such as porcelain gallbladder, gallbladder polyps, congenital biliary cysts, and abnormal pancreaticobiliary duct junction are associated with higher risk of cancer of the gallbladder. In these patients, obstructive jaundice is the most common symptom and often presents in the context of advanced disease. Abdominal pain may be an accompanying feature.

Ampullary Carcinoma

Periampullary tumors originate from the pancreas, duodenum, distal CBD, or the structures of the ampullary (ampulla of Vater) complex. Primary ampullary tumors are rare, with an incidence of approximately four to six cases per million population (Goodman and Yamamoto 2007; Albores-Saavedra et al. 2009). However, compared to any other site of small intestine, neoplastic transformation of the intestinal mucosa occurs more commonly near the ampulla. The average age at diagnosis of sporadic ampullary carcinomas is 60–70 years (O'Connell et al. 2008). Ampullary tumors can occur sporadically or in the setting of a genetic syndrome such as hereditary polyposis syndromes. The common presenting symptom of ampullary carcinoma is obstructive jaundice. Additional symptoms may include occult gastrointestinal bleeding, diarrhea due to fat malabsorption (steatorrhea), mild weight loss, and fatigue.

Role of ERCP in the Diagnosis and Management of Distal Biliary Obstruction

Depending on the nature and type of malignancy, the principle objective is to provide both diagnostic and therapeutic solutions. A diagnostic procedure such as EUS with FNA or ERCP with brushings is often needed. Presently, EUS has largely replaced ERCP for the diagnosis of pancreatic head adenocarcinoma, and thus, preoperative ERCP is not required unless there is evidence of distal biliary obstruction or cholangitis.

ERCP findings suggestive of a pancreatic head cancer include stricture of both bile and pancreatic ducts with an upstream dilation (i.e., double duct sign). Unresectable malignant diseases may need therapeutic endoscopy such as ERCP with biliary stenting. In geriatric patients with distal malignant biliary obstruction, a randomized control trial has shown that endoscopic stent placement has been associated with significantly reduced procedure-related mortality (3% vs. 14%) and fewer complication rates (11% vs. 29%) compared to surgery (Smith et al. 1994). ERCP with pancreatic duct brush cytology and biopsy may be required for evaluation of suspicious bile duct or pancreatic duct strictures or after nondiagnostic EUS-FNA. Although the specificity of brush cytology and biopsy approaches 100%, the sensitivity is only 15–50% for brush cytology and 33–50% for biopsy.

In recent years, a single operator cholangioscopy system (Spyglass, Boston Scientific) has become very popular and is widely used in the setting of indeterminate or complex biliary stricture disease. This procedure involves a cholangioscope being inserted through the therapeutic channel of a duodenoscope and advanced directly into the bile duct. Cholangioscopy provides information regarding location and extent of a biliary stricture. This may help to differentiate between an often-challenging dilemma of a malignant (such as cholangiocarcinoma) and benign biliary stenosis (such as primary sclerosing cholangitis, IgG4-related sclerosing cholangitis, or inflammatory strictures). Concurrent tissue sampling of the biliary strictures can be obtained by biliary brush cytology or cholangioscopy-guided intraductal biliary biopsy (Fig. 5b). Although biliary brushings are the most commonly performed tissue diagnostic technique, a combination of brush cytology and cholangioscopy-guided intraductal biopsy increases the sensitivity in diagnosing malignant biliary strictures compared to the diagnostic methods alone (Navaneethan et al. 2015). Recently, a second-generation digital Spyglass (Boston Scientific) has become available which provides a wider angle of view with significant improvement in the image quality. In addition, the diagnostic yield of ERCP can be improved by subjecting tissue samples to fluorescence in situ hybridization (FISH) and flow cytometry techniques. Probe-based confocal laser endomicroscopy (pCLE; Cellvizio, Mauna Kea Technologies) is another novel technology that enables real-time high-resolution histological analysis of the targeted tissue during ERCP and may raise the diagnostic yield of ERCP in the setting of a biliary stricture (Taunk et al. 2017). Unfortunately, FISH and pCLE are not widely available and require further validation for routine clinical practice.

Stent placement during the ERCP is a standard method of palliating biliary obstruction especially distal biliary strictures. Significantly lower complication rates (24% vs. 46%) have been reported when using fully covered self-expanding metal stents (FCSEMS) compared to plastic stents in patients with obstructive jaundice in the palliation of advanced pancreatic cancer (Tol et al. 2016). Additionally, a recent meta-analysis demonstrated the superiority of metal stents over plastic stents for distal as well as proximal malignant biliary obstruction (Sawas et al. 2015).

Dilated Pancreatic Duct

The average dimension of the pancreatic duct (PD) varies among patients and largely depends on the location within the pancreas. The main PD diameter is approximately 3–4 mm in the head, 2–3 mm in the body, and 1–2 mm in the tail. Pancreatic ductal dilatation refers to the ductal dimension when it exceeds the accepted upper limit of normal at each anatomic location. Nevertheless, age must be considered when interpreting pancreatic duct size. In a study consisting of 136 older subjects, 31 (22.8%) were noted to have definite pathology (Hastier et al. 1998). Comparing the remaining 105 older patients with the control group (patients younger than 50 years), the mean main PD diameter (in millimeters) was larger in the head (5.3 vs. 3.3), body (3.7 vs. 2.3), and tail (2.6 vs. 1.6) ($p < 0.05$). The PD diameter also increased significantly in each of the age cohorts (70–79, 80–89, and 90–99 years). Only 33 out of 105 (31.4%) of the older patients had duct diameters within defined normal limits. The majority (63.3%) of the older patients has global dilatation of the PD, but in a minority, it was confined to the head and/or body (Hastier et al. 1998).

Etiologies of pancreatic ductal dilatation can be broadly classified into those associated with benign versus malignant conditions. Certain benign conditions associated with PD dilatation include chronic pancreatitis (with and without pancreatic stones or strictures), papillary stenosis (secondary to inflammation or stones, chronic narcotics, HIV/AIDs, prior endoscopic intervention such as sphincterotomy and ampullectomy, embolization of periampullary or pancreatic head arteries), iatrogenic (e.g., stent-induced stricture, stricture of surgical anastomosis), pancreatic divisum, pancreatic necrosis disrupting of the

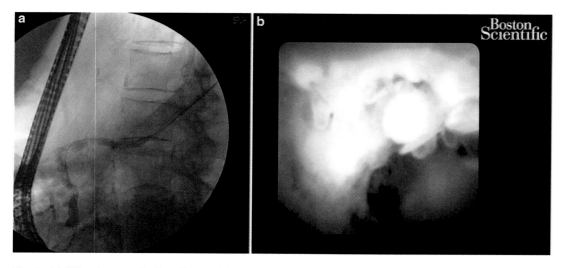

Fig. 6 (**a**) Dilated pancreatic duct diagnosed by cholangiogram. (**b**) Visualization of pancreatic duct through direct pancreatoscopy in the same patient

pancreatic duct, cystic fibrosis, age-related, and idiopathic. Alternatively, malignant lesions such as pancreatic adenocarcinoma, ampullary adenoma or carcinoma, intraductal pancreatic mucinous neoplasm (IPMN), and rarely metastatic disease to the pancreas may be associated with pancreatic ductal dilatation.

Non-invasive diagnostic studies such as pancreatic protocol CT scan and MRCP provides a significant amount of information in evaluating the pancreaticobiliary anatomy and has effectively replaced ERCP in the evaluation of pancreatic ductal dilatation. EUS provides further diagnostic information by assessment of the pancreatic parenchyma, identification of masses or strictures, and evaluation of adjacent vasculature and lymph nodes.

The role of ERCP solely as a diagnostic tool for evaluation of pancreatic ductal dilatation is limited especially when equally effective noninvasive or less invasive modalities are available. However, ERCP with sphincter of Oddi manometry is an exception, where ERCP can provide diagnostic value in assessing the underlying sphincter hypertension. Visualization of the pancreatic duct through direct pancreatoscopy is a relatively new field of endoscopy which can be used to differentiate the main duct from side

branch IPMN, define the extent of duct involvement, and provide tissue samples for histopathologic diagnosis (Fig. 6a, b).

Endoscopic therapies are aimed toward the relief of obstructive component and restoration of the normal flow of pancreatic juice to the duodenum. Such endoscopic therapies include pancreatic sphincterotomy (major or minor), pancreatic duct stricture dilatation, pancreatic duct stone removal (often with extracorporeal shock wave lithotripsy or ESWL), pancreatic stent placement, pseudocyst drainage, and endoscopic necrosectomy.

Summary

- Age alone should not be used as a contraindication for therapeutic ERCP in the older adults.
- Therapeutic success rates of ERCP in the older patients are comparable to the success rates in younger patients.
- Increasing age appears to be protective against post-ERCP pancreatitis, although patients with advanced age are more prone to cardiopulmonary and sedation-related complications.
- Biliary obstruction secondary to choledocholithiasis is the most frequent indication of

ERCP in the older patients. ERCP is indicated in patients who meet the high-risk criteria for having a choledocholithiasis, i.e., a CBD stone visualized in the US or cross-sectional imaging, cholangitis, a combination of total bilirubin level higher than 4 mg/dL and a dilated CBD (>6 mm) on US.

- In patients with gallstone pancreatitis, ERCP should be restricted to patients who present with biliary sepsis or obstructive jaundice.
- In patients with malignant obstruction, the principle objective is to provide both diagnostic and therapeutic solutions. A diagnostic procedure such as EUS with FNA or ERCP with brushings is often needed. Presently, EUS has largely replaced ERCP for the diagnosis of pancreatic head adenocarcinoma, and thus, preoperative ERCP is not required unless there is evidence of distal biliary obstruction or cholangitis. Stent placement during the ERCP is a standard method of palliating biliary obstruction.

References

Albores-Saavedra J, Schwartz AM, Batich K, et al. Cancers of the ampulla of Vater: demographics, morphology, and survival based on 5,625 cases from the SEER program. J Surg Oncol. 2009;100:598–605.

Ali M, Ward G, Staley D, et al. A retrospective study of the safety and efficacy of ERCP in octogenarians. Dig Dis Sci. 2011;56:586–90.

American Cancer Society. Cancer facts and figures. 2012. https://www.cancer.org/research/cancer-facts-statistics.html

Andriulli A, Loperfido S, Napolitano G, et al. Incidence rates of post-ERCP complications: a systematic survey of prospective studies. Am J Gastroenterol. 2007; 102:1781–8.

ASGE Standards of Practice Committee, Maple JT, Ben-Menachem T, et al. The role of endoscopy in the evaluation of suspected choledocholithiasis. Gastrointest Endosc. 2010;71:1–9.

ASGE Standards of Practice Committee, Chandrasekhara V, Early DS, et al. Modifications in endoscopic practice for the elderly. Gastrointest Endosc. 2013;78:1–7.

ASGE Standards of Practice Committee, Khashab MA, Chithadi KV, et al. Antibiotic prophylaxis for GI endoscopy. Gastrointest Endosc. 2015;81:81–9.

ASGE Standards of Practice Committee, Acosta RD, Abraham NS, et al. The management of antithrombotic agents for patients undergoing GI endoscopy. Gastrointest Endosc. 2016;83:3–16.

ASGE Standards of Practice Committee, Chandrasekhara V, Khashab MA, et al. Adverse events associated with ERCP. Gastrointest Endosc. 2017; 85:32–47.

ASGE Standards of Practice Committee, Buxbaum JL, Abbas Fehmi SM, et al. ASGE guideline on the role of endoscopy in the evaluation and management of choledocholithiasis. Gastrointest Endosc. 2019;89: 1075–105.e15.

Ashton CE, McNabb WR, Wilkinson ML, et al. Endoscopic retrograde cholangiopancreatography in elderly patients. Age Ageing. 1998;27:683–8.

Bachar GN, Cohen M, Belenky A, et al. Effect of aging on the adult extrahepatic bile duct: a sonographic study. J Ultrasound Med. 2003;22:879–82; quiz 883–5.

Baron TH, Fleischer DE. Past, present, and future of endoscopic retrograde cholangiopancreatography: perspectives on the National Institutes of Health consensus conference. Mayo Clin Proc. 2002;77:407–12.

Behlul B, Ayfer S, Sezgin V, et al. Safety of endoscopic retrograde cholangiopancreatography in patients 80 years of age and older. Prz Gastroenterol. 2014;9:227–31.

Bergquist A, von Seth E. Epidemiology of cholangiocarcinoma. Best Pract Res Clin Gastroenterol. 2015;29:221–32.

Boss GR, Seegmiller JE. Age-related physiological changes and their clinical significance. West J Med. 1981;135:434–40.

Cariani G, Di Marco M, Roda E, et al. Efficacy and safety of ERCP in patients 90 years of age and older. Gastrointest Endosc. 2006;64:471–2.

Chan FKL, Goh KL, Reddy N, et al. Management of patients on antithrombotic agents undergoing emergency and elective endoscopy: joint Asian Pacific Association of Gastroenterology (APAGE) and Asian Pacific Society for Digestive Endoscopy (APSDE) practice guidelines. Gut. 2018;67:405–17.

Chen YK, Pleskow DK. SpyGlass single-operator peroral cholangiopancreatoscopy system for the diagnosis and therapy of bile-duct disorders: a clinical feasibility study (with video). Gastrointest Endosc. 2007;65:832–41.

Chong VH, Yim HB, Lim CC. Endoscopic retrograde cholangiopancreatography in the elderly: outcomes, safety and complications. Singapore Med J. 2005;46: 621–6.

Clarke GA, Jacobson BC, Hammett RJ, et al. The indications, utilization and safety of gastrointestinal endoscopy in an extremely elderly patient cohort. Endoscopy. 2001;33:580–4.

Cohen LB, Hightower CD, Wood DA, et al. Moderate level sedation during endoscopy: a prospective study using low-dose propofol, meperidine/fentanyl, and midazolam. Gastrointest Endosc. 2004;59:795–803.

Cotton PB, Blumgart LH, Davies GT, et al. Cannulation of papilla of Vater via fiber-duodenoscope. Assessment of retrograde cholangiopancreatography in 60 patients. Lancet. 1972;1:53–8.

Daradkeh S, Tarawneh E, Al-Hadidy A. Factors affecting common bile duct diameter. Hepatogastroenterology. 2005;52:1659–61.

Day LW, Lin L, Somsouk M. Adverse events in older patients undergoing ERCP: a systematic review and meta-analysis. Endosc Int Open. 2014;2:E28–36.

DiSario JA. Endoscopic balloon dilation of the sphincter of Oddi for stone extraction in the elderly: is the juice worth the squeeze? Gastrointest Endosc. 2008;68:483–6.

Dollhopf M, Larghi A, Will U, et al. EUS-guided gallbladder drainage in patients with acute cholecystitis and high surgical risk using an electrocautery-enhanced lumen-apposing metal stent device. Gastrointest Endosc. 2017;86:636–43.

Dong SQ, Singh TP, Zhao Q, et al. Sphincterotomy plus balloon dilation versus sphincterotomy alone for choledocholithiasis: a meta-analysis. Endoscopy. 2019;51:763.

Enns R, Eloubeidi MA, Mergener K, et al. ERCP-related perforations: risk factors and management. Endoscopy. 2002;34:293–8.

Fisher L, Fisher A, Thomson A. Cardiopulmonary complications of ERCP in older patients. Gastrointest Endosc. 2006;63:948–55.

Fleisher LA, Beckman JA, Brown KA, et al. ACCF/AHA focused update on perioperative beta blockade incorporated into the ACC/AHA 2007 guidelines on perioperative cardiovascular evaluation and care for noncardiac surgery: a report of the American College of Cardiology Foundation/American Heart Association task force on practice guidelines. Circulation. 2009; 120:e169–276.

Freeman ML. Adverse outcomes of ERCP. Gastrointest Endosc. 2002a;56:S273–82.

Freeman ML. Adverse outcomes of endoscopic retrograde cholangiopancreatography. Rev Gastroenterol Disord. 2002b;2:147–68.

Freeman ML, Nelson DB, Sherman S, et al. Complications of endoscopic biliary sphincterotomy. N Engl J Med. 1996;335:909–18.

Fritz E, Kirchgatterer A, Hubner D, et al. ERCP is safe and effective in patients 80 years of age and older compared with younger patients. Gastrointest Endosc. 2006;64: 899–905.

Garewal D, Powell S, Milan SJ, et al. Sedative techniques for endoscopic retrograde cholangiopancreatography. Cochrane Database Syst Rev. 2012; CD007274.

Giampieri M. Communication and informed consent in elderly people. Minerva Anestesiol. 2012;78:236–42.

Glenn F, Hays DM. The age factor in the mortality rate of patients undergoing surgery of the biliary tract. Surg Gynecol Obstet. 1955;100:11–8.

Go AS, Hylek EM, Phillips KA, et al. Prevalence of diagnosed atrial fibrillation in adults: national implications for rhythm management and stroke prevention: the AnTicoagulation and Risk Factors in Atrial Fibrillation (ATRIA) Study. JAMA. 2001;285:2370–5.

Goodman MT, Yamamoto J. Descriptive study of gallbladder, extrahepatic bile duct, and ampullary cancers in the United States, 1997–2002. Cancer Causes Control. 2007;18:415–22.

Harness JK, Strodel WE, Talsma SE. Symptomatic biliary tract disease in the elderly patient. Am Surg. 1986; 52:442–5.

Hastier P, Buckley MJ, Dumas R, et al. A study of the effect of age on pancreatic duct morphology. Gastrointest Endosc. 1998;48:53–7.

Hayee B, Dunn J, Loganayagam A, et al. Midazolam with meperidine or fentanyl for colonoscopy: results of a randomized trial. Gastrointest Endosc. 2009;69:681–7.

Hosking MP, Warner MA, Lobdell CM, et al. Outcomes of surgery in patients 90 years of age and older. JAMA. 1989;261:1909–15.

Hui CK, Liu CL, Lai KC, et al. Outcome of emergency ERCP for acute cholangitis in patients 90 years of age and older. Aliment Pharmacol Ther. 2004;19:1153–8.

Ito Y, Tsujino T, Togawa O, et al. Endoscopic papillary balloon dilation for the management of bile duct stones in patients 85 years of age and older. Gastrointest Endosc. 2008;68:477–82.

Jee SL, Jarmin R, Lim KF, et al. Outcomes of early versus delayed cholecystectomy in patients with mild to moderate acute biliary pancreatitis: a randomized prospective study. Asian J Surg. 2018;41:47–54.

Karsenti D, Coron E, Vanbiervliet G, et al. Complete endoscopic sphincterotomy with vs. without large-balloon dilation for the removal of large bile duct stones: randomized multicenter study. Endoscopy. 2017;49:968–76.

Katsinelos P, Paroutoglou G, Kountouras J, et al. Efficacy and safety of therapeutic ERCP in patients 90 years of age and older. Gastrointest Endosc. 2006;63:417–23.

Katsinelos P, Paroutoglou G, Chatzimavroudis G, et al. Endoscopic sphincterotomy for acute relapsing pancreatitis associated with periampullary diverticula: a long-term follow-up. Acta Gastroenterol Belg. 2007;70:195–8.

Katsinelos P, Kountouras J, Chatzimavroudis G, et al. Outpatient therapeutic endoscopic retrograde cholangiopancreatography is safe in patients aged 80 years and older. Endoscopy. 2011;43:128–33.

Kawai K, Akasaka Y, Murakami K, et al. Endoscopic sphincterotomy of the ampulla of Vater. Gastrointest Endosc. 1974;20:148–51.

Koklu S, Parlak E, Yuksel O, et al. Endoscopic retrograde cholangiopancreatography in the elderly: a prospective and comparative study. Age Ageing. 2005;34:572–7.

Koziel D, Gluszek-Osuch M, Suliga E, et al. Elderly persons with acute pancreatitis – specifics of the clinical course of the disease. Clin Interv Aging. 2019;14:33–41.

Laasch HU, Martin DF. Management of benign biliary strictures. Cardiovasc Intervent Radiol. 2002;25: 457–66.

Lukens FJ, Howell DA, Upender S, et al. ERCP in the very elderly: outcomes among patients older than eighty. Dig Dis Sci. 2010;55:847–51.

Luo H, Zhao L, Leung J, et al. Routine pre-procedural rectal indometacin versus selective post-procedural rectal indometacin to prevent pancreatitis in patients undergoing endoscopic retrograde cholangiopancreatography: a multicentre, single-blinded, randomised controlled trial. Lancet. 2016;387:2293–301.

MacMahon M, Walsh TN, Brennan P, et al. Endoscopic retrograde cholangiopancreatography in the elderly: a single unit audit. Gerontology. 1993;39:28–32.

Maitin-Casalis N, Neeman T, Thomson A. Protective effect of advanced age on post-ERCP pancreatitis and unplanned hospitalisation. Intern Med J. 2015;45:1020–5.

Margiotta SJ Jr, Willis IH, Wallack MK. Cholecystectomy in the elderly. Am Surg. 1988;54:34–9.

Masci E, Toti G, Mariani A, et al. Complications of diagnostic and therapeutic ERCP: a prospective multicenter study. Am J Gastroenterol. 2001;96:417–23.

McCune WS, Shorb PE, Moscovitz H. Endoscopic cannulation of the ampulla of Vater: a preliminary report. Ann Surg. 1968;167:752–6.

Mitchell RM, O'Connor F, Dickey W. Endoscopic retrograde cholangiopancreatography is safe and effective in patients 90 years of age and older. J Clin Gastroenterol. 2003;36:72–4.

Moon JH, Ko BM, Choi HJ, et al. Direct peroral cholangioscopy using an ultra-slim upper endoscope for the treatment of retained bile duct stones. Am J Gastroenterol. 2009;104:2729–33.

Muravchick S. The elderly outpatient: current anesthetic implications. Curr Opin Anaesthesiol. 2002;15:621–5.

Naess IA, Christiansen SC, Romundstad P, et al. Incidence and mortality of venous thrombosis: a population-based study. J Thromb Haemost. 2007;5:692–9.

Nassar Y, Richter S. Management of complicated gallstones in the elderly: comparing surgical and non-surgical treatment options. Gastroenterol Rep (Oxf). 2019;7:205–11.

Navaneethan U, Njei B, Lourdusamy V, et al. Comparative effectiveness of biliary brush cytology and intraductal biopsy for detection of malignant biliary strictures: a systematic review and meta-analysis. Gastrointest Endosc. 2015;81:168–76.

Nojkov B, Cappell MS. Safety and efficacy of ERCP after recent myocardial infarction or unstable angina. Gastrointest Endosc. 2010;72:870–80.

O'Connell JB, Maggard MA, Manunga J Jr, et al. Survival after resection of ampullary carcinoma: a national population-based study. Ann Surg Oncol. 2008;15:1820–7.

Oi I. Fiberduodenoscopy and endoscopic pancreato-cholangiography. Gastrointest Endosc. 1970;17:59–62.

Parekh PJ, Buerlein RC, Shams R, et al. An update on the management of implanted cardiac devices during electrosurgical procedures. Gastrointest Endosc. 2013;78:836–41.

Patai A, Solymosi N, Mohacsi L, et al. Indomethacin and diclofenac in the prevention of post-ERCP pancreatitis: a systematic review and meta-analysis of prospective controlled trials. Gastrointest Endosc. 2017;85:1144–56.e1.

Patel K, Li F, Luthra A, et al. Acute biliary pancreatitis is associated with adverse outcomes in the elderly: a propensity score-matched analysis. J Clin Gastroenterol. 2019;53:e291–7.

Petersen BT, Hussain N, Marine JE, et al. Endoscopy in patients with implanted electronic devices. Gastrointest Endosc. 2007;65:561–8.

Platt TE, Smith K, Sinha S, et al. Laparoscopic common bile duct exploration; a preferential pathway for elderly patients. Ann Med Surg (Lond). 2018;30:13–7.

Rahib L, Smith BD, Aizenberg R, et al. Projecting cancer incidence and deaths to 2030: the unexpected burden of thyroid, liver, and pancreas cancers in the United States. Cancer Res. 2014;74:2913–21.

Riphaus A, Stergiou N, Wehrmann T. Sedation with propofol for routine ERCP in high-risk octogenarians: a randomized, controlled study. Am J Gastroenterol. 2005;100:1957–63.

Riphaus A, Stergiou N, Wehrmann T. ERCP in octogenerians: a safe and efficient investigation. Age Ageing. 2008;37:595–9.

Rodriguez-Gonzalez FJ, Naranjo-Rodriguez A, Mata-Tapia I, et al. ERCP in patients 90 years of age and older. Gastrointest Endosc. 2003;58:220–5.

Saluja SS, Sharma R, Pal S, et al. Differentiation between benign and malignant hilar obstructions using laboratory and radiological investigations: a prospective study. HPB (Oxford). 2007;9:373–82.

Sawas T, Al Halabi S, Parsi MA, et al. Self-expandable metal stents versus plastic stents for malignant biliary obstruction: a meta-analysis. Gastrointest Endosc. 2015;82:256–67.e7.

Sethi S, Sethi N, Wadhwa V, et al. A meta-analysis on the role of rectal diclofenac and indomethacin in the prevention of post-endoscopic retrograde cholangiopancreatography pancreatitis. Pancreas. 2014;43:190–7.

Siegel JH, Kasmin FE, Cohen SA. Endoscopic retrograde cholangiopancreatography treatment of cholecystitis: possible? Yes; practical?? Diagn Ther Endosc. 1994;1:51–6.

Smith AC, Dowsett JF, Russell RC, et al. Randomised trial of endoscopic stenting versus surgical bypass in malignant low bile duct obstruction. Lancet. 1994;344:1655–60.

Sugiyama M, Atomi Y. Endoscopic sphincterotomy for bile duct stones in patients 90 years of age and older. Gastrointest Endosc. 2000;52:187–91.

Taunk P, Singh S, Lichtenstein D, et al. Improved classification of indeterminate biliary strictures by probe-based confocal laser endomicroscopy using the Paris criteria following biliary stenting. J Gastroenterol Hepatol. 2017;32:1778–83.

Thomopoulos KC, Vagenas K, Assimakopoulos SF, et al. Endoscopic retrograde cholangiopancreatography is safe and effective method for diagnosis and treatment of biliary and pancreatic disorders in octogenarians. Acta Gastroenterol Belg. 2007;70:199–202.

Tol JA, van Hooft JE, Timmer R, et al. Metal or plastic stents for preoperative biliary drainage in resectable pancreatic cancer. Gut. 2016;65:1981–7.

Trust MD, Sheffield KM, Boyd CA, et al. Gallstone pancreatitis in older patients: are we operating enough? Surgery. 2011;150:515–25.

Veitch AM, Vanbiervliet G, Gershlick AH, et al. Endoscopy in patients on antiplatelet or anticoagulant therapy, including direct oral anticoagulants: British Society of Gastroenterology (BSG) and European Society of Gastrointestinal Endoscopy (ESGE) guidelines. Gut. 2016;65:374–89.

Wallner BK, Schumacher KA, Weidenmaier W, et al. Dilated biliary tract: evaluation with MR cholangiography with a T2-weighted contrast-enhanced fast sequence. Radiology. 1991;181:805–8.

Wan J, Ren Y, Zhu Z, et al. How to select patients and timing for rectal indomethacin to prevent post-ERCP pancreatitis: a systematic review and meta-analysis. BMC Gastroenterol. 2017;17:43.

Yang XM, Hu B. Endoscopic sphincterotomy plus large-balloon dilation vs endoscopic sphincterotomy for choledocholithiasis: a meta-analysis. World J Gastroenterol. 2013;19:9453–60.

Yang C, Zhao Y, Li W, et al. Rectal nonsteroidal anti-inflammatory drugs administration is effective for the prevention of post-ERCP pancreatitis: an updated meta-analysis of randomized controlled trials. Pancreatology. 2017;17:681–8.

Yasui T, Takahata S, Kono H, et al. Is cholecystectomy necessary after endoscopic treatment of bile duct stones in patients older than 80 years of age? J Gastroenterol. 2012;47:65–70.

Yun DY, Han J, Oh JS, et al. Is endoscopic retrograde cholangiopancreatography safe in patients 90 years of age and older? Gut Liver. 2014;8:552–6.

Wireless Capsule Endoscopy

41

Anwar Dudekula and C. S. Pitchumoni

Contents

A. Dudekula
Division of Gastroenterology and Hepatology, Department
of Internal Medicine, Saint Peter's University Hospital/
Rutgers-RWJ Medical School, New Brunswick, NJ, USA
e-mail: meetanwar@gmail.com

C. S. Pitchumoni (✉)
Department of Medicine, Robert Wood Johnson School of
Medicine, Rutgers University, New Brunswick, NJ, USA

Department of Medicine, New York Medical College,
Valhalla, NY, USA

Division of Gastroenterology, Hepatology and Clinical
Nutrition, Saint Peters University Hospital, New
Brunswick, NJ, USA
e-mail: pitchumoni@hotmail.com

© Springer Nature Switzerland AG 2021
C. S. Pitchumoni, T. S. Dharmarajan (eds.), *Geriatric Gastroenterology*,
https://doi.org/10.1007/978-3-030-30192-7_35

Abstract

The small intestine except for the duodenum and terminal ileum was always considered a black box for routine endoscopic examination until the discovery of wireless capsule endoscopy (WCE), also known as wireless video endoscopy (WVE) or video capsule endoscopy (VCE). In the last two decades, WCE has been established as a valuable test for routine imaging of the small intestine in all age groups. It is a safe and relatively comfortable procedure to perform that can provide useful information in the diagnosis of small bowel conditions. In the older adult, WCE is valuable in diagnosing lesions of active small intestinal bleeding as well as chronic low-grade bleeding lesions causing chronic iron deficiency anemia. The rare complication of the procedure is retained capsule but is not related to an older age. Pill colonoscopy is under study but is a procedure with a great promise in the older adult.

Keywords

Wireless capsule endoscopy · Indications for wireless capsule endoscopy · NSAID ulcers · Arteriovenous malformations · Iron deficiency anemia · Crohn's disease · Drug-induced enteropathy · Olmesartan · NSAIDs · Small bowel tumors · Lymphoma · Celiac disease · Indeterminate colitis · Familial adenomatosis polyposis · Peutz-Jeghers syndrome · Retained capsule

Abbreviations

AV	Arteriovenous malformation
CAP	Chronic abdominal pain
CD	Crohn's disease
CECDAI	Capsule Endoscopy Crohn's Disease Activity Index
CeD	Celiac disease
CTE	Computed tomography enterography
DBE	Double-balloon enteroscopy
EGD	Esophagogastroduodenoscopy
GIB	Gastrointestinal bleeding
IC	Indeterminate colitis
IDA	Iron deficiency anemia
MRE	Magnetic resonance enterography
OGIB	Obscure gastrointestinal bleeding
PCCE	PillCam colon capsule endoscopy
PCCE	PillCam colon capsule endoscopy
PE	Push enteroscopy
RCT	Randomized controlled trial
SB	Small bowel
SBB	Small bowel bleeding
SBE	Single-balloon enteroscopy
SE	Spiral enteroscopy
WCE	Wireless video capsule endoscopy

Introduction

Since wireless capsule endoscopy (WCE) was introduced in the year 2000 by Paul Swan, much experience has accumulated (Moglia et al. 2009; Moglia and Cuschieri 2009; Eliakim 2010; Mark Feldman and Brandt 2016; Tee and Kaffes 2010). The first capsule manufactured by as PillCam® SB (Given Imaging, Yokneam, Israel) was an 11×26 mm capsule-shaped camera powered by two batteries to allow a total transit time of 7–8 h, sufficient often to reach the cecum having imaged the entire small bowel (SB). Improved technology has further extended battery life to provide increased imaging time (11 h for the MiroCam™ (IntroMedic (Seoul,

Korea)) (Moglia et al. 2009). Once removed from its magnetic holder, the disposable capsule is activated; it contains four light-emitting diodes (MiroCam™ and EndoCapsule™ each with six light-emitting diodes) to illuminate the bowel lumen, an antenna, and two metal oxide semiconductor cameras to transmit the images to an external device for analysis and storage. A radio frequency band signal captures the images by the capsule. The images are transmitted to a recording unit worn by the patient around the waist. Following the examination, the recording unit is connected to a computer to review the images (Moglia and Cuschieri 2009).

Role for Wireless Capsule Endoscopy

Traditional procedures, esophagogastroduodenoscopy (EGD), and colonoscopy, available to us for more than five decades, do not permit a complete evaluation of SB which was hence considered the "black box" of the GI tract. Therefore, many lesions of the SB could not be visualized and promptly treated. The advent of WCE is a major advancement that has filled the void and permits complete noninvasive evaluation of SB. The clinical conditions that escaped diagnosis included bleeding lesions of the SB (causative factors for acute and chronic anemia), neoplastic diseases of the SB, and inflammatory disorders of SB. Before the advent of WCE, the options available to evaluate the SB were barium studies, which were not helpful in the diagnosis of acute bleeding lesions and lacked sensitivity in evaluating SB tumors, ulcerations, and AV malformations. Other options available were invasive procedures such as angiography and single and double enteroscopy, which are expensive and time-consuming. These procedures lacked sensitivity and required prolonged intravenous sedation not well tolerated by older adults. WCE is painless and noninvasive, has an excellent capacity to visualize the entire SB mucosa, and identifies acute and chronic bleeding lesions with practically no complications. WCE has shed new light on our knowledge of small bowel disorders (Eliakim 2010) (Table 1).

Table 1 Indications for Wireless Capsule Endoscopy

Indications (Akin et al. 2012; Cellier et al. 2005; Cobrin et al. 2006; Culliford et al. 2005; Gastineau et al. 2012; Haanstra et al. 2015; Petroniene et al. 2005; Committee et al. 2013)
1. Small bowel bleeding (occult and overt)
2. Iron deficiency anemia
3. Rebleeding in patients with known small bowel AVM
4. Diagnosis of suspected Crohn's disease (CD)
5. To assess the extent, disease activity and mucosal healing in a patient with known CD
6. Evaluation for small bowel CD recurrence after surgical treatment
7. Diagnosis of small bowel tumors
8. Diagnosis of celiac disease
9. Evaluate any abnormal small bowel imaging
Relative indications (Akin et al. 2012; Cellier et al. 2005; Cobrin et al. 2006; Culliford et al. 2005; Gastineau et al. 2012; Haanstra et al. 2015; Petroniene et al. 2005)
1. Assess mucosal healing in CD
2. Assess bowel injury with NSAID usage
3. Evaluate abdominal pain of unclear etiology
4. Evaluation of indeterminate colitis
5. Screen for polyps in patients with familial polyposis syndromes such as Peutz-Jeghers syndrome, familial adenomatous polyposis
6. Assess for small bowel tumors in Lynch syndrome
7. Assess GI complications (acute cellular rejection, gastrointestinal dysfunction, etc.) after a small bowel transplant

Currently, at least five companies manufacture WCE for visualization of the esophagus and colon (Table 2). Also, a WCE, specifically designed for use in CD patients with SB involvement, is available.

WCE in Specific Diseases

Small Bowel Bleeding: Overt and Occult

Gastrointestinal bleeding (GIB) is a common and perplexing problem encountered by gastroenterologists. The entity of obscure gastrointestinal bleeding (OGIB) is by definition GIB of unclear etiology after a negative EGD and colonoscopy. It is estimated that upper GIB, lower GIB, and obscure GIB account for 50%, 40%, and 10%, respectively,

Table 2 Specifications of currently available WCE systems. (**Adapted from** (Hosoe et al. 2019))

WCE	Manufacturer	Size (mm)		Weight (g)	Battery life (h)	Field of view (degree)	Communication
		Length	Diameter				
PillCam SB3	Medtronic	26.2	11.4	3	$\geq$11	156	Radiofrequency communication
EndoCapsule 10	Olympus	26	11	3.3	12	160	Radiofrequency communication
MiroCam	IntroMedic	24.5	10.8	3.25–4.7	12	170	Radiofrequency communication
OMOM Capsule2	Jinshan	25.4	11	4.5	$\geq$10	165	Radiofrequency communication
CapsoCam SV-1	CapsoVision	31	11	3.8	15	360	No communication (stored inside the capsule)

of the total GIB cases (Mark Feldman and Brandt 2016). With the use of WCE, balloon enteroscopy, and spiral enteroscopy, the cause of bleeding can be detected in the majority of these patients to originate from the SB (bleeding from the ampulla of Vater to the ileocecal valve – terminal ileum) (Tee and Kaffes 2010; Pennazio et al. 1995; Chong et al. 1994). Small bowel bleeding (SBB) is classified as "overt" when there is a clinical manifestation of GIB such as hematochezia or melena and "occult" when there is a positive fecal occult blood test with or without iron deficiency anemia (IDA) (Raju et al. 2007a, b; Gerson et al. 2015) (Fig. 1).

SBB, in the older adult, is most commonly from ulcers due to NSAID use, vascular ectasia, followed by tumors of the SB, and of uncertain origin (Lewis and Swain 2002; Ell et al. 2002; Mylonaki et al. 2003; Adler et al. 2004). Establishing a diagnosis for SBB can be difficult and incurs cost and time; extensive testing including SB radiology, EGD, push enteroscopy (PE) (to visualize SB mucosa 50–100 cm distal to the ligament of Treitz), balloon-assisted enteroscopy, and colonoscopy often fails to demonstrate the bleeding source (Saperas et al. 2007; Leung and Graham 2010; Friedman 2004; Triester et al. 2005). In a study of 911 patients with suspected SBB (Lepileur et al. 2012), WCE identified the lesion (thought to be responsible for the bleeding) in 56% of patients. In this study, the etiology was felt to be as follows: SB AVM (22%), SB ulceration (10%), SB tumors (7%),

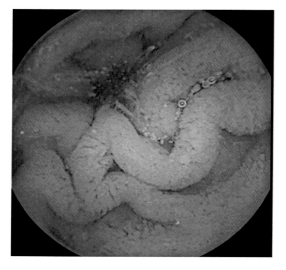

Fig. 1 Normal duodenum

varices (3%), esophagogastric lesions (11%), and colonic AVM (2%) (Mata et al. 2004) (Fig. 2 and Table 3).

The etiology of SBB is in part dependent on age (Table 4). Patients (>40 years of age or more) are likely to have NSAID-induced ulcers, AVM, Dieulafoy's lesions, or SB neoplasms compared to younger patients (<40 years of age) (Gerson et al. 2015). Currently, the most common indication for WCE is suspected SBB in a hemodynamically stable patient after an adequate and unrevealing EGD (or PE)/colonoscopy and after the extra-gastrointestinal source of bleeding has been ruled out (Gerson et al. 2015; Liao et al. 2010). In hemodynamically unstable patients, WCE is not the preferred option, WCE will unnecessarily delay the diagnosis, and angiography is the test of choice (Fig. 3).

WCE is more effective than PE in detecting a cause of SBB (Triester et al. 2005; Lewis and Swain 2002; Ell et al. 2002; Mylonaki et al. 2003; Adler et al. 2004; Mata et al. 2004). The yield by WCE is higher for any SB findings (63%) compared to PE (26%) and barium studies (8%) (Triester et al. 2005), a procedure that has become nearly obsolete. The yield ranges from 30 to 70 percent depending on the definition of a

positive finding (due to varied diagnostic accuracy for various causes of SBB) and type of the bleeding investigated (Triester et al. 2005; Lepileur et al. 2012; Liao et al. 2010; Lewis and Swain 2002; Ell et al. 2002; Scapa et al. 2002; Hartmann et al. 2005; Koulaouzidis et al. 2012a, b; Laine et al. 2010; Park et al. 2010; Pennazio et al. 2004). In a randomized controlled trial (RCT), WCE first, before PE, was felt to be a more effective strategy than vice versa (de Leusse et al. 2007). In one study, patients with SBB were randomized to WCE first versus PE first, followed by WCE or PE, respectively, if the initial study was negative. WCE first strategy had significantly higher diagnostic yield compared to PE first (50% vs. 24%; p < 0.05) and also reduced the percentage of patients requiring PE (25% vs. 79%; p < 0.05) (de Leusse et al. 2007) (Fig. 4).

Technological advances in the endoscopy field led to the introduction of double-balloon enteroscopy (DBE; Fujifilm Corp., Tokyo, Japan) in 2004, single-balloon enteroscopy (SBE; Olympus Medical Systems, Tokyo, Japan) in 2007, and spiral enteroscopy (SE; Spirus Medical, LLC, West Bridge, MA) in 2007. These devices enable extensive evaluation of SB (Wadhwa et al. 2015). Although there are no prospective randomized controlled trials (RCT) comparing WCE and DBE, a meta-analysis showed a similar diagnostic yield (61.7 vs. 55.5%; p = 0.16)(Teshima et al. 2011). Another study demonstrated a higher diagnostic yield with SBE compared to WCE (73.6 vs. 47.5%; p < 0.01) (Ooka et al. 2016). But the

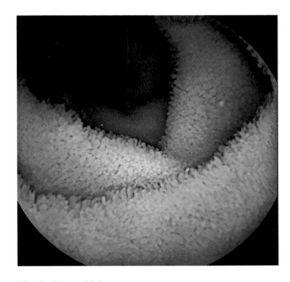

Fig. 2 Normal jejunum

Table 3 Contraindications by manufacturer. (**Adapted from** (Bandorski et al. 2016))

	PillCam SB3	EndoCapsule 10	MiroCam	CapsoCam SV-1	OMOM Capsule2
Manufacturer	Medtronic	Olympus	IntroMedic	CapsoVision	Jinshan
Known or suspected GI obstruction, fistula, or small bowel diverticulosis	x	x	x	x	x
Motility disorder (slow gastric emptying)		x	x	x	
Swallowing disorder (dysphagia)	x	x	x	x	x
Cardiac pacemaker and other implanted electromedical devices		x	x	x	
Strong electromagnetic fields		x	x	x	
Inability to endure capsule retrieval surgery		x			x
Inability to communicate sufficiently			x		
Concomitant heart disease or epilepsy			x		

Table 4 Causes of small bowel bleeding

Common causes		Rare causes (in all age groups)
Under age 40 years	*Over age 40 years*	
Inflammatory bowel disease	NSAID ulcers	Small bowel varices and/or portal hypertensive enteropathy
Meckel diverticulum	Angioectasia	Amyloidosis
Dieulafoy's lesions	Dieulafoy's lesions	Blue rubber bleb nevus syndrome
Neoplasia	Neoplasia	Pseudoxanthoma elasticum
Polyposis syndromes	IBD	Hereditary hemorrhagic telangiectasia (Osler-Weber-Rendu syndrome)
		Kaposi sarcoma with AIDS
		Plummer-Vinson syndrome
		Ehlers-Danlos syndrome
		Inherited polyposis syndromes (FAP, Peutz-Jeghers)
		Malignant atrophic papulosis
		Hematobilia
		Aortoenteric fistula
		Hemosuccus entericus
		Henoch-Schonlein purpura

Adapted from ACG Clinical Guideline: Diagnosis and Management of Small Bowel Bleeding. Am J Gastroenterol 2015; 110:1265

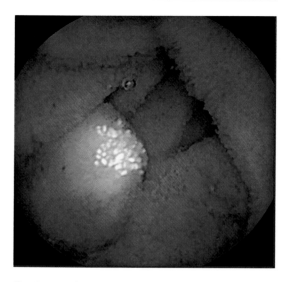

Fig. 3 Lymphangiectasia

results of this study should be interpreted critically as WCE was performed before SBE in 28.5% of the SBE group and as WCE before balloon enteroscopy is known to increase its diagnostic and therapeutic yield (Teshima et al. 2011; Fry et al. 2009). Also, the percentage of patients with overt bleeding was high in SBE followed by the WCE group (80.8 vs. 58.4%). The authors feel that WCE is not competing with and balloon enteroscopy but rather complementary to each other. WCE can guide the direction of the insertion of balloon enteroscopy and increase the yield and accuracy. In a prospective study, DBE only after a positive WCE result for SBB, the diagnostic yield was 75% (Kaffes et al. 2007; Li et al. 2009). In this

study, they adopted an anal approach to DBE if the capsule transit time from the pylorus to the lesion was >60% of the total transit time (from the pylorus to the ileocecal valve) and the accuracy of selecting the correct insertion route was 100%. Based on the ACG guidelines, WCE is the first-line procedure for patients with suspected SBB (who are hemodynamically stable), and balloon enteroscopy should be attempted if SB lesion is strongly suspected based on the clinical presentation and WCE findings (Gerson et al. 2015) (Fig. 5).

Factors associated with increased yield are advancing age, male sex, increasing transfusion requirement, inpatient status, and presence of connective tissue disorder (Lepileur et al. 2012; Robinson et al. 2011; Shahidi et al. 2012). Patients with overt SBB yield positive WCE results (Pennazio et al. 2004; Ge et al. 2007). Chronic bleeding, ongoing anticoagulation therapy, liver comorbidities, severe anemia, and performing the study within 1–2 weeks from the prior bleeding episode increase the diagnostic yield of WCE (Bresci et al. 2005; Esaki et al. 2010; Estevez et al. 2006; May et al. 2005; Parikh et al. 2011; Sidhu et al. 2009). In SBB, the diagnostic yield of WCE is highest when performed as close as possible to the bleeding episode, followed by yield in patients with overt GIB and lowest in occult GIB (Lepileur et al. 2012; Pennazio et al. 2004; Singh

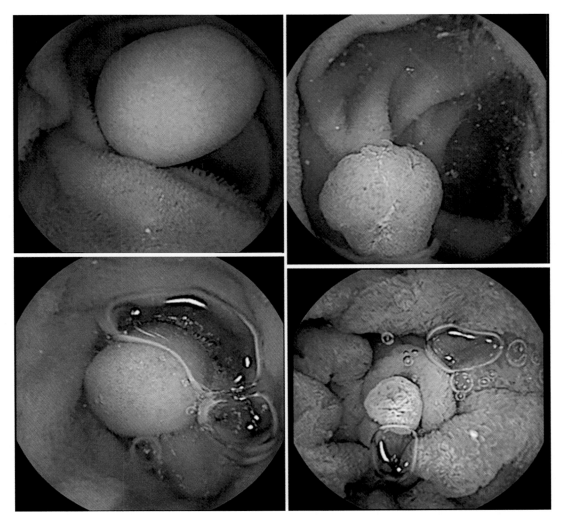

Fig. 4 SI polyp. A 72-year-old man presented with diffuse abdominal pain and chronic diarrhea. CT scan of the abdomen and colonoscopy performed 5 months ago were negative. WCE demonstrates incidental small bowel polyp

et al. 2013; Schlag et al. 2015). Sing and associates (Singh et al. 2013) demonstrated increased detection of active GIB, rate of therapeutic intervention, and decreased length of stay when WCE is performed earlier (<72 h vs. >72 h) (Singh et al. 2013) (Fig. 6).

Multiple studies have reported a favorable impact of WCE in patients with SBB. For example, Pennazio and associates reported the resolution of bleeding in 87% of patients after treatment based on the findings of the WCE (Pennazio et al. 2004). Other studies have confirmed Pennazio's observation (Estevez et al. 2006; Hindryckx et al. 2008; Katsinelos et al. 2011). Although favorable

outcomes (absence of rebleeding) were reported in the short term, the data on long-term outcomes are not clear. In an Italian study, a positive WCE study had a greater rebleeding rate than a negative study (45.1 vs. 16.4%; p < 0.001). However, in some Korean studies, cumulative rebleeding rates were similar regardless of the WCE findings (Park et al. 2010; Koh et al. 2013; Min et al. 2014). These differences in the long-term outcomes are explained based upon the WCE findings from Western and Eastern countries (Carey et al. 2007; Lai et al. 2006); ulcer/erosion and AVM were the most common in Korean and Western studies, respectively (Carey et al. 2007; Lai et al.

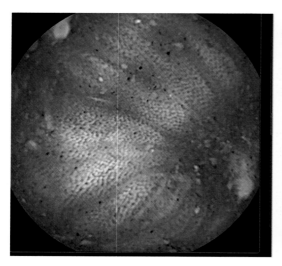

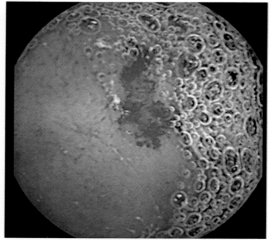

Fig. 5 Melanosis coli. A 73-year-old woman with chronic constipation on anthracene laxatives, underwent WCE, which reveals dark colored mucosa due to melanosis coli (proximal colon is occasionally visible on WCE)

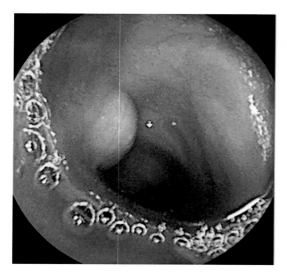

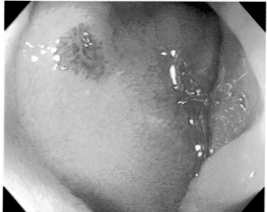

Fig. 7 AVM. An 80-year-old man presented with severe anemia. An EGD and colonoscopy were negative. WCE demonstrated AVM in jejunum

Drug-Induced Enteropathy

Enteropathy is caused by various medications such as Olmesartan, immunosuppressive drugs (Imuran and CellCept), antibiotics (Neomycin), anti-inflammatory conditions (CD, collagenous sprue, tropical sprue, radiation enteritis, eosinophilic gastroenteritis), infections (small intestinal bacterial overgrowth, giardiasis), and HIV enteropathy. NSAIDs are extensively used as anti-inflammatory analgesics, and 90% of the prescriptions are in patients over 65 years old (Tai and McAlindon 2018). There is a 40% increase in the over-the-counter NSAID use from 2005 to 2010 (Zhou et al. 2014). NSAID-related enteropathy is

Fig. 6 SI lipoma. A 64-year-old male underwent WCE for IDA, and it showed a subepithelial lesion compatible with lipoma

2006; Xin et al. 2011). AVM, due to its multifocal nature, has a higher rebleeding rate than ulcer (Min et al. 2014). The findings of WCE do not directly influence the long-term outcomes, but it plays an important role in selecting patients for additional interventions (Fig. 7).

on the rise and accounts for 1–2% of serious gastrointestinal outcomes (ulceration, perforation, bleeding) (Maiden et al. 2005). NSAID-related upper gastrointestinal events such as gastroduodenal ulcer bleeding and perforation can be prevented with concomitant PPI usage, especially in patients with a high risk of upper gastrointestinal events ($\geq$65 years, history of peptic ulcer disease, use of bisphosphonates, SSRIs, corticosteroids, anticoagulants) (Tai and McAlindon 2018; Lanas et al. 2009). NSAID-related SB injury is distinct from gastroduodenal disease, partially because gastric acid does not play a role in its pathogenesis (Hunt et al. 2009). Non-oral NSAIDs can also cause enteropathy due to enterohepatic circulation/re-exposure of toxic NSAID glucuronides. The pathogenesis is felt to be multifactorial: mucosal inflammation, increased permeability (due to cellular gut barrier function), and changes in the intestinal microbiome (Petruzzelli et al. 2007; Tanaka et al. 2002; Takeuchi 2014). NSAIDs increase gastrointestinal permeability 12 h following administration; inflammatory changes of the SB are visible through WCE within 10 days of ingesting NSAIDs (Maiden et al. 2005). WCE reveals mucosal injuries such as mucosal erythema, breaks, subepithelial hemorrhages, erosions, and ulcerations. Serious complications of NSAID use include diaphragm-like strictures (diaphragm disease, Fig. 8) and small bowel perforations (Maiden et al. 2005). IDA is the most common presentation of NSAID-induced enteropathy, which is often painless due to the analgesic property of the medication.

Small Bowel Tumors

Although the small intestine is the longest part of the gastrointestinal tract and occupies more than 90% of the surface of the gastrointestinal tract, it has low tumorigenic property (Cheung et al. 2016). SB tumors represent 3–6% of all gastrointestinal malignancies, with adenomas and mesenchymal tumors being the most common ones, whereas neuroendocrine tumors, adenocarcinoma, lymphoma, and sarcoma are the most common malignant tumors (Swain 2005; Fleischer 2005). SB tumors

have vague clinical presentations, resulting in a delay in diagnosis and a less favorable prognosis. Hence, special attention needs to be paid to a high-risk group for SB tumors such as those with follicular lymphoma, metastatic neuroendocrine tumor, malignant melanoma, long-standing SB celiac disease (at risk of adenocarcinoma and small bowel T-cell lymphoma), and inherited polyposis syndromes. Also, SB tumors should be considered in the differential diagnosis of patients with OGIB, vague abdominal pain, and nausea/vomiting/weight loss. The findings are difficult to interpret; caution should be exercised in diagnosing SB tumors by WCE. Innocent bulgings can be interpreted as a mass with ill-defined borders. The diagnostic yield of MRE and CTE was similar to WCE (Girelli et al. 2011). In another study of SB disease including SB tumors, CD, and others, the specificity of MRE was higher than WCE (0.97 vs. 0.84, p = 0.047), whereas sensitivity was similar (0.79 vs. 0.74, p = 0.591). The authors of a recent manuscript concluded that we cannot determine any superiority of one examination over the other among MRE/CTE/WCE for evaluation of SB tumors (Cheung et al. 2016). In studies, SB tumor detection is usually performed in an enriched sample with a high clinical suspicion rather than for general indication, thereby explaining the high rate of tumor diagnosis (47%) (Mitsui et al. 2009). WCE may miss tumors located in duodenum and proximal jejunum due to rapid transit. Also, subepithelial tumors with intact overlying mucosa may be missed. SBE often fails to achieve complete SB examination and has risk from procedure and sedation-related complications. Hence, SBE should be used to confirm the diagnosis of SB lesions by visualization and histology, whereas WCE/MRE/CTE are likely first-line diagnostic modalities to detect SB lesions.

Evaluation of Celiac Disease

In the past, celiac disease (CeD) was considered to be a disorder diagnosed in children and younger adults. The growing interest in its incidence has led to the diagnosis of CeD in those mild/atypical symptoms. Thus, an analogy of iceberg was

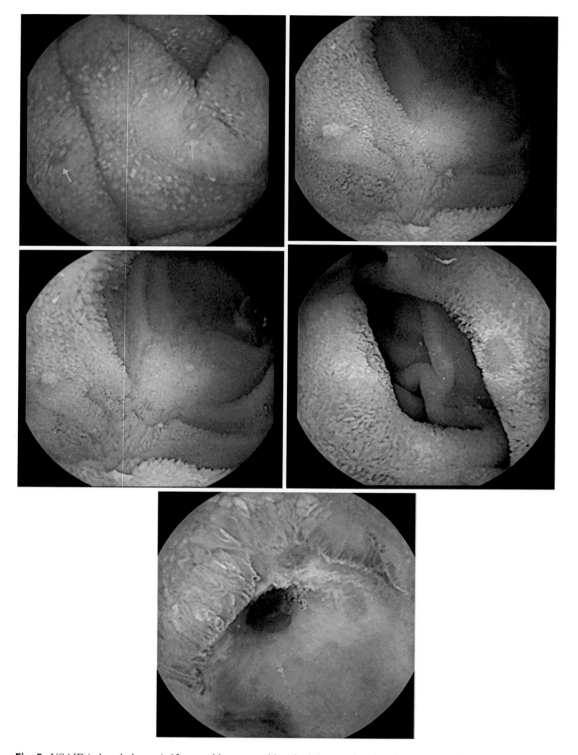

Fig. 8 NSAID induced ulcers. A 65-year-old woman with arthralgias, on chronic NSAIDs, presenting with severe IDA and WCE shows multiple ulcers and a circumferential/diaphragmatic ulcer

suggested for CeD, where a small portion of patients with classic symptoms are diagnosed, whereas the majority of asymptomatic individuals or subjects with atypical symptoms remain undiagnosed and untreated. Currently, it is felt to be a disease detected at any age, primarily due to the development of reliable serological tests and advent of endoscopy techniques to obtain duodenal biopsies. It may present with mild/atypical symptoms such as weakness, anemia, reduced appetite indigestion, and old age which should not be blamed empirically without proper investigation. Thus, we have a compelling case to diagnose CeD at any age to avoid long-term complications such as osteopenia/osteoporosis, T-cell lymphoma, and autoimmune disorders. The gold standard in the diagnosis of CeD is histopathology of the small bowel (Ludvigsson et al. 2014). Some of the features of celiac disease are scalloping of the folds, villous atrophy, mosaic appearance, and layering of mucosal folds (Tukey et al. 2009). These changes are better visualized in WCE than by conventional endoscopy due to a wider angle of view, better magnification, underwater navigation, and lack of insufflation (Fig. 9).

Crohn's Disease and WCE

Although CD and ulcerative colitis (UC) are grouped under inflammatory bowel disorders (IBD), they are mostly the diseases of the younger age group. But 10–30% of patients living with IBD are over the age of 60, either living with IBD or developing it as an older adult. Among older adults worldwide, the incidence of CD and UC is 3/100000 and 3–11/100000 respectively. The incidence decreased with each subsequent decade after the age of 60, with 25% of individuals being diagnosed in their 70s and 10% being diagnosed in their 80s. In patients with IBD, the SB is involved in approximately 70% of Crohn's disease patients, and CD is limited to ileum alone in 27% of patients (Kopylov et al. 2015a). In many cases, CD may involve SB proximal to terminal ileum, which is not accessible by conventional ileocolonoscopy. Hence, a normal ileocolonoscopy does not necessarily exclude

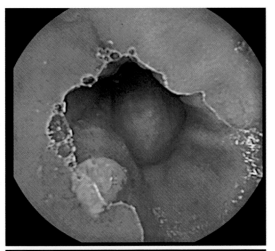

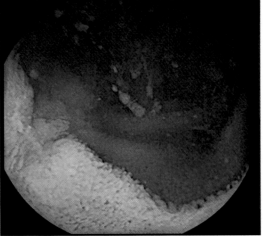

Fig. 9 CD – ileal ulcer. A 64-year-old women with chronic abdominal pain, without any NSAID usage, presenting with ileal ulcers (on WCE) concerning for CD

CD. Also, occasionally, the ileum cannot be visualized properly, and ileocolonoscopy and radiological investigations can be inconclusive, whereas WCE allows for direct inspection of SB mucosa and detection of subtotal mucosal changes. Furthermore, extensive SB CD and proximal SB CD are known risk factors for worse long-term prognosis, higher risk of surgery, the risk for future relapse, and increased risk for complications (Zallot and Peyrin-Biroulet 2012; Lazarev et al. 2013; Flamant et al. 2013). Hence, WCE is an effective tool to aid the diagnosis (rather than invasive tests such as balloon

enteroscopy) in patients with symptoms suggestive of CD with normal upper endoscopy and
colonoscopy (a more clinically relevant scenario)
(Enns et al. 2017). It is also helpful in determining
the extent of disease, evaluation of patients with
indeterminate colitis, and response to anti-inflammatory therapy and to assess for postoperative
disease recurrence in well-selected patients.
(Eliakim 2010; Enns et al. 2017; Swain 2005;
Fleischer 2005) (Fig. 10).

The diagnostic yield of WCE in suspected
Crohn's disease ranges from 40% to 70%
(Eliakim 2010; Liao et al. 2010; Fleischer 2005;
Kornbluth et al. 2005), but it is unclear whether
abnormalities detected are always clinically relevant. A recent meta-analysis demonstrated superior diagnostic yield of WCE compared to SB
radiography and enteroclysis and is comparable
to CTE and MRE (Choi et al. 2017). In the study
in suspected or newly diagnosed CD patients,
sensitivity and specificity of WCE (100,91%)
were higher compared to CTE (81,85%) and
MRE (76,85%), respectively (Jensen et al.
2011). Conversely, WCE findings have a high
negative predictive value (97%) in patients with
SB CD (Tukey et al. 2009). In one study of CD
patients, those with jejunal lesions on WCE were
at higher risk for disease relapse (Flamant et al.

2013). The European Society of Gastrointestinal
Endoscopy recommends the usage of validated
activities scores (Lewis score and Capsule Endoscopy CD Activity Index [CECDAI] Tables 4, 5
and 6) to facilitate prospective WCE endoscopy
follow-up for longitudinal assessment of clinical
course in patients with SB CD in response to

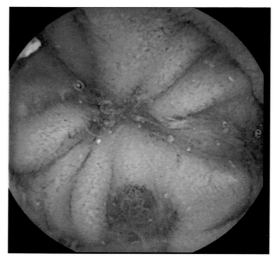

Fig. 10 Metastatic angiosarcoma. A 76-year-old male
presenting with lower GI bleeding due to metastatic
angiosarcoma, diagnosed on WCE

Table 5 Capsule endoscopy Lewis score

Parameter	Descriptor	Longitudinal extent	Descriptor
Villous appearance (worst-affected tertile)	Normal (0) Edematous (1)	Short segment (8) Long segment (12) Whole tertile (20)	Single (1) Patchy (14) Diffuse (17)
Ulcers (worst-affected tertile)	None (0) Single (3) Few (5) Multiple (10)	Short segment (5) Long segment (10) Whole tertile (15)	< ¼ (9) ¼–½ (12) >½ (18)
Stenosis (whole study)	None (0) Single (14) Multiple (20)	Ulcerated (24) Nonulcerated (2)	Traversed (7) Not traversed (10)

Small bowel is divided into tertiles according to transit time
Core total (in worst-affected tertile): villous appearance x extent x descriptor + ulcers x extent x size + stenosis x ulcerated x traversed
Short segment, < 10%; long segment, 11–50%; whole tertile, > 50%
Ulcers: single (1), few (2–7), multiple (≥8)
Ulcer descriptor (size): the proportion of capsule picture filled by largest ulcer
Lewis score
a)<135➔ clinically insignificant inflammation
b)135–790➔ mild inflammation
c)≥ 790➔ moderate-severe inflammation

Table 6 Capsule Endoscopy Crohn's Disease Activity Index **(CECDAI)**

Parameter	Score	Descriptor
Inflammation score		
	0	None
	1	Mild-moderate (edema/hyperemia/denudation)
	2	Severe (edema/hyperemia/denudation)
	3	Bleeding, exudate, erosion, aphthae, ulcer <0.5 cm
	4	Pseudopolyp, ulcer 0.5–2 cm
	5	Ulcer >2 cm
Extent of disease score		
	0	None
	1	Single segment (focal disease)
	2	2–3 segments (patchy disease)
	3	>3 segments (diffuse disease)
Stricture score		
	0	None
	1	Single, traversed
	2	Multiple, traversed
	3	Obstruction

CECDAI: Proximal segment (Axb + C) + distal segment (Axb + C)

Score range: 0–36

Clinical or endoscopic remission: CECDAI <4

medical therapy. The Lewis score is a measure of inflammatory activity, and the magnitude of score may play a role in assessing the likelihood of CD accounting for the lesions noted on WCE (Monteiro and Boal Carvalho 2015; Rosa et al. 2012) (Fig. 11).

The current treatment paradigm (treat-to-target) focuses on reversing the inflammation and mucosal healing and thus limiting the disease progression and bowel damage. Mucosal healing does not parallel with normalization of biochemical markers and clinical remission and has been demonstrated in multiple studies (Kopylov et al. 2015a, b; Hall et al. 2014; Efthymiou et al. 2008). In a study by Kopylov et al. (Kopylov et al. 2015a), mucosal healing was demonstrated by WCE in only 15.4% of patients with clinical remission. The lack of mucosal healing on WCE resulted in changes in disease management in 64% (Lorenzo-Zuniga et al. 2010; Long et al. 2011) and provided an explanation for patient symptomatology not explained by a normal ileocolonoscopy (Dussault et al. 2013; Kim et al. 2017). The Canadian WCE guidelines and European guidelines recommend WCE in CD patients signs/symptomatology not explained by ileocolonoscopy or other imaging modalities (Enns et al. 2017; Annese et al. 2013). Thereby, WCE has an evolving role to assess mucosal healing and evaluating unexplained symptomatology in CD patients.

Indeterminate colitis (IC) refers to IBD cases (~ 15%), with colonic involvement, difficult to differentiate between CD and UC by colonoscopy, or on histological examination of the resection specimen in up to 15% of those patients undergoing colectomy (Guindi and Riddell 2004). Nearly 30% of these patients are reclassified as CD later on during the disease course (Eliakim 2007). The latter observation has clinical implications, especially in patients thought to have UC and are being considered for colectomy. The findings of erosions or ulcers in the small bowel may result in management from surgical to a more intensive medical therapy (Loftus Jr. 2004). In our opinion, every UC patient being considered for elective colectomy should get WCE to avoid inappropriate colectomy. The rates of pouch failure are higher in patients with CD patients compared to UC and IC (Oresland et al. 2015). In summary, WCE has a major role in assessing SB involvement and if required to reclassify IC and or UC as CD (Maunoury et al. 2007).

WCE is more effective than ileocolonoscopy in detecting disease recurrence and may be a reasonable choice for postsurgical surveillance in patients when ileocolonoscopy is contraindicated/or terminal ileum cannot be intubated at all or if the patient refuses an endoscopic evaluation (Papay et al. 2013; Pons Beltran et al. 2007). Some authors recommend WCE 6 months to 1 year after ileocecal resection to detect recurrence, depending on the presence of risk factors (De Cruz et al. 2012).

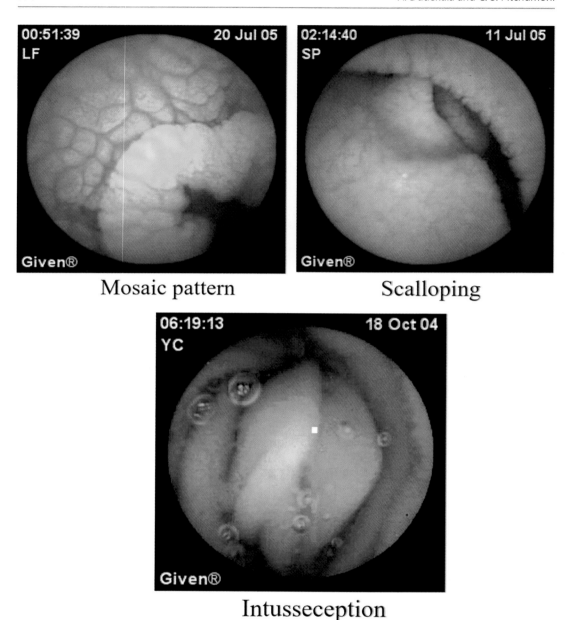

Fig. 11 Celiac disease. A 76-year-old male with IDA underwent WCE, which showed intestinal features consistent with celiac disease

A limitation of WCE is the lack of definitive diagnostic criteria for CD. WCE findings such as mucosal erythema, edema, ulcerations, and erosions are nonspecific and present in up to 15 percent of normal individuals and two-thirds of patients with NSAID-induced enteropathy (Bar-Meir 2006; Sidhu et al. 2010). For this

reason, patients undergoing WCE are advised to avoid taking NSAIDs for 4 weeks prior to the procedure (Pennazio et al. 2015). Physicians will need to be cognizant of the fact that SB enteropathies such as SB lymphoma, radiation enteropathy, intestinal tuberculosis, Behcet's disease, and enteropathy related to HIV-associated opportunistic infections share similar mucosal appearance on WCE (Bar-Meir 2006).

Patients with known CD are at increased risk of retention of capsule compared to those with suspected Crohn's disease (5 to 13 versus 1 to 2%, respectively) (Kornbluth et al. 2005; Cheifetz and Lewis 2006). Agile patency capsule (Given Imaging, Yokneam, Israel) approved by the FDA in 2006,reliably predicts safe capsule endoscopy (Spada et al. 2005). The passage of the agile capsule in the stool by the patient and the absence of radio frequency signal detected by a handheld scanner or absence of the capsule on abdominal radiography almost exclude an obstructing lesion and a safe subsequent real capsule endoscopy (Spada et al. 2005; McAlindon et al. 2010).

Surveillance of Inherited Polyposis Syndromes

SB polyps occur in more than 75% of familial adenomatosis polyposis (FAP) and Peutz-Jeghers syndrome (Enns et al. 2017). In patients with FAP, duodenal adenomatosis develops and increases the risk of cancer with age. The cumulative lifetime risk of duodenal adenomatosis is 88%, and the cumulative incidence of cancer is 18% at 75 years of age (Bulow et al. 2012). Spigelman's staging is a predictor for malignant changes in duodenal adenomatosis (Spigelman et al. 1989). Up to 70% of patients with FAP have adenomatous polyps in jejunum and ileum, but in contrast to duodenal adenomatosis, malignancy is seldom reported. WCE/CTE/MRE can be considered to detect polyps in the rest of the SB, but clinical relevance is yet to be established. In Peutz-Jeghers syndrome, polyps present early in life as intussusception and anemia and progress to cancer later in life. Hence, SB surveillance is needed, either by WCE/MRE (Enns et al. 2017). For smaller polyps, WCE has better sensitivity than MRE, but for larger polyps (> 1 cm), both have equal sensitivity (Postgate et al. 2009). SB screening is recommended every 3 years if polyps are found during the initial examination from the age of 8 years or earlier if the patient is symptomatic (Beggs et al. 2010).

Chronic Abdominal Pain

Chronic abdominal pain (CAP) is a common gastrointestinal complaint, present in up to 21% of population (Quigley et al. 2006; Sandler et al. 2000; Townsend et al. 2005), is a common indication for gastroenterology clinic visits, and yet can be a diagnostic challenge due to varied etiologies ranging from benign and functional disorders to malignancy and inflammatory diseases (IBD) (Hulisz 2004; Middleton and Hing 2006; Myer et al. 2013). Patients with unexplained CAP undergo a series of examinations including ultrasound of abdomen, radiography, EGD, and colonoscopy. The role of WCE remains unclear. Studies evaluating the diagnostic yield of WCE in CAP patients are limited, inconsistent, performed mostly in tertiary care referral centers, and report a wide diagnostic yield (4–44%) (Makins and Blanshard 2006; Qvigstad et al. 2006; Xue et al. 2015). In a meta-analysis of 21 studies with 1520 patients, the yield of WCE for chronic abdominal pain is 21% with inflammatory (78%) and tumors (9%) being most common lesions (Xue et al. 2015). Overall, WCE is a noninvasive diagnostic tool in evaluating patients with unexplained CAP, with a limited diagnostic yield, and among patients with positive findings, change in management is likely limited to those with a history of CD (Egnatios et al. 2015).

Special Considerations of WCE in the Older Adult

The most common indication for WCE in the older adult is obscure or occult gastrointestinal bleeding, whereas in the younger adult, it is used to evaluate suspected SB CD and chronic diarrhea of unknown origin (Papadopoulos et al. 2008).

The failure rate of WCE in the general population is about 20%, similar to that observed in the older adult (Papadopoulos et al. 2008). A major difference between the younger (age < 65) and older age group (age > 65) is the SB transit time, which influences completion of the procedure (Papadopoulos et al. 2008). One way to overcome prolonged transit time or impaired swallowing in the older adult is to place the capsule beyond the pylorus with the assistance of an upper gastrointestinal endoscope (Yachimski and Friedman 2008). Another consideration is the interference of signal transmission with the concomitant use of cardiac pacemakers or other implanted electromechanical devices (such as pacemaker), a common scenario in the older adult (Payeras et al. 2005) (Dirks et al. 2008). These problems appear to be more perception than reality (Moglia et al. 2009) (Liao et al. 2010) (Payeras et al. 2005) (Dirks et al. 2008). Furthermore, there is potential for inadequate visualization due to poor preparation in older adults with impairments and concern for capsule retention. Dysphagia and dementia can also be a hindrance to performing WCE in elderly.

Contraindications for WCE

An important concern with WCE is the potential retention of the capsule within the gastrointestinal tract (Swain 2005) (Cheifetz and Lewis 2006) (Lewis 2005). Capsule retention may occur in patients with (a) prior abdominal surgery and (b) intestinal obstruction (Liao et al. 2010) (Lewis 2005) (Papadakis et al. 2005). In the event the capsule is not spontaneously excreted and cannot be removed endoscopically, surgery may be required (Cheifetz and Lewis 2006). The risk of capsule retention and impaction increases with the concerns above when the capsule gets lodged in a narrowed segment of SB and causes further obstruction. The retention rate is about 1%; most patients are asymptomatic and have a partial obstruction or symptomatic complete intestinal obstruction (Fleischer 2005). Capsule retention in Crohn's disease can reach 8% (Eliakim 2010). Failure of the passage of the capsule is an acceptable outcome in patients if it demonstrates a site of obstruction when surgery to remove the capsule results in clinical improvement for which the WCE was originally performed (Cheifetz and Lewis 2006).

Absolute contraindications include clinical or radiographic evidence of gastrointestinal obstruction, active and extensive Crohn's disease with or without the presence of strictures, and extensive intestinal diverticulosis (Liao et al. 2010).

Limitations of Capsule Endoscopy

There are a few limitations for WCE. The expected life span of the battery is a maximum of 8 h and 45 min. About 10–20% of capsules do not reach the cecum; here battery failure can cause inadequate visualization of SB pathology (Tatar et al. 2006). Battery failure is more common in patients with delayed gastric emptying or when the capsule sits in the stomach for over 1.5 h (Liao et al. 2010). Image quality may be influenced by the presence of bile, poor bowel preparation, or residual barium from previous radiographic studies. Up to 40% of all lesions can be missed due to inability to control the velocity or direction of the capsule passage (Papadakis et al. 2005). Furthermore, the images are not in real time; therefore on-the-spot treatment and histopathologic confirmation of the findings are not possible (Papadakis et al. 2005).

Preparation

Although WCE can be performed after an overnight fast and an empty stomach without intestinal cleansing, a bowel preparation enhances the visualization of the mucosa, increases the likelihood of a complete cecal examination, and prevents smudging of the camera lens (Eliakim 2010), (Gerson 2009). A half-day bowel preparation using polyethylene glycol (PEG) enhances the quality and diagnostic yield (Moglia et al. 2009). The ingested capsule passively travels through the gastrointestinal tract, while the cameras in the capsule capture images at two to three color frames per second (Moglia et al. 2009). The capsule is evacuated, usually 24–48 h later, with stool (Eliakim 2010). A complete examination of the SB is possible in over 80% of patients (Liao et al. 2010), (Van Gossum et al. 2009).

Other Capsule Endoscopic Procedures

Although esophageal and colon capsules are FDA approved, their usage is limited and is yet to gain widespread acceptance.

Esophageal WCE

Esophageal WCE is a noninvasive unsedated imaging technique for visualization of the esophagus. In a meta-analysis, pooled sensitivity and specificity for the diagnosis of Barret's esophagus were moderate, 77% and 86%, respectively (Bhardwaj et al. 2009). It can be utilized to detect esophageal varices (Karatzas et al. 2018) and esophagitis. Esophageal WCE has FDA approval for evaluation of esophageal varices and esophagitis but not for Barrett's esophagus.

Colon Capsule

Optical colonoscopy is still regarded as the gold standard test for CRC prevention as it allows for both diagnostic and therapeutic intervention for premalignant lesions and unequivocally demonstrated benefit in CRC screening/surveillance. Still, the acceptance of colonoscopy for CRC screening remains far from optimal due to concerns regarding adverse events, privacy, implications of work-related absence, and invasive nature of the procedure. The PillCam colon capsule (PCCE) is minimially invasive, can be performed at patients' homes without any privacy concerns, does not require sedation, and has significant potential to improve compliance for CRC screening. This is currently approved by the European Society for Gastrointestinal Endoscopy (ESGE) for average-risk CRC screening and also for high-risk screening in patients who refuse colonoscopy or have a contraindication for colonoscopy (Spada et al. 2012). In the USA, FDA has approved it as an adjunctive test in those with a prior incomplete colonoscopy and in the evaluation of patients with suspected lower GI bleeding (Rex et al. 2017). The test is not yet approved as an option for average-risk CRC screening. Compared to colonoscopy, PCCE has similar adenoma detection rate and colon completion rate but lower specificity (Spada et al. 2016) (Rex et al. 2015) (van Rijn et al. 2006). CT colonography is currently recommended as one of the options for average-risk CRC screening in patients who have a prior incomplete colonoscopy, as well as those with contraindications or unwilling to undergo colonoscopy. Studies comparing PCCE with CT colonography showed comparable results for sensitivity and specificity to polyp detection (Rondonotti et al. 2014). However, PCCE had a significantly higher reading time compared to CT colonography (62.8 30.8 mins vs. 18.5 7.3 min) (Rondonotti et al. 2014). Preliminary studies have showed PCCE as an effective tool for the assessment of disease activity and mucosal healing. But inability to biopsy and risk of retention are prohibiting its widespread usage (Hall et al. 2015) (Shi et al. 2015). PCCE requires a more rigorous bowel preparation compared to optical colonoscopy due to lack of ability to irrigate, suction, and insufflate. This may be the biggest limiting factory in patients' acceptance of the procedure.

Elements of Capsule Report

A good wireless capsule endoscopy report should include data on the following.

Indication for the study, patient demographics, comorbidities, prior h/o abdominal surgery, h/o anticoagulant and NSAID use, capsule system used, duration of the study, quality of bowel preparation, identification key landmarks, and gastric emptying and oro-cecal transit time are optional findings of limited use, pertinent findings in SB, and incidental findings in the stomach and proximal colon (if observed), adverse effects, diagnosis, and potential recommendations.

Key Points

Wireless Capsule Endoscopy (WCE)

1. WCE is a novel, noninvasive method of visualizing the entire small bowel (SB), which was considered inaccessible by routine endoscopy.

2. In contrast to other conventional endoscopies, WCE is solely a diagnostic procedure with no feasibility for biopsy or therapeutic capability.

3. WCE is a tool to detect bleeding sites in the small bowel as a cause of anemia in the older adults, tumors of the SB, Crohn's disease (CD), and nonsteroidal ulcers.

4. WCE is helpful in patients with acute occult gastrointestinal bleeding where the bleeding site is not seen by conventional endoscopies.

5. Older adults with dysphagia may rarely encounter difficulty swallowing the capsule.

6. Previous gastric surgery and gastroparesis may pose a delay in the WCE exiting the stomach, and endoscopic placement of the capsule in the duodenum may be needed.

7. The complications are rare. Capsule retention may occur rarely and occasionally need for surgical removal of the retained capsule.

References

Adler DG, Knipschield M, Gostout C. A prospective comparison of capsule endoscopy and push enteroscopy in patients with GI bleeding of obscure origin. Gastrointest Endosc. 2004;59(4):492–8. PubMed PMID: 15044884.

Akin E, Demirezer Bolat A, Buyukasik S, Algin O, Selvi E, Ersoy O. Comparison between capsule endoscopy and magnetic resonance enterography for the detection of polyps of the small intestine in patients with familial adenomatous polyposis. Gastroenterol Res Pract. 2012;2012:215028. PubMed PMID: 22518115. Pubmed Central PMCID: 3296287.

Annese V, Daperno M, Rutter MD, Amiot A, Bossuyt P, East J, et al. European evidence based consensus for endoscopy in inflammatory bowel disease. J Crohns Colitis. 2013;7(12):982–1018. PubMed PMID: 24184171.

Bandorski D, Kurniawan N, Baltes P, Hoeltgen R, Hecker M, Stunder D, et al. Contraindications for video capsule endoscopy. World J Gastroenterol. 2016;22(45):9898–908. PubMed PMID: 28018097. Pubmed Central PMCID: 5143757.

Bar-Meir S. Review article: capsule endoscopy – are all small intestinal lesions Crohn's disease? Aliment Pharmacol Ther. 2006;24(Suppl 3):19–21. PubMed PMID: 16961739.

Beggs AD, Latchford AR, Vasen HF, Moslein G, Alonso A, Aretz S, et al. Peutz-Jeghers syndrome: a systematic review and recommendations for management. Gut. 2010;59(7):975–86. PubMed PMID: 20581245.

Bhardwaj A, Hollenbeak CS, Pooran N, Mathew A. A meta-analysis of the diagnostic accuracy of esophageal capsule endoscopy for Barrett's esophagus in patients with gastroesophageal reflux disease. Am J Gastroenterol. 2009;104(6):1533–9. PubMed PMID: 19491867.

Bresci G, Parisi G, Bertoni M, Tumino E, Capria A. The role of video capsule endoscopy for evaluating obscure gastrointestinal bleeding: usefulness of early use. J Gastroenterol. 2005;40(3):256–9. PubMed PMID: 15830284.

Bulow S, Christensen IJ, Hojen H, Bjork J, Elmberg M, Jarvinen H, et al. Duodenal surveillance improves the prognosis after duodenal cancer in familial adenomatous polyposis. Color Dis: Off J Assoc Coloproctology G B Irel. 2012;14(8):947–52. PubMed PMID: 21973191.

Carey EJ, Leighton JA, Heigh RI, Shiff AD, Sharma VK, Post JK, et al. A single-center experience of 260 consecutive patients undergoing capsule endoscopy for obscure gastrointestinal bleeding. Am J Gastroenterol. 2007;102(1):89–95. PubMed PMID: 17100969.

Cellier C, Green PH, Collin P, Murray J. ICCE. ICCE consensus for celiac disease. Endoscopy. 2005;37(10): 1055–9. PubMed PMID: 16189790.

Cheifetz AS, Lewis BS. Capsule endoscopy retention: is it a complication? J Clin Gastroenterol. 2006;40(8):688–91. PubMed PMID: 16940879. Epub 2006/08/31. eng.

Cheung DY, Kim JS, Shim KN, Choi MG. Korean gut image study G. the usefulness of capsule endoscopy for small bowel tumors. Clin Endoscopy. 2016;49(1):21–5. PubMed PMID: 26855919. Pubmed Central PMCID: 4743724.

Choi M, Lim S, Choi MG, Shim KN, Lee SH. Effectiveness of capsule endoscopy compared with other diagnostic modalities in patients with small bowel Crohn's disease: a meta-analysis. Gut liver. 2017;11(1):62–72. PubMed PMID: 27728963. Pubmed Central PMCID: 5221862.

Chong J, Tagle M, Barkin JS, Reiner DK. Small bowel push-type fiber optic enteroscopy for patients with occult gastrointestinal bleeding or suspected small bowel pathology. Am J Gastroenterol. 1994;89(12):2143–6. PubMed PMID: 7977230.

Cobrin GM, Pittman RH, Lewis BS. Increased diagnostic yield of small bowel tumors with capsule endoscopy. Cancer. 2006;107(1):22–7. PubMed PMID: 16736516.

Committee AT, Wang A, Banerjee S, Barth BA, Bhat YM, Chauhan S, et al. Wireless capsule endoscopy. Gastrointest Endosc. 2013;78(6):805–15. PubMed PMID: 24119509.

Culliford A, Daly J, Diamond B, Rubin M, Green PH. The value of wireless capsule endoscopy in patients with complicated celiac disease. Gastrointest Endosc. 2005;62(1):55–61. PubMed PMID: 15990820.

De Cruz P, Kamm MA, Prideaux L, Allen PB, Desmond PV. Postoperative recurrent luminal Crohn's disease: a systematic review. Inflamm Bowel Dis. 2012;18 (4):758–77. PubMed PMID: 21830279.

de Leusse A, Vahedi K, Edery J, Tiah D, Fery-Lemonnier E, Cellier C, et al. Capsule endoscopy or push enteroscopy for first-line exploration of obscure gastrointestinal bleeding? Gastroenterology. 2007;132(3):855–62; quiz 1164-5. PubMed PMID: 17324401.

Dirks MH, Costea F, Seidman EG. Successful video-capsule endoscopy in patients with an abdominal cardiac pacemaker. Endoscopy. 2008;40(1):73–5.. PubMed PMID: 18161651. Epub 2007/12/29. eng.

Dussault C, Gower-Rousseau C, Salleron J, Vernier-Massouille G, Branche J, Colombel JF, et al. Small bowel capsule endoscopy for management of Crohn's disease: a retrospective tertiary care Centre experience. Dig Liver Dis: Off J Ital Soc Gastroenterolo Ital Assoc Study Liver. 2013;45(7):558–61. PubMed PMID: 23238033.

Efthymiou A, Viazis N, Mantzaris G, Papadimitriou N, Tzourmakliotis D, Raptis S, et al. Does clinical response correlate with mucosal healing in patients with Crohn's disease of the small bowel? A prospective, case-series study using wireless capsule endoscopy. Inflamm Bowel Dis. 2008;14(11):1542–7. PubMed PMID: 18521929.

Egnatios J, Kaushal K, Kalmaz D, Zarrinpar A. Video capsule endoscopy in patients with chronic abdominal pain with or without associated symptoms: a retrospective study. PLoS One. 2015;10(4):e0126509. PubMed PMID: 25893440. Pubmed Central PMCID: 4404061.

Eliakim R. The impact of wireless capsule endoscopy on gastrointestinal diseases. South Med J. 2007;100(3): 235–6. PubMed PMID: 17396720.

Eliakim R. Video capsule endoscopy of the small bowel. Curr Opin Gastroenterol. 2010;26(2):129–33. PubMed PMID: 20145540. Epub 2010/02/11. eng.

Ell C, Remke S, May A, Helou L, Henrich R, Mayer G. The first prospective controlled trial comparing wireless capsule endoscopy with push enteroscopy in chronic gastrointestinal bleeding. Endoscopy. 2002;34(9):685–9. PubMed PMID: 12195324.

Enns RA, Hookey L, Armstrong D, Bernstein CN, Heitman SJ, Teshima C, et al. Clinical practice guidelines for the use of video capsule endoscopy. Gastroenterology. 2017;152(3):497–514. PubMed PMID: 28063287.

Esaki M, Matsumoto T, Yada S, Yanaru-Fujisawa R, Kudo T, Yanai S, et al. Factors associated with the clinical impact of capsule endoscopy in patients with overt obscure gastrointestinal bleeding. Dig Dis Sci. 2010;55(8):2294–301. PubMed PMID: 19957038.

Estevez E, Gonzalez-Conde B, Vazquez-Iglesias JL, de Los Angeles Vazquez-Millan M, Pertega S, Alonso PA, et al. Diagnostic yield and clinical outcomes after capsule endoscopy in 100 consecutive patients with obscure gastrointestinal bleeding. Eur J Gastroenterol Hepatol. 2006;18(8):881–8. PubMed PMID: 16825907.

Flamant M, Trang C, Maillard O, Sacher-Huvelin S, Le Rhun M, Galmiche JP, et al. The prevalence and outcome of jejunal lesions visualized by small bowel capsule endoscopy in Crohn's disease. Inflamm Bowel Dis. 2013;19(7):1390–6. PubMed PMID: 23552764.

Fleischer D. Capsule imaging. Clin Gastroenterol Hepatol. 2005;3(7 Suppl 1):S30–2. PubMed PMID: 16012992. Epub 2005/07/14. eng.

Friedman S. Comparison of capsule endoscopy to other modalities in small bowel. Gastrointest Endosc Clin N Am. 2004;14(1):51–60. PubMed PMID: 15062380. Epub 2004/04/06. eng.

Fry LC, Mönkemüller K, Neumann H, Von Arnim U, Bellutti M, Malfertheiner P. Capsule endoscopy (CE) increases the diagnostic yield of double balloon Enteroscopy (DBE) in patients being investigated for obscure gastrointestinal bleeding (OGIB). Gastrointest Endosc. 2009;69(5):AB190.

Gastineau S, Viala J, Caldari D, Mas E, Darviot E, Le Gall C, et al. Contribution of capsule endoscopy to Peutz-Jeghers syndrome management in children. Dig Liver Dis: Off J Ital Soc Gastroenterolo Ital Assoc Study Liver. 2012;44(10):839–43. PubMed PMID: 22795616.

Ge ZZ, Chen HY, Gao YJ, Hu YB, Xiao SD. Best candidates for capsule endoscopy for obscure gastrointestinal bleeding. J Gastroenterol Hepatol. 2007;22 (12):2076–80. PubMed PMID: 18031363.

Gerson LB. Preparation before capsule endoscopy: the value of the purge. Gastroenterology. 2009;137 (3):1166–8; discussion 8. PubMed PMID: 19635602. Epub 2009/07/29. eng.

Gerson LB, Fidler JL, Cave DR, Leighton JA. ACG clinical guideline: diagnosis and management of small bowel bleeding. Am J Gastroenterol. 2015;110 (9):1265–87; quiz 88. PubMed PMID: 26303132.

Girelli CM, Porta P, Colombo E, Lesinigo E, Bernasconi G. Development of a novel index to discriminate bulge from mass on small-bowel capsule endoscopy. Gastrointest Endosc. 2011;74(5):1067–74; quiz 115 e1-5. PubMed PMID: 21907982.

Guindi M, Riddell RH. Indeterminate colitis. J Clin Pathol. 2004;57(12):1233–44. PubMed PMID: 15563659. Pubmed Central PMCID: 1770507.

Haanstra JF, Al-Toma A, Dekker E, Vanhoutvin SA, Nagengast FM, Mathus-Vliegen EM, et al. Prevalence of small-bowel neoplasia in lynch syndrome assessed by video capsule endoscopy. Gut. 2015;64(10):1578–83. PubMed PMID: 25209657.

Hall B, Holleran G, Chin JL, Smith S, Ryan B, Mahmud N, et al. A prospective 52 week mucosal healing assessment of small bowel Crohn's disease as detected by capsule endoscopy. J Crohns Colitis. 2014;8(12):1601–9. PubMed PMID: 25257546.

Hall B, Holleran G, McNamara D. PillCam COLON 2((c)) as a pan-enteroscopic test in Crohn's disease. World J Gastrointestinal Endoscopy. 2015;7(16):1230–2. PubMed PMID: 26566430. Pubmed Central PMCID: 4639745.

Hartmann D, Schmidt H, Bolz G, Schilling D, Kinzel F, Eickhoff A, et al. A prospective two-center study comparing wireless capsule endoscopy with intraoperative enteroscopy in patients with obscure GI bleeding. Gastrointest Endosc. 2005;61(7):826–32. PubMed PMID: 15933683.

Hindryckx P, Botelberge T, De Vos M, De Looze D. Clinical impact of capsule endoscopy on further strategy and long-term clinical outcome in patients with obscure bleeding. Gastrointest Endosc. 2008;68 (1):98–104. PubMed PMID: 18291382.

Hosoe N, Takabayashi K, Ogata H, Kanai T. Capsule endoscopy for small-intestinal disorders: current status. Dig Endosc: Off J Jpn Gastroenterological Endoscopy Soc. 2019;31(5):498–507. PubMed PMID: 30656743.

Hulisz D. The burden of illness of irritable bowel syndrome: current challenges and hope for the future. J Manag Care Pharm : JMCP. 2004;10(4):299–309. PubMed PMID: 15298528.

Hunt RH, Lanas A, Stichtenoth DO, Scarpignato C. Myths and facts in the use of anti-inflammatory drugs. Ann Med. 2009;41(6):423–37. PubMed PMID: 19430988.

Jensen MD, Nathan T, Rafaelsen SR, Kjeldsen J. Diagnostic accuracy of capsule endoscopy for small bowel Crohn's disease is superior to that of MR enterography or CT enterography. Clin Gastroenterol Hepatol. 2011;9(2):124–9. PubMed PMID: 21056692.

Kaffes AJ, Siah C, Koo JH. Clinical outcomes after double-balloon enteroscopy in patients with obscure GI bleeding and a positive capsule endoscopy. Gastrointest Endosc. 2007;66(2):304–9. PubMed PMID: 17643704.

Karatzas A, Konstantakis C, Aggeletopoulou I, Kalogeropoulou C, Thomopoulos K, Triantos C. Non-invasive screening for esophageal varices in patients with liver cirrhosis. Ann Gastroenterol. 2018;31(3):305–14. PubMed PMID: 29720856. Pubmed Central PMCID: 5924853.

Katsinelos P, Chatzimavroudis G, Terzoudis S, Patsis I, Fasoulas K, Katsinelos T, et al. Diagnostic yield and clinical impact of capsule endoscopy in obscure gastrointestinal bleeding during routine clinical practice: a single-center experience. Med Princ Pract: Int J Kuwait Univ, Health Sci Cent. 2011;20(1):60–5. PubMed PMID: 21160216.

Kim Y, Jeon SR, Choi SM, Kim HG, Lee TH, Cho JH, et al. Practice patterns and clinical significance of use of capsule endoscopy in suspected and established Crohn's disease. Intestinal Res. 2017;15(4):467–74. PubMed PMID: 29142514. Pubmed Central PMCID: 5683977.

Koh SJ, Im JP, Kim JW, Kim BG, Lee KL, Kim SG, et al. Long-term outcome in patients with obscure gastrointestinal bleeding after negative capsule endoscopy. World J Gastroenterol. 2013;19(10):1632–8. PubMed PMID: 23539070. Pubmed Central PMCID: 3602481.

Kopylov U, Yablecovitch D, Lahat A, Neuman S, Levhar N, Greener T, et al. Detection of small bowel mucosal healing and deep remission in patients with known small bowel Crohn's disease using biomarkers, capsule endoscopy, and imaging. Am J Gastroenterol. 2015a;110(9):1316–23. PubMed PMID: 26215531.

Kopylov U, Nemeth A, Koulaouzidis A, Makins R, Wild G, Afif W, et al. Small bowel capsule endoscopy in the management of established Crohn's disease: clinical impact, safety, and correlation with inflammatory biomarkers. Inflamm Bowel Dis. 2015b;21(1):93–100. PubMed PMID: 25517597.

Kornbluth A, Colombel JF, Leighton JA, Loftus E. ICCE. ICCE consensus for inflammatory bowel disease. Endoscopy. 2005;37(10):1051–4. PubMed PMID: 16189789.

Koulaouzidis A, Rondonotti E, Giannakou A, Plevris JN. Diagnostic yield of small-bowel capsule endoscopy in patients with iron-deficiency anemia: a systematic review. Gastrointest Endosc. 2012a;76(5):983–92. PubMed PMID: 23078923.

Koulaouzidis A, Yung DE, Lam JH, Smirnidis A, Douglas S, Plevris JN. The use of small-bowel capsule endoscopy in iron-deficiency anemia alone; be aware of the young anemic patient. Scand J Gastroenterol. 2012b;47(8-9):1094–100. PubMed PMID: 22852553.

Lai LH, Wong GL, Chow DK, Lau JY, Sung JJ, Leung WK. Long-term follow-up of patients with obscure gastrointestinal bleeding after negative capsule endoscopy. Am J Gastroenterol. 2006;101(6):1224–8. PubMed PMID: 16771942.

Laine L, Sahota A, Shah A. Does capsule endoscopy improve outcomes in obscure gastrointestinal bleeding? Randomized trial versus dedicated small bowel radiography. Gastroenterology. 2010;138(5):1673–80 e1; quiz e11-2. PubMed PMID: 20138043. Epub 2010/02/09. eng.

Lanas A, Garcia-Rodriguez LA, Polo-Tomas M, Ponce M, Alonso-Abreu I, Perez-Aisa MA, et al. Time trends and impact of upper and lower gastrointestinal bleeding and perforation in clinical practice. Am J Gastroenterol. 2009;104(7):1633–41. PubMed PMID: 19574968.

Lazarev M, Huang C, Bitton A, Cho JH, Duerr RH, McGovern DP, et al. Relationship between proximal Crohn's disease location and disease behavior and surgery: a cross-sectional study of the IBD genetics consortium. Am J Gastroenterol. 2013;108(1):106–12. PubMed PMID: 23229423. Pubmed Central PMCID: 4059598.

Lepileur L, Dray X, Antonietti M, Iwanicki-Caron I, Grigioni S, Chaput U, et al. Factors associated with diagnosis of obscure gastrointestinal bleeding by video capsule enteroscopy. Clin Gastroenterol Hepatol. 2012;10(12):1376–80. PubMed PMID: 22677574.

Leung WK, Graham DY. Obscure gastrointestinal bleeding: where do we go from here? Gastroenterology. 2010;138(5):1655–8. PubMed PMID: 20332043. Epub 2010/03/25. eng.

Lewis B. How to prevent endoscopic capsule retention. Endoscopy. 2005;37(9):852–6. PubMed PMID: 16116537. Epub 2005/08/24. eng.

Lewis BS, Swain P. Capsule endoscopy in the evaluation of patients with suspected small intestinal bleeding: results of a pilot study. Gastrointest Endosc. 2002;56 (3):349–53. PubMed PMID: 12196771.

Li X, Chen H, Dai J, Gao Y, Ge Z. Predictive role of capsule endoscopy on the insertion route of double-balloon enteroscopy. Endoscopy. 2009;41(9):762–6. PubMed PMID: 19662592.

Liao Z, Gao R, Xu C, Li ZS. Indications and detection, completion, and retention rates of small-bowel capsule endoscopy: a systematic review. Gastrointest Endosc. 2010;71(2):280–6. PubMed PMID: 20152309. Epub 2010/02/16. eng.

Loftus EV Jr. Capsule endoscopy for Crohn's disease: ready for prime time? Clin Gastroenterol Hepatol. 2004;2(1):14–6. PubMed PMID: 15017627.

Long MD, Barnes E, Isaacs K, Morgan D, Herfarth HH. Impact of capsule endoscopy on management of inflammatory bowel disease: a single tertiary care center experience. Inflamm Bowel Dis. 2011;17(9):1855–62. PubMed PMID: 21830264. Pubmed Central PMCID: 3116981.

Lorenzo-Zuniga V, de Vega VM, Domenech E, Cabre E, Manosa M, Boix J. Impact of capsule endoscopy findings in the management of Crohn's disease. Dig Dis Sci. 2010;55(2):411–4.. PubMed PMID: 19255845.

Ludvigsson JF, Bai JC, Biagi F, Card TR, Ciacci C, Ciclitira PJ, et al. Diagnosis and management of adult coeliac disease: guidelines from the British Society of Gastroenterology. Gut. 2014;63(8):1210–28. PubMed PMID: 24917550. Pubmed Central PMCID: 4112432.

Maiden L, Thjodleifsson B, Theodors A, Gonzalez J, Bjarnason I. A quantitative analysis of NSAID-induced small bowel pathology by capsule enteroscopy. Gastroenterology. 2005;128(5):1172–8. PubMed PMID: 15887101. Epub 2005/05/12. eng.

Makins R, Blanshard C. Guidelines for capsule endoscopy: diagnoses will be missed. Aliment Pharmacol Ther. 2006;24(2):293–7. PubMed PMID: 16842455.

Mark Feldman LSF, Brandt LJ. Sleisenger & Fordtran's gastrointestinal and liver disease : pathophysiology, diagnosis, management. 10th ed. Philadelphia: Saunders; 2016.

Mata A, Bordas JM, Feu F, Gines A, Pellise M, Fernandez-Esparrach G, et al. Wireless capsule endoscopy in patients with obscure gastrointestinal bleeding: a comparative study with push enteroscopy. Aliment Pharmacol Ther. 2004;20(2):189–94. PubMed PMID: 15233699.

Maunoury V, Savoye G, Bourreille A, Bouhnik Y, Jarry M, Sacher-Huvelin S, et al. Value of wireless capsule endoscopy in patients with indeterminate colitis (inflammatory bowel disease type unclassified). Inflamm Bowel Dis. 2007;13(2):152–5. PubMed PMID: 17206697.

May A, Wardak A, Nachbar L, Remke S, Ell C. Influence of patient selection on the outcome of capsule endoscopy in patients with chronic gastrointestinal bleeding. J Clin Gastroenterol. 2005;39(8):684–8. PubMed PMID: 16082277.

McAlindon ME, Sanders DS, Sidhu R. Capsule endoscopy: 10 years on and in the frontline. Frontline Gastroenterolo. 2010;1:82–7.

Middleton KR, Hing E. National Hospital Ambulatory Medical Care Survey: 2004 outpatient department summary. Adv Data. 2006;23(373):1–27. PubMed PMID: 16841784.

Min YW, Kim JS, Jeon SW, Jeen YT, Im JP, Cheung DY, et al. Long-term outcome of capsule endoscopy in obscure gastrointestinal bleeding: a nationwide analysis. Endoscopy. 2014;46(1):59–65. PubMed PMID: 24254387.

Mitsui K, Tanaka S, Yamamoto H, Kobayashi T, Ehara A, Yano T, et al. Role of double-balloon endoscopy in the diagnosis of small-bowel tumors: the first Japanese multicenter study. Gastrointest Endosc. 2009;70(3):498–504. PubMed PMID: 19555947.

Moglia APA, Cuschieri A. Capsule endoscopy. BMJ. 2009;339:796–9.

Moglia A, Menciassi A, Dario P, Cuschieri A. Capsule endoscopy: progress update and challenges ahead. Nat Rev Gastroenterol Hepatol. 2009;6(6):353–62. PubMed PMID: 19434097. Epub 2009/05/13. eng.

Monteiro S, Boal Carvalho P, Dias de Castro F, Magalhaes J, Machado F, Moreira MJ, et al. Capsule endoscopy: diagnostic accuracy of Lewis score in patients with suspected Crohn's disease. Inflamm Bowel Dis. 2015;21(10):2241–6. PubMed PMID: 26197449.

Myer PA, Mannalithara A, Singh G, Singh G, Pasricha PJ, Ladabaum U. Clinical and economic burden of emergency department visits due to gastrointestinal diseases in the United States. Am J Gastroenterol. 2013;108(9):1496–507. PubMed PMID: 23857475.

Mylonaki M, Fritscher-Ravens A, Swain P. Wireless capsule endoscopy: a comparison with push enteroscopy in patients with gastroscopy and colonoscopy negative gastrointestinal bleeding. Gut. 2003;52(8):1122–6. PubMed PMID: 12865269. Pubmed Central PMCID: 1773749.

Ooka S, Kobayashi K, Kawagishi K, Kodo M, Yokoyama K, Sada M, et al. Roles of capsule endoscopy and single-balloon Enteroscopy in diagnosing unexplained gastrointestinal bleeding. Clin Endosc. 2016;49(1):56–60. PubMed PMID: 26855925. Pubmed Central PMCID: 4743720.

Oresland T, Bemelman WA, Sampietro GM, Spinelli A, Windsor A, Ferrante M, et al. European evidence based consensus on surgery for ulcerative colitis. J Crohns Colitis. 2015;9(1):4–25. PubMed PMID: 25304060.

Papadakis KA, Lo SK, Fireman Z, Hollerbach S. Wireless capsule endoscopy in the evaluation of patients with suspected or known Crohn's disease. Endoscopy. 2005;37(10):1018–22. PubMed PMID: 16189777. Epub 2005/09/29. eng.

Papadopoulos AA, Triantafyllou K, Kalantzis C, Adamopoulos A, Ladas D, Kalli T, et al. Effects of ageing on small bowel video-capsule endoscopy examination. Am J Gastroenterol. 2008;103(10):2474–80. PubMed PMID: 18759823. Epub 2008/09/02. eng.

Papay P, Ignjatovic A, Karmiris K, Amarante H, Milheller P, Feagan B, et al. Optimising monitoring in the management of Crohn's disease: a physician's perspective. J Crohns Colitis. 2013;7(8):653–69. PubMed PMID: 23562672.

Parikh DA, Mittal M, Leung FW, Mann SK. Improved diagnostic yield with severity of bleeding. J Dig Dis. 2011;12(5):357–63. PubMed PMID: 21955428.

Park JJ, Cheon JH, Kim HM, Park HS, Moon CM, Lee JH, et al. Negative capsule endoscopy without subsequent enteroscopy does not predict lower long-term rebleeding rates in patients with obscure GI bleeding. Gastrointest Endosc. 2010;71(6):990–7. PubMed PMID: 20304392.

Payeras G, Piqueras J, Moreno VJ, Cabrera A, Menendez D, Jimenez R. Effects of capsule endoscopy on cardiac pacemakers. Endoscopy. 2005;37 (12):1181–5.. PubMed PMID: 16329014. Epub 2005/12/06. eng.

Pennazio M, Arrigoni A, Risio M, Spandre M, Rossini FP. Clinical evaluation of push-type enteroscopy. Endoscopy. 1995;27(2):164–70. PubMed PMID: 7601049.

Pennazio M, Santucci R, Rondonotti E, Abbiati C, Beccari G, Rossini FP, et al. Outcome of patients with obscure gastrointestinal bleeding after capsule endoscopy: report of 100 consecutive cases. Gastroenterology. 2004;126(3):643–53. PubMed PMID: 14988816.

Pennazio M, Spada C, Eliakim R, Keuchel M, May A, Mulder CJ, et al. Small-bowel capsule endoscopy and device-assisted enteroscopy for diagnosis and treatment of small-bowel disorders: European Society of Gastrointestinal Endoscopy (ESGE) clinical guideline. Endoscopy. 2015;47(4):352–76. PubMed PMID: 25826168.

Petroniene R, Dubcenco E, Baker JP, Ottaway CA, Tang SJ, Zanati SA, et al. Given capsule endoscopy in celiac disease: evaluation of diagnostic accuracy and interobserver agreement. Am J Gastroenterol. 2005;100(3):685–94. PubMed PMID: 15743369.

Petruzzelli M, Vacca M, Moschetta A, Cinzia Sasso R, Palasciano G, van Erpecum KJ, et al. Intestinal mucosal damage caused by non-steroidal anti-inflammatory drugs: role of bile salts. Clin Biochem. 2007;40 (8):503–10. PubMed PMID: 17321514.

Pons Beltran V, Nos P, Bastida G, Beltran B, Arguello L, Aguas M, et al. Evaluation of postsurgical recurrence in Crohn's disease: a new indication for capsule endoscopy? Gastrointest Endosc. 2007;66(3):533–40. PubMed PMID: 17725942.

Postgate A, Hyer W, Phillips R, Gupta A, Burling D, Bartram C, et al. Feasibility of video capsule endoscopy in the management of children with Peutz-Jeghers syndrome: a blinded comparison with barium enterography for the detection of small bowel polyps. J Pediatr Gastroenterol Nutr. 2009;49(4):417–23. PubMed PMID: 19543117.

Quigley EM, Locke GR, Mueller-Lissner S, Paulo LG, Tytgat GN, Helfrich I, et al. Prevalence and management of abdominal cramping and pain: a multinational survey. Aliment Pharmacol Ther. 2006;24(2):411–9. PubMed PMID: 16842469.

Qvigstad G, Hatlen-Rebhan P, Brenna E, Waldum HL. Capsule endoscopy in clinical routine in patients with suspected disease of the small intestine: a 2-year prospective study. Scand J Gastroenterol. 2006;41(5): 614–8. PubMed PMID: 16638706.

Raju GS, Gerson L, Das A, Lewis B, American Gastroenterological A. American Gastroenterological Association (AGA) institute medical position statement on obscure gastrointestinal bleeding. Gastroenterology. 2007a;133(5):1694–6. PubMed PMID: 17983811.

Raju GS, Gerson L, Das A, Lewis B, American GA. American Gastroenterological Association (AGA) institute technical review on obscure gastrointestinal bleeding. Gastroenterology. 2007b;133 (5):1697–717. PubMed PMID: 17983812.

Rex DK, Adler SN, Aisenberg J, Burch WC Jr, Carretero C, Chowers Y, et al. Accuracy of capsule colonoscopy in detecting colorectal polyps in a screening population. Gastroenterology. 2015;148(5):948–57 e2. PubMed PMID: 25620668.

Rex DK, Boland CR, Dominitz JA, Giardiello FM, Johnson DA, Kaltenbach T, et al. Colorectal Cancer screening: recommendations for physicians and patients from the U.S. multi-society task force on colorectal cancer. Am J Gastroenterol. 2017;112(7):1016–30. PubMed PMID: 28555630.

Robinson CA, Jackson C, Condon D, Gerson LB. Impact of inpatient status and gender on small-bowel capsule endoscopy findings. Gastrointest Endosc. 2011;74 (5):1061–6. PubMed PMID: 21924720.

Rondonotti E, Borghi C, Mandelli G, Radaelli F, Paggi S, Amato A, et al. Accuracy of capsule colonoscopy and computed tomographic colonography in individuals with positive results from the fecal occult blood test. Clin Gastroenterol Hepatol. 2014;12(8):1303–10. PubMed PMID: 24398064.

Rosa B, Moreira MJ, Rebelo A, Cotter J. Lewis score: a useful clinical tool for patients with suspected Crohn's disease submitted to capsule endoscopy. J Crohns Colitis. 2012;6(6):692–7. PubMed PMID: 22398099.

Sandler RS, Stewart WF, Liberman JN, Ricci JA, Zorich NL. Abdominal pain, bloating, and diarrhea in the United States: prevalence and impact. Dig Dis Sci. 2000;45(6):1166–71. PubMed PMID: 10877233.

Saperas E, Dot J, Videla S, Alvarez-Castells A, Perez-Lafuente M, Armengol JR, et al. Capsule endoscopy versus computed tomographic or standard angiography for the diagnosis of obscure gastrointestinal bleeding. Am J Gastroenterol. 2007;102(4):731–7. PubMed PMID: 17397406. Epub 2007/04/03. eng.

Scapa E, Jacob H, Lewkowicz S, Migdal M, Gat D, Gluckhovski A, et al. Initial experience of wireless-capsule endoscopy for evaluating occult gastrointestinal bleeding and suspected small bowel pathology. Am J Gastroenterol. 2002;97(11):2776–9. PubMed PMID: 12425547.

Schlag C, Menzel C, Nennstiel S, Neu B, Phillip V, Schuster T, et al. Emergency video capsule endoscopy in patients with acute severe GI bleeding and negative upper endoscopy results. Gastrointest Endosc. 2015;81(4):889–95. PubMed PMID: 25432532.

Shahidi NC, Ou G, Svarta S, Law JK, Kwok R, Tong J, et al. Factors associated with positive findings from capsule endoscopy in patients with obscure gastrointestinal bleeding. Clin Gastroenterol Hepatol. 2012;10(12):1381–5. PubMed PMID: 22975384.

Shi HY, Ng SC, Tsoi KK, Wu JC, Sung JJ, Chan FK. The role of capsule endoscopy in assessing mucosal inflammation in ulcerative colitis. Expert Rev Gastroenterol Hepatol. 2015;9(1):47–54. PubMed PMID: 24966092.

Sidhu R, Sanders DS, Kapur K, Leeds JS, McAlindon ME. Factors predicting the diagnostic yield and intervention in obscure gastrointestinal bleeding investigated using capsule endoscopy. J Gastrointest Liver Dis: JGLD. 2009;18(3):273–8. PubMed PMID: 19795019.

Sidhu R, Brunt LK, Morley SR, Sanders DS, McAlindon ME. Undisclosed use of nonsteroidal anti-inflammatory drugs may underlie small-bowel injury observed by capsule endoscopy. Clin Gastroenterol Hepatol. 2010;8(11):992–5. PubMed PMID: 20692369.

Singh A, Marshall C, Chaudhuri B, Okoli C, Foley A, Person SD, et al. Timing of video capsule endoscopy relative to overt obscure GI bleeding: implications from a retrospective study. Gastrointest Endosc. 2013;77 (5):761–6. PubMed PMID: 23375526.

Spada C, Spera G, Riccioni M, Biancone L, Petruzziello L, Tringali A, et al. A novel diagnostic tool for detecting functional patency of the small bowel: the given patency capsule. Endoscopy. 2005;37(9):793–800. PubMed PMID: 16116528. Epub 2005/08/24. eng.

Spada C, Hassan C, Galmiche JP, Neuhaus H, Dumonceau JM, Adler S, et al. Colon capsule endoscopy: European Society of Gastrointestinal Endoscopy (ESGE) guideline. Endoscopy. 2012;44(5):527–36. PubMed PMID: 22389230.

Spada C, Pasha SF, Gross SA, Leighton JA, Schnoll-Sussman F, Correale L, et al. Accuracy of first- and second-generation Colon capsules in endoscopic detection of colorectal polyps: a systematic review and meta-analysis. Clin Gastroenterol Hepatol. 2016;14 (11):1533–43 e8. PubMed PMID: 27165469.

Spigelman AD, Williams CB, Talbot IC, Domizio P, Phillips RK. Upper gastrointestinal cancer in patients with familial adenomatous polyposis. Lancet. 1989;2 (8666):783–5. PubMed PMID: 2571019.

Swain P. Wireless capsule endoscopy and Crohn's disease. Gut. 2005;54(3):323–6. PubMed PMID: 15710975. Pubmed Central PMCID: 1774425. Epub 2005/02/16. eng.

Tai FWD, McAlindon ME. NSAIDs and the small bowel. Curr Opin Gastroenterol. 2018;34(3):175–82.. PubMed PMID: 29438118.

Takeuchi K. Prophylactic effects of prostaglandin E2 on NSAID-induced enteropathy-role of EP4 receptors in its protective and healing-promoting effects. Curr Opin Pharmacol. 2014;19:38–45. PubMed PMID: 25063918.

Tanaka A, Hase S, Miyazawa T, Ohno R, Takeuchi K. Role of cyclooxygenase (COX)-1 and COX-2 inhibition in nonsteroidal anti-inflammatory drug-induced intestinal damage in rats: relation to various pathogenic events. J Pharmacol Exp Ther. 2002;303(3):1248–54. PubMed PMID: 12438549.

Tatar EL, Shen EH, Palance AL, Sun JH, Pitchumoni CS. Clinical utility of wireless capsule endoscopy: experience with 200 cases. J Clin Gastroenterol. 2006;40(2):140–4. PubMed PMID: 16394875. Epub 2006/01/06. eng.

Tee HP, Kaffes AJ. Non-small-bowel lesions encountered during double-balloon enteroscopy performed for obscure gastrointestinal bleeding. World J Gastroenterol. 2010;16(15):1885–9. PubMed PMID: 20397267. Pubmed Central PMCID: 2856830.

Teshima CW, Kuipers EJ, van Zanten SV, Mensink PB. Double balloon enteroscopy and capsule endoscopy for obscure gastrointestinal bleeding: an updated meta-analysis. J Gastroenterol Hepatol. 2011;26(5):796–801. PubMed PMID: 21155884.

Townsend CO, Sletten CD, Bruce BK, Rome JD, Luedtke CA, Hodgson JE. Physical and emotional functioning of adult patients with chronic abdominal pain: comparison with patients with chronic back pain. J Pain: Off J Am Pain Soc. 2005;6(2):75–83. PubMed PMID: 15694873.

Triester SL, Leighton JA, Leontiadis GI, Fleischer DE, Hara AK, Heigh RI, et al. A meta-analysis of the yield of capsule endoscopy compared to other diagnostic modalities in patients with obscure gastrointestinal bleeding. Am J Gastroenterol. 2005;100(11):2407–18. PubMed PMID: 16279893. Epub 2005/11/11. eng.

Tukey M, Pleskow D, Legnani P, Cheifetz AS, Moss AC. The utility of capsule endoscopy in patients with suspected Crohn's disease. Am J Gastroenterol. 2009;104(11):2734–9. PubMed PMID: 19584828.

Van Gossum A, Munoz-Navas M, Fernandez-Urien I, Carretero C, Gay G, Delvaux M, et al. Capsule endoscopy versus colonoscopy for the detection of polyps and cancer. N Engl J Med. 2009;361(3):264–70. PubMed PMID: 19605831. Epub 2009/07/17. eng.

van Rijn JC, Reitsma JB, Stoker J, Bossuyt PM, van Deventer SJ, Dekker E. Polyp miss rate determined by tandem colonoscopy: a systematic review. Am J Gastroenterol. 2006;101(2):343–50. PubMed PMID: 16454841.

Wadhwa V, Sethi S, Tewani S, Garg SK, Pleskow DK, Chuttani R, et al. A meta-analysis on efficacy and safety: single-balloon vs. double-balloon enteroscopy. Gastroenterolo Report. 2015;3(2):148–55. PubMed PMID: 25698560. Pubmed Central PMCID: 4423464.

Xin L, Liao Z, Jiang YP, Li ZS. Indications, detectability, positive findings, total enteroscopy, and complications of diagnostic double-balloon endoscopy: a systematic review of data over the first decade of use. Gastrointest Endosc. 2011;74(3):563–70. PubMed PMID: 21620401.

Xue M, Chen X, Shi L, Si J, Wang L, Chen S. Small-bowel capsule endoscopy in patients with unexplained chronic abdominal pain: a systematic review. Gastrointest Endosc. 2015;81(1):186–93. PubMed PMID: 25012561.

Yachimski PS, Friedman LS. Gastrointestinal bleeding in the elderly. Nat Clin Pract Gastroenterol Hepatol. 2008;5(2):80–93. PubMed PMID: 18253137. Epub 2008/02/07. eng.

Zallot C, Peyrin-Biroulet L. Clinical risk factors for complicated disease: how reliable are they? Dig Dis. 2012;30(Suppl 3):67–72. PubMed PMID: 23295694.

Zhou Y, Boudreau DM, Freedman AN. Trends in the use of aspirin and nonsteroidal anti-inflammatory drugs in the general U.S. population. Pharmacoepidemiol Drug Saf. 2014;23(1):43–50. PubMed PMID: 23723142.

Gastrointestinal Radiology: A Case-Based Presentation

42

Judith K. Amorosa and C. S. Pitchumoni

Contents

The chapter is a revision (Amorosa and Pitchumoni 2012).

J. K. Amorosa (✉)
Robert Wood Johnson School of Medicine, Rutgers
University, New Brunswick, NJ, USA

Faculty Development and Academic Affairs, Department
of Radiology, RUTGERS Robert Wood Johnson Medical
School, Rutgers University, New Brunswick, NJ, USA

University Radiology Group, East Brunswick, NJ, USA
e-mail: amorosa@rutgers.edu;
judith.amorosa@univrad.com

C. S. Pitchumoni (✉)
Department of Medicine, Robert Wood Johnson School of
Medicine, Rutgers University, New Brunswick, NJ, USA

Department of Medicine, New York Medical College,
Valhalla, NY, USA

Division of Gastroenterology, Hepatology and Clinical
Nutrition, Saint Peters University Hospital, New
Brunswick, NJ, USA
e-mail: pitchumoni@hotmail.com

© Springer Nature Switzerland AG 2021
C. S. Pitchumoni, T. S. Dharmarajan (eds.), *Geriatric Gastroenterology*,
https://doi.org/10.1007/978-3-030-30192-7_36

Abstract

The utility of various endoscopic procedures to visualize the entire gastrointestinal tract (esophagogastroduodenoscopy, wireless capsule endoscopy, and colonoscopy) complements the value of many advanced imaging procedures such as abdominal ultrasound, computerized axial tomography (CT scan), and magnetic resonance imaging (MRI). When properly used, modern imaging techniques substantially help in the early diagnosis of intra-abdominal conditions and assess the severity of several gastrointestinal, pancreatic, and hepatobiliary emergencies. It is essential to be aware of the appropriate indications and the relatively small contraindications to minimize the abuse of the procedures, reduce the cost of care, and avoid overdiagnosis of incidental abnormalities related to an older age. The major contraindication for the techniques is the rare but occasionally life-threatening reaction and renal failure secondary to IV dye. To achieve a balance between the misuse and use with indications, one should be familiar with the American College of Radiology (ACR) guidelines. In this chapter, we have addressed some of the issues and provided images of educational value to the practicing physician.

Keywords

Achalasia · Zenker's diverticula · Carcinoma of the esophagus · Linitis plastica · Gastric cancer · Gastroparesis · GIST tumor · Enteritis · Small intestinal obstruction · Free air · Perforated viscus · Cecal cancer · Sigmoid cancer · Ischemic colitis · Pneumatosis intestinalis · Portal venous air · Diverticulitis · Hepatic metabolism · Intestinal distention · Acute cholecystitis · Gallstones · Porcelain gallbladder · Cystic tumor of the pancreas · Pancreatic cancer · Pancreatic pseudocyst · Walled-off necrosis (WON) · Necrotizing pancreatitis · Infected pancreatic necrosis · Hepatic abscess · Hepatic carcinoma · Computerized axial tomography (CT scan) magnetic resonance cholangiography · Magnetic resonance pancreatic-cholangiography (MRCP) and abdominal ultrasound

Introduction

Dramatic developments have occurred in gastrointestinal (GI) imaging in the past four decades. Two Nobel Prize–winning discoveries followed the discovery of abdominal ultrasound imaging of internal organs, the versatile computed tomography (CT) and magnetic resonance imaging (MRI). What was once a diagnostic imaging technique advanced to "interventional radiology" (IR), referring to a range of methods relying on radiological imaging to target therapy precisely. IR in many instances replaced not only traditional surgery but the minimally invasive procedures resulted in lower costs and better outcomes. During the same period, the field of gastrointestinal endoscopy also advanced. What was only an imaging procedure of the upper (esophagus, stomach, and duodenum) as well as the lower gastrointestinal tract (predominantly the colon) has introduced many endoscopic therapies. The two major fields of radiology and gastrointestinal endoscopy are currently well integrated; the specialties complement each other in early diagnosis and therapeutic choices.

Appropriate Use of Imaging Modalities

In most cases, when appropriately used, the imaging techniques aid in early diagnosis, exclusion of critical disorders, and in assessing the severity of diseases (Iglehart 2006). The distinction between the two major diagnostic specialties, i.e., radiology or endoscopy is blurred. Older adults, in particular, are beneficiaries. Previously older adults were excluded from open or laparoscopic surgical procedures because of age or comorbidities but currently benefit from the new IR therapeutic endoscopy approach (Ray et al. 2017).

Along with the changes, traditional radiology using barium studies fell into disrepute and is currently replaced by the wide use of abdominal sonogram, CT scan, and MRI. The senior radiologists lament the near demise of barium studies. Many believe that barium studies still have a clear advantage over endoscopy for evaluating submucosal and extrinsic mass lesions and diagnosing several postoperative complications (e.g., perforation and obstruction). Fluoroscopic studies with water-soluble contrast material followed by barium are ideal for showing these leak sites and locations (Levine et al. 2008).

Acute abdominal pain is a frequent presentation in older adults, severity ranging from benign to life threatening and is a common diagnostic dilemma. As discussed in another chapter in the book, abdominal pain is a significant diagnostic challenge because of the delay in older adult tending to seek medical attention, the atypical presentations, presence of coexisting diseases, and atypical physical examination findings (Marco et al. 1998). Although economists criticized the increasing cost of care, emergency medicine studies emphasize the importance of early, liberal imaging in the older population with undifferentiated abdominal pain (Marco et al. 1998). The indication for the study and the nature of the study chosen should be appropriate.

The use of ultrasound over CT for right upper quadrant pain is emphasized by the American College of Radiology. In all other instances, CT abdomen has been widely accepted as a valuable imaging modality to evaluate patients with abdominal pain in the emergency department. In assessing any patient with abdominal pain, clinicians emphasize the need for a good history and physical examination before diagnostic tests. In many instances, older adults' unique problems exclude the advantages of a good history and physical examination. Patients may have dementia or anxiety states, precluding a good record. Physical examination in the older adult may be impossible or misleading with many pre-existing conditions. Appropriate and prompt use of Imaging studies can be considered an extension of a physical examination that markedly improves diagnostic accuracy. The early use of CT scanning in evaluating abdominal pain has been accepted based on increased diagnostic certainty, and reduces morbidity and mortality and decreases hospital length of stay. It expedites the admission process (Brenton et al. 2014). The growth in medical imaging over the past few decades has yielded unquestionable benefits to older patients.

Contrast Versus Noncontrast CT Abdomen

The two vexing questions of clinicians are whether to request a noncontrast or contrast-enhanced CT, whether oral contrast will suffice, or IV contrast is essential. An oral contrast agent is used for bowel opacification and is generally a barium and water-soluble iodinated solution. Ingestion of a large volume of contrast material may be difficult or nearly impossible in many older adults and may delay a diagnosis and treatment (Anderson et al. 2009). That the patient has not finished drinking the oral contrast is a frustrating complaint of the ER nurse. However, current research studies support performing CT scans of the abdomen and pelvis without the need for positive oral contrast in most clinical situations (Kielar et al. 2016).

Concern in Using IV Contrast

The concern with the use of IV contrast is the associated increased risk of nephrotoxicity (ACR – Manual on Contrast Media 2012. https://www. acr.org/-/media/ACR/Files/Clinical-Resources/ContrastMedia). A history of multiple drug allergies and asthma increases the risk. Whenever allergy is a consideration, ACR recommends administration of prednisone, 50 mg orally 13, 7, and 1 h before contrast administration; plus diphenhydramine, 50 mg intravenously, intramuscularly, or orally 1 h before contrast administration. A second concern is potential nephrotoxicity. In those with a history of mild to moderate reactions to intravenous contrast agents premedication with antihistamines and corticosteroids is required. The renal status is assessed by a baseline serum creatinine level obtained within a month before administering intravenous contrast agents. Metformin-associated nephrotoxicity and lactic acidosis (MALA) following intravenous contrast media is a concern. Many older adults may be on metformin for type 2 diabetes. Metformin use is likely to increase. Therefore, metformin use should be discontinued when IV contrast is administered and resumed only after careful reevaluation and monitoring of renal status (American College of Radiology. ACR manual on contrast media: version 8 2012. http://www.acr.org/~/media/ACR/Documents/PDF/QualitySafety/Resources/Contrast%20Manual/FullManual.pdf).

Magnetic Resonance Imaging (MRI)

Despite many recent technical advances, the lengthy examination and interpretation times, as well as higher costs, represent barriers to the use (Canellas et al. 2019). The recent development of abbreviated, efficient, and precise MRI protocols represent a growing trend across radiology practices, but are useful for chronic problems. A serious problem is the danger of MRI in older adults with several cardiac implantable electronic devices. The electronic components of pacemakers or an implanted defibrillator can interact dangerously with a large magnet. Even patients forget that they have these devices implanted years earlier. Markedly obese persons may not fit comfortably inside a traditional MRI device. CT scans are cheaper, faster, do not cause claustrophobia, and thus may be a better choice in an emergency. Older adults and their caregivers should be aware of their medical histories and provide information to imaging professionals related to any implanted devices.

Appropriate Use of Imaging

There is a growing concern that medical technology advances are one of the primary drivers of the increase in health-care costs (Iglehart 2006,). The availability of many imaging studies coupled with the uncertainty in diagnosing the cause of abdominal pain in older adults results in overuse and even abuse of the studies. To achieve a balance between the overuse, misuse, and underuse of imaging studies, one should be familiar with the American College of Radiology (ACR) guidelines. Many clinicians request imaging procedures possess little knowledge about the techniques or possible alternative strategies that may yield the same or better information at a reduced cost or with less risk to the patient. Whenever possible, the examining physicians should obtain the history of previous imaging examinations the patients might have undergone to ensure that studies are not duplicated. Duplicate studies are frequent and contribute to medical imaging overutilization (Emanuel et al. 2008).

Although appropriateness criteria are available for many imaging applications, knowledge about them is not widespread or the criteria are ignored. We emphasize the need to be familiar with the American College of Radiology (ACR) Appropriateness Criteria® (AC) for imaging guidelines that rank the most appropriate test for multiple clinical conditions, based on the location of abdominal pain. The ACR Appropriateness Criteria (ACR AC) are evidence-based guidelines created by the American College of Radiology (American College of Radiology. ACR Appropriateness Criteria®. [accessed April 21, 2018]. Available at: http://bit.ly/2NDAbmN). The various guidelines are evidence based for specific clinical conditions reviewed annually by a multidisciplinary expert panel). The practicing clinician should be familiar with the American College of Radiology Appropriateness Criteria and is well advised to refer to the guidelines when in doubt.

A summary of the guidelines is provided here. The summary cites the relevant studies. In the original section by the ACR, there is a list of inappropriate reviews also. For the sake of brevity, we have excluded the list of problematic studies. The ACR guidelines cover various topics. They include: acute nonlocalized abdominal pain, acute pancreatitis, chronic liver disease, colorectal cancer screening, crohn disease, dysphagia, imaging of mesenteric ischemia, left lower quadrant pain–suspected diverticulitis, liver lesion – initial characterization, nonvariceal upper gastrointestinal bleeding, palpable abdominal mass-suspected neoplasm, pancreatic cyst, pretreatment staging of colorectal cancer, right lower quadrant pain–suspected appendicitis, right upper quadrant pain, staging of pancreatic ductal adenocarcinoma, suspected small-bowel obstruction, and jaundice.

A few general principles in performing a CT examination of the abdomen in the older adult are as follows (Rawson et al. 2013). Although there is no direct interaction between metformin and IV radiologic contrast agents, the fact that metformin is actively excreted through the kidneys raises concerns of metformin clearance and metabolic acidosis. The US Food and Drug Administration advises that metformin therapy should be withheld for an IV contrast administration and 48 h afterward, and resumed only after reevaluation of renal status (i.e., return to baseline serum creatinine level) (Figs. 1, 2, 3, 4, 5, 6, 7, 8, 9, 10, 11, 12, 13, 14, 15, 16, 17, 18, 19, 20, 21, 22, 23, 24, 25, 26, 27, 28, 29, 30, 31, 32, 33, 34, 35, 36, 37, 38, 39, and 40).

The following tables are adapted from the ACR criteria (American College of Radiology. ACR Appropriateness Criteria®. [accessed April 21, 2018]. Available at: http://bit.ly/2NDAbmN); the information in the tables are summaries and not full guidelines. The readers are advised to refer to the full text (Tables 1, 2, 3, and 4).

Key Points

1. Modern imaging techniques such as abdominal ultrasound (AUS), computerized axial tomography (CT scan), magnetic resonance imaging (MRI) help in early diagnosis of intra-abdominal conditions, exclusion of critical disorders, and in assessing the severity of gastrointestinal, pancreatic, and hepatobiliary diseases.
2. Endoscopy and imaging studies are complementary.
3. Although traditional radiology using barium studies is replaced mainly by modern imaging techniques, there are limited indications for barium studies. Fluoroscopic studies with water-soluble contrast material are ideal for showing gastrointestinal leaks.
4. The concern with the use of IV contrast is because of the increased risk of nephrotoxicity (ACR 127 – Manual on Contrast Media 2012. https://www.128acr.org/-/media/ACR/Files/Clinical-Resources/129Contrast Media).
5. A history of multiple drug allergies and asthma increases the risk for reaction to IV contrast agents.
6. A serious problem with the use of MRI in older adults is that many may use several cardiac implantable electronic devices. The electronic components can interact dangerously with a large magnet in the MRI machine.
7. To achieve a balance between the overuse, misuse, and underuse of imaging studies, one should be familiar with the American College of Radiology (ACR) guidelines.
8. Although there is no direct interaction between metformin and IV radiologic contrast agents, metformin is actively excreted through the kidneys and raises concerns of metformin clearance and metabolic acidosis.
9. The practicing clinician should be familiar with the American College of Radiology Appropriateness Criteria.
10. The pictures illustrate the most common gastrointestinal disorders with a few classic findings, but the examples are not complete.

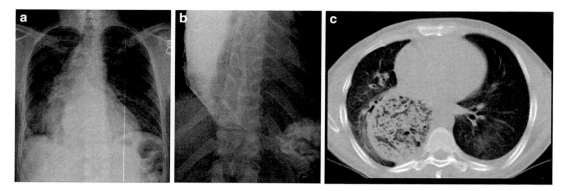

Fig. 1 A 73-year-old woman is evaluated for progressive dysphagia, for solid foods and liquids. She has frequent episodes of regurgitation of undigested food and weight loss. (**a**) PA chest X-ray shows a mass density along the entire right mediastinum (white arrows). (**b**) Axial CT with pulmonary window setting through the lower chest shows particulate material in a distended esophagus. (**c**) Barium esophagogram shows distended esophagus demonstrating beak like narrowing in its distal portion in the area of achalasia. Diagnosis: Achalasia (Vaezi et al. 2013)

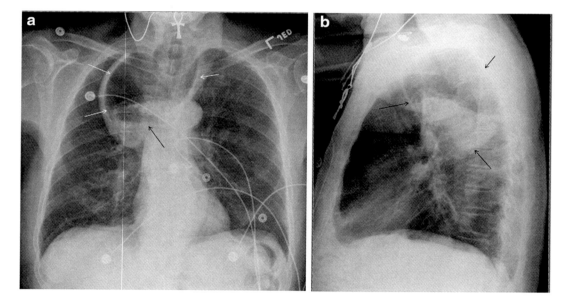

Fig. 2 A 90-year-old man presents with halitosis and otherwise asymptomatic. (**a**) PA chest X-ray shows a large air- fluid (black arrow) containing structure (white arrows) in the upper chest. (**b**) Lateral chest X-ray shows the air-fluid containing structure (black arrows) to be in the superior posterior portion of the chest. This is a large Zenker's diverticulum filled with food. Diagnosis: Zenker's diverticulum (Le Mouel and Fumery 2007)

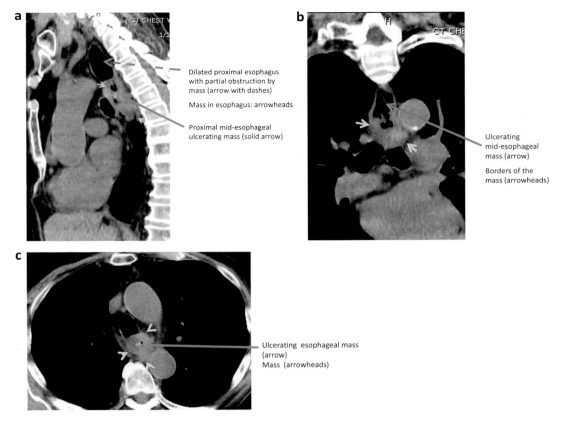

Fig. 3 (a–c) **82-year-old patient with dysphagia. (a)
Sagittal reconstructed chest CT image through the
mid-chest.** Dilated proximal esophagus with partial
obstruction by mass (arrow with dashes). Mass in esophagus: arrowheads. Proximal mid-esophageal ulcerating
mass (solid arrow). **(b) Coronal reconstructed CT scan**
of the Chest through the posterior mediastinum. Ulcerating mid-esophageal mass (arrow). Borders of the mass
(arrowheads). **(c) Axial CT chest image at the Level just
above the carina (arrowheads).** Ulcerating esophageal
mass (arrow). Mass (arrowheads)

Fig. 4 An 80-year-old man
is evaluated for a 3-month
history of progressive, dull,
constant, non-radiating
epigastric pain. The patient
has had weight loss with
early satiety and nausea.
Axial oral contrast-
enhanced CT image at the
level of the gastric fundus
shows a thick infiltrating
mass (white arrows) which
surrounds the irregular
contrast filled lumen.
Diagnosis: Gastric cancer

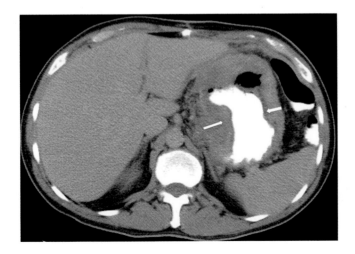

Fig. 5 A 70-year-old woman with long-standing, hard to control type 2 diabetes mellitus is evaluated for a 6-month history of nausea, vomiting, early satiety, and postprandial bloating. Supine abdominal image shows distended, air-filled stomach. Diagnosis: Gastroparesis (Camilleri et al. 2018)

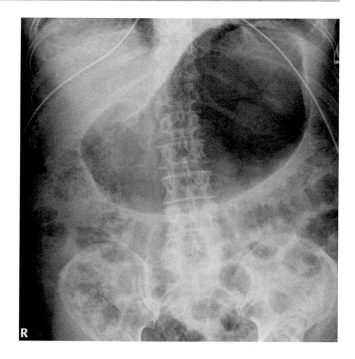

Fig. 6 A 67-year-old man with left upper quadrant abdominal pain, early satiety, and vomiting. Axial oral contrast-enhanced CT image shows contrast in the fundus, a large mass displacing the fundus. The mass contains low density material (probably necrotic tumor. Gastrointestinal stromal tumor GIST

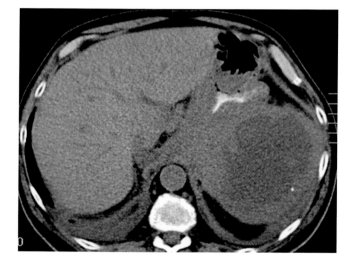

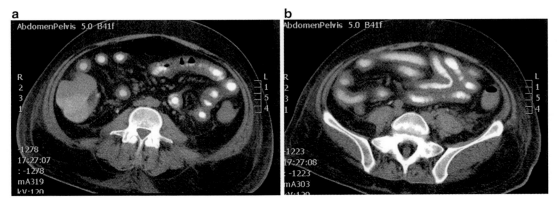

Fig. 7 A 74-year-old woman after returning from a trip developed severe diarrhea and crampy abdominal pain. (**a**, **b**) Axial oral contrast-enhanced CT images in the lower abdomen/upper pelvis level shows diffuse small bowel, predominantly ileal wall thickening without definite obstruction. Diagnosis: Enteritis (Murphy et al. 2015)

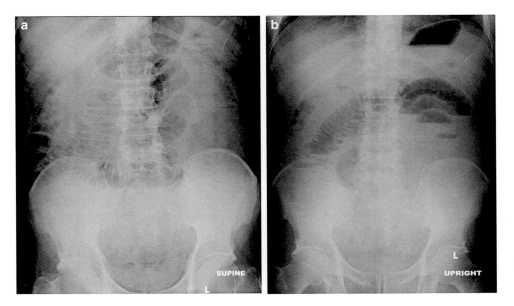

Fig. 8 A 69-year-old man with a history of prior abdominal surgery presents with abdominal distention. (**a**) Supine abdominal image shows distended loops of bowel in the mid abdomen with circumferential markings (valvulae conniventes) indicating the presence of distended small bowel loops. Some air is present in the colon, suggesting the diagnosis of partial small bowel obstruction (SBO). (**b**) Erect, upright abdominal image shows no free air, air fluid levels in the distended small bowel loops are present. Diagnosis: Partial small bowel obstruction

Fig. 9 A 68-year-old woman presents with acute abdominal pain. Supine abdominal image shows previous cholecystectomy and free air. Bowel loops are seen with air on both sides of the intestinal wall (termed the Rigler sign) (black arrow); the area of lucency depicts extra luminal air (asterisks). This is difficult to detect, warranting confirmation with a left lateral decubitus or erect image. Diagnosis: Free air in the peritoneal cavity

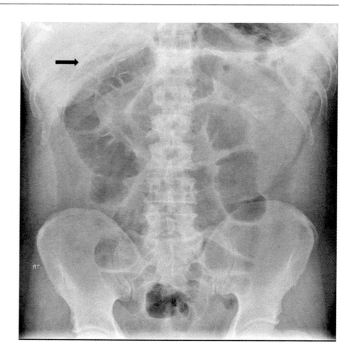

Fig. 10 A 77-year-old man with iron deficiency anemia. Axial oral and intravenous contrast-enhanced CT image through the lower abdomen shows a mass in the cecum (white arrow). Diagnosis: Cecal carcinoma

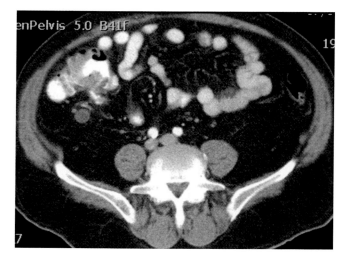

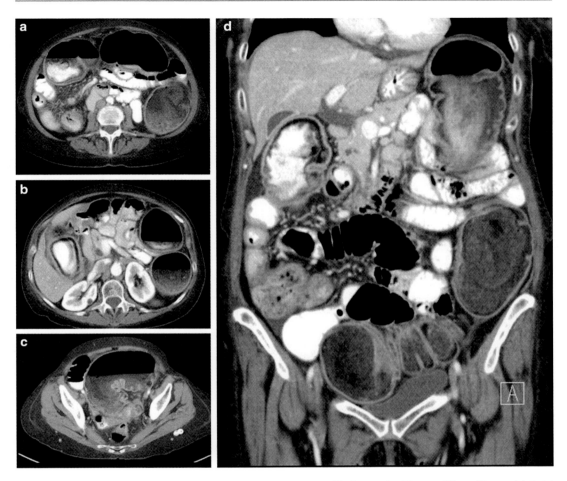

Fig. 11 A 68-year-old woman with distended abdomen and severe constipation. (**a**) Axial oral and intravenous contrast-enhanced CT image through the upper abdomen shows the markedly distended colon. (**b**) Axial oral and intravenous contrast-enhanced CT image through the mid abdomen shows distended, fecal material filled colon. The contrast filled normal caliber small bowel loops. (**c**) Axial oral and intravenous contrast-enhanced CT image through the lower pelvic level shows the distended sigmoid colon and the collapsed rectum. (**d**) Coronal reconstructed CT image through the mid abdomen shows the colonic distention. Diagnosis: Cancer, sigmoid colon, with obstruction

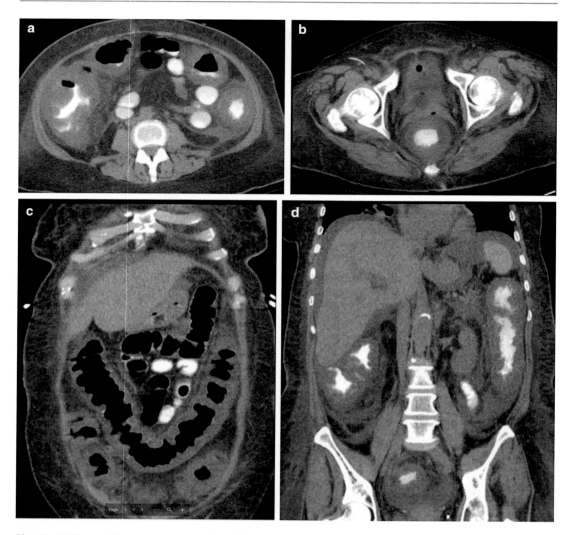

Fig. 12 A 72-year-old man on treatment for malignancy developed severe bloody diarrhea in the last 48 h. (**a**) Axial oral contrast-enhanced CT image through the mid abdomen demonstrates marked thickening of the ascending and descending colon. (**b**) Coronal reconstructed CT image through the anterior shows markedly thickened colonic wall; note that air is present in the nondependent portion of the colon. (**c**) Coronal reconstructed CT image through the posterior abdomen (see vertebrae) shows colonic wall thickening, and of note, contrast in the dependent portion of the colon. (**d**) Axial oral contrast-enhanced CT image through the lower pelvis shows markedly thickened rectal mucosa. Diagnosis: Severe colitis *C. difficle* (Guerri et al. 2019)

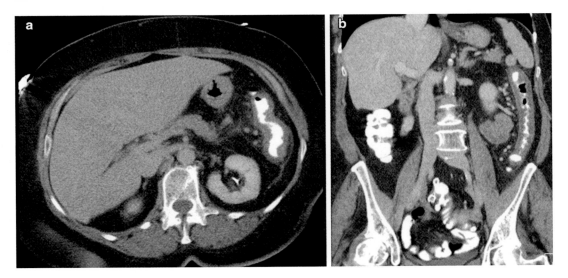

Fig. 13 An 82-year-old man presents with bloody diarrhea. He has a history of coronary artery disease and hyperlipidemia. (**a**) Axial oral and intravenous contrast-enhanced image through the upper abdomen shows at the level of the splenic flexure thick colonic wall suggestive of ischemic colitis. (**b**) Coronal reconstructed image through the mid to posterior abdomen shows a thickened descending colonic wall, with a normal cecum. Diagnosis: Ischemic colitis (Demetriou et al. 2020)

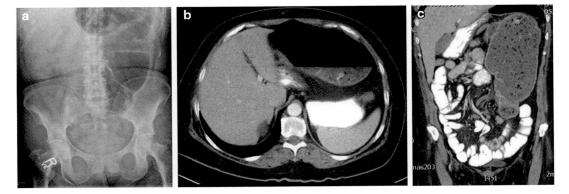

Fig. 14 A 65-year-old woman presents with acute diffuse abdominal pain. (**a**) Supine abdominal image shows a markedly distended air-filled structure in the area of the stomach, with prominent haustral markings. (**b**) Axial oral and intravenous contrast-enhanced image through the upper abdomen shows contrast filled gastric fundus and air and fecal material level in a more anterior structure (*fat containing right adrenal mass, reflecting an adenoma). (**c**) Coronal reconstructed image through the anterior abdomen shows markedly distended cecum filled with fecal material located in the mid to left upper abdomen. Diagnosis: Cecal volvulus (Hasbahceci et al. 2012)

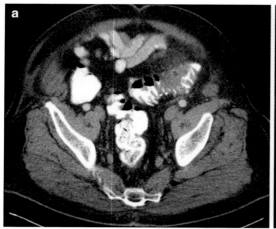

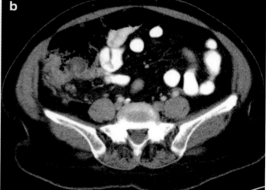

Fig. 15 An 83-year-old man with fever, leukocytosis, left lower quadrant (LLQ) abdominal pain, and tenderness. (**a**) Axial oral and intravenous contrast-enhanced CT image through the mid pelvis with enlargement (inset) shows abnormal sigmoid colon with multiple diverticula. An intramural abscess is apparent, with soft tissue density and an air pocket. Adjacent to the abnormal sigmoid is in filtration of pericolic fat. (**b**) Coronal reconstructed CT image shows the abnormal sigmoid with an intramural abscess with air. Diagnosis: Diverticulitis with abscess (Bates et al. 2018)

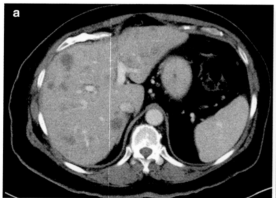

Fig. 16 A 77-year-old man with anemia and RUQ abdominal pain. (**a**) Axial oral and intravenous contrast-enhanced CT image through the upper abdomen shows multiple focal liver lesions. (**b**) Axial oral and intravenous contrast-enhanced CT image through the lower abdomen shows a mass (white arrows) in the cecum. An enlarged mesenteric lymph node is visible (black arrow). Diagnosis: Cecal carcinoma with hepatic metastases

Fig. 17 A 73-year-old man presents with acute abdominal pain. Erect, upright PA (frontal) chest X-ray shows air (black arrow) under the diaphragms indicating free air in the peritoneal cavity, usually from a perforated viscus. Diagnosis: Perforated viscus

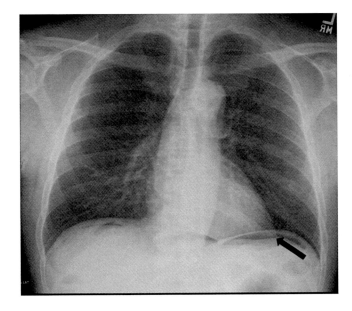

Fig. 18 A 65-year-old woman with prior colectomy now presents with abdominal pain and distension. Supine abdominal image shows surgical clips in the pelvis and distended small bowel loops. Diagnosis: Intestinal obstruction

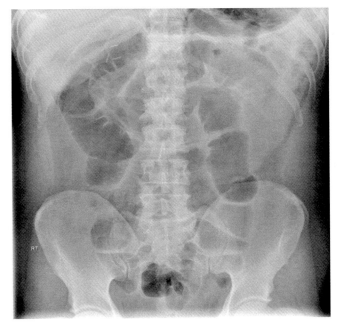

Fig. 19 A 78-year-old woman with prior radiation therapy presents with foul smelling vaginal discharge. Lateral rectal image during gastrographin enema via rectal tube (T) shows a fistulous communication (black arrow) between the rectum (R) and vagina (V). Diagnosis: Rectovaginal fistula

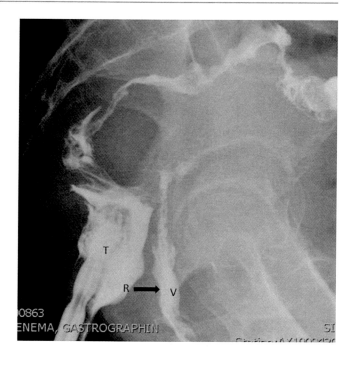

Fig. 20 A 67-year-old woman with a history of previous cholecystectomy has recurrent symptoms of biliary colic. Right upper quadrant ultrasound sagittal image shows a dilated CBD (common bile duct) with two round confirming stones in the CBD (choledocholithiasis). Diagnosis: Choledocholithiasis

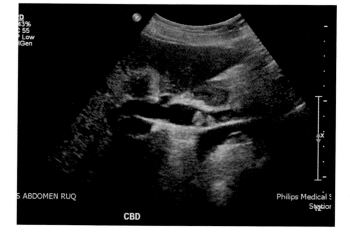

Fig. 21 A 72-year-old woman with RUQ abdominal pain. Hepatobiliary scan shows excretion of the radioactive tracer into the biliary tree and into the duodenum and more distal small bowel. Gallbladder is not seen, indicating occluded cystic duct due to inflammation. Diagnosis: Acute cholecystitis

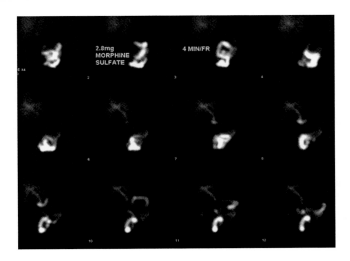

Fig. 22 A 77-year-old woman known to have gallstones presents with RUQ abdominal pain for about 6 weeks; she is afebrile. Oral and intravenous contrast-enhanced CT image through the gallbladder shows thick gallbladder wall (about 6 mm), intermittent gallbladder wall calcification (white arrows), two gallstones, and a mass (black arrows) protruding into the gallbladder lumen. Diagnosis: Gallstones and gallbladder cancer (Sharma et al. 2017)

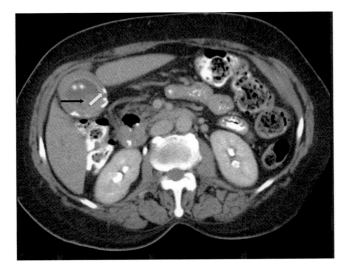

Fig. 23 A 67-year-old woman presents with postprandial RUQ abdominal pain that radiates to her right shoulder accompanied by fever, nausea, and vomiting. Axial oral and intravenous contrast administration through the upper abdomen shows gallbladder wall thickening. Diagnosis: Acute cholecystitis

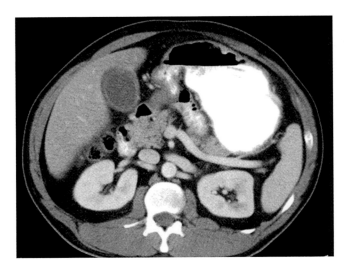

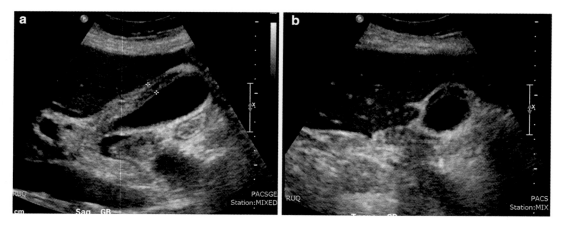

Fig. 24 A 79-year-old man with sepsis, severe RUQ abdominal pain, and tenderness. (**a**) Sagittal real-time ultrasound shows thick gallbladder wall (6 mm) (asterisks).

(**b**) Transverse real-time ultrasound shows thick gallbladder wall (6 mm). Diagnosis: Acute cholecystitis

Fig. 25 A 65-year-old woman with RUQ abdominal pain and tenderness. Right upper quadrant decubitus ultrasound image shows multiple echogenic foci with acoustic shadowing (black arrows) within the gallbladder; these are gallstones (white arrow). Diagnosis: Gallstones

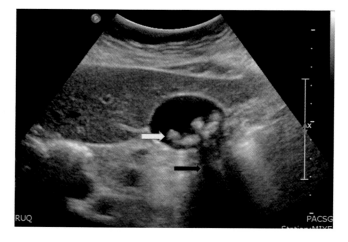

Fig. 26 Porcelain Gallbladder. A rare finding often seen more often in elderly females (Female to male preponderance of 5:1). In the past, it was believed to be associated with gallbladder malignancy. Recent studies have shown 6% increased risk of developing adenocarcinoma in patchy mucosal calcification type as compared with complete intramural type (Stephen and Berger 2001)

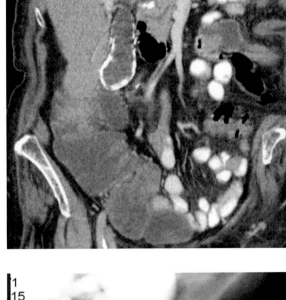

Fig. 27 A 65-year-old woman presents with jaundice. Spot image during ERCP shows catheter (white thin arrow) traversing biliary stricture; a dilated proximal CBD (thick arrow) is present. Diagnosis: CBD stricture. (Courtesy of Satya Kastuar, MD. Saint Peters University Hospital) (Nakai et al. 2020)

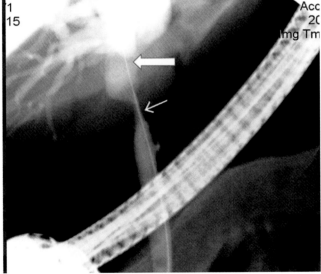

Fig. 28 A 75-year-old patient, incidental detection of a pedunculated gallbladder polyp (Wiles et al. 2017)

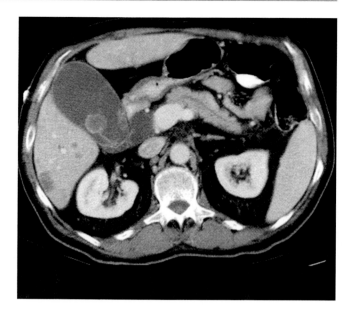

Fig. 29 A 68-year-old woman with a history of cholecystectomy, now status post-ERCP. Erect image of the upper abdomen demonstrates air in the biliary tree (solid black arrow), biliary stent in the CBD, surgical clips for cholecystectomy, and moderately distended stomach. Diagnosis: Air in the biliary tree; stent in place

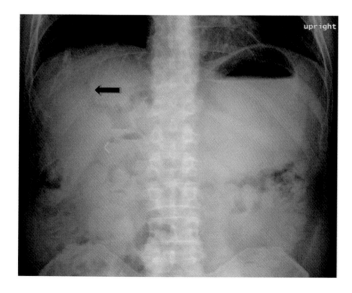

Fig. 30 A 70-year-old woman presents with RUQ abdominal pain and abnormal LFTs. Spot image during ERCP shows the endoscope through which a wire (black arrow) has been introduced into the biliary system. There are three stones (labeled 1, 2, 3) in the dilated CBD. Diagnosis: CBD stones. (Courtesy of Satya Kastuar, MD. Saint Peters, University Hospital)

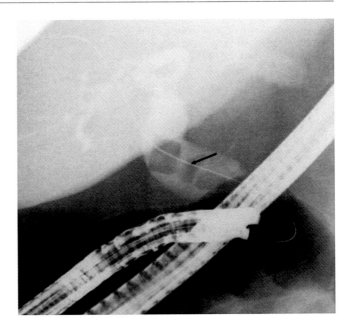

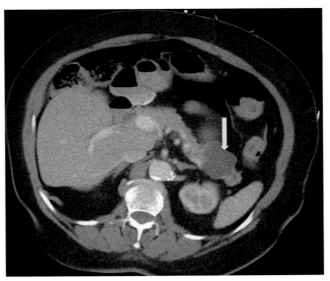

Fig. 31 A 76-year-old asymptomatic man had a chest CT as part of evaluation to exclude lung cancer because of a long history of smoking. On a prior image of that CT a pancreatic mass was suspected, so a dedicated CT abdomen and pelvis was done. Axial intravenous contrast-enhanced CT image at the level of the body and tail of the pancreas shows a 3.5 cm multilobulated mass (white arrow) with low attenuation material (40 HU – soft tissue density, not fluid) with enhancing borders, suggesting a cystic tumor. Diagnosis: Cystic tumor, tail of pancreas (Abdelkader et al. 2020)

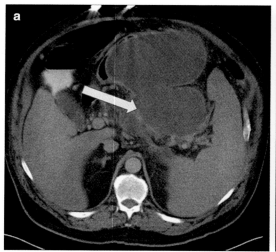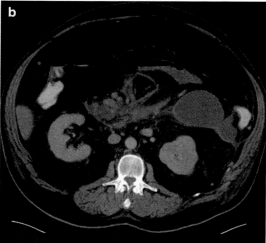

Fig. 32 A 65-year-old man with a history of chronic pancreatitis and severe abdominal pain with vomiting. (**a**) Axial oral and intravenous contrast-enhanced CT image through the upper abdomen shows a large fluid collection anterior to the area of the pancreas; a definite normal pancreas is not identifiable. This collection is displacing the stomach (white arrow). (**b**) Axial oral and intravenous contrast-enhanced CT image through the level of the kidneys demonstrates fluid beyond the tail of the pancreas in the retroperitoneal space; the collection is in the anterior pararenal space. Diagnosis: Pseudocyst of the pancreas (Foster et al. 2016)

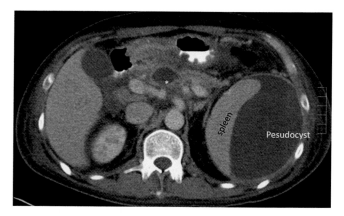

Fig. 33 A 65-year-old man with LUQ abdominal pain. Axial oral and intravenous enhanced CT image through the upper abdomen shows subcapsular fluid collection in the spleen and a small fluid collection (asterisk) in the body of the pancreas with some inflammatory changes anteriorly. Small amount of fluid (white circles) is noted around the head of the pancreas. The recent classification of acute pancreatitis redefines the nomenclature. Diagnosis: Pancreatic pseudocyst (Banks et al. 2013)

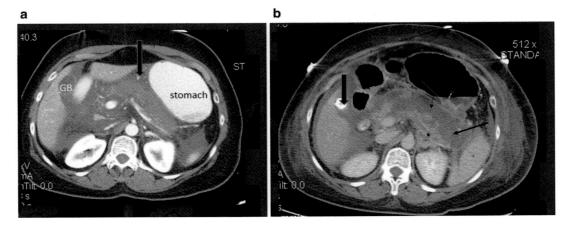

Fig. 34 A 69-year-old woman with severe upper abdominal pain and hypotension. (**a**) On day 1: axial oral and intravenous contrast-enhanced CT image through the upper abdomen shows relative lack of enhancement of the pancreas. There is peripancreatic fluid and ascites (solid black arrows). A gallstone is not visualized within the GB (gallbladder). (**b**) On day 9: axial oral and intravenous contrast-enhanced CT image through the upper abdomen shows necrosis of most of the pancreas; only small portions of the pancreas are identifiable (black arrows). Fluid density is seen in the pancreatic bed. There is splenic venous thrombosis (black arrowhead). On this image a gallstone is visible (black arrow). Diagnosis: Severe acute necrotizing pancreatitis

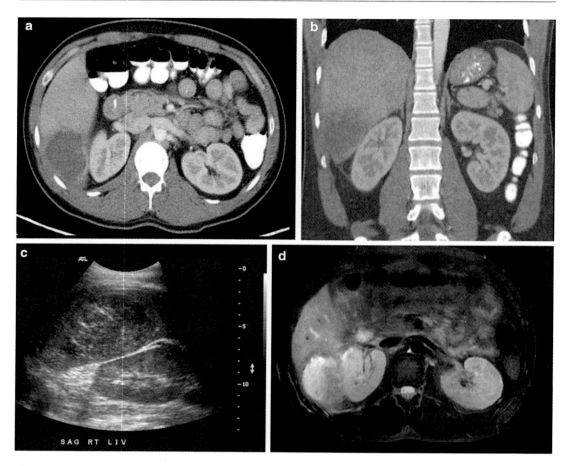

Fig. 35 A 65-year-old woman with fever and RUQ abdominal pain. (**a**) Axial oral and intravenous contrast-enhanced CT image through the mid abdomen shows a focal mass in the right lobe of the liver with low attenuation and slightly irregular border. (**b**) Coronal reconstructed CT image through the posterior abdomen shows a focal mass in the right lobe of the liver. (**c**) Right upper quadrant ultrasound sagittal image shows a complex mass in the liver. (**d**) Magnetic resonance imaging was done to further clarify the nature of this mass and confirmed an enhancing mass suggestive of an abscess. Diagnosis: Hepatic abscess (Khim et al. 2019)

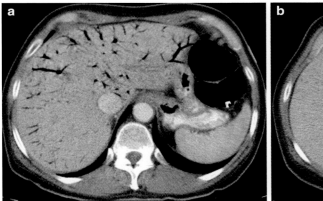

Fig. 36 A 69-year-old man with hepatic encephalopathy. (**a**) Axial intravenous contrast-enhanced CT image through the upper abdomen shows a mass in the liver (black arrows). The liver is small and irregular-cirrhotic. There is splenomegaly; small amount of ascites and large right pleural effusion (white circles), and varices (black circle). (**b**) Sagittal ultrasound image shows the liver mass (white arrows) to be complex consistent with hepatocellular carcinoma. Diagnosis: Hepatic carcinoma

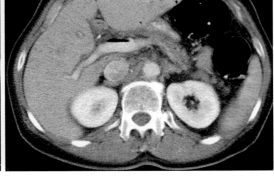

Fig. 37 A 72-year-old man with severe abdominal pain and bloody diarrhea. Axial oral and intravenous contrast-enhanced CT image through the level of the upper abdomen shows air in the portal venous system. Axial oral and intravenous contrast-enhanced CT image through the level of the portal vein shows air-contrast level in the portal vein (black arrow). Axial oral and intravenous contrast-enhanced CT image through the level of the kidneys shows air in the superior mesenteric vein (black arrow). Axial oral and intravenous contrast-enhanced CT image with pulmonary window setting shows air in the bowel wall, suggesting pneumatosis intestinalis (black arrows). Diagnosis: Pneumatosis intestinalis and portal venous air

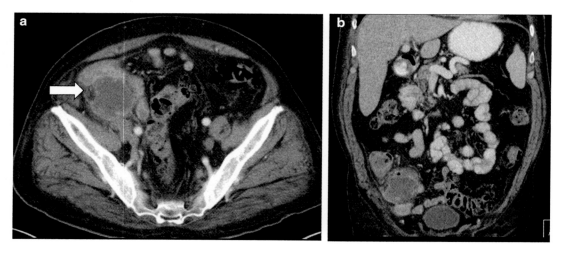

Fig. 38 An 89-year-old man presents with fever, nausea, vomiting, and severe RLQ abdominal pain. (**a, b**) Axial and coronal oral and intravenous contrast-enhanced CT images in the lower abdomen demonstrate a soft tissue mass with fluid and air (white arrow) adjacent to the cecum. The features suggest a perforated appendiceal abscess. Diagnosis: Appendiceal abscess

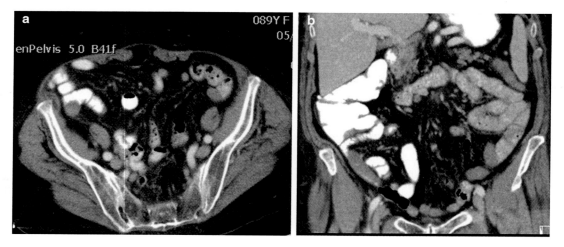

Fig. 39 An 89-year-old woman with RLQ abdominal pain and tenderness. (**a, b**) Axial and coronal oral and intravenous contrast-enhanced CT images through the lower abdomen and pelvis show a dilated appendix, indicative of acute, but not perforated appendicitis (white arrows). Diagnosis: Acute appendicitis

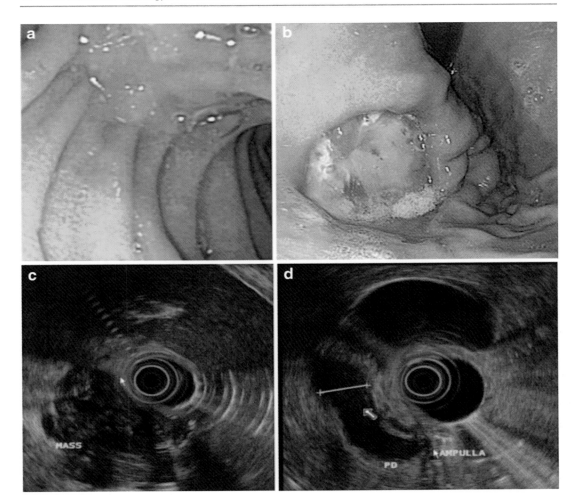

Fig. 40 A 74-year-old man presents with chronic relapsing pancreatitis, weight loss, and steatorrhea. (**a**) Endoscopic view of the major papilla shows a fish mouth papilla secreting mucinous material. (**b**) Retroflexion reveals a deep ulcer in the fundus with mucous adherent to ulcer base. This is secondary to a direct extension to the gastric fold by a malignant intraductal papillary mucinous tumor (IPMT). (**c**) EUS: markedly expanded main pancreatic duct by a heterogeneous head of pancreas mass with irregular borders containing mucinous material. (**d**) EUS: head of pancreas with markedly dilated main pancreatic duct and echogenic material within the duct consistent with mucin. The duct does not manifest any strictures. Diagnosis: Malignant intraductal papillary mucinous tumor. (Courtesy of Hazar Michael, MD. Robert Wood Johnson University Hospital)

Table 1 Acute nonlocalized abdominal pain and fever. No recent surgery. Initial imaging (Summarized from American College of Radiology ACR Appropriateness Criteria)

Procedure	Appropriateness category
CT abdomen and pelvis with IV contrast	**Usually appropriate**
MRI abdomen and pelvis without and with IV contrast	May be appropriate
US abdomen	May be appropriate
CT abdomen and pelvis without IV contrast	May be appropriate
MRI abdomen and pelvis without IV contrast	May be appropriate
CT abdomen and pelvis without and with IV contrast	May be appropriate

Table 2 Acute nonlocalized abdominal pain and fever. Postoperative patient. Initial imaging (Summarized from American College of Radiology ACR Appropriateness Criteria)

Procedure	Appropriateness category
CT abdomen and pelvis with IV contrast	**Usually appropriate**
MRI abdomen and pelvis without and with IV contrast	May be appropriate
US abdomen	May be appropriate
CT abdomen and pelvis without IV contrast	May be appropriate
MRI abdomen and pelvis without IV contrast	May be appropriate
CT abdomen and pelvis without and with IV contrast	May be appropriate

Table 3 Acute nonlocalized abdominal pain. Neutropenic patient. Initial imaging (Summarized from American College of Radiology ACR Appropriateness Criteria)

Procedure	Appropriateness category
CT abdomen and pelvis with IV contrast	**Usually appropriate**
CT abdomen and pelvis without IV contrast	May be appropriate
MRI abdomen and pelvis without and with IV contrast	May be appropriate
US abdomen	May be appropriate
MRI abdomen and pelvis without IV contrast	May be appropriate
CT abdomen and pelvis without and with IV contrast	May be appropriate

Table 4 Acute nonlocalized abdominal pain. Not otherwise specified. Initial imaging (Summarized from American College of Radiology ACR Appropriateness Criteria)

Procedure	Appropriateness category
CT abdomen and pelvis with IV contrast	**Usually appropriate**
CT abdomen and pelvis without IV contrast	Usually appropriate
MRI abdomen and pelvis without and with IV contrast	Usually appropriate
US abdomen	May be appropriate
MRI abdomen and pelvis without IV contrast	May be appropriate
CT abdomen and pelvis without and with IV contrast	May be appropriate

Usually appropriate: Indicated with a favorable risk-benefit ratio for patients, printed in Bold type
May be appropriate. The specified clinical scenarios may be indicated as an alternative to imaging procedures or treatments with a more favorable risk-benefit ratio

References

Abdelkader A, Hunt B, Hartley CP, et al. Cystic lesions of the pancreas: differential diagnosis and cytologic-histologic correlation. Arch Pathol Lab Med. 2020;144(1): 47–61. https://doi.org/10.5858/arpa.2019-0308-RA. Epub 2019 Sep 20. PMID: 31538798

American College of Radiology (2012) ACR manual on contrast media: version 8. http://www.acr.org/~/media/ACR/Documents/PDF/QualitySafety/Resources/Contrast%20Manual/FullManual.pdf. Accessed 21 Nov 2012.

American College of Radiology. ACR appropriateness criteria®. Available at: http://bit.ly/2NDAbmN.

Amorosa JK, Pitchumoni CS. Gastrointestinal radiology. In: Pitchumoni CS, Dharmarajan TS, editors. Geriatric gastroenterology. 1st ed. New York: Springer; 2012. p. 227–247.

Anderson SW, Soto JA, Lucey BC, et al. Abdominal 64-MDCT for suspected appendicitis: the use of oral and IV contrast material versus IV contrast material only. AJR Am J Roentgenol. 2009;193(5):1282–8.

Banks PA, Bollen TL, Dervenis C. Classification of acute pancreatitis – 2012: revision of the Atlanta classification and definitions by international consensus. Gut. 2013;62:102–11.

Bates DDB, Fernandez MB, Ponchiardi C, et al. Surgical management in acute diverticulitis and its association with multi-detector C.T., modified Hinchey classification, and clinical parameters. Abdom Radiol (NY). 2018;43 (8):2060–5. https://doi.org/10.1007/s00261-017-1422-y.

Camilleri M, Chedid V, Ford AC. Gastroparesis. Nat Rev Dis Primers. 2018;4(1):41. https://doi.org/10.1038/s41572-018-0038-z. PMID: 30385743

Canellas R, Rosenkrantz AB, Taouli B, et al. Radiographics. 2019;39(3):744–58.

Demetriou G, Nassar A, Subramonia S. The pathophysiology, presentation and management of ischaemic colitis: a systematic review. World J Surg. 2020;44:927–38.

Emanuel EJ, Fuchs VR. The perfect storm of overutilization. JAMA. 2008;299(23):2789–91.

Foster BR, Jensen KK, Bakis G, Shaaban AM, Coakley FV. Revised Atlanta classification for acute pancreatitis: a pictorial essay. Radiographics. 2016;36(3):675–87. https://doi.org/10.1148/rg.2016150097.

Guerri S, Danti G, Frezzetti G, et al. Clostridium difficile colitis: CT findings and differential diagnosis. Radiol Med. 2019;124(12):1185–98. https://doi.org/10.1007/s11547-019-01066-0.

Hasbahceci M, Basak F, Alimoglu O. Cecal volvulus. Indian J Surg. 2012;74(6):476–9. https://doi.org/10.1007/s12262-012-0432-9.

Iglehart JK. The new era of medical imaging: progress and pitfalls. N Engl J Med. 2006;354(26):2822–8.

Khim G, Em S, Mo S, Townell N. Liver abscess: diagnostic and management issues found in the low resource setting. Br Med Bull. 2019;132(1):45–52. https://doi.org/

10.1093/bmb/ldz032. PMID: 31836890; PMCID: PMC6992887

Kielar A, Patlas MN, Katz DS. Oral contrast for C.T in patients with acute non-traumatic abdominal and pelvic pain: what should be its current role? Emerg Radiol. 2016;23(5):477–81. https://doi.org/10.1007/s10140-016-1403-4.

Levine MS, Rubesin SE, Laufer I. Barium esophagography: a study for all seasons. Clin Gastroenterol Hepatol. 2008;6:11–25. 2015 April 1;91 (7):452–9

Marco CA, Schoenfeld CN, Keyl PM, Menkes ED, Doehring MC. Abdominal pain in geriatric emergency patients: variables associated with adverse outcomes. Acad Emerg Med. 1998;5:1163–8.

Mouel JL, Fumery M. Zenker's diverticuum. N Engl J Med. 2007;377:e31. https://doi.org/10.1056/NEJMicm1701620.

Murphy KP, Twomey M, McLaughlin PD, et al. Imaging of ischemia, obstruction and infection in the abdomen. Radiol Clin N Am. 2015;53(4):847–69. https://doi.org/10.1016/j.rcl.2015.02.008. ix–x. PMID: 26046514

Nakai Y, Isayama H, Wang HP, et al. International consensus statements for endoscopic management of distal biliary stricture. J Gastroenterol Hepatol. 2020;35(6): 967–79. https://doi.org/10.1111/jgh.14955. Epub 2020 Jan 10. PMID: 31802537; PMCID: PMC7318125

Rawson JV, Pelletier AL. When to order contrast-enhanced CT. Am Fam Physician. 2013;88(5):312–6.

Ray D, Srinivasan I, Tang, et al. Complementary roles of interventional radiology and therapeutic endoscopy in gastroenterology. World J Radiol. 2017;9(3):97–111.

Sharma A, Sharma KL, Gupta A. Gallbladder cancer epidemiology, pathogenesis and molecular genetics: recent update. World J Gastroenterol. 2017;23(22): 3978–98. https://doi.org/10.3748/wjg.v23.i22.3978. PMID: 28652652; PMCID: PMC5473118

Stephen AE, Berger DL. Carcinoma in the porcelain gallbladder: a relationship revisited. Surgery. 2001;129(06): 699–703.

Systermans BJ, Devitt PG. Computed tomography in acute abdominal pain: an overused investigation? ANZ J Surg. 2014;84:155–9.

Vaezi MF, Pandolfino JE, Vela MF. ACG clinical guideline: diagnosis and management of achalasia. Am J Gastroenterol. 2013;108:1238–49.

Wiles R, Thoeni RF, Barbu ST, et al. Management and follow-up of gallbladder polyps : joint guidelines between the European Society of Gastrointestinal and Abdominal Radiology (ESGAR), European Association for Endoscopic Surgery and other Interventional Techniques (EAES), International Society of Digestive Surgery - European Federation (EFISDS) and European Society of Gastrointestinal Endoscopy (ESGE). Eur Radiol. 2017;27(9):3856–66. https://doi.org/10.1007/s00330-017-4742-y. Epub 2017 Feb 9

Imaging in Clinical Geriatric Gastroenterology

43

David Hirschl, Melanie Moses, and Rona Orentlicher

Contents

Abstract

Medical imaging is a continuously evolving field which is increasingly utilized for the diagnosis, characterization, and follow-up of innumerable physiological processes. This chapter presents a selection of imaging findings frequently encountered in disease processes of the geriatric gastrointestinal tract. The cases are organized in anatomical order from the esophagus down the alimentary tract and also include a few entities of extraintestinal organs that could be confused with gastrointestinal diseases. The disorders included are those most commonly seen in the geriatric population. They are presented utilizing the imaging modality that most commonly and effectively aids in the diagnosis, along with the typical findings that can be seen. The chapter will help readers better understand the strengths of medical imaging, as well as the modalities that should be considered for delineation of the diverse pathology of gastrointestinal tract disorders in older adults. In addition, key imaging findings that are illustrated in the chapter will help aid in the diagnosis of gastrointestinal disorders in the geriatric population, providing a means to guide subsequent therapy.

Keywords

Imaging for gastrointestinal disorders · Radiology and GI disorders · Imaging for GI disorders · Geriatric imaging · Geriatric radiology · Ultrasound · Magnetic resonance imaging · X-ray · Ultrasound · CT · MRI · Fluoroscopy · Imaging for dysphagia · Isotope scan for gastric emptying · Barium swallow for esophageal disorder · CT scan of abdomen for diagnosis of GI disorders · Air under the diaphragm · Imaging for misplaced feeding tubes · Dislodged feeding tubes · Gastrointestinal stromal tumor · Gastric ulcer · Duodenal ulcer · Diverticular disease · Hepatic cysts · Ultrasound for cysts in the liver · CT abdomen for cystic disease · Hepatic cavernous angioma · Hepatic tumors · Hepatic metastases · Hepatobiliary scan · Gallbladder

D. Hirschl (✉) · M. Moses · R. Orentlicher
Albert Einstein College of Medicine, Montefiore Medical Center, Bronx, NY, USA
e-mail: dhirschl@montefiore.org;
mmoses@montefiore.org; rorentli@montefiore.org

stones · Choledocholithiasis · Biliary sludge · Porcelain gallbladder · Cysts of the liver · Jaundice · Abdominal pain · Abdominal aortic aneurysm · Perforated viscus · Mesenteric vascular ischemia · Perforated viscus · Pneumatosis · Pneumoperitoneum · Colon cancer

Introduction

The diagnostic evaluation of older patients can be challenging. As people age there is a general increase in chronic illness and comorbidities. In addition, older adults may be more prone to acute illness due to infection, which could be more debilitating than in a younger patient. Initial evaluation in the older adult begins with history and physical exam that may be inconclusive or misleading. Communication barriers as a result of neurological disorders associated with aging, including cognitive decline, dementia, memory loss, or stroke, may hinder an adequate history. Furthermore, physical barriers such as immobility, combativeness, contracture, and movement disorders may complicate or confound a physical assessment. Infection can be difficult to diagnose. Characteristic fever and elevated white blood cell count may not always be present. Symptomatic presentations may be less specific due to change in mental status, or malaise. An added complexity is that older patients more often have medical devices such as percutaneous gastrostomy or suprapubic tubes that can be a source of infection or complication.

Due to potential compromise of the patient history and physical examination, and even the decreased sensitivity of laboratory tests, radiological imaging is often essential to make the correct diagnosis in older adults.

The images from multiple cases presented in this chapter include various common conditions throughout the gastrointestinal tract in anatomical order. A few disease entities of neighboring structures that can be mistaken for gastrointestinal disease are included. Diagnosis of gastrointestinal disorders in geriatric patients is often made radiographically, using computerized tomography, ultrasound, fluoroscopy, magnetic resonance imaging, and nuclear medicine imaging. The imaging modality used is the most effective for making the diagnosis. Characteristic imaging findings are delineated. Although fluoroscopy is essential to evaluate motility and often necessary to evaluate patency of bowel, as well as placement and position of tubes, CT is the most utilized modality due to its ready availability, rapid scan time, and ease of use, especially in patients in poor medical condition. In addition, CT is often optimal for evaluation because of its range of coverage, ability to evaluate vascular flow, and delineate structures due to its high contrast resolution, as well as mitigate motion artifact due to the rapid scan time. Additional modalities are often complementary, but can be the test of choice to make the diagnosis. As imaging technologies continue to evolve it may be challenging to choose the most appropriate examination for a particular clinical situation.

The American College of Radiology has developed a set of evidence-based recommendations called Appropriateness Criteria to aid clinicians in imaging study decision making. It can be accessed at: https://www.acr.org/Clinical-Resources/ACR-Appropriateness-Criteria (Figs. 1–81).

Key Points

- Imaging findings in common and uncommon pathologic processes affecting the gastrointestinal system are presented.
- Images are acquired using the most appropriate imaging modality for the pathologic process being investigated.
- Readers are urged to refer to the American College of Radiology appropriateness criteria when unsure of which imaging modality to use in various clinical scenarios.

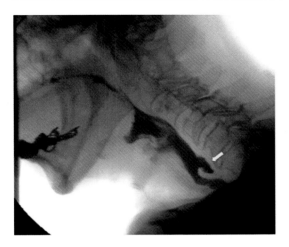

Fig. 1 Zenker's diverticulum in a 91-year-old male with dysphagia and cough on thin liquids. Modified barium swallow demonstrates a posterior outpouching at the junction of the hypopharynx and esophagus (white arrow)

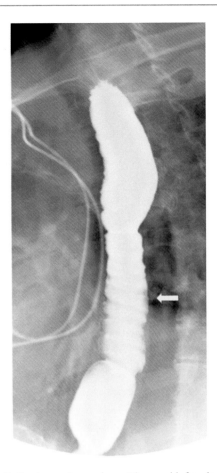

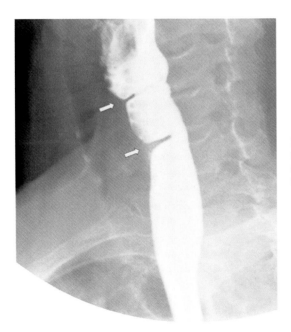

Fig. 3 Presbyesophagus in a 76-year-old female with difficulty swallowing. Barium swallow reveals severe dysmotility with poor stripping wave and extensive tertiary, nonpropulsive contractions (white arrow)

Fig. 2 Esophageal webs in an 86-year-old female with dysphagia. Barium swallow demonstrates two hypopharyngeal and cervical thin fold of tissues (white arrows)

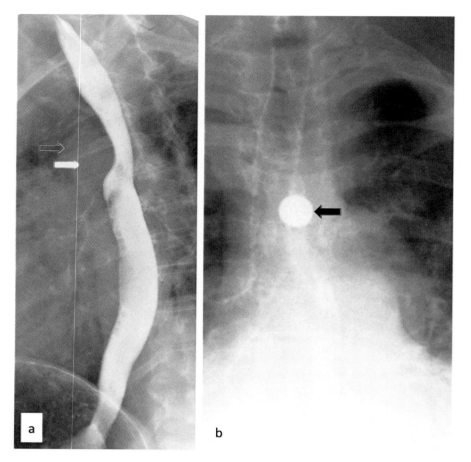

Fig. 4 Esophageal narrowing from ectatic aortic arch in a 90-year-old male with dysphagia. (**a**) Barium swallow-esophageal narrowing at the level of a prominent, ectatic aortic arch (white arrow). (**b**) A barium pill is impacted just proximal to the narrowing (black arrow)

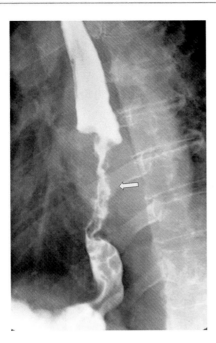

Fig. 5 Esophageal carcinoma in a 78-year-old male with severe dysphagia. Barium swallow demonstrates a 6 cm stricture along the mid esophagus with overhanging edges superiorly and mucosal irregularities (white arrow)

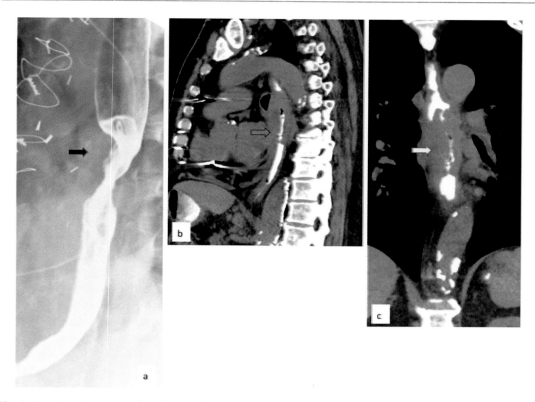

Fig. 6 Esophageal carcinoma in a 78-year-old male with dysphagia. (**a**) Esophagram – irregular stricture along the mid/distal esophagus (black arrow). (**b, c**) CT scan – sagittal and coronal projections: irregular mural thickening and overhanging edges with significant luminal narrowing

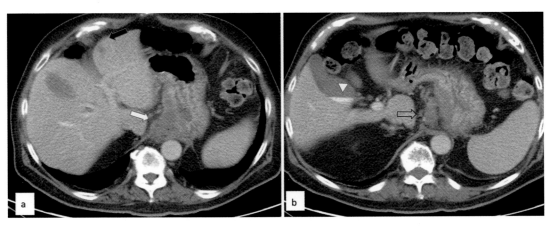

Fig. 7 Metastatic esophageal carcinoma in an 82-year-old female with dysphagia. Contrast enhanced abdominal CT scan: (**a**) soft tissue mass involving the distal esophagus and GE junction (white arrow). Hypodensity in the left hepatic lobe consistent with esophageal metastatic disease (black arrow). (**b**) More inferior image demonstrates peri-gastric lymphadenopathy (clear arrow) and incidental layering gallbladder sludge (arrowhead)

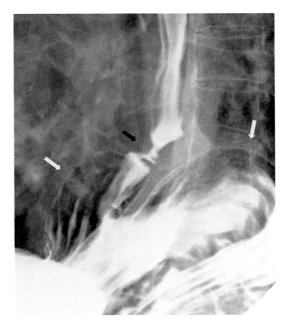

Fig. 8 Sliding hiatal and paraesophageal hernias in an 81-year-old female with heartburn. Upper GI series utilizing barium reveals a portion of gastric body and antrum above the diaphragm (white arrows). A stricture at the gastro-esophageal junction, may be result of instrumentation (black arrow)

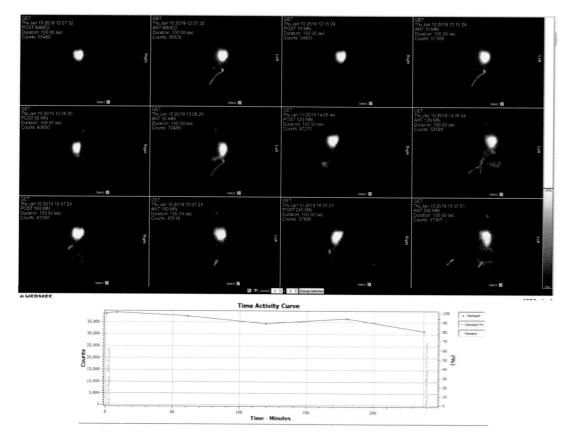

Fig. 9 Gastroparesis in a 66-year-old male with diabetes. Tc-99m labeled sulfur colloid liquid is administered through a gastrostomy tube. Sequential images obtained over the abdomen for 4 hours shows significant delay in gastric emptying, with calculated 81% of activity in the stomach at 4 h (Normal: 0–10%)

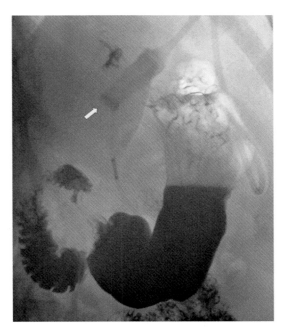

Fig. 10 Bariatric surgery in a 67-year-old female with laparoscopic adjustable banding procedure. Fluoroscopic exam with ingested barium demonstrates band (white arrow) in good position. A small hiatal hernia is seen

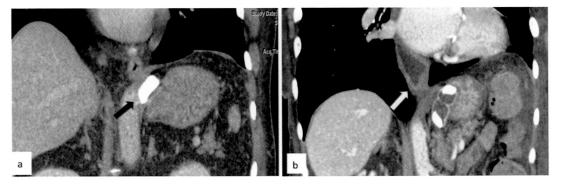

Fig. 11 (**a**) Normal lap band procedure in a 66-year-old male with no symptoms. Coronal CT with lap band (black arrow) in normal position. (**b**) Lap band maladjustment in a 65-year-old female with vomiting and food intolerance. Coronal CT reveals dilatation of the distal esophagus (white arrow) proximal to a lap band that is too tight

Fig. 12 A 66-year-old female status post gastric bypass surgery. CT scan, coronal view, reveals a Roux- en-Y procedure with patent gastrojejunal and jejunal-jejunal anastomoses (arrows)

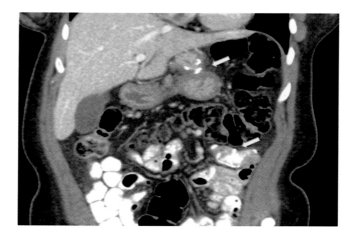

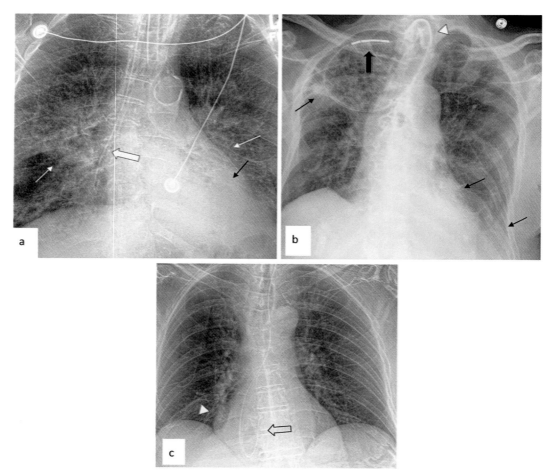

Fig. 13 Malpositioned feeding tubes: (**a**) Feeding tube tip within a right lower lobe bronchus (white arrow). Endotracheal tube in good position. Bilateral pneumonias (thin white arrows) with large left lower lobe consolidation (thin black arrow). (**b**) Feeding tube tip within the right upper pleural space (black arrow). Tracheostomy tube present (arrowhead). Bilateral infiltrates and left pleural effusion (thin arrows). (**c**) Feeding tube tip coiled in a large hiatal hernia (clear arrow). Air and fluid within hernia seen along cardiac border (arrowhead)

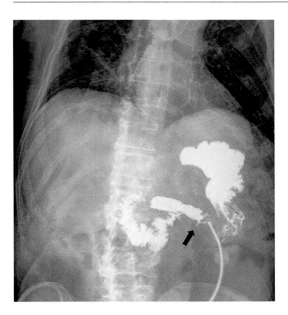

Fig. 14 Normal gastrostomy tube position in an 86-year-old male with dislodged tube which was replaced at the patient's bedside. Frontal radiograph of the abdomen acquired after instilling contrast (Gastrografin) into gastrostomy tube to confirm appropriate positioning. Imaging shows the tip of the catheter to be in the pylorus (black arrow). Contrast is seen in the stomach and duodenum. No extraluminal extravasation is seen

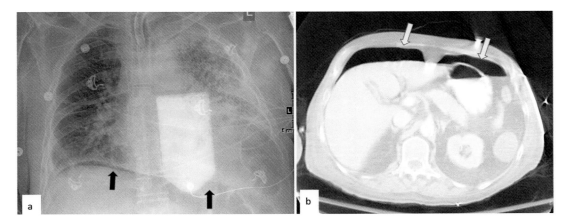

Fig. 15 Free intraperitoneal air related to PEG leak in a 68-year-old male, status post lung transplant. (**a**) Air seen below the diaphragms causing a continuous diaphragm sign (black arrows). (**b**) CT scan, axial view, demonstrates free air along the anterior abdomen (white arrows)

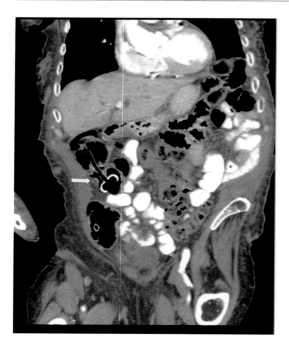

Fig. 16 Dislodged feeding tube in an 86-year-old female. Contrast enhanced CT, coronal view, showing the feeding tube with bumper in the ascending colon (white arrow)

Fig. 17 Dislodged gastrostomy in a 72-year-old male. CT of the abdomen (axial bone windows) demonstrating a dislodged bumper style gastrostomy tube in the left anterior abdominal wall. Note the asymmetric thickening of the wall indicative of a collection (white arrow)

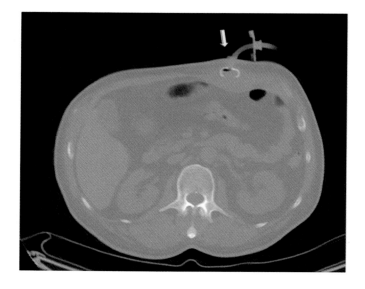

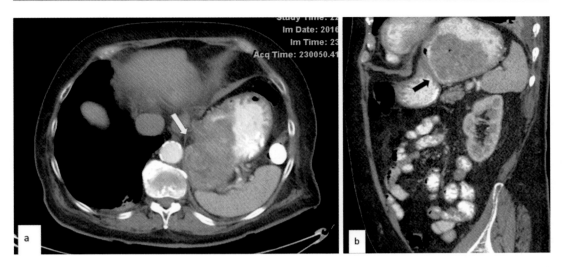

Fig. 18 Invasive gastric adenocarcinoma in a 74-year-old female with vomiting. Abdominal CT with oral and IV contrast. (**a**) Axial view: large polypoid soft tissue mass in the gastric fundus (white arrow). (**b**) Sagittal view: soft tissue mass occupying a large portion of the gastric lumen (black arrow)

Fig. 19 Gastrointestinal stromal tumor (GIST) in a 68-year-old with abdominal pain and bloating. Contrast enhanced CT scan, axial view, reveals a large hypodense mass arising from the stomach (white arrow)

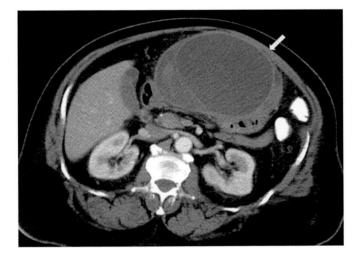

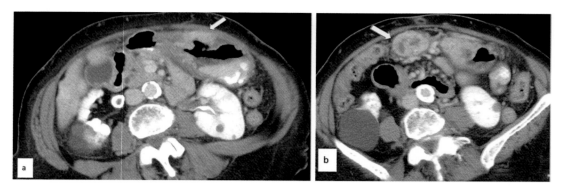

Fig. 20 Malignant gastric ulcer with metastatic lymph-adenopathy in a 77-year-old female with abdominal pain. Contrast enhanced CT scan, axial views, reveals (**a**) large malignant ulcer along anterior gastric fundus with associated wall thickening (white arrow) and (**b**) a necrotic lymph node in the anterior mesentery (white arrow)

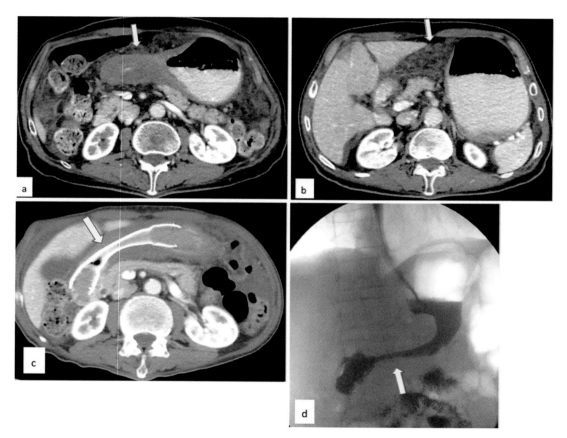

Fig. 21 Metastatic gastric adenocarcinoma in a 75-year-old male. CT scan of the abdomen shows (**a**) a distended partially obstructed stomach due to wall thickening in the distal body and antrum (white arrow) and (**b**) peritoneal carcinomatosis in the gastrohepatic region (white arrow). A gastroduodenal stent was placed and demonstrates patency on (**c**) CT and (**d**) fluoroscopy (white arrows)

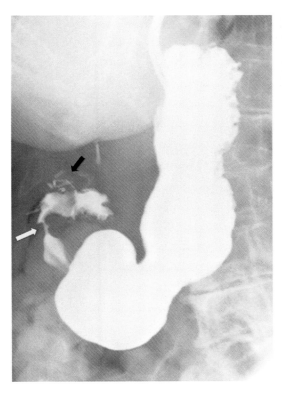

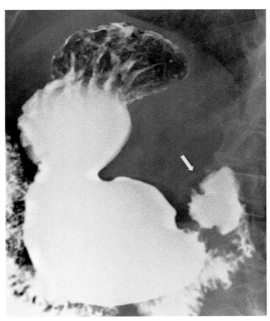

Fig. 23 Chronic changes of peptic ulcer disease in a 74-year-old male. Double contrast upper gastrointestinal series under fluoroscopic guidance reveals a cloverleaf shaped deformity of the duodenal bulb (white arrow)

Fig. 22 Duodenal ulcer in an 88-year-old female with abdominal pain. Single contrast upper gastrointestinal series under fluoroscopic guidance reveals narrowing of the pyloric channel with small ulcer and deformity of the duodenal bulb (white arrow). Right upper quadrant surgical clips (black arrow), status post cholecystectomy

Fig. 24 Gastric ulcer in a 75-year-old with abdominal pain. Upper GI series under fluoroscopic guidance reveals benign appearing ulcer at the antrum (white arrow) with a small leak of contrast (black arrow)

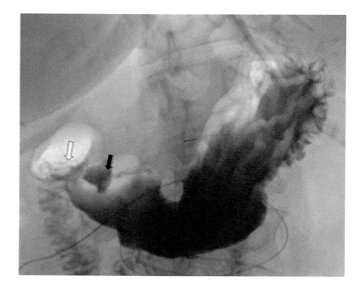

Fig. 25 Duodenal diverticulum in a 75-year-old female with abdominal pain. Upper GI series demonstrates a small diverticulum along the third portion of the duodenum (black arrow)

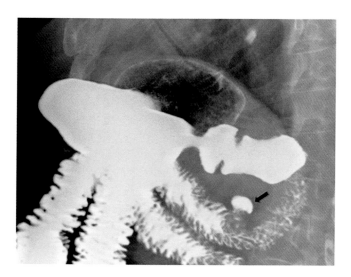

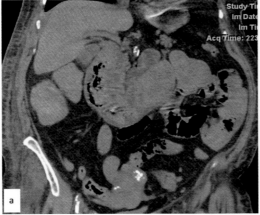
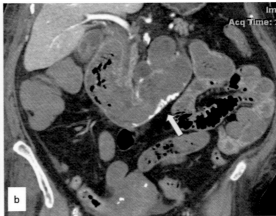

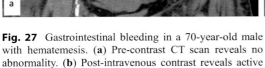

Fig. 26 Duodenal ulcer in an 84-year-old female from a nursing home admitted for an upper GI bleed. On endoscopy, a 2.5 cm ulcer crater with adherent clot was seen in the medial duodenal wall. The duodenum appears normal (white arrow) in Aug 2016 on a CT scan for abdominal pain (**a**). A CT scan performed without IV contrast on Sept 16, 2019, (**b**) shows an air filled ulcer crater (white arrow). A CT scan with IV contrast on Sept 23, 2019, (**c**) shows a layering hypodensity compatible with fluid in the ulcer (white arrow)

Fig. 27 Gastrointestinal bleeding in a 70-year-old male with hematemesis. (**a**) Pre-contrast CT scan reveals no abnormality. (**b**) Post-intravenous contrast reveals active extravasation of vascular contrast in third and fourth segments of duodenum (white arrow)

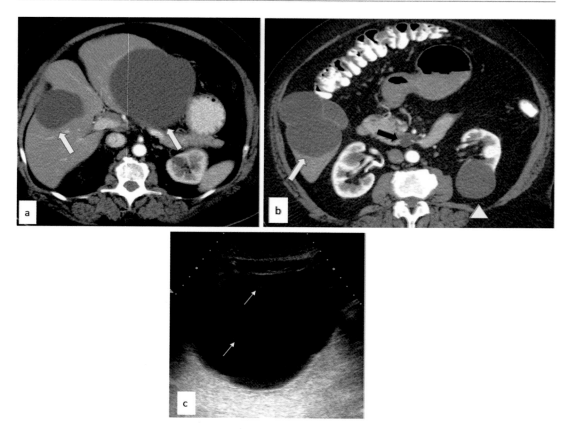

Fig. 28 Hepatic cysts in a 79-year-old female. Contrast enhanced CT scan: (**a**) round low attenuation lesions are seen (white arrows). (**b**) An inferior hepatic cyst demonstrates thin septations (white arrow). Additional cysts in the uncinate process of the pancreas are stable compared to prior studies going back twelve years (black arrow). A cyst is also seen in the left kidney (arrowhead). (**c**) Abdominal ultrasound. An image of the largest cyst shows posterior acoustic enhancement. Internal echoes appear artifactual (white arrows)

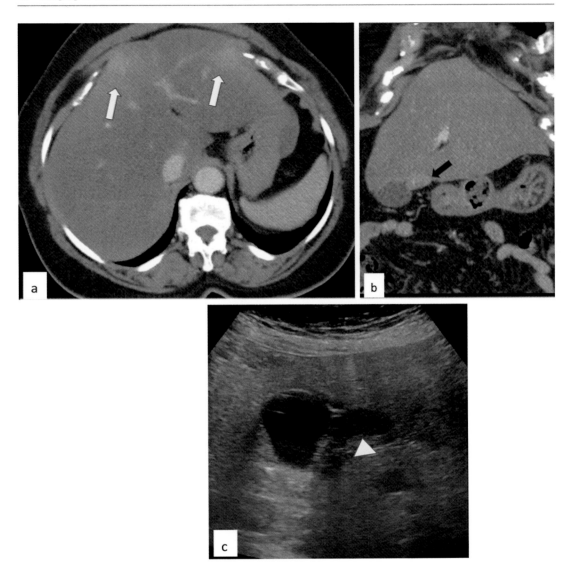

Fig. 29 Fatty infiltration of the liver in a 69-year-old male with elevated liver enzymes. (**a**) Post-contrast CT scan, axial view. Low density liver consistent with fatty infiltration. Areas of focal fatty sparing seen as increased density along the periphery of the liver (white arrows). (**b**) Post-contrast CT scan, coronal view. Area of focal fatty sparing is seen in the region of the gallbladder fossa (black arrow). (**c**) RUQ ultrasound. Focal fatty sparing correlates with a hypoechoic area seen near the gallbladder two weeks earlier (arrowhead)

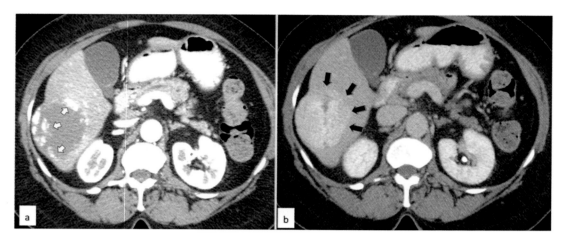

Fig. 30 Hepatic cavernous hemangioma in a 67-year-old female. Post-contrast CT scan: (**a**) Arterial phase- hemangioma reveals characteristic peripheral nodular enhancement (white arrows). (**b**) Delayed venous phase-hemangioma reveals characteristic filling in of contrast (black arrows)

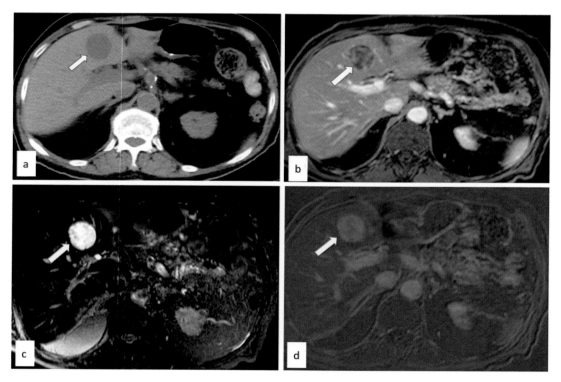

Fig. 31 Right thigh sarcoma with single hepatic metastatic lesion in an 82-year-old male. Abdominal MRI: (**a**) the lesion is hypodense on non-contrast CT (white arrow), (**c**) hyperintense on T2 (white arrow), and (**b**) enhances on contrast enhanced MR. Subtraction image (**d**) reveals internal enhancement. The imaging is characteristic of malignancy

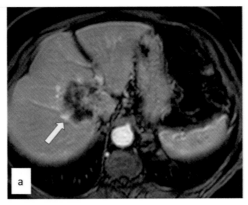

July 2019

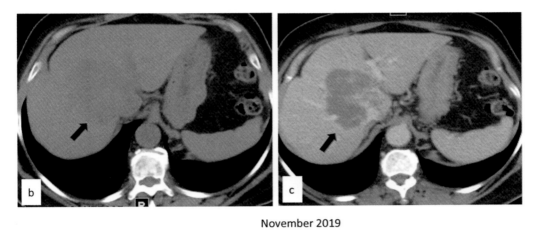

November 2019

Fig. 32 Enlarging cholangiocarcinoma in a 69-year-old female. (**a**) Abdominal MRI with contrast from July 2019 shows a central peripherally enhancing hypointense mass surrounding the intrahepatic IVC and portal veins (white arrow). (**b, c**) Abdominal CT without and with contrast from Nov 2019 again shows enhancement of the hypodense mass and interval enlargement (black arrows)

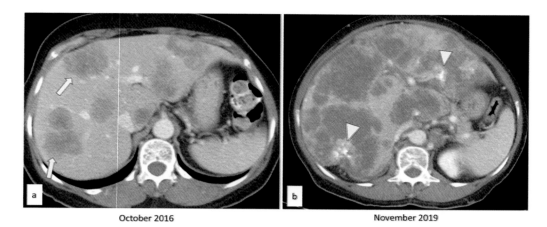

October 2016   November 2019

Fig. 33 Progression of liver metastases from colon carcinoma in a 63-year-old male. Contrast enhanced CT scans, three years apart (**a**, **b**). On the earlier study (**a**), multiple hypoenhancing lesions are consistent with metastatic disease (examples-white arrows). On the later study (**b**), lesions have increased in size and number. Several lesions have calcified and retracted from the liver capsule (arrowheads)

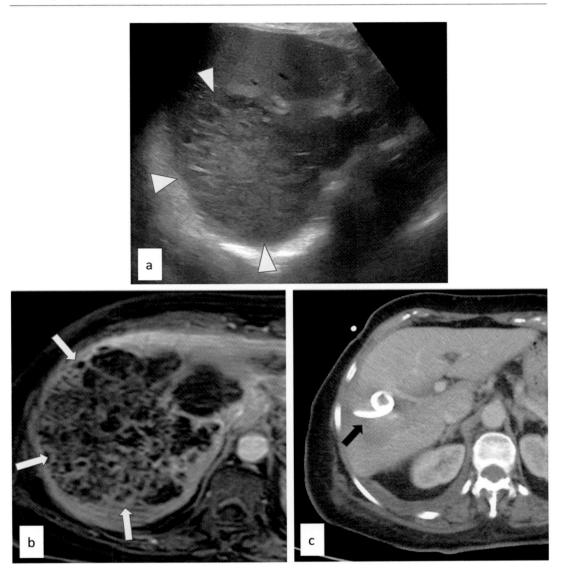

Fig. 34 Hepatic abscess in a 74-year-old female with transaminitis. (**a**) Abdominal ultrasound shows a heterogeneous hepatic mass with ill-defined margins (arrowheads). (**b**) Liver MRI, post-gadolinium T1-weighted image, three days later, shows a complex mass with multiple enhancing septations (white arrow), compatible with an abscess. (**c**) The lesion is significantly smaller after treatment with a drainage catheter (black arrow)

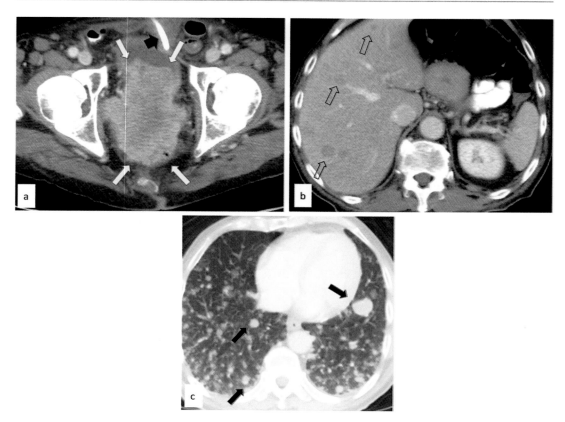

Fig. 35 Metastatic rectal cancer and prostate cancer in a 74-year-old male. Abdominal and pelvic CT scan: (**a**) Axial view of the pelvis shows a lobulated mass that replaces the prostate and seminal vesicles, invades the anterior rectal wall and bladder, and extends along the urogenital tract (white arrows). There is a suprapubic catheter (black arrow). (**b**) Axial view of the liver reveals faint hypodensities with vague rim enhancement consistent with metastases (clear arrows). (**c**) Axial view of the chest with lung windows reveals multiple round pulmonary metastases (black arrows)

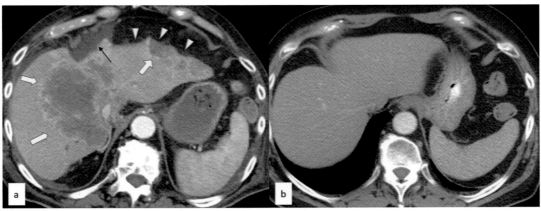

July 2019   December 2010

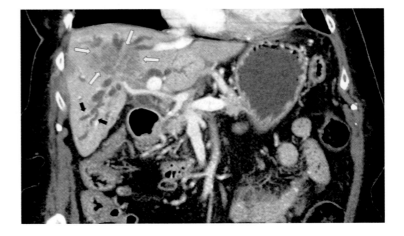

Fig. 36 An 84-year-old male with multiple hepatic hypodense lesions with peripheral vascularity and capsular retraction (arrowheads), consistent with metastases (**a**). The CT scan also shows a small amount of loculated perihepatic ascites (thin arrow). An ultrasound (**c**) shows a heterogeneous liver with a large hypoechoic mass (arrows) surrounding the intrahepatic IVC (arrowhead). The liver is normal on a prior CT scan from Dec 2010 (**b**)

Fig. 37 Klatskin tumor in a 70-year-old male with abdominal pain. Coronal contrast enhanced CT of the abdomen shows a central hypodense mass (white arrows) in the liver causing ductal dilatation (black arrows) of both the right and left biliary tree

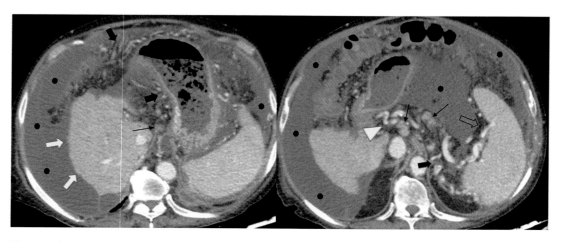

Fig. 38 Liver cirrhosis in a 74-year-old male with a history of alcoholism. The liver is nodular and shrunken (white arrows). There are abundant perigastric and perisplenic collaterals (black arrows). The spleen is enlarged (clear arrow). The main portal vein is attenuated and there are multiple peripancreatic collaterals, consistent with cavernous transformation (arrowhead). There is moderate ascites (black stars) and periportal adenopathy (thin black arrows)

Fig. 39 Gallstones in a 75-year-old male with right upper quadrant pain. Abdominal ultrasound demonstrates highly reflective echogenic foci within the gallbladder lumen with prominent posterior acoustic shadowing consistent with stones (white arrow)

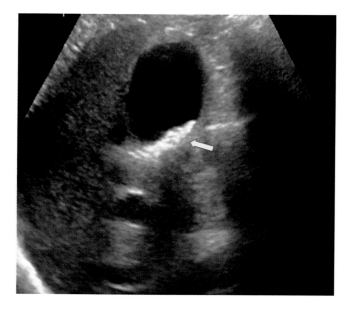

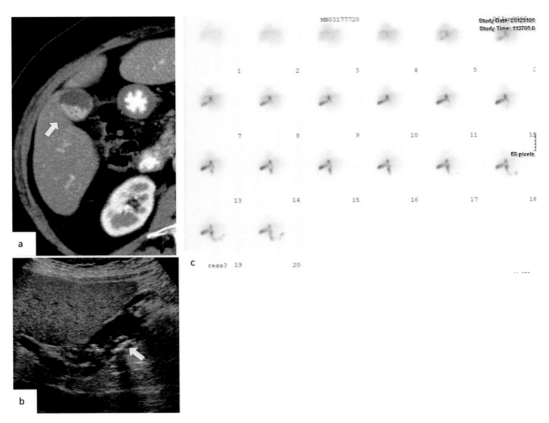

Fig. 40 A 76-year-old female with multiple gallbladder stones and sludge seen on CT (**a**) and ultrasound (**b**) (white arrows). A hepatobiliary scan performed with Tc-99m labeled BRIDA (**c**) shows a patent cystic duct with no evidence of acute cholecystitis. There was, however, an abnormally low ejection fraction consistent with gallbladder dyskinesia

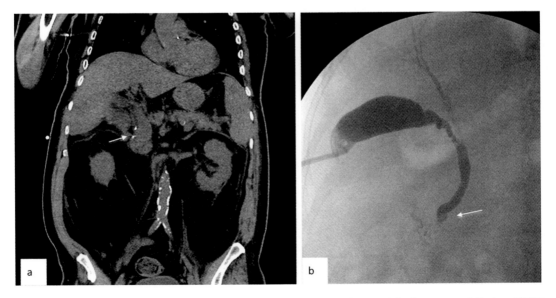

Fig. 41 Choledocolithiasis. Coronal CT (**a**) shows two small calculi (white arrow) in the common bile duct (CBD). Cholangiogram (**b**) shows a filling defect in the distal CBD (thin arrow)

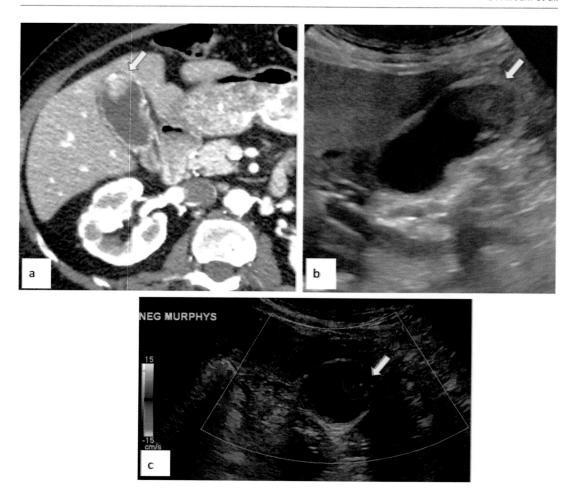

Fig. 42 A 76-year-old female with a mass in the gallbladder fundus consistent with gallbladder carcinoma. A contrast enhanced CT scan of the abdomen (**a**) shows an enhancing mass (white arrow). There is also irregularity and abnormal enhancement of the gallbladder wall. Ultrasound of the abdomen (**b**) from two months prior shows an echogenic mass in the gallbladder fundus, which correlates with the CT finding. Color Doppler (**c**) shows flow within the mass (white arrow), compatible with internal vascularity

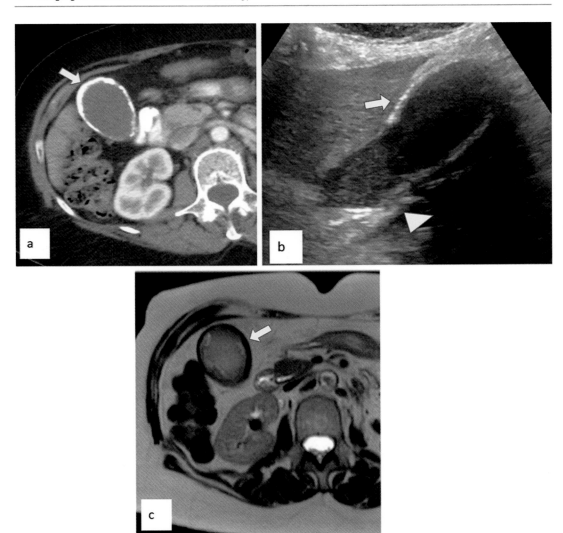

Fig. 43 A 69-year-old female with an incidental porcelain gallbladder. The CT scan (**a**) shows peripheral calcification outlining the gallbladder (white arrow). There is relative increased density within the gallbladder lumen compatible with sludge. The ultrasound (**b**) shows an echogenic thin line in the gallbladder wall (white arrow) with posterior acoustic shadowing (arrowhead). Gallbladder sludge is better seen on the ultrasound. MRI (**c**) signal in the gallbladder wall is compatible with calcification. Signal within the gallbladder is compatible with sludge

Fig. 44 Acute
cholecystitis. Axial contrast
enhanced CT of the
abdomen demonstrating a
hydropically distended
gallbladder with mucosal
thickening and surrounding
stranding indicating the
presence of inflammation
(white arrows)

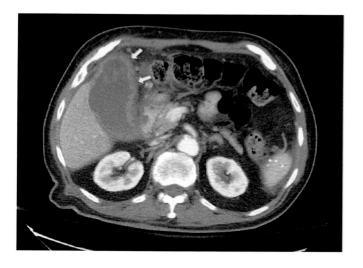

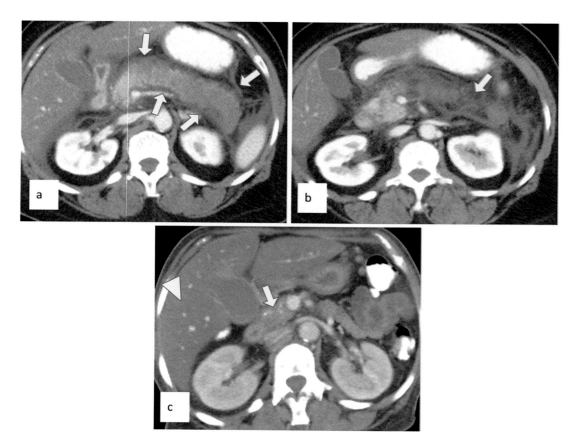

Fig. 45 A 63-year-old female with acute pancreatitis. Contrast enhanced CT. There is enlargement of the gland and peripancreatic fluid, with thickening of the adjacent fascia (**a**, **b**) (arrows). Three years later, the pancreas is normal in size and there are punctate calcifications in the head (arrow), compatible with chronic pancreatitis (**c**). There is also diffuse fatty infiltration of the liver (arrowhead)

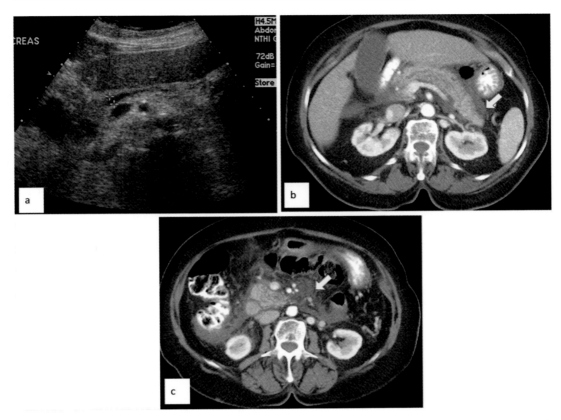

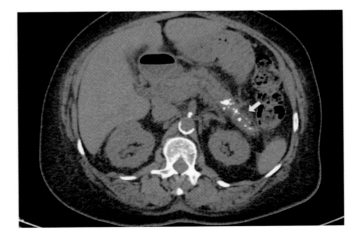

Fig. 46 An 87-year-old male with acute pancreatitis. Ultrasound (**a**) showed mild dilatation of the pancreatic duct. Labs showed an elevated lipase. CT scan (**b, c**) showed peripancreatic fluid (arrows) and mild pancreatic ductal dilatation

Fig. 47 Chronic pancreatitis. CT scan without oral or IV contrast – 65-year-old female with persistent abdominal pain. Extensive calcifications within the pancreatic body and tail (arrow)

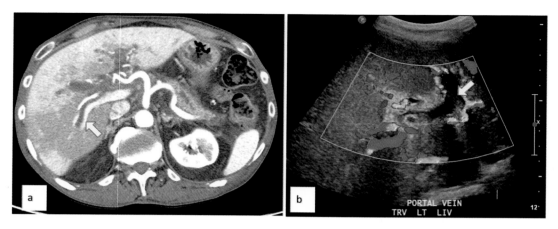

Fig. 48 Portal vein thrombosis in a 71-year-old female with abdominal pain. Contrast enhanced CT (**a**) shows a filling defect extending into the right portal vein (arrow) with associated geographic hypoenhancement of the right hepatic lobe. Ultrasound (**b**) shows lack of color flow in the portal vein (arrow)

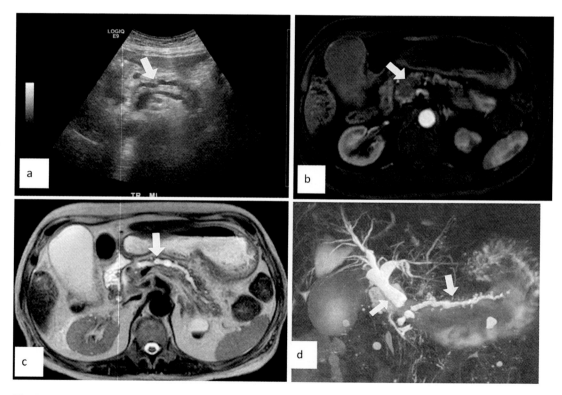

Fig. 49 A 79-year-old male with weight loss, epigastric pain, and hyperbilirubinemia. Ultrasound (**a**) shows pancreatic ductal dilatation (arrow). MRI (**b, c**) revealed a hypointense pancreatic mass that proved to be malignant and pancreatic ductal dilatation (arrows). MRCP (**d**) shows biliary and pancreatic ductal dilatation (arrows)

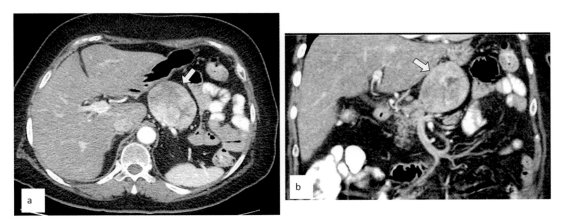

Fig. 50 A 73-year-old female with pancreatic neuroendocrine tumor. Contrast enhanced axial CT (**a**) and coronal CT (**b**) show a well-circumscribed heterogeneously enhancing mass in the mesentery (white arrows)

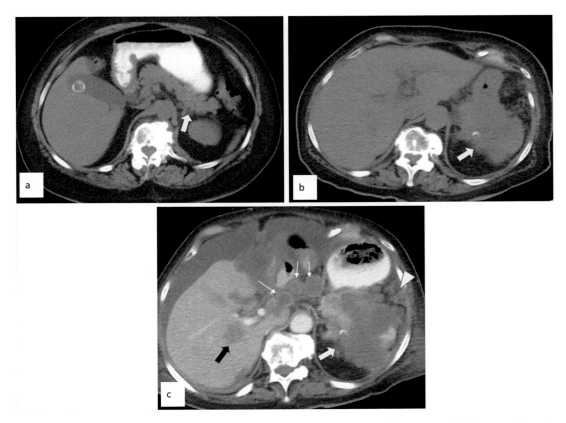

Fig. 51 A 74-year-old male with metastatic pancreatic cancer. (**a**) On a prior non-contrast CT scan from Sept 2012, the pancreas (white arrow) was normal. (**b**) A large mass is in the tail of the pancreas in Sep 2019, on a CT scan performed for RUQ pain and worsening liver function tests (white arrow). (**c**) Two months later on a contrast enhanced CT scan, there is diffuse metastatic disease with peripancreatic and periportal adenopathy (thin white arrows), ascites, liver mets (black arrow), an enlarging heterogeneous necrotic pancreatic mass (white arrow), and peritoneal implants (arrowhead)

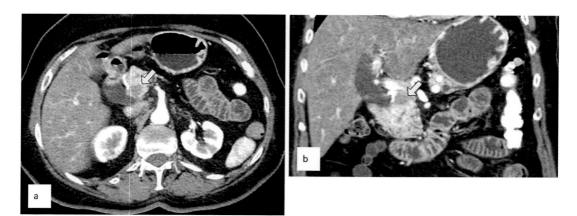

Fig. 52 An 86-year-old female with abdominal pain, jaundice, and scleral icterus had a negative ERCP at an outside hospital and was transferred for further work up. CT scan, axial and coronal images (**a**, **b**), shows a hypodense mass in the head of the pancreas (white arrows). FNA revealed a well-differentiated adenocarcinoma in a background of intraductal papillary mucinous neoplasm

Fig. 53 Superior mesenteric artery (SMA) thrombus. Axial contrast enhanced CT of the abdomen shows a filling defect in the SMA (white arrow)

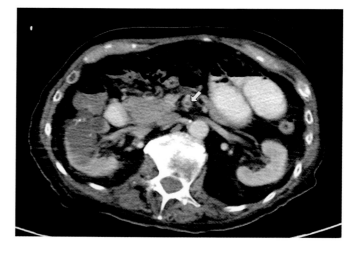

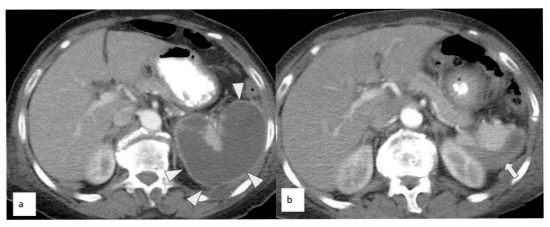

August 29, 2016   January 18, 2017

Fig. 54 A 74-year-old female with a large splenic infarct. The patient presented with new atrial fibrillation and bilateral deep vein thrombosis. Axial contrast enhanced CT (**a**) demonstrates diffuse hypoenhancement of the spleen (arrowheads). The spleen is lobulated and mildly atrophic five months later (**b**) (white arrow)

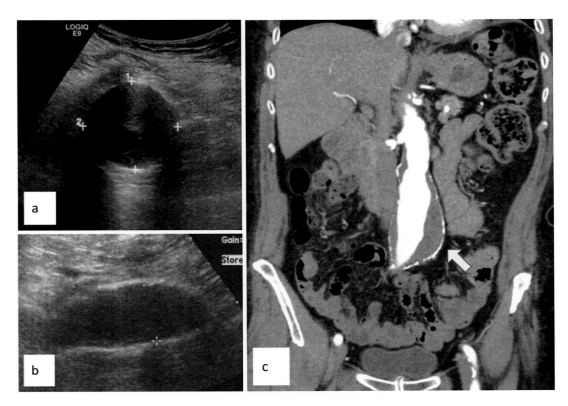

Fig. 55 Infrarenal abdominal aortic aneurysm (AAA) in a 74-year-old female. Ultrasound is the recommended screening method (**a**, **b**). The AAA in this patient measures 4.5 cm in greatest AP dimension (measured in **a**, **b**). There is peripheral thrombus better seen on the CT scan, coronal view (**c**), performed with intravenous contrast for presurgical evaluation (white arrow)

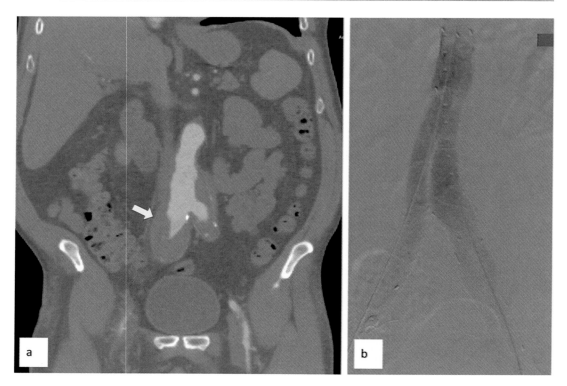

Fig. 56 Abdominal aortic aneurysm (AAA). A coronal image from a contrast enhanced CT (**a**) shows a dilated irregular abdominal aorta with mural thrombus (white arrow). Disease extends into the common iliac arteries bilaterally. Intraoperative angiogram (**b**) showing endovascular repair with placement of an aorto-bi iliac endograft

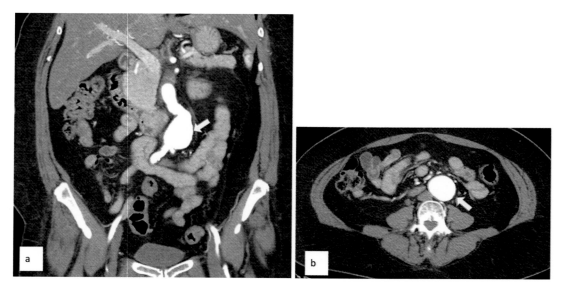

Fig. 57 A 78-year-old with an infrarenal abdominal aortic aneurysm. Coronal (**a**) and axial (**b**) images from a CTA show a tortuous and aneurysmal aorta (arrows)

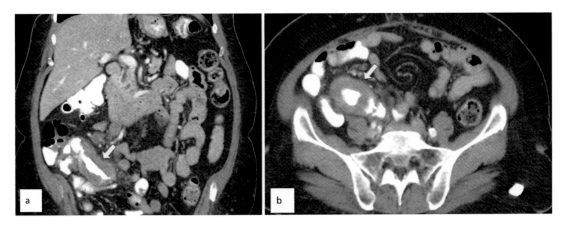

Fig. 58 Small bowel lymphoma: 76-year-old female with diffuse abdominal pain. Coronal (**a**) and axial (**b**) images from a CT scan demonstrate marked circumferential thickening of the terminal ileal wall (arrow). The bowel is not obstructed

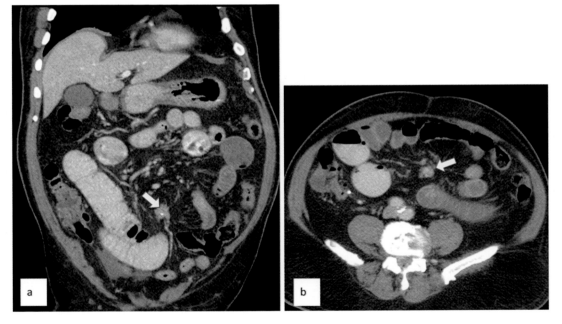

Fig. 59 Carcinoid in an 81-year-old male with abdominal pain. Coronal (**a**) and axial (**b**) images from a CT scan with oral and IV contrast show focal enhancing nodularity with spiculated borders (white arrows) in the mesentery. The findings are characteristic for carcinoid which was diagnosed at surgery

Fig. 60 An 87-year-old with small bowel obstruction secondary to an incarcerated incisional hernia. An axial CT scan image demonstrates a fluid filled segment of bowel with wall thickening and submucosal edema within the subcutaneous soft tissues of the anterior abdominal wall (white arrow). There is an adjacent Richter's hernia (arrowhead). Multiple small bowel loops are dilated

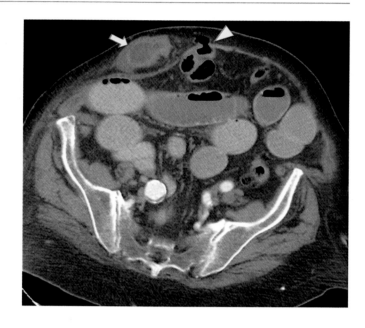

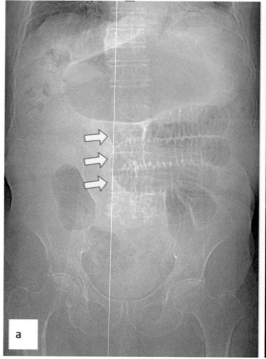
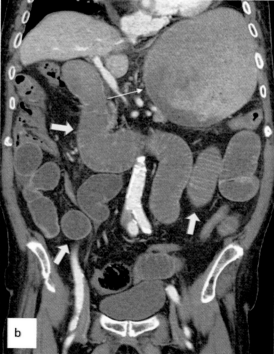

Fig. 61 Small bowel obstruction in an 85-year-old male with diabetes and dementia. The patient presented with vomiting and three days of abdominal pain. CT scan scout view (**a**) reveals multiple dilated small bowel loops in a stepladder appearance (white arrows). A coronal image (**b**) shows multiple dilated fluid filled small bowel loops which resolved with conservative treatment. The stomach is distended (thin white arrow)

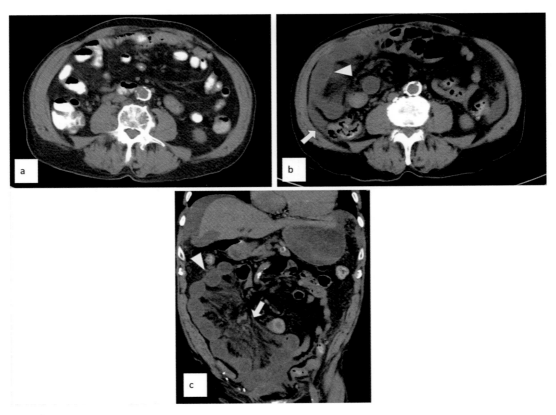

Fig. 62 An 82-year-old male with acute onset lower abdominal pain. Non-contrast CT, axial and coronal views (**b**, **c**), show mesenteric edema and ascites (white arrows), and fluid filled loops of bowel (arrowhead). Prior axial CT (**a**) at a comparable level (top left image) shows normal appearing mesenteric fat

Fig. 63 Acute appendicitis with microperforation in an 84-year-old female who presented with abdominal pain and rectal bleeding. A coronal CT scan image reveals a thick walled appendix with surrounding fatty infiltration and fluid (white arrow). Extraluminal air is consistent with focal perforation (arrowhead)

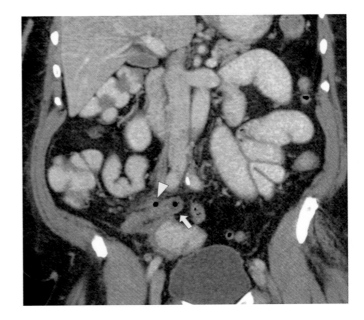

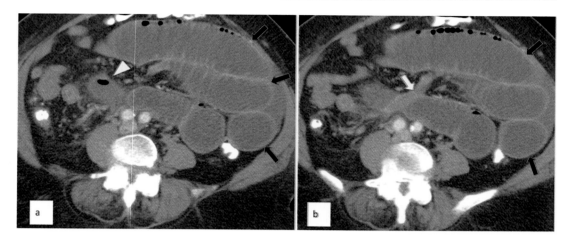

Fig. 64 An 84-year-old female with acute appendicitis. CT scan, axial views (**a**, **b**), reveals multiple dilated, fluid filled small bowel loops (black arrows) secondary to an inflammatory stricture (white arrow) from a fluid and air filled periappendicular abscess (arrowhead)

Fig. 65 A 74-year-old female with abdominal pain has splenomegaly (white arrow) and upper abdominal adenopathy (black arrows) on an axial CT scan image, consistent with known T-cell lymphoma

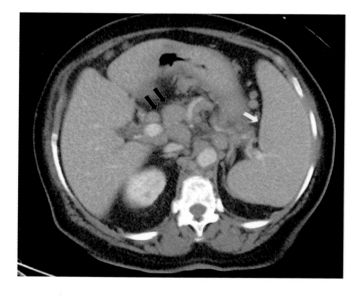

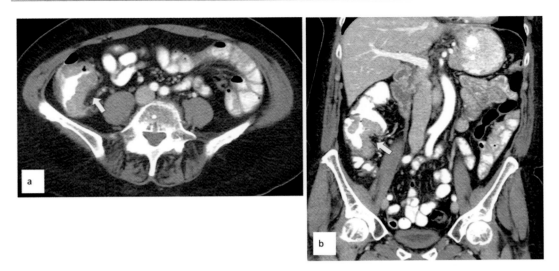

Fig. 66 A 67-year-old presents with unexplained weight loss. A cecal mass is seen on colonoscopy. CT scan, axial and coronal views (**a**, **b**), demonstrates focal, irregular wall thickening of the cecal wall, consistent with carcinoma (white arrows)

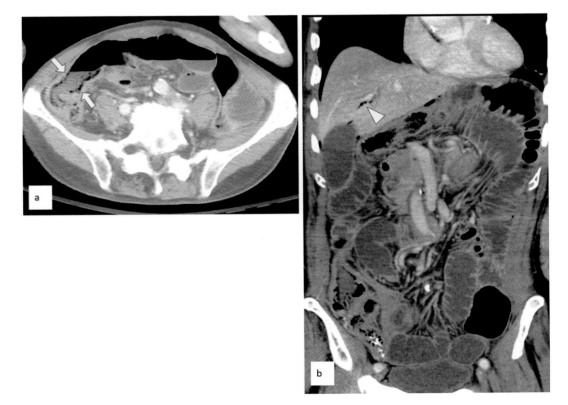

Fig. 67 Colonic pneumatosis with associated portal venous gas in a patient with ischemic bowel. Contrast enhanced axial CT (**a**) shows air on both dependent and nondependent aspects of the cecum (white arrows), consistent with pneumatosis which can be seen with ischemic or infarcted bowel. Coronal reformats (**b**) show air in portal venous branches of segment 4B of the liver (arrowhead). There are multiple fluid filled small bowel loops compatible with an ileus

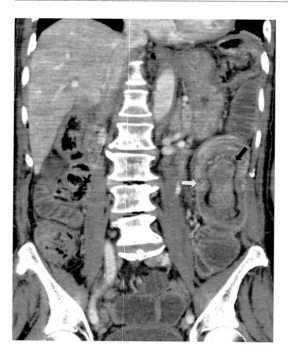

Fig. 68 Colo-colonic intussusception in a 75-year-old with acute abdominal pain. Coronal images from a contrast enhanced CT show a large intussusception of the descending colon (white arrow). Note bowel with surrounding fat, black on CT, surrounded again by bowel. Internal enhancement is suggestive of a colonic mass as a lead point (black arrow)

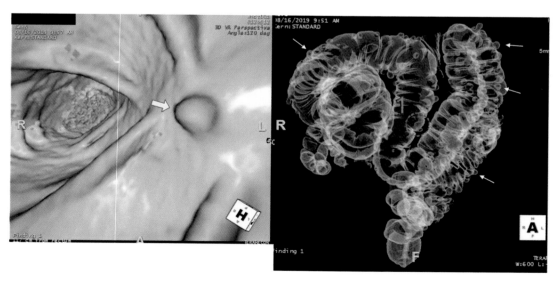

Fig. 69 Screening colonoscopy was incomplete due to severe sigmoid diverticulosis in this 69-year-old. 3D reformatted images from a CT colonography demonstrate an 11 mm polyp in the mid transverse colon (white arrow, red circle). Multiple colonic diverticula are seen on the 3D reformats (e.g., thin white arrows)

Fig. 70 Uncomplicated diverticulitis of the descending colon. Axial non-contrast CT of the abdomen showing stranding and haziness in the pericolonic fat of the descending colon (white arrow)

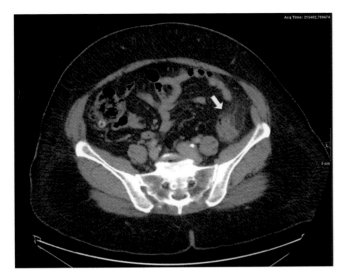

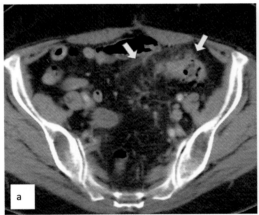 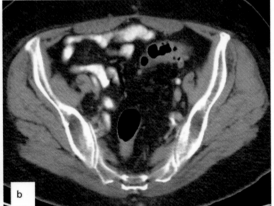

Fig. 71 Acute diverticulitis in a 71-year-old female with lower abdominal pain. CT scan with oral and IV contrast (**a**) demonstrates sigmoid wall thickening and mesenteric fat stranding and edema (white arrows). There is no drainable collection. Follow-up CT scan (**b**) for recurrent abdominal pain 3 months later shows complete resolution of acute inflammatory changes

Fig. 72 An 85-year-old with MALToma (mucosa associated lymphoid tissue), a type of lymphoma on an axial image of a contrast enhanced CT scan (white arrow). There is mass effect on the bladder (black arrow)

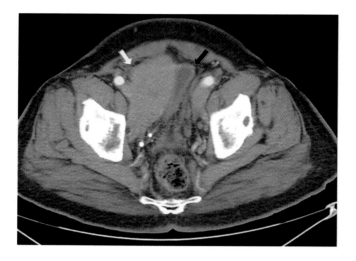

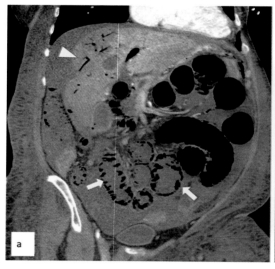

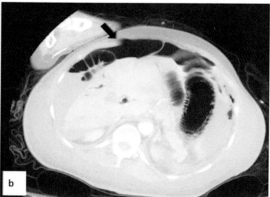

Fig. 73 A 67-year-old female admitted with cardiac arrest, developed abdominal distension and projectile vomiting after 5 weeks in intensive care. CT scan, coronal view (**a**) and axial view with lung window (**b**), shows pneumoperitoneum (black arrow), intestinal pneumatosis (white arrows), and portal venous air (arrowhead) consistent with bowel ischemia and, or infarction. There is also ascites

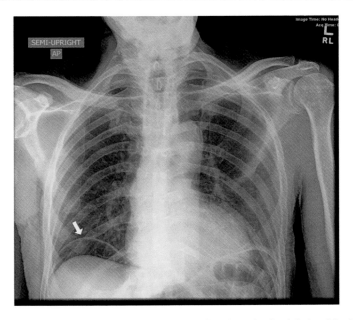

Fig. 74 Pneumoperitoneum. Chest X-ray, frontal view, showing free air under the right hemidiaphragm (white arrow)

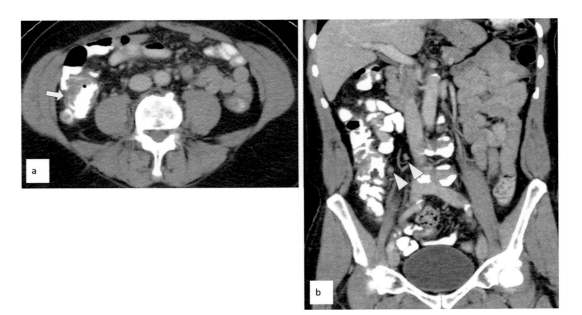

Fig. 75 A 69-year-old male with a history of a right colonic mass presents for evaluation. On a CT scan with oral and IV contrast, axial (**a**) and coronal (**b**) images, a right colonic mass (white arrow) is above the ileocecal valve without obstruction. Pericolonic lymph nodes along the mesenteric border (arrowheads) are suspicious for local spread of disease

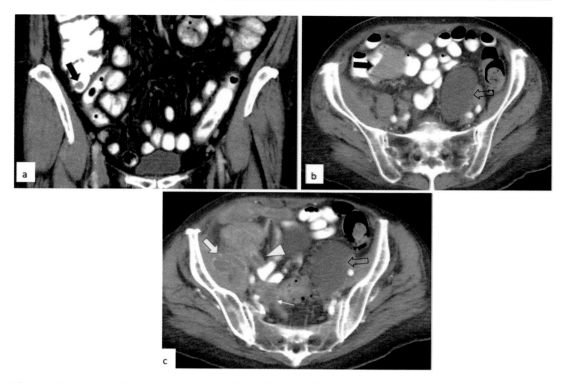

Fig. 76 Enlarging cecal mass in a 91-year-old female. A small cecal polyp (black arrow) was seen on a CT scan in 2010 (coronal image: (**a**) nine years later, the patient presents with abdominal pain and a 4 cm soft tissue cecal mass (black arrow) (axial images: **b**, **c**). The mass obstructs the appendix which is distended with fluid and demonstrates wall thickening and enhancement (arrowhead). The mass extends outside of the cecum to involve the peritoneum and the iliacus muscle. Heterogeneous hypodensity and enhancement in the iliacus is compatible with an abscess (white arrow). A right internal iliac mass is consistent with adenopathy (thin arrow). An incidental slowly growing left adnexal mass measures 7 cm (clear arrow)

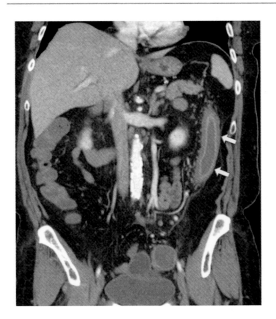

Fig. 77 A 69-year-old male with recurrent ischemic colitis involving the left colon. A coronal CT image shows diffuse wall thickening of the descending colon with mucosal enhancement (white arrows) compatible with colitis

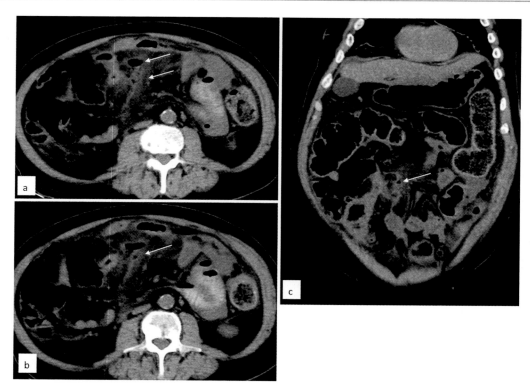

Fig. 78 A 74-year-old male presented to the ER with acute diverticulitis. CT scan, axial (**a**, **b**) and coronal views (**c**), shows focal narrowing and wall thickening in the sigmoid colon, without obstruction. A contained abscess with air and fluid in the adjacent mesentery (thin arrows) formed secondary to local perforation

Fig. 79 A 78-year-old presents with lower abdominal pain. Contrast enhanced CT scan, axial view, reveals acute sigmoid diverticulitis with abscess formation (white arrow)

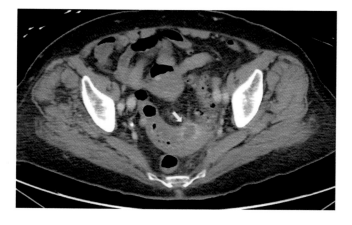

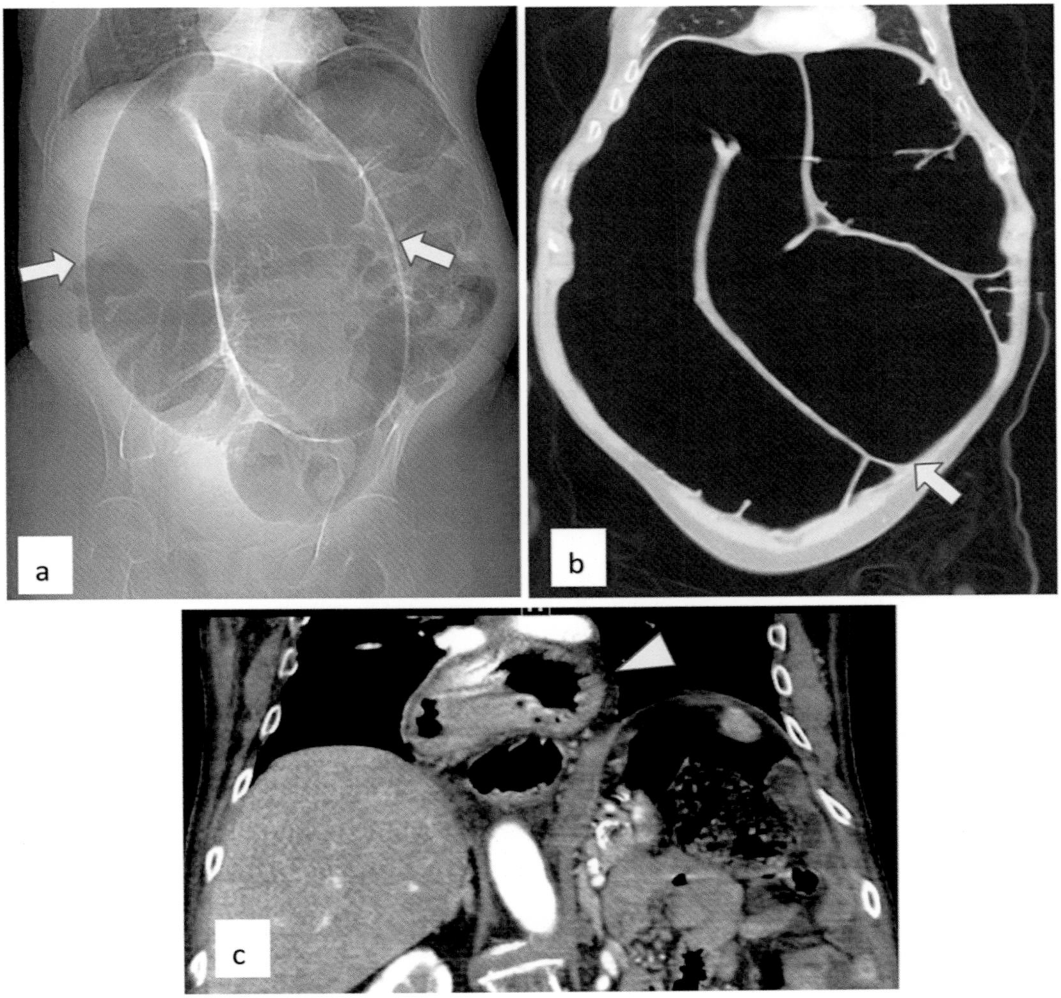

Fig. 80 A 69-year-old male with abdominal distention has a partial sigmoid volvulus. CT scan, scout view (**a**), reveals the classic coffee bean sign of sigmoid volvulus (white arrow). Coronal view (**b**) reveals distended sigmoid colon in a coffee bean appearance (white arrow). Coronal view of the upper abdomen (**c**) reveals an incidental large hiatal hernia (arrowhead)

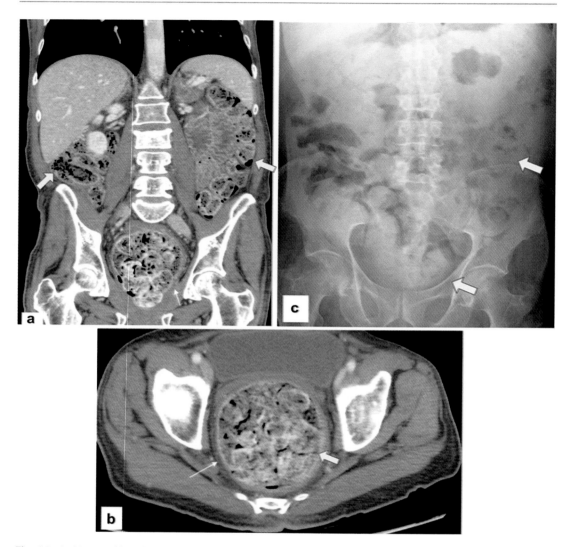

Fig. 81 A 65-year-old male presents to the emergency room with abdominal pain and no bowel movements for several days. CT scan, coronal and axial views (**a**, **b**), and an abdominal x-ray (**c**) show abundant stool throughout the colon and rectum (white arrows), compatible with constipation. There is wall thickening of the rectum and perirectal fat stranding consistent with stercoral colitis (thin arrows)

Advanced Imaging of Geriatric Gastrointestinal Pathology

Fernanda Samara Mazzariol

Contents

Abstract

Gastrointestinal disorders are common in the old; evaluation may utilize one of several available imaging modalities. These include plain abdominal radiographs, fluoroscopic exams, ultrasonography, computed tomography, nuclear medicine scans, and magnetic resonance imaging, each with its own specific applications. In this chapter, we will discuss the applications of magnetic resonance cholangiopancreatography (MRCP), CT colonography, and the imaging of gastrointestinal hemorrhage.

Keywords

CT colonography · MRCP · CT scan · Gastrointestinal bleeding · CT angiogram · Conventional angiography · Acute mesenteric ischemia · Chronic mesenteric ischemia

Introduction

Gastrointestinal ailments in the elderly may affect any part of the gastrointestinal tract from the mouth to the anus and its associated glands.

F. S. Mazzariol (✉)
Radiology, New York Presbyterian Hospital/Weill Cornell Medicine, New York, NY, USA
e-mail: fem9021@med.cornell.edu;
fmazzariolgunduz@gmail.com

© Springer Nature Switzerland AG 2021
C. S. Pitchumoni, T. S. Dharmarajan (eds.), *Geriatric Gastroenterology*,
https://doi.org/10.1007/978-3-030-30192-7_37

While discussion of the appropriate imaging work up of all geriatric gastrointestinal diseases is beyond the scope of this chapter, it is important for the geriatric gastroenterologist to understand the available imaging modalities, their applicability, and pitfalls. The American College of Radiology provides evidence-based guidelines to assist the referring physician in making the most appropriate imaging or treatment decision for specific clinical conditions. Evaluation of biliary and pancreatic diseases may start with ultrasonography but often requires CT scan and MRI/MRCP for a comprehensive evaluation. CT colonography has emerged as alternative or replacement to optical colonoscopy for screening and diagnosis of colonic polyps and cancer due to its tolerability and noninvasive nature, and it is particularly suited to the elderly. The aging population is at an increased risk for gastrointestinal bleeding due to an increased incidence of chronic diseases and greater drug consumption. Timely imaging and image-guided therapy can help decrease geriatric gastrointestinal hemorrhage mortality. In this chapter, we will discuss the applications of magnetic resonance cholangiopancreatography (MRCP), CT colonography, and the imaging of gastrointestinal hemorrhage.

Magnetic Resonance Cholangiopancreatography (MRCP)

MRCP imaging is the mainstay for diagnosis of biliary and pancreatic pathology and helps guide tissue sampling and interventions performed via endoscopic retrograde pancreatography (ERCP). The main indication for MRCP, with or without intravenous contrast, is evaluation of biliary obstruction. Biliary obstruction in the elderly can be caused by stone disease (Fig. 1a, b), malignant or benign strictures (Fig. 2a, b). MRCP is also used to evaluate patients presenting with cholangitis and acute pancreatitis, evaluate and follow-up pancreatic cystic lesions (Fig. 3) and tumors, and to assess exocrine pancreatic function (Palmucci et al. 2017; Manfredi and Pozzi 2016).

CT Colonoscopy

The American Cancer Society (ACS) 2018 recommendation for colorectal cancer (CRC) screening for patients with average risk is high sensitivity stool-based test or visual examination starting at age 45 (qualified recommendation). The ACS strongly recommends CRC screening

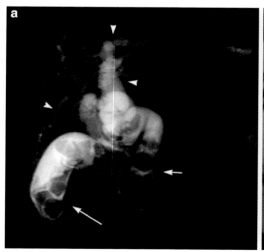
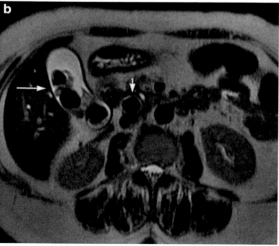

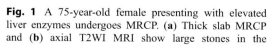

Fig. 1 A 75-year-old female presenting with elevated liver enzymes undergoes MRCP. (**a**) Thick slab MRCP and (**b**) axial T2WI MRI show large stones in the gallbladder (long arrow) and common bile duct (short arrow) and biliary ductal dilatation (arrowheads)

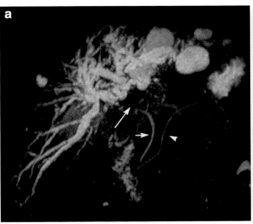
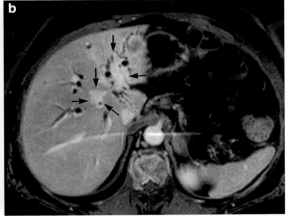

Fig. 2 A 67-year-old male presents with painless jaundice. (**a**) Thick slab MRCP shows intrahepatic biliary ductal dilatation with short segment of non-visualization of the ducts in the porta hepatis (long arrow) and marked intrahepatic biliary ductal dilatation. The normal common bile duct (short arrow) and pancreatic duct are visualized (arrowhead). (**b**) Axial post-contrast T1WI shows ill-defined enhancing masses in the porta hepatis (between arrows) causing biliary obstruction consistent with cholangiocarcinoma, Klatskin tumor

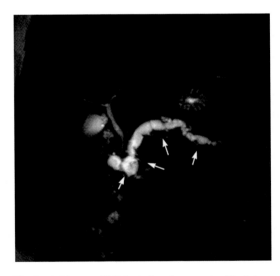

Fig. 3 A 76-year-old diabetic female presents with abdominal pain. CT scan (not shown) showed atrophic pancreas and marked dilatation of main pancreatic duct. MRCP shows dilated pancreatic duct (arrows) most consistent with main duct intraductal papillary mucinous neoplasia (IPMN) of the pancreas. The patient underwent ERCP with sampling of duct fluid. Cytology identified mucin in the fluid without high-grade cellular dysplasia, confirming main duct IPMN

starting at age 50 and older. Average risk adults in good health and with life expectancy greater than 10 years should continue colorectal screening until age 75. CRC screening options for stool based tests are: (a) fecal immunochemical test every year, (b) high-sensitivity guaiac-based fecal occult blood test every year, or (c) multitarget stool DNA test every 3 years. A positive fecal exam should be followed promptly by visual examination. CRC screening options for visual examinations are: (a) conventional optical colonoscopy (COC) every 10 years, (b) CT colonoscopy (CTC) every 5 years, or (c) flexible sigmoidoscopy every 5 years. Between ages 76 and 85, screening should be individualized based on patient's preference, life expectancy, health status, and prior screening history. The ACS discourages CRC screening after age 85 (Wolf et al. 2018).

COC limitations include need for sedation and potential risk of bleeding and perforation in 0.1–0.3% of patients. Failure to complete COC ranges from 5% to 10%. An incomplete COC exam can be followed by a same day or interval CTC. In the geriatric population, CTC can be the exam of choice as contraindications for sedation and instrumentation due to severe cardiopulmonary disease or use of anticoagulation medication may be more prevalent (Yucel et al. 2008; Kim et al. 2010).

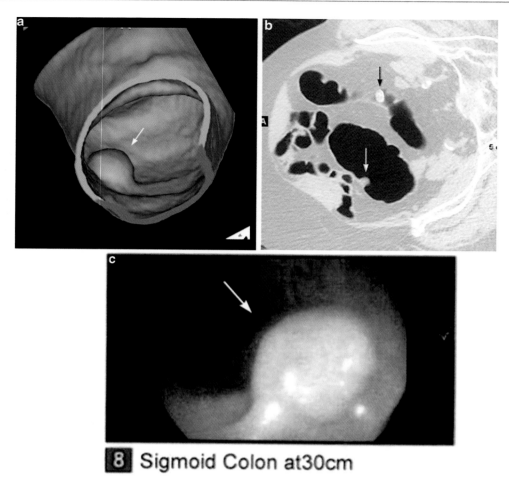

Sigmoid Colon at30cm

Fig. 4 A 71-year-old morbidly obese female with contra-indication for anesthesia underwent CTC. (**a**) 3-D cube view shows a 1.5 cm sessile sigmoid polyp (white arrow) and a tagged stool pellet (black arrow). (**b**) 2-D right lateral decubitus view of the polyp (arrow). Patient underwent COC for polyp removal. (**c**) Endoscopic view of the polyp (arrow). Pathology revealed a tubular adenoma with focal villous architecture

Adequate colonic cleansing, fecal tagging, and colonic distention are prerequisites to a successful CTC. Bowel cleansing may be challenging in the elderly. A study found that limited colonic preparation is sufficient to exclude mass and polypoid lesions greater than 1 cm (Keeling et al. 2010) (Fig. 4a–c).

The adenoma-carcinoma sequence and "de novo" carcinogenesis are two proposed pathways for colorectal cancer development, although controversial in importance (Bedenne et al. 1992). Most small polyps found on colonoscopy are not adenomatous and the incidence of cancer in small polyps is rare (Aldridge and Simson 2001; Nusko et al. 1997). CTC cannot differentiate adenomatous from hyperplastic polyp. Small polyp measurement can vary slightly between CTC, COC, and pathology specimens with CTC measurement closest to the true dimension of the polyp (Summers 2010). Flat adenomas, lesions with height less than 50% of its width, and lesions less than 2 mm raised from the mucosa are more difficult and sometimes impossible to detect on CTC. CTC screening can also detect colonic and extra-colonic cancers in addition to other significant disease in one of 200 asymptomatic adults (Pickhardt et al. 2010). Early detection and treatment of cancers may contribute to favorable outcomes.

COC is the gold standard for colorectal cancer screening allowing for immediate tissue sampling. CTC is the alternative visual exam when COC is incomplete or cannot be performed (Pickhardt et al. 2019; Johnson 2009).

Acute Gastrointestinal (GI) Bleeding

In patients presenting with acute gastrointestinal bleeding, once hemodynamic instability is managed and achieved, radiographic exams can localize, characterize, and treat bleeding lesions. Endoscopy is the initial diagnostic and therapeutic modality in acute GI bleeding (Millward 2008), particularly upper GI bleeding, happening above the ligament of Treitz. Radiologic exams play a greater role in the diagnosis of lower GI bleeding. Bleeding must be active at the time of imaging for radiographic diagnosis. CT angiography (CTA) and conventional catheter angiography (CA) are the exams of choice in hemodynamically unstable patients because they can determine the precise location of bleeding and treat the bleeding lesion. Radionuclide imaging is often used for hemodynamically stable patients with slow intermittent bleeding.

Radionuclide Imaging (Scintigraphy)

In this exam, a radioactive nuclide agent is bound to the patient's red blood cells (RBC), injected in the patient and imaged with a gamma camera. Scintigraphy can detect bleeding rates as low as 0.04–0.1 ml/min, is noninvasive, and generally well tolerated. The imaging can be performed up to 18–24 h after injection of the labeled RBC. Positive scintigraphy increases the diagnostic yield of CA (Gunderman et al. 1998; Ng et al. 1997).

Diagnosis of bleeding is made by intraluminal manifestation of the radiotracer with increased intensity over time and demonstration of movement in the GI tract during dynamic acquisition of data (Holder 2000) (Fig. 5).

Scintigraphy may be time consuming and precise anatomic localization of bleeding is not always possible. The reported accuracy varies from 40% to 100%, and therefore, surgical interventions, particularly segmental intestinal resections, are rarely performed on the basis of scintigraphy findings alone (Hammond et al. 2007).

Catheter-Directed Angiography (CA)

Bleeding rates as low as 0.5 ml/min can be detected with accurate anatomic localization and treatment can be performed with high success rates. In variceal or non-variceal upper GI bleeding, CA is used less frequently due to higher yield from EGD for diagnosis and treatment (Hastings 2000; Murata et al. 2006; Barkun et al. 2010). CA is used when EGD is not available, if bleeding cannot be controlled using EGD (Andersen and Duvnjak 2010) and for poor surgical candidates (Millward 2008).

Most commonly, lower GI bleeding in the geriatric population is due to colonic diverticulosis and angiodysplasia. Treatment by superselective catheter embolization, usually with microcoils (Funaki et al. 2001; Funaki 2004), is effective and has low complication rates. Small bowel is a less frequent site of lower GI bleed, and angioectasia is the most common cause (Fig. 6). Sources of bleeding in the small bowel are more difficult to diagnose and patient outcomes can be poor (Prakash and Zuckerman 2003). If bowel resection is entertained, microcatheter infusion of methylene blue stain or a microcoil can be used to limit the extent of bowel resection.

Extravasation of contrast into the bowel lumen is diagnostic of active bleeding. Indirect findings of bleeding are pseudoaneurysm, arterial venous fistula, hyperemia, neovascularity, and extravasation of contrast into a confined space.

Fig. 5 A 74-year-old male with GI bleeding of unknown location was evaluated with scintigraphy. Multiple sequential images show bleeding with activity localizing in the stomach (short arrow) and progressing to the small bowel (arrowhead)

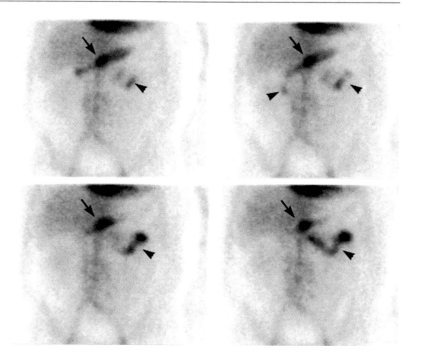

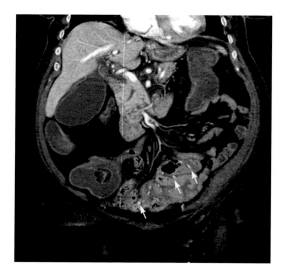

Fig. 6 CT angiogram of a 76-year-old female with end-stage renal disease presenting with massive GI bleeding. CT coronal reformatted image showing angioectasia of the small bowel evidenced by several focally dilated arteries along the small bowel wall (arrows). No active bleeding was demonstrated during CTA. Patient recovered with conservative treatment and the diagnosis was confirmed later with double-balloon endoscopy

Disadvantages of CA include, high cost, invasiveness, associated risk of catheter related and vascular access complications, utilization of iodinated contrast material and false negative exam related to intermittent bleeding, bleeding below detectable rates, and variant vascular anatomy.

CT Angiography (CTA)

CTA localization accuracy is comparable to CA (Wells et al. 2018; Yoon et al. 2006a; b; Zink et al. 2008; Kuhle and Sheiman 2000, 2003; Sabharwal et al. 2006). A noncontrast CT scan to detect preexisting hyperdense material in the bowel lumen is followed by contrast enhanced CTA. CTA diagnosis is made by detection of contrast material in the bowel lumen. Pitfalls include poor CTA technique, bowel mucosal enhancement, which can be interpreted as bleeding, and preexisting high attenuation material (often oral contrast) in the bowel lumen, which decreases CTA accuracy. Although CTA involves radiation

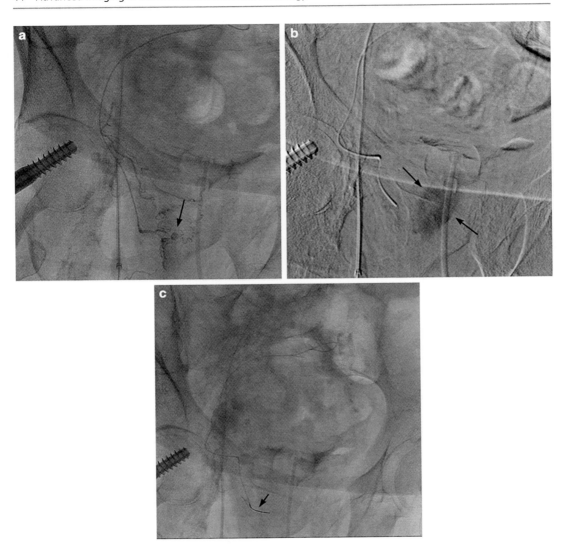

Fig. 7 An elderly patient with rectal bleeding. (**a**) Super-selective angiography showing contrast extravasation into the rectal lumen (arrow). (**b**) Increased contrast pooling in the rectal lumen (between arrows). (**c**) Microcoil embolization (arrow) of the rectal artery branches feeding the bleeding lesion

exposure and use of iodinated intravenous contrast material, it is less invasive than CA. The information obtained by CTA regarding etiology and site of bleeding, and delineation of vascular anatomy are important to plan patient management and are very helpful to guide CA interventions (Fig. 7).

CTA is rapid, safe, sensitive, easy to perform, and readily available. Many institutions use CTA to triage patient presenting with lower GI bleeding (Laing et al. 2007; Lee et al. 2009; Artigas et al.

2013) to facilitate a focused CA intervention and spare an invasive intervention for patients without active bleeding (Fig. 8).

Acute Mesenteric Ischemia and Chronic Mesenteric Insufficiency

Acute mesenteric ischemia is caused by arterial occlusive disease, venous occlusive disease, strangulation/obstruction, and hypoperfusion

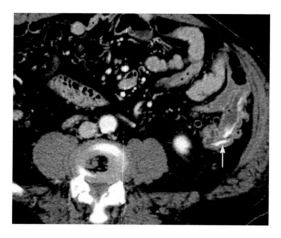

Fig. 8 CTA showing acute GI bleed in an elderly patient with diverticulosis. Axial image shows contrast pooling in the lumen of the left colon (arrow) from a bleeding diverticulum

associated with nonocclusive vascular disease. CT findings vary depending on the cause of ischemia. In patients with chronic arterial insufficiency of the intestines, known as abdominal angina, CTA is used to determine the degree of atherosclerotic stenosis of celiac and superior mesenteric arteries and evaluate collateral circulation and to exclude other cause of intestinal ischemia such as malignancy, median arcuate ligament syndrome, aneurysm, or dissection.

CA is the preferred modality to treat abdominal angina. CTA evaluates the bowel wall, mesentery, and vessels in a single exam. The two main limitations of CTA are lack of dynamic visualization of the flow pattern and difficulty in determining degree of stenosis in heavily calcified vessels. Bowel wall is thickened when ischemia is caused by venous occlusion and reperfusion. In occlusive arterial ischemia with or without bowel infarction, the bowel wall may be paper thin due to lack of edema and may demonstrate hemorrhage. After contrast administration, poor enhancement is specific but not sensitive for bowel infarction. Hyper-enhancement of the bowel can also be seen with ischemia. Gas in the bowel wall (pneumatosis intestinalis) and portomesenteric venous gas in the presence of mesenteric ischemia indicate transmural infarction. The bowel is often dilated due to interruption of peristalsis and may contain fluid particularly in venous occlusive disease and strangulation. Ascites and mesenteric fat stranding represent transudation of fluid (Furukawa et al. 2009; Ofer et al. 2009).

Once the etiology of acute mesenteric ischemia and abdominal angina has been established, the treatment may be with open surgery or with catheter-directed thrombolysis, balloon angioplasty, and stent placement.

Key Points

- MRCP imaging is the mainstay for diagnosis of biliary and pancreatic pathology and is also used for planning of ERCP or percutaneous guided interventions.
- Conventional optical colonoscopy is the gold standard for colorectal cancer screening allowing for immediate tissue sampling. CT colonography is the alternative visual test and can be performed when optical colonoscopy is incomplete or cannot be performed due to contraindications for sedation or instrumentation.
- In hemodynamically unstable patients with acute lower GI bleeding, CTA and CA are the exams of choice for diagnosis and treatment. Radionuclide imaging is the initial exam for hemodynamically stable patients with slow and/or intermittent bleeding.
- CTA and CA are used for diagnosis of acute mesenteric ischemia and abdominal angina. CTA can evaluate the bowel wall, mesentery, and vessels in a single examination.
- Percutaneous balloon angioplasty and stent placement are the preferred treatment of abdominal angina.

References

Aldridge AJ, Simson JH. Histological assessment of colorectal adenomas by size: are polyps less than 10 mm in size clinically important? Eur J Surg. 2001;167:777–81.

Andersen P, Duvnjak S. Endovascular treatment of non varicael acute arterial upper gastrointestinal bleeding. World J Radiol. 2010;2(7):257–61.

Artigas J, Marti M, Soto J, et al. Multidetector CT angiography for acute gastrointestinal bleeding; technique and findings. Radiographics. 2013;33:1453–70.

Barkun AN, Bardou M, Kuipers EJ, et al. International consensus recommendations on the management of patients with nonvaricael upper gastrointestinal bleeding. Ann Intern Med. 2010;152(2):101–13.

Bedenne L, Faivre J, Boutron MC, Piard F, Cauvin JM, Hillon P. Adenoma-carcinoma sequence or "de novo" carcinogenesis. Cancer. 1992;69:883–8.

Funaki B. Superselective embolization of lower gastrointestinal hemorrhage: a new paradigm. Abdom Imaging. 2004;29:434–8.

Funaki B, Kostic J, Lornz J, Ha T, Yip D, Rosenblum J, Leef J, Straus C, Zaleski G. Superselective microcoil embolization of colonic hemorrhage. AJR. 2001;177:829–36.

Furukawa A, Kanasaki S, Naoaki K, et al. CT findings of acute mesenteric ischemia from various causes. AJR. 2009;192:408–16.

Gunderman R, Leef J, Ong K, et al. Scintigraphic screening prior to visceral arteriography in acute lower gastrointestinal bleeding. J Nucl Med. 1998;39:1081–3.

Hammond K, Beck D, Hicks T, Timmcke A, Whitlow C, Margolin D. Implications of negative technetium 99-labeled red blood cell scintigraphy in patients presenting with lower gastrointestinal bleeding. Am J Surg. 2007;193:404–8.

Hastings G. Angiographic localization and transcatheter treatment of gastrointestinal bleeding. Radiographics. 2000;20:1160–8.

Holder L. Radionuclide imaging in the evaluation of acute gastrointestinal bleeding. Radiographics. 2000;20:1153–9.

Johnson C. CT colonography: coming of age. AJR. 2009;193:1239–42.

Keeling A, Slattery M, Leong S, McCarthy E, Susanto M, Lee M, Morrin M. Limited-preparation CT colonography in frail elderly patients: a feasibility study. AJR. 2010;194:1279–87.

Kim D, Pickhardt P, Hanson M, Hinshaw J. CT colonography: performance and program outcome measures in an older screening population. Radiology. 2010;254:493–500.

Kuhle WG, Sheiman RG. The sensitivity of helical CT in detecting active colonic hemorrhage (abstr). J Vasc Interv Radiol. 2000;11(Suppl):208.

Kuhle WG, Sheiman RG. Detection of active colonic hemorrhage with use of helical CT: findings in a swine model. Radiology. 2003;228(3):743–52.

Laing C, Tobias T, Rosenblum D, Banker W, Tseng L, Tamrkin S. Acute gastrointestinal bleeding: emerging role of multidepector CT angiography and review of current imaging techniques. Radiographics. 2007;27:1055–70.

Lee S, Welman CJ, Ramsay D. Investigation of acute lower gastrointestinal bleeding with 16 and 64-slice multidetector CT. J Med Imaging Radiat Oncol. 2009;53:56–63.

Manfredi R, Pozzi R. Secretin enhanced MR imaging of the pancreas. Radiology. 2016;279:29–43.

Millward S. ACR appropriateness criteria on treatment of acute nonvaricael gastrointestinal tract bleeding. J Am Coll Radiol. 2008;5(4):550–4.

Murata S, Tajima H, Fukunaga T, Abe Y, Niggemann P, Onozawaga S, Kumazaki T, Kurramochi M, Kuramoto K. Management of pancreaticoduodenal artery aneurysms: results of superselective transcatheter embolization. AJR. 2006;187:290–8.

Ng DA, Opelka FG, Beck DE, et al. Predictive value of Tc99m-labeled red blood cell scintigraphy for positive angiogram in massive lower gastrointestinal hemorrhage. Dis Colon Rectum. 1997;40:471–7.

Nusko G, Mansmann U, Altendorf-Hofmann A, Groitl H, Wittekind C, Hahn EG. Risk of invasive carcinoma in colorectal adenomas assessed by size and site. Int J Colorectal Dis. 1997;12:267–71.

Ofer A, Abadi S, Nitechi S, et al. Multidetector CT angiography in the evaluation of acute mesenteric ischemia. Eur Radiol. 2009;19:24–30.

Palmucci S, Roccasalva F, Piccoli M et al. Contrast-enhanced magnetic resonance cholangiography: practical tips and clinical indication for biliary disease management. Gastroenterol Res Pract. 2017; Article ID 2403012, 11 pages. https://doi.org/10.1155/2017/2403012.

Pickhardt P, Kim D, Meiners R, et al. Colorectal and extracolonic cancers detected at screening CT colonography in 10286 asymptomatic adults. Radiology. 2010;255:83–8.

Pickhardt P, Correale L, Hassan C. Positive predictive value for colorectal lesions at CT colonography: analysis of factors impacting results in a large screening cohort. AJR. 2019;213:W1–8.

Prakash C, Zuckerman G. Acute small bowel bleeding: a distinct entity with significant different economic implications compared with GI bleeding from other locations. Gastrointest Endosc. 2003;58:330–5.

Sabharwal R, Vladica P, Chou R, Law P. Helical CT in the diagnosis of acute lower gastrointestinal haemorrhage. Eur J Radiol. 2006;58:273–9.

Summers R. Polyp size measurement at CT colonography: what do we know and what do we need to know? Radiology. 2010;255:707–20.

Wells M, Hansel S, Bruining D, et al. CT for evaluation of acute gastrointestinal bleeding. Radiographics. 2018;38:1089–107.

Wolf A, Fontham ETH, Church TR, et al. Colorectal cancer screening for average-risk adults: 2018 guideline update from the American Cancer Society. CA Cancer J Clin. 2018;68:250–81.

Yoon W, Jeong YY, Kim JK. Acute gastrointestinal bleeding: contrast enhanced MDCT. Abdom Imaging. 2006a;31:1–8.

Yoon W, Jeong Y, Shin S, Lim H, Song S, Jang N, Kim J, Kang H. Acute massive gastrointestinal bleeding: detection and localization with arterial phase multi-detector row helical CT. Radiology. 2006b;239:160–7.

Yucel C, Lev-Toaff A, Moussa N, Durrani H. CT colonography for incomplete or contraindicated optical colonoscopy in older patients. AJR. 2008;190:145–50.

Zink SI, Ohki SK, Stein B, Zambuto DA, Rosenberg RJ, Choi JJ, Tubbs DS. Noninvasive evaluation of active lower gastrointestinal bleeding: comparison between contrast-enhanced MDCT and 99mTc-labeled RBC scintigraphy. AJR. 2008;191:1107–14.

Laboratory Testing in Older Adults: Indications, Benefits, and Harms

45

T. S. Dharmarajan and C. S. Pitchumoni

Contents

T. S. Dharmarajan (✉)
Department of Medicine, Division of Geriatrics,
Montefiore Medical Center, Wakefield Campus, Bronx,
NY, USA

Department of Medicine, Albert Einstein College of
Medicine, Bronx, NY, USA

Department of Medicine, New York Medical College,
Valhalla, NY, USA
e-mail: dharmarajants@yahoo.com

C. S. Pitchumoni
Department of Medicine, Robert Wood Johnson School of
Medicine, Rutgers University, New Brunswick, NJ, USA

Department of Medicine, New York Medical College,
Valhalla, NY, USA

Division of Gastroenterology, Hepatology and Clinical
Nutrition, Saint Peters University Hospital, New
Brunswick, NJ, USA
e-mail: pitchumoni@hotmail.com

© Springer Nature Switzerland AG 2021
C. S. Pitchumoni, T. S. Dharmarajan (eds.), *Geriatric Gastroenterology*,
https://doi.org/10.1007/978-3-030-30192-7_38

Abstract

Laboratory testing trends have changed from a tendency to ordering numerous laboratory tests in the past to the current approach in requesting tests selectively and on an individualized basis. The number of tests ordered, the type of tests requested, the costs involved, and the value provided ultimately define in large measure the quality and cost of care provided. Multiple and repetitive laboratory testing is not proven to be of value and escalates costs of healthcare. Older adults manifest multi-morbidity and accordingly are subject to cumbersome and needless testing. Selective testing has value in the screening for disease, in evaluating the stage of disease, and in determining management strategies or their efficacy. Test results may yield a diagnosis, but there may be no specific treatment available for the disorder. The asymptomatic patient with abnormal test results is always an enigma. Test results may provide satisfaction in yielding a diagnosis, but there may be no specific treatment available for the disorder. Age by itself is not associated with significant alterations in laboratory test results. Marked deviations in test results usually indicate the presence of underlying disease or a response to therapy. Testing trends prior to a surgical procedure must be tailored to history, physical examination, comorbidity, and the procedure. Results of laboratory testing may be influenced by several factors, including use of medications, both prescribed and over the counter. Routine repeat testing of common tests does not offer advantage over a single run. Discussing the indications and value of testing with the patient is the first step; decision for testing must relate to benefits outweighing any disadvantages.

Keywords

Laboratory testing · Elective testing · Routine testing · Cost-effective testing · Value of testing · Preoperative testing · Needless testing · Benefits of testing · Harms of testing · False-positive results · False-negative results · Repeat testing · Homocysteine · Ferritin · Albumin · Liver function tests · Pancreatic function tests · Lipid levels · Prothrombin time · Vitamin D levels · Testing for *Clostridium difficile* · Testing for celiac disease · Antinuclear antibody · Thyroid function · B12 assay · Folate assay · Hemoglobin · Hematocrit · Creatinine · Blood urea nitrogen · Electrolytes · Fecal occult blood tests · Testing for celiac disease · Testing for diabetes mellitus · HbA1c measurements · Lipid levels · Vitamin D assay · Prothrombin time · PT · PTT · Platelet counts · INR · Analytical methods in the clinical laboratory

Introduction

The number of tests we order, the type of tests we order, the costs of testing, and the value provided ultimately define in large measure the quality and cost of care provided. In the era of escalating healthcare costs, every step taken in the provision of care, including laboratory tests both indicated and questionable, comes under scrutiny as part of the quality of care rendered. While we recognize the relevance and role of laboratory tests in healthcare, providers need to be cognizant of the benefits, risks, and costs of routine or standard batteries of tests. Caution needs to be exercised in solely utilizing age-based criteria as the reason to choose tests in the geriatric age group, especially in the asymptomatic older adult or prior to a minor surgical procedure. As stated in an editorial, "the tests that we order define us" (Mandell 2019).

In general, it is more likely that test results may be abnormal as one ages and in particular in the very old population, who are more likely to have subclinical or apparent comorbidity (Hepner 2009). As more tests are performed, the odds of obtaining an abnormal result increases, posing implications for both patient and provider. False-positive tests contribute to further testing and escalation of costs (Fleisher 2001). The costs of paying for routine tests ordered based on age alone may no longer be paid for by insurance companies. In the past several years, there have been changes in the approach to ordering of tests (and diagnostic imaging procedures) due to economic pressures, with a trend toward "indicated" rather than routine testing (Fleisher 2001). Tests do not, often times, provide the information that the physician seeks; in many cases, the results may be irrelevant to diagnosis or management.

The Emergence of Laboratory Testing

The sophistication of diagnostic testing has advanced substantially over centuries. From what was bedside medicine in the middle ages and the period when physicians made a diagnosis solely on observations based on visual and auditory approaches, the clinical laboratory has developed to modern, sophisticated methods that provide accurate information rapidly.

The emergence of laboratory testing effectively used at primary healthcare level significantly improves diagnosis and treatment outcomes and is incorporated into routine clinical practice (Carter et al. 2012). At the same time many measures have been placed in the clinical laboratory to improve quality of testing; an example is the introduction of International Standards Organization (ISO) relating to the validation and verification of method performance; in fact, there are practical guides to validate and verify analytical laboratory methods (Pum 2019). As healthcare budgets are under constant pressure globally to lower costs of care, it is essential to ensure that efficiency gains are achieved by reducing laboratory error rate; thus quality indicators play a crucial role and allow for performance assessment; the indicators largely relate to laboratory errors (Tsai et al. 2019).

Additionally, the benefits of point-of-care testing are being now evaluated. A point-of-care testing program is helpful if it ensures that testing will result in an actionable management decision, which may confirm a diagnosis, referral, use of specific treatment, or some other action (Engel et al. 2015). A large study in India suggested rapid tests were not necessarily translated into practical treatment decisions, undermining the potential for benefit from the program (Engel et al. 2015). An example of testing for a common disorder is the utility of HbA1c for diabetes mellitus. Laboratory-based HbA1c testing is now recommended for diagnosing diabetes, a disorder common in older people, and for the monitoring of glycemic status, although it must be emphasized that there is wide variability in the performance of point-of-care HbA1c testing devices and commercially available models, which limit their value (O'Brien and Sacks 2019). Thus, testing should not be used to establish a diagnosis of diabetes unless the test is validated as accurate (O'Brien and Sacks 2019).

Is Old Age a Reason to Perform Laboratory Tests?

It is generally accepted that advancing age is associated with increasing comorbidity. Does this alone justify routine screening, especially in the asymptomatic older adult? In a study of 544 surgical patients over age 70, the prevalence of abnormal electrolyte values and thrombocytopenia was small (0.5–5%); the prevalence of abnormal hemoglobin, creatinine, and glucose was higher at 12%, 10%, and 7% respectively, but did not predict adverse outcomes (Dzankic et al. 2001). The authors concluded that routine testing for hemoglobin, creatinine, glucose, and electrolytes, on the basis of age alone, may not be indicated (Dzankic et al. 2001). Laboratory values used for screening by insurers were not significantly influenced by age alone; most abnormalities arose from health impairments, rather than the age factor (Carter et al. 2012). However, the cost-effectiveness is greater in older age, as there is a better likelihood of disease being detected (Pokorski 1990). These statements must be weighed against the probability that disease detected by testing will modify management (Fleisher 2001), justifying the test. Whether an inadequate history in a cognitively impaired person or an atypical presentation in an older person will justify the use of tests is debatable (Pokorski 1990). One often uses the rationale that more testing is attempted in older persons because of difficulties in obtaining a good history due to the presence of impaired cognition or sensorium; perhaps in such situations, it may be justifiable in ordering specific tests focused on an age-based presentation, as addressed below.

Modified reference values exist for some tests in the over 65 age group (Bourdel-Marchasson et al. 2010). An example is the erythrocyte sedimentation rate, which increases minimally with age. It may be difficult to determine promptly, or ahead of time, the specific tests that will provide significant yield in older people with multi-morbidity, causing an increase in the number of tests ordered (Keiso 1990). A focused history on the use of prescribed and over-the-counter medications including supplement use may be relevant to decision-making; the intake of supplements influences common laboratory test results such as platelet counts, hemoglobin, prothrombin time, vitamin D, and calcium levels, among others. Evaluating the medication list becomes relevant in the era of polypharmacy, a common, addressable issue encountered in the geriatric population. The National Health and Nutrition Examination Survey (NHANES) data indicates that about half the older adults consume an inappropriately excessive number of medications and supplements; several drugs and supplements influence laboratory result values (Kantor et al. 2015). For example, use of metformin or PPIs may cause B12 deficiency; protease inhibitors may increase triglyceride levels, and isoniazid may cause liver enzyme abnormalities.

Manifestations Must Determine the Need for Tests

In general, tests are done on the basis of symptoms or signs, to rule out underlying disease, to understand the severity of a disorder, to monitor the progress or prognosis of the illness, and to assess the effectiveness of treatment. What constitutes normal or a range of accepted values is rarely an ideal scenario; laboratory values are determined by a reference population factoring age, gender, race and other variables (Pokorski 1990).

Most laboratory values in older adults fall in the normal range; significant deviations or abnormal values must raise suspicion for disease (Coodley 1989). Among the common abnormalites noted in a study involving alkaline phosphatase, serum phosphorus, low creatinine clearance without an alteration of serum creatinine, abnormalities in glucose, and deficiencies in vitamins and albumin, many abnormalities indicated the presence of disease or the effect of a drug, rather than suggest a result of aging (Coodley 1989). Interestingly, data from common blood laboratory tests demonstrated that metabolic abnormalities are associated with global cognitive changes in older people, as evident by psychological testing; they included hyperglycemia, hypernatremia, hyperkalemia, low hemoglobin, and elevated creatinine, BUN, and white blood cell counts (Bruce et al. 2009). Additionally, several common test values are neglected. An example is a frequently ordered test, the complete blood cell count (CBC); underutilized components of the CBC include red blood cell distribution width, platelet volume, and nucleated red blood cell count (May et al. 2019). These results have much value for diagnosis, prognosis, and outcomes in older adults and may signify a serious underlying disorder (May et al. 2019). When a test is requested, it is incumbent on the provider to verify the entire results and take appropriate action. Yet, older adults in good health with mild anemia and a low MCV count but a high normal RBC count reflect a thalassemia trait but are extensively tested for chronic blood loss or the rare possibility of celiac disease in the older adult. And finally, a large number of tests ordered are often not verified or followed through, suggesting the questionable value of these tests in management.

Unwanted Testing May Carry Risks More than Benefits

Three important questions should be asked before requesting a test. Is the test relevant to the patient's health? Is there is a reason for the test? Does the test have potential to influence management? A screening program for the old in a rural practice found that although a few patients benefited from blood tests carried out during screening of older adults, and it was academically stimulating, the benefits were not worth the effort; and there was reservation of the impact of testing on the quality of life (Edwards 1991). Daily routine testing in the sick hospitalized older adult, a common practice without evidence for benefit, may lead to significant blood loss and iatrogenic anemia with hemodynamic changes; the results were higher transfusion requirements and a negative influence on mortality (Adiga et al. 2003). In a study, healthcare providers who were made aware of the costs of phlebotomy did order tests more appropriately and brought on savings for the hospital, leave alone benefits to the patient

(Stuebing and Miner 2011). Clinicians should realize that there are diagnostic tests which will not change following therapy and return of prognostic markers. For example, in the evaluation of macrocytic anemia, intrinsic factor antibodies are diagnostic of pernicious anemia, but will not alter management with B12 administration, yet the antibody testing may be repeated multiple times. Similarly testing for serum amylase or lipase in a patient suspected to have acaute pancreatitis is not required on a daily basis. The ritualistic testing of stool samples for ova and parasites in all patients with diarrhea has the poorest diagnostic yield and yet is one of the most overused tests ordered with little understanding of the clinical utility in modern times (Mohapatra et al. 2018).

Unfortunately laboratory test results are not always simple to interpret; results may be positive, negative, or inconclusive. A positive or abnormal test indicates that the disorder is present; a negative or normal test means that the disorder is not present; an inconclusive test is neither positive nor negative. A false-positive test suggests that a disorder is present, when in reality it is not; a false-negative test does not detect the disorder when in reality it is present. Even in the healthy adult, there is a likelihood that 1 in 20 tests ordered may be abnormal (5%) in the absence of an evident underlying abnormality (Pokorski 1990). For a panel of 20 tests, the chances are that there is a 64% chance of at least one abnormal test (Macpherson 1993). This may lead to "labeling" of the patient with a disorder that may or may not be significant. Thus more testing has the potential to cause anxiety for the patient (and provider). Interestingly, if anesthesiologists ordered tests prior to a procedure, instead of primary physicians and surgeons, there appeared a significant reduction in costs without an increase in complications (Finegan et al. 2005).

The question of an increase in liability for not requesting a test is a common consideration, at least in the minds of providers. Legal concerns are often sufficient reason for providers to request routine laboratory tests. Although there may be a legal risk for failure to order a test and make a diagnosis in the first place, the risk may be greater when ordering a laboratory test and not following

Table 1 Factors that influence interpretation of test results

Use of prescribed and "over-the-counter" drugs
Supplements
Herbals
Fasting or fed state
False-negative tests
False-positive tests

Reproduced from the original work by the same authors: Dharmarajan TS, Pitchumoni CS. Laboratory tests in older adults: Indications, interpretations, issues. In Pitchumoni CS, Dharmarajan TS eds. Geriatric Gastroenterology, First edition. Springer, New York, 2012; 261–269

Table 2 Additional concerns about laboratory testing in the elderly

Costs of testing and willingness to undergo testing
Repeat testing for inconsistent results
Unwarranted repeated blood draws and resultant anemia
Legal implications of overlooking an abnormal test result
Fears and emotions associated with testing, especially dementia
Hematomas, local injuries associated with fragile skin and veins

Reproduced from the original work by the same authors: Dharmarajan TS, Pitchumoni CS. Laboratory tests in older adults: Indications, interpretations, issues. In Pitchumoni CS, Dharmarajan TS eds. Geriatric Gastroenterology, First edition. Springer, New York, 2012; 261–269

up in a timely fashion with required actions based on the abnormal results (Hepner 2009; Macpherson 1993). Laboratory test results must be acknowledged by the provider and reports attested in the medical record by the provider. Documentation must include normal and abnormal findings; critical test results warrant immediate action and appropriate, timely communication to the patient, along with documentation of results and actions taken. In summary, it is recommended and desirable that the provider who orders a test follows up with the test results in a timely manner (Tables 1 and 2).

The following discussion arbitrarily divides laboratory tests into those *commonly or routinely* considered in all patients undergoing examination (or a procedure) irrespective of the history and physical examination, as opposed to those tests selected on the basis of a *specific or individualized* reason. The discussion does not cover every available test.

Common or Routine Tests

Hemoglobin and Hematocrit

Hemoglobin and hematocrit are among the useful routine tests. A study comparing two groups of men and women around 44 ± 0.9 years to 63 ± 0.9 years found significant differences with aging in hemoglobin levels, typically a decline, MCV (increase or decrease), and alterations in the indices; also observed were differences in ferritin values (Martin et al. 2001). The most common causes of microcytosis are iron deficiency and thalassemia trait. Anemia is a common multifactorial disorder in the geriatric age group. Based on the WHO definition, anemia is present in 10% of those over 65 years and in 20% of the over 85 year group in the community, increasing to 48–63% of nursing home patients (Patel 2008). Even more important, based on the National Health and Nutritional Examination Survey (NHANES) data, two thirds of anemia have a discernible cause from simple laboratory testing; a third of cases are due to a nutritional basis involving iron, B12, and folate deficiency in variable combinations, a third has anemia of chronic disease, and in the last third, routine tests do not provide an explanation (Guralnik et al. 2004). Thus laboratory tests provide a clue to the etiology of two thirds of older adults with anemia. The impact of anemia on organ dysfunction cannot be underestimated; it is an added risk factor component in heart disease, diabetes, and cerebrovascular disease and a predictor of mortality (Patel 2008; Dharmarajan and Dharmarajan 2007; Dharmarajan et al. 2005). A study of the 65+ age group revealed 12% to have iron deficiency anemia; many with unexplained anemia were "suspicious for myelodysplastic syndrome" (Price et al. 2011). There exists a strong association between anemia and gastrointestinal disease, a common disorder outlined in another chapter.

Ferritin, Transferrin Saturation, B12, and Folate

While ferritin is a useful marker for body iron stores in the stable community patient, it tends to be elevated in the ill patient (acute phase reactant), when ferritin values require cautious interpretation (Knovich et al. 2009). Ferritin should be interpreted in conjunction with health status, along with serum iron levels, iron binding capacity, and transferrin saturation (Coyne 2006). At times the markers may be inadequate to guide iron therapy (Ferrari et al. 2011), especially in the setting of iron deficiency anemia coexisting with chronic disease or inflammation (Dharmarajan et al. 2005). In the NHANES I study, elevated transferrin saturation was associated with elevated mortality in over 2% of adults; but data from NHANES III suggested that ferritin and transferrin saturation are not associated with morality in those people not taking iron supplements and without a baseline history of cardiovascular disease or cancer (Menke et al. 2012).

The need to evaluate folate and B12 status must be individualized based on clinical manifestations, history of prior illness, gastrointestinal resective surgical procedures (partial gastrectomy, bariatric surgery, and ileectomy), dietary habits (vegan or vegetarian), and chronic use of certain medications (e.g., PPIs, metformin) along with consideration for hematological indices (May et al. 2019). Both these nutrients can be low in older adults and in several gastrointestinal disorders affecting sites between the stomach and terminal ileum (detailed in another chapter). At this time testing for B12 and folate is not recommended among the routine initial panel of tests but may be indicated if the patient is anemic. An exception would be the older adult who has had a gastric surgical procedure (such as bariatric surgery), when iron and B12 deficiency follow invariably; in such patients, testing must also address ferrokinetics and B12 status (Dharmarajan et al. 2005).

Renal Function

Serum creatinine by itself is an unreliable indicator of renal function in the old. Although the creatinine level would be commonly expected to rise with age or a disease-related decline in renal function, the value may nevertheless remain normal as a result of coexisting age-associated sarcopenia. Thus, instead of using the serum

creatinine as a marker, a better approach would be to utilize an acceptable formula that estimates glomerular filtration rate (eGFR). Because of the high prevalence of CKD in geriatric age groups, precise estimates of renal function and staging are relevant, especially for appropriate dosing of drugs, when pharmacokinetics are dependent on renal function and further, to also assess stage of kidney disease. Particularly in the frail elderly, such estimates are invaluable. The choices of formulae include the Cockcroft-Gault equation, Modification of Diet in Renal Disease Study, and the newer Chronic Kidney Disease Epidemiology Collaboration Initiative Equation (Dharmarajan and Dharmarajan 2007). The three formulae do not provide identical values in older adults; in other words, they do not concur (Michels et al. 2010; Dharmarajan et al. 2012). It may be best to use a given formula in a particular patient to monitor renal function test results over time.

Blood urea nitrogen (BUN) levels are influenced by multiple causes. Levels are elevated in acute and chronic kidney disease, volume depletion, heart failure, gastrointestinal bleeding, dietary factors, obstructive uropathy, and following the use of medications such as steroids and diuretics; on the other hand, low BUN levels occur in chronic liver disease. In the presence of renal disease, one must also routinely assess for electrolyte abnormalities.

Liver Function

While the liver demonstrates much resilience with age, there are cellular hallmarks of aging that do occur through alterations of the genome and epigenome and dysregulation of mitochondrial function (Hunt et al. 2019). While the aging process of the liver is largely not clear, data from a Netherlands study suggest that liver function deteriorates with age (Cieslak et al. 2016). In a study of 1673 men aged over 70 years, alanine transaminase (ALT) was lower in older participants; older age, frailty, and low albumin were associated with reduced survival; low ALT was associated with frailty (Le Couteur et al. 2010a).

Liver function tests (LFTs) include a panel of tests: liver enzymes, bilirubin, and hepatic synthetic measures (prothrombin time and albumin). About 1–4% of asymptomatic patients manifest abnormal tests (Krier and Ahmed 2009). As many as 14.7% of a Chinese population had abnormal LFTs, the most common causes being metabolic syndrome, nonalcoholic fatty liver disease, and alcoholism (Zhang et al. 2011). Nonalcoholic fatty liver disease is a common cause of abnormal AST and ALT worldwide, especially in affluent nations, increasing with the growing obesity epidemic (Vernon et al. 2011).

Liver function tests are a panel, and not all are true tests of liver function; a better terminology is liver injury tests. True liver function tests are serum albumin levels and prothrombin time. Abnormalities may not reflect liver disease (Coates 2011; Coyne 2006). A focused history and physical examination are a foundation for appropriate testing (Hunt et al. 2019). Enzyme levels vary with gender, ethnicity, and age. Abnormal LFTs are commonly encountered in asymptomatic patients during routine visits and consultations; a cost-effective and systematic approach is recommended for their interpretation. Even the excessive use of certain vitamins, such as vitamin A may influence LFTs. Higher mortality was demonstrated in a study of 560,000 life insurance applicants, in those with higher levels of AST, ALT, and GGT (Pinkham and Krause 2009). On the other hand, low ALT activity was also a predictor of reduced survival, mediated by its association with frailty and increasing age (Le Couteur et al. 2010b).

Serum Albumin

Screening for protein energy malnutrition at an early stage allows interventions to be more successful (Omran and Morley 2000). The value of serum albumin level is immense; levels reflect not only nutritional status but may also relate to renal and hepatic function, gastrointestinal disease, and catabolic states. In an orthogeriatric unit, nearly 450 elderly with hip fractures demonstrated better functional independence with normoalbuminemia at admission and at discharge (Mizrahi et al. 2007). Hypoalbuminemia is a predictor of poor outcome or mortality in many gastrointestinal disorders such

as *C.difficile* colitis, acute pancreatitis, ulcerative colitis, and other organ involvement such as decompensated heart failure or kidney disease with proteinuria (Uthamalingam et al. 2010) and colon cancer prior to surgery (Lai et al. 2011).

Serum Lipids

Measurements of total cholesterol and its fractions (high density, low density, very low density) and triglycerides are now considered standard screening tests in adults. While they need to be repeated to monitor impact of therapy, multiple testing in the geriatric population appears associated with multiple providers, independent of indications and comorbidity, as demonstrated in a study of over 1.15 million Medicare beneficiaries (Goodwin et al. 2011). Hyperlipidemia is common in older people and undoubtedly a treatable risk factor for vascular disease. Measurements of serum cholesterol fractions and triglycerides are indicated for screening; repeat testing is indicted to monitor the response to therapy and for adjusting dosage of medications used in management (Grundy et al. 2018). Unfortunately, although the tests are repeated, the results are not always acted upon to titrate statin medication dosage, which negate the value of the testing (Table 3).

The frequency of ordering unnecessary routine tests in a hospital (or other) setting was reduced by imparting education to those in training regarding indications for testing and costs involved, in conjunction with frequent reminders (Faisal et al. 2018). The study demonstrated a drop in testing by 50% and was associated with a shorter length of hospital stay (Faisal et al. 2018). Practicing physicians stand to benefit by using a similar strategy.

Specific or Individualized Tests

On the other hand, specific testing may be indicated based on an individual's history and physical examination. Specific tests are not requested in all patients and are best tailored to each individual.

Table 3 Common or "routine" tests (Fleisher 2001; Pokorski 1990; Coodley 1989; May et al. 2019; Macpherson 1993; Martin et al. 2001; Dharmarajan et al. 2012; Krier and Ahmed 2009)

Hemoglobin
Anemia: prevalence 10% of community adults over age 65, 20% over 85
Laboratory tests can delineate an etiology in two thirds of anemics
Creatinine and BUN
Renal function declines with age; but serum creatinine may remain normal in spite of decline in kidney function (effect of sarcopenia)
Calculate eGFR to assess renal function, using an acceptable formula
BUN: non-specific and increased by several causes: renal failure, volume depletion, heart failure, gastrointestinal bleeding, dietary causes, medication effect (steroids), and obstructive uropathy
BUN may be lower in liver disease
Electrolytes
Abnormal in the presence of renal disease, gastrointestinal volume losses, heart failure, and medication effect
Abnormalities may result from hepatic or pulmonary disease
Albumin and pre-albumin:
Lower levels in liver disease, gastrointestinal or renal protein losses, and malnutrition
Are acute negative phase reactant; deconditioning or illness associated with lower albumin levels
Cholesterol, total and fractions, triglycerides
Considered as standard screen in all adults
Frequency of testing relates to levels, cardiovascular risk and to determine management
Liver function
Abnormal tests are common, even in asymptomatic adults
Interpretation may need specialist consultation
Medication history is helpful
Prothrombin time and APTT
Dictated by bleeding or clotting history and presence of liver disease
Use of anticoagulants, antiplatelet agents, herbals, and alcoholism
Erythrocyte sedimentation rate
Marginal increase with age, more in females than in males
Non-specific and increases with many illnesses

Reproduced from the original work by the same authors: Dharmarajan TS, Pitchumoni CS. Laboratory tests in older adults: Indications, interpretations, issues. In Pitchumoni CS, Dharmarajan TS eds. Geriatric Gastroenterology, First edition. Springer, New York, 2012; 261–269

Fecal Occult Blood Testing (FOBT)

Colorectal cancer (CRC) is the fourth most common cancer diagnosed among adults and the second leading cause of death from cancer (Wolf et al. 2018). CRC screening is detailed in a separate chapter. The American Cancer Society 2018 guideline update suggests that adults aged 45 years and older with an average risk for CRC undergo regular screening with either a high-sensitivity stool-based test or a structural visual examination, based on patient preference and test availability (Wolf et al. 2018). Regular screening of adults aged 50 years and older is currently a strong recommendation. Options for laboratory testing include fecal immunochemical test annually; high-sensitivity, guaiac-based fecal occult blood test annually; and multi-target DNA test every 3 years (Wolf et al. 2018). All positive screening tests are required to be followed by colonoscopy.

The stool occult blood test has been utilized for reasons other than CRC screening; in a study most patients were not suitable candidates due to contraindications for testing, leading to further needless investigations (Soin et al. 2019). The use of a single dose of oral aspirin prior to fecal immunochemical testing did not increase test sensitivity for detecting colorectal neoplasms (versus placebo) in a study of 2422 patients, mean age 59.6 years (Brenner et al. 2019). Anticoagulant or aspirin therapy, commonly used in older adults, does not affect the positive predictive value of an immunological fecal occult blood test in those undergoing CRC screening, as noted in a cohort case-controlled study (Mandelli et al. 2011). Even immunochemical FOBT appears associated with false-negative results. Improvements in stool DNA tests relating to sensitivity for CRC and the use of fecal immunochemical tests have evolved over the years. Data from a longitudinal cohort of patients over age 70 suggests that the net burden could be decreased by better targeting FOBT screening and follow-up to healthy older adults; those with the best life expectancy were less likely to experience a net burden (Kistler et al. 2011).

A guidance statement from the American College of Physicians suggests the following approach to screening for CRC in asymptomatic average risk adults (Qaseem et al. 2019). Clinicians must screen for CRC in average risk adults between 50 and 75 years. They must select the screening test based on a discussion of benefits, harms, costs, and patient preferences; screening intervals are fecal immune-chemical testing or high-sensitivity guaiac-based fecal occult bleed testing every 2 years, colonoscopy every 10 years, or flexible sigmoidoscopy every 10 years plus fecal immunochemical testing every 2 years. Discontinue screening for CRC in average risk adult older than 75 years or those with a life expectancy of less than 10 years (Qaseem et al. 2019). Additional details are provided in the chapter on colon cancer.

Screening for Celiac Disease

Celiac disease (CD) is not uncommon, yet is an under-recognized disorder in older adults. It is an inflammatory disease triggered by dietary gluten in those with a genetic tendency; the best noted genetic susceptibilities are class II human leucocyte antigen (HLA) genes HLA-DQ2 and DQ8 (Brown et al. 2019). Genetic testing is possible through laboratories to evaluate a patient or identify family members at risk. HLA genetic testing carries a low positive predictive value but a high negative predictive value, which suggests the need for appropriate testing and proper test result interpretation (Brown et al. 2019). In the appropriate patient, if HLA typing and clinical presentation favor the diagnosis of celiac disease, a biopsy may not be necessary (Gulseraen et al. 2019). The European Society for the Study of Coeliac Disease guideline has provided recommendations; there appears to be a marked increase in the prevalence of CD, and many are undiagnosed (Al-Toma et al. 2019). Testing must be performed on a gluten-containing diet. Most CD patients (90–95%) carry the HLA-DQ2.5 heterodimers, encoded by the DQA1*05 and DQB1*02 alleles; the rest carry HLA-DQ8.

Testing for IGA-antigliadin antibodies has been used for a long time and is reasonably accurate (sensitivity 85% and specificity 90%), when there is a high pretest prevalence of CD, but not a good test for the general population (Al-Toma et al. 2019). Serum IgA antibodies to tissue transglutaminase (TG2) are increased in active disease (except when IgA deficient); a related anti-endomysial IgA antibody is similar in sensitivity and specificity at around 95% (Al-Toma et al. 2019; van der Windt et al. 2010). The following should be tested: adults with symptoms, signs, and malabsorption; first-degree relatives of a patient with celiac disease; HLA-matched siblings, parents, and children especially; a lower likelihood for second-degree relatives; and type 1 diabetes mellitus (Al-Toma et al. 2019); they may be screened through a blood test or cheek swab for HLA DQ2 or HLA DQ8, by polymerase chain reaction; their absence makes celiac disease highly unlikely (negative predictive value 100%) (van der Windt et al. 2010; Rostom and Dube 2005).

Because of the high incidence of CD in association with type 1 diabetes mellitus (7%), Down syndrome (16%), autoimmune diseases, inflammatory bowel diseases, and those with unexplained elevation of liver enzymes, besides first-degree relatives with the disease, screening for CD is highly recommended (Al-Toma et al. 2019). On the other hand, the US Preventive Services Task Force has concluded that that current evidence is insufficient to assess the balance of benefits and harms of screening for celiac disease in asymptomatic patients (Bibbibns-Domingo 2017).

Screening for Diabetes

With an increase in life expectancy and the prevalence of obesity, there is a higher likelihood that older patients will have type 2 diabetes (T2D). The 2019 American Diabetes Association guidelines suggest that screening for T2D is indicated at age 45 years and additionally in the presence of overweight or obese status, history of T2D in a first-degree relative, presence of cardiovascular disease or hypertension, and other settings (Riddle 2019). The major difference of note is in management, where less stringent HbA1c targets are set for older people; targets are tailored to patient setting (community versus institutions), coexisting morbidity, and remaining years of life expectancy (Riddle 2019). HbA1c has largely replaced the glucose tolerance test and is the mainstay for monitoring glucose control. Fundamental to good diagnostic testing is standardization with defined reference materials and measurement procedures (Wilson et al. 2009; English and Lenters-Westera 2018). Frequency of monitoring is important; based on the degree of control (good versus poor), the guidelines suggest every 3 or 6 months (Riddle 2019). However, testing every 6 months may be as effective as quarterly testing and compared to four tests a year; more than four tests were associated with lower likelihood of achieving targets, with two or three tests giving similar likelihoods as 4 per year (Duff et al. 2018). HbA1c testing at the point of care offers an opportunity for improvement of diabetes care but needs to be conducted with stringent quality assurance processes (Kenealy et al. 2019). HbA1c testing is currently used less frequently than glucose testing for screening but is far more likely to result in a clinical diagnosis of prediabetes and diabetes (Evron et al. 2019).

Acute Pancreatitis

Data covering 1996–2005 suggests an increase in the incidence of acute pancreatitis, in part because of the increased testing for pancreatic enzymes; the proportion of ED visits resulting in an inpatient discharge diagnosis of acute pancreatitis appears to be going up (Yadav et al. 2011). Serum amylase and lipase are relevant in this context, although both are non-specific especially when the elevations are less than three times the upper normal (Yadav et al. 2002). Amylase levels rise and decline rapidly and may not be helpful in those patients who have delay in getting to the hospital; presently serum lipase is preferred in view of its high sensitivity and specificity (Muniraj et al. 2015). Overdiagnosis of acute pancreatitis is likely in view of false-positive

elevations in many patients with diabetes. Underdiagnosis is also likely if proper diagnostic testing is not done when the history of abdominal pain is unclear as is the case of older adults with dementia. C-reactive protein is a non-specific acute phase reactant and is useful in older people when diagnosis is not readily apparent. The approach to testing is detailed in the chapter of acute pancreatitis.

Testing for Bleeding and Coagulation

Routine coagulation testing may have a higher yield if based on a perceived risk of coagulopathy in those on warfarin or heparin or with liver disease (Martin and Beardsell 2012; Thachil 2008). In complex situations such as disseminated intravascular coagulation, when several bleeding and clotting parameters are abnormal, not a single test appears sufficiently accurate to establish or reject the diagnosis (Levi and Meijers 2011). For coagulation monitoring, an initial history for clotting or bleeding history should be obtained, followed by appropriate testing should the history be suggestive (Kistler et al. 2011). The change in paradigm is the increasing use of an evidence-based approach based on bleeding history and awareness of limitations of routine coagulation tests to guide management in the event of massive bleeding (Kozek-Langenecker 2010). It is prudent to obtain a history of herbal and supplement use, as several of these products influence bleeding and clotting parameters; the simultaneous use of medications with herbal supplements such as garlic, ginger, ginkgo biloba, feverfew, saw palmetto, and ginseng can influence the INR (Abad et al. 2010; Wittkowsky 2008).

Vitamin D Status

Status of vitamin D (25-hydroxy D) appears relevant in older adults who are vulnerable to deficiency, based on the many predispositions such as restricted mobility to indoors; poor intake of supplements, fish, and fortified products such as dairy; malabsorption and malnutrition; use of medications that influence metabolism of vitamin D (e.g., anticonvulsants);

chronic liver disease; chronic kidney disease; inflammatory bowel disease; gait abnormalities and falls; and generalized unexplained musculoskeletal or bone pain with or without fractures. For vitamin D measurement to add value, the test may be used in conjunction with calcium, phosphorus, and alkaline phosphatase levels (Rosen 2011). Laboratory testing for vitamin D has increased dramatically in the USA since 2008 largely due to an awareness of vitamin D status and its links to health (Kennel et al. 2010; Manson et al. 2017). This has reached such an extent that the government and laboratories have placed stringent requirements or indications for testing, as opposed to routine screening in most patients. There is considerable disagreement regarding the interpretations of serum concentrations of 25(OH)D and as to what is normal or optimal good health versus deficiency; cutoff points have not been developed by a scientific consensus process. Based on its review of data regarding vitamin D requirements, the Institute of Medicine concluded that 25 (OH) D levels ≥ 20 ng/ml are generally considered adequate for bone and overall health in healthy individuals (NIH office of Dietary Supplements 2019).

Testing for *Clostridium difficile*

The topic is detailed in a separate chapter. An appropriate selection of tests must be made between enzyme immunoassays for toxin A and B, which are less sensitive than either glutamate dehydrogenase immunoassays (GDH) or the nucleic acid amplification test (NAATs). Tests vary in sensitivity and specificity and are associated with overdiagnosis (owing to detection of *C. difficile* carriers) or underdiagnosis due to lower sensitivity; multistep testing may be an option (Collins and Riley 2018; Gupta et al. 2018).

Laboratory Testing in Rheumatology

Autoimmune diseases are common with no age group exempt. However, the tests lack sensitivity and standardization and include false positives and negatives (Meroni and Schur 2010). In fact, false-positive antinuclear antibodies (ANA) without disease are far more common than systemic lupus, particularly in older age. Besides low titer positivity that is common in the geriatric patient, medications such as hydralazine, anticonvulsants, and isoniazid give a positive test, as also non-viral hepatitis and primary biliary cirrhosis; drug-induced lupus is not uncommon, and in such cases the ANA testing must be followed by additional tests (Hossain et al. 2019). Laboratory tests in rheumatology are useful but have limitations; it is necessary to be practical and select evidence-based guidance on requesting and interpreting selected tests including rheumatoid factor, ANA, human leukocyte antigen-B27, anti-neutrophil cytoplasmic antibody, and others (Suresh 2019). Often, the negative test provides far more value in rheumatological diagnosis (Suresh 2019).

Homocysteine

Homocysteine levels are increased in several settings including aging, chronic kidney disease, hypothyroidism, and vitamin B12, folate, and B6 deficiencies, suggesting that the test is far from specific. Routine testing for homocysteine is not warranted including in inflammatory bowel disease; although 13% of all inflammatory bowel disease patients had elevated levels, the authors concluded that routine testing is not warranted and there was no correlation between levels and disease activity (Vagianos and Berstein 2012). Providers need to be knowledgeable about the application and interpretation of elevated homocysteine levels and that although levels are elevated in B12 and folate deficiency, the values are not specific to the nutrient status (Fei et al. 2017). On the other hand, the assessment of vitamin B12 and folate status is frequently indicated in patients with cognitive impairment and gait speed abnormalities and in the presence of anemia of nutrient deficiency in older people (Fei et al. 2017; Vidoni et al. 2017). The B vitamins have been detailed in other chapters (Table 4).

Table 4 Individualized or "specific" tests (Knovich et al. 2009; Coyne 2006; Ferrari et al. 2011; Soin et al. 2019; Qaseem et al. 2019; Al-Toma et al. 2019; Riddle 2019; Muniraj et al. 2015; Heindl 2010; Kennel et al. 2010; Collins and Riley 2018; Meroni and Schur 2010; Vidoni et al. 2017)

Antinuclear antibody
Is positive with illnesses, e.g., systemic lupus, scleroderma, etc.
Can be drug-induced (anticonvulsants, hydralazine, isoniazid)
Positive ANA in low titers common in the old
Ferrokinetics
Serum iron, total iron binding capacity, ferritin
Used in conjunction with transferrin saturation, indicator of iron availability
Ferritin is an acute phase reactant, falsely elevated in inflammation
B12 and folic acid:
Deficiencies are common and occur in up to 25% of the older adults
B12 levels in borderline range are hard to interpret and may require homocysteine and methylmalonic acid assays to confirm
Additional tests help determine the specific etiology of B12 deficiency: such as intrinsic factor antibodies for pernicious anemia
Vitamin D status:
25 hydroxy D levels are index of vitamin D status
Predisposition: diet, restricted mobility, lack of sun exposure, age
Low calcium levels may be suggestive of vitamin D deficiency
Guidelines regarding screening vary; they do not call for routine screening
Tests for pancreatic function
Amylase levels rise and decline rapidly, unhelpful in delayed presentations
Serum lipase preferred in view of its high sensitivity and specificity
Tests for celiac disease, an entity that is generally underdiagnosed
Serum IgA antibodies to tissue transglutaminase (TG2) (except when IgA deficient); a related anti-endomysial IgA antibody is similar in sensitivity and specificity at around 95%
Select patients screened through a blood test or cheek swab for HLA DQ2 or HLA DQ8 by PCR; their absence makes celiac disease unlikely (negative predictive value 100%)
Thyroid function
Tests are commonly abnormal from thyroid and non-thyroid illness
Initial screen: thyroid-stimulating hormone, free thyroxine (T4)
Guidelines regarding screening and frequency vary
C-reactive protein
Non-specific marker of inflammation
Homocysteine and methylmalonic acid assays do not provide a specific diagnosis in most situations but are helpful where B12 levels are borderline
Urinalysis and/or culture
In those with diabetes, renal disease, polyuria, infection, abdominal pain, etc.
Fecal tests:
Fecal immunochemical tests
High-sensitivity guaiac-based fecal occult blood tests
Multi-targeted DNA test
Clostridium difficile infection-associated disease
Tests for malabsorption
Tests for parasitic or bacterial infection

Reproduced from the original work by the same authors: Dharmarajan TS, Pitchumoni CS. Laboratory tests in older adults: Indications, interpretations, issues. In Pitchumoni CS, Dharmarajan TS eds. Geriatric Gastroenterology, First edition. Springer, New York, 2012; 261–269

Selecting Tests Prior to a Procedure

As a general rule, the best approach to choosing tests prior to an elective surgical or gastrointestinal (GI) procedure is to make the selection based on a comprehensive history, physical examination, morbidity, type of procedure, and an awareness of the current and recently prescribed medications, including over-the-counter preparations, herbals, and ophthalmic preparations. History is targeted to relevant aspects of the procedure to be performed; for example, is the procedure just endoscopy or endoscopy plus biopsy and excision of lesions? Is there likely to be significant blood loss? Is there an available prior history of outcomes following previous surgery?

There is an ongoing trend toward less testing and obtaining only relevant tests in contrast to the past when several tests were routinely ordered in all patients. As an example, an electrocardiogram and urinalysis were requested in all patients in the past even for minor procedures, in contrast to selectively ordering tests today based on the patient profile and procedure involved.

In a study of 19,557 older adults, over 9000 patients underwent cataract surgery without routine testing, compared to a similar number on routine testing. Routine medical testing did not measurably increase the safety of surgery (Schein et al. 2000). Although it was not pertinent to a gastrointestinal procedure, valuable lessons were provided from the study. Far more was expected from the physician's physical assessment compared to the yield of laboratory testing (Roizen 2000). The results may be extrapolated to several low risk procedures. More than 30 years of evidence suggests that a focused history and physical examination and minimal selective laboratory tests may be the best approach, with costs optimized by this approach (Richman 2010). A healthy older adult in good functional state, undergoing evaluation for inguinal hernia surgery, requires little by way of testing; in such cases there is minimal need for prothrombin time and partial thromboplastin time, as they are clinically insignificant for the concerned procedure, unless the patient is on medications that alter the values or there is evidence of abnormal liver function or

history of a bleeding or clotting disorder (Richman 2010).

After adjustment for age and comorbidities, serum albumin level was a predictor of postoperative complications in the elderly with hip fracture (Lee et al. 2009). Although a predictor, little can be done to substantially change low albumin levels prior to impending surgery. In a study, hypoalbuminemia, acute renal injury, and a high white cell count were nevertheless present in 11%, 24%, and 33% of 70+-year-old persons tested prior to surgery, where only 47% had all the tests performed (Achuthan et al. 2011).

Routine repeat testing of critical values of hemoglobin, platelet count, white blood cell count, prothrombin time, and activated partial thromboplastin time do not offer advantage over a single run (Toll et al. 2011). If repeating testing has limited value, does timing matter? Timing of endoscopic retrograde cholangiopancreatography and association of laboratory values with clinical outcomes (death or organ failure) was evaluated in a Japanese study (Schwed et al. 2016). White blood cell count over 20,000 cells/μl and elevated bilirubin were independent prognostic factors for adverse outcomes (Schwed et al. 2016).

Erythrocyte sedimentation rate is a useful nonspecific test in some illnesses, with higher values typically seen in anemia and inflammatory states; however, low sedimentation rates are noted in heart failure, a common disorder in older adults. Marginal increase in the sedimentation rates also occur with age (Keiso 1990). Thus, requesting the sedimentation rate routinely does not add value prior to a procedure.

Data does not provide an optimal strategy on improving the diagnostic tests used in intensive care units (ICU) and their impact on outcomes. An open-label prospective study indicated that a decrease in the overall number of tests per ICU-patient-days was possible after an educational approach; the total costs of the tests decreased, and no secondary effect from the intervention was observed; thus senior committed physicians can effectively contribute to this quality improvement process (Clouzeau et al. 2019). While laboratory testing is an integral tool in the management of patients in the ICU, there is a trade-off in the selection and timing of lab tests and utility of clinical decision-making at a specific time;

Table 5 Pre-procedure testing (Pokorski 1990; Bourdel-Marchasson et al. 2010; Keiso 1990; Kantor et al. 2015; Coodley 1989; Bruce et al. 2009; May et al. 2019; Martin and Beardsell 2012; Thachil 2008; Levi and Meijers 2011; Heindl 2010; Kozek-Langenecker 2010)

General:
The approach must be to individualize tests based on a comprehensive history and physical examination
Review all medications: prescribed, topical, ophthalmic, herbals, and supplements; include over-the-counter medications
Laboratory tests do not require repeat testing if performed in the recent past and the patient's clinical status remains unchanged
In the healthy, asymptomatic older adult
Hematological
Hemoglobin level if anemic and/or blood loss is expected
Complete blood count generally not required
Platelet counts if indicated by history, examination, or medication intake
Renal, electrolyte, and metabolic
Serum creatinine and blood urea nitrogen
Blood glucose; screen if warranted for prediabetes and diabetes
Electrolytes generally indicated (e.g., in CKD, diuretic, laxative, ACE inhibitor, and other medication use)
Coagulation parameters, if suggested by history and/or examination
In the older adult with comorbidity:
Chest radiographs, electrocardiogram, and additional tests based on age and comorbidity; individualize accordingly
CKD: tests for renal function and electrolytes
Diabetes type 2: evaluate for end organ damage
Heart disease: specialized cardiac testing as indicated
Liver function, with a history of alcoholism or chronic liver disease
Bleeding history: history of medication use (anticoagulants, aspirin, herbals) and alcohol intake; individualize tests for liver function, platelet counts, bleeding, and clotting parameters
Blood type and cross match: in anemia and anticipated blood loss

Reproduced from the original work by the same authors: Dharmarajan TS, Pitchumoni CS. Laboratory tests in older adults: Indications, interpretations, issues. In Pitchumoni CS, Dharmarajan TS eds. Geriatric Gastroenterology, First edition. Springer, New York, 2012; 261–269

experiments show that a policy can reduce frequency of lab tests and optimize timing to minimize information redundancy (Cheng et al. 2019) (Table 5).

Preoperative Hematological Assessment

Preoperative hematological assessment has changed over the years. The 2018 Frankfurt Consensus Conference on Blood Management made several clinical recommendations, regarding the diagnosis and management of preoperative anemia; key points are outlined in Table 6 (Mueller et al. 2019). Mild anemia, a marker of most gastrointestinal diseases, is not an indication for blood transfusion. Preoperative blood transfusion is potentially lifesaving in specific circumstances, but inappropriate blood transfusion can also be an independent risk factor for adverse patient outcomes. The key recommendations from the conference are that the diagnosis and management of preoperative anemia are crucial and iron-deficient anemia must be treated with iron supplementation; the red blood cell transfusion threshold for critically ill, clinically stable patients is <7 g/dL, for cardiac surgery <7.5 g/dl, and for hip fractures and cardiovascular disease <8 g/dl; for acute GI

Table 6 Preoperative anemia and management. (Recommendations from the 2018 Frankfurt Consensus Conference) (Mueller et al. 2019)

Defined preoperative anemia and its management
RBC transfusion thresholds
Critically ill, clinically stable: hgb <7 g/dl
Undergoing cardiac surgery: hgb <7.5 g/dl
Hip fractures and CVD or risks: hgb <8 g/dl
Acute GI bleeding: hgb 7–8 g/dl
Detect and manage preoperative anemia early, prior to surgery
Use iron supplements to reduce red cell transfusion rate in those with iron deficiency anemia undergoing elective surgery
Do not use erythropoiesis-stimulating agents routinely for pre-op anemia
Consider short-acting erythropoietins plus iron to reduce transfusions in patients with hgb <13 g/dl undergoing major orthopedic surgery

bleeding, the Hgb concentration of 7–8 g/dl is relatively well-defined, although the quality of evidence is moderate to low (Mueller et al. 2019) (Table 6).

The United Kingdom National Institute for Health and Care Excellence updated their guidelines, but there was lack of consensus in the requirements for pre-op investigations, suggesting that several tests with a low probability of altering pre-op management are being undertaken in low-risk patients despite national guidelines in the UK and USA (Dhatariya and Wiles 2016). Interestingly, improving diabetes control or tight control made little difference to outcomes, and those without diabetes preoperatively benefited the most, versus those who had diabetes (Dhatariya and Wiles 2016).

Monitoring of perioperative coagulation includes assessing individual bleeding risk (through history) prior to surgery and accordingly ordering laboratory testing if perioperative bleeding is anticipated; although coagulation tests are to be ordered in those with bleeding risk, limitations exist with the tests being poor predictors of bleeding and mortality (Fowler and Perry 2015). Tests should be interpreted with caution. In general, preoperative anemia, blood loss, and allogenic blood transfusions are associated with higher postoperative morbidity and mortality; approaches should address these concerns (Munoz et al. 2016; Munoz et al. 2015). When feasible, preoperative anemia, which is common, must be detected at least 4 weeks prior to the procedure and addressed through use of iron, B12, folic acid, or an erythropoietic agent (Munoz et al. 2015).

Testing prior to endoscopy is detailed in another chapter. Generally, the principles of testing may follow the suggested approaches outlined above. There is insufficient data to determine the benefit of routine laboratory testing before endoscopy procedures (Levy et al. 2008). In the absence of evidence for a bleeding disorder or coagulopathy, the prothrombin time, INR, and partial thromboplastin time neither predict nor correlate with procedural bleeding. In fact, when bleeding does occur, it is more often in those with normal coagulation factors in absence of clinical risk factors (Levy et al. 2008).

Data-based outcomes from select studies relating to the value, pros, and cons of laboratory testing in the peri-procedure period are provided in Table 7 (Keshavan and Swamy 2016; Lakomkin et al. 2016; Mata-Miranda Mdel et al. 2016; Reazaul Karim et al. 2018; Karimian et al.

Table 7 Pre-procedure testing and outcomes (Keshavan and Swamy 2016; Lakomkin et al. 2016; Mata-Miranda Mdel et al. 2016; Reazaul Karim et al. 2018; Karimian et al. 2018; Harley et al. 2019; Howell et al. 2019; Guttikonda et al. 2019)

Comparison and costs (Keshavan and Swamy 2016)
Tertiary care hospital. 163 patients, 984 tests
515 tests (52%) un-indicated, 7 were abnormal
Additional costs incurred 63% of total costs
Pre-op labs, wasted dollars (Lakomkin et al. 2016)
Orthopedic trauma, 56,336 patients, hip fractures
Outcomes: cardiac and septic shock
Abnormal preoperative platelet and bilirubin values predicted poor outcomes
Lab tests for surgery referrals (Mata-Miranda Mdel et al. 2016)
Determine percent of unnecessary lab test and unnecessary expenses in pre-op assessment
In 65% of patients (n = 175), unnecessary tests were requested; in 25% were not requested the tests they needed
Only 10% of patients were requested tests in accordance with criteria
Pre-op lab tests and anesthesia (Karim et al. 2018)
414 patients: study of pre-op tests to identify hidden problems
Majority (57.2%) had at least one abnormal routine test result, but only 1.8% abnormal tests had significant impact
The NNI to find a significant impact was over 20
Elevated pre-op HgbA1c and complications in nondiabetic patients (Karimian et al. 2018)
Six observational studies to study pre-op HbA1c levels in nondiabetics and post-op complications
Two studies noted increased postoperative infection rates
Four studies correlated between pre-op HbA1c levels and post-op complications rates in nondiabetic patients; two noted no difference
Only one study noted higher mortality rates with suboptimal HbA1c
Suboptimal pre-op HbA1c in nondiabetics predicts post-op complications and is modifiable
Pre-op screening for coagulopathy (Harley et al. 2019)

(continued)

Table 7 (continued)

| 1143 elective neurosurgical patients, where INR and aPTT was done |
| Cost of coagulation testing was $68,009 |
| Limited value in indiscriminate laboratory coagulation testing |
| Routine complete blood counts and clinical impact (Howell et al. 2019) |
| 484 patients who underwent primary total knee arthroplasty |
| 25 patients needed transfusion following surgery (5.2%) |
| Risk of transfusions was 5.2 times higher in those with pre-op anemia |
| Daily CBCs are unnecessary if the first post-op lab does not prompt intervention; those anemic pre-op should obtain a post-op blood count |
| Pre-op lab testing, NICE (National Institute of Clinical Excellence) guidelines, compared to current practice (Guttikonda et al. 2019) |
| Tertiary referral center, 385 patients, 16 investigations looked at |
| Almost no agreement of current practice with NICE guidelines |
| Most tests overprescribed; costs up, none with impact on clinical care |

2018; Harley et al. 2019; Howell et al. 2019; Guttikonda et al. 2019).

Ultimately, ordering a test requires taking into consideration the likelihood that a patient has specific disorders prior to the order, along with an understanding of the accuracy of tests and as to how they will change management (Redberg et al. 2011). Having a discussion with the patient is the first step; the decision for testing must relate to benefits from testing outweighing any disadvantages. No test, not even a noninvasive one, is benign; often less is more (Redberg et al. 2011).

Key Points

- Although a large number of laboratory tests are available as screening options, the best approach would be to individualize testing for each patient based on history and physical examination.
- Significant laboratory abnormalities do not occur solely from aging.

- Marked deviations in test results usually indicate the presence of underlying disease or a response to therapy.
- Abnormal test results in older people likely indicate underlying disease; repeat testing to clarify has limited value.
- Test results are influenced by several factors, including gender, race, fasting or fed state and patient's list of medications and supplements.
- The probability of abnormal test results increases in older adults, in large part due to underlying comorbidity or medication effect.
- Pre-procedure testing is best guided by a focused history and examination, current medication list, and planned procedure.
- A large number of tests have a low probability of altering preoperative management and are not indicated in low-risk patients.
- In the hospital setting, judicious ordering of tests is recommended; the approach is associated with lower costs and negative consequences.
- Blood management guidelines suggest thresholds for transfusion in the preoperative period and the need to recognize and treat anemia that can be treated prior to surgery, for example, iron deficiency.
- Test results must be followed up by providers; abnormal test results need to be acknowledged and addressed.
- The number of tests ordered, the type of tests requested, the costs involved, and the value provided ultimately define in large measure the quality and cost of care provided.

References

Abad MJ, Bedoya LM, Bermejo P. An update on drug interactions with the herbal medicine ginkgo biloba. Curr Drug Metab. 2010;11(2):171–81.

Achuthan S, Smirk A, Keeble A, Leslie K. Perioperative mortality score: data collection and cost. Anaesth Intensive Care. 2011;39(2):274–8.

Adiga GU, Dharmarajan TS, Dutcher JP. Iatrogenic anemia in hospitalized older adults: impact on mortality. J Am Geriatr Soc. 2003;51:S212.

Al-Toma A, Volta U, Auricchio R, et al. European Society for the Study of Celiac Disease (ESsCD) guideline for coeliac disease and other gluten-related disorders. United European Gastroenterol J. 2019;7(5):583–613.

Bibbibns-Domingo K. Screening for celiac disease. US preventive services task force recommendation statement. JAMA. 2017;317:1252–7.

Bourdel-Marchasson I, Laksir H, Puget E. Interpreting routine biochemistry in those aged over 65 years: a time for change. Maturitas. 2010;66(1):39–45.

Brenner H, Calderazzo S, Seufferlein T, et al. Effect of a single aspirin dose prior to fecal immunochemical testing on test sensitivity for detecting advanced colorectal neoplasms: a randomized clinical trial. JAMA. 2019;321(17):1686–92.

Brown NK, Guandalini S, Semrad C, Kupfer SS. A clinician's guide to celiac disease HLA genetics. Am J Gastroenterol. 2019;114(10):1587–92. https://doi.org/10.14309/ajg.0000000000000310.

Bruce JM, Harrington CJ, Foster S, Westervelt HJ. Common laboratory values are associated with cognition among older inpatients referred for neuropsychological testing. Clin Neuropsychol. 2009;23(6):909–25.

Carter JY, Lema OE, Wangai MW, et al. Laboratory testing improves diagnosis and treatment outcomes in primary health care facilities. Afr J Lab Med. 2012;1(1):8. https://doi.org/10.4102/ajlm,v1i1.8.

Cheng L-F, Prasad N, Engelhardt BE. An optimal policy for patient laboratory tests in intensive care units. Pac Symp Biocomput. 2019;24:320–31.

Cieslak KP, Baur O, Verheji J, et al. Liver function declines with increased age. HPB (Oxford). 2016;18 (8):691–6.

Clouzeau B, Caujolle M, San-Miguel A, et al. The sustainable impact of an educational approach to improve the appropriateness of laboratory test orders in the ICU. PLoS One. 2019;14(5):e0214802. https://doi.org/10.1371/journal.pone.0214802.

Coates P. Liver function tests. Aust Fam Physician. 2011;40(3):113–5.

Collins DA, Riley TV. Clostridium difficile guidelines. Clin Infect Dis. 2018;67(10):1639. https://doi.org/10.1093/cid/ciy249.

Coodley EL. Laboratory tests in the elderly. What is abnormal? Postgrad Med. 1989;85(1):333–8.

Coyne D. Iron indices: what do they really mean? Kidney Int Suppl. 2006;101:S4–8.

Dharmarajan TS, Dharmarajan L. Anemia in older adults: an indicator requiring evaluation. Fam Pract Recertification. 2007;29(6):16–26.

Dharmarajan TS, Pitchumoni CS. Laboratory tests in older adults: indications, interpretations, issues. In: Pitchumoni CS, Dharmarajan TS, editors. Geriatric gastroenterology. 1st ed. New York: Springer; 2012. p. 261–9.

Dharmarajan TS, Pais W, Norkus EP. Does Anemia matter? Anemia, morbidity and mortality in older adults: need for greater recognition. Geriatrics. 2005;60 (12):22–9.

Dharmarajan TS, Yoo J, Russell RO, Norkus EP. Chronic kidney disease staging in nursing home and community older adults: does the choice of Cockcroft-Gault, modification of diet in renal disease study, or the chronic kidney disease epidemiology collaboration initiative equations matter? J Am Med Dir Assoc. 2012;13:151–5.

Dhatariya KK, Wiles MD. Pre-operative testing guidelines: a NICE try but not enough. Anaesthesia. 2016;71:1391–407.

Duff CJ, Solis-Trapala I, Driskell OJ, et al. The frequency of testing for glycated haemoglobin, HbA1c, is linked to the probability of achieving target levels in patients with suboptimally controlled diabetes mellitus. Clin Chem Lab Med. 2018;57(2):296–304.

Dzankic S, Pastor D, Gonzalez C, Leung JM. The prevalence and predictive value of abnormal preoperative laboratory tests in elderly surgical patients. Anesth Analg. 2001;93:301–8.

Edwards Y. Usefulness of blood tests carried out during screening of the elderly population in one practice. Br J Gen Pract. 1991;41:496–8.

Engel N, Ganesh G, Patil M, et al. Point-of-care testing in India: missed opportunities to realize the true potential of point-of-care testing programs. BMC Health Serv Res. 2015;15:550. https://doi.org/10.1186/s12913-015-1223-3.

English E, Lenters-Westera E. HbA1c method performance: the great success story of global standardization. Crit Rev Clin Lab Sci. 2018;55(6):408–19.

Evron JM, Herman WH, McEwen LN. Changes in screening practices for prediabetes and diabetes since the recommendation for hemoglobin A1c testing. Diabetes Care. 2019;42(4):576–84.

Faisal A, Andres K, Rind JAK, et al. Reducing the number of unnecessary routine laboratory tests through education of internal medicine residents. Postgrad Med J. 2018;94(1118):716–9.

Fei MA, Tianfeng W, Jiangang Z, et al. Plasma homocysteine and serum folate and vitamin B12 levels in mild cognitive impairment and Alzheimer's disease: a case controlled study. Nutrients. 2017;9(7):725.

Ferrari P, Kulkarni H, Dheda S, et al. Serum iron markers are inadequate for guiding iron repletion in chronic kidney disease. Clin J Am Soc Nephrol. 2011;6(1):77–83.

Finegan BA, Rashiq S, McAlister FA, O'Connor P. Selective ordering of preoperative investigations by anesthesiologists reduces the number and costs of tests. Can J Anaesth. 2005;52:575–80.

Fleisher LA. Routine laboratory testing in the elderly: is it indicated? Anesth Analg. 2001;93:249–50.

Fowler A, Perry DJ. Laboratory monitoring of haemostasis. Anaesthesia. 2015;70(1):68–72.

Goodwin JS, Asrabadi A, Howrey B, et al. Multiple measurement of serum lipids in the elderly. Med Care. 2011;49(2):225–30.

Grundy SM, Stone NJ, Bailey AL, et al. Guideline on the management of blood cholesterol. A report of the American College of Cardiology/American Heart Association task force on clinical practice guidelines. J Am Coll Cardiol. 2018; https://doi.org/10.1016/j.jacc.2018.11.003.

Gulseraen YD, Adiloglu AK, Yucel M, et al. Comparison of non-invasive tests with invasive tests in the diagnosis of celiac disease. J Clin Lab Anal. 2019;33(3):e22722.

Gupta A, Cifu AS, Khanna S. Diagnosis and treatment of Clostridium difficile infection. JAMA. 2018;320:10–1.

Guralnik JM, Eisenstaedt RS, Ferrucci L, et al. Prevalence of anemia in persons 65 years and older in the United States: evidence for a high rate of unexplained anemia. Blood. 2004;104(8):2263–8.

Guttikonda N, Nileshwar A, Rao M, Sushma TK. Preoperative laboratory testing - comparison of National Institute of Clinical Excellence guideline with current practice- an observational study. J Anaesthesiol Clin Prarmacol. 2019;35(2):227–30.

Harley S, Abussuud Z, Wickremesekera A, et al. Preoperative screening for coagulopathy in elective neurosurgical patients in Wellington regional hospital and survey of practice across Australia and New Zealand. J Clin Neurosci. 2019;6:201–5.

Heindl B. Perioperative coagulation monitoring – medical and economic aspects. Anaesthesiol Intensivmed Norfallmed Schmerzther. 2010;45(5):292–6.

Hepner DL. The role of testing in the preoperative evaluation. Cleve Clin J Med. 2009;76(4):S22–7.

Hossain N, Lebelt AS, Dharmarajan TS. Unexplained chronic skin lesions in an older male! Consider the iatrogenic factor: hydralazine induced cutaneous lupus! Int J Geriatr Gerontol. 2019;3:120. https://doi.org/10.29011/2577-0748.100020.

Howell EP, Dildow BJ, Karas V, et al. Clinical impact of routine complete blood counts following total knee arthroplasty. J Arthroplast. 2019;34(7S):S168–72.

Hunt NJ, Woo S, Lockwood GP, et al. Halls of aging in the liver. Comput Struct Biotechnol J. 2019;17:1151–61.

Kantor ED, Rehm CD, Haas JS, et al. Trends in prescription drug use among adults in the United States from 1999–2012. JAMA. 2015;314:1818–31.

Karimian N, Niculiseanu P, Amar-Zifkin A, et al. Association of elevated pre-operative hemoglobin A1c and post-operative copmplicaions in non-diabetic patients: a systematic review. World J Surg. 2018;42(1):61–72.

Keiso T. Laboratory values in the elderly. Are they different? Emerg Med Clin North Am. 1990;8(2):241–54.

Kenealy T, Herd G, Musaad S, Wells S. HbA1c screening in the community: lessons for safety and quality management of a point of care programme. Prim Care Diabetes. 2019;13(2):170–5.

Kennel KA, Mathew TD, Hurley DL. Vitamin D deficiency in adults: when to test and how to treat. Mayo Clin Proc. 2010;85(8):752–8.

Keshavan NH, Swamy CM. Pre-operative laboratory testing: a prospective study on comparison and cost analysis. Indian J Anaesth. 2016;60(11):838–42.

Kistler CE, Kirby KA, Lee D, et al. Long term outcomes following positive fecal occult blood test results in older adults: benefits and harms. Arch Intern Med. 2011;171(15):1344–51.

Knovich MA, Store JA, Coffman LG, et al. Ferritin for the clinician. Blood Rev. 2009;23(3):95–104.

Kozek-Langenecker SA. Perioperative coagulation monitoring. Best Pract Res Clin Anaesthesiol. 2010;24(1):27–40.

Krier M, Ahmed A. The asymptomatic outpatient with abnormal liver function tests. Clin Liver Dis. 2009;13(2):167–77.

Lai CC, You JF, Yeh CY, et al. Low preoperative serum albumin in colon cancer: a risk factor for poor outcome. Int J Color Dis. 2011;26(4):473–81.

Lakomkin N, Sathiyakumar V, Dodd AC, et al. Pre-operative labs: wasted dollars or predictors of post-operative cardiac and septic events in orthopedic trauma patients? Injury. 2016;47(6):1217–21. https://doi.org/10.1016/j.injury.2016.03.004.

Le Couteur DG, Blyth FM, Creasey HM, et al. The association of alanine transaminase with aging, frailty and mortality. J Gerontol A Biol Sci Med Sci. 2010a;65A(7):712–7.

Le Couteur DG, Blyth FM, Creasey HM, et al. The association of alanine transaminase with aging and morality. J Gerontol A Biol Med Sci. 2010b;65(7):712–7.

Lee HP, Chang YY, Jean YH, Wang HC. Importance of serum albumin level in the preoperative tests conducted in elderly patients with hip fracture. Injury. 2009;40(7):756–9.

Levi M, Meijers JC. DIC: which laboratory tests are most useful. Blood Rev. 2011;25(1):33–7.

Levy MJ, Anderson MA, Baron TH, et al. Position statement on routine laboratory testing before endoscopic procedures. Gastrointest Endosc. 2008;68(5):827–32.

Macpherson DS. Preoperative laboratory testing: should any tests be "routine" before surgery? Med Clin North Am. 1993;77(2):289–308.

Mandell BF. The tests that we order define us. Cleve Clin J Med. 2019;86(3):150.

Mandelli G, Radaelli F, Paggi S, et al. Anticoagulant or aspirin treatment does not affect the positive predictive value of an immunological fecal occult blood test in patients undergoing colorectal cancer screening: results from a nested in a cohort case-controlled study. Eur J Gastroenterol Hepatol. 2011;23(4):323–6.

Manson J, Bassuk SS, Buring JE. Vitamin D, calcium and cancer. Approaching daylight? JAMA. 2017;317:1217–8.

Martin D, Beardsell I. Is routine coagulation testing necessary in patients presenting to the emergency department with chest pain? Emerg Med J. 2012;29(3):184–7.

Martin H, Langenhan K, Huth M, et al. Clinical laboratory diagnosis and aging. 3: evaluation of a study of aging – complete blood and urine status. Z Gerontol Geriatr. 2001;3493:183–91.

Mata-Miranda Mdel P, Cano-Matus N, Rodriguez-Murrieta M, et al. Unnecessary routine laboratory tests in patients referred for surgical services. Cir Cir. 2016;84(2):121–6.

May JE, Marques MB, Reddy VVB, Gangaraju R. Three neglected numbers in the CBC: the RDW, MPV and NRBC count. Cleve Clin J Med. 2019;86:167–72.

Menke A, Muntner P, Fernandez-Real JM, Gualiar E. The association of biomarkers of iron status with mortality in US adults. Nutr Metab Cardiovasc Dis. 2012;22(9):734–40.

Meroni PL, Schur PH. ANA screening: an old test with new recommendations. Ann Rheum Dis. 2010;69(8):1420–2.

Michels WM, Grootendorst DC, Verduijn M, et al. Performance of the Cockcroft-Gault, MDRD and new CKD-EPI formulas in relation to GFR, age and body size. Clin J Am Soc Nephrol. 2010;5:1003–9.

Mizrahi EH, Fleissig Y, Arad M, et al. Admission testing and functional outcome of elderly hip fracture patients: is it important? Aging Clin Exp Res. 2007;19(4):284–9.

Mohapatra S, Singh DP, Alcid D, Pitchumoni CS. Beyond O and P times three. Am J Gastroenterol. 2018;113(6):805–18.

Mueller MM, Remoortel HV, Meybohm P, et al. Patient blood management recommendations from the 2018 Frankfurt consensus conference. JAMA. 2019;321(100):983–97.

Muniraj T, Dang S, Pitchumoni CS. Pancreatitis or not? Elevated lipase and amylase in ICU patients. J Crit Care. 2015;30(6):1370–5. [cited 2018 Dec 24].

Munoz M, Gomes-Ramirez S, Campos A, et al. Pre-operative anemia: prevalence, consequences and approaches to management. Blood Transfus. 2015;13:370–9.

Munoz M, Gomes-Ramirez S, Kozek-Langeneker S. Pre-operative hematological assessment in patients scheduled for major surgery. Anaesthesia. 2016;71(1):19–28.

NIH office of Dietary Supplements. Vitamin D fact sheet for health care professionals. Updated August 67, 2019. https://ods.od.nih.gov/factsheets/VitaminD-Health Professional

O'Brien MJ, Sacks DB. Point-of-care hemoglobin A1c. JAMA. 2019;322:1404–5.

Omran ML, Morley JE. Assessment of protein energy malnutrition in older persons, part II: laboratory evaluation. Nutrition. 2000;16(2):131–40.

Patel KV. Epidemiology of anemia in older adults. Semin Hematol. 2008;45(4):210–7.

Pinkham CA, Krause KJ. Liver function tests and mortality in a cohort of life insurance applicants. J Insur Med. 2009;41(3):170–7.

Pokorski RJ. Laboratory values in the elderly. J Insur Medicine. 1990;22(2):117–9.

Price EA, Mehra R, Homes TH, Schrier SL. Anemia in older persons: etiology and evaluation. Blood Cells Mol Dis. 2011;46(2):159–65.

Pum J. A practical guide to validation and verification of analytical methods I the clinical laboratory. Adv Clin Chem. 2019;90:215–81.

Qaseem A, Crandall CJ, Mustafa RA, et al. Screening for colorectal cancer in asymptomatic average-risk adults: a guidance statement from the American College of Physicians. Ann Intern Med. 2019;171:643–54.

Reazaul Karim HM, Prakash A, Sahoo SK, et al. Abnormal routine pre-operative test results and their impact on anaesthetic management: an observational study. Indian J Anaesth. 2018;62(1):23–8.

Redberg R, Katz M, Grady D. Diagnostic tests: another frontier for less is more. Arch Intern Med. 2011;172:619.

Richman DV. Ambulatory surgery: how much testing do we need? Anesthesiol Clin. 2010;28(2):185–97.

Riddle MC. Standards of Medical Care in Diabetes – 2019. Diabetes Care. 2019;42:S1–S186.

Roizen MF. More preoperative assessment by physicians and less by laboratory tests. N Engl J Med. 2000;342:204–5.

Rosen CJ. Vitamin D insufficiency. N Engl J Med. 2011;364:248–54.

Rostom A, Dube C. Conney et al. the diagnostic accuracy of serologic tests for celiac disease: a systematic review. Gastroenterology. 2005;128:538–46.

Schein OD, Katz J, Bass EB, et al. The value of routine preoperative medical testing before cataract surgery. N Engl J Med. 2000;342:168–75.

Schwed AC, Boggs MM, Xuan-Binh D, et al. Association of admission laboratory values and the timing of endoscopic retrograde cholangiopancreatography with clinical outcomes in acute cholangitis. JAMA Surg. 2016;151(11):1039–45.

Soin S, Akanbi O, Ahmed A, et al. Use and abuse of fecal occult blood tests: a community hospital experience. BMC Gastroenterol. 2019;19(1):161. https://doi.org/10.1186/s12876-010-1079-9.

Stuebing EA, Miner TJ. Surgical vampires and rising health care expenditure: reducing the cost of daily phlebotomy. Arch Surg. 2011;146(5):524–7.

Suresh E. Laboratory tests in rheumatology: a rational approach. Cleve Clin J Med. 2019;86(3):198–210.

Thachil J. Relevance of clotting tests in liver disease. Postgrad Med. 2008;84(990):177–81.

Toll AD, Lir JM, Gulati G, et al. Does routine repeat testing of critical values offer any advantage over single testing? Arch Pathol Lab Med. 2011;135(4):440–4.

Tsai ER, Tintu AN, Demirtas D, et al. A critical review of laboratory performance indicators. Crit Rev Clin Lab Sci. 2019;56(7):458–71.

Uthamalingam S, Kandala J, Daley M, et al. Serum albumin and mortality in acutely decompensated heart failure. Am Heart J. 2010;160(6):1149–55.

Vagianos K, Berstein CN. Homocysteinemia and B vitamin status among adult patients with inflammatory bowel disease: a one year prospective follow-up study. Inflamm Bowel Dis. 2012;18(4):718–24.

van der Windt DA, Jellema P, Mulder CJ, et al. Diagnostic testing for celiac disease among patients with abdominal symptoms, a systematic review. JAMA. 2010;303:1738–46.

Vernon G, Baranova A, Younossi ZM. Systematic review: the epidemiology and natural history of non-alcoholic fatty liver disease and non-alcoholic steatohepatitis in adults. Aliment Pharmacol Ther. 2011;34(3):274–85.

Vidoni ML, Gabreil KP, Luo ST, et al. Vitamin B12 and homocysteine associations with gait speed in older adults: the Baltimore longitudinal study of aging. J Nutr Health Aging. 2017;21(10):1321–8.

Wilson SE, Lipscombe LL, Rosella LC, Manuel DG. Trends in laboratory testing for diabetes in Ontario, Canada 1995–2005: a population-based study. BMC Health Serv Res. 2009;9:41.

Wittkowsky AK. Dietary supplements, herbs and oral anticoagulants: the nature of the evidence. J Thromb Thrombolysis. 2008;25(1):72–7.

Wolf AMD, Fontham ETH, Church TR, et al. Colorectal cancer screening for average-risk adults: 2018 guideline update from the American Cancer Society. CA Cancer J Clin. 2018;68(4):25–281.

Yadav D, Agarwal N, Pitchumoni CS. A critical evaluation of laboratory tests in acute pancreatitis. Am J Gastroenterol. 2002;97:1309–18.

Yadav D, Ng B, Saul M, Kennard ED. Relationship of serum pancreatic enzyme testing trends with the diagnosis of acute pancreatitis. Pancreas. 2011;40(3):383–9.

Zhang H, He SM, Sun J, et al. Prevalence and etiology of abnormal liver function tests in an adult population in Jilin, China. Int J Med Sci. 2011;8(3):254–62.

Gastrointestinal Pathology in the Older Adult

46

Noam Harpaz, Mohammad Raoufi, and Hongfa Zhu

Contents

Abstract

This chapter is aimed at acquainting the clinician with pathological aspects of gastrointestinal disorders. The chapter offers an overview of the pathology of diverse disease entities that are likely to be encountered in the geriatric population. The technological advances that now provide nearly unlimited direct access to tissues via endoscopy and endoscopic ultrasound throughout the digestive system for diagnostic sampling have made familiarity with pathological diagnosis an indispensable part of health-care delivery. The image-based format of this chapter provides the clinician a broad but easily digestible overview of the essential gross and microscopic pathological features of entities involving the entire gastrointestinal system, including hepatobiliary disorders, utilizing classical illustrations that are readily reviewed and retained.

Keywords

Gastrointestinal pathology · Esophagus · Stomach · Small intestine · Large intestine · Pancreas · Liver · Cancer · Inflammatory diseases

N. Harpaz (✉)
Department of Pathology, Molecular and Cell-Based Medicine, Icahn School of Medicine at Mount Sinai, New York, NY, USA
e-mail: noam.harpaz@mountsinai.org

M. Raoufi
Department of Pathology and Laboratory Medicine, Henry Ford Health System, Detroit, MI, USA
e-mail: raoufim@gmail.com

H. Zhu
Hackensack Pathology Associates, Hackensack University Medical Center, Hackensack, NJ, USA
e-mail: Hongfa.Zhu@hackensack.meridian.org

Introduction

The spectrum of gastrointestinal pathology is diverse and extensive, affecting all sites of the gastrointestinal tract. Current advances in technology and in diagnostic histopathological modalities including utility of high-resolution endoscopy, endoscopic ultrasound, and fine-needle biopsy enable targeted biopsies, enhanced diagnostic yield, and high-level accuracy of histopathological diagnosis in the geriatric patient. In conjunction with a comprehensive history and clinical examination, the role for histopathology in the diagnosis of numerous classical and newer gastrointestinal disorders has become readily possible in older adults, with minimally invasive diagnostic procedures. Precise histopathological diagnosis offers the opportunity for tailored therapy. Along with clinical examination, laboratory testing, and imaging, where applicable, direct access to tissues of the gastrointestinal system and diagnostic sampling have enabled precise histopathological diagnosis. This is indispensable for diagnosis in current health-care delivery.

The chapter offers a sampling of histopathological figures of several gastrointestinal disorders that are prevalent in older adults; the figures

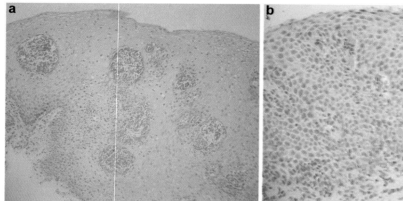

Fig. 1 Reflux esophagitis. Reflux esophagitis presents a variety of different but overlapping microscopic manifestations. (Left) In this biopsy, the squamous esophageal mucosa features prominent dilated capillaries, or vascular lakes, corresponding endoscopically to mucosal erythema. The surrounding squamous cells are swollen and contain densely eosinophilic cytoplasm. This squamous "ballooning" is caused by intracellular leakage of plasma protein across chemically injured cell membranes. (Right) Biopsy of another patient with reflux esophagitis showing basal cell hyperplasia, reflecting increased cell turnover, and scattered eosinophils

Fig. 2 Candida esophagitis. Candida esophagitis, a cause of odynophagia, presents microscopically as pseudomembranes consisting of fungal spores, pseudohyphae, and desquamated squamous cells. The fungi are best seen with special stains such as this silver impregnation stain. (Inset) Endoscopically, the pseudomembranes present as whitish mucosal plaques

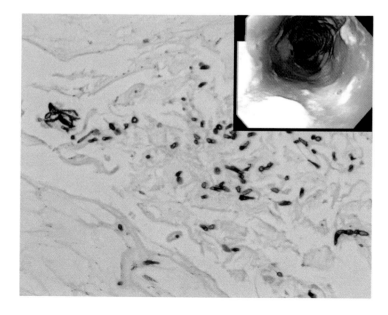

are accompanied by succinct, comprehensive descriptions to enable clinicians develop an understanding of the pathological essentials of the disorder (Figs. 1, 2, 3, 4, 5, 6, 7, 8, 9, 10, 11, 12, 13, 14, 15, 16, 17, 18, 19, 20, 21, 22, 23, 24, 25, 26, 27, 28, 29, 30, 31, 32, 33, 34, 35, 36, 37, 38, 39, 40, 41, 42, 43, 44, 45, 46, 47, 48, 49, 50, 51, 52).

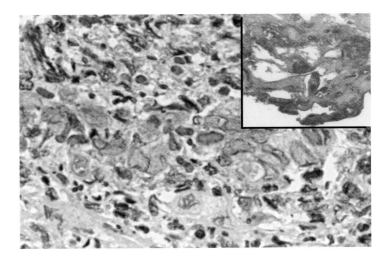

Fig. 3 Herpes esophagitis. Herpes esophagitis, another cause of odynophagia, presents endoscopically as mucosal vesicles and erosions. Microscopically, one observes desquamated squamous cells with single or multiple "ground glass" nuclei characterized by grayish central pallor. (Inset) Immunoperoxidase stain for herpes antigen

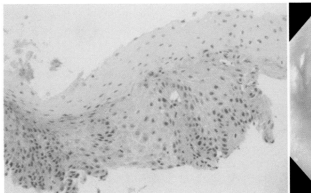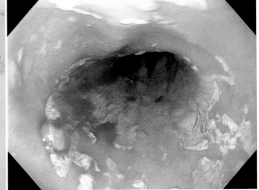

Fig. 4 Sloughing esophagitis. Sloughing esophagitis, also known as esophagitis dissecans superficialis, is an idiopathic, clinically innocuous disorder characterized by desquamation of superficial squamous epithelium. (Left) Histologically one sees a superficial layer of pale, parakeratotic, partially necrotic squamous mucosa which contrasts with the deeper viable mucosa, resulting in a distinctive "two-tone" appearance. (Right) Endoscopically, there are white patches corresponding to partially detached mucosa

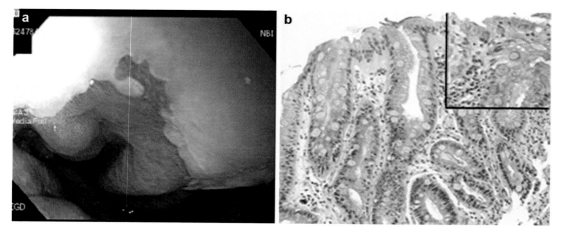

Fig. 5 Barrett's esophagus. Barrett's esophagus is defined as metaplastic columnar-lined mucosa which extends cephalad at least 1 cm from the gastroesophageal junction. It is estimated to occur in approximately 10% of individuals with chronic gastroenteric reflux. (Left) Short-segment Barrett's esophagus, observed with narrow band imaging, featuring an irregular tongue of dark mucosa that extends into the tubular esophagus. (Right) The metaplastic columnar epithelium consists of cells with micro-vesicular cytoplasm interspersed with goblet cells with a single large mucin vacuole. (Inset) Alcian Blue stain highlights the goblet cells, helping to distinguish them from gastric surface cells

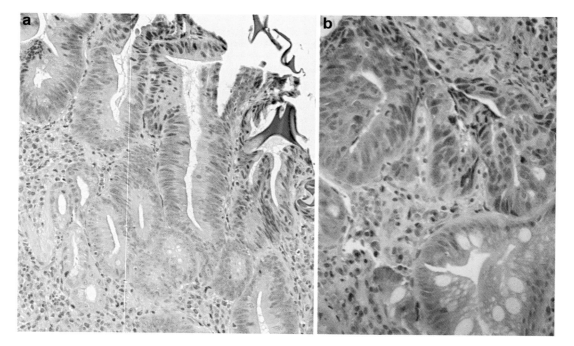

Fig. 6 Barrett's dysplasia. Barrett's dysplasia is a neo-plastic change that precedes the development of esopha-geal adenocarcinoma. (Left) Low-grade dysplasia is characterized by glandular and surface epithelium with darkly stained, crowded nuclei. The nuclei have a parallel configuration and are mostly confined to the base of the cells. (Right) High-grade dysplasia features epithelial cells with disorderly, stratified nuclei that occupy a large pro-portion of the cytoplasm

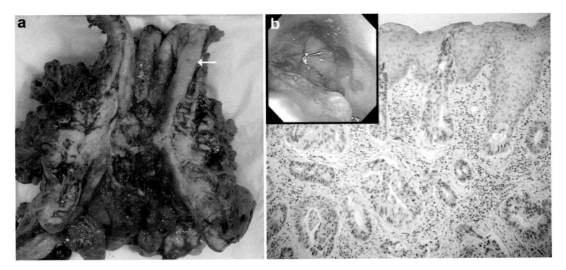

Fig. 7   Barrett's adenocarcinoma. Esophageal adenocarcinoma occurs in a subset of patients with Barrett's esophagus at a rate estimated at 2-5% per decade. (Left) Esophagectomy specimen containing an ulcerated, stricturing mass which invades transmurally into the surrounding soft tissue. Arrow highlights the squamocolumnar junction. (Right) Another tumor consisting microscopically of malignant glands invading into the esophageal wall. The overlying squamous mucosa has re-grown following previous ablation of dysplastic Barrett's mucosa by photodynamic therapy. (Inset) Protuberant mass arising in partially columnar-lined esophagus

Fig. 8   Eosinophilic Esophagitis. Squamous mucosa of esophagus with superficial infiltration and sloughing of eosinophils. Inset shows transverse esophageal rings, or so-called trachealization, resulting from submucosal fibrosis

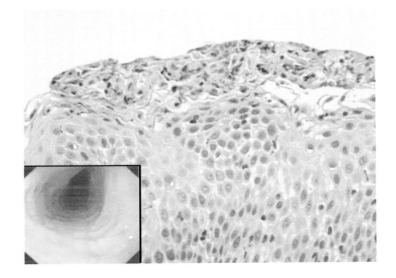

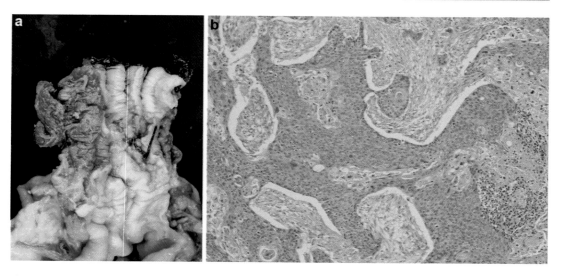

Fig. 9 Esophageal squamous cell carcinoma. Squamous cell carcinoma in a patient who presented with dysphagia and weight loss. (Left) Esophagectomy specimen with ulcerated tumor mass surrounded above and below by squamous mucosa. (Right) Microscopically, the tumor consists of solid sheets of cohesive tumor cells. Scattered groups of keratinized tumor cells appear as dyscohesive eosinophilic cells

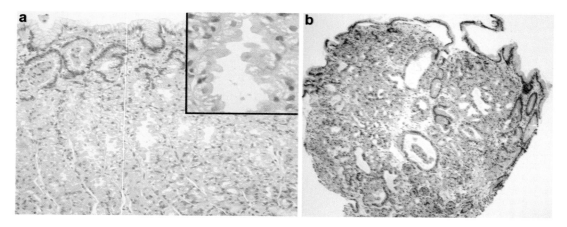

Fig. 10 Hypergastrinemia. Hypergastrinemia, usually associated with chronic use of proton pump inhibitors or less commonly with Zollinger-Ellison syndrome, causes striking hyperplasia of the gastric parietal cells. (Left) The oxyntic glands have dilated lumens lined by abundant parietal cells. (Inset) The parietal cells are enlarged and vacuolated and protrude into the lumen, producing a sawtooth profile. (Right) Chronic use of PPIs also results in single or multiple gastric fundic gland polyps that consist of cystically dilated foveolar and oxyntic-lined glands with increased parietal cells

Fig. 11 Iron pill gastropathy. Deposition of therapeutic iron, a potential cause of erosive gastritis, presents microscopically as subsurface basophilic- and gold-colored deposits (arrows). (Inset) The iron particles can be highlighted with Perl's Prussian blue stain

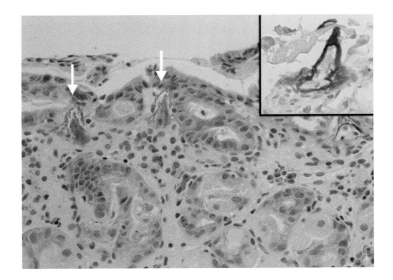

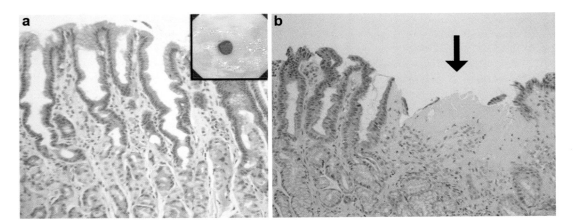

Fig. 12 Other chemical gastropathies. (Left) Bile reflux gastropathy presents microscopically with corkscrew-shaped foveolae lined by mucin-deficient, basophilic columnar epithelium. (Inset) Endoscopically, the gastric mucosa is erythematous and covered with bile-tinged secretions. (Right) NSAID-associated erosive gastritis. The mucosa contains a discrete erosion covered by fibrinous exudate (arrow). The adjacent intact foveolae are similar to those in bile reflux gastropathy

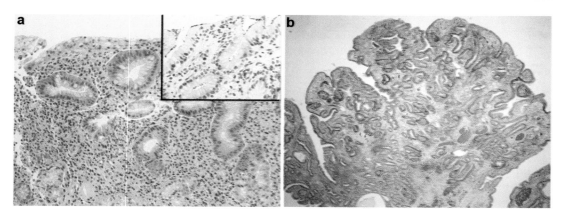

Fig. 13 Chronic gastritis. (Left) *H. pylori*-associated gastritis featuring dense mononuclear inflammatory cell infiltrates. (Inset) Immunoperoxidase stain highlights the slender bacilli attached to the gastric surface epithelium. (Right) Hyperplastic gastric polyp. These polyps occur singly or multiply in the setting of chronic gastritis. They consist microscopically of tortuous, dilated gastric foveolae surrounded by expanded, chronically inflamed stroma

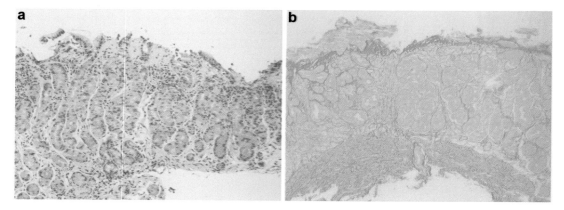

Fig. 14 Collagenous gastritis. An uncommon idiopathic gastritis that causes chronic dyspepsia and which occurs alone or in conjunction with collagenous colitis, collagenous sprue, or other autoimmune diseases. (Left) Gastric mucosa with subepithelial collagen deposition. (Inset) The gastric mucosa is typically nodular. (Right) The collagen band can be highlighted with Sirius picric red stain. Alternative stains include tenascin, Masson's trichrome, and Epstein van Gieson

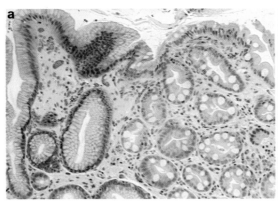
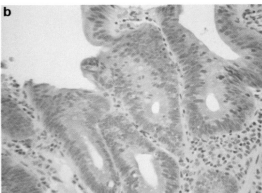

Fig. 15 Precursors of gastric cancer. (Left) Intestinal metaplasia, seen in the right side of this biopsy, presents as replacement of the gastric columnar cells by goblet cells and enteric columnar cells. Precancerous molecular alterations may begin at this stage. (Right) Dysplasia, an intermediate stage in the progression to gastric cancer, is characterized by glandular and surface epithelium with dark-staining, crowded, elliptical nuclei

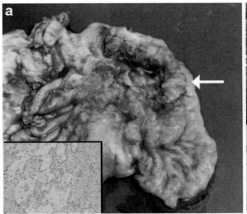
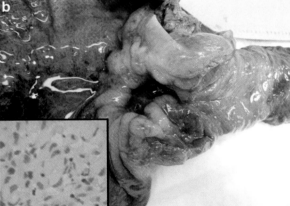

Fig. 16 Gastric adenocarcinoma. (Left) Large, ulcerated tumor occupying the gastric antrum. (Inset) Microscopically, the tumor consists of malignant, partially formed glands and is classified as "intestinal" or "tubular." (Right) Ulcerated tumor occupying the pylorus. (Inset) Microscopically, the tumor consists of signet ring cells, i.e., dyscohesive cells with mucin vacuoles and peripherally displaced crescentic nuclei, and is classified as "diffuse" or "poorly cohesive."

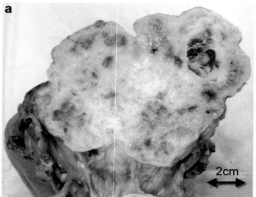

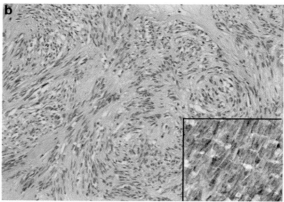

Fig. 17 GIST. Gastrointestinal stromal tumors (GISTs) may arise throughout the gastrointestinal tract or abdomen. They vary with respect to malignant potential from essentially benign to highly malignant, the distinction depending mainly on location, size, and mitotic activity. (Left) 8 cm GIST of low malignant potential protruding from the serosal aspect of the stomach. The cut surface reveals a well-circumscribed, gray-white, mostly solid mass. (Right) Microscopically, the tumor consists of whorls of uniform spindle cells with absent mitotic figures. (Inset) Immunohistochemical expression of the c-Kit tyrosine-protein kinase (CD117) occurs in the great majority of GISTs and helps distinguish them from other spindle cell tumors

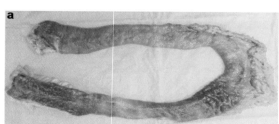

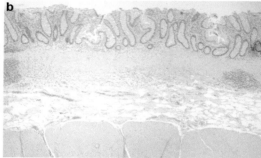

Fig. 18 Ulcerative colitis. (Left) Colon resection specimen featuring diffuse attenuation of the mucosal folds and scattered regions of erythema and nodularity. (Right) Postinflammatory changes in quiescent ulcerative colitis include skewed crypt architecture and fibrous thickening of the muscularis mucosae

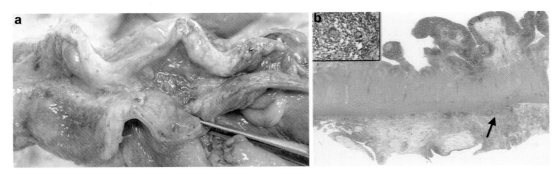

Fig. 19 Crohn's disease. (Left) Small intestinal segment with Crohn's disease manifested by multiple strictures, thickened wall and ulcerated mucosa. (Right) Crohn's colitis featuring ulceration, inflammatory polyps and transmural chronic inflammation. Note the markedly thickened subserosal layer with lymphoid follicles and granulomas (arrow and inset)

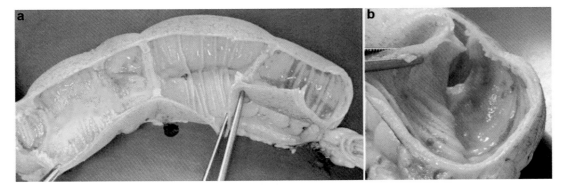

Fig. 20 NSAID-associated enteropathy. Excessive use of NSAIDs may result in enteric erosions or, less commonly, formation of intestinal diaphragms. (Left) Segment of small intestine with multiple transverse septa. (Right) Close-up view of diaphragm with central lumen

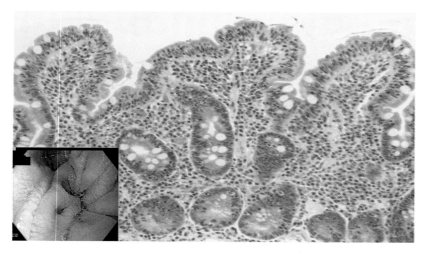

Fig. 21 Celiac disease. Celiac disease in older patients may account for symptoms of weight loss, diarrhea, iron deficiency anemia, or early-onset osteoporosis. Additionally, it predisposes to lymphoma and other malignancies. The most sensitive though not necessarily specific microscopic feature is an increased number of intraepithelial lymphocytes, usually accompanied by a dense infiltrate of mononuclear inflammatory cells in the lamina propria. Villous blunting, elongated crypts, and mitotically active crypt epithelium are common but not essential features, especially in patients with mild symptoms. All the above features are present in the example shown. Celiac disease may be mimicked by various other conditions including infections, autoimmune enteritis, food sensitivities, drug reactions, etc. As a result, serological and possibly HLA testing are an integral part of the evaluation. (Inset) Endoscopically, scalloping of the small intestinal mucosa is a clue to the diagnosis of celiac disease, albeit not a specific feature

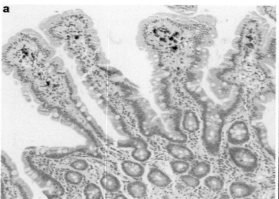
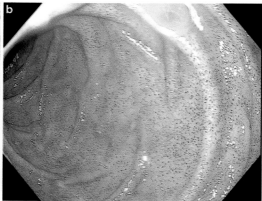

Fig. 22 Pseudomelanosis duodeni. (Left) This idiopathic, asymptomatic disorder presents endoscopically as spotty mucosal pigmentation. (Right) The upper villous lamina propria contains brownish pigment deposits which are composed of iron, sulfur, and other metallic substances

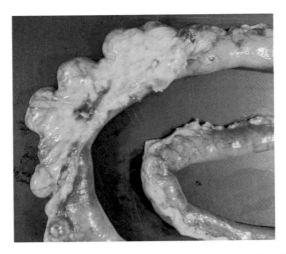

Fig. 23 Small intestinal diverticulosis. Small intestinal diverticulosis, a potential cause of bacterial overgrowth and malabsorption syndrome, usually occurs in elderly patients. Multiple bulging diverticula are seen along the mesenteric insertion

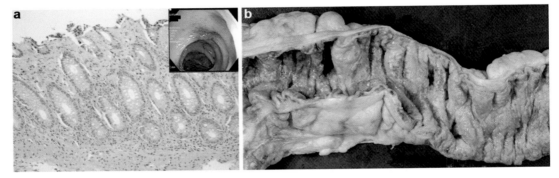

Fig. 24 Ischemic colitis. Ischemic colitis can vary greatly in clinical severity, mild cases affecting the mucosa and more severe cases involving progressively deeper layers of the colonic wall. (Left) Mild ischemia in a patient with abdominal pain and rectal bleeding presenting endoscopically with mucosal petechia and red-brown discoloration. (Inset) Microscopically, the colonic crypts, especially near the surface, are narrowed and depleted of goblet cells, and the lamina propria is eosinophilic due to leakage of plasma protein from damaged capillaries. (Right) Moderately severe ischemic colitis with extensive ulceration but no evidence of peritonitis

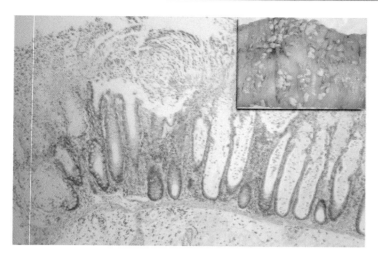

Fig. 25 Antibiotic-associated colitis. Pseudomembranous colitis, the most severe manifestation of antibiotic-associated colitis, presents microscopically with dilated, mucin-filled colonic crypts and overlying mucosuppurative exudates that appear to spew forth from a necrotic surface. On the far left, nearly the entire thickness of the mucosa has been effaced by necrosis. (Inset) Resected colon containing tan, plaque-like pseudomembranes each surrounded by a halo of erythema. Although *C. difficile* accounts for most cases of pseudomembranous colitis, other bacterial pathogens including *Shigella*, enterohemorrhagic *E. coli*, and *K. oxytoca* can have similar manifestations

Fig. 26 Melanosis coli. Abuse of laxatives may result in melanosis coli, a dark-brown mucosal pigmentation, manifested in this case by a "leopard skin" pattern. (Inset) Microscopically, the mucosa contains clusters of histiocytes with brown cytoplasmic lipofuscin pigment, a breakdown product of apoptotic epithelial cells

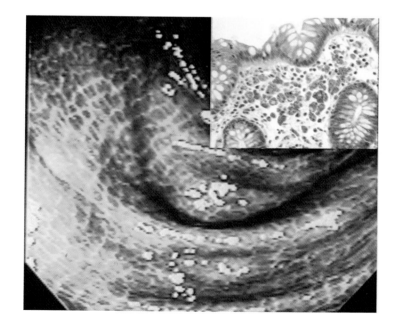

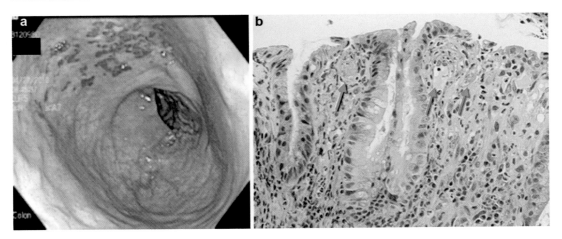

Fig. 27   Radiation proctitis. Radiation proctitis following pelvic radiotherapy in a patient presenting with rectal pain and bleeding. (Left) Endoscopic findings include localized or diffuse hyperemia, petechia, or telangiectasias. (Right) Microscopically, the mucosa contains dilated, thrombosed subsurface capillaries (arrows)

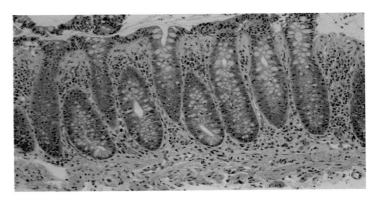

Fig. 28   Collagenous colitis. Collagenous colitis, a cause of non-bloody diarrhea, cramping, or abdominal pain affecting mainly older women. The colon is usually endoscopically normal or near-normal. Microscopically, normal crypt architecture is maintained, but the lamina propria contains increased mononuclear inflammatory cells. The diagnostic feature is a subepithelial band of eosinophilic collagen that entraps capillaries and inflammatory cells. Frequently, intraepithelial lymphocytes are present in the surface and crypts

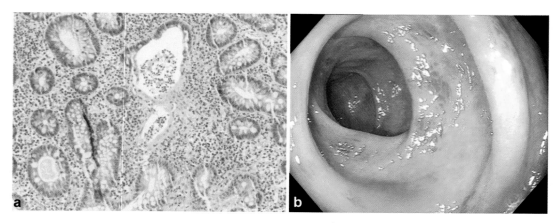

Fig. 29 Immune checkpoint therapy-associated colitis. Colitis associated with immune checkpoint inhibitor therapy is increasingly common. It can mimic IBD or ischemic, autoimmune, or microscopic colitis. (Left) Active chronic inflammation with crypt abscesses and dense mononuclear inflammatory cells. (Right) Endoscopic view shows patchy mucosal erythema

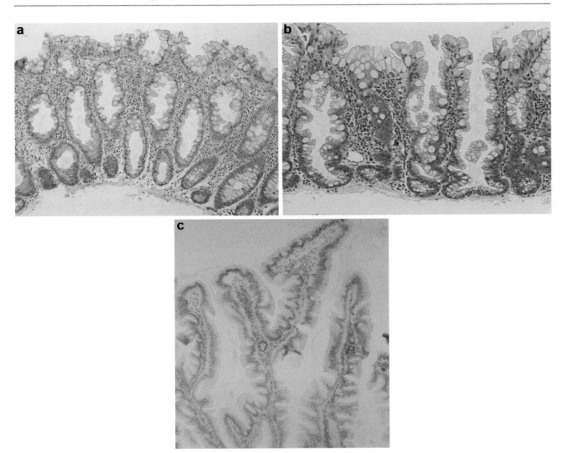

Fig. 30 Serrated colorectal polyps. Serrated colorectal polyps affect similar demographic groups as conventional colorectal polyps, the great majority arising from middle age and beyond. (a) Hyperplastic polyp. This tends to be quite small and is usually situated in the distal colorectum. Microscopically, the upper portion of the crypts is expanded and has a serrated luminal profile which becomes tapered and circular basally. (b) Sessile serrated lesion. This polyp tends to be larger and more frequently right-sided than hyperplastic polyps. Microscopically, the crypts are hyperserrated along their entire length, and some have a flat base that extends laterally forming an inverted T. (c) Traditional serrated adenoma. This polyp also tends to be large and occurs in the distal colorectum. The epithelium is dysplastic and features eosinophilic cytoplasm and crowded, elongated nuclei. Sessile serrated lesions and traditional serrated adenomas are both considered precancerous

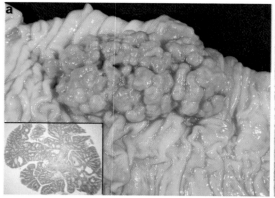

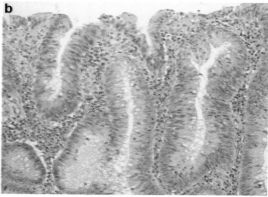

Fig. 31 Colorectal adenoma. Colorectal adenomas occur anywhere in the colorectum and vary greatly in size and configuration. The likelihood of harboring cancer is directly related to their size, multiplicity, and severity of histologic dysplasia. (Left) Large, sessile colorectal adenoma. (Inset) Microscopically, this portion of the adenoma consists of crowded tubular structures. (Right) The lining epithelium, seen at high magnification, consists of dysplastic columnar epithelial cells with crowded, elongated, dark-staining nuclei

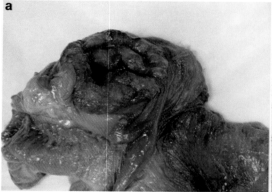

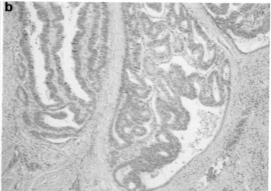

Fig. 32 Colorectal cancer. (Left) Protuberant cecal adenocarcinoma with granular, hemorrhagic surface. (Right) Typical histological appearance of colorectal cancer featuring columnar cells with a gland-within-gland arrangement and surrounding fibrotic stroma

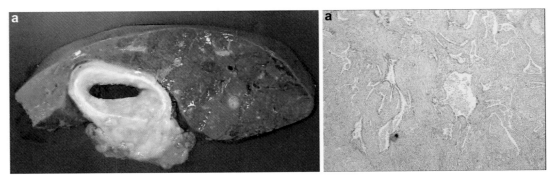

Fig. 33 Gallbladder adenocarcinoma - extrahepatic cholangiocarcinoma. (Left) Liver with cholangiocarcinoma of gallbladder. The wall is circumferentially thickened and replaced by a scirrhous, white tumor. (Right) Microscopically, the tumor consists of large, irregularly shaped glands surrounded by reactive fibrous stroma

Fig. 34 Diverticulitis. Diverticulitis of the sigmoid colon complicated by a mesenteric abscess (white arrow) communicating with a diverticulum (black arrow)

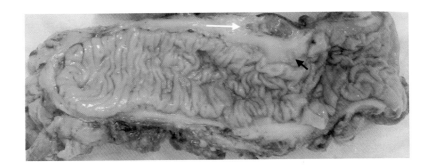

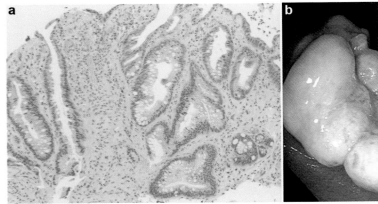
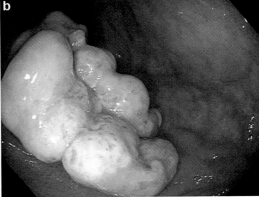

Fig. 35 Solitary rectal ulcer syndrome. This inflammatory lesion results from internal rectal or rectosigmoid intussusception and causes chronic constipation. It can present as an ulcer, firm plaque, or polyp that can closely mimic malignancy. (Left) Rectal mucosa expanded by fibromuscular lamina propria with numerous subepithelial capillaries and lined by non-dysplastic epithelium. (Right) Polypoid mucosa mimicking a neoplasm

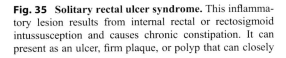

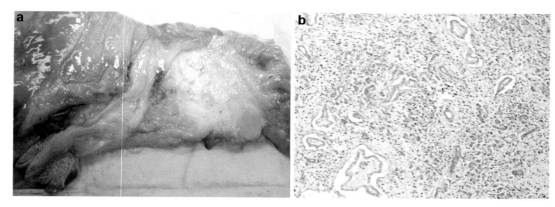

Fig. 36 Pancreatic adenocarcinoma. (Left) Scirrhous white mass in the pancreatic head impinging on the duodenum adjacent to the common bile duct. (Right) Microscopically, the pancreatic parenchyma is replaced by pleomorphic invasive glands and fibroinflammatory stroma

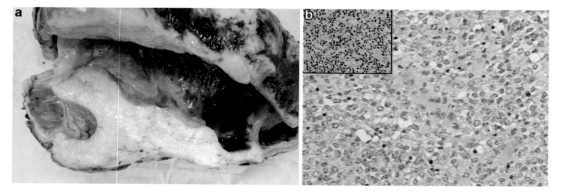

Fig. 37 Extranodal lymphoma. Extranodal lymphomas arise most frequently in the gastrointestinal tract. (Left) Small intestine with diffuse large B cell lymphoma presenting as an ileal tumor mass. Cut section reveals fleshy tan ("fish flesh") parenchyma that replaces the intestinal wall. (Right) Microscopically, the tumor consists of large, atypical monomorphous cells. (Inset) Immunostain for Pax-5, a transcription factor specific for B lymphocytes

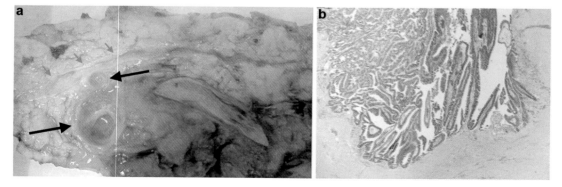

Fig. 38 Intraductal papillary mucinous neoplasm. (Left) Pancreas containing two mucin-filled, cystically-dilated branches of the main pancreatic duct (arrows). (Right) Cystic cavity containing villiform epithelium proliferation

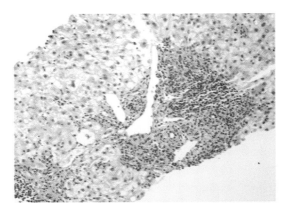

Fig. 39 Autoimmune hepatitis. Autoimmune hepatitis. Liver needle biopsy with lobular and portal lymphoplasmacytic inflammatory cell infiltrates, interface hepatitis, and hepatocyte necrosis

Fig. 40 Hepatocellular carcinoma. Hepatocellular carcinoma may present diverse histological appearances. This example features trabecular architecture and bile secretions (arrows). (Inset) Caudate lobectomy specimen with well-demarcated, slightly green tumor nodule that is grossly diagnostic of HCC

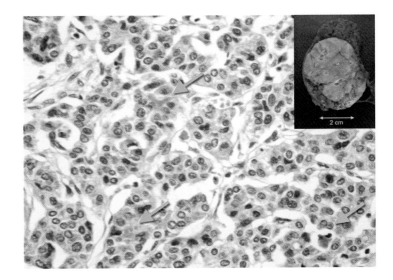

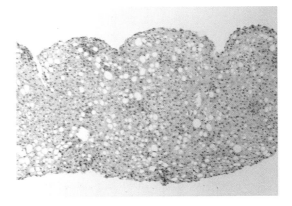

Fig. 41 Steatohepatitis. Steatohepatitis is characterized microscopically by large droplet steatosis, ballooning hepatocyte degeneration, and mild lobular inflammation

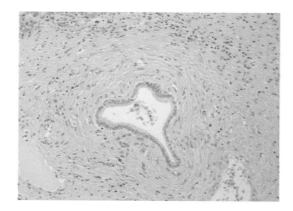

Fig. 42 Primary sclerosing cholangitis. Biliary tract in primary sclerosing cholangitis shows periductal "onion-skin" fibrosis

Fig. 43 Intrahepatic cholangiocarcinoma. Liver with intrahepatic cholangiocarcinoma. Microscopically, the hepatic tissue is invaded by well-differentiated adenocarcinoma. (Inset) Segmentectomy with main tumor mass (arrow) and satellite nodules featuring scalloped, infiltrative borders, and central necrosis

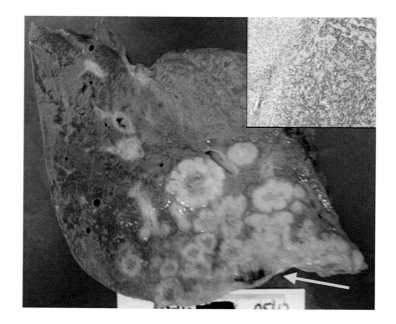

Fig. 44 Metastatic colon cancer. Segmental liver resection with isolated metastasis of colonic adenocarcinoma. Macroscopically, the yellow-grey color, central fibrosis and irregular, infiltrative borders are typical of such lesions

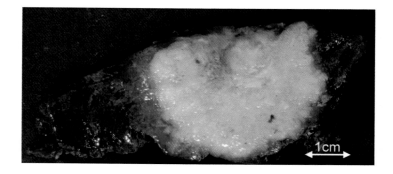

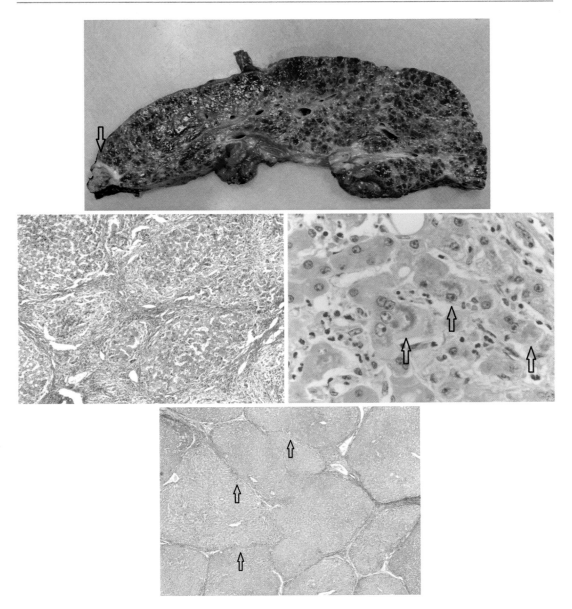

Fig. 45 Alcohol cirrhosis. (Top) Liver explant containing treated hepatocellular carcinoma (arrow) in a background of micronodular cirrhosis secondary to alcohol abuse. (Middle left) Microscopically, the parenchyma is composed of regenerative hepatocyte lobules surrounded by fibrous septa (trichrome stain). (Middle right) Hepatocytes with Mallory-Denke hyaline (arrow). (Bottom) Abstinence from alcohol can result in histological regression characterized by thin, incomplete septa (arrow)

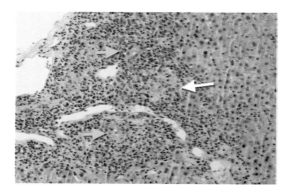

Fig. 46 Primary biliary cirrhosis. Primary biliary cirrhosis. This liver biopsy shows lymphoplasmacytic inflammation of portal tracts, bile ductular damage (yellow arrows), and periductular granulomatous reaction (white arrow)

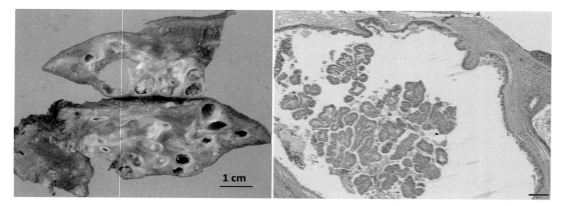

Fig. 47 Intraductal papillary tumor of bile duct. (Left) This lesion is characterized by multiple cystically dilated intraductal spaces and is sometimes associated with invasive carcinoma analogously to pancreatic intraductal papillary mucinous neoplasm. (Right) Microscopic appearance of dilated cystic space containing papillary epithelial proliferation

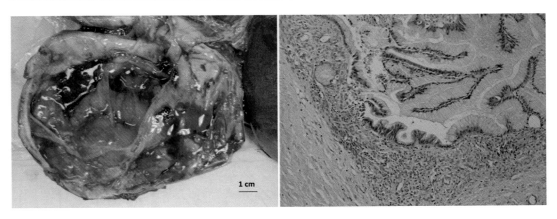

Fig. 48 Pancreatic mucinous cystic neoplasm. (Left) This multiloculated cystic pancreatic lesion ("cyst in cyst") with mucoid contents is premalignant. (Right) Microscopically, it features tall columnar mucinous epithelium surrounded by ovarian-type spindle cell stroma

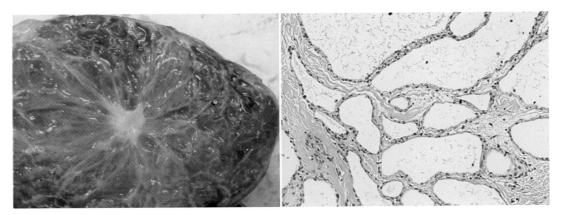

Fig. 49 Pancreatic serous cystadenoma. Pancreatic serous cystadenoma. This tumor is slow-growing, almost invariably benign, and usually arises in the pancreatic tail, thus rarely causing jaundice. (Left) Well-circumscribed tumor featuring central scar and radiating fibrous septa. (Right) Microscopic features include numerous small cysts lined by a single layer of cuboidal or flat epithelial cells with clear cytoplasm and small, uniform nuclei

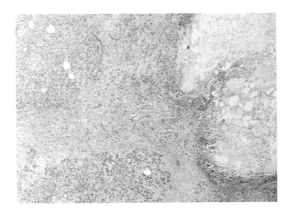

Fig. 50 Chronic pancreatitis. Chronic pancreatitis is manifested microscopically by atrophy of the acinar and ductal pancreatic tissues associated with chronic inflammation and fibrosis. The pale regions on the right correspond to fat necrosis

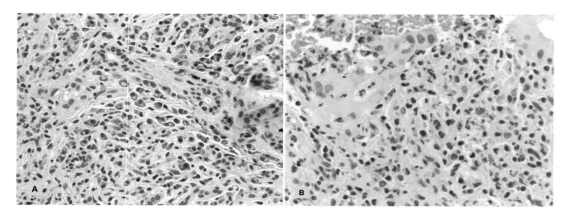

Fig. 51 Autoimmune pancreatitis. Also known as IgG4-related disease, this rare benign condition can mimic pancreatic cancer clinically. It can be subclassified into two types. (Left) Type 1 features diffuse lymphoplasmacytic infiltrates, diffuse enlargement of the pancreas radiologically, and elevation of serum IgG4. (Right) Type 2 is often associated with inflammatory bowel disease and is characterized histologically by granulocytic epithelial lesions (arrow). Both types respond well to steroid therapy

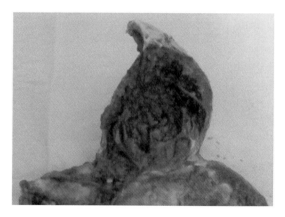

Fig. 52 Pancreatic pseudocyst. Pancreatic pseudocyst, consisting of a fibrous wall without any epithelial lining, results from cystic necrosis of pancreatic and surrounding soft tissues in the setting of acute pancreatitis. The inner surface of this resected cyst is bloodstained due to intracystic hemorrhage

Part VIII

Motility Disorders

Oropharyngeal Dysphagia

47

Custon Nyabanga, Abraham Khan, and Rita M. Knotts

Contents

Abstract

Oropharyngeal dysphagia (OD) is defined as difficulty in moving a food bolus from the mouth to the upper esophagus and disproportionately affects the older population. There are a multitude of potential etiologies of OD, and current diagnostic testing modalities utilized to decipher the cause of OD in an individual geriatric patient include videofluoroscopic swallow studies, nasopharyngolaryngoscopy, fiber-optic endoscopic evaluation of swallowing, high-resolution manometry, as well as functional lumen imaging probe technology. Determining the particular etiology of OD in a patient can direct appropriate treatment. Management options for OD range from noninvasive swallow exercises and rehabilitative techniques targeted to the underlying pathophysiology to invasive therapy to the upper esophageal sphincter or non-oral feeding. A careful diagnostic evaluation with meticulous attention to the underlying mechanism of OD can allow a practitioner to weigh risks and benefits of suitable treatment options for older patients affected with OD.

C. Nyabanga
Department of Medicine, NYU Langone Health, NYU School of Medicine, New York, NY, USA
e-mail: Custon.Nyabanga@nyulangone.org

A. Khan (✉) · R. M. Knotts
Division of Gastroenterology. Department of Medicine, NYU Langone Health, NYU School of Medicine, New York, NY, USA
e-mail: Abraham.Khan@nyulangone.org;
Rita.Knotts@nyulangone.org

© Springer Nature Switzerland AG 2021
C. S. Pitchumoni, T. S. Dharmarajan (eds.), *Geriatric Gastroenterology*,
https://doi.org/10.1007/978-3-030-30192-7_40

Keywords

Oropharyngeal dysphagia · Presbyphagia ·
Cricopharyngeus · Upper esophageal
sphincter · Striatal muscle dysfunction ·
Oropharyngeal dysphagia · Esophageal
dysphagia · Deglutition · Stroke ·
Malnutrition · Dehydration · Aspiration ·
Cranial nerves V, VII, and XII · Cervical
osteophytes · Cricopharyngeus ·
Cerebrovascular accident · Plummer-Vinson
syndrome · Amyotrophic lateral sclerosis ·
Guillain-Barré syndrome · Myasthenia gravis ·
Sjogren's syndrome · Rheumatoid arthritis ·
Periodontal disease · Shaker head lift exercise ·
Tongue-to-palate resistance training (TPRT) ·
Mendelsohn maneuver

Introduction

Dysphagia disproportionately affects the older
population and can result in grave morbidity,
mortality, and increased healthcare costs (Khan
et al. 2014; Wirth et al. 2016). Dysphagia is
defined as impaired preparation and transfer of
liquid or solid food bolus from the mouth into
the stomach (Hawkey et al. 2012). The disorder
is classified anatomically into oropharyngeal or
esophageal dysphagia, typically delineated
by the upper esophageal sphincter (UES).
Oropharyngeal dysphagia (OD), also referred
to as transfer dysphagia, is the difficulty in
moving a food bolus from the mouth to the
upper esophagus and is further subdivided into
disorders of the oral and pharyngeal phases
(Hawkey et al. 2012; Matsuo and Palmer 2008).

Presbyphagia describes the normal physiologic
changes in deglutition that occur with aging in
an otherwise healthy adult, which certainly may
augment the risk of dysphagia-related complications in adults with other comorbidities (Humbert
and Robbins 2008). OD is more common among
adults over the age of 65, and an estimated
12–33% of independent community dwellers
and more than 50% of healthcare facility-
domiciled elderly have abnormal deglutition
(Wirth et al. 2016; Roy et al. 2007; Lin et al.

2002; Serra-Prat et al. 2011). In the United States
alone, it is estimated that at least 13% of adults
over the age of 65 are affected by dysphagia, and 1
in 25 overall adults will develop dysphagia every
year (Sura et al. 2012; Patel et al. 2018;
Bhattacharyya 2014). As such, dysphagia has
been increasingly recognized as a geriatric syndrome that has implications for health outcomes
and quality of life (Roy et al. 2007; Chen et al.
2009). Many affected patients are unaware of
initial symptoms, and thus the disorder often
goes unrecognized until further progression
when complications arise (Clave and Shaker
2015; Serra-Prat et al. 2012).

When dysphagia is unrecognized or untreated,
there can be deleterious consequences ranging
from malnutrition, dehydration, aspiration
which can ultimately precipitate a decline in
patient outcomes, morbidity, mortality, and longer
hospital stays (Patel et al. 2018; Altman 2011;
Andrade et al. 2018). Thus, in this respect
dysphagia may represent a surrogate marker for
disease severity. Patients with OD are more likely
to incur higher inpatient costs and are often
discharged to long-term care facilities, leading to
a substantial cost burden to the healthcare system
(Patel et al. 2018; Attrill et al. 2018). Thus, prompt
recognition and screening for OD can ultimately
lead to a reduction in overall associated complications and costs.

Mechanism of Swallow: Oropharyngeal Phase

To understand the etiology and pathogenesis of
OD, it is essential to outline normal physiology
and mechanics of swallowing. The oropharyngeal
phase of swallowing is subdivided into two distinct phases, the oral preparatory and the pharyngeal phase, and involves structures of the mouth,
pharynx, and UES (Hawkey et al. 2012; Dodds
et al. 1990). The phases are tightly coordinated
processes between areas of the central nervous
system (CNS), peripheral nervous system, anatomic structures of the oropharynx and larynx,
and the respiratory system (Clave and Shaker
2015). This complex coordination ensures safe

and efficient delivery of a food bolus from the mouth to the upper esophagus. The process involves mostly involuntary and reflexive inputs from the swallowing centers within the brain stem, projected through the motor and premotor cortex (Shaw and Martino 2013; Inoue 2015).

The oral preparatory phase is mostly voluntary and involving cranial nerves V, VII, and XII, with the autonomic nervous system controlling saliva secretion to facilitate the oral breakdown of food (Dodds et al. 1990; Ertekin and Aydogdu 2003; Lund 1991). Liquid boluses are placed in the anterior mouth with the tongue pushed against the soft palate to avoid aspiration before the oropharyngeal swallow response is triggered. Solid boluses are broken down to appropriate size via mastication, with coordinated tongue and cheek action to move the food onto the molars (Shaw and Martino 2013; Sasegbon and Hamdy 2017). To contain food within the oral cavity, the facial muscles seal the lips and close the anterior and lateral sulci. The contraction of the palatoglossus muscle depresses the soft palate against the base of the tongue to prevent premature leakage of food contents into the oropharynx, thereby preventing aspiration (Shaw and Martino 2013; Dodds 1989). The tongue then directs the chewed and mixed bolus posteriorly, and elevation of the tongue in the direction of the hard palate then propels the bolus through the fauces and into the oropharynx prior to swallowing (Palmer et al. 2000). During this time there are a simultaneous elevation of the soft palate and contraction of the superior pharyngeal constrictors, which seal the nasopharynx to prevent nasal regurgitation (Shaw and Martino 2013; Azpeitia Arman et al. 2019).

The pharyngeal phase is mostly involuntary, involving cranial nerves V, IX, X, and XII, and lasting close to 1 s in normal individuals (Dodds et al. 1990; Ertekin and Aydogdu 2003). Once the bolus reaches the pharynx, the contact initiates the pharyngeal phase of the swallow. The initial reaction is the cessation of respiration for airway protection during pharyngeal peristalsis (Sasegbon and Hamdy 2017; Shaker et al. 1990). Closure of the nasopharyngeal inlet and contractions of the superior constrictor muscle advance the bolus through the pharynx and into the esophagus (Azpeitia Arman et al. 2019). The larynx and hyoid are simultaneously pulled upward and anteriorly, while the epiglottis moves downward and posteriorly to allow the bolus to pass over the larynx without penetration into the trachea (Shaw and Martino 2013; Pearson Jr et al. 2012). The concurrent relaxation of the cricopharyngeus muscle then allows for the bolus to pass through the UES and into the upper esophagus (Ertekin and Aydogdu 2002).

OD thus occurs when there are mechanical, structural, or neuromuscular perturbations to the structures that are involved in both the voluntary and in the involuntary aspects of the oropharyngeal swallow phases (Wirth et al. 2016; Sasegbon and Hamdy 2017; Rommel and Hamdy 2016; Smukalla et al. 2017). Oftentimes, the presenting symptoms and exam findings can give insight into determining the underlying etiology.

Pathophysiology of Oropharyngeal Dysphagia

Dysphagia is a consequence of neuromuscular (central and/or peripheral) and mechanical pathologies which may prohibit the involuntary and voluntary components of deglutition (Table 1). The etiology of OD is diverse and varies based on the defect in the underlying pathophysiology. For a food bolus to be swallowed safely without risk of aspiration, appropriate size, consistency, and lubrication must be achieved by coordinated processes before food can be mobilized for an effective swallow.

Anterior cervical osteophytes and cervical spine curvature abnormalities can cause or contribute to OD in older adults. Through mechanical compression of pharyngeal and UES tissues/musculature, mass effect, inflammation, and spasms can lead to significant OD that is often overlooked on initial workup (Ferreira et al. 2019; Abdel-Aziz et al. 2018). Cervical esophageal webs, idiopathic or in the case of Plummer-Vinson syndrome, can result in OD (Allen et al. 2011). Mass effect from oropharyngeal, thyroid, or parathyroid neoplasms needs to be ruled out in patients with evidence of narrowing of the pharyngeal lumen on evaluation.

Table 1 Causes of Oropharyngeal dysphagia

Mechanical disorders	Neuromuscular disorders
Cervical osteophytes	Amyloidosis
Cervical spine	Amyotrophic lateral
abnormalities	sclerosis
Cricopharyngeal	Cerebral palsy
achalasia, bar, rings, and	Cushing's syndrome
stenosis	Dementia
Esophageal stricture	Dermatomyositis
Oropharyngeal and	Drugs (botulinum toxin,
laryngeal neoplasm	procainamide, cytotoxins,
Pharyngoesophageal	amiodarone, alcohol,
diverticula or pouches	statins)
Pharyngoesophageal webs	Guillain-Barré syndrome
(PVS)	Head trauma
Thyroid neoplasms	Huntington's disease
Thyromegaly	Hyperthyroidism
	Hypothyroidism
	Malignancy of the central
	nervous system
	Metabolic encephalopathy
	Mixed connective tissue
	disease
	Multiple sclerosis
	Muscular dystrophy
	Myasthenia gravis
	Paraneoplastic syndromes
	Parkinson's disease
	Polymyositis
	Sjogren's syndrome
	Stroke
	Tabes dorsalis
	Wilson's disease

Postsurgical and postradiation therapy changes can also cause damage to the neuromuscular swallow structures, presenting with significant OD (King et al. 2016).

OD can be the primary manifestation of systemic autoimmune diseases. Common disorders associated with OD include Sjogren's syndrome, granulomatosis with polyangiitis, pemphigus and pemphigoid, rheumatoid arthritis, systemic lupus erythematosus, and inflammatory myopathies (Anis and Soliman 2013). Though diagnosis is most common in the fourth and fifth decades of life, these disorders are often encountered among the elderly and contribute to dysphagia. The pathophysiology involves salivary gland dysfunction, painful oral ulcerations, blisters, and soft tissue nodular disease, resulting in odynophagia and muscle paralysis (Amos et al. 2016). Rheumatoid arthritis affects several neck joints including

cricoarytenoid joints causing acute tenderness, joint ankylosis, and vocal cord immobility which places patients at risk for aspiration (Ebert and Hagspiel 2011). Inflammatory myopathies affect both striated and smooth muscles of the oropharynx resulting in poor contraction and increased transit time predisposing the patient to increased risk for OD.

Neurologic control of swallowing involves complex sensorimotor integration with cortical and subcortical structures, interwoven to control the voluntary and involuntary components of deglutition (Leopold and Daniels 2010). Sensory input results in the activation of this network. Thus a stroke involving the cerebral hemispheres or brain stem is frequently associated with dysphagia (Yang et al. 2015). Functional MRI studies have demonstrated a left-to-right hemispheric shift in neural activation during each phase of deglutition (Teismann et al. 2009). Although swallowing laterality has been studied, the exact mechanism is unclear, and there is variability of dysphagia after a cerebrovascular accident (Yang et al. 2015). In stroke patients, lesions in the left hemisphere predominantly affect the oral stage of swallowing, while lesions on the right affect the pharyngeal phase of swallow (Suntrup-Krueger et al. 2017; Suntrup et al. 2015; Daniels et al. 1996). Size and lateralization of stroke lesions have implications on the significance and prognosis of resulting dysphagia. Lateralization of the swallow control makes it likely for recovery of function post-unilateral stroke, with studies showing that the unaffected side compensates for contralateral loss (Hamdy et al. 2000). Thus in neurodegenerative diseases such as Parkinson's, swallow deficits may be well compensated for until the late stages of the disease (Suntrup et al. 2013). In contrast, bilateral damage from disease processes such as amyotrophic lateral sclerosis may predispose to more permanent dysphagia with a lower likelihood for recovery (Teismann et al. 2011). In addition to central neurologic lesions, peripheral disease processes such as ENT malignances and peripheral neuropathies can affect the efferent and afferent pathways of the complex swallow pathways resulting in dysphagia. It is therefore paramount to identify candidates with underlying neurologic lesions that can benefit from early interventions to facilitate recovery.

Poor oral health has been linked with malnutrition, decreased cognitive function, and increased dependence in activities of daily living in the old (Pu et al. 2017). A lower number of teeth and periodontal disease contribute to poor mastication and dysphagia, resulting in food avoidance, malnutrition, and debility in older adults (Hildebrandt et al. 1997; Ikebe et al. 2012). The number of "functional tooth units" as well as the distribution of teeth are vital to the maintenance of oral function (Naka et al. 2014). Periodontal disease can impair regulation of masticatory forces due to faulty mechanoreceptive innervation. In the setting of periodontitis, pain can limit effective forces of mastication rendering the forces inefficient, leading to dysphagia (Johansson et al. 2006; Borges Tde et al. 2013). The negative effects of periodontitis and caries have been linked to poor masticatory performance and quality of life in the geriatric population (Borges Tde et al. 2013; Ortega et al. 2014). Correcting edentulism with correctly fitting denture wear improves mastication and swallow efficiency (Furuta et al. 2013; Okabe et al. 2016). Xerostomia or oral dryness is common in the old. The prevalence of xerostomia and salivary gland hypofunction increases with age and is associated with both systemic disease and local factors (Millsop et al. 2017; Anil et al. 2016). Along with age-related atrophy of salivary glands, the elderly are likely to have comorbidities or require medications whose side effects often impair saliva production (Anil et al. 2016; Peyron et al. 2017; Percival et al. 1994; Schein et al. 1999). Causes of xerostomia include the side effects of radiation therapy or chemotherapy; however, there are a host of commonly prescribed drugs that also contribute including those with anticholinergic activity, sympathomimetics, benzodiazepines, and diuretics which may trigger volume depletion (Millsop et al. 2017; Anil et al. 2016; Wolff et al. 2017). Even iron supplementation can have oral mucosal toxicity leading to pain and has been associated with deglutition disorders (Liabeuf et al. 2014). Lubrication is essential to formation of a food bolus, and thus xerostomia makes it difficult to gather food into a bolus with consistency and viscosity that is safe for swallow. As a consequence of dry mouth, there is an increased risk for developing oropharyngeal infections, dental caries, ulcers, and functional difficulties that impair swallowing (Napenas and Rouleau 2014; Eyigor et al. 2017). Chemotherapy and radiation therapies lead to mucosal and muscular cellular damage and inflammation leading to reduced barrier function, resulting in trauma and infections that impair normal oropharyngeal swallowing (King et al. 2016). Fibrosis and atrophy of the oropharyngeal musculature from radiation therapy can result in edema, fibrosis, and loss of elasticity, leading to strictures, deformities, and impaired contraction which may alter bolus propulsion mechanisms (Dornfeld et al. 2007; Sanguineti et al. 2007).

The tongue plays an important role in coordinating sensory and motor activities involved in the oral and pharyngeal phases of swallowing (Robbins et al. 1995; Tamine et al. 2010). It is integral in delivering food particles from the front of the mouth to the molars, mixing the food bolus with saliva for appropriate consistency. The tongue also crushes food against the hard palate, gathers particles ready for swallow into a bolus, and cleans the mouth and teeth of food particles after the swallow. Reduced lingual pressures have been linked to natural aging and have been shown to be a consequence of reduced muscle mass and CNS changes, further increasing the vulnerability of the elderly to recover from any potential compromise in neuromuscular function such as cerebrovascular events or neurodegenerative disorders (Robbins et al. 1995). A suboptimal preparatory phase can be seen with an impaired lingual, jaw, and other oropharyngeal muscles in disease states such as Parkinson's disease, cerebrovascular disease, dementia, as well as other neurodegenerative disorders, placing these individuals at risk for choking and/or aspiration (Tamine et al. 2010).

Age significantly impacts mechanoreceptors and chemoreceptors of the mouth and affects oropharyngeal perceptions of food bolus characteristics. Disruption of afferent sensory information severely impedes the cortical control of swallowing (Wirth et al. 2016). Given components of swallow physiology rely on the inputs of these receptors, misperception of food bolus viscosity has been linked to dysphagia in the elderly (Smith et al. 2006).

Safe pharyngoesophageal transit of a food bolus requires coordinated relaxation of the cricopharyngeus muscle, anterior-superior displacement of the hyoalaryngo-cricoids-complex by the contraction of the suprahyoid and thyrohyoid muscles, and compliant UES muscles (Wirth et al. 2016). Abnormalities in any of those components can lead to a reduction in the maximal opening of the UES resulting in the retention of pharyngeal residue and aspiration (Dejaeger et al. 1997). Cricopharyngeal dysfunction may be due to incoordination as well as reduction in maximal opening of the UES during deglutition and flow across the sphincter. The main function of the UES is to protect against the reflux of food into the airways and to prevent the entry of air into the digestive tract (Sivarao and Goyal 2000). In a small study comparing healthy young and older adults, suboptimal UES opening muscle contraction and decreased sphincter compliance were linked to decreased UES cross-sectional area which may contribute to presbyphagia (Kern et al. 1999). Dysfunctional UES opening as a cause of OD is a factor in a number of disorders that affect older persons. In Parkinson's disease, pharyngeal constrictor muscle atrophy leads to slow bolus transition, while fast-to-slow fiber-type transformation in the cricopharyngeal sphincter muscles can lead to increased sphincter tone that contributes to dysphagia in these patients (Mu et al. 2012). Identification of UES dysfunction, through tools such as videofluoroscopic swallowing study (VFSS) and high-resolution manometry, is essential to the diagnosis and management of OD, which will be discussed later in this chapter.

In addition to insults to the complex neuromuscular system as precipitants of OD, it is important to recognize alternative causes of dysphagia including sarcopenic dysphagia. Sarcopenia is defined by a progressive and generalized loss of skeletal muscle mass and strength (Cruz-Jentoft

et al. 2019). The understanding of sarcopenia especially in the elderly is an evolving field of research with a now greater understanding that sarcopenic dysphagia can be caused by several factors including deterioration in activity-, disease-, and nutrition-related sarcopenia of the whole body and swallowing-related muscles. This, in effect, leads to a decline in the functional reserves of the muscles required to carry out effective deglutition (Fujishima et al. 2019; Wakabayashi 2014). Disuse atrophy in this setting plays an important role as older adults without preexisting dysphagia can develop dysphagia after hospitalization with restricted oral intake, especially when placed *nil* per os *due to concerns for aspiration (*Maeda et al. 2017*;* Jardine et al. 2018*)*. Sarcopenic dysphagia should be diagnosed in the presence of whole-body sarcopenia and is therefore distinguished from neuromuscular etiologies that could lead to dysphagia (Fujishima et al. 2019). Risk factors for this condition include malnutrition, low activities of daily living, and skeletal muscle loss, which suggests that preventative measures with early therapy and nutritional support may significantly impact this population (Fujishima et al. 2019).

Screening and Diagnosis

Early recognition of swallowing difficulty should be a priority in hospitalized geriatric patients and especially in those with neurological injury or a combination of oral and pharyngeal abnormalities. In addition, patients with clinical symptoms suggestive of OD should go through an evaluation with validated screening tools that can facilitate early recognition and avoid adverse complications of undetected OD. Common manifestations of OD include coughing, choking, nasal regurgitation, and/or neuromuscular and neurodegenerative pathologies (Table 2). A comprehensive and accurate swallowing assessment is essential in clinical decision-making regarding oral vs. non-oral means of nutrition, which in itself has significant implications for healthcare outcomes, costs, and discharge disposition (Park et al. 2017a; Johansen et al. 2004).

Table 2 Symptoms suggestive of oropharyngeal dysphagia

Difficulty initiating swallow	Coughing
Food spillage from lips or drooling	Choking
	Dysphonia
Nasopharyngeal regurgitation	Avoidance of certain consistencies
The sensation of residual food in the throat	Weight loss
	Recurrent pneumonia
Piecemeal swallows	Prolonged meal duration
Chronic low-level secretions	

Diagnosis of OD is a multidisciplinary process involving speech pathology, otolaryngology, gastroenterology, neurology, and radiology. In those with suspected OD, the initial step is screening with a physical exam and clinically validated tools including swallow assessment (Rommel and Hamdy 2016). The initial assessment of OD generally involves a bedside examination and assessment of feeding status, mental status, and breathing status. This is then followed by an assessment of the oropharyngeal musculature, reflexes, and trial of a bolus feed. The evaluation involves the use of validated questionnaires and surveys to facilitate in evaluating progression, timing, and burden of symptoms. Physical exam should incorporate assessment of neurological, nutritional, functional, and respiratory status. A thorough medical examination by a specialist, often an otolaryngologist, neurologist, or gastroenterologist, is performed to further delineate underlying pathology. This is often followed by a clinical oral examination performed by a speech and language pathologist assessing the oropharyngeal structures, cranial nerves, and voice articulation while incorporating standardized dysphagia assessment tools. A trial of different food consistencies and bolus sizes is performed in the appropriate patient to assess the risk of aspiration and penetration.

Optimal screening can identify those requiring further evaluation and has been shown to reduce sequelae of OD including enteral feeding tube dependence, pneumonia, and death (Hinchey et al. 2005). Complete assessments can be performed by a speech and language pathologist and, if unavailable, a provider trained in the use of the validated tools (Palli et al. 2017). A wide range of screening tools have been validated for OD, but their effectiveness and applicability, given the heterogeneity of underlying pathology and comorbidities, still require further validation (Smith et al. 2018; O'Horo et al. 2015). The screening tools include the Eating Assessment Tool (EAT-10), the Gugging Swallowing Screen (GUSS), the Standardized Swallowing Assessment (SSA), and the Mann Assessment of Swallowing Ability (MASA) (O'Horo et al. 2015; Trapl et al. 2007; Belafsky et al. 2008; Ohira et al. 2017; Park et al. 2015; Perry and Love 2001). These tools have been shown to reliably identify eating and swallowing disorders with the ability to predict development of dysphagia sequelae. The EAT-10 is a simple, self-administered survey that can be used to both diagnose severity of dysphagia and monitor for treatment response (Belafsky et al. 2008). The test is simple, takes about 2 min, and can be administered in a variety of settings. The GUSS is a bedside test with 100% sensitivity for aspiration, originally developed for dysphagia screening in acute stroke (Trapl et al. 2007). Though easy to administer, the test has a low specificity of 50–63% but remains a reliable and convenient screening tool for the elderly in nursing homes (Park et al. 2015). The SSA was originally validated in the poststroke population but has been adopted for use as a bedside screening tool with high sensitivity and specificity (Park et al. 2015; Perry and Love 2001). The MASA is another screening tool with high sensitivity for predicting aspiration and pharyngeal retention among dependent older adults (Ohira et al. 2017; Park et al. 2015). The original MASA cutoff points validated for post-acute stroke assessment had to be redefined to reduce the number of false negative diagnoses in the assessment of dependent elderly (Ohira et al. 2017). These tests can oftentimes miss silent aspiration and do not give detailed information on the nature and extent of pathology or insight on the appropriate management approach. It is thus necessary to follow with an instrumental test that would verify the impressions of the bedside evaluation and direct appropriate therapy (Murry and Carrau 2012).

Instrumental Evaluation of Swallow

A videofluoroscopic swallowing study (VFSS) or the modified barium swallow involves dynamic radiologic video imaging of the oropharyngeal swallow complex with the subject swallowing a radiopaque food bolus (Azpeitia Arman et al. 2019) (Table 3). The procedure involves having the patient in an upright position with X-ray imaging from the lateral and anteroposterior positions observed on a monitor by a radiologist and a speech and language pathologist (Gates et al. 2006). Different sizes and consistencies of radiopaque barium-based boluses are administered while recording detailed functional anatomy and/

Table 3 Diagnostic testing modalities for oropharyngeal dysphagia

Test	Utility
Videofluoroscopic swallowing study (VFSS)	Radiologic video imaging of the oropharyngeal swallow complex Assessment of functional and structural anatomy during deglutition. Noninvasive
Nasopharyngolaryngoscopy	Assessment of structural anatomy. Can identify masses, secretions, or food residue No radiation exposure, no risk of barium aspiration, portable
Fiber-optic endoscopic evaluation of swallowing (FEES)	Various solid and liquid consistencies provided with endoscopic visualization Functional, structural, and sensory assessment of deglutition. Can identify food residue and pooled secretions No radiation exposure, no risk of barium aspiration, portable
High-resolution manometry	Functional assessment of musculature
Functional lumen imaging probe (EndoFLIP)	Distensibility of the UES No radiation exposure, no risk of barium aspiration, can be used during endoscopy

or pathology of the oral, pharyngeal, laryngeal, and upper esophageal structures during deglutition (Palmer et al. 2000). Qualitative assessment of aspects of swallow, i.e., lip seal, oral transit, tongue-soft palate seal, soft palate-superior constrictor muscle seal, propulsive phase, hyoid and laryngeal movements, or epiglottic tilt, can therefore be performed (Azpeitia Arman et al. 2019). The variations in bolus consistency and volume allow for evaluation of the subject's response to different consistencies and the extent of retention or aspiration. The information obtained makes it possible to design individualized diets that can minimize dysphagia and its sequelae (Palmer et al. 2000). The images obtained are often evaluated by an interdisciplinary team, involving a radiologist and a speech and language pathologist. Though regarded as the gold standard for evaluating direct aspiration, the technique is limited by the use of radiation, non-physiologic bolus, and the qualitative nature of the assessment (Palmer et al. 2000; Rommel and Hamdy 2016). In addition, there is high interpreter variability, and results from VFSS have poor correlation with sequelae of OD such as pneumonia and mortality (Rommel and Hamdy 2016). Some quantitative assessments, including the timing of opening and closure of the glossopharyngeal junction, velopharyngeal junction, laryngeal vestibule, and UES, can provide additional information on the quality of airway protection. These measurements are often not part of the routine clinical VFSS due to low intra-rater and inter-rater reliability (Baijens et al. 2013).

Fiber-optic endoscopic evaluation of swallowing (FEES) involves the use of a flexible laryngoscope to directly view pharyngeal and laryngeal structures during the process of deglutition and movement as well as delivery of various foods and liquids (Hiss and Postma 2003; Leder and Murray 2008). The procedure involves introducing the laryngoscope transnasally and advancing toward the pharynx and positioned to visualize the tongue base, pharynx, and larynx (Murry and Carrau 2012). The subject swallows different amounts of dye-infused food and liquid consistencies, and movement of the tongue base, pharynx, and larynx can be visualized as the bolus transits. The procedure allows for direct pharyngeal dysphagia assessment and can be used to guide rehabilitative interventions to promote safe deglutition (Leder and Murray 2008). At the time of epiglottic tilting and maximal pharyngeal closure, visualization of these structures is lost, and thus the entire swallow process is never visualized with FEES. Regardless, the intra-rater and inter-rater reliability is very high for the procedure compared to VFSS. The reliance on subjective and qualitative assessment is a limitation for the procedure though the incorporation of validated rating scales utilized in describing the endoscopy findings can make the finding more clinically relevant in guiding care. Involuntary closure of the vocal cords in response to laryngeal stimulation (laryngeal adductor reflex) with air boluses delivered from the tip of the laryngoscope can be assessed with FEES and is a good measure of involuntary airway protection. FEES is well validated and tolerated, and its convenience as a bedside procedure without radiation exposure makes it a versatile technique that can be applied to all patient demographics.

High-resolution manometry (HRM) is currently utilized and has been extensively validated in the diagnosis and management of esophageal dysphagia. Although its use in OD, specifically examining the integrity of the UES, has been described extensively, the data examining specific metrics and clinical implications are not as robust. A typical HRM solid catheter has 36 circumferential pressure sensors at 1–2 cm intervals extending from the hypopharynx to the stomach, which capture and measure the pressures generated along the entire length simultaneously (Clouse and Staiano 1991). Esophageal pressure topography plots are then generated that represent esophageal motility and sphincter function on color-coded, pressure-space-time plots (Carlson and Pandolfino 2015). Although HRM provides precise pharyngeal pressure information, it has yet to be applied to routine clinical practice as the assessment method for OD. HRM can provide biomechanical swallowing information in patients with OD, which can potentially help guide therapeutic interventions (Cock and Omari 2017). The anatomical landmarks for HRM

parameters are velopharynx (VP), tongue base (TB), epiglottis, low pharynx (LP), and UES (Ryu et al. 2015). Measurements that are utilized include the rise time and duration of the VP and TB regions; UES basal pressure (UES-BP) or pre-deglutitive basal pressure, which assesses UES tonic contractility; and UES integrated relaxation pressure (UES-IRP), which measures the extent of maximal UES relaxation over a 0.2 s period during swallowing (Sivarao and Goyal 2000; Cock and Omari 2017; Park et al. 2017b). Intra-bolus pressure (IBP), a measure of pharyngeal propulsive forces and luminal diameter, is also vital to the understanding of etiology of oropharyngeal dysphagia as this takes into account the maximum distension of the hypopharynx. Therefore, an elevated IBP may be indicative of restrictive flow or resistance in the setting of structural pathology or sensory dysregulation leading to failure to accommodate appropriately for bolus size, leading to incomplete pharyngeal transition and residue (Wirth et al. 2016; Cock and Omari 2017).

The functional lumen imaging probe (FLIP) utilizes high-resolution impedance planimetry during volume-controlled distention to measure luminal cross-sectional area in relation to pressure, in order to assess the distensibility along an axial plane with a metric referred to as the distensibility index (DI) measured in $mm^2/mmHg$ (Pandolfino et al. 2013; Kwiatek et al. 2010; Hirano et al. 2017). The EndoFLIP impedance planimetry system consists of a 24-cm-long, 3-mm-outer diameter catheter with a highly compliant balloon. This catheter is typically inserted alongside the endoscope and positioned under direct vision. Majority of research thus far has focused on the esophagogastric junction; however this catheter has also been used to examine the UES. Regan et al. studied the utility of EndoFLIP among healthy volunteers to assess UES distensibility, diameter, and pressure at rest, during swallowing and voluntary maneuvers. This group displayed comparable results to VFSS but remarked that it was limited in its ability to display luminal shape of the UES region. This group also found that EndoFLIP may be a safe and valuable tool to evaluate pharyngoesophageal segment distensibility and pharyngoesophageal segment opening among patients who have undergone total laryngectomy. Further research is required to support the use of EndoFLIP in the diagnostic algorithm of OD (Regan et al. 2013; Regan et al. 2015).

Clinical Management of Oropharyngeal Dysphagia

When OD involves cricopharyngeus dysfunction, treatment should target the underlying cause, but largely consists of augmenting muscle opening. This can be accomplished by dilation, decreasing tone or relaxation through botulinum toxin injection or disruption of the muscle by myotomy. Kocdor et al. performed a systemic review examining each of these treatment modalities among patients with cricopharyngeal dysfunction and found that there appeared to be a greater success rate among patients who underwent myotomy, particularly with an endoscopic approach over botulinum toxin injection (78% vs. 69%); however myotomy had similar outcomes to dilation (73%) (Kocdor et al. 2016). All methods of treatment had similar safety outcomes. Practically, risks and expected benefits of each option should be weighed individually in a patient with OD.

OD management often involves compensatory and rehabilitative efforts to speed up recovery and facilitate safe swallow by preventing aspiration and ensuring proper bolus transit (Wirth et al. 2016; Murry and Carrau 2012). The goal of therapy is to achieve adequate safe nutrition and hydration while minimizing complications of OD, especially morbidity associated with aspiration events (Wirth et al. 2016). If there is an identifiable cause, i.e., thyroid disease, malignancy, or autoimmune disease, treatment of the underlying condition should take precedence (Shaker 2013). In most instances, and especially in the geriatric patient, OD becomes a multifactorial disorder, and therefore rehabilitative efforts to ensure safe swallow and adequate nutrition become the mainstay therapies. The approach remains multidisciplinary with a speech and language pathologist (SLP), dietician, nurse, and qualified physician involvement (Murry and Carrau 2012).

Compensatory swallow therapy involves oropharyngeal neuromotor stimulatory exercises to strengthen muscles and optimize the oral and pharyngeal phases of swallow (Murry and Carrau 2012). The therapies do not require the patient to physiologically swallow a food bolus, but the participant should be cognitively intact, able to follow simple instructions, and motivated to practice independently. Though there is limited evidence to suggest efficacy, these oral motor exercises are aimed at improving strength, awareness, and control of food bolus as it transits through the oropharynx (Murry and Carrau 2012; Shaker 2013). Exercises to augment labial opening and closure, tongue pressure, mandible strength, and sensory awareness have been shown to be efficacious in both normal and poststroke patients with OD (Robbins et al. 2007). In a small study utilizing the videofluoroscopic dysphagia scale, bedside self-exercise therapy was shown to be effective in improving oropharyngeal swallow in post-stroke patients (Cho et al. 2017). The Shaker head lift exercise, a head lift maneuver developed to improve UES opening ability during swallow through suprahyoid muscle strengthening and thyrohyoid muscle shortening, has been shown to reduce aspiration in older patients with OD (Shaker et al. 1997; Mepani et al. 2009). Tongue-to-palate resistance training (TPRT) in stroke patients with dysphagia was also shown to improve swallow function (Kim et al. 2017).

Tongue and labial rehabilitation may facilitate in improving bolus manipulation, preparation, and oral clearance, but vocal closure is paramount in preventing aspiration during the swallow. Implementation of vocal fold training and laryngeal elevation techniques, such as Lee Silverman Voice Treatment (LSVT), has been shown to increase the valving ability of vocal cords and prevent aspiration in individuals with dysphagia following CVA (Fox et al. 2006). LSVT can be implemented in appropriately chosen patients, but there is a lack of controlled trials to validate its clinical application in all patients with dysphagia. Strengthening of non-swallow expiration and submental muscles has also been shown to improve speech production, cough, and swallow in individuals with dysphagia (Murry and Carrau 2012; Shaker 2013). Expiratory muscle strength training (EMST) is a technique that utilizes a one-way device to block expiratory air flow until a certain pressure threshold is reached and was shown in a trial to improve swallow function in Parkinson's disease patients with dysphagia at 4 weeks of follow-up (Troche et al. 2010). The response to these therapies may be varied owing to the heterogeneity of the underlying causes and appropriateness of individuals for the treatment of choice. There is a lack of well-designed clinical studies to validate immediate or long-term efficacy of these exercise maneuvers in the reduction of clinically relevant outcomes such as pneumonia, nutritional status, or quality of life (QoL) (Murry and Carrau 2012; Langmore and Pisegna 2015; Bath et al. 2018).

Swallow rehabilitation therapy combines the use of different food bolus consistencies and application of swallow maneuvers, postural adjustments, and compensatory exercises to improve swallow quality (Murry and Carrau 2012). Participants are required to have a baseline ability to safely swallow small amounts of physiologic foods or liquids. There are data showing improved swallowing and aspiration reduction in individuals who implement swallow postures, i.e., side lying, head back, chin down, head rotation, and head tilt while swallowing (Wirth et al. 2016; Sura et al. 2012). These maneuvers have reported the benefit of increased UES opening, decreased aspiration, better bolus transit, and reduced oropharyngeal swallow residue (Solazzo et al. 2012; Logemann et al. 1994). Swallow maneuvers including supraglottic swallow, super supraglottic swallow, and effortful swallow and the Mendelsohn maneuver can also be incorporated as rehabilitative strategies to reduce aspiration, increase pharyngeal pressure, facilitate UES relaxation, and reduce residue (Sura et al. 2012; Murry and Carrau 2012; Carnaby et al. 2006). Currently, the data available for both swallow postures and maneuvers are based on inadequately powered studies and lack generalizability (Murry and Carrau 2012; Langmore and Pisegna 2015; Bath et al. 2018). When applied to patients with dysphagia, these maneuvers need to be

followed with objective measures of swallow improvement to assess for a benefit at an individual basis (Sura et al. 2012; Shaker 2013).

Given the most common source of bacteria in the upper gastrointestinal tract is the mouth, the initial step in preventing aspiration pneumonia is effective oral hygiene (Shaker 2013). Patients with OD should ensure adequate oral care through brushing teeth and/or mouth rinsing with frequent dentist visits to minimize the amount of oral bacteria buildup (Logemann et al. 2013).

Thickening of liquids is believed to help control speed, direction, duration, and clearance of bolus, but there is lack of evidence to support its effect on health outcomes related to dysphagia (Robbins et al. 2002; Kaneoka et al. 2017). Though nectar thick is the most frequently utilized consistency, only honey thick and ultra-thick liquid consistencies have been shown to reduce aspiration events (Garcia et al. 2005; Kuhlemeier et al. 2001). Thickened liquids are intolerable for most patients, and hence there is a higher prevalence of poor adherence leading to decreased fluid intake and complications of dehydration (Garcia et al. 2005; Logemann et al. 2008). Implementation of alternative approaches such as the Frazier Water Protocol, where individuals with dysphagia can drink water between meals, can potentially help decrease rates of dehydration in these individuals (Panther et al. 2008). The protocol is derived from a single-center study, and is yet to be validated, but has been shown to safely achieve hydration goals and improve quality of life in the elderly with OD (Sura et al. 2012; Panther et al. 2008).

Similar to liquid thickening, solid food texture modification lacks robust data to support its role in reducing aspiration and improving nutrition and overall QoL in those with OD (Wirth et al. 2016). Inconsistencies in terminology and definitions of the different textures make it difficult to generalize findings from the few studies that exist (Sura et al. 2012). The recommendations to modify food texture are based on best practice guidelines rather than well-designed clinical trials (Andersen et al. 2013). In a recent systemic review aimed at investigating the role of liquid and solid food modification in adults with OD, the scarcity of clinical studies investigating these interventions became apparent. There was no literature that addressed the effects of using texture-modified food consistencies as a compensatory strategy to facilitate safe and efficient intake of foods among adults with OD. Nevertheless, the authors propose that nectar-thickened and honey-thickened liquids, also described as slightly or mildly thick liquids, should only be used as a compensatory strategy to facilitate the intake of liquids in adults with oropharyngeal dysphagia (OD), as there is an unclear benefit with regard to risk of pneumonia and laryngeal penetration. The authors were in favor of offering modified food consistencies for patients with OD, noting that different levels of texture are frequently utilized in this setting based on individual patient assessment (Beck et al. 2018). In addition, most patients have been shown to prefer non-modified foods, and texture modification has been linked with decreased food intake, leading to undernutrition and decreased QoL (Beck et al. 2018; O'Keeffe 2018). Given the paucity of data on long-term benefits of texture modification in patients with OD, providers, therefore, need to partner with their patients and make individualized informed decisions with a common goal of maximizing nutrition and QoL (Wirth et al. 2016; Sura et al. 2012; Beck et al. 2018).

When all compensatory and rehabilitative maneuvers fail to meet individual caloric goals, non-oral nutrition is the ultimate and last resort option for an individual with OD (Sura et al. 2012; Shaker 2013). For most patients, this includes the utilization of artificial feeds through a nasogastric tube (NGT) or a percutaneous endoscopic gastrostomy (PEG) tube (Wirth et al. 2016). Choice of non-oral feeds depends on the prognosis and extent of nutritional deficit in the individual patient. Artificial enteral feeding is generally recommended for a patient who has failed to meet half of their nutritional demand for longer than 10 days or those without nutritional intake for longer than 3 days (Volkert et al. 2019). Artificial enteral feeds ensure adequate nutrition, thereby preventing cognitive decline, maintaining robust immune status, and promoting wound healing in appropriately chosen individuals with OD (Shlisky

et al. 2017; Chandra 1997; Hengstermann et al. 2007). One review looking at use of NGT and PEG tube feeding in elderly patients with OD from head and neck tumor or chemotherapy-induced mucositis found PEG tube feeding to be associated with better overall QoL compared to NGT (Bozzetti 2015). Though both NGT and PEG feeding were associated with improved QoL, there was no clinically significant weight gain or improvement in mortality. Another study showed lower complications associated with PEG tube compared to NGT feeding, but both methods had comparable nutritional and clinical outcomes at 4-month follow-up (Jaafar et al. 2019). In elderly patients with advanced dementia, evidence suggests a lack of benefit of enteral feeding in improving QoL, preventing aspirations, and prolonging life (Sampson et al. 2009; Finucane et al. 1999). A small study on poststroke elderly patients with dysphagia also showed negative impact of prolonged NGT placement on swallow outcomes when assessed by VFSS (Wang et al. 2019). In addition, post-procedure complications, including site infection, tube malfunction, and increased reflux, may increase hospitalizations with implications on overall prognosis and mortality (Wirth et al. 2016; Sura et al. 2012). Therefore, the impact of non-oral nutrition on patients QoL should be carefully evaluated as this may have negative psychosocial implications including depression and social withdrawal in some individuals (Sura et al. 2012; Martin et al. 2012). In the appropriately chosen individual with OD, non-oral nutrition remains an important alternative, but care should be taken to choose the appropriate patient who would have expected long-term benefits from the intervention.

Key Points

- At least 13% of adults over the age of 65 are affected by dysphagia.
- Oropharyngeal dysphagia occurs when there are mechanical, structural, or neuromuscular insults to the structures that are involved in both the voluntary oral phase and in the involuntary pharyngeal phase of deglutition.

- Clinical symptoms typically seen in OD include coughing, choking, nasal regurgitation, or recurrent pneumonia.
- The initial assessment of OD generally involves a bedside history and physical examination and assessment of feeding status, mental status, and breathing status.
- A clinical oral examination performed by a speech and language pathologist assessing the oropharyngeal structures, cranial nerves, and voice articulation is vital to assess possible areas of pathology.
- A videofluoroscopic swallowing study (VFSS) or the modified barium swallow involves dynamic radiologic imaging of the oropharyngeal swallow utilizing different sizes and consistencies and is the gold standard for diagnosis of OP dysphagia and aspiration.
- Fiber-optic endoscopic evaluation of swallowing (FEES) utilizes a flexible laryngoscope to directly view pharyngeal and laryngeal structures during swallowing and structural pathology.
- High-resolution manometry (HRM) and the endoscopic functional lumen imaging probe (EndoFLIP) can be helpful in the functional assessment of oropharyngeal musculature and distensibility of the upper esophageal sphincter, but further study is required to support the diagnostic utility of these tools.
- When OD involves cricopharyngeus dysfunction, management should target the underlying cause, which could include dilation, botulinum toxin injection, or myotomy.
- Swallow therapy involves oropharyngeal neuromotor stimulatory exercises to strengthen muscles and optimize the oral and pharyngeal phases of swallow but requires patients to be cognitively intact and able to follow instructions.
- When deglutitive rehabilitation fails, non-oral means of nutrition can be considered based on patient prognosis.

References

Abdel-Aziz M, Azab N, El-Badrawy A. Cervical osteophytosis and spine posture: contribution to swallow disorders and symptoms. Curr Opin Otolaryngol Head Neck Surg. 2018;26(6):375–81.

Allen JE, et al. Posterior cricoid region fluoroscopic findings: the posterior cricoid plication. Dysphagia. 2011;26(3):272–6.

Altman KW. Dysphagia evaluation and care in the hospital setting: the need for protocolization. Otolaryngol Head Neck Surg. 2011;145(6):895–8.

Amos J, Baron A, Rubin AD. Autoimmune swallowing disorders. Curr Opin Otolaryngol Head Neck Surg. 2016;24(6):483–8.

Andersen UT, et al. Systematic review and evidence based recommendations on texture modified foods and thickened fluids for adults (≥18 years) with oropharyngeal dysphagia. e-SPEN J. 2013;8(4):e127–34.

Andrade PA, et al. The importance of dysphagia screening and nutritional assessment in hospitalized patients. Einstein (Sao Paulo). 2018;16(2):eAO4189.

Anil S, et al. Xerostomia in geriatric patients: a burgeoning global concern. J Investig Clin Dent. 2016;7(1):5–12.

Anis MM, Soliman AM. Autoimmune swallowing disorders. Ear Nose Throat J. 2013;92(12):538–42.

Attrill S, et al. Impact of oropharyngeal dysphagia on healthcare cost and length of stay in hospital: a systematic review. BMC Health Serv Res. 2018;18(1):594.

Azpeitia Arman J, et al. Videofluoroscopic evaluation of normal and impaired oropharyngeal swallowing. Radiographics. 2019;39(1):78–9.

Baijens L, Barikroo A, Pilz W. Intrarater and interrater reliability for measurements in videofluoroscopy of swallowing. Eur J Radiol. 2013;82(10):1683–95.

Bath PM, Lee HS, Everton LF. Swallowing therapy for dysphagia in acute and subacute stroke. Cochrane Database Syst Rev. 2018;10:Cd000323.

Beck AM, et al. Systematic review and evidence based recommendations on texture modified foods and thickened liquids for adults (above 17 years) with oropharyngeal dysphagia – an updated clinical guideline. Clin Nutr. 2018;37(6 Pt A):1980–91.

Belafsky PC, et al. Validity and reliability of the Eating Assessment Tool (EAT-10). Ann Otol Rhinol Laryngol. 2008;117(12):919–24.

Bhattacharyya N. The prevalence of dysphagia among adults in the United States. Otolaryngol Head Neck Surg. 2014;151(5):765–9.

Borges Tde F, et al. Changes in masticatory performance and quality of life in individuals with chronic periodontitis. J Periodontol. 2013;84(3):325–31.

Bozzetti F. Tube feeding in the elderly cancer patient. Nutrition. 2015;31(4):608–9.

Carlson DA, Pandolfino JE. High-resolution manometry in clinical practice. Gastroenterol Hepatol (N Y). 2015;11(6):374–84.

Carnaby G, Hankey GJ, Pizzi J. Behavioural intervention for dysphagia in acute stroke: a randomised controlled trial. Lancet Neurol. 2006;5(1):31–7.

Chandra RK. Nutrition and the immune system: an introduction. Am J Clin Nutr. 1997;66(2):460s–3s.

Chen PH, et al. Prevalence of perceived dysphagia and quality-of-life impairment in a geriatric population. Dysphagia. 2009;24(1):1–6.

Cho YS, et al. Effects of bedside self-exercise on oropharyngeal swallowing function in stroke patients with dysphagia: a pilot study. J Phys Ther Sci. 2017;29 (10):1815–6.

Clave P, Shaker R. Dysphagia: current reality and scope of the problem. Nat Rev Gastroenterol Hepatol. 2015;12 (5):259–70.

Clouse RE, Staiano A. Topography of the esophageal peristaltic pressure wave. Am J Phys. 1991;261(4 Pt 1):G677–84.

Cock C, Omari T. Diagnosis of swallowing disorders: how we interpret pharyngeal manometry. Curr Gastroenterol Rep. 2017;19(3):11.

Cruz-Jentoft AJ, et al. Sarcopenia: revised European consensus on definition and diagnosis. Age Ageing. 2019;48(1):16–31.

Daniels SK, et al. Lesion site in unilateral stroke patients with dysphagia. J Stroke Cerebrovasc Dis. 1996;6 (1):30–4.

Dejaeger E, et al. Mechanisms involved in postdeglutition retention in the elderly. Dysphagia. 1997;12(2):63–7.

Dodds WJ. The physiology of swallowing. Dysphagia. 1989;3:171–8.

Dodds WJ, Stewart ET, Logemann JA. Physiology and radiology of the normal oral and pharyngeal phases of swallowing. AJR Am J Roentgenol. 1990;154 (5):953–63.

Dornfeld K, et al. Radiation doses to structures within and adjacent to the larynx are correlated with long-term diet- and speech-related quality of life. Int J Radiat Oncol Biol Phys. 2007;68(3):750–7.

Ebert EC, Hagspiel KD. Gastrointestinal and hepatic manifestations of rheumatoid arthritis. Dig Dis Sci. 2011;56(2):295–302.

Ertekin C, Aydogdu I. Electromyography of human cricopharyngeal muscle of the upper esophageal sphincter. Muscle Nerve. 2002;26(6):729–39.

Ertekin C, Aydogdu I. Neurophysiology of swallowing. Clin Neurophysiol. 2003;114(12):2226–44.

Eyigor S, et al. Evaluation of swallowing functions in patients with Sjogren's syndrome. Dysphagia. 2017;32(2):271–8.

Ferreira JMS, et al. Oropharyngeal dysphagia as an uncommon manifestation of an osteoarticular disease. BMJ Case Rep. 2019;12(1):e227411.

Finucane TE, Christmas C, Travis K. Tube feeding in patients with advanced dementia: a review of the evidence. JAMA. 1999;282(14):1365–70.

Fox CM, et al. The science and practice of LSVT/LOUD: neural plasticity-principled approach to treating individuals with Parkinson disease and other neurological disorders. Semin Speech Lang. 2006;27(4):283–99.

Fujishima I, et al. Sarcopenia and dysphagia: position paper by four professional organizations. Geriatr Gerontol Int. 2019;19(2):91–7.

Furuta M, et al. Interrelationship of oral health status, swallowing function, nutritional status, and cognitive ability with activities of daily living in Japanese elderly people receiving home care services due to physical disabilities. Community Dent Oral Epidemiol. 2013;41 (2):173–81.

Garcia JM, Chambers ET, Molander M. Thickened liquids: practice patterns of speech-language pathologists. Am J Speech Lang Pathol. 2005;14(1):4–13.

Gates J, Hartnell GG, Gramigna GD. Videofluoroscopy and swallowing studies for neurologic disease: a primer. Radiographics. 2006;26(1):e22.

Hamdy S, et al. Organization and reorganization of human swallowing motor cortex: implications for recovery after stroke. Clin Sci (Lond). 2000;99(2):151–7.

Hawkey CJ, et al. Textbook of clinical gastroenterology and hepatology. Hoboken: Wiley; 2012.

Hengstermann S, et al. Nutrition status and pressure ulcer: what we need for nutrition screening. JPEN J Parenter Enteral Nutr. 2007;31(4):288–94.

Hildebrandt GH, et al. Functional units, chewing, swallowing, and food avoidance among the elderly. J Prosthet Dent. 1997;77(6):588–95.

Hinchey JA, et al. Formal dysphagia screening protocols prevent pneumonia. Stroke. 2005;36(9):1972–6.

Hirano I, Pandolfino JE, Boeckxstaens GE. Functional lumen imaging probe for the management of esophageal disorders: expert review from the clinical practice updates committee of the AGA institute. Clin Gastroenterol Hepatol. 2017;15(3):325–34.

Hiss SG, Postma GN. Fiberoptic endoscopic evaluation of swallowing. Laryngoscope. 2003;113(8):1386–93.

Humbert IA, Robbins J. Dysphagia in the elderly. Phys Med Rehabil Clin N Am. 2008;19(4):853–66.. ix-x

Ikebe K, et al. Masticatory performance in older subjects with varying degrees of tooth loss. J Dent. 2012;40 (1):71–6.

Inoue M. The neural mechanisms underlying swallowing. Brain Nerve. 2015;67(2):157–68.

Jaafar MH, et al. Long-term nasogastric versus percutaneous endoscopic gastrostomy tube feeding in older asians with dysphagia: a pragmatic study. Nutr Clin Pract. 2019;34(2):280–9.

Jardine M, Miles A, Allen J. Dysphagia onset in older adults during unrelated hospital admission: quantitative videofluoroscopic measures. Geriatrics. 2018;3(4):66.

Johansen N, et al. Effect of nutritional support on clinical outcome in patients at nutritional risk. Clin Nutr. 2004;23(4):539–50.

Johansson AS, Svensson KG, Trulsson M. Impaired masticatory behavior in subjects with reduced periodontal tissue support. J Periodontol. 2006;77 (9):1491–7.

Kaneoka A, et al. A systematic review and meta-analysis of pneumonia associated with thin liquid vs. thickened liquid intake in patients who aspirate. Clin Rehabil. 2017;31(8):1116–25.

Kern M, et al. Comparison of upper esophageal sphincter opening in healthy asymptomatic young and elderly volunteers. Ann Otol Rhinol Laryngol. 1999;108 (10):982–9.

Khan A, Carmona R, Traube M. Dysphagia in the elderly. Clin Geriatr Med. 2014;30(1):43–53.

Kim HD, et al. Tongue-to-palate resistance training improves tongue strength and oropharyngeal swallowing function in subacute stroke survivors with dysphagia. J Oral Rehabil. 2017;44(1):59–64.

King SN, et al. Pathophysiology of radiation-induced dysphagia in head and neck cancer. Dysphagia. 2016;31(3):339–51.

Kocdor P, Siegel ER, Tulunay-Ugur OE. Cricopharyngeal dysfunction: a systematic review comparing outcomes of dilatation, botulinum toxin injection, and myotomy. Laryngoscope. 2016;126(1):135–41.

Kuhlemeier KV, Palmer JB, Rosenberg D. Effect of liquid bolus consistency and delivery method on aspiration and pharyngeal retention in dysphagia patients. Dysphagia. 2001;16(2):119–22.

Kwiatek MA, et al. Esophagogastric junction distensibility assessed with an endoscopic functional luminal imaging probe (EndoFLIP). Gastrointest Endosc. 2010;72 (2):272–8.

Langmore SE, Pisegna JM. Efficacy of exercises to rehabilitate dysphagia: a critique of the literature. Int J Speech Lang Pathol. 2015;17(3):222–9.

Leder SB, Murray JT. Fiberoptic endoscopic evaluation of swallowing. Phys Med Rehabil Clin N Am. 2008;19 (4):787–801.. viii-ix

Leopold NA, Daniels SK. Supranuclear control of swallowing. Dysphagia. 2010;25(3):250–7.

Liabeuf S, et al. Ulceration of the oral mucosa following direct contact with ferrous sulfate in elderly patients: a case report and a review of the French National Pharmacovigilance Database. Clin Interv Aging. 2014;9:737–40.

Lin LC, et al. Prevalence of impaired swallowing in institutionalized older people in Taiwan. J Am Geriatr Soc. 2002;50(6):1118–23.

Logemann JA, et al. Effects of postural change on aspiration in head and neck surgical patients. Otolaryngol Head Neck Surg. 1994;110(2):222–7.

Logemann JA, et al. A randomized study of three interventions for aspiration of thin liquids in patients with dementia or Parkinson's disease. J Speech Lang Hear Res. 2008;51(1):173–83.

Logemann JA, et al. Aging effects on oropharyngeal swallow and the role of dental care in oropharyngeal dysphagia. Oral Dis. 2013;19(8):733–7.

Lund JP. Mastication and its control by the brain stem. Crit Rev Oral Biol Med. 1991;2(1):33–64.

Maeda K, Takaki M, Akagi J. Decreased skeletal muscle mass and risk factors of sarcopenic dysphagia: a prospective observational cohort study. J Gerontol A Biol Sci Med Sci. 2017;72(9):1290–4.

Martin L, Blomberg J, Lagergren P. Patients' perspectives of living with a percutaneous endoscopic gastrostomy (PEG). BMC Gastroenterol. 2012;12:126.

Matsuo K, Palmer JB. Anatomy and physiology of feeding and swallowing: normal and abnormal. Phys Med Rehabil Clin N Am. 2008;19(4):691–707, vii

Mepani R, et al. Augmentation of deglutitive thyrohyoid muscle shortening by the Shaker exercise. Dysphagia. 2009;24(1):26–31.

Millsop JW, Wang EA, Fazel N. Etiology, evaluation, and management of xerostomia. Clin Dermatol. 2017;35 (5):468–76.

Mu L, et al. Altered pharyngeal muscles in Parkinson disease. J Neuropathol Exp Neurol. 2012;71(6): 520–30.

Murry T, Carrau RL. Clinical management of swallowing disorders. San Diego: Plural Publishing, Inc.; 2012.

Naka O, Anastassiadou V, Pissiotis A. Association between functional tooth units and chewing ability in older adults: a systematic review. Gerodontology. 2014;31(3):166–77.

Napenas JJ, Rouleau TS. Oral complications of Sjogren's syndrome. Oral Maxillofac Surg Clin North Am. 2014;26(1):55–62.

Ohira M, et al. Evaluation of a dysphagia screening system based on the Mann Assessment of Swallowing Ability for use in dependent older adults. Geriatr Gerontol Int. 2017;17(4):561–7.

O'Horo JC, et al. Bedside diagnosis of dysphagia: a systematic review. J Hosp Med. 2015;10(4):256–65.

Okabe Y, et al. Swallowing function and nutritional status in Japanese elderly people receiving home-care services: a 1-year longitudinal study. J Nutr Health Aging. 2016;20(7):697–704.

O'Keeffe ST. Use of modified diets to prevent aspiration in oropharyngeal dysphagia: is current practice justified? BMC Geriatr. 2018;18(1):167.

Ortega O, et al. Oral health in older patients with oropharyngeal dysphagia. Age Ageing. 2014;43(1): 132–7.

Palli C, et al. Early dysphagia screening by trained nurses reduces pneumonia rate in stroke patients: a clinical intervention study. Stroke. 2017;48(9):2583–5.

Palmer JB, Drennan JC, Baba M. Evaluation and treatment of swallowing impairments. Am Fam Physician. 2000;61(8):2453–62.

Pandolfino JE, et al. Distensibility of the esophagogastric junction assessed with the functional lumen imaging probe (FLIP) in achalasia patients. Neurogastroenterol Motil. 2013;25(6):496–501.

Panther K, A.P. Development, A. American Speech-Language-Hearing. Frazier water protocol: safety, hydration, and quality of life. Rockville: American Speech-Language-Hearing Association; 2008.

Park YH, et al. Dysphagia screening measures for use in nursing homes: a systematic review. J Korean Acad Nurs. 2015;45(1):1–13.

Park YE, et al. Impact and outcomes of nutritional support team intervention in patients with gastrointestinal disease in the intensive care unit. Medicine (Baltimore). 2017a;96(49):e8776.

Park CH, et al. Ability of high-resolution manometry to determine feeding method and to predict aspiration pneumonia in patients with dysphagia. Am J Gastroenterol. 2017b;112(7):1074–83.

Patel DA, et al. Economic and survival burden of dysphagia among inpatients in the United States. Dis Esophagus. 2018;31(1):1–7.

Pearson WG Jr, et al. Structural analysis of muscles elevating the hyolaryngeal complex. Dysphagia. 2012;27(4):445–51.

Percival RS, Challacombe SJ, Marsh PD. Flow rates of resting whole and stimulated parotid saliva in relation to age and gender. J Dent Res. 1994;73(8):1416–20.

Perry L, Love CP. Screening for dysphagia and aspiration in acute stroke: a systematic review. Dysphagia. 2001;16(1):7–18.

Peyron MA, et al. Age-related changes in mastication. J Oral Rehabil. 2017;44(4):299–312.

Pu D, et al. Indicators of dysphagia in aged care facilities. J Speech Lang Hear Res. 2017;60(9):2416–26.

Regan J, et al. A new evaluation of the upper esophageal sphincter using the functional lumen imaging probe: a preliminary report. Dis Esophagus. 2013;26 (2):117–23.

Regan J, et al. Endoflip(R) evaluation of pharyngo-oesophageal segment tone and swallowing in a clinical population: a total laryngectomy case series. Clin Otolaryngol. 2015;40(2):121–9.

Robbins J, et al. Age effects on lingual pressure generation as a risk factor for dysphagia. J Gerontol A Biol Sci Med Sci. 1995;50(5):M257–62.

Robbins J, et al. Defining physical properties of fluids for dysphagia evaluation and treatment. Perspect Swallowing Swallowing Disord (Dysphagia). 2002;11 (2):16–9.

Robbins J, et al. The effects of lingual exercise in stroke patients with dysphagia. Arch Phys Med Rehabil. 2007;88(2):150–8.

Rommel N, Hamdy S. Oropharyngeal dysphagia: manifestations and diagnosis. Nat Rev Gastroenterol Hepatol. 2016;13(1):49–59.

Roy N, et al. Dysphagia in the elderly: preliminary evidence of prevalence, risk factors, and socio-emotional effects. Ann Otol Rhinol Laryngol. 2007;116(11):858–65.

Ryu JS, Park DH, Kang JY. Application and interpretation of high-resolution manometry for pharyngeal dysphagia. J Neurogastroenterol Motil. 2015;21(2):283–7.

Sampson EL, Candy B, Jones L. Enteral tube feeding for older people with advanced dementia. Cochrane Database of Systematic Reviews 2009, Issue 2. Art. No.: CD007209. https://doi.org/10.1002/14651858.CD007209.pub2.

Sanguineti G, et al. Dosimetric predictors of laryngeal edema. Int J Radiat Oncol Biol Phys. 2007;68 (3):741–9.

Sasegbon A, Hamdy S. The anatomy and physiology of normal and abnormal swallowing in oropharyngeal dysphagia. Neurogastroenterol Motil. 2017;29(11). https://doi.org/10.1111/nmo.13100. Epub 2017 May 25

Schein OD, et al. Dry eye and dry mouth in the elderly: a population-based assessment. Arch Intern Med. 1999;159(12):1359–63.

Serra-Prat M, et al. Prevalence of oropharyngeal dysphagia and impaired safety and efficacy of swallow in independently living older persons. J Am Geriatr Soc. 2011;59(1):186–7.

Serra-Prat M, et al. Oropharyngeal dysphagia as a risk factor for malnutrition and lower respiratory tract infection in independently living older persons: a population-based prospective study. Age Ageing. 2012;41 (3):376–81.

Shaker R. Manual of diagnostic and therapeutic techniques for disorders of deglutition. New York: Springer; 2013.

Shaker R, et al. Coordination of deglutitive glottic closure with oropharyngeal swallowing. Gastroenterology. 1990;98(6):1478–84.

Shaker R, Kern M, Bardan E. Augmentation of deglutitive upper esophageal sphincter opening in the elderly by exercise. Am J Phys. 1997;272:G1518–22.

Shaw SM, Martino R. The normal swallow: muscular and neurophysiological control. Otolaryngol Clin N Am. 2013;46(6):937–56.

Shlisky J, et al. Nutritional considerations for healthy aging and reduction in age-related chronic disease. Adv Nutr. 2017;8(1):17–26.

Sivarao DV, Goyal RK. Functional anatomy and physiology of the upper esophageal sphincter. Am J Med. 2000;108(Suppl 4a):27s–37s.

Smith CH, et al. Oral and oropharyngeal perceptions of fluid viscosity across the age span. Dysphagia. 2006;21 (4):209–17.

Smith EE, et al. Effect of dysphagia screening strategies on clinical outcomes after stroke: a systematic review for the 2018 guidelines for the early management of patients with acute ischemic stroke. Stroke. 2018;49 (3):e123–8.

Smukalla SM, et al. Dysphagia in the elderly. Curr Treat Options Gastroenterol. 2017;15(3):382–96.

Solazzo A, et al. Investigation of compensatory postures with videofluoromanometry in dysphagia patients. World J Gastroenterol. 2012;18(23):2973–8.

Suntrup S, et al. Evidence for adaptive cortical changes in swallowing in Parkinson's disease. Brain. 2013;136(Pt 3):726–38.

Suntrup S, et al. The impact of lesion location on dysphagia incidence, pattern and complications in acute stroke. Part 1: dysphagia incidence, severity and aspiration. Eur J Neurol. 2015;22(5):832–8.

Suntrup-Krueger S, et al. The impact of lesion location on dysphagia incidence, pattern and complications in acute stroke. Part 2: oropharyngeal residue, swallow and cough response, and pneumonia. Eur J Neurol. 2017;24(6):867–74.

Sura L, et al. Dysphagia in the elderly: management and nutritional considerations. Clin Interv Aging. 2012;7:287–98.

Tamine K, et al. Age-related changes in tongue pressure during swallowing. J Dent Res. 2010;89 (10):1097–101.

Teismann IK, et al. Time-dependent hemispheric shift of the cortical control of volitional swallowing. Hum Brain Mapp. 2009;30(1):92–100.

Teismann IK, et al. Cortical processing of swallowing in ALS patients with progressive dysphagia – a magnetoencephalographic study. PLoS One. 2011;6 (5):e19987.

Trapl M, et al. Dysphagia bedside screening for acute-stroke patients: the Gugging Swallowing Screen. Stroke. 2007;38(11):2948–52.

Troche MS, et al. Aspiration and swallowing in Parkinson disease and rehabilitation with EMST: a randomized trial. Neurology. 2010;75(21):1912–9.

Volkert D, et al. ESPEN guideline on clinical nutrition and hydration in geriatrics. Clin Nutr. 2019;38(1): 10–47.

Wakabayashi H. Presbyphagia and sarcopenic dysphagia: association between aging, sarcopenia, and deglutition disorders. J Frailty Aging. 2014;3(2):97–103.

Wang ZY, Chen JM, Ni GX. Effect of an indwelling nasogastric tube on swallowing function in elderly post-stroke dysphagia patients with long-term nasal feeding. BMC Neurol. 2019;19(1):83.

Wirth R, et al. Oropharyngeal dysphagia in older persons – from pathophysiology to adequate intervention: a review and summary of an international expert meeting. Clin Interv Aging. 2016;11:189–208.

Wolff A, et al. A guide to medications inducing salivary gland dysfunction, Xerostomia, and subjective sialorrhea: a systematic review sponsored by the world workshop on oral medicine VI. Drugs R D. 2017;17(1):1–28.

Yang S, Choi KH, Son YR. The effect of stroke on pharyngeal laterality during swallowing. Ann Rehabil Med. 2015;39(4):509–16.

Gastroparesis in Older Adults

48

Richard W. McCallum, Ashish Malhotra,
Marco A. Bustamante Bernal, and Luis O. Chavez

Contents

R. W. McCallum (✉) · M. A. Bustamante Bernal
Department of Internal Medicine, Texas Tech University
Health Science Center, El Paso, TX, USA

Department of Internal Medicine, Division of
Gastroenterology, Texas Tech University Health Science
Center, El Paso, TX, USA
e-mail: richard.mccallum@ttuhsc.edu

A. Malhotra
Department of Gastroenterology and Hepatology, Seton
Hall University of Health and Medical Sciences,
Paterson, NJ, USA

L. O. Chavez
Department of Internal Medicine, Texas Tech University
Health Science Center, El Paso, TX, USA

© Springer Nature Switzerland AG 2021
C. S. Pitchumoni, T. S. Dharmarajan (eds.), *Geriatric Gastroenterology*,
https://doi.org/10.1007/978-3-030-30192-7_41

Abstract

Gastroparesis is a debilitating condition in which delayed gastric emptying is associated with a constellation of symptoms (nausea, vomiting, boating, abdominal pain, etc.) in the absence of mechanical obstruction. Gastric motility changes with aging; however, significant impairment of gastric emptying is not a normal physiologic aging process. Different causes may contribute to gastroparesis in the older population. The most common etiologies in all subgroups of ages are diabetes, idiopathic, and postsurgical, but certain common disorders (medication side effects and neurological conditions) in the geriatric population warrant special emphasis. Management involves dietary modifications, combinations of antiemetics and prokinetics cautiously selected to minimize likelihood of adverse events. Other treatment options should be cautiously selected in this particular population.

Keywords

Gastroparesis diagnosis · Gastric motility · Geriatric population · Gastroparesis management

Introduction

Gastroparesis is a chronic symptomatic disorder characterized by evidence of gastric retention or delayed emptying in the absence of mechanical obstruction (Parkman et al. 2004). The normal process of gastric emptying is achieved by the participation and synchronization of the nervous system (parasympathetic and sympathetic), smooth muscle cells, neurons, and interstitial cells of Cajal. Abnormalities in any of these components can lead to gastric emptying delay (Camilleri et al. 2013).

Epidemiology

The true prevalence of gastroparesis is difficult to ascertain given the relatively poor correlation of symptoms with gastric emptying (GE), the need to apply a diagnostic test in a community setting, and the fact that many patients with gastroparesis may not even seek health care or be referred to gastroenterologists (Talley et al. 2006; Soykan et al. 1998). In a study out of Olmsted County, USA, the age-adjusted incidence per 100,000 person-years of definite gastroparesis was 2.5 for men and 9.8 for women and the age-adjusted prevalence was 9.6 and 37.8 for men and women, respectively (Jung et al. 2009). The incidence of definite gastroparesis increased significantly with advancing age with a peak incidence of 10.5 per 100,000 in patients ≥60 years of age.

The overall survival for gastroparesis patients is significantly reduced when compared to their age/gender-specific expected survival. Hospitalizations related to gastroparesis have been increasing in the USA, with economic impact (Wang et al. 2007).

Normal Gastric Motility

The proximal portion of the stomach (fundus, cardia) mainly serves as the reservoir for food. Nutrients can be ingested without a rise in the intragastric pressure (Ahluwalia et al. 1996).

Three main mechanisms involved in the regulation of this function are the receptive relaxation, accommodation, and enterogastric reflexes (Mizumoto et al. 1997). The distal part of the stomach (primarily the antrum) acts as the "grinder." To achieve this function, the slow waves, controlled by the interstitial cells of Cajal, also known as the pacemaker cells, coordinate the postprandial fed pattern that leads to emptying of digestive solids when particle size is <5 mm. Contractions associated with the migrating motor complex (MMC) empty indigestible solids soon after solid food digestion is completed and during fasting between meals and at night (Hinder and Kelly 1977; Meyer et al. 1981). The physical nature of the food, such as the particle size, fat, and calorie content, and various neurohormonal factors influence the rate of GE. The glucose-regulating hormones such as glucagon-like peptide (GLP-1), hormones released with fat and protein intake such as cholecystokinin (CKK), peptide YY, and secretin slow GE while motilin and ghrelin levels are increased with meals and augment gastric motility (Morgan and Szurszewski 1980; Hirst and Edwards 2004). Solid particles empty in three phases over 3–4 h. An initial lag phase, where food is stored in the proximal stomach; next it gets triturated and churned in a milieu of acid, pepsin, and mucous, as the antral contractions propel particles against a closed pylorus, and finally is followed by the propellant phase of relatively constant emptying where food particles are pushed out of the stomach once the particle size is <5 mm (Meyer et al. 1981; Camilleri 2006; Hunt and Pathk 1960). Noncaloric and minimally caloric liquids empty faster, but increased caloric content may slow down the emptying rate (McCallum 1989). For example, the caloric supplement "Ensure" (1 cal./cc) empties very similarly to a standardized eggbeater meal.

Effects of Aging on Gastric Motility

In general, gastric motility is regarded as being relatively preserved during healthy aging. However, studies on the effect of aging on GE have yielded some conflicting results (Evans et al. 1981; Horowitz et al. 1984; Madsen and Graff 2004; Kupfer et al. 1985). This is largely due to various study limitations, such as, choice of tests for GE being less than ideal, and heterogeneous study population including those with significant comorbidities.

It has been demonstrated that healthy aging is associated with decreased perception of stomach distension and reduced gastric tone late in the postprandial period; however, there are no significant changes in gastric compliance. Overall gastric emptying is mildly delayed in the older population, without any clinical significance (Kuo et al. 2007; Rayner et al. 2000).

The mechanisms underlying the slowing of GE with aging are uncertain. Autonomic nerve dysfunction is more common in older subjects but its correlation with slower GE is poor (Clarkston et al. 2006). It remains unclear if there is derangement of gastric electrical rhythm with aging, but there is no data indicating any loss of interstitial cells of Cajal with aging. Neurohormonal changes such as increased plasma CCK (both fasting and postprandial), decreased plasma ghrelin, decreased mucosal prostaglandins, pepsin, and bicarbonate levels have been reported in the elderly, which may affect gastric motility and digestive function (Kuo et al. 2007). A decrease in gastric acid secretion associated with aging may decrease the efficiency of trituration of solids and hence will mildly and subtly slow gastric emptying. This aspect as well as other possible attributing factors will be summarized in the following section on "Etiologies."

Etiologies

The potential underlying causes for gastroparesis are numerous (Table 1). Any disease that can alter motor or sensory pathways of the stomach can potentially cause or contribute to gastroparesis. Idiopathic, diabetes, and postsurgical/vagotomy are the three main etiologies for gastroparesis, accounting for almost 80% of the cases (Soykan et al. 1998).

Certain common disorders in the geriatric population warrant special emphasis:

Table 1 Etiology of gastroparesis

Neuromuscular disorders

Central nervous system disorders: *Parkinson's disease,* brainstem tumors, multiple sclerosis

Peripheral neuromuscular disorders: Muscular dystrophy, Guillain-Barré syndrome, acute dysautonomia. Myasthenia gravis

Others: *Amyloidosis,* visceral neuropathies, visceral myopathies

Endocrine disorders

Diabetes mellitus[a]

Hypothyroidism

Hypoparathyroidism

Hypoadrenalism

Metabolic disorders

Uremia

Chronic liver disease

Paraneoplastic/cancer-related syndromes

Gastrointestinal disorders

Gastroesophageal reflux disease

Atrophic gastritis with or without pernicious anemia

Acute viral gastroenteritis (cytomegalovirus)

Acute/chronic gastritis

Idiopathic intestinal pseudo-obstruction

Pancreatitis

Mesenteric ischemia

Autoimmune/collagen vascular disorders

Systemic sclerosis

Scleroderma

Dermatomyositis

Polymyositis

Mixed connective tissue disease

Systemic lupus erythematosus

Postsurgical disorders[a]

Vagotomy

Antireflux operations

Roux en Y syndrome

Trauma

Head injury, spinal cord injury

Psychogenic disorders

Anorexia nervosa, stress

Medications (Table 2)

Idiopathic/infectious[a]

Viral (cytomegalovirus, Epstein-Barr, Norwalk, and herpes simplex virus)

Causes are common in older adults (*Italicized*)

[a]Represents most common causes of gastroparesis (diabetes mellitus, postsurgical disorders, idiopathic/infectious)

1. *Neurological diseases*: The most common central nervous system disorder that affects GE is Parkinson's disease (PD). In a prospective study, it was shown that 88% of patients with PD have delayed GE (Rayner et al. 2000). There are two components of gastrointestinal

(GI) dysfunction in PD. First, PD is associated with striatal muscle dysfunction, affecting primarily the oropharynx, proximal esophagus, and the anal canal. Second, dysfunction can involve the smooth muscle and autonomic and/or enteric nervous system (ENS) with a more global adverse impact on GI motility (Goetze et al. 2006). Although there are a large causes for peripheral neuropathies, few affect the stomach (Table 1). Amyloidosis is another entity to consider. In a large retrospective series of patients with primary amyloidosis, only 0.4%, however, were found to have delayed GE (Menke et al. 1993). Other conditions that may delay GE by affecting the extrinsic neural components (vagus nerve) are brainstem strokes and primary dysautonomias. Myasthenia gravis has been reported to cause gastroparesis secondary to a subacute autonomic failure, hence ptosis and dysphagia should be a clinical tip off to consider this entity.

2. *Endocrine disorders*: The prevalence of diabetes mellitus (DM) increases with age and is one of the most common causes of impaired motility. Normal aging is associated with mild impaired glucose tolerance. This is considered secondary to increased peripheral insulin resistance, decreased beta cell function, and possibly delayed postprandial suppression of hepatic gluconeogenesis (Kuo et al. 2007). In the Western world, it is estimated that at least 20% of the population age 65 and above have DM, with the majority being type 2 (Kuo et al. 2007). Furthermore, disordered gastric motor function may affect nutrient delivery to the small bowel and thus cause fluctuations in blood glucose levels (O'Mahony et al. 2002). Between 20% and 40% of patients with DM developed dysfunction of the autonomic nervous system, contributing to delay in GE (Kuo et al. 2007). Furthermore, hyperglycemia alone causes acute disruption of gastric motility even when the autonomic nervous system is intact, as in diabetic ketoacidosis (McCallum 1989). Motor abnormalities and diabetic gastroparesis include abnormal intragastric distribution

of food, reduced occurrence of the antral component of the MMC, antral dilation, and electrical dysrhythmias (Kuo et al. 2007). These abnormalities may be secondary to extrinsic autonomic denervation (as above), hyperglycemia per se, and/or direct involvement of the ENS and enteric muscle (Quigley 2002). Hormonal factors including CCK, peptide YY, amylin, and secretin tightly regulate GE and their upper regulation could contribute to retardation of gastric motility (Kuo et al. 2007). Hypothyroidism increases with old age and may affect GI motility. Hypothyroidism may be associated with pernicious anemia and decreased gastric acid secretion with further decrease in gastric motility. Hypothyroidism is associated with slowing of motor activity throughout the GI tract, especially the small and large bowel rather than in the stomach (Ebert 2010). Glucocorticoids play a role in normal motility function, thus hypoadrenalism is also associated with gastric dysmotility. In patients with adrenal insufficiency and gastroparesis, corticosteroid replacement therapy has been shown to restore gastric motor function (Krishna and report 1996).

3. *Renal disease*: The prevalence of chronic kidney disease (CKD) increases exponentially in older adults (Lindeman 1990). CKD, regardless of its etiology, is associated with symptoms of impaired gastric motility such as bloating, nausea, and vomiting. Patient with diabetic nephropathy have increased predilection for gastroparesis (Dumitrascu et al. 1995).

4. *Paraneoplastic/cancer-related syndromes*: The prevalence of cancer is high in older adults (Smith et al. 2009). Paraneoplastic syndromes caused by cancer cells that express conditions mimicking neuronal tissues results in an autoimmune/inflammatory neuropathy of the ENS. A study demonstrated that sera containing anti-neuronal antibodies inhibited contractions of the circular muscle (Lucchinetti et al. 1998; Hejazi et al. 2009). Small cell cancer of the lung is the most common cause, with cancer of the prostate, pancreas, and breast, lymphoma, and melanoma less common (Lucchinetti et al. 1998; Hejazi et al. 2009). Neuronal invasion by

tumor and side effects of chemotherapy may also contribute to delayed GE (Hejazi et al. 2009). Occult malignancy should be suspected in the presence of anti-Hu antibodies and unexplained gastroparesis, particularly in an older individual with accompanying weight loss.

5. *Achlorhydria*: Elderly patients may have decreased gastric acid secretion, chronic atrophic gastritis, and pernicious anemia (Carmel et al. 2001). Atrophic gastritis may be the final stage of Helicobacter pylori infection with diffuse gastritis involving the proximal stomach and antrum; patients with atrophic gastritis can have delayed GE. The two main mechanisms hypothesized are: (1) impaired trituration due to low gastric acid and pepsin secretion and (2) thinner smooth muscle, reported in pernicious anemia (McCallum 1989; Minami and McCallum 1984). A study with dual-isotope technique in a patient with achlorhydria due to atrophic gastritis and pernicious anemia showed that GE of solids was delayed but liquid emptying was preserved (Halvorsen et al. 1973). Excessive gastric acid as in Zollinger-Ellison syndrome is associated with accelerated GE (McCallum 1989).

6. *Medications*: In the older population, medications may be the most common cause of slowing of gastric emptying. Many subclasses of medications that are routinely prescribed to the aged adults have a direct effect on gastric motility. Narcotic pain medications act on mu opiate receptors and have a slowing effect on gastric, small bowel, and colonic motility. Additionally, opioids may reduce the effectiveness of medications used to treat gastroparesis (Jehangir and Parkman 2017). Other medications that may delay gastric motility are tricyclic antidepressants, calcium channel blockers, dopamine agonists, glucagon-like peptide (GLP)-1 agonists or analogues among others. Table 2 illustrates common medications by subgroups that could delay gastric motility (psychiatric, cardiovascular, hormonal, and gastrointestinal drugs) (Veevers and Oxberry 2017; Bouras et al. 2008; Linnebjerg et al. 2008; Giron et al. 2001).

Table 2 Medications that cause delayed gastric emptying

Cardiovascular/respiratory drugs
Calcium channel antagonist (nifedipine, diltiazem, verapamil)
Potassium
Beta adrenergic agonists
Gastrointestinal drugs
Aluminum hydroxide
Proton pump inhibitors
Anticholinergic/antispasmodics (hyoscyamine, dicyclomine)
Psychiatric/neurologic drugs
Tricyclics (amitriptyline, nortriptyline, etc.)
Phenothiazines
Levodopa
Dopamine agonists
Hormonal drugs
Synthetic estrogen
Somatostatin (octreotide)
GLP analog (exenatide or pramlintide)
Narcotics
Opioids (morphine, fentanyl, hydromorphone, codeine, etc.)

7. *Connective Tissue Diseases*: Patients with Raynaud's phenomenon, systemic lupus erythematosus, and scleroderma may have gastric muscle layer involvement and delayed gastric emptying (Weston et al. 1998).

8. Previous surgeries: Patients that underwent gastrointestinal surgeries may present with gastroparesis. Vagal injury may occur with fundoplication for hiatal hernia, Billroth II gastrectomy, and Roux-en-Y gastric bypass. Patients with obesity surgery where a "gastric sleeve" method was used are also candidates for delayed gastric emptying. Any past history of peptic ulcer that required surgery should be investigated, since the vagus nerve could be involved.

Clinical Presentation

Gastroparesis may present with constellation of symptoms. Some patients may present with debilitating nausea and vomiting, and in others, it may be a more indolent disease with early satiety, postprandial fullness, abdominal

distention or even weight loss, and decreased appetite (Hasler 2007).

In one study, nausea, vomiting, bloating, and early satiety were reported by 92%, 84%, 75%, and 60%, respectively, and abdominal pain in 46% (Soykan et al. 1998). Succussion splash may be elicited as a sign of retained gastric contents (solid and liquid). Heartburn may be the main symptom of gastroparesis. Gastroesophageal reflux is facilitated by fundic distention which increases the rate of transient lower esophageal sphincter relaxation (Hasler 2007). Although some patients with gastroparesis with frequent vomiting lose weight and develop malnutrition, others are overweight or obese through consumption of a liquid diet (Bizer et al. 2005). Phytobezoars may complicate gastroparesis. Retained food seen during an upper endoscopy may be early sign. Gastric ulcer and pyloric outlet obstruction are complications of bezoars. Elimination of bezoars is accomplished by endoscopic destruction and lavage; enzymatic digestion; and dietary exclusion of foods rich in indigestible residue. Variably delayed GE in diabetics may lead to unpredictable nutrient delivery to the small bowel, with erratic glycemic control; this can be a clinical "tip-off" for gastroparesis (Kuo et al. 2007).

Differential Diagnosis

Vomiting associated with gastroparesis must be differentiated from regurgitation due to reflux disease or rumination syndrome, episodic vomiting seen in cyclic vomiting syndrome, and abdominal pain with vomiting and superior mesenteric artery syndrome (Park and Camilleri 2006). Vomiting typically occurs 1–2 h or longer following a meal, with older food contents being identified. Since functional dyspepsia and rapid GE may have similar clinical manifestations, a standardized 4-h GE scintigraphy test may help differentiate the disorders (Delegado-Aros et al. 2004). The symptomatic spectrum of small intestinal bacterial overgrowth (SIBO) and gastroparesis has significant overlap. Patients may have bloating, early satiety, and upper abdominal discomfort in both. The two disorders can coexist in older adults due to hypoacidity promoting bacterial colonization of the small bowel; awareness of this relationship helps management (Reddymasu and McCallum 2010).

Diagnostic Approach

Initial Evaluation

A detailed history and physical examination are critical to understand the severity of the disease, underlying etiologies and exclude disorders with similar presentation. A review of medications that delay GE is important (Table 2). Symptoms may vary based on the etiology, and the most common symptoms are nausea, vomiting, and abdominal pain; however, bloating, early satiety, and postprandial fullness are also reported.

Evaluate for Etiologies and Complications

Blood tests for diabetes, uremia, thyroid and parathyroid disease, pernicious anemia, and serologic studies for connective tissue disorders (in particular scleroderma) and serum protein electrophoresis for amyloidosis may help identify potential causes of gastroparesis. Especially with new onset symptoms of gastroparesis and weight loss, serologic markers for paraneoplastic syndromes should be considered. They includes type I anti-neuronal nuclear antibody (specifically), anti-Hu antibodies, anti-Purkinje cells cytoplasmic antibody, and ganglionic nicotinic acetylcholine receptor antibody (De Giorgio et al. 2004). Serum electrolytes to rule out hypokalemia and contraction alkalosis, a blood count to exclude anemia and serum protein and albumin as a nutritional marker, are indicated.

Exclude Mechanical Obstruction

Most patients with suspected gastroparesis require upper endoscopy or radiographic imaging to exclude mechanical obstruction, such as compression of the distal duodenum, which can be explained by superior mesenteric artery syndrome or as early manifestation of pancreatic cancer compressing the third portion of the duodenum. Adhesions due to a prior surgery, ulcer disease and pyloric obstruction need to be considered. The presence of retained food in the stomach after overnight fasting in the absence of mechanical obstruction on endoscopy is suggestive of gastroparesis. Computed tomographic enterography or Magnetic resonance enterography may be used to rule out mechanical obstruction.

Confirm Delayed GE

A gastric emptying test is required to establish a definite diagnosis of gastroparesis. GE of a solid phase meal by scintigraphy is considered the gold standard as it quantifies the emptying of a physiologic, caloric meal that can assess the motor function of the stomach. An international scintigraphy method has been established with 99 mTc-sulfur colloid labeled, low-fat meal consisting of scrambled egg substitute, two slices of bread, strawberry jam, and water (Tougas et al. 2000; Abell et al. 2008). Images are taken at 0, 1, 2, 3, and 4 h after the test meal ingestion. Gastroparesis is confirmed when >60% at 2 h or >10% at 4 h of gastric content is found using the abovementioned technique. The severity of delayed GE can be classified as mild (10–15%), moderate (15–35%), and severe (>35%); however, the symptom severity is not directly correlated with the rate of gastric emptying. In those with diabetes, blood glucose should be measured prior to the test and recorded in the report. If the glucose level is more than 275 mg/dL, it should be lowered with insulin and/or that test be rescheduled (Abell et al. 2008). Ideally, the patient should also be instructed to stop antisecretory drugs such as proton pump inhibitors for 5–7 days, prokinetics at least for 72 h, and narcotics for at least 24 h prior to the test. Smoking and marijuana also delay gastric emptying.

Table 3 Evaluation and testing for gastroparesis

Evaluation	Test	Description
Exclude mechanical obstruction	Upper gastrointestinal endoscopy	Test used to visualize any mechanical obstruction. All symptomatic patients need to be evaluated for any obstruction
	CT or MR enterography	Used to exclude any intrinsic or extrinsic mechanical bowel obstruction such as a mass or superior mesenteric syndrome
	Upper gastrointestinal barium radiograph	Used when not able to obtain CT/MR, provides information regarding mucosal abnormalities
Assess gastric motor function	Scintigraphic gastric emptying	Gold standard for diagnosis and cost-effective. Results classify as mild, moderate, severe based on the extent of gastric retention at 4 h
	Wireless motility capsule	Alternative approach for assessing gastric motor function. This test can measure pH, temperature, and phasic pressure amplitudes
	13 C breath testing	Noninvasive, avoids radiation exposure. Measures expiratory 13-CO_2 after ingestion of a stable isotope labeled meal
Test to establish etiology	Laboratory studies	Test that may aid on establishing a diagnosis based on clinical suspicion: Fasting glucose, hbA1C, serum total protein, albumin, TSH, ANA, etc.
	Antroduodenal manometry	Aids to distinguish between myopathic process versus neuropathic process
	Autonomic testing	If neuropathic etiology is suspected, this test may distinguish central vs. peripheral lesion or neuropathy.
Other (used as research tools)	Electrogastrogram	Changes in frequency and amplitude of postprandial electrical signal are seen in idiopathic and diabetic gastroparesis
	SPECT	Single photon emission computed tomography assess postprandial gastric accommodation
	Full-thickness gastric and small bowel intestinal biopsy	Convey histologic abnormalities such as fibrosis, inflammation, reduced number of interstitial cells of Cajal. Aids to confirm an organic etiology

The wireless motility capsule (WMC) is an alternative test used to evaluate gastric motility. The advantage of using the WMC is that it avoids radiation and it can relay additional information such as phasic pressure amplitudes and pH which may help to rule out a myopathic disorder (Lee et al. 2018).

Other tests that assess the myoelectric function of the stomach and may yield information to establish the etiology of gastroparesis are listed in Table 3.

Treatment

Diet and Lifestyle Modifications

Although there are no prospective, randomized control trials comparing dietary treatments for gastroparesis, a low-fat, low-fiber diet of small portions and frequent feedings are often recommended (Parkman et al. 2010). High-fiber food requires effective antral motility, and in patients with impaired GE, fiber can increase the risk for bezoar formation (Parrish 2007; Sanders 2004; Whitson et al. 2008). Large volumes of food not only slow GE but aggravate the early satiety often present. Patients are advised to chew foods well since the antrum's grinding capability is compromised. The patient should remain upright in an effort to use the effect of gravity to move food from fundus to antrum and to decrease postprandial reflux (Parkman et al. 2010). Alcohol, smoking, and carbonated beverages should be restricted as they contribute to decrease GE.

Pharmacological Therapy

Antiemetics: Antiemetic therapy may help to achieve rapid symptomatic relief (Table 4) (Reddymasu and McCallum 2009). There are no

Table 4 Classification, doses, and adverse reactions of commonly used antiemetic agents in gastroparesis

Class name	Agent	Mode of action	Usual dose	Side effects
Phenothiazine	Prochlorperazine	D2 receptor antagonist	Start with 5–10 mg 3 times daily or 5–25 mg as required every 12 h as rectal suppository	Extrapyramidal effects, rarely jaundice
Anti-serotoninergic	Ondansetron (others: Granisetron, Dolasteron)	Serotonin 5-HT 3 receptor antagonist	4–80 mg 3 times daily as required	Constipation with regular use
Anticholinergic	Scopolamine	Muscarinic M1 receptor antagonist	1 mg every 3 days	Drowsiness, headache, dry mouth, glaucoma, or bladder dysfunction
Phenothiazine	Promethazine	Histamine H1 receptor antagonist	12.5–25 mg 3 times daily as required or intramuscular	Drowsiness, headache, dry mouth, bowel, or bladder dysfunction
Benzodiazepine	Lorazepam	Anti-GABA effect	0.5–1 mg as required	Sedation
Neurokinin antagonist	Aprepitant	Neurokinin receptor-1 antagonist	40 mg once daily as required	Weakness, bowel dysfunction, reduced efficacy for OCP
Cannabinoids	Dronabinol	Acts on cannabinoid receptors with multiple central nervous system effects	2.5–5 mg twice a day as required	Dependence or abuse potential, somnolence, euphoria

studies to guide the management of nausea in patients with gastroparesis, and most of the antiemetics should be used with caution in older adults. Phenothiazines are less expensive; however, its use is limited due to central nervous system side effects and QT interval prolongation. 5HT3 antagonists (ondansetron 4–8 mg orally every 8 h) and antihistamines (Diphenhydramine 12.5 mg orally or IV every 6–8 h) are used to treat patients with persistent nausea and vomiting (Camilleri et al. 2013; Reddymasu and McCallum 2009). The use of higher doses of antihistamines may exert the potential anticholinergic effect and may worsen gastric emptying (Reddymasu and McCallum 2009). The geriatric population is vulnerable to drug toxicity and drug interactions, and hence special caution is advised with the concomitant use of antiemetics and prokinetics. 5HT3 antagonists are not recommended in patients with electrolyte disturbances or with underlying arrhythmias.

Scopolamine patch or promethazine, either oral or rectal suppository, may alleviate continuous nausea. Other alternative options for symptomatic relief that lack randomized trials are dronabinol (synthetic cannabinoid) and aprepitant (neurokinin receptor-1 antagonist). Dronabinol may improve the quality of life by improving oral intake in patients with ongoing nausea and vomiting.

Pain control and psychopharmacology: Mechanisms involved in the pathogenesis of pain include (but not limited to) visceral hyperalgesia, coexistent inflammatory/cytokine reactions, and dysmotility (Parkman et al. 2010). A logical step would be to empathize with the patient. NSAIDs like ketorolac and indomethacin may have a role, but given their ulcerogenic potential, require caution (Hasler et al. 1995). Tricyclic antidepressants (amitriptyline), selective serotonin reuptake inhibitors (paroxetine), and antiepileptics (gabapentin) help control neuropathic pain and reduced visceral perception (Reddymasu and McCallum 2009). Tramadol, an opiate antagonist, with limited effect on mu receptors has little impact on gastric transit if used in low doses of 50 mg once or twice daily; however, higher doses do have motility effects (Mauer et al. 1996). It also has the added benefit of lack of addictive potential with prolonged use. Acupuncture and biofeedback should also be considered as increased anxiety is present in these patients due to visceral hypersensitivity. Mirtazapine, an antidepressant, has been used in refractory gastroparesis to provide symptomatic relief, improving appetite in patients with nausea and depression. The serotonin reuptake antidepressants have not been effective. Restoration of euglycemia and correction of electrolytes and fluid balance help GE.

Exacerbating factors: Medications that delay GE (Table 2) should be discontinued or limited if possible.

Drugs to augment GE/prokinetics (Tables 5 and 6): Prokinetic agents mainly used to treat gastroparesis are metoclopramide and domperidone (McCallum et al. 1983). Both agents are equally effective in reducing the symptoms of diabetic gastroparesis particularly nausea and vomiting. Adverse CNS effects are more severe and more common with metoclopramide and include somnolence and confusion (Patterson et al. 1999). Chronic use of metoclopramide has

been linked to tremor and rigidity referred to as a "Parkinson's-like effect" and tardive dyskinesia, which includes involuntary and repetitive movements of the face, tongue, and body. Those prone include diabetics, female gender, and older adults (Pasricha et al. 2006). Metoclopramide has received a black box warning. Although the original food and drug administration (FDA) approval of medication was for up to 6 weeks, chronic use entails monitoring for adverse events. When starting treatment with metoclopramide in a liquid formulation, a low dose (5 mg before meals and bedtime) should be titrated up to the lowest effective dose. In patients unable to tolerate oral metoclopramide, parental routes can be used. Domperidone is not approved in the USA but can be obtained by filing for an investigational new drug application to the FDA in obtaining local IRB approval. The responsibility for initiating this agent lies on focusing on the electrocardiogram where the QT interval needs to be less than 475 ms for females and less than 450 ms in males and potassium levels to be maintained in the normal range. Some compounding pharmacies in the USA provide the drug. The usual effective

Table 5 Classification, doses, and adverse reactions of commonly used prokinetic agents in gastroparesis

Name of the drug	Mode of action	Doses	Adverse effects
Metoclopramide	D2 dopamine receptor antagonist, antiemetic action also contributes to relief	Start with 5 mg orally 3 times daily, usual 15–20 mg 3 times daily, 15 min before meals, can be used IM, SC, or IV	Anxiety, depression, galactorrhea, extrapyramidal side effects, and tardive dyskinesia
Domperidone	D2 dopamine receptor antagonist	Start with 5 mg 3 times daily, usual 15–20 mg 3 times daily, 15 min before meals	Anxiety, depression, galactorrhea, extrapyramidal side effects, and tardive dyskinesia. (less common than metoclopramide)
Erythromycin	Motilin receptor agonist	40–250 mg 3 times daily, 15 min before meals	Abdominal cramping, loss of appetite, potential for many drug interactions, tachyphylaxis develops rapidly
Cisapride	5 HT4 serotonin receptor agonist	10–20 mg 3 times daily, 15 min before meals	Diarrhea, potential for cardiac dysrhythmia, under strict compassionate use protocol approved by IRB as otherwise not available in the USA
Bethanechol	Muscarinic receptor agonist	10–20 mg 3 times daily, 15 min before meals	Cholinergic side effects, efficacy against symptoms unclear, side effects are dose-limiting
Pyridostigmine	Acetylcholine esterase inhibitors	30 mg 4 times daily	Cholinergic side effects, unclear efficacy

Table 6 Practical approach to gastroparesis management in the elderly

	Mild gastroparesis	Moderated gastroparesis	Severe gastroparesis
Criteria	Symptoms relatively easily controlled, able to maintain weight and nutrition, gastric retention of 11–20%	Moderate symptoms with partial control with pharmacological agents, able to maintain nutrition with dietary adjustments, rare hospital admissions, gastric retention 21–40%	Refractory symptoms despite medical therapy inability to maintain nutrition via oral route, frequent ER visits or hospitalizations, gastric retention of more than 40%
Dietary modifications	Homogenized foods, frequent small feedings, decrease fat content, decrease fiber content	As in mild, rare use of nutritional or caloric supplementation (Ensure, boost)/enteral access	As in mild plus routine use of nutrition or caloric supplementation (Ensure, boost)
Enteral access	Never	Rarely	Usually required for venting or feeding purposes
Pharmacologic treatment	Antiemetic (promethazine) or prokinetic (metoclopramide before meals) required on as-needed basis (when symptomatic)	May require daily therapy with prokinetics and symptomatic as needed management with antiemetics; if nausea or vomiting severe, may need drugs and suspension form (metoclopramide) or rectal suppositories (such as Phenergan suppositories)	Usually daily metoclopramide therapy 10 mg half an hour before each meal or domperidone 10–20 mg 3 times daily half an hour before each meal; daily antiemetic and may require intravenous forms (ondansetron) during severe symptom attacks
Nonpharmacologic treatment	Not needed	Not needed	Gastrostomy tube decompression, parenteral nutrition, and or compassionate use of gastric neurostimulation device

Modified from data found in Abell et al. (2008) and Camilleri (Reddymasu and McCallum 2009)

dose is 20 mg 4 times per day (before meals and bedtime); start with 10 mg three times a day, but sometimes the maximal dose of 30 mg 4 times per day is necessary. Domperidone has no or minimal penetration of the blood–brain barrier, and hence the only real side effects relate to elevation of prolactin-induced breast enlargement and/or tenderness in approximately 5% of patients. Additionally, patients need follow-up in 3 months to assess the QT interval by electrocardiogram.

Erythromycin is a motilin receptor agonist that promotes gastric propulsive contractions and fundus contractility. It can be given orally, preferably as liquid, in a dose of 150–250 mg up to three times a day for <4 weeks at a time to minimize concern for tachyphylaxis, which develops with chronic use (Reddymasu and McCallum 2009). It is the most effective IV prokinetic agent; its use is indicated mainly for acute exacerbations. Side effects include ototoxicity, QT prolongation, and some gastrointestinal toxicity (nausea, vomiting, abdominal pain, and diarrhea). Azithromycin is another macrolide that promotes antral motility with longer half-life and less gastrointestinal side effects; however, it also has increase risk of arrhythmias.

The FDA approved prucalopride (5HT4 agonist) for constipation; it is also used for patients with gastroparesis as an "off label" medication showing improvement in symptoms and gastric emptying (Myint et al. 2018).

Histamine 2 receptor antagonists, particularly nizatidine, are also partial choline esterase inhibitors and accelerate gastric emptying and thus can be used to augment emptying of meals at night particularly in patients with severe gastroesophageal reflux symptoms (Reddymasu and McCallum 2009).

Role of Botulinum Toxin

Although safe, endoscopic injection of botulinum toxin type A into the pylorus has shown little to no effect for symptom relief (Arts et al. 2007; Freiedenberg et al. 2008). There is the possibility that improved techniques with the use of ultrasonography may improve outcomes in patients with refractory gastroparesis but at this time it cannot be recommended as a treatment approach (Gilsdorf et al. 2017).

Role of Feeding/Venting Tubes

Up to 30% of patients are refractory to pharmacological therapy and require hospitalizations (Syed et al. 2005). Endoscopic therapy or surgical procedures for establishing a feeding jejunostomy may be required where weight loss, nutrition, and hydration are major challenges. Feeding jejunostomy in upper GI motility disorders reduces hospitalization rate during the first year after placement by providing an access for efficient nutrition with enteral supplementation bypassing the non-emptying stomach (Colemont and Camilleri 1989). A nasogastric tube is placed to achieve gastric decompression in acute exacerbations but is only short term. A nasojejunal/duodenal tube maybe used for a trial of feedings prior to the placement of a jejunostomy for long-term feedings. The role of a venting gastrostomy tube is not recommended in "standard" gastroparesis but may be required in the setting of gastroparesis plus intestinal pseudo obstruction.

Gastric Electrical Stimulation

Open label study suggests that the gastric electrical stimulation (GES) therapy leads to improvement in symptoms in idiopathic, diabetic, and postsurgical gastroparesis (Familoni et al. 1997; McCallum et al. 1998; Abell et al. 2002; Forster et al. 2001; McCallum et al. 2011). The mechanism of symptom relief is through activation of afferent pathways controlling CNS centers for nausea and vomiting. Gastric emptying is generally unchanged. A single center study reported significant improvement in 43% of 151 patients in a 1.4 year mean follow-up (Heckert et al. 2016). Three clinical parameters have been shown to predict a favorable clinical response with GES: (1) diabetic and past gastric surgery or past vagotomy settings rather than idiopathic gastroparesis, (2) nausea/vomiting rather than abdominal pain as a primary symptom, and (3) independence from narcotic analgesics prior to stimulator implantation (Maranki et al. 2008). GES provides better symptom relief mainly in diabetic gastroparesis (Van der Voort et al. 2005). In the report of the most extensive series to date where patients were followed up to 10 years with GES and gastroparesis, many patients were in the 60–70 years age range and overall had a sustained response of about 50% symptomatic improvement with the Enterra neurostimulation device (McCallum et al. 2011). Complications included infection of the subcutaneous pocket and about 5% of patients over time, electrode dislodgment, electrode erosion into the stomach, and bowel obstruction from the wires (Anand et al. 2007; Abell et al. 2003).

Role of Pyloroplasty

Pyloroplasty is being utilized as an adjunct to GES or as a "stand alone." It improves gastric emptying and may provide symptomatic relief by more than 70%. No increase in morbidity has been reported with its concomitant use of stimulator and pyloroplasty. Good clinical outcomes have been reported with pyloroplasty alone (Davis et al. 2017). The technique improves gastric emptying and reduces symptoms such as bloating, nausea, and vomiting. Controversy exists if the combination of GES and pyloroplasty has better outcomes than the surgical technique by itself. Endoscopic pyloromyotomy is a recent alternative for laparoscopic pyloroplasty; two prospective studies utilizing the "gastric per-oral endoscopic pyloromyotomy" reported clinical improvement in more than 70% of the patients with idiopathic, diabetic, and postsurgical gastroparesis. In both studies, there was a significant improvement of gastric emptying (Davis et al. 2017). The improved surgical and endoscopic techniques are providing alternative options for patients with refractory gastroparesis.

Chronic Constipation and Gastric Emptying

Gastroparesis in the setting of chronic constipation is a result of a reflex gastric tone inhibition by colonic distension. Abnormalities in gastric emptying studies may arise secondary to chronic constipation. Decreased colonic motility is not a natural physiologic result of aging. The high prevalence of chronic constipation in the older adult population is due to multiple factors such as decreased ambulation, polypharmacy, comorbidities, and decreased water and fiber intake (Shahid et al. 2012; Zikos et al. 2019). Treatment should be multimodal, include diet and lifestyle modifications, and an individualize approach to each patient. The improvement of colonic motility in the elderly population indirectly improves the gastric emptying (Shahid et al. 2012; Zikos et al. 2019).

Table 6 summarizes a practical approach to gastroparesis management in older adults.

Key Points

- The gut ages well and in most cases gastric motility is preserved.
- Gastroparesis is a motor disorder of the stomach with a myriad of clinical manifestations and specific etiologies related to the geriatric setting.
- The "gold standard" for diagnosis is confirmation of delayed GE, defined as >10% retention, on a standardized 4-h scintigraphic test utilizing a low-fat (2%) eggbeater meal, after careful exclusion of mechanical obstruction.
- Medication induced effects on gastric motility must always be a consideration.
- Treatment involves combinations of antiemetics and prokinetics cautiously selected to minimize likelihood of adverse events.

- Chronic constipation should be addressed because it can sabotage attempts to improve gastric emptying.
- The combination of gastric electrical stimulation and pyloroplasty is the current "gold" standard for treating gastroparesis not responding to all medical measures.

References

Abell TL, Van Cutsem E, Abrahamsson H, et al. Gastric electrical stimulation in intractable symptomatic gastroparesis. Digestion. 2002;66:204–12.

Abell T, McCallum RW, Hocking M, et al. Gastric electrical stimulation for medically refractory gastroparesis. Gastroenterology. 2003;125:421–8.

Abell TL, Camilleri M, Donohoe K, et al. Consensus recommendations for gastric emptying scintigraphy: a joint report of the American Neurogastroenterology and Motility Society and Society of Nuclear Medicine. Am J Gastroenterol. 2008;103:753–63.

Ahluwalia NK, Thompson DG, Barlow J. Effect of distension and feeding on phasic changes in human proximal gastric tone. Gut. 1996;39:757–61.

Anand C, Al- Juburi A, Familoni B, et al. Gastric electric stimulation is safe and effective: a long-term study in patients with refractory gastroparesis in three reginal centers. Digestion. 2007;75:83–9.

Arts J, Holvoet L, Caenepeel P, et al. Clinical trial: a randomized-controlled crossover study of intrapyloric injection of botulinum toxin in gastroparesis. Aliment Pharmacol Ther. 2007;26:1251–8.

Bizer E, Harrell S, Koopman J, et al. Obesity is common in gastroparesis despite nausea, vomiting, and early satiety. Gastroenterology. 2005;128:M1895.

Bouras EP, Talley NJ, Camilleri M, et al. Effects of amitriptyline on gastric sensorimotor function and postprandial symptoms in healthy individuals: a randomized, double-blind, placebo-controlled trial. Am J Gastroenterol. 2008;103:2043.

Camilleri M. Integrated upper gastro-intestinal response to food intake. Gastroenterology. 2006;131:640–58.

Camilleri M, Parkman HP, Shafi MA, et al. Clinical guideline: management of gastroparesis. Am J Gastroenterol. 2013;108:18.

Carmel R, Aurangzeb I, Qian D. Associations of food-cobalamin malabsorption with ethnic origin, age, Helicobacter pylori infection, and serum markers of gastritis. Am J Gastroenterol. 2001;96:63–70.

Clarkston WK, Pantano MM, Morley JE, et al. Predictors of gastric emptying in Parkinson's disease. Neurogastroenterol Motil. 2006;18:369–75.

Colemont LJ, Camilleri M. Chronic intestinal pseudo-obstruction: diagnosis and treatment. Mayo Clin Proc. 1989;64:60–70.

Davis BR, Sarosiek I, Bashashati M, et al. The long-term efficacy and safety of pyloroplasty combined with gastric electrical stimulation therapy in gastroparesis. J Gastrointest Surg. 2017;21(2):222–7.

De Giorgio R, Guerrini S, Barbara G, et al. Inflammatory neruopathies of the enteric nervous system. Gastroenterology. 2004;126(7):1872–83.

Delegado-Aros S, Camilleri M, Cremonnini F, et al. Contributions of gastric volumes and gastric emptying to meal size and post meal symptoms in functional dyspepsia. Gastroenterology. 2004;127(6):1685–94.

Dumitrascu DL, Barnet J, Kirschner T, et al. Antral emptying of semisolid meal measured by real-time ultrasonography in chronic renal failure. Dig Dis Sci. 1995;40:636–44.

Ebert EC. The thyroid and the gut. J Clin Gastroenterol. 2010;44(6):402–6.

Evans MA, Triggs EJ, Cheung M, et al. Gastric emptying rate in the elderly: implications for drug therapy. J Am Geriatr Soc. 1981;29(5):201–5.

Familoni BO, Abell TL, Voeller G, et al. Electrical stimulation at a frequency higher than basal rate in human stomach. Dig Dis Sci. 1997;42:885–91.

Forster J, Sarosiek I, Delcore R, et al. Gastric pacing is a new surgical treatment for gastroparesis. Am J Surg. 2001;182:676–81.

Freiedenberg FK, Palit A, Parkman HP, Hanlon A, Nelson D. Botulinum toxin A for the treatment of delayed gastric emptying. Am J Gastroenterol. 2008;103:416–23.

Gilsdorf D, Volckmann E, Brickley A, et al. Pyloroplasty offers relief of postfundoplication gastroparesis in patients who improved after botulinum toxin injection. J Laparoendosc Adv Surg Tech A. 2017;27(11):1180–4.

Giron MS, Wang HX, Bernsten C, et al. The appropriateness of drug use in an older non-demented and demented population. J Am Geriatr Soc. 2001;49:277–83.

Goetze O, Nikodem AB, Weizcorek J, et al. Predictors of gastric emptying in Parkinson's disease. Neurogastroenterol Motil. 2006;18:369–75.

Halvorsen L, Dotevall G, Walan A. Gastric emptying in patients with achlorhydia or hyposecretion of hydrochloric acid. Scand J Gastroenterol. 1973;8(5):395–9.

Hasler WL. Gastroparesis: symptoms, evaluation and treatment. Gastroenterol Clin N Am. 2007;36(3):619–47.

Hasler WL, Soudah HC, Dulai G, et al. Mediation of hyperglycemia-evoked gastric slow-wave dysrhythmias by endogenous prostaglandins. Gastroenterology. 1995;108(3):727–36.

Heckert J, Sankineni A, Hughes WB, et al. Gastric electric stimulation for refractory gastroparesis: a prospective analysis of 151 patients at a single center. Dig Dis Sci. 2016;61(1):168–75.

Hejazi RA, Zhang D, McCallum RW. Gastroparesis, pseudoachalasia and impaired intestinal motility as paraneoplastic manifestations of small cell lung cancer. Am J Med Sci. 2009;338(1):69–71.

Hinder RA, Kelly K. Human gastric pacesetter potential. Site of origin, spread, and response to gastric transection and proximal gastric vagotomy. Am J Surg. 1977;133:29–33.

Hirst GD, Edwards FR. Role of interstitial cells of Cajal in the control of gastric motility. J Pharmacol Sci. 2004;96:1–10.

Horowitz M, Maddern GJ, Chatterton BE, et al. Changes in gastric emptying rates with age. Clin Sci (Lond). 1984;67(2):213–8.

Hunt JN, Pathk JD. The osmotic effects of some simple molecules and ions on gastric emptying. J Physiol. 1960;154:254–69.

Jehangir A, Parkman HP. Chronic opioids in gastroparesis: relationship with gastrointestinal symptoms, healthcare utilization and employment. World J Gastroenterol. 2017;23(40):7310–20.

Jung HK, Choung RS, Locke GR III, et al. The incidence, prevalence, and outcomes of patients with gastroparesis in Olmsted County, Minnesota, from 1996 to 2006. Gastroenterology. 2009;136:1225–33.

Krishna AY, report BLSJC. reversible gastroparesis inn patients with hypopituitary disease. Am J Med Sci. 1996;312(1):43–5.

Kuo P, Rayner CK, Horowitz M. Gastric emptying, diabetes and aging. Clin Geriatr Med. 2007;23: 785–808.

Kupfer RM, Heppell M, Haggith JW, et al. Gastric emptying and small-bowel transit rate in the elderly. J Am Geriatr Soc. 1985;33(5):340–3.

Lee AA, Rao S, Nguyen LA, et al. Validation of diagnostic and performance characteristics of the wireless motility capsule in patients with suspected gastroparesis. Clin Gastroenterol Hepatol. 2018. pii: S1543-3565(18) 31381-8.

Lindeman RD. Overview: renal physiology and pathophysiology of aging. Am J Kidney Dis. 1990;16:275–82.

Linnebjerg H, Park S, Kothare PA, et al. Effect of exenatide on gastric emptying and relationship to postprandial glycemia in type 2 diabetes. Regul Pept. 2008;151:123.

Lucchinetti CF, Kimmel DW, Lennon VA. Paraneoplastic and oncologic profiles of patients seropositive for type 1 antineuronal nuclear autoantibodies. Neurology. 1998;50:652–7.

Madsen JL, Graff J. Effects of ageing on gastrointestinal motor function. Age Ageing. 2004;33(2):154–9.

Maranki JL, Lytes V, Meilahn JE, et al. Predictive factors for clinical improvement with Enterra gastric electric stimulation treatment for refractory gastroparesis. Dig Dis Sci. 2008;53(8):2072–8.

Mauer AH, Krevsky B, Knight LC, et al. Opioid and opioid like drug effects on whole-gut transit measured by scintigraphy. J Nucl Med. 1996;37(5):818–22.

McCallum RW. Motor function of stomach in health and disease. In: Sleisenger MH, Fordtran JS, editors. Gastrointestinal disease: pathophysiololgy, diagnosis, management, vol. 1. 4th ed. Philadephia: Saunders; 1989. p. 675–713.

McCallum RW, Ricci DA, Rakatansky H, et al. A multi-center placebo controlled clinical trial of oral metoclopramide in diabetic gastroparesis. Diabetes Care. 1983;6:463–7.

McCallum RW, Chen JD, Lin Z, et al. Gastric pacing improves emptying and symptoms in patients with gastroparesis. Gastroenterology. 1998;114:456–61.

McCallum RW, Lin Z, Forster J, et al. Gastric electrical stimulation improves outcomes in patients with gastroparesis for up to 10 years. Clin Gastroenterol Hepatol. 2011;9:314–9.

Menke DM, Kyle RA, Fleming CR, et al. Symptomatic gastric amyloidosis in patients with primary systemic amyloidosis. Mayo Clin Proc. 1993;68:763–7.

Meyer JH, Ohashi H, Jehn D, Thomson JB. Size of liver particles emptied from the human stomach. Gastroenterology. 1981;80:1489–96.

Minami H, McCallum RW. The physiology and pathophysiology of gastric emptying in humans. Gastroenterology. 1984;86(6):1592–610.

Mizumoto A, Monchiki E, Suzuki H, Tanaka T, Itoh Z. Neuronal control of motility changes in the canine lower esophageal sphincter and stomach in response to meal ingestion. J Smooth Muscle Res. 1997;33:211–22.

Morgan KG, Szurszewski JH. Mechanisms of phasic and tonic actions of pentagastrin on canine gastric smooth muscle. J Physiol. 1980;30:229–42.

Myint AS, Rieders B, Tashkandi M, et al. Current and emerging therapeutic options for gastroparesis. Gastroenterol Hepatol (N Y). 2018;14(11):639–45.

O'Mahony D, O'Leary P, Quigley EMM. Aging and intestinal motility a review of factors that affect intestinal motility in the aged. Drugs Aging. 2002;19(7):515–27.

Park MI, Camilleri M. Gastroparesis: clinical update. Am J Gastroenterol. 2006;101:1129–39.

Parkman HP, Hasler WL, Fisher RS. American Gastroenterological Association technical review on the diagnosis and treatment of gastroparesis. Gastroenterology. 2004;127:1592–622.

Parkman HP, Camilleri M, Farrugia G, et al. Gastroparesis and functional dyspepsia: excerpts from the AGA/ANMS meeting. Neurogastroenterol Motil. 2010;22:113–33.

Parrish CR. Nutrition concerns for the patient with gastroparesis. Curr Gastroenterol Rep. 2007;9:295–302.

Pasricha PJ, Pehlivanov A, Sugumar A, et al. Drug insight: from disturbed motility to disordered movement – a review of the clinical benefits and medicolegal risks of metoclopramide. Nat Clin Pract Gastroenterol Hepatol. 2006;3:138–48.

Patterson D, Abell T, Rothstein R, et al. A double-blind multicenter comparison of domperidone and metoclopramide in the treatment of diabetic patients with symptoms of gastroparesis. Am J Gastroenterol. 1999;94:1230–4.

Quigley EMM. Gastric motility and sensation in health and disease. In: Feldman M, Friedman L, Sleisenger M, editors. Sleisenger and Fortran's gastrointestinal and liver disease. 14th ed. New York: Mosby; 2002.

Rayner CK, MacIntosh CG, Chapman IM, et al. Effects of age on proximal gastric motor and sensory function. Scand J Gastroenterol. 2000;35(10):1041–7.

Reddymasu SC, McCallum RW. Pharmacotherapy of gastroparesis. Expert Opin Pharmacother. 2009;10(3):469–84.

Reddymasu SC, McCallum RW. Small intestinal bacterial overgrowth in gastroparesis: are there any predictors? J Clin Gastroenterol. 2010;44:e8–13.

Sanders MK. Bezoars: from mystical charms to medical and nutritional management. Pract Gastroenterol. 2004; XXVIII:37.

Shahid S, Ramzan Z, Maurer AH, et al. Chronic idiopathic constipation: more than a simple colonic transit disorder. J Clin Gastroenterol. 2012;46(2):150–4.

Smith BD, Smith GL, Hurria A, et al. Future of cancer incidence in the United States: burdens upon an aging, changing nation. J Clin Oncol. 2009; 27:2758–65.

Soykan I, Sivri B, Sarosiek I, et al. Demography, clinical characteristics, psychological and abuse profiles, treatment, and long-term follow-up of patients with gastroparesis. Dig Dis Sci. 1998; 43:2398–404.

Syed AA, Rattansingh A, Furtado SD. Current perspectives on management of gastroparesis. J Postgrad Med. 2005;51:54–60.

Talley NJ, Locke GR III, Lahr BD, et al. Functional dyspepsia, delayed gastric emptying, and impaired quality of life. Gut. 2006;55:933–9.

Tougas G, Eaker EY, Abell TL, et al. Assessment of gastric emptying using a low fat meal: establishment of international control values. Am J Gastroenterol. 2000;95:1496–62.

Van der Voort IR, Becker JC, Dietl KH, et al. Gastric electrical stimulation results in improved metabolic control in diabetic patients suffering from gastroparesis. Exp Clin Endocrinol Diabetes. 2005; 113(1):38–42.

Veevers AE, Oxberry SG. Ranitidine: forgotten drug of delayed gastric emptying. BMJ Support Palliat Care. 2017;7(3):255–7.

Wang YR, Fisher RS, Parkman HP. Gastroparesis-related hospitalizations in the United States: trends, characteristics, and outcomes, 1995–2004. Am J Gastroenterol. 2007;103:313–22.

Weston S, Thumshirn M, Wiste J, Camilleri M. Clinical and upper gastrointestinal motility features in systemic sclerosis and related disorders. Am J Gastroenterol. 1998;93:1085.

Whitson BA, Kandaswamy R, Sutherland DER. Diabetic gastroparesis associated bezoar resolution via colalysis. Clin Transpl. 2008;22:242–4.

Zikos TA, Kamal AN, Neshatian L, et al. High prevalence of slow transit constipation in patients with gastroparesis. Neurogastroenterol Motil. 2019; 25(2):267–75.

Gastroesophageal Reflux Disease and Complications

49

Adharsh Ravindran and Prasad G. Iyer

Contents

A. Ravindran
Department of Internal Medicine, University at Buffalo,
Buffalo, NY, USA
e-mail: Ravindran.adharsh@gmail.com

P. G. Iyer (✉)
Division of Gastroenterology and Hepatology, Mayo
Clinic, Rochester, MN, USA
e-mail: iyer.prasad@mayo.edu

© Springer Nature Switzerland AG 2021
C. S. Pitchumoni, T. S. Dharmarajan (eds.), *Geriatric Gastroenterology*,
https://doi.org/10.1007/978-3-030-30192-7_42

Abstract

Gastroesophageal reflux disease (GERD) and its complications such as esophagitis, Barrett's esophagus, and esophageal adenocarcinoma are more prevalent in the elderly compared to the young. This is likely due to the higher prevalence of risk factors and hyposensitivity to symptoms in this age group, which makes diagnosis and treatment more challenging. In this chapter we focus on the epidemiology, etiopathogenesis, diagnosis, and management (medical and surgical) of GERD and its complications in the elderly. Diagnosis of GERD is made by a combination of clinical features (identification of risk factors and esophageal and extraesophageal symptoms) and investigations (such as ambulatory pH monitoring and endoscopy). The mainstay of treatment is a combination of lifestyle modifications and medications (predominantly proton pump inhibitors and histamine receptor antagonists). Surgery is usually reserved for those with refractory symptoms and complications not responding to medications. We also address some of the current misconceptions on the adverse effects attributed to proton pump inhibitors in the literature and provide recommendations on their appropriate and judicious use.

Keywords

Reflux · Heartburn · Regurgitation · Proton pump inhibitors · Barrett's esophagus · Esophageal adenocarcinoma · Ambulatory pH monitoring · Complications

Introduction

Gastroesophageal reflux disease (GERD) is defined as a condition that develops when the reflux of stomach contents causes troublesome symptoms and/or complications (Vakil et al. 2006). It is a condition that is fairly common among people of all ages, races, and genders. Older adults appear to be at a higher risk of morbidity from GERD due to the additional comorbidities and risk factors that play a role in the development and progression of the disease. GERD is a multifactorial disorder that can have diverse clinical presentations and complications of varying severity. The recognition of this condition in older adults warrants early diagnosis and treatment to prevent progression of the disease into precancerous and cancerous conditions like esophagitis, Barrett's esophagus, and esophageal adenocarcinoma (EAC). Elderly patients are also at risk of developing extraesophageal complications with chronic GERD. Additionally, medical treatment of GERD with proton pump inhibitors (PPI) and histamine-2-receptor antagonists (H2RAs) is more cost-effective compared to nonmedical management options for manifestations of GERD. However, it is also important to recognize that over or inappropriate use of these medications in the old is prevalent. Hence, understanding the nature and severity of GERD and personalizing the management of this condition in each individual are critical.

Epidemiology

GERD symptoms are highly prevalent in the general population worldwide (Table 1). Population studies have shown that one out of five individuals experience heartburn or acid regurgitation on a weekly basis and two out of five experience heartburn or acid regurgitation at least once a month (Locke et al. 1997). The prevalence of GERD worldwide appears to be increasing with higher rates in the Americas and Europe. A population-based study reported an overall increase in prevalence of reflux symptoms from 10–20% in 2005 to 18–27% in 2014 in North America (El-Serag et al. 2014). Factors such as obesity, eradication of

Table 1 GERD prevalence estimates in global population (El-Serag et al. 2014)

Geographical area	Prevalence rates
North America	18–28%
South America	23%
Europe	9–26%
Middle East	9–33%
Australia	12%
East Asia	3–8%

H. pylori infection, and other lifestyle and genetic factors could be related to this rise in prevalence. Several large population studies have demonstrated that there is no significant increase in GERD symptoms with age; despite that, the prevalence of esophagitis is significantly higher in older compared to younger subjects (Pilotto et al. 2006). However, the actual prevalence of GERD in the elderly is probably higher given the low perception of symptoms and manifestations in this population. Epidemiologic data consistently support the view that as people age, the severity of reflux esophagitis increases, whereas symptoms are attenuated and become less typical (Becher and Dent 2011). Indeed, a large epidemiological study from the USA reported that age was an important risk factor for the development of severe forms of GERD, in addition to male gender, white ethnicity, and hiatus hernia (Johnson and Fennerty 2004).

Etiopathogenesis of GERD

Reflux in the general population is not always pathologic (Crookes 2006). Physiologic reflux can occur immediately after consumption of food or can occur at night. This is usually asymptomatic and brief and resolves on its own without need for medical management. Pathologic reflux is usually symptomatic, commonly presenting with acid reflux or heartburn symptoms with or without endoscopic evidence of esophageal mucosal inflammation. The factors that influence progression from physiologic reflex GERD include imbalances between acid production, acid clearance, and mucosal defense in the esophagus (Boeckxstaens et al. 2014).

Acid Production

Although reducing the gastric acidity is the mainstay of management in GERD, it is rarely associated with increased acid production. More often than not, development of GERD is multifactorial except in conditions like Zollinger-Ellison syndrome (Moore et al. 2013), atrophic gastritis with hypergastrinemia (Phan et al. 2015; Dacha et al. 2015), and *H. pylori* infection (Phan et al. 2015; Dacha et al. 2015) where the pathogenesis is primarily from acid hypersecretion. In addition to increased acid levels, the acidity of the secretions is also associated with gastric and esophageal mucosal injury (Goldberg et al. 1970). Gastric secretions with pH less than 4 have been associated with mucosal damage that can cause GERD and peptic ulcer disease (PUD) (Hunt 1999). Presence of enzymes like pepsin and trypsin and bile acids in the refluxate can also potentiate symptomatic GERD and esophagitis even at normal acid levels (Powell 1981).

Acid Clearance

Acid in the esophagus as a result of normal physiologic reflux is normally cleared by a combination of peristalsis and alkaline saliva. Peristalsis pushes acid into the stomach, while ingested saliva mixes and neutralizes the remaining acid. Hence, impaired peristalsis or reduced salivation can lead to an increase in the duration of acid exposure in the esophagus, increasing the risk of mucosal injury.

Impaired Peristalsis

Impaired peristalsis could be related to ineffective emptying of acid into the stomach or reflux of gastric contents back into the esophagus. This is commonly seen in patients with low lower esophageal sphincter (LES) pressure. LES pressure is lower in older adults, which in turn can lead to increased esophageal acid exposure and incomplete acid clearance (Kahrilas et al. 1988; Lee et al. 2007).

Impaired esophageal body peristalsis as seen in achalasia can also present with symptoms of heartburn and GERD. Achalasia is more common in the older age group with a mean age at diagnosis of 50 years; further, incidence increases with age (Wadhwa et al. 2017). Hiatal hernias, more common in the elderly over the age of 65, are associated with increased retrograde acid flow due to anatomic shortening of esophagus with swallowing. This further leads to increase in frequency and duration of esophageal acid exposure, thereby causing GERD (Kishikawa et al. 2017). Interestingly, a recent study from Japan revealed that increased gastric acid secretion, with or without symptomatic GERD, independently induced development of hiatal hernias. The exactly pathophysiology is poorly understood, but it is likely related to recurrent inflammation and healing occurring with acid exposure causing acid-induced esophageal shortening which promotes proximal herniation of the stomach into the thorax (Kishikawa et al. 2017).

Salivary Hyposecretion or Dysfunction

Saliva, with a normal alkaline pH between 6.3 and 7.6 (Baliga et al. 2013), is a natural buffer for refluxed gastric acid when it is swallowed. Patients with chronic xerostomia have been shown to experience increased acid exposure to the esophageal mucosa due to ineffective buffering of refluxed gastric acid, compared to those with intact saliva production (Korsten et al. 1991).

The rate and composition of salivary secretion have been studied to show an age-related decline. This age-related salivary dysfunction places older people at risk for xerostomia-related adverse effects (Dodds et al. 2005). In smokers, one of the mechanisms is related to salivary hyposecretion and dysfunction that lead to xerostomia and, hence, a delayed clearance of refluxed gastric acid. In addition, saliva in smokers has lower levels of titratable base than non-smokers, which leads to ineffective neutralization of acid (Petrusic et al. 2015).

Mucosal Defense

The esophageal mucous layer acts as an epithelial barrier against the harmful effects of acid. Integrity of this layer is important in the development of GERD. Several factors can influence integrity of the mucosal barrier such as age, lifestyle, nutritional status, medications, and pre-existing injuries from instrumentation. Any break in the continuity of this barrier exposes the esophagus to corrosive effects of acid which in turn can result in GERD, esophagitis, ulceration, or rarely perforation.

Increased Intra-Abdominal Pressure

An increase in the intra-abdominal pressure can cause elevated intragastric pressure. This further leads to increase in gastroesophageal reflux to incorporate the pressure gradient. Obesity has been studied to have a strong association with GERD due to a mechanical rise in intra-abdominal pressure. The prevalence of obesity among the elderly has been steadily rising. Data from CDC showed that more than one-third of adults over 65 years of age were obese between 2007 and 2010 with the prevalence being higher between 65 and 74 years (Fakhouri et al. 2012). Obesity is also associated with an increased risk of developing hiatal hernia which in turn can result in acid reflux and heartburn. Drugs and lifestyle are important risk factors for development of GERD. Alcohol, smoking, and certain foods (fatty food, citrus fruits, spicy food, caffeine, carbonated drinks, and chocolate) have strong association with GERD (Table 3).

Table 3 contains a list of commonly used medications that are associated with GERD.

Clinical Features

Reflux or regurgitation and heartburn are the most common presentations of GERD. But patients with GERD need not necessarily have one of these symptoms. Some may not have any symptoms of GERD but can have endoscopic evidence of erosive esophagitis. This is more common in the elderly due to their relative hyposensitivity to perceiving acid reflux.

Heartburn is defined as a burning sensation in the anterior chest (substernal or retrosternal). It usually begins behind the sternum and radiates upward to the throat and neck. This is one of the most common presentations of GERD in all age groups especially in the elderly with comorbidities and polypharmacy (Vallot et al. 2011; Moshkowitz et al. 2011; Furuta et al. 2012). Heartburn is commonly experienced in the postprandial period but can be experienced during sleep or rest also in older subjects.

Regurgitation is the reflux of gastric contents including acid and undigested or partially digested food through the esophagus into the mouth and characterized as a bitter or sour tasting fluid. This is more common in people with low LES tone and obesity due to the mechanical effects of intra-abdominal pressure that can increase the tendency for upward flow from the stomach.

In patients with chronic GERD, the acidic content can eventually damage the esophageal barrier and lead to erosive esophagitis. Recurrent esophagitis can cause strictures, presenting as dysphagia to solid foods with food getting stuck in the lower esophagus. The evidence is unclear with regard to the presence of typical and atypical GERD symptoms between the elderly and non-elderly population as many other factors are involved in the pathogenesis and progression of GERD, such as presence of mucosal breaks and degree of esophagitis (Furuta et al. 2012).

Not all patients with symptomatic GERD will present with acid reflux and heartburn. Some of the atypical presentations of GERD in the old are non-cardiac or atypical chest pain that may mimic angina, asthma, dysphagia, globus sensation in the throat, chronic cough, laryngitis (hoarseness), dental erosions, and recurrent pulmonary aspiration (Vakil et al. 2006; Raiha et al. 1992).

Complications

Although GERD is a common condition in all ages, diagnosis and timely management are imperative in preventing its progression to complications. The complications could be due to the local progression of mucosal injury (esophageal) or due to systemic effects from worsening reflux (extraesophageal).

Esophageal Complications

Esophageal complications occur as a series of events that unfold from untreated and worsening reflux.

– Erosive esophagitis: The esophageal mucosa is injured with repeated or long-term exposure to the acidic refluxate. The mucosa eventually develops inflammation as cytokines and other inflammatory factors are released, resulting in erosive esophagitis. Some of these patients may not have symptoms of GERD (Lee et al. 2015). Erosive esophagitis is an endoscopic diagnosis, and the severity is proportional to the extent of mucosal injury, compliance to medical treatment, and pre-existing mucosal defects (Table 5). Figure 1 shows mucosal erosions in erosive esophagitis. A subset of patients may present with chronic regurgitation or heartburn symptoms without endoscopic evidence of esophagitis but may have histologic evidence of esophageal injury characterized by basal cell hyperplasia. This condition is termed non-erosive reflux disease (NERD) (Dellon et al. 2014).

– Esophageal strictures: As a consequence of erosive esophagitis-related damage and healing in the setting of chronic GERD, the esophageal mucosa can undergo morphologic and histologic changes leading to the formation of strictures in the distal esophagus. Repetitive damage and healing initiates fibrin and collagen deposition that further leads to fibrosis and scar formation. This distal scarring results in shortening of the length of the esophagus and narrowing of the lumen. Strictures may be seen in the elderly from chronic inflammation over the years. Management of strictures requires mechanical dilation of the lumen along with acid suppressive therapy to prevent recurrence (Ravich 2017; Adler and Siddiqui 2017). Esophageal strictures can also occur in patients undergoing endoscopic management for esophageal varices, Barrett's esophagus, or early-stage esophageal adenocarcinoma (EAC) which usually involves tissue coagulation using bipolar cautery, sclerotherapy, band

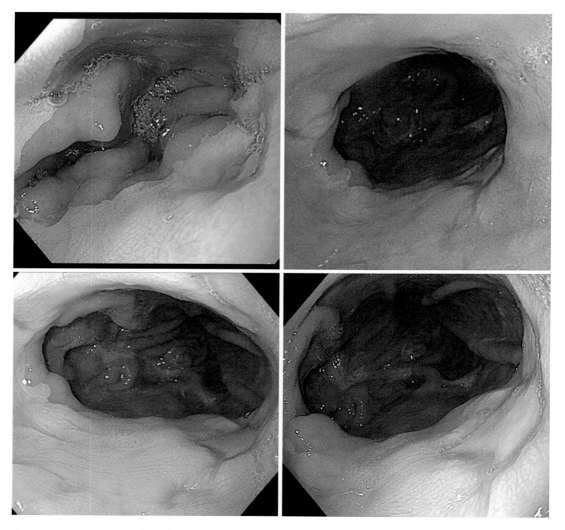

Fig. 1 Endoscopic images of erosive esophagitis

ligation, or radiofrequency ablation (Reilly et al. 1984; Stier et al. 2016).

– Barrett's esophagus: The esophagus is normally lined by stratified squamous epithelium that provides adequate protection from acid injury. The gastric mucosa is lined by columnar epithelium that helps with the secretory activities of the stomach. The site of transition from esophageal squamous to gastric columnar cells is termed the squamocolumnar junction (SCJ). In patients with chronic GERD, the repetitive irritation of esophageal squamous epithelium at the GEJ can lead to metaplastic change at the lower

esophagus to columnar epithelium. This columnar epithelial metaplasia in the distal esophagus with intestinal metaplasia on histology is called Barrett's esophagus, a disorder associated with an increased risk of progression to EAC. Barrett's esophagus progresses to EAC via the development of dysplasia (low grade and high grade). Hence screening for the detection of BE and endoscopic surveillance for the detection of dysplasia are recommended. If dysplasia is detected on histology, endoscopic ablation is recommended to reduce the risk of progression to EAC (Shaheen et al. 2016).

– Esophageal adenocarcinoma: Incidence of EAC has been rising steadily in Western countries with strong predominance in Caucasian males. Risk factors like smoking, older age, central obesity, and Barrett's esophagus that are commonly associated with chronic GERD have been associated with a higher risk of progression to EAC (Rubenstein et al. 2011). Early-stage EAC can be successfully treated endoscopically.

Extraesophageal Complications

GERD has been associated with many extra-esophageal complications in the elderly. This is common due to the synergism between GERD and coexisting comorbidities that pose higher risk in the geriatric population. In patients with asthma, untreated GERD may trigger asthma exacerbations. The mechanism for these triggers could be related to bronchoconstriction from increased vagal tone with acid exposure, airway hyper-reactivity, and micro-aspiration of gastric refluxate. Treatment of GERD symptoms in asthmatic patients may lower exacerbation rates (Field and Sutherland 1998).

One of the very common atypical presentations of GERD in older adults is non-cardiac chest pain or pseudoangina. It can appear as a retrosternal, mid-sternal, or epigastric pain or tightness which mimics angina. In geriatric patients with comorbidities and risk factors for cardiac disease, it is important to rule out acute coronary syndrome (ACS) with EKG and serial troponins before the symptoms can safely be attributed to GERD (Barboi et al. 2016).

Other less common extraesophageal complications are chronic laryngitis, laryngeal stenosis, chronic cough, bronchitis, and aspiration pneumonia. Furthermore, in bedridden patients and patients under palliative care, the risk of developing pulmonary complications such as recurrent aspiration is higher due to underlying swallowing impairment, esophageal dysphagia, loss of esophageal peristalsis, and impaired LES contraction (Palmer et al. 2000) (Table 2).

GERD has been shown to have a strong association with sleep disorders. A high prevalence of symptomatic GERD was noticed in patients with

Table 2 Complications of gastroesophageal reflux disease (Chait 2010)

Esophageal	Erosive esophagitis
	Esophageal stricture
	Barrett's esophagus
	Esophageal adenocarcinoma
Extraesophageal	Atypical non-cardiac chest pain
	Globus sensation
	Pharyngitis
	Sinusitis
	Dental erosions
	Hoarseness
	Laryngitis
	Vocal cord granulomas
	Subglottic stenosis
	Laryngeal cancer
	Chronic cough
	Asthma
	Pulmonary fibrosis
	Aspiration pneumonia

Table 3 List of commonly used medications that may be associated with GERD

Decrease LES pressure	Directly injure esophageal mucosa	Delay gastric emptying
Anticholinergics	Antiretroviral agents	Anticholinergics
Barbiturates	Ascorbic acid	Calcium channel blocker
Benzodiazepines	Aspirin	Clonidine
Beta-agonists	Bisphosphonates	Dopamine agonists
Caffeine	Doxycycline	Lithium
Calcium channel blockers	Ferrous sulfate	Narcotics
Dopamine	Phenytoin	Nicotine
Ethanol	Potassium chloride	Progesterone
Estrogen	Propranolol	
Nitrates	NSAIDs	
Progesterone	Tetracycline	
Theophylline	Trimethoprim–sulfamethoxazole	
	Quinidine	

severe obstructive sleep apnea (OSA). Although obesity is a confounding factor and could be a major contributor to both GERD and OSA, treatment of OSA with CPAP has shown to be beneficial for OSA and GERD symptoms in some patient populations (Green et al. 2003; Shaker and Magdy 2016). Symptomatic GERD is also known to cause conscious and unconscious arousals at night that leads to poor quality of sleep and disruptive sleep patterns. This nocturnal increase in GERD intensity is likely due to the increased acid exposure time at night. However, good sleep quality with minimal disruptions has also been studied to relieve GERD symptoms. In a study involving patients with erosive esophagitis, patients had a significant decrease in lag time to onset of symptoms and an overall increase in intensity rating during sleep-deprived nights as compared to the nights with good sleep (Jung et al. 2010; Schey et al. 2007).

Diagnosis

GERD is usually diagnosed based on clinical presentation with typical symptoms of acid reflux or heartburn. Sometimes patients can present with atypical symptoms like chronic cough, atypical non-cardiac chest pain, globus sensation, or nocturnal wheezing. In such cases, it is imperative to rule out other conditions that could be causing these symptoms before a diagnosis of GERD can be established. In some patients, GERD can present as chest pain indistinguishable from the pain of angina. In such cases, complete cardiac workup should be performed, particularly in those with cardiovascular risk factors. An upper gastrointestinal endoscopy is not always needed to diagnose GERD (particularly in the presence of typical symptoms); however, it may be needed in patients with suspected complications of GERD like esophagitis, Barrett's esophagus, and EAC. In patients with chronic GERD refractory to PPI therapy, upper GI endoscopy with biopsy can be considered to rule out alternate diagnoses such as eosinophilic esophagitis and achalasia. Eosinophilic esophagitis (EE), an inflammatory condition of the esophagus caused by eosinophilic infiltration of the esophageal mucosa, can also present with GERD-like symptoms. EE has a bimodal incidence with high incidence in adults and elderly (Trifan et al. 2016).

Gastroenterologists and geriatricians should have high suspicion of EE in adults and elderly presenting with chronic persistent heartburn and dysphagia refractory to PPI use. Endoscopic examination and biopsies are essential in these patients to diagnose EE.

An endoscopic examination is also mandatory in patients with chronic GERD who develop alarm symptoms such as gastrointestinal bleeding, anemia dysphagia, odynophagia, and weight loss. It is also essential to first exclude cardiac causes of chest discomfort before considering GERD as the diagnosis.

Ambulatory pH monitoring which involves the placement of a pH sensor in the distal esophagus to measure the intra-esophageal pH over 24–48 h may be needed to confirm the diagnosis of GERD in those with a negative endoscopic exam or those not responding to a therapeutic trial with PPIs. Ambulatory pH monitoring also allows the correlation of symptoms experienced by the patient with intra-esophageal pH. This can be done in two ways: first, placing the sensor transnasally with a thin tube containing a sensor 5 cm proximal to the lower esophageal sphincter, which is retained for 24 h, or, second, deploying the sensor endoscopically and retaining for 48–96 h (Bravo pH monitoring) (Ang et al. 2010). The test can be performed on or off medications to answer appropriate questions: off medications, does the patient have GERD, and on medications, do the patient's symptoms on medications correlate with persistent uncontrolled reflux?

Management

Lifestyle Management

The goals of treatment of GERD are essentially the same in all adults and include symptom relief, healing of erosive esophagitis, and prevention and management of complications. Lifestyle modification is an important first step in the management of GERD. Food-induced reflux and heartburn are one of the most important and reversible causes of GERD. Spicy foods have been known to increase risk of symptomatic GERD from direct irritation of esophageal mucosa. Capsaicin, a neurotoxin found in red pepper, has been shown to delay gastric emptying, thereby increasing the risk of reflux (Milke et al. 2006; Choe et al. 2017). Foods rich in fat may also increase esophageal acid exposure by delaying gastric emptying and increasing frequency of transient lower esophageal sphincter relaxation (tLESRs). Similarly, peppermint and chocolate may induce reflux symptoms by reducing the LES pressure. Beverages such as coffee, tea, soda, tomato, and citrus juice, which are either acidic or can stimulate gastric acid production, contribute to heartburn (Dore et al. 2008). Table 4 contains a list of commonly consumed beverages and their pH.

Table 4 Commonly consumed beverages and their pH (Reddy et al. 2016)

Drink	pH
Tap water	7.20
Milk	6.90
Dasani Regular	5.03
Vitamin Water Zero	3.10
Perrier Carbonated Mineral Water	5.25
Arizona Diet Green Tea	3.29
Starbucks Medium Roast	5.11
Lemon Juice	2.25
Canada Dry Club Soda	5.24
Canada Dry Ginger Ale	2.82
Rockstar Energy Drink	2.84
A&W Root Beer	4.27
Monster Energy	3.48
Coca-Cola	2.37
Pepsi	2.39
Red Bull	3.43
Gatorade Orange	2.99
Powerade Orange	2.73
Diet Coca-Cola	3.10
Coca-Cola Zero	2.96
Dr. Pepper	2.88
Ocean Spray Cranberry	2.56
Minute Maid Orange Juice	2.85
Minute Maid Lemonade	2.57
Tropicana 100% Apple Juice	3.50
Tropicana 100% Orange Juice	3.80
Tropicana Lemonade	2.70
Welch's 100% Grape Juice	3.38
V8 Vegetable Juice	4.23

Smoking has been shown to increase distal esophageal exposure time through the effect on the LES, while alcohol may precipitate GERD by increasing acid secretion, reducing LES pressure, increasing spontaneous LES relaxations, and impairing esophageal motility and gastric emptying (Festi et al. 2009).

However, a systemic review that evaluated the literature from 1975 to 2004 revealed no evidence supporting an improvement in GERD symptoms after cessation of smoking, alcohol, and other dietary interventions (Kaltenbach et al. 2006). In the same study, only reduction of excess weight and elevation of the head of the bed were shown to benefit patient symptoms, but neither prevented complications. Additionally ensuring a 3- to 4-h interval between the last meal of the day and bedtime is also helpful in helping with nocturnal symptoms, particularly regurgitation. A careful review of the patient's current medications, and where possible, avoidance of drugs known to worsen GERD, is also prudent (Table 3). Weight loss has also been shown to improve GERD symptoms and should be recommended. Body posture and positioning during sleep are one of the simple, yet important ways to reduce nocturnal GERD symptoms. Studies have shown improvement in nocturnal heartburn and reflux with keeping the head end elevated during sleep (Khan et al. 2012). A more recent study that tested body posture during sleep revealed that people who slept with their left side down had significantly lesser GERD symptoms than right. This difference is likely due to collection of gastric contents close to GE junction with right lateral position, thereby promoting reflux and GERD, whereas the gastric contents are collected in the dependent part of the stomach while lying on left lateral position (Person et al. 2015).

Antacids

Antacids are available over the counter and promptly act by neutralizing gastric acid. Simethicone is added to many formulations and provides an additional physical barrier to acid. These measures help self-treat mild, infrequent heartburn symptoms and provide rapid relief; however, they do not heal erosive esophagitis, nor prevent complications (Behar et al. 1975). Furthermore, antacids require frequent dosing and should be used with caution in older adults due to the potential risk of salt overload, calcinosis and calcium nephrolithiasis, constipation, diarrhea, and drug interactions. Alginate-antacid combinations have been widely used in management of reflux symptoms. They have also been proven to reduce the incidence of acid reflux episodes (Yuan et al. 2016). This can be used in combination with acid suppressive therapy in patients with GERD refractory to PPI monotherapy. Sucralfate, a commonly used agent in management of gastric and duodenal ulcers, has also shown to have benefit in GERD and reflux esophagitis by promoting tissue healing as a result of providing mucosal protection (Laitinen et al. 1985).

Histamine-2-Receptor Antagonists

Acid secretion by gastric parietal cells is stimulated by acetylcholine, histamine, and gastrin. Histamine-2-receptor antagonists (H2RAs) reduce acid secretion by competing for histamine receptors on parietal cells. They are more effective in controlling nocturnal as compared with meal-related acid secretion because the parietal cell is stimulated postprandially by gastrin and by acetylcholine (Lipsy et al. 1990). Compared to placebo, H2RAs significantly decreased heartburn, although symptoms are rarely abolished. The overall esophagitis healing rates with H2RAs rarely exceed 60% following 12 weeks of treatment, even when higher doses were used (Wang et al. 2005). H2RAs are relatively safe with a side effect rate of about 4%, most being minor and reversible. However, cimetidine and to a lesser degree ranitidine can inhibit the P450 cytochrome system causing drug interactions, which requires monitoring of other medications taken simultaneously. When used intermittently, H2RAs can be effective in blocking nocturnal acid reflux. When used daily, tolerance develops and the benefit diminishes. Hence an intermittent drug holiday may be of benefit in those patients who use the medication regularly.

Proton Pump Inhibitors

PPIs provide meal-stimulated and nocturnal gastric acid inhibition of the parietal cell regardless of any stimuli and to a significantly greater degree than H2Ras and are currently the cornerstone of treatment of GERD. Compared to H2RAs, PPIs promote a greater degree and more sustained duration of acid suppression. In a recent Cochrane review involving 4032 patients in 26 RCT trials, PPIs were superior to H2RAs in healing esophagitis at 4–8 weeks with a number to treat of 3 (Khan et al. 2007). Currently, there are seven PPIs available in the market with similar therapeutic efficacies; however, large studies comparing PPIs found a greater therapeutic advantage to using esomeprazole in severe LA grade C/D esophagitis (Metz et al. 2000). A recommended regimen in patients with confirmed esophagitis is a 2-month course of daily PPI with expected cure rates over 90%. However, GERD is a chronic disease, and most elderly will require long-term maintenance therapy. The relapse rate can be as high as 90% annually after discontinuation of PPIs (Pilotto et al. 2003). Relapse rates increase following the abrupt discontinuation of a PPI due to oxyntic cell hyperplasia (Niklasson et al. 2010). Tapering off the PPI over 3–4 weeks may reduce relapse. PPIs are widely used with high effectiveness and safety in the old. Common side effects include diarrhea including predisposition to *Clostridium difficile* infection, abdominal pain, constipation, osteoporosis, hypomagnesemia, and headache which are rarely limiting and typically respond to dose reduction or discontinuation of the medication. When PPIs are ineffective, an alternate diagnosis should be sought for (Table 4).

PPI-Clopidogrel Interaction

Following widespread use of antiplatelet therapy, upper gastrointestinal bleeding (UGI) has emerged as a common and often life-threatening complication. Prophylactic co-administration of PPIs significantly reduces bleeding risk; however, some studies have questioned the safety of this

Table 5 The Los Angeles classification of erosive esophagitis (Lundell et al. 1999)

Grade A	One (or more) mucosal break no longer than 5 mm that does not extend between the tops of two mucosal folds
Grade B	One (or more) mucosal break more than 5 mm long that does not extend between the tops of two mucosal folds
Grade C	One (or more) mucosal break that is continuous between the tops of two or more mucosal folds but which involves less than 75% of the circumference
Grade D	One (or more) mucosal break which involves at least 75% of the esophageal circumference

approach. Clopidogrel, a prodrug, undergoes CYP2C19- dependent activation in the liver. Ex vivo studies suggest that PPIs, such as omeprazole, competitively inhibit the CYP2C19 enzyme, thereby interfering with activation of clopidogrel and decrease its antiplatelet effect (Gilard et al. 2008). The FDA issued a warning regarding the concomitant use of clopidogrel and PPIs. However subsequent studies have not revealed any substantial increase in cardiac events in patients taking PPIs with clopidogrel, and hence this potential interaction is not thought to be clinically relevant. Other drug-drug interactions are mentioned in Table 5.

Potential Adverse Effects of Chronic PPI Use

PPI Use and Pneumonia

Gastric acid is an important barrier to colonization and infection by invading pathogens. Attenuation of this acidity results in increased bacterial colonization of the upper aerodigestive tract, providing a plausible mechanism as to why patients on PPIs or H2RAs might be at increased risk of pneumonia. Studies designed to clarify this risk have shown contradictory results. A recent large US-based population study did not observe an increased risk of community-acquired pneumonia (CAP) in older adults on PPI and H2RAs (Dublin et al. 2010). On the other hand, several studies demonstrate a slight trend toward an association

between PPI use and pneumonia, with a higher risk for PPIs over H2RAs (Fohl and Regal 2011; Laheij et al. 2004). However, the association between CAP and PPI use is stronger with acute than with chronic PPI use. Indeed, a meta-analysis of eight observational studies showed significant association of CAP with recent initiation of PPI (<7 days and <30 days) (Eom et al. 2011). This appears to be inconsistent with a biological effect and more suggestive of confounding. Therefore, the use of PPIs should be limited to situations where the indications are clear, and in such cases, they must be used in the lowest effective dose and for the shortest duration.

PPI Therapy and Enteric Infections

Potent inhibition of gastric acid can reduce the antiseptic benefit of gastric acid and lead to a proliferation and increased enteric exposure to ingested pathogenic bacteria. Enteric infections including *Salmonella*, *Campylobacter*, and *Shigella* are more prevalent in those on PPIs (Leonard et al. 2007). More importantly, an increased incidence of *Clostridium difficile* infections has been reported with PPI administration, with a doubling in the incidence of infections (Dial et al. 2004; Wright et al. 2008). The duration of PPI treatment was found to be an independent risk factor in one study, with the incidence of infection increasing from 5 to 23% in those on PPI therapy for over 6 months (Dalton et al. 2009).

Therefore, a risk-benefit evaluation is necessary prior to initiating antisecretory therapy in those at high risk of developing enteric infections (e.g., hospitalized patients on antibiotics, frail and elderly, immunosuppressed). In such patients, preventative measures may be utilized.

PPIs, Osteoporosis, and Fractures

PPIs may interfere with calcium absorption, a process dependent on gastric acidity. In turn, this leads to a decline in bone loss and increased risk of fractures (Wright et al. 2008). Several retrospective studies suggest that a higher dose and duration of PPI use conferred an increased risk, the largest odds ratio being 1.92 (1.16–3.18) after 7 years of PPI use (Kaye and Jick 2008). The studies have shown that the drop in bone density scores is comparable over time between those on and not on PPIs. Additionally, the use of chronic high-dose PPIs was not shown to increase the incidence of fractures in a population-based study (Kumar et al. 2017). Nevertheless, the FDA has recently issued a warning regarding the possible link between PPI use and increased fracture risk. In those who require high-dose, long-term PPIs, osteoporosis and fall risk should be assessed, and the use of medications revised as appropriate. This includes the use of calcium supplements, vitamin D, and/or bisphosphonates. In the elderly, with osseointegrated dental implants, PPI use has shown to have higher risk of dental implant failures (Wu et al. 2017; Chrcanovic et al. 2017). Impaired intestinal calcium absorption linked with PPI use leads to decreased serum calcium levels. Proton pumps (H^+/K^+ ATPase) have also been found to be located in osteoclast cells (Costa-Rodrigues et al. 2013). PPI use can lead to inhibition of these proton pumps leading to inhibition of osteoclastic activity and thereby bone and dental remodeling.

PPI, AKI, and CKD

Both acute and chronic uses of PPI have been associated with renal injury. Acute use (3–4 weeks into starting PPI) has been associated with biopsy-proven acute interstitial nephritis (AIN) (Muriithi et al. 2014; Sampathkumar et al. 2013). This effect is usually not dose-dependent and can result in serious kidney damage. Chronic use of PPI in the elderly has been associated with development of CKD. In a large study involving the VA population in New York with a mean age of 56 years, 24.4% of the population developed CKD with chronic PPI use (Arora et al. 2016). The mechanism for development of CKD is likely due to the cumulative damage to kidneys caused by undiagnosed and untreated subclinical AIN

from chronic PPI use. It is important to understand mechanisms of renal injury in patients with acute and chronic PPI use to prevent irreversible damage. Although there are no current guidelines to monitor renal function with PPI use, it is reasonable to monitor GFR annually in patients who require chronic PPI.

PPI and Gastric Cancer

Chronic PPI use was previously studied to have a significant association with new onset gastric cancers. The pathogenesis was assumed as a result of hypergastrinemia from chronic PPI use. It was also seen in this study that more than 25% of people over the age of 60 were on chronic PPI. However, the study was limited due to lack of information on underlying *H. pylori* infection that is a major confounding factor (Poulsen et al. 2009). In a recent study in China, chronic PPI use after eradication of *H. pylori* infection was found to result in higher incidence of gastric cancers. This study had limitation in generalizability beyond the Chinese population, where incidence rates are already high (Cheung et al. 2018). Currently, the evidence to provide a strong causal relationship between PPI use and gastric cancers is limited and needs additional study.

Endoscopic Therapy

Although PPIs have remained the mainstay management of GERD, a proportion of patients with erosive and non-erosive reflux disease fail to respond to PPI therapy. Minimally invasive endoscopic therapies have been used in PPI-resistant patients who may not wish to proceed with antireflux surgery. Some of the antireflux endoscopic therapies used in the management of GERD in the USA are radiofrequency ablation and transoral incisionless fundoplication (Nabi and Reddy 2016; Rouphael et al. 2018). Long-term data on symptom control and acid reflux control after these procedures are awaited.

Antireflux Surgery

Performed in expert hands, antireflux surgery can potentially eliminate GERD by increasing basal LES pressure, decreasing episodes of tLESRs, and inhibiting complete LES relaxation. Long-term maintenance studies comparing medical therapy with antireflux surgery have demonstrated either similar clinical efficacy or significantly better control of GERD symptoms postsurgery (Oelschlager et al. 2008; Galmiche et al. 2011). Therefore, patients with typical or atypical GERD symptoms well controlled on PPIs desiring alternative therapy or patients with volume regurgitation and aspiration symptoms not controlled on PPIs may benefit from surgery. Currently, the two most popular procedures, performed laparoscopically through the abdomen, are the Nissen 360° fundoplication and the Toupet partial fundoplication. Postoperative mortality is rare (<1%), but a variety of complications occur with relative frequency after antireflux surgery, including dysphagia, gas-bloat syndrome, and post-vagotomy symptoms. Perhaps far more concerning is the high recurrence rate of GERD symptoms after antireflux surgery (Galmiche et al. 2011).

Several studies have observed that laparoscopic fundoplication-related mortality or morbidity does not increase in older adults compared to younger counterparts (Brunt et al. 1999; Wang et al. 2008). Therefore, the healthy older adult should not be refused antireflux surgery solely on the basis of age. Best results are obtained by experienced surgeons in high-volume centers who report recurrence of symptoms in only 10–15% of patients; long-term studies suggest that 60% of patients are back on acid-suppressive medication 5–15 years later. Furthermore, fundoplication procedure is difficult to perform in morbidly obese patients, and the rate of failure is high in comparison to non-obese patients. In this subset of patients, bariatric surgery may provide better results in controlling and curing GERD symptoms. Certain bariatric surgeries like gastric banding and Roux-en-Y gastric bypass have shown to alleviate GERD symptoms, while sleeve gastrectomy has shown to worsen manifestations (El-Hadi et al. 2014). Prior to antireflux surgery, endoscopy must be performed to identify Barrett's esophagus and exclude stricture, dysplasia, or carcinoma. Motility studies in selected patients can identify ineffective esophageal peristalsis or diagnose a motility disorder which may alter management. Although not routinely indicated, barium esophagogram can help define a nonreducible hiatal hernia and a shortened esophagus which may entail additional surgical maneuvers. In the subset of patients with erosive esophagitis not responding to PPI therapy or those with non-erosive GERD, 24-h pH testing is necessary to confirm the diagnosis (Fass et al. 1994).

Overall, PPIs seem to be a safe therapy in the elderly, while antireflux or bariatric surgery may be safe and effective in a subset of older adults with GERD (Poh et al. 2010).

Key Points

- GERD is a common condition caused by reflux of gastric contents into the esophagus causing troublesome symptoms and related complications.
- It is a multifactorial disorder with diverse clinical presentations. Symptom severity may vary from person to person.
- Factors influencing GERD are imbalances in acid production, acid clearance, integrity of the gastroesophageal junction reflux barrier, and esophageal mucosal defense.
- Complications of GERD may be esophageal or extraesophageal.
- Important esophageal complications include esophagitis, strictures, Barrett's esophagus, and esophageal adenocarcinoma.
- Some of the extraesophageal complications include asthma, non-cardiac chest pain, chronic cough, chronic laryngitis, and pneumonia.
- Diagnosis is usually based on clinical presentation. Endoscopic diagnosis may be required in chronic, refractory GERD and to rule out esophageal complications. Ambulatory pH monitoring can help confirm excessive distal esophageal acid/non-acid exposure.

- Proton pump inhibitors are the mainstay in management of symptomatic GERD.
- Management therapies include lifestyle changes, medical management, and endoscopic and surgical management.

References

Adler DG, Siddiqui AA. Endoscopic management of esophageal strictures. Gastrointest Endosc. 2017;86:35–43. https://doi.org/10.1016/j.gie.2017.03.004.

Ang D, et al. To Bravo or not? A comparison of wireless esophageal pH monitoring and conventional pH catheter to evaluate non-erosive gastroesophageal reflux disease in a multiracial Asian cohort. J Dig Dis. 2010;11:19–27. https://doi.org/10.1111/j.1751-2980.2009.00409.x.

Arora P, et al. Proton pump inhibitors are associated with increased risk of development of chronic kidney disease. BMC Nephrol. 2016;17:112. https://doi.org/10.1186/s12882-016-0325-4.

Baliga S, Muglikar S, Kale R. Salivary pH: a diagnostic biomarker. J Indian Soc Periodontol. 2013;17:461–5. https://doi.org/10.4103/0972-124X.118317.

Barboi OB, et al. Extradigestive manifestations of gastroesophageal reflux disease: demographic, clinical, biological and endoscopic features. Rev Med Chir Soc Med Nat Iasi. 2016;120:282–7.

Becher A, Dent J. Systematic review: ageing and gastro-oesophageal reflux disease symptoms, oesophageal function and reflux oesophagitis. Aliment Pharmacol Ther. 2011;33:442–54. https://doi.org/10.1111/j.1365-2036.2010.04542.x.

Behar J, Sheahan DG, Biancani P, Spiro HM, Storer EH. Medical and surgical management of reflux esophagitis. A 38-month report of a prospective clinical trial. N Engl J Med. 1975;293:263–8. https://doi.org/10.1056/NEJM197508072930602.

Boeckxstaens G, El-Serag HB, Smout AJ, Kahrilas PJ. Symptomatic reflux disease: the present, the past and the future. Gut. 2014;63:1185–93. https://doi.org/10.1136/gutjnl-2013-306393.

Brunt LM, Quasebarth MA, Dunnegan DL, Soper NJ. Is laparoscopic antireflux surgery for gastroesophageal reflux disease in the elderly safe and effective? Surg Endosc. 1999;13:838–42.

Chait MM. Gastroesophageal reflux disease: important considerations for the older patients. World J Gastrointest Endosc. 2010;2:388–96. https://doi.org/10.4253/wjge.v2.i12.388.

Cheung KS, et al. Long-term proton pump inhibitors and risk of gastric cancer development after treatment for Helicobacter pylori: a population-based study. Gut. 2018;67:28–35. https://doi.org/10.1136/gutjnl-2017-314605.

Choe JW, et al. Foods inducing typical gastroesophageal reflux disease symptoms in Korea. J Neurogastroenterol Motil. 2017;23:363–9. https://doi.org/10.5056/jnm16122.

Chrcanovic BR, Kisch J, Albrektsson T, Wennerberg A. Intake of proton pump inhibitors is associated with an increased risk of dental implant failure. Int J Oral Maxillofac Implants. 2017;32:1097–102. https://doi.org/10.11607/jomi.5662.

Costa-Rodrigues J, Reis S, Teixeira S, Lopes S, Fernandes MH. Dose-dependent inhibitory effects of proton pump inhibitors on human osteoclastic and osteoblastic cell activity. FEBS J. 2013;280:5052–64. https://doi.org/10.1111/febs.12478.

Crookes PF. Physiology of reflux disease: role of the lower esophageal sphincter. Surg Endosc. 2006;20(Suppl 2):S462–6. https://doi.org/10.1007/s00464-006-0039-y.

Dacha S, Razvi M, Massaad J, Cai Q, Wehbi M. Hypergastrinemia. Gastroenterol Rep (Oxf). 2015;3:201–8. https://doi.org/10.1093/gastro/gov004.

Dalton BR, Lye-Maccannell T, Henderson EA, Maccannell DR, Louie TJ. Proton pump inhibitors increase significantly the risk of Clostridium difficile infection in a low-endemicity, non-outbreak hospital setting. Aliment Pharmacol Ther. 2009;29:626–34. https://doi.org/10.1111/j.1365-2036.2008.03924.x.

Dellon ES, Jensen ET, Martin CF, Shaheen NJ, Kappelman MD. Prevalence of eosinophilic esophagitis in the United States. Clin Gastroenterol Hepatol. 2014;12:589–596.e581. https://doi.org/10.1016/j.cgh.2013.09.008.

Dial S, Alrasadi K, Manoukian C, Huang A, Menzies D. Risk of Clostridium difficile diarrhea among hospital inpatients prescribed proton pump inhibitors: cohort and case-control studies. CMAJ. 2004;171:33–8.

Dodds MW, Johnson DA, Yeh CK. Health benefits of saliva: a review. J Dent. 2005;33:223–33. https://doi.org/10.1016/j.jdent.2004.10.009.

Dore MP, et al. Diet, lifestyle and gender in gastro-esophageal reflux disease. Dig Dis Sci. 2008;53:2027–32. https://doi.org/10.1007/s10620-007-0108-7.

Dublin S, et al. Use of proton pump inhibitors and H2 blockers and risk of pneumonia in older adults: a population-based case-control study. Pharmacoepidemiol Drug Saf. 2010;19:792–802. https://doi.org/10.1002/pds.1978.

El-Hadi M, Birch DW, Gill RS, Karmali S. The effect of bariatric surgery on gastroesophageal reflux disease. Can J Surg. 2014;57:139–44.

El-Serag HB, Sweet S, Winchester CC, Dent J. Update on the epidemiology of gastro-oesophageal reflux disease: a systematic review. Gut. 2014;63:871–80. https://doi.org/10.1136/gutjnl-2012-304269.

Eom CS, et al. Use of acid-suppressive drugs and risk of pneumonia: a systematic review and meta-analysis. CMAJ. 2011;183:310–9. https://doi.org/10.1503/cmaj.092129.

Fakhouri TH, Ogden CL, Carroll MD, Kit BK, Flegal KM. Prevalence of obesity among older adults in the United States, 2007–2010. NCHS Data Brief. 2012;(106):1–8.

Fass R, Mackel C, Sampliner RE. 24-hour pH monitoring in symptomatic patients without erosive esophagitis who did not respond to antireflux treatment. J Clin Gastroenterol. 1994;19:97–9.

Festi D, et al. Body weight, lifestyle, dietary habits and gastroesophageal reflux disease. World J Gastroenterol. 2009;15:1690–701.

Field SK, Sutherland LR. Does medical antireflux therapy improve asthma in asthmatics with gastroesophageal reflux?: a critical review of the literature. Chest. 1998;114:275–83.

Fohl AL, Regal RE. Proton pump inhibitor-associated pneumonia: not a breath of fresh air after all? World J Gastrointest Pharmacol Ther. 2011;2:17–26. https://doi.org/10.4292/wjgpt.v2.i3.17.

Furuta K, et al. Comparisons of symptoms reported by elderly and non-elderly patients with GERD. J Gastroenterol. 2012;47:144–9. https://doi.org/10.1007/s00535-011-0476-9.

Galmiche JP, et al. Laparoscopic antireflux surgery vs esomeprazole treatment for chronic GERD: the LOTUS randomized clinical trial. JAMA. 2011;305:1969–77. https://doi.org/10.1001/jama.2011.626.

Gilard M, et al. Influence of omeprazole on the antiplatelet action of clopidogrel associated with aspirin: the randomized, double-blind OCLA (Omeprazole CLopidogrel Aspirin) study. J Am Coll Cardiol. 2008;51:256–60. https://doi.org/10.1016/j.jacc.2007.06.064.

Goldberg HI, Dodds WJ, Montgomery C, Baskin SA, Zboralske FF. Controlled production of acute esophagitis. Experimental animal model. Investig Radiol. 1970;5:254–6.

Green BT, Broughton WA, O'Connor JB. Marked improvement in nocturnal gastroesophageal reflux in a large cohort of patients with obstructive sleep apnea treated with continuous positive airway pressure. Arch Intern Med. 2003;163:41–5. https://doi.org/10.1001/archinte.163.1.41.

Hunt RH. Importance of pH control in the management of GERD. Arch Intern Med. 1999;159:649–57.

Johnson DA, Fennerty MB. Heartburn severity underestimates erosive esophagitis severity in elderly patients with gastroesophageal reflux disease. Gastroenterology. 2004;126:660–4.

Jung HK, Choung RS, Talley NJ. Gastroesophageal reflux disease and sleep disorders: evidence for a causal link and therapeutic implications. J Neurogastroenterol Motil. 2010;16:22–9. https://doi.org/10.5056/jnm.2010.16.1.22.

Kahrilas PJ, Dodds WJ, Hogan WJ. Effect of peristaltic dysfunction on esophageal volume clearance. Gastroenterology. 1988;94:73–80.

Kaltenbach T, Crockett S, Gerson LB. Are lifestyle measures effective in patients with gastroesophageal reflux disease? An evidence-based approach. Arch Intern Med. 2006;166:965–71. https://doi.org/10.1001/archinte.166.9.965.

Kaye JA, Jick H. Proton pump inhibitor use and risk of hip fractures in patients without major risk factors. Pharmacotherapy. 2008;28:951–9. https://doi.org/10.1592/phco.28.8.951.

Khan M, Santana J, Donnellan C, Preston C, Moayyedi P. Medical treatments in the short term management of reflux oesophagitis. Cochrane Database Syst Rev. 2007:CD003244. https://doi.org/10.1002/14651858.CD003244.pub2.

Khan BA, et al. Effect of bed head elevation during sleep in symptomatic patients of nocturnal gastroesophageal reflux. J Gastroenterol Hepatol. 2012;27:1078–82. https://doi.org/10.1111/j.1440-1746.2011.06968.x.

Kishikawa H, et al. Association between increased gastric juice acidity and sliding hiatal hernia development in humans. PLoS One. 2017;12:e0170416. https://doi.org/10.1371/journal.pone.0170416.

Korsten MA, et al. Chronic xerostomia increases esophageal acid exposure and is associated with esophageal injury. Am J Med. 1991;90:701–6.

Kumar S, et al. Incidence and predictors of osteoporotic fractures in patients with Barrett's oesophagus: a population-based nested case-control study. Aliment Pharmacol Ther. 2017;46:1094–102. https://doi.org/10.1111/apt.14345.

Laheij RJ, et al. Risk of community-acquired pneumonia and use of gastric acid-suppressive drugs. JAMA. 2004;292:1955–60. https://doi.org/10.1001/jama.292.16.1955.

Laitinen S, et al. Sucralfate and alginate/antacid in reflux esophagitis. Scand J Gastroenterol. 1985;20:229–32. https://doi.org/10.3109/00365528509089662.

Lee J, et al. Effects of age on the gastroesophageal junction, esophageal motility, and reflux disease. Clin Gastroenterol Hepatol. 2007;5:1392–8. https://doi.org/10.1016/j.cgh.2007.08.011.

Lee SP, et al. The clinical course of asymptomatic esophageal candidiasis incidentally diagnosed in general health inspection. Scand J Gastroenterol. 2015;50:1444–50. https://doi.org/10.3109/00365521.2015.1057519.

Leonard J, Marshall JK, Moayyedi P. Systematic review of the risk of enteric infection in patients taking acid suppression. Am J Gastroenterol. 2007;102:2047–56; quiz 2057. https://doi.org/10.1111/j.1572-0241.2007.01275.x.

Lipsy RJ, Fennerty B, Fagan TC. Clinical review of histamine2 receptor antagonists. Arch Intern Med. 1990;150:745–51.

Locke GR 3rd, Talley NJ, Fett SL, Zinsmeister AR, Melton LJ 3rd. Prevalence and clinical spectrum of gastroesophageal reflux: a population-based study in Olmsted County, Minnesota. Gastroenterology. 1997;112:1448–56.

Lundell LR, et al. Endoscopic assessment of oesophagitis: clinical and functional correlates and further validation of the Los Angeles classification. Gut. 1999;45:172–80. https://doi.org/10.1136/gut.45.2.172.

Metz DC, et al. Oral and intravenous dosage forms of pantoprazole are equivalent in their ability to suppress gastric acid secretion in patients with gastroesophageal reflux disease. Am J Gastroenterol. 2000;95:626–33. https://doi.org/10.1111/j.1572-0241.2000.01834.x.

Milke P, Diaz A, Valdovinos MA, Moran S. Gastroesophageal reflux in healthy subjects induced by two different species of chilli (Capsicum annum). Dig Dis. 2006;24:184–8. https://doi.org/10.1159/000090323.

Moore AR, Varro A, Pritchard M. Zollinger-Ellison syndrome. Gastrointest Nurs. 2013;10 https://doi.org/10.12968/gasn.2012.10.5.44.

Moshkowitz M, Horowitz N, Halpern Z, Santo E. Gastroesophageal reflux disease symptoms: prevalence, sociodemographics and treatment patterns in the adult Israeli population. World J Gastroenterol.

2011;17:1332–5. https://doi.org/10.3748/wjg.v17.i10.
1332.

Muriithi AK, et al. Biopsy-proven acute interstitial nephritis, 1993-2011: a case series. Am J Kidney Dis.
2014;64:558–66. https://doi.org/10.1053/j.ajkd.2014.
04.027.

Nabi Z, Reddy DN. Endoscopic management of gastroesophageal reflux disease: revisited. Clin Endosc.
2016;49:408–16. https://doi.org/10.5946/ce.2016.133.

Niklasson A, Lindstrom L, Simren M, Lindberg G,
Bjornsson E. Dyspeptic symptom development after
discontinuation of a proton pump inhibitor: a double-
blind placebo-controlled trial. Am J Gastroenterol.
2010;105:1531–7. https://doi.org/10.1038/ajg.2010.81.

Oelschlager BK, et al. Long-term outcomes after laparoscopic antireflux surgery. Am J Gastroenterol.
2008;103:280–7; quiz 288. https://doi.org/10.1111/
j.1572-0241.2007.01606.x.

Palmer JB, Drennan JC, Baba M. Evaluation and treatment
of swallowing impairments. Am Fam Physician.
2000;61:2453–62.

Person E, Rife C, Freeman J, Clark A, Castell DO. A novel
sleep positioning device reduces gastroesophageal
reflux: a randomized controlled trial. J Clin
Gastroenterol. 2015;49:655–9. https://doi.org/10.1097/
MCG.0000000000000359.

Petrusic N, Posavac M, Sabol I, Mravak-Stipetic M. The
effect of tobacco smoking on salivation. Acta Stomatol
Croat. 2015;49:309–15. https://doi.org/10.15644/
asc49/4/6.

Phan J, Benhammou JN, Pisegna JR. Gastric hyper-
secretory states: investigation and management. Curr
Treat Options Gastroenterol. 2015;13:386–97. https://
doi.org/10.1007/s11938-015-0065-8.

Pilotto A, Leandro G, Franceschi M. Ageing & Acid-
Related Disease Study, G. Short- and long-term therapy
for reflux oesophagitis in the elderly: a multi-centre,
placebo-controlled study with pantoprazole. Aliment
Pharmacol Ther. 2003;17:1399–406.

Pilotto A, et al. Clinical features of reflux esophagitis in
older people: a study of 840 consecutive patients. J Am
Geriatr Soc. 2006;54:1537–42. https://doi.org/10.1111/
j.1532-5415.2006.00899.x.

Poh CH, Navarro-Rodriguez T, Fass R. Review: treatment
of gastroesophageal reflux disease in the elderly. Am
J Med. 2010;123:496–501. https://doi.org/10.1016/j.
amjmed.2009.07.036.

Poulsen AH, et al. Proton pump inhibitors and risk of
gastric cancer: a population-based cohort study. Br
J Cancer. 2009;100:1503–7. https://doi.org/10.1038/
sj.bjc.6605024.

Powell DW. Barrier function of epithelia. Am J Phys.
1981;241:G275–88. https://doi.org/10.1152/ajpgi.1981.
241.4.G275.

Raiha IJ, Impivaara O, Seppala M, Sourander
LB. Prevalence and characteristics of symptomatic gas-
troesophageal reflux disease in the elderly. J Am Geriatr
Soc. 1992;40:1209–11.

Ravich WJ. Endoscopic management of benign esophageal strictures. Curr Gastroenterol Rep. 2017;19:50.
https://doi.org/10.1007/s11894-017-0591-8.

Reddy A, Norris DF, Momeni SS, Waldo B, Ruby JD. The
pH of beverages in the United States. J Am Dent Assoc.
2016;147:255–63. https://doi.org/10.1016/j.adaj.2015.
10.019.

Reilly JJ Jr, Schade RR, Van Thiel DS. Esophageal function after injection sclerotherapy: pathogenesis of
esophageal stricture. Am J Surg. 1984;147:85–8.

Rouphael C, Padival R, Sanaka MR, Thota
PN. Endoscopic treatments of GERD. Curr Treat
Options Gastroenterol. 2018;16:58–71. https://doi.
org/10.1007/s11938-018-0170-6.

Rubenstein JH, Scheiman JM, Sadeghi S, Whiteman D,
Inadomi JM. Esophageal adenocarcinoma incidence in
individuals with gastroesophageal reflux: synthesis
and estimates from population studies. Am
J Gastroenterol. 2011;106:254–60. https://doi.org/10.
1038/ajg.2010.470.

Sampathkumar K, Ramalingam R, Prabakar A, Abraham
A. Acute interstitial nephritis due to proton pump inhibitors. Indian J Nephrol. 2013;23:304–7. https://doi.org/
10.4103/0971-4065.114487.

Schey R, et al. Sleep deprivation is hyperalgesic in patients
with gastroesophageal reflux disease. Gastroenterology.
2007;133:1787–95. https://doi.org/10.1053/j.gastro.200
7.09.039.

Shaheen NJ, Falk GW, Iyer PG, Gerson LB, American
College of Gastroenterology. ACG clinical guideline:
diagnosis and management of Barrett's esophagus. Am
J Gastroenterol. 2016;111:30–50; quiz 51. https://doi.
org/10.1038/ajg.2015.322.

Shaker A, Magdy M. Frequency of obstructive sleep apnea
(OSA) in patients with gastroesophageal reflux disease
(GERD) and the effect of nasal continuous positive airway pressure. Egypt J Chest Dis Tu. 2016;65:797–803.
https://doi.org/10.1016/j.ejcdt.2016.02.011.

Stier MW, Konda VJ, Hart J, Waxman I. Post-ablation
surveillance in Barrett's esophagus: a review of the
literature. World J Gastroenterol. 2016;22:4297–306.
https://doi.org/10.3748/wjg.v22.i17.4297.

Trifan A, et al. Eosinophilic esophagitis in an octogenarian:
a case report and review of the literature. Medicine
(Baltimore). 2016;95:e5169. https://doi.org/10.1097/
MD.0000000000005169.

Vakil N, et al. The Montreal definition and classification of
gastroesophageal reflux disease: a global evidence-
based consensus. Am J Gastroenterol. 2006;101:
1900–20; quiz 1943. https://doi.org/10.1111/j.1572-
0241.2006.00630.x.

Vallot T, Coudsy B, Becq J. Clinical characteristics and
management of Gastro Esophageal Reflux Disease
(GERD) in elderly patients consulting a general practitioner. Gastroenterology. 2011;140:S-252. https://doi.
org/10.1016/S0016-5085(11)61013-5.

Wadhwa V, Thota PN, Parikh MP, Lopez R, Sanaka
MR. Changing trends in age, gender, racial distribution

and inpatient burden of achalasia. Gastroenterology Res. 2017;10:70–7. https://doi.org/10.14740/gr723w.

Wang WH, et al. Head-to-head comparison of H2-receptor antagonists and proton pump inhibitors in the treatment of erosive esophagitis: a meta-analysis. World J Gastroenterol. 2005;11:4067–77.

Wang W, Huang MT, Wei PL, Lee WJ. Laparoscopic anti-reflux surgery for the elderly: a surgical and quality-of-life study. Surg Today. 2008;38:305–10. https://doi.org/10.1007/s00595-007-3619-0.

Wright MJ, Proctor DD, Insogna KL, Kerstetter JE. Proton pump-inhibiting drugs, calcium homeostasis, and bone health. Nutr Rev. 2008;66:103–8. https://doi.org/10.1111/j.1753-4887.2008.00015.x.

Wu X, et al. Proton pump inhibitors and the risk of osseointegrated dental implant failure: a cohort study. Clin Implant Dent Relat Res. 2017;19:222–32. https://doi.org/10.1111/cid.12455.

Yuan YZ, et al. Alginate antacid (Gaviscon DA) chewable tablets reduce esophageal acid exposure in Chinese patients with gastroesophageal reflux disease and heartburn symptoms. J Dig Dis. 2016;17:725–34. https://doi.org/10.1111/1751-2980.12406.

Part IX

Signs and Symptoms

Abdominal Pain

50

C. S. Pitchumoni and T. S. Dharmarajan

Contents

C. S. Pitchumoni (✉)
Department of Medicine, Robert Wood Johnson School of
Medicine, Rutgers University, New Brunswick, NJ, USA

Department of Medicine, New York Medical College,
Valhalla, NY, USA

Division of Gastroenterology, Hepatology and Clinical
Nutrition, Saint Peters University Hospital, New
Brunswick, NJ, USA
e-mail: Medicinepitchumoni@hotmail.com;
pitchumoni@hotmail.com

T. S. Dharmarajan
Department of Medicine, Division of Geriatrics,
Montefiore Medical Center, Wakefield Campus, Bronx,
NY, USA

Department of Medicine, Albert Einstein College of
Medicine, Bronx, NY, USA

Department of Medicine, New York Medical College,
Valhalla, NY, USA
e-mail: dharmarajants@yahoo.com

Abstract

Abdominal pain is a common problem in the geriatric population. Assessment is challenging in this age group because of the difficulty in obtaining a satisfactory history due to the presence of comorbid processes including impaired cognition, delirium, physical or other disabilities. It is generally more likely that the older patient with abdominal pain may have a serious underlying disorder. Older patients presenting to the emergency department (ED) with abdominal pain have a greater likelihood of requiring hospitalization and perhaps surgery. The importance of rapid assessment, use of appropriate tests, and early surgical consultation where indicated may be instrumental in improving outcomes. A focused physical examination is important. A combination of approaches in pain management based on current guidelines will help address pain. The geriatric patient has unique and differing

© Springer Nature Switzerland AG 2021
C. S. Pitchumoni, T. S. Dharmarajan (eds.), *Geriatric Gastroenterology*,
https://doi.org/10.1007/978-3-030-30192-7_43

pharmacokinetics and dynamics with regard to use of medications, including analgesics, and is thereby prone to adverse drug effects. Older adults are additionally subject to polypharmacy and consequent drug–drug or drug–disease interactions. The traditional indicators of disease in the younger individual may be lacking in the older adult, making it pivotal to consider a wide differential diagnosis during evaluation. A multidisciplinary approach may be helpful in tackling abdominal pain in the geriatric patient.

Keywords

Lactate · Dementia · Aspirin · Pancreatitis · Anemia · Abdominal pain in the old · Atypical presentations in the old · Abdominal pain and differential diagnosis · Causes of abdominal pain in older adults · Abdominal pain and outcomes in the old · Abdominal pain and time to diagnosis in the old

Introduction

Older adults commonly suffer both acute and chronic abdominal pain. Nearly half the over-65-year age group presenting to the emergency department with abdominal pain require hospitalization and as many as a third require surgical intervention (Yeh and McNamara 2007; Kizer and Vassar 1998; Brewer et al. 1976). Geriatric patients differ in that the majority of older individuals manifest comorbidity; many are incapable of expressing themselves adequately or describe their complaints appropriately to the physician to facilitate assessment, evaluation, and execute diagnostic procedures (Herr and Garand 2001).

Pain is considered as a "sixth sense" apart from the five senses of sight, sound, smell, taste, and touch, whereby the faculty of pain warns the patient of impending danger or presence of injury (Cervo et al. 2009). The patient deprived of the ability to perceive pain may be in grave peril. Sadly this may be the situation in some elderly patients. On the other hand, appropriate assessment of pain by the provider, once considered

routine in healthcare and important enough to be termed a fifth vital sign (along with temperature, pulse, blood pressure, and respiratory rate) and has no longer been given the importance it received once (Scher et al. 2018).

Abdominal pain, similar to other painful disorders, negatively impairs the older patients' quality of life. Impaired cognitive function, sleep disturbance, impaired functional abilities, and diminished socialization are some factors that affect quality of life. Further, abdominal pain in the older adult may be ominous; the overall mortality for older adults attending the emergency department with the chief complaint of abdominal pain exceeds 10% (Yeh and McNamara 2007; Herr and Garand 2001).

Addressing the special concerns of pain in general in older adults, the American Geriatrics Society published clinical practice guidelines specific for the assessment and management of pain, and the American Medical Doctors Association published clinical practice guidelines for the management of pain in long-term care settings (AGS Panel on Pharmacological Management of Persistent Pain in Older Persons 2009; Hanlon et al. 2010; AGS Clinical Practice Committee 1997).

Assessment of Pain

There may be a misconception among some patients and providers that aches and pains are a part of aging. It is also erroneous to believe that older individuals perceive less pain than the young. It is important that providers understand the barriers in the assessment of pain in geriatric patients. The older patient and caregiver may dismiss pain for several reasons: belief that is a natural consequence of aging; the desire not to be a burden to the caregiver, family, or nursing staff; fear of dreadful disease and impending death; fear of hospitalizations, diagnostic studies; and finally costs of health care (Martinez and Mattu 2006; Lyon and Clark 2006; Burg and Francis 2005; Bjoro and Herr 2008; McCleane 2008; Makhana 2011; Dempsey 2010). The current best indicator of the pain experience is the patient's own report, including the intensity of pain and its impact on function or activities of daily living (AGS Panel on Pharmacological Management of Persistent Pain in Older Persons 2009).

Communication barriers add to the burden in evaluating pain. Many older adults suffer from impaired cognitive, sensory-perceptual, and motor abilities posing difficulty in communication. Patients with dementia, delirium, stroke, and aphasic syndromes encounter communication barriers; further, language and cultural background may compound difficulties in pain assessment.

Abdominal pain in the geriatric age group is common and potentially serious, besides being an under-recognized problem. Comprehensive assessment of abdominal pain in the older adult is a clinical art that cannot be replaced by endoscopic and imaging procedures or the finding an "incidentaloma." Recognition and proper understanding of pain is often a key to diagnosis. A focused history from the patient and/or caregiver is the most important initial step to determine the choice of diagnostic studies that may be cost effective and useful, taking into account the unique problems in obtaining a history in the cognitively impaired. In such cases, a separate interview from the caregiver or staff member is warranted. The approach should be to not only look but also to listen to the patient, as in the case of gastroesophageal reflux disease (GERD), and use validated scales as indicated (Manias et al. 2011; Andrade et al. 2011; Bardhan and Berghofer 2007).

Several instruments or tools have been tested and used for pain assessment, including the Visual Analog Scale, Faces Pain Scale, Short-Form McGill Pain questionnaire, and Pain Assessment in Advanced Dementia Tool; they help in practice to improve pain assessment and management (Manias et al. 2011). On the other hand, assessment of pain in the demented older adult is different. Patients with early Alzheimer's disease may have pain discriminatory capacity and weaker emotional and affective experience of pain, but in advanced cases, it may be difficult or even impossible to determine the presence of pain (Andrade et al. 2011). Here, a systematic

approach requires three steps: direct questioning (self-report), direct behavioral observation, and interview with caregiver/informant (Andrade et al. 2011). In the nursing home residents with dementia, the use of a Certified Nursing Assistant Pain Assessment Tool (CPAT) has proved useful and observes five categories of facial expression, behavior, mood, body language, and activity tool to arrive at a score of 0–5 (Cervo et al. 2009). Pain perception can also vary with the type of dementia and criteria adopted (Carlino et al. 2010). A multidisciplinary approach may help better deal with demented patients presenting with abdominal pain.

Several of the challenges encountered in the diagnosis of abdominal pain in the older are listed in Table 1. An approach to the evaluation and the importance of history are cited in Tables 2 and 3 (Yeh and McNamara 2007; Kizer and Vassar 1998; Brewer et al. 1976; Herr and Garand 2001; Martinez and Mattu 2006; Lyon and Clark 2006; Burg and Francis 2005; Bjoro and Herr 2008; McCleane 2008; Makhana 2011; Dempsey 2010; Bruckenthal 2008).

Causes of Abdominal Pain

It is beyond the scope of this chapter to discuss individual conditions causing abdominal pain. Causes of abdominal pain may be gastrointestinal or non-gastrointestinal in origin. Non-gastrointestinal causes may be cardiac, genitourinary, musculoskeletal, dermal, metabolic, thoracic, or spinal; they must be part of the differential diagnosis of abdominal pain in the older adult (Table 4).

Biliary tract disease accounts for almost 25% of cases of abdominal pain in the older adult, followed by nonspecific pain, malignancy, intestinal obstruction, complicated peptic ulcer, incarcerated hernias, diverticulitis, and appendicitis. Chronic disorders may also present with intermittent exacerbations. Internal hernia, adhesion, volvulus, Crohn's disease, porphyria, diabetic neuropathy, irritable bowel syndrome (IBS), chronic mesenteric ischemia, metastatic cancer, chronic pancreatitis, psychiatric causes, and the

Table 1 Challenges in the diagnosis of abdominal pain in older adults (Yeh and McNamara 2007; Kizer and Vassar 1998; Brewer et al. 1976; Herr and Garand 2001; Cervo et al. 2009; Scher et al. 2018; AGS Panel on Pharmacological Management of Persistent Pain in Older Persons 2009; Hanlon et al. 2010; AGS Clinical Practice Committee 1997; Martinez and Mattu 2006; Lyon and Clark 2006; Burg and Francis 2005; Bjoro and Herr 2008; McCleane 2008; Makhana 2011; Dempsey 2010; Bruckenthal 2008; Chang and Wang 2007; Sanson and O'Keefe 1996; Bugliosi et al. 1990; Rothrock and Greenfield 1992; Telfer et al. 1998; de Dombal 1994; Birnbaum and Jeffrey 1998; Frauenfelder et al. 2000; Glasgow and Mulvihill 2010; Cotton et al. 2011)

Physiological changes
Decrease in pain perception Delayed presentation to provider or ED Atypical presentations
History taking
Decreased hearing Impaired memory Dementia Decreased ability to speak Fear of diagnosis Fear of losing independence Fear of financial loss Psychiatric disorders Comprehension difficulties Language barriers
Effect of concurrent medications
NSAIDs: Blunting of pain, risk of peptic ulcer, anemia Narcotic use: Blunting of pain and sensorium Digoxin, colchicine, metformin, aspirin, NSAIDs cause abdominal pain Beta blockers: Blunt cardiac response and mask tachycardia Anticholinergics: Antihistamines, antispasmodics, antipsychotics, and antidepressants Drugs that cause constipation: Iron, sucralfate, antacids, anticholinergics, and calcium channel blockers
Physical examination
Normothermic/hypothermic in the presence of infection Tachycardia may be blunted Tachypnea disproportionate to pain Decreased pain perception/tenderness Decreased rebound and guarding
Comorbid conditions
Diabetes may blunt pain May mask the acute problem Rapid deterioration in the presence of organ dysfunction
Laboratory values
White cell count may be normal or low even in the presence of infection
Imaging studies
Plain X-ray abdomen: General usefulness limited but helpful for evaluation of free air and intestinal obstruction

(continued)

Table 1 (continued)

Ultrasound: Useful to diagnose abdominal aortic aneurysm (AAA), gallstones Findings may be obscured by body habitus, bowel gas CT: Useful, but incidental findings may lead to overdiagnosis

Table 2 Suggested steps in the evaluation of abdominal pain (Herr and Garand 2001; Martinez and Mattu 2006; Lyon and Clark 2006; Burg and Francis 2005; Bjoro and Herr 2008; McCleane 2008; Makhana 2011; Dempsey 2010)

Anticipate difficulties in obtaining a complete history
Additional history from family members or caregivers may be helpful
Repeat vital signs often
Auscultation of abdomen before percussion/palpation
Listen to bowel sounds/bruits
Perform all of the following routine tests
White blood cell count including differential Hemoglobin and hematocrit Electrolytes including serum calcium and phosphorus Serum creatinine and BUN Liver function tests Amylase/lipase Thyroid function
Imaging studies – Select study individualized to patient
Plain film of abdomen (KUB) Abdominal sonography CT of abdomen Chest X-ray
Cardiac evaluation
EKG: Generally recommended
Second-line tools
Blood gas Blood and urine culture Angiography Nuclear scan MRI

effects of medications are examples. Organizing the differential diagnosis into categories (inflammatory, obstructive, vascular, and other) provides a framework for history, physical examination, and diagnostic studies (Ragsdale and Southerland 2011). Despite the difficulties in evaluating abdominal pain (in the elderly) for the primary care physician and the subspecialists, the goals of clinical assessment are similar and are detailed in several excellent reviews (Bjoro and Herr 2008; McCleane 2008; Makhana 2011;

Table 3 Points to elicit in the history of abdominal pain

Location
Character
Radiation
Onset
Duration
Periodicity
Tempo/chronology
Aggravating factors
Relieving factors
Associated features
Past medical/surgical history
Family and social history
Detailed medication history
History of occult or evident alcohol consumption

Table 4 Non-gastrointestinal causes of abdominal pain as part of differential diagnosis (Salkin 1997; Chang and Wang 2007; Sanson and O'Keefe 1996; Bugliosi et al. 1990; Rothrock and Greenfield 1992; Telfer et al. 1998; de Dombal 1994; Birnbaum and Jeffrey 1998; Frauenfelder et al. 2000; Glasgow and Mulvihill 2010; Cotton et al. 2011)

Genitourinary	Kidney stones Pyelonephritis Acute or chronic urinary retention
Cardiovascular	Aortic dissection Aortic aneurysm Unstable angina Acute myocardial infarction Pulmonary embolism
Respiratory	Pneumonia
Gynecological	Ovarian rupture
Musculoskeletal	Inguinal/ventral hernia, strangulated Osteomyelitis Paraspinal abscess Radiculitis Vertebral disorders Muscle injury
Metabolic	DKA Uremia Hyperparathyroidism Porphyria Addison's disease
Heavy metal poisoning	Lead poisoning with herbal medicines
Neurocutaneous	Herpes zoster Injection abscess (in diabetics)

Dempsey 2010; Manias et al. 2011; Andrade et al. 2011; Bardhan and Berghofer 2007; Carlino et al. 2010; Bruckenthal 2008; Ragsdale and Southerland 2011; Crane and Talley 2007; Barie and Eachempati 2010; Morley 2007; Ozden and Gurses 2007; Cangemi and Picco 2009; Touzios and Dozois 2009; Cartwright and Knudson 2008).

An experience with the *acute abdomen* in subjects of mean age 78 years over 4 years revealed that the most common reasons for emergency surgery in the group were mechanical bowel obstruction (45%), perforation (18%), and strangulated hernia (18%); mesenteric ischemia was the most important cause of fatal outcome; the study concluded that acute abdomen is a frequent cause of death requiring vigilance and early attention (Costamagna et al. 2009). The following summarizes selected painful abdominal disorders in the geriatric patient.

1. Cholecystitis: Cholelithiasis increases with age, with the severity of gallstone disease much higher with age. Unlike in the young, more than half the older patients with acute cholecystitis do not have nausea, vomiting, or fever (Martinez and Mattu 2006). Even with complications such as gall bladder empyema, gangrene, or frank perforation, a third may be afebrile (Morrow et al. 1978). Leukocytosis is absent in 30–40% along with normal liver function tests. The accuracy of sonographic Murphy's sign does not decline even with premedication with opioid drugs (Nelson et al. 2004). There is an increased incidence of acalculous cholecystitis, a fact not appreciated readily on ultrasound (Shuman 1984). With a high clinical suspicion for cholecystitis, and a negative ultrasound, HIDA scan is to be performed.

2. Peptic ulcer disease: There is an increased incidence of NSAID-induced peptic ulcer disease in the geriatric population, particularly in women who tend to consume more analgesics than men on a chronic basis for back pain. NSAID-induced peptic ulcers are likely to be painless because of the analgesic property of the medication but often cause low-grade

bleeding resulting in iron deficiency anemia. Perforated peptic ulcer may be the initial manifestation of peptic ulcer. The onset of abdominal pain may not be acute, and abdominal rigidity may be absent (Fenyo 1982). Plain radiographs of the abdomen may not show free intraperitoneal air in nearly 40% of patients unless a lateral film is obtained (McNamara 1996).

3. Pancreatitis: The incidence of pancreatitis increases as age advances, with the most common etiology being gallstone disease. The mortality increases as age advances. The disease may present initially solely with systemic inflammatory response syndrome. Although an early CT scan in the younger patient with acute pancreatitis may not be necessary, the threshold for performing a CT scan in the older patient should be low (Martinez and Mattu 2006).

4. Diverticular disease: The incidence of the disorder increases with age. Few disorders are obviously more prevalent with age, diverticular disease being one of them. With ischemic colitis also increasing in prevalence, differentiating from diverticular hemorrhage becomes relevant, as management differs. Further complications of diverticular disease such as diverticulitis are common. Diverticulitis manifests as left lower quadrant pain, along with fever and leukocytosis. Diverticulitis may be complicated by a fistula to the bladder or uterus.

Juxtapapillary duodenal diverticulitis is nonspecific in clinical presentation with abdominal pain, nausea, vomiting, and fever. CT imaging may suggest a duodenal mass or abscess; early diagnosis may help prevent complications such as perforation. Free perforation, rare in the younger population, occurs more often in the elderly.

5. Appendicitis: The incidence of appendicitis in older adults is much lower than in the young, but nevertheless, it does occur with a mortality ranging from 4% to 8%. The diagnosis of appendicitis in the elderly is often missed, with half of all cases already perforated at time of diagnosis. Fever, anorexia, right lower quadrant pain, and leukocytosis are evident in less than a third, and one-quarter may have no right lower quadrant tenderness. CT scan of the abdomen is mandatory in the evaluation of a patient with suspected appendicitis, along with early surgical consultation (McNamara 1996; Gupta and Dupuy 1997; Storm-Dickerson and Horratas 2003).

6. Mesenteric ischemia: The symptoms of acute mesenteric ischemia are nonspecific. The classic triad of abdominal pain, gut emptying, and underlying cardiac disease is found in a minority of cases. Leukocytosis is notable along with some degree of metabolic acidosis and elevated lactate. Physical examination is often nonrevealing. Abdominal tenderness, peritoneal signs, and bloody stools are late occurrences. Hyperamylasemia should not be mistaken for acute pancreatitis. CT is the imaging test of choice. However, angiography is the gold standard (Meyer et al. 1998; Glenister and Corke 2004).

7. Splenic infarction: This entity is a rare cause of acute abdominal pain in the old and especially seen in those with primary antiphospholipid antibodies syndrome; CT scan of the abdomen helps diagnosis (Rossato et al. 2009).

8. Ruptured abdominal aortic aneurysm (AAA): Because of sudden onset of back pain radiating toward the groin associated with microscopic hematuria, AAA is often confused with renal colic. Other conditions which mimic ruptured AAA include diverticulitis, GI bleeding from aortoenteric fistula, and acute coronary syndrome. The diagnosis of AAA should be excluded in any patient who has syncope or hypertension in combination with abdominal or back pain, and especially in the presence of vascular disease (Martinez and Mattu 2006). The U.S. Preventive Services Task Force (USPSTF) recommends a one-time screening for AAA by ultrasonography in men aged 65 years or older in those who have ever smoked; the recommendation is to selectively screen men aged 65–75 years who have never smoked; screening is not

offered for women who have never smoked; and evidence is insufficient to determine benefits and harms of screening in women who have ever smoked (Guirguis-Blake et al. 2014). Patients with peripheral arterial disease and peripheral aneurysms who present with abdominal pain deserve consideration for dissecting aneurysm. In a patient with suspected AAA bleed, the preferred imaging is a CT scan or MRI, in contrast to ultrasound that is used for screening. Hypotension is absent in nearly 65% of cases. Atypical presentations of ruptured AAA are not uncommon (Marston et al. 1992; Salkin 1997).

9. Bowel obstruction: Small bowel obstruction (SBO) occurs secondary to adhesions consequent to prior abdominal surgery. SBO is characterized by sudden, sharp, periumbilical pain, bilious vomiting suggestive of high gut obstruction, and feculent emesis low gut obstruction. Hyperactive bowel sounds and audible rushes are suggestive physical examination findings. Large bowel obstruction is often a consequence of left-sided colon cancer, diverticulitis, or volvulus.

10. Hernia: Femoral and inguinal hernia tend to be overlooked. In particular, in older obese women, the inguinal regions escape physical examination; hence, examination for hernias should be performed in the supine and if possible, the upright position; CT or MRI scan can establish the diagnosis (van de Langenberg et al. 2008).

11. Drug-induced pain is associated with a high prevalence of polypharmacy. Commonly incriminated drugs include NSAIDs, aspirin, erythromycin, colchicines, drugs associated with acute pancreatitis, and antibiotics associated with *Clostridium difficile* colitis (Dang et al. 2002).

12. Unusual causes: Physical examination should include the abdomen, inguinal regions, and the back in evaluation of abdominal pain. Herpes zoster as the cause of pain may be evident by the presence of vesicles or crusting. Pain in herpes can precede the onset of rash, making it a difficult diagnosis, and be concurrent with or appear after the rash subsides, the last one termed postherpetic neuralgia. Older adults may be unaware of the rash as they do not routinely look at the back, emphasizing the importance of a thorough physical examination. Besides herpes, causes of abdominal pain encountered in the geriatric patient include pyelonephritis, renal colic, and hepatic or subphrenic abscess. Hence the need for physicians to entertain a broad differential diagnosis, in the setting of an inadequate to no history (Chang and Wang 2007; Sanson and O'Keefe 1996; Bugliosi et al. 1990; Rothrock and Greenfield 1992; Telfer et al. 1998; de Dombal 1994; Birnbaum and Jeffrey 1998; Frauenfelder et al. 2000; Glasgow and Mulvihill 2010; Cotton et al. 2011).

Figure 1 provides an overview of abdominal pain.

Dealing with Abdominal Pain

As the geriatric patient may be hypotensive, obtunded or even hypothermic, portending a serious illness, speed of diagnosis is vital in managing abdominal pain. In addition to routine pulse oximetry, oxygen, and cardiac monitoring in those with acute abdominal pain, intravenous access is essential. Surgical consultation is best entertained early rather than too late. As already stated, the liberal utility of ultrasound and CT may be a consideration (Dang et al. 2002). Further, the patient may have to be placed on "nothing by mouth orders" until a diagnosis is apparent.

Pain management is multifactorial and involves psychological and physical methods, and drugs (including NSAIDs, opioids, antispasmodics, regional, and epidural analgesia), in conjunction with risk-benefit assessment (Makhana 2011). A detailed approach to pharmacology of pain is essayed in a guideline from the American Geriatrics Society (AGS Panel on Pharmacological Management of Persistent Pain in Older Persons 2009). Although older adults are generally at higher risk of adverse drug reactions, analgesics and pain-modulating drugs are still safe and effective, when comorbidities are carefully

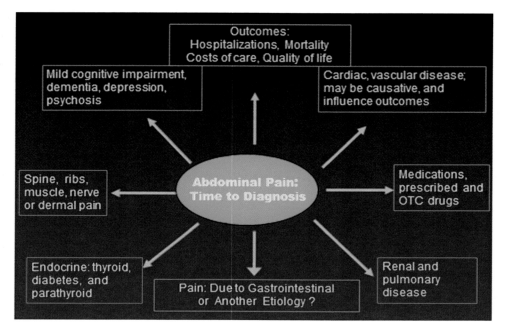

Fig. 1 Abdominal pain in the Geriatric setting

considered (AGS Panel on Pharmacological Management of Persistent Pain in Older Persons 2009). Age-associated differences in perception of pain, effect, sensitivity, pharmacokinetics and dynamics, and adverse effects must be understood by the provider with regard to use of analgesics.

A study on the influence of gender on emergency department management and outcomes in geriatric abdominal pain in those aged 70 years and over demonstrated no difference in diagnoses and management between men and women; however, men had a higher rate of death within 3 months (Gardner et al. 2010). Further, patients over age 80 years appear 17% less likely than the <65 year group to receive analgesia for abdominal pain in the emergency department and also less likely to receive opioids (Mills et al. 2011). A systematic PubMed and Cochrane analysis of data over 18 years suggests a dearth of data on the effect of pain treatment in those with dementia and agitation (Husebo et al. 2011), indicating the need for more studies.

A common under-recognized cause of typically, chronic abdominal pain is abdominal wall pain; its etiology varies; endless search for a cause

of intra-abdominal pain will be fruitless as the pain is not visceral in origin (Sweetser 2019).

In the emergency department, unenhanced CT alone appears accurate and associated with high degrees of inter-reader agreement for clinical triage of patients older than 75 years with acute abdominal pain presenting to the ED. In this study of 208 consecutive patients, men and women, average 85.4 years, diagnostic accuracy ranged from 64% to 68% for unenhanced CT, and from 68% to 71% for both unenhanced and contrast enhanced CT, with the conclusion that unenhanced CT alone is accurate and has a high degree of inter-reader agreement in the ED setting (Barat et al. 2019).

Key Points

- Abdominal pain in the geriatric population is a challenging problem in view of its common occurrence and difficulty in diagnosis.
- Nearly 50% of older adults with abdominal pain who present at the ED require hospitalization; surgical intervention is required in about a third.

- Abdominal pain is not a natural consequence of aging.
- Difficulties in obtaining an adequate history, communication barriers, and medication effects confound the pathology and interfere with early diagnosis of the etiology.
- Physical examination findings may be absent, not evident or may be atypical.
- Physical examination may appear benign even in the presence of life-threatening conditions such as aneurysm rupture or mesenteric ischemia.
- Comorbid diseases, especially dementia, may blunt or confuse the clinical picture.
- Pain assessment in dementia should depend on observations and examination rather than the patient's complaints.
- Laboratory values may not be abnormal despite a critical illness.
- In those presenting with upper abdominal discomfort or "indigestion," cardiac causes of pain (such as angina or pericardial disease) must be excluded.
- Patients with appendicitis may not manifest leukocytosis and elevated amylase may not mean pancreatitis.
- More than half the elderly with acute cholecystitis do not have nausea, vomiting, or fever.
- NSAID-induced peptic ulcers are common in older adults and associated with no pain, rather may present with severe anemia.
- Appendicitis, although rare, may present with no fever, anorexia, right lower quadrant pain, or leukocytosis.
- CT scan of the abdomen has to be liberally used in the evaluation of abdominal pain.
- The traditional indicators of disease in the younger individual may be lacking in the older adult, making it pivotal to consider a wide differential diagnosis during evaluation (Leuthauser and McVane 2016).

References

AGS Clinical Practice Committee. Management of cancer pain in older patients. J Am Geriatr Soc. 1997;45:1273.

AGS Panel on Pharmacological Management of Persistent Pain in Older Persons. Pharmacological management of persistent pain in older persons. J Am Geriatr Soc. 2009;57:1331–46.

Andrade DC, Faria JW, Caramelli P, et al. The assessment and management of pain in the demented and non-demented elderly patient. Arq Neuropsiquiatr. 2011;69(2-B):387–94.

Barat M, Paisant A, Calame P, et al. Unenhanced CT for clinical triage of elderly patients presenting to the emergency department with acute abdominal pain. Diagn Interv Imaging. 2019;110:pii: S2211-5684(19)30115-9. (ahead of print).

Bardhan KD, Berghofer P. Look-but also listen! ReQuest: an essay on a new validated scale to assess the outcomes of GERD treatment. Digestion. 2007;75(Suppl 1):87–100.

Barie PS, Eachempati SR. Acute acalculous cholecystitis. Gastroenterol Clin N Am. 2010;39:343–57.

Birnbaum BA, Jeffrey RB Jr. CT and sonographic evaluation of acute right lower quadrant abdominal pain. Am J Roentgenol. 1998;170:361–71.

Bjoro K, Herr K. Assessment of pain in the nonverbal or cognitively impaired older adult. Clin Geriatr Med. 2008;24:237–62.

Brewer BJ, Goldern GT, Hitch DC, Rudolf LE, Wangensteen SL. Abdominal pain. An analysis of 1,000 consecutive cases in a University Hospital emergency room. Am J Surg. 1976;131:457–78.

Bruckenthal P. Assessment of pain in the elderly adult. Clin Geriatr Med. 2008;24:213–6.

Bugliosi TF, Meloy TD, Vukov LF. Acute abdominal pain in the elderly. Ann Emerg Med. 1990;19:1383–6.

Burg M, Francis L. Acute abdominal pain in the elderly. Emerg Med. 2005;37:8–12.

Cangemi JR, Picco MF. Intestinal ischemia in the elderly. Gastroenterol Clin N Am. 2009;38:527–40.

Carlino E, Benedetti F, Rainero I, et al. Pain perception and tolerance in patients with frontotemporal dementia. Pain. 2010;151(3):783–9.

Cartwright SL, Knudson MP. Evaluation of acute abdominal pain in adults. Am Fam Physician. 2008;77:971–8.

Cervo FA, Bruckenthal P, Chen JJ, et al. Pain assessment in nursing home residents with dementia: psychometric properties and clinical utility of the CAN pain assessment tool. J Am Med Dir Assoc. 2009;10:505–10.

Chang C, Wang S. Acute abdominal pain in the elderly. Int J Gerontol. 2007;1:77–82.

Costamagna D, Pipitone Federico NS, Erra S, et al. Acute abdomen in the elderly. A peripheral general hospital experience. G Chir. 2009;30(6–7):315–22.

Cotton D, Taichman D, Williams S. In the clinic: herpes zoster. Ann Intern Med. 2011;154:ITC-1–14.

Crane SJ, Talley NJ. Chronic gastrointestinal symptoms in the elderly. Clin Geriatr Med. 2007;23:721–34.

Dang C, Aguilera P, Dang A, Salem L. Acute abdominal pain. Geriatrics. 2002;57:30–42.

de Dombal FT. Acute abdominal pain in the elderly. J Clin Gastroenterol. 1994;19:331–5.

Dempsey DT. Chapter 26: Stomach. In: Brunicardi FC, Andersen DK, Billiar TR, Dunn DL, Hunter JG, Matthews JB, Pollock RE, editors. Schwartz's principles of surgery. 9th ed. New York: McGraw-Hill; 2010. http://www.accessmedicine.com/content.aspx?aID=503024.

Fenyo G. Acute abdominal disease in the elderly: experience from two series in Stockholm. Am J Surg. 1982;143:751–4.

Frauenfelder T, Wildermuth S, Marineck B, Boehm T. Nontraumatic emergent abdominal vascular conditions: advantages of multi-detector row CT and three-dimensional imaging. Radiographics. 2000;24: 481–96.

Gardner RL, Almeida R, Maselli JH, Auerbach A. Does gender influence emergency department management and outcomes in geriatric abdominal pain? J Emerg Med. 2010;39(3):275–81.

Glasgow RE, Mulvihill SJ. Acute abdominal pain. In: Fledman M, Friedman LS, Brandt LJ, editors. Sleisenger and Fordtran's gastrointestinal and liver disease. 8th ed. Philadelphia: Saunders Elsevier; 2010. p. 87–98.

Glenister KM, Corke CF. Infarcted intestine: a diagnostic void. ANZ J Surg. 2004;74:260–5.

Guirguis-Blake JM, Beil TL, Senger CA, Whitlock EP. Ultrasonography screening for abdominal aortic aneurysms: a systemic evidence review for the U.S. Prev Serv Task Force. 2014;160:321–9.

Gupta H, Dupuy DE. Advances in imaging of the acute abdomen. Surg Clin North Am. 1997;77:1245–63.

Hanlon JT, Perers S, Sevick MA, et al. Pain and its treatment in older nursing home hospice/palliative care residents. J Am Med Dir Assoc. 2010;11:579–83.

Herr KA, Garand L. Assessment and measurement of pain in older adults. Clin Geriatr Med. 2001;17:457–78.

Husebo BS, Ballard C, Aarsland D. Pain treatment of agitation in patients with dementia: a systematic review. Int J Geriatr Psychiatry. 2011;26(10):1012–8.

Kizer KW, Vassar MJ. Emergency department diagnosis of abdominal disorders in the elderly. Am J Emerg Med. 1998;16:357–62.

Leuthauser A, McVane B. Abdominal pain in the geriatric patient. Emerg Med Clin North Am. 2016;34(2): 363–75.

Lyon C, Clark DC. Diagnosis of acute abdominal pain in older patients. Am Fam Physician. 2006;74: 1537–44.

Makhana GK. Understanding and treating abdominal pain and spasms in organic gastrointestinal diseases: inflammatory bowel diseases and biliary diseases. J Clin Gastroenterol. 2011;45:S89–93. (Proceedings from the Pan-European conference on irritable bowel syndrome, 10 Dec 2010, Vienna).

Manias E, Gibson SJ, Finch S. Testing an educational nursing intervention for pain assessment and management of older people. Pain Med. 2011;12 (8):1199–215.

Marston WA, Ahlquist R, Johnson G Jr, et al. Misdiagnosis of ruptured abdominal aortic aneurysms. J Vasc Surg. 1992;16:859–68.

Martinez JP, Mattu A. Abdominal pain in the elderly. Emerg Med Clin North Am. 2006;74:371–88.

McCleane G. Pain perception in the elderly patient. Clin Geriatr Med. 2008;24:203–11.

McNamara RM. Acute abdominal pain. In: Sanders AB, editor. Emergency care of the elder person. St. Louis: Beverly Cracom Publications; 1996. p. 219–43.

Meyer T, Klein P, Schweiger H, et al. How can the prognosis of acute mesenteric artery ischemia be improved? Results of a retrospective analysis [German]. Zentralbl Chir. 1998;123:230–4.

Mills AM, Edwards JM, Shofer FS, et al. Analgesia for older adults with abdominal pain or back pain in the emergency department. West J Emerg Med. 2011;12(1):43–50.

Morley JE. Constipation and irritable bowel syndrome in the elderly. Clin Geriatr Med. 2007;23:823–32.

Morrow DJ, Thompson J, Wilson SE. Acute cholecystitis in the elderly. Arch Surg. 1978;113:1149–52.

Nelson BP, Senecal EL, Prak T, et al. Opioid analgesia in the elderly: is the diagnosis of gallbladder pathology hindered. Ann Emerg Med. 2004;44(S4):S89.

Ozden N, Gurses B. Mesenteric ischemia in the elderly. Clin Geriatr Med. 2007;23:871–87.

Scher C, Meador L, Van Cleabe JH. Moving beyond pain as the fifth vital sign and patient satisfaction scores to improve pain care in the 21st century. Pain Manage Nurs. 2018;19:125–9.

Ragsdale L, Southerland L. Acute abdominal pain in the older adult. Emerg Med Clin North Am. 2011;29(2): 429–48.

Rossato M, Paccagnella M, Burei M, et al. Splenic infarction: a rare cause of acute abdominal pain presenting in an older patient with primary antiphospholipid antibodies syndrome. Intern Emerg Med. 2009;4(6):531–3.

Rothrock SG, Greenfield RH. Acute abdominal pain in the elderly: clue to identify serious illness. Part 2: diagnosis and management of common disorder. Emerg Med Rep. 1992;13:185–92.

Salkin MS. Abdominal aortic aneurysm: avoiding failure to diagnose. ED Leg Lett. 1997;8:67–78.

Sanson TG, O'Keefe KP. Evaluation of abdominal pain in the elderly. Emerg Med Clin North Am. 1996;14:615–27.

Shuman WP. Low sensitivity of sonography and cholescintigraphy in acalculous cholecystitis. Am J Roentgenol. 1984;143(3):531–4.

Storm-Dickerson TL, Horratas MC. What have we learned over the past 20 years about appendicitis in the elderly? Am J Surg. 2003;185:198–201.

Sweetser S. Abdominal wall pain: a common clinical problem. Mayo Clin Proc. 2019;94(2):347–55.

Telfer S, Fenyo G, Holt PR, de Dombal FT. Acute abdominal pain in patients over 50 years of age. Scand J Gastroenterol Suppl. 1998;144:47–50.

Touzios JG, Dozois EJ. Diverticulosis and acute diverticulitis. Gastroenterol Clin N Am. 2009;38:513–25.

van de Langenberg R, Scheltinga MR, Streukens SA, et al. Elderly women with abdominal pain due to an incarcerated "femoral hernia". Ned Tijdschr Geneeskd. 2008;152(29):1597–601.

Yeh E, McNamara RM. Abdominal pain. Clin Geriatr Med. 2007;23:255–70.

Functional Abdominal Pain

51

Douglas A. Drossman and Jill K. Deutsch

Contents

Abstract

The centrally mediated disorders of gastrointestinal pain including centrally mediated abdominal pain syndrome (CAPS) are distinguished from other functional gastrointestinal disorders (FGIDs), now termed disorders of gut-brain interaction (DGBIs), by the greater contribution of the central nervous system (CNS) in producing pain symptoms relative to the contribution of gut motility disorders that may cause pain. While these disorders are less common than other DGBIs such as irritable bowel syndrome (IBS) or functional dyspepsia (FD), their impact on quality of life is significant. Older adults present as a unique population vulnerable to DGBIs and CAPS, whose pain symptoms and management should be approached somewhat differently compared to their younger cohort. The approach to elderly patients with chronic

D. A. Drossman
Division of Gastroenterology and Hepatology, University of North Carolina, Center for Education and Practice of Biopsychosocial Care and Drossman Gastroenterology PLLC, Chapel Hill, NC, USA
e-mail: doug@drossmancenter.com

J. K. Deutsch (✉)
Section of Digestive Diseases – Department of Internal Medicine, Yale University School of Medicine – Yale New Haven Hospital, New Haven, CT, USA
e-mail: jill.deutsch@yale.edu

© Springer Nature Switzerland AG 2021
C. S. Pitchumoni, T. S. Dharmarajan (eds.), *Geriatric Gastroenterology*,
https://doi.org/10.1007/978-3-030-30192-7_99

abdominal pain should focus on a thorough history and physical exam, looking for "alarm" features or "red flag" symptoms. Evaluations should be limited to those which might help provide an alternate explanation for these "alarm" features, if they are present. Diagnostic failures in disorders of centrally mediated abdominal pain are rare due to the relatively benign but protracted course of chronic pain conditions; the likelihood of morbid conditions presenting with such an extended course of pain is exceedingly low, once evaluation for "red flag" symptoms is complete. Treatment then focuses on pain modulation using centrally acting neuromodulators, either alone or in combination with psychotherapy such as cognitive behavioral therapy (CBT), mindfulness-based strategies, or hypnotherapy. Most importantly, older adults benefit from entering a therapeutic partnership with their provider to achieve improvement of symptoms by recognizing CAPS as the unifying diagnosis.

Keywords

Functional gastrointestinal disorders (FGIDs) · Disorders of gut-brain interaction (DGBIs) · Centrally mediated abdominal pain syndrome (CAPS), Centrally acting neuromodulators · Cognitive behavioral therapy (CBT) · Gut-directed hypnotherapy

Centrally Mediated Abdominal Pain Syndrome (CAPS)

Introduction

Renaming the Syndrome

Centrally mediated abdominal pain syndrome (CAPS) was formerly known as functional abdominal pain syndrome (FAPS) based on Rome III. By 2016 with the publication of Rome IV, it became apparent that the pain generated in this syndrome has a strong central component (Whorwell et al. 2016), more than in many of the other DGBIs. Consistent with this, with the

publication of Rome IV, the entirety of functional GI disorders was renamed to disorders of gut-brain interaction (DGBIs) based on the emerging scientific knowledge within neurogastroenterology that suggested gut-brain dysregulation played a significant role in symptom generation; this will be discussed later in the section on pathophysiology. Additionally, this new terminology is significantly less stigmatizing to the large patient population who suffer from chronic pain and other gastrointestinal disorders.

The Rome IV diagnostic criteria for CAPS can be found in Table 1 (Whorwell et al. 2016). The hallmark feature of CAPS is chronic pain as the predominant complaint with few or no other associated gastrointestinal complaints; thus the pain is unrelated to food intake or defecation. This distinguishes it from other DGBIs such as functional dyspepsia (FD) and irritable bowel syndrome (IBS). The pain is described as constant, near constant, or frequently recurrent for at least 6 months before the diagnosis (Keefer et al.

Table 1 Diagnostic criteria for centrally mediated abdominal pain syndrome (CAPS) (Whorwell et al. 2016)

Diagnostic criteria[a] for centrally mediated abdominal pain syndrome (CAPS)[b]	Must include all of the following:
	1. Continuous or nearly continuous abdominal pain
	2. No or only occasional relationship of pain with physiological events (i.e., eating, defecation, or menses)[c]
	3. Pain limits some aspect of daily functioning[d]
	4. The pain is not feigned
	5. Pain is not explained by another structural or functional gastrointestinal disorder or other medical condition

[a]Criteria fulfilled for the past 3 months with symptom onset at least 6 months before the diagnosis
[b]CAPS is typically associated with psychiatric comorbidity, but there is no specific profile that can be used for diagnosis
[c]Some degree of gastrointestinal dysfunction may be present
[d]Daily function could include impairments in work, intimacy, social/leisure, family life, and caregiving for self or others

2016). The pain cannot be explained by other structural or metabolic disorders within the gastrointestinal system or related findings attributed to other abdominal organs such as those of the reproductive and genitourinary systems. Furthermore, patients frequently describe their pain in "emotional" terms along with other somatic complaints related to fibromyalgia and chronic fatigue syndrome (Keefer et al. 2016). Psychological distress is an important risk factor in the development of DGBIs, and this distress can perpetuate or exacerbate pain; furthermore, there are mechanistic data to support a relationship between stress and increased pain reports via activation of CNS pain modulatory regions. Clinicians should recognize CAPS is often associated with a significant loss of quality of life.

Older adults, over the age of 65 years, present a unique challenge to clinicians in the realm of disorders of gut-brain interaction, especially centrally mediated abdominal pain syndrome. It is well established that pain thresholds are elevated in older adults; thus CAPS may present atypically. The diagnostic challenges in older patients can be clouded by presence of cognitive impairment or dementia, but a thorough set of differentials is considered later in this chapter. Furthermore, treatment may be challenging in older patients due to interactions of neuromodulators with other medications or limited by significant side effects; a thorough approach to the safe treatment of symptoms with neuromodulators and psychotherapy follows.

Epidemiology

While centrally mediated abdominal pain syndrome has been regarded as an uncommon condition, its prevalence has been difficult to elucidate due to lack of additional signs and symptoms to confirm this symptom-based diagnosis combined with an extensive group of differential diagnoses and limited diagnostic modalities available. The diagnosis of CAPS is relatively new in comparison with the other DGBIs, making retrospective chart and literature review challenging. Additionally, methods to report disease prevalence include collecting data from patient surveys which may overestimate symptoms or from members of the medical community who may dismiss CAPS as a disorder of "drug-seeking or malingering" behavior.

In a US householder survey using Rome I criteria, the self-reported prevalence of chronic abdominal pain was 2.2% (Drossman et al. 1993). As mentioned above, given the self-reported method of data collection, the true prevalence is likely lower. A large Canadian survey reported the prevalence of FAPS (now CAPS) at 0.5% (Thompson et al. 2002). In other countries, surveys detail similarly low rates of CAPS when patients with IBS are removed from the population due to a similarly overlapping constellation of symptoms.

Women more commonly report chronic abdominal pain than men in the US householder survey (Drossman et al. 1993), though rates are similarly reported in the Canadian study (Thompson et al. 2002). The prevalence of CAPS peaks in the fourth decade of life (35–44 years in the US householder survey) and declines with age (Drossman et al. 1993). It is unclear why the prevalence of CAPS declines with age. Patients with CAPS have high healthcare resource utilization, having visited a physician four times more frequently than people without abdominal pain (Drossman et al. 1993). In an Australian study, 75.9% of patients with CAPS consulted a physician, and half of them saw a physician 1 to 3 times per year (Koloski et al. 2002). In a UK-based study, CAPS patients required 5.7 consultant visits and 6.4 endoscopic or imaging exams and underwent 2.7 surgical interventions over a 7-year follow-up period (Maxton and Whorwell 1992).

Pathophysiology

As described above, the hallmark feature of CAPS is pain not associated with contribution from visceral or somatic factors; the International Association for the Study of Pain defines pain as "an unpleasant sensory and emotional experience associated with actual or potential tissue damage, or described in terms of such damage" (International Association for the Study of Pain IASP 2017). CAPS does not fit easily into the traditional categories of neuropathic or inflammatory pain, rather alterations in modulatory and motivational pain play a major role in both the generation and perpetuation of pain in CAPS. There have been no definitive neuropsychological or nerve studies reported in CAPS patients; thus most of the information provided here is derived from studies in patients with various other chronic pain syndromes.

The central nervous system receives input from the enteric nervous system that is combined with cognitive, emotional, and other sensory information for conscious interpretation. This central integration is thought to occur within the anterior insular cortex. Neuroimaging studies in irritable bowel syndrome (IBS) show abnormality in the central processing of pain signals with functional and structural abnormalities noted in sensory (mid-cingulate, insular, and somatosensory cortices, and thalamus), emotional arousal (anterior cingulate cortex, amygdala), and prefrontal cortical modulatory regions. Modulation of descending pain regulatory pathways in the brainstem by these cortical regions can lead to exaggerated sensitivity to both noxious and innocuous stimuli. The descending pain regulatory pathways (opioidergic and noradrenergic) originate in distinct brainstem regions and are activated in response to noxious stimuli. They modulate dorsal horn (spinal cord) excitability and can therefore determine how much of a peripheral afferent input from the gut can ascend to the brain.

It is thought that the phasic, physiological, and visceral afferent input from the gut plays a lesser role in symptom generation in CAPS when compared to IBS. In CAPS, altered visceral sensitivity appears to be less important as a trigger for chronic pain than behavioral factors associated with an exaggerated anticipatory response to potential pain. Thus, once central sensitization is established, symptoms of pain can persist in the absence of ongoing abnormal peripheral stimulation or can worsen with minimal stimulation. CAPS can thus be characterized by alterations in descending pain modulation from the brainstem; it has been speculated that patients with chronic pain syndromes may have compromised ability to activate inhibitory controls from the brainstem. In effect, in patients with CAPS, there is greater central disinhibition or a failure of the CNS to downregulate incoming visceral signals to a greater degree than increased afferent (visceral) signaling. This has implications for treatment targets focused on central rather than peripheral, or visceral gut-related, targets.

Psychology of Abdominal Pain

Psychological distress is an important factor in the development of disorders of gut-brain interaction. When considering abdominal pain burden in the general population, both anxiety and depression independently predict pain reporting, particularly in women (Walter et al. 2013). Similarly, veterans who screen positive for post-traumatic stress disorder (PTSD) are more likely to report abdominal pain even after controlling for depression, age, injury, and gender (Moeller-Bertram et al. 2014).

Anxiety may worsen the impairment associated with CAPS as it manifests in uncontrollable worry around the meaning of abdominal pain. This tends to perpetuate anxiety and pain symptoms. Inflexible problem-solving, which often drives worry, has been noted in patients with DGBIs (Cheng et al. 2000). This highlights patients' (with DGBIs) inability to use a healthy range of coping skills. There is strong empirical support for the importance of pain catastrophizing (Leung 2012), fear-avoidance behavior (Esteve and Ramirez-Maestre 2013), self-efficacy (Saunders 2004), lack of perceived control (Muller et al. 2012), and passive pain coping (McCracken and Eccleston 2003) on pain experience. This highlights the potential use of psychological interventions for the management of CAPS.

Evaluation of the Patient

Medical History

Taking a thorough history and performing a detailed physical examination remain the cornerstone of diagnosis for CAPS where pain is the central feature. Asking open-ended questions will allow the patient to detail their pain more elaborately and feel their concerns are heard.

This approach, however, may make it challenging for the clinician to tease out the patient's most bothersome symptoms. A useful strategy to understand the most salient features of the history is to correlate patients' nonverbal cues with the history obtained through interview; this is helpful especially in older patients who experience a higher pain threshold and may not be able to reliably express signs or symptoms of underlying disease processes. Drossman has published extensively on patient communication and emphasizes the positive impact of good communication skills which can, in turn, improve disclosure of meaningful information, promote greater patient adherence, reduce symptom severity and emotional distress, and improve psychological parameters and better overall clinical outcomes (Drossman 2013).

It is of utmost importance to ascertain the duration of the patient's painful symptoms; the pain of CAPS is long-standing, whereas acute abdominal pain has a different approach to history taking, diagnostic evaluation, and therapy. Additionally, looking for "red flag" or "alarm" features including unintentional weight loss, nausea with vomiting, change in bowel habits including diarrhea, presence of blood in the stool, and new onset of symptoms in the elderly is a key component to a thorough medical history.

Emotional terms, for example, "agonizing," "unbearable," and "like a knife stabbing from the inside," are often the key descriptors of the pain character and intensity in CAPS; this relates to the central nervous system's contribution to the pain experience (Whorwell et al. 2016). The location of the pain is not precise, rather encompassing a large anatomic region; it is often described as constant, nearly constant, or frequently recurring. The pain is not, or is less commonly, associated with eating or bowel movements. The pain is often associated with loss of daily functioning, for example, absenteeism from work. Finally, patients with pain characteristic of CAPS often complain of other painful extraintestinal conditions including fibromyalgia. Many patients with CAPS also fulfill diagnostic criteria for the comorbid psychological diagnoses of anxiety, depression, and somatization;

however, patients with CAPS frequently do not associate these diagnoses with their pain. Clinicians should feel comfortable to ask patients a detailed history of potential psychosocial contributors to pain including sensitive questions regarding sexual history and history of abuse as well as of eating disorders.

A unique feature of the history, especially in older adults, is that a family's interaction with the patient can have a major impact on illness. A spouse or child may assume responsibility for reporting the patient's history. This can interrupt the patient's own narrative or redirect the discussion away from a key area and subsequently lead the patient to passively withdraw from the interview. While the family member's contribution to the interview may reflect concern and a desire to be involved in healthcare for their elderly family member, it may interfere with implementing an effective diagnostic and treatment strategy for the patient.

Physical Exam

Important information can be obtained with a thorough physical examination. Once again, it is especially useful to correlate a patient's nonverbal cues, for example, their ability to move around the exam room or onto the examination table, with reports of "severe, constant pain." Evaluation of vital signs may reveal "alarm" features such as fever, tachycardia, or hypertension which are more suggestive of either an acute or alternate cause of pain. A visual inspection of the abdominal wall may reveal numerous surgical scars, suggestive of a long history of pain leading to often unnecessary surgical procedures or rash indicative of herpes zoster infection (this may be misleading if the rash has not yet become evident or has resolved but the pain is in the same dermatomal distribution, thus suggesting postherpetic neuralgia). Jaundice in the setting of abdominal pain may indicate biliary pathology. Ecchymoses in unusual locations, such as on the abdominal wall or flanks, should raise the clinician's suspicion for falls or abuse. The patient should be asked to point to the location of greatest pain with one finger; the inability to do so in CAPS is aligned with evidence of a disorder of gut-brain interaction.

Auscultation of the abdomen can elucidate a bruit suggestive of vascular insufficiency. Palpation may reveal a "closed-eyes sign" in which the patient with CAPS winces with eyes closed, opposite to that of a patient with acute abdominal pain who keeps his eyes open in fearful anticipation of the examination (Whorwell et al. 2016). Masses including pulsatile aortic aneurysm, guarding, tenderness, and organ abnormalities may be palpated. Particularly painful areas, whether from visceral etiology or more superficial pathologies such as musculoskeletal or dermatologic diagnoses, may be elucidated as well. Evaluation for abdominal wall pain by assessing for the presence of Carnett's sign should be a standard feature of the abdominal physical examination. Carnett's sign is evaluated by extending the thighs while raising the head to the chest to contract abdominal musculature; a positive Carnett's sign indicates the etiology of abdominal pain is secondary to the abdominal wall, where the pain is increased with rectus contraction. A negative or absent Carnett's sign would imply visceral pain; however, like the "closed-eyes sign," patients with CAPS may indicate pain is worse with contraction of the rectus muscles out of attribution that pain may worsen with increased abdominal muscle tension. The remainder of the physical examination should focus on evaluation for other pathology which may lead to abdominal pain. Keep in mind that the physical exam may be limited by the presence of cognitive impairment or dementia in the elderly or the administration of pain medication, which may mask response to pain.

Diagnostics

Diagnostic testing in patients with chronic abdominal pain syndrome should be limited to rule out organic etiologies of pain as suggested by the history and physical exam. As mentioned above, "red flag" or "alarm" features should trigger additional evaluation with routine laboratory testing to rule out inflammation and evidence of GI blood loss. Imaging should be obtained in patients who may have underlying vascular disease, bowel obstruction, or unintentional weight loss. Endoscopic and colonoscopic evaluation should be reserved for patients with evidence of GI blood loss.

In the absence of "alarm" features or diagnostic abnormalities on laboratory, imaging, or endoscopic examinations, the diagnosis of CAPS is highly likely if the diagnostic criteria are met. Pursuing unnecessary testing will instill a notion to the patient and patient's family that a diagnosis is being missed and may encourage a patient to seek care elsewhere. Rather, it is important for the clinician to reinforce that CAPS is the most likely diagnosis and that additional testing will not add to or change a diagnosis and the focus should shift away from investigation to treatment and management of bothersome symptoms.

Differential Diagnoses

For the most part, the diagnostic evaluations do not differ in the older population compared to the younger cohort; there are, however, some key differences related to the differential diagnoses. Abdominal pain in the elderly with higher pain thresholds, where pain is present for up to a few weeks, may represent the subacute onset of potentially life-threatening conditions such as myocardial infarction, pneumonia, small bowel obstruction (especially in those with prior abdominal surgery), appendicitis, diverticulitis, or even perforation with peritonitis. As mentioned, auscultation for bruit is helpful to elucidate presence of abdominal aneurysm and especially in the older population, vascular compromise leading to chronic mesenteric ischemia. This should be considered if the patient offers a history of postprandial abdominal pain, sitophobia, and weight loss. Internal hernias, for example, Spigelian hernia, in addition to sigmoid or other gastrointestinal volvulus, may present with subacute abdominal pain. Change in bowel habits with concurrent abdominal pain may represent an advanced and atypical presentation of colorectal or other gastrointestinal malignancy. Pelvic pain may implicate urogynecological diseases (such as pyelonephritis or abscess); in older women, any abnormal gynecological bleeding should be considered as an "alarm" feature, and a thorough gynecological evaluation should be pursued. Furthermore, presence of uterine or ovarian gynecologic malignancy may present with abdominal pain and bloating. As mentioned in the physical examination section above, abdominal wall pain due to entrapment of an anterior cutaneous branch of one or more thoracic intercostal nerves may be elucidated by the presence of Carnett's sign. Finally, other disorders of gut-brain interaction should be considered especially if pain is intermittent and modified by eating or defecation, for example, in irritable bowel syndrome or if the pain is predominantly located in the epigastrium such as in functional dyspepsia or right upper quadrant as in biliary disease.

If the medical history and physical exam do not correlate, the clinician's level of suspicion for feigned pain should be raised. A factitious disorder or malingering relates to false or grossly exaggerated symptoms with the intention of secondary gain. Feigned pain, in addition to physical abuse, may be suspected in the older population especially in the presence of strained family or caretaker dynamics.

Treatment

General Principles of Treatment

The management of CAPS can be challenging but is founded most importantly on an effective patient-physician relationship, as shown in Fig. 1 (Whorwell et al. 2016). Following a treatment plan where setting clear and realistic treatment goals and basing treatment decisions on symptom severity is pivotal. Patients must be ready to enter a therapeutic relationship with a clinician in which the patient shares in the responsibility; creating continuity of care is paramount to a successful therapeutic relationship. The clinician should listen actively, offer empathy, ask open-ended questions with matching body language, validate the patient's feelings, educate the patients about their condition, and maintain boundaries (Keefer et al. 2016; Drossman 2013). Perhaps one of the most underestimated features of entering into a mutually beneficial therapeutic relationship with patients is that these patients are not necessarily looking for a cure as much as wanting their clinician to listen, show interest and concern, to not abandon them, and to offer support and a sense of hope (Drossman 2013). The management approach should further encompass a

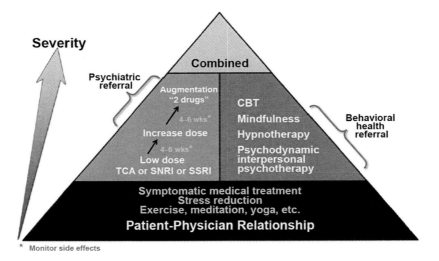

Fig. 1 Management of CAPS relies on a strong patient-physician relationship, early incorporation of behavioral health strategies, pharmacologic therapies, and referral to mental health specialists when appropriate. (Permission obtained from Douglas A. Drossman for reprint Keefer et al. 2016)

combination of options including stress reduction techniques and exercise, behavioral health, pharmacologic therapies, and referral to a mental health provider if needed.

Centrally Acting Neuromodulators

Clinical studies for pharmacologic therapies in CAPS are limited, so treatment recommendations are extrapolated from studies pertaining to other disorders of gut-brain interaction. Antidepressants, particularly those which target serotonin and norepinephrine, are helpful in treating chronic painful disorders; they are also useful to treat comorbid depression. The basis for prescription of this class of medications is to reduce afferent signals from the gut and to downregulate incoming visceral pain signals going to the central nervous system. A newer understanding of the role of these medications in patients with chronic pain relates to CNS neuroplasticity and the value of these agents in promoting neurogenesis. There has been a strong relationship between degree of improvement in

severe depression and levels of brain-derived neurotrophic factor (BDNF), a precursor of brain neuronal growth (Brunoni et al. 2008). This would suggest that patients with chronic abdominal pain can benefit from antidepressants for symptom improvement but also for re-establishment of neuronal functioning to recover pain regulation. It also raises the hypothesis that neurogenesis may occur in the enteric nervous system as well as in the CNS (Drossman 2009).

In the older population with chronic abdominal pain syndrome, it is important to consider what other medications the patient is already prescribed and the potential interactions the following therapies may have. Furthermore, the relatively benign side effect profile of many of these medications may be exaggerated or intolerable in older patients, though interestingly, the side effects most commonly reported after initiation of pharmacotherapy for DGBIs relates to concurrent anxiety rather than true side effects from the medications themselves (Drossman 2009). Table 2 details some important features of the pharmacotherapies described below.

Table 2 Centrally acting neuromodulators, their mechanisms of action, clinical indications, side effect profiles, and dosage for treatment of patients with CAPS (Drossman et al. 2018)

Drug class	Mechanism of action	Clinical indication	Side effects	Drugs/dose
Tricyclic antidepressants	Presynaptic serotonin and norepinephrine reuptake inhibition. Inhibition of postsynaptic 5-HT$_2$, 5-HT$_3$, H$_1$, M1, α_1 and presynaptic α_2 receptors	Chronic abdominal pain; best documented for IBS but also epigastric pain syndrome	Drowsiness, xerostomia, constipation, sexual dysfunction, arrhythmia, weight gain	Amitriptyline, imipramine, desipramine, nortriptyline. 25–100 (–150) mg qd
Serotonin and norepinephrine reuptake inhibitors	Presynaptic serotonin and norepinephrine reuptake inhibition	Extrapolated data for abdominal pain based on data for fibromyalgia, headache, and back pain	Nausea, fatigue, agitation, dizziness, liver dysfunction	Duloxetine (30–90 mg qd), milnacipran (50–100 mg bid), venlafaxine (for pain 150–225 mg qd)
Selective serotonin reuptake inhibitors	Presynaptic serotonin reuptake inhibition	Anxiety, phobias, obsessive-compulsive disorder in patients with CAPS	Diarrhea, insomnia, agitation, headaches, weight loss, sexual dysfunction	Citalopram (10–40 mg qd), escitalopram (5–20 mg qd), fluoxetine (10–40 mg qd), paroxetine (10–40 mg qd), sertraline (50–150 mg qd)
Atypical antipsychotics	D$_2$ receptor antagonism. Various 5-HT$_{2A}$ antagonism, 5-HT$_{1A}$ agonism, H$_1$, α_1, α_2, M1 receptor antagonism	Augmentation for abdominal pain and improved sleep in those with CAPS	Sedation, dizziness, weight gain leading to hyperlipidemia and diabetes	Aripiprazole (2.5–7.5 mg qd), quetiapine (25–200 mg qd)

Tricyclic antidepressants (TCAs; amitriptyline, nortriptyline, desipramine, doxepin, and trimipramine) are commonly used to treat chronic pain conditions, for example, fibromyalgia, postherpetic neuralgia, and diabetic neuropathy. The dose administered for pain control is typically much lower than that needed to achieve antidepressant effects, suggesting that the analgesic effect of TCAs is unrelated to the antidepressant effect. A study by Halpert and colleagues suggested that in IBS, improvement in pain with desipramine was not related to blood levels of medication dose (Halpert et al. 2005). In a recent meta-analysis, 186 (42.7%) of 436 patients assigned to receive TCA therapy reported unimproved IBS symptoms compared with 224 (63.8%) of 351 allocated to placebo; this suggests a relative risk of no improvement in IBS symptoms of 0.65 and a calculated number needed to treat of 4.5 (Ford et al. 2019). One can conclude that therapy with TCAs is therefore effective in the treatment of IBS. The most common side effects related to TCA use are due to anticholinergic and antihistaminic properties and include sedation, constipation, urinary retention, xerostomia, and hypotension; these side effects often limit the utility of TCAs in the elderly population. Due to TCA effects on cardiac sodium channels, baseline EKG should be checked, and patients should be advised on the overdose potential of these medications.

Selective serotonin-norepinephrine reuptake inhibitors (SNRIs; duloxetine, venlafaxine, desvenlafaxine, and milnacipran) are increasingly being used to treat chronic painful conditions in addition to their use in treatment of depression. There have been no studies looking at the effects of SNRIs on improvement of CAPS symptoms (Törnblom and Drossman 2018), but their theoretical use has been proven anecdotally. Dose ranges vary based on level of norepinephrine reuptake inhibition. For example, duloxetine can be used at usual dose ranges, but venlafaxine requires higher doses (at least 200 mg/day) because the norepinephrine effect does not occur in lower doses. SNRIs have relatively few side effects compared with TCAs; most commonly nausea is described which subsides after the first few weeks of use. We favor the use of SNRIs over

TCAs in the older population with CAPS due to the more favorable side effect profile.

Selective serotonin reuptake inhibitors (SSRIs) do not have as robust of an analgesic effect when compared to TCAs and SNRIs due to their lack of norepinephrine reuptake inhibition. This class of medications should be reserved for patients where anxiety, depression, or psychological impairment is a significant contributor to symptoms. Doses used are typical for the doses used to treat concurrent depression or anxiety (Törnblom and Drossman 2018). 45.5% of patients (80 of 176) assigned to receive SSRI therapy for IBS reported unimproved symptoms following therapy compared to 67.2% of patients (121 of 180) allocated to placebo with a RR of no improvement in symptoms of 0.68; this yields a number needed to treat of 5 (Ford et al. 2019). Again, this suggests SSRIs appear to be at least somewhat effective in the treatment of IBS. Side effects of SSRIs include nausea and diarrhea in addition to sexual dysfunction.

Atypical antipsychotics should be considered in patients with CAPS refractory to usual pharmacologic therapy with SNRIs or TCAs or in those elderly patients where use of these first-line agents is limited. Quetiapine has been most extensively studied for use in other chronic painful conditions such as migraine headaches and fibromyalgia due to its complex mechanism of action involving norepinephrine reuptake inhibition (Törnblom and Drossman 2018). In two studies, quetiapine has been shown to be superior to placebo to improve pain in fibromyalgia (McIntyre et al. 2014) but inferior to amitriptyline (Calandre et al. 2014) and in another study was shown to have benefit when added to a TCA or SNRI for treatment of refractory gastrointestinal pain (Grover et al. 2009). In a 2009 pilot study of a small group of patients with severe DGBIs (which can represent up to 20% of patients with DGBIs), over half of the patients who remained on quetiapine experienced marked improvement in their overall functioning, coping skills, sleep, and mood (Grover et al. 2009). However, given its complex mechanism of action and effects on multiple other neurotransmitters, it is often used as augmentation therapy at low doses (25–100 mg) in conjunction with other neuromodulators. It does, however, have the potential to cause extrapyramidal symptoms, sedation, and weight gain. Furthermore, there is a relative contraindication to using atypical antipsychotics such as quetiapine in the elderly with comorbid dementia due to elevated risk of cerebrovascular complications including stroke.

Other pharmacologic therapies which have been shown to have benefit in patients with chronic abdominal pain are a subset of peripherally acting medications. These include the delta ligand agents pregabalin and gabapentin, the tetracyclic antidepressant mirtazapine, aripiprazole, and the anticonvulsants carbamazepine and lamotrigine.

Psychotherapy

It is well established that the biopsychosocial model for management of chronic pain should be at the forefront of the clinician's mind when investigating patients with chronic abdominal pain. Psychological factors can amplify the experience of pain. The discovery of psychological underpinnings to a patient's pain complaints can often be targeted with specific psychological therapies. The use of psychotherapies targets functional areas such as coping, reappraising maladaptive cognition, and cognitively adapting to loss and trauma. Brain imaging studies have shown that psychological interventions work in the prefrontal or cognitive areas (Goldapple et al. 2004), whereas antidepressants work in subcortical areas such as the anterior cingulate cortex and insula to improve connectivity to prefrontal and other cortical areas. One of the primary advantages of behavioral therapies is that the clinician then eliminates the risk of polypharmacy or medication side effects from pharmacotherapy described above. There is no evidence to suggest that the older population with DGBIs are any less likely to respond to or benefit from psychological therapies compared to younger patients.

The current psychotherapies that have shown relevance to CAPS include cognitive behavioral therapy (CBT), hypnosis, and more recently, mindfulness-based behavioral interventions. A recent meta-analysis demonstrated a relative risk of no improvement in global IBS symptoms with the use of psychological therapies at 0.69 with a number needed to treat of 4 (Ford et al. 2019). This data suggest that CBT, relaxation therapy, multicomponent psychological therapy, hypnotherapy, and dynamic psychotherapy were all more effective than placebo or controls in the treatment of IBS (Ford et al. 2019).

Cognitive behavioral therapy is a commonly employed technique for treatment of disorders of gut brain interaction with the most robust data in IBS as well as other painful conditions such as fibromyalgia. It assumes that specific skills deficits lead to maladaptive behaviors and that these behaviors can be remediated through practical, short-term skills-based interventions. The first component of CBT involves psychoeducation where patients learn how to gain control over their pain and how various cognitive processes and behaviors alter the pain experience. The second component includes skills training where the psychologist teaches relaxation exercises (e.g., diaphragmatic breathing or progressive muscle relaxation), setting pace, and distraction techniques, among others. The final component of CBT is challenging negative or maladaptive thoughts including pain catastrophizing and unhelpful worry. A similar intervention also studied for patients with IBS, psychodynamic interpersonal therapy (PIT), focuses on an individual's emotional state rather than his thought process in CBT (Guthrie et al. 1991).

Gut-directed hypnotherapy has proven efficacy to improve symptoms of IBS, though may be less effective for patients with CAPS. In patients with CAPS, hypnotherapy has been shown to improve negative cognition and improve anxiety and depression.

Mindfulness-based stress reduction (MBSR), developed by Jon Kabat-Zinn, strives to improve one's ability to regulate attention toward what is happening in the moment without interpretation of the events, thoughts, or feelings (Kabat-Zinn 1982). Kabat-Zinn's approach allows the patient to separate the sensation of pain from their response by accepting the pain as it is. This allows the patient to reduce negative emotions or fears which often serve to amplify the pain.

Other Interventions

Many patients choose to seek nontraditional approaches to obtain relief from bothersome symptoms. In the elderly population especially, patients may be accustomed to certain anecdotal practices for relief of pain, may be fearful of potential side effects or interactions with pharmacotherapy, and may be unwilling to engage in psychological therapies due to the time they require. In general, these peripherally based treatment approaches are not as helpful but may be used especially in conjunction with the therapies described above. It is relevant for the clinician to consider these alternate approaches as they allow the patient to feel they have gained some control over their symptoms and that the clinician understands the patient's point of view on treatment strategies. Acupuncture has shown conflicting results in several clinical trials in the control of gastrointestinal pain (Lembo et al. 2009). Yoga has shown clear benefit to patients with IBS-related abdominal pain (Schumann et al. 2016). Finally, the use of heat pads or wraps is commonly seen in patients with gastrointestinal pain, but there are no studies to support this.

Key Points

- Chronic abdominal pain syndrome (CAPS) should be distinguished from irritable bowel syndrome (IBS) and other disorder of gut-brain interaction as it is characterized primarily by pain which is not modified by eating or defecation.
- CAPS is an underrecognized entity among the disorders of gut-brain interaction.
- Patients with CAPS are thought to have alterations in descending pain modulation and compromised ability to activate inhibitory controls from the brainstem.
- Psychological distress is an important factor in the development of chronic abdominal pain syndrome.

- A careful medical history and physical examination should be performed by clinicians in an elderly population where history may be masked by family members or patients with dementia and physical examination can indicate alternate diagnoses.
- The biopsychosocial model should guide clinicians to develop a strong therapeutic relationship with patients who suffer from CAPS.
- Pharmacotherapy with centrally acting neuromodulators and psychological therapies are the mainstay of treatment for CAPS.
- Older adults may be unwilling or unable to take centrally acting neuromodulators due to side effects or interactions with other medications.
- Elderly patients may be unable to participate in psychological interventions due to limitations of cognition, time, or ability to see trained mental health professionals.

References

Brunoni AR, Lopes M, Fregni F. A systematic review and meta-analysis of clinical studies on major depression and BDNF levels: implications for the role of neuroplasticity in depression. Int J Neuropsychopharmacol. 2008;11(8):1169–80.

Calandre EP, Rico-Villademoros F, Galan J, Molina-Barea R, Vilchez JS, Rodriguez-Lopez CM, et al. Quetiapine extended-release (Seroquel-XR) versus amitriptyline monotherapy for treating patients with fibromyalgia: a 16-week, randomized, flexible-dose, open-label trial. Psychopharmacology. 2014;231(12):2525–31.

Cheng C, Hui W, Lam S. Perceptual style and behavioral pattern of individuals with functional gastrointestinal disorders. Health Psychol. 2000;19(2):146–54.

Drossman DA. Beyond tricyclics: new ideas for treating patients with painful and refractory functional gastrointestinal symptoms. Am J Gastroenterol. 2009;104(12):2897–902.

Drossman DA. 2012 David sun lecture: helping your patient by helping yourself – how to improve the patient-physician relationship by optimizing communication skills. Am J Gastroenterol. 2013;108(4):521–8.

Drossman DA, Li Z, Andruzzi E, Temple RD, Talley NJ, Thompson WG, et al. U.S. householder survey of functional gastrointestinal disorders. Prevalence, sociodemography, and health impact. Dig Dis Sci. 1993;38(9):1569–80.

Drossman DA, Tack J, Ford AC, Szigethy E, Tornblom H, Van Oudenhove L. Neuromodulators for functional gastrointestinal disorders (Disorders of Gut-Brain

Interaction): a Rome foundation working team report. Gastroenterology. 2018;154(4):1140–71.e1.

Esteve R, Ramirez-Maestre C. Pain fear avoidance and pain acceptance: a cross-sectional study comparing their influence on adjustment to chronic pain across three samples of patients. Ann Behav Med. 2013;46(2):169–80.

Ford AC, Lacy BE, Harris LA, Quigley EMM, Moayyedi P. Effect of antidepressants and psychological therapies in irritable bowel syndrome: an updated systematic review and meta-analysis. Am J Gastroenterol. 2019;114(1):21–39.

Goldapple K, Segal Z, Garson C, Lau M, Bieling P, Kennedy S, et al. Modulation of cortical-limbic pathways in major depression: treatment-specific effects of cognitive behavior therapy. Arch Gen Psychiatry. 2004;61(1):34–41.

Grover M, Dorn SD, Weinland SR, Dalton CB, Gaynes BN, Drossman DA. Atypical antipsychotic quetiapine in the management of severe refractory functional gastrointestinal disorders. Dig Dis Sci. 2009;54(6):1284–91.

Guthrie E, Creed F, Dawson D, Tomenson B. A controlled trial of psychological treatment for the irritable bowel syndrome. Gastroenterology. 1991;100(2):450–7.

Halpert A, Dalton CB, Diamant NE, Toner BB, Hu Y, Morris CB, et al. Clinical response to tricyclic antidepressants in functional bowel disorders is not related to dosage. Am J Gastroenterol. 2005;100(3):664–71.

International Association for the Study of Pain IASP. Terminology. Washington, DC: International Association for the Study of Pain; 2017. Updated 14 Dec 2017. Available from: https://www.iasp-pain.org/terminology?navItemNumber=576#Pain

Kabat-Zinn J. An outpatient program in behavioral medicine for chronic pain patients based on the practice of mindfulness meditation: theoretical considerations and preliminary results. Gen Hosp Psychiatry. 1982;4(1): 33–47.

Keefer L, Drossman DA, Guthrie E, Simren M, Tillisch K, Olden K, et al. Centrally mediated disorders of gastrointestinal pain. Gastroenterology. 2016;150:1408.

Koloski NA, Talley NJ, Boyce PM. Epidemiology and health care seeking in the functional GI disorders: a population-based study. Am J Gastroenterol. 2002;97(9):2290–9.

Lembo AJ, Conboy L, Kelley JM, Schnyer RS, McManus CA, Quilty MT, et al. A treatment trial of acupuncture in IBS patients. Am J Gastroenterol. 2009;104(6): 1489–97.

Leung L. Pain catastrophizing: an updated review. Indian J Psychol Med. 2012;34(3):204–17.

Maxton D, Whorwell P. Use of medical resources and attitudes to health care of patients with "chronic abdominal pain". Br J Med Econ. 1992;2:75–9.

McCracken LM, Eccleston C. Coping or acceptance: what to do about chronic pain? Pain. 2003;105(1–2): 197–204.

McIntyre A, Paisley D, Kouassi E, Gendron A. Quetiapine fumarate extended-release for the treatment of major depression with comorbid fibromyalgia syndrome: a double-blind, randomized, placebo-controlled study. Arthritis Rheumatol (Hoboken). 2014;66(2):451–61.

Moeller-Bertram T, Afari N, Mostoufi S, Fink DS, Johnson Wright L, Baker DG. Specific pain complaints in Iraq and Afghanistan veterans screening positive for post-traumatic stress disorder. Psychosomatics. 2014;55(2):172–8.

Muller L, Korsgaard H, Ethelberg S. Burden of acute gastrointestinal illness in Denmark 2009: a population-based telephone survey. Epidemiol Infect. 2012;140(2):290–8.

Saunders D. Coping with chronic pain: what can we learn from pain self-efficacy beliefs? J Rheumatol. 2004;31(6):1032–4.

Schumann D, Anheyer D, Lauche R, Dobos G, Langhorst J, Cramer H. Effect of yoga in the therapy of irritable bowel syndrome: a systematic review. Clin Gastroenterol Hepatol. 2016;14(12):1720–31.

Thompson WG, Irvine EJ, Pare P, Ferrazzi S, Rance L. Functional gastrointestinal disorders in Canada: first population-based survey using Rome II criteria with suggestions for improving the questionnaire. Dig Dis Sci. 2002;47(1):225–35.

Törnblom H, Drossman DA. Psychotropics, antidepressants, and visceral analgesics in functional gastrointestinal disorders. Curr Gastroenterol Rep. 2018;20(12): 58.

Walter SA, Jones MP, Talley NJ, Kjellstrom L, Nyhlin H, Andreasson AN, et al. Abdominal pain is associated with anxiety and depression scores in a sample of the general adult population with no signs of organic gastrointestinal disease. Neurogastroenterology and motility: the official journal of the European gastrointestinal motility. Society. 2013;25(9):741–e576.

Whorwell PJ, Keefer L, Drossman D, Guthrie E, Simren M, Tillisch K, et al. Centrally mediated disorders of gastrointestinal pain. IV ed. Drossman DA, Chang L, Chey WD, Kellow J, Tack J, Whitehead WE, editors. Raleigh: Rome Foundation; 2016.

Gas, Belching, Bloating, and Flatulence: Pathogenesis, Evaluation, and Management

C. S. Pitchumoni, Debra R. Goldstein, and Cynthia L. Vuittonet

Contents

C. S. Pitchumoni
Department of Medicine, Robert Wood Johnson School of Medicine, Rutgers University, New Brunswick, NJ, USA

Department of Medicine, New York Medical College, Valhalla, NY, USA

Division of Gastroenterology, Hepatology and Clinical Nutrition, Saint Peters University Hospital, New Brunswick, NJ, USA
e-mail: pitchumoni@hotmail.com

D. R. Goldstein (✉)
Department of Gastroenterology, Saint Peters University Hospital, New Brunswick, NJ, USA

Rutgers University School of Medicine, New Brunswick, NJ, USA
e-mail: dgoldstein@saintpetersuh.com

C. L. Vuittonet
Director of Addiction Medicine, Jewish Renaissance Medical Center, Perth Amboy, NJ, USA
e-mail: cvuittonet@gmail.com

© Springer Nature Switzerland AG 2021
C. S. Pitchumoni, T. S. Dharmarajan (eds.), *Geriatric Gastroenterology*,
https://doi.org/10.1007/978-3-030-30192-7_44

Abstract

Over the past 10 years, there has been a development of criteria that defines functional gastrointestinal disorders and the significance of their symptoms based on motility disturbance, visceral hypersensitivity, altered mucosal and immune function, altered gut microbiota, and altered central nervous system processing. The gastrointestinal manifestations related to these functional disorders are belching, bloating, and food intolerance. The topic of food intolerance is an extensive one and difficult to study properly. The major components of food intolerance that contribute to clinical symptoms are lactose, fructose, sorbitol, and high FODMAPs (fermentable oligosaccharides, disaccharides, monosaccharides, and polyols). In the older adult, prior to considering their symptoms as functional, it is crucial to evaluate the patient for alarm symptoms as these functional symptoms may be due to organic disease.

Keywords

Belching · Bloating · Flatus/flatulence · Nitrogen · Oxygen · Carbon dioxide · Hydrogen · Methane · Abdominal distention · Visceral hypersensitivity · Rapid intestinal transit · Bacterial fermentation · Short-chain fatty acids · Lactose intolerance · Fructose intolerance · Disaccharidase deficiency · Oligosaccharide · Raffinose · Stachyose · Legume · Maldigestion · Malabsorption · IBS · SIBO · Hydrogen breath testing · Probiotic · Prokinetic · a-galactosidase · B-galactosidase

Introduction

For millennia, physicians and laypersons alike have been intrigued by intestinal gas. The topic of gaseousness, familiar to all, has not always been afforded proper scientific respect. In the past century, though, many analyses have been made of the physiology and composition of intestinal gas (Kalantar-Zadeh et al. 2019). These intestinal gases have been identified as carbon dioxide, hydrogen, methane, and sulfur-containing compounds. They are generated by the chemical and metabolic actions of the gut microbiota via fermentation of undigested dietary substances in the colon.

In the last 10 years, there has been an increased focus on gaseousness and the clinical, nutritional, and pathophysiological implications. There are three recent areas of research exploring the clinical symptoms that arise from gaseousness. The first area of research was established by the Rome III criteria which culminated in the definition of functional gastrointestinal disorders and clarified the clinical significance of functional symptoms in the absence of structural disease (Drossman 2006). The more recent Rome IV criteria expanded upon this concept and separated the group of functional disorders based on gastrointestinal symptoms: motility disturbance, visceral hypersensitivity, altered mucosal and immune function, altered gut microbiota, and altered central nervous system processing (Drossman and Hasler 2016). The second advance is the exploration of the gut microbiota and the implications that it has on health and disease

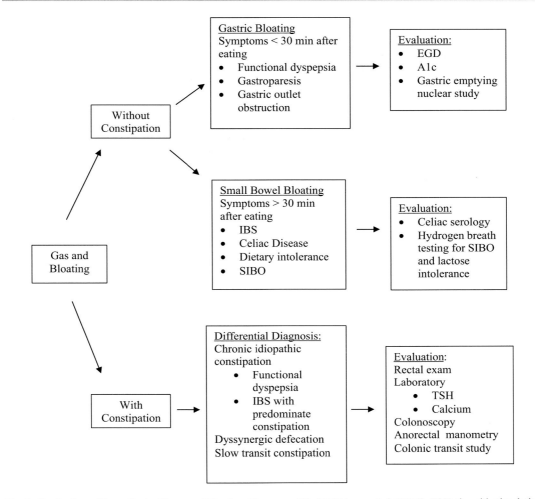

Fig. 1 Evaluation of the patient with gas and bloating. Figure modified Wilkinson et al. (2019). TSH, thyroid-stimulating hormone; A1c, hemoglobin A1c as a marker of diabetes

(Collins 2014). The third advance relates to the management of functional gastrointestinal disorders, particularly the role that undigested carbohydrates play on the gut (Scaldaferri et al. 2013).

This chapter will discuss the pathogenesis, evaluation, and management of gaseousness as it pertains to the elderly population (Fig. 1). This chapter will first discuss the physiology of intestinal gases. Then we will give a brief overview of the passage of gas through the various segments of the intestinal tract, followed by a review of the components of intestinal gas. Attention will then

be turned to common clinical gastrointestinal syndromes, to associated topics in the field of gas, and to problems unique to older people, to provide insights into medical management options.

Background

The major symptoms of gas are abdominal bloating and belching or eructation (Simrén 2009). These symptoms may occur with or without vague chronic symptoms of abdominal pain or altered bowel habits. The symptoms can sometimes flare and cause significant distress to patients. Often the manifestations are related to functional gastrointestinal disorders (FGID) and historically are not evaluated by many diagnostic studies (Weinberg 1998). There used to be a notion that FGID is a diagnosis of exclusion, but it is not. Often the practicing gastroenterologist performs diagnostic testing if alarm symptoms are present (Table 1) (Weinberg 1998; Wilkinson et al. 2019). However, older age alone can be considered alarming and warrant diagnostic testing to exclude organic disorders that require prompt treatment. Anyone of the three, belching, bloating, and flatulence, or a combination of one or more carries with it a unique pathophysiology, either organic or functional and differing implications for management.

The management of intestinal gas in the geriatric population is even more challenging than in the younger population (Almario et al. 2017). Communication of complaints may be compromised due to cognitive impairments. Signs and symptoms are frequently the result of both polypharmacy and underlying chronic illnesses. In the older population, pharmacologic intervention may be limited by a greater proclivity to untoward effects. Therefore, it is appropriate that this topic is reviewed in a text dedicated to geriatrics, with proper attention given to factors in the older

population that complicate diagnosis and treatment.

Gas in the Gastrointestinal Tract

Physiology of Intestinal Gas

Intestinal gas can affect gut physiology and ultimately contribute to symptoms. Prior to understanding the clinical implications from gaseousness, it is crucial to have an understanding of the physiology of gas. The predominate intestinal gases are nitrogen (N_2), carbon dioxide (CO_2), hydrogen (H_2), and methane CH_4, The composition of flatus is variable influenced by the composition of diet and gut microbiota (Kalantar-Zadeh et al. 2019; Azpiroz and Levitt 2010). In the colon, most of the oxygen is removed, and the amount of carbon dioxide is increased. *Methane production is confined to the colon, and most of it is absorbed into the portal blood for delivery to the lungs* (Table 2).

Nitrogen

The act of swallowing air introduces atmospheric air into the gastrointestinal system. The nitrogen (N_2) content of the GI tract approximates that of swallowed air, with only a small amount sourced by bacterial metabolism (Tomlin et al. 1991). Nitrogen is a relatively insoluble gas and diffuses poorly from the gut. Diffusion of N_2 will occur if

Table 1 Alarming symptoms that should prompt further evaluation for potentially serious causes of gas, bloating, and belching (Wilkinson et al. 2019)

Alarm symptoms
Acute abdominal pain associated with bloating
Abdominal mass
Dysphagia
Extreme diarrhea symptoms
Fever
Family history of colon, gastric, ovarian, or pancreatic cancer
Gastrointestinal bleeding
Jaundice
Lymphadenopathy
New-onset symptoms in patients 55 years and older
Odynophagia
Tenesmus
Unintentional weight loss
Vomiting

Table 2 Composition and sources of intestinal gas

	Location	Composition	Source
Belching	Supragastric Gastric	N_2 CO_2 O_2	Air swallowing Transfer dysphagia Ill-fitting dentures Usage of straws to drink fluids Anxiety Postnasal drip
Flatus	Intestinal lumen	N_2 O_2 H_2 CH_2 HCO_3 CO_2	Bacteria (microbiota) Dietary residue

the partial pressure of nitrogen oxide (pNO_2) in the bowel lumen falls below that of blood (Montalto et al. 2009). The fall of pNO_2 has been known to occur after the ingestion of a meal rich in fiber. For example, if one consumes a meal rich in indigestible oligosaccharides, then oligosaccharides come in contact with intestinal bacteria resulting in a rapid production of carbon dioxide (CO_2), hydrogen (H_2), and methane (CH_4) (Scaldaferri et al. 2013; Montalto et al. 2009).

Carbon Dioxide

Gas is also produced via acid within the intestinal lumen. Intestinal acid is delivered via gastric acid secretion and may result in the production of over 600 ml of CO_2 (Kalantar-Zadeh et al. 2019). Fatty acid hydrolysis can produce several liters of CO_2 secondary to the large quantities of bicarbonate secreted in the saliva, mucus, bile, and pancreatic juice (Stephen and Cummings 1980; Gasbarrini et al. 2008) – bacterial fermentation results in increased bicarbonate and subsequent CO_2 (Montalto et al. 2009). Due to an absorptive coefficient and active transport mechanisms, most of this CO_2 is absorbed as it passes down the intestinal tract and does not appear in flatus (Montalto et al. 2009).

Hydrogen

The percentage of hydrogen gas (H_2) that is present in the gastrointestinal tract is highly variable and depends in part upon the bacterial population within the intestinal lumen (Tomlin et al. 1991). The presence of hydrogen gas fluctuates with available substrates, such as undigestible disaccharides and oligosaccharides (Rumessen and Gudmand-Høyer 1988; Rao 1997). Hydrogen is also a by-product of malabsorptive states and conditions associated with bacterial overgrowth (Roccarina et al. 2010). Colonic bacteria containing alpha-D-galactopyranoside, an enzyme absent in humans, readily digest the oligosaccharides stachyose and raffinose which liberates hydrogen gas (Levitt 1969). Other colonic bacteria rapidly consume the hydrogen that is liberated by these organisms (Levitt et al. 1987). The hydrogen gas that is not consumed is

either excreted per rectum or absorbed in the portal circulation and excreted by the lungs (Scaldaferri et al. 2013).

Methane

Methane gas (CH_4), interestingly, is not present in all individuals. Its production depends upon both highly anaerobic conditions and favored bacterial flora (Tomlin et al. 1991). Two-thirds of adults over 10 years of age are CH_4 "nonproducers." The production of CH_4 is dependent more upon the concentration of CH_4-producing bacteria in the gut rather than upon a particular substrate (Montalto et al. 2009). Recent literature supports a reciprocal relationship between the presence of CH_4 and delayed transit states (Kunkel et al. 2011). The excretion of methane alone in constipation-predominant irritable bowel syndrome (IBS) patients has been demonstrated in breath testing with a positive predictive value of 100%, compared to the diarrhea-predominant IBS patients who were found to be mainly hydrogen excreters (Roccarina et al. 2010; Levitt and Ingelfinger 1968). Both CH_4 and H_2 are combustible gases that may be explosive when present with oxygen. Interestingly, mannitol, once used to prepare patients for colonoscopy, was reported to cause accumulation of potentially explosive concentrations of hydrogen (>4.1%) and/or methane (>5%), producing a combustible mixture (Avgerinos et al. 1984; Mansueto et al. 2015; El-Salhy and Gundersen 2015).

Oxygen contained in swallowed air is utilized by bacteria along the entire course of the intestinal tract. Oxygen is diffused readily into the circulation where it is bound by hemoglobin; little backward diffusion takes place; therefore, the resulting partial pressure of oxygen (pO_2) in the flatus is only 1–2 mm Hg (Montalto et al. 2009; Roccarina et al. 2010). The pO_2 of feces is less than that of flatus; therefore, creating an environment favoring the growth of fastidious anaerobic bacteria is thus formed (Tomlin et al. 1991; Onyenekwe et al. 2000). Since N_2, CO_2, H_2, CH_4, and O_2 are all odorless gases, there must be other trace gases to account for the odor of flatus (Goldstein and Pitchumoni 2012). Less than 1% of flatus is composed of ammonia, hydrogen sulfide, methanethiol,

Fig. 2 Belching is defined as an audible escape of air from the esophagus into the pharynx. Belching can be further categorized as either supragastric or gastric (Katzka 2013)

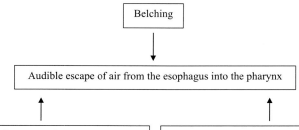

dimethylsulfide, indole, skatole, mercaptans, volatile amines, and short-chain fatty acids (Tomlin et al. 1991). The human nose is able to detect gases in concentration as low as 1:100,000,000 (Suarez et al. 1997). As some of these gases are absorbed from the bowel lumen and then excreted by the lungs, they may contribute to the characteristics and individual odor of breath and also to the phenomenon of so-called extra-oral halitosis (Tangerman and Winkel 2010). Intestinal bacteria produce several sulfur-containing compounds that cause the distasteful odor. The human nose can detect hydrogen sulfide in concentrations as low as one-half part per billion, so passing even a very small amount of flatus may be associated with a foul odor (Fernández-Bañares et al. 2006).

Sources of Intestinal Gas

The methods of measuring intestinal gas are not discussed in this chapter, but they include both direct and indirect techniques. The source of gas in the gastrointestinal tract varies based on the anatomical location (Fig. 2). The average person generates 0.6–1.8 L of gas per day (Weinberg 1998). Gas is often found in either the stomach or large intestine (Serra et al. 2001). In the stomach, gas is mostly air that has been swallowed (exogenous) during eating or drinking (Rao 1997). The gas in the stomach is therefore composed mostly of oxygen, nitrogen, and carbon dioxide and similar in ratio to that of atmospheric air (78% nitrogen, 21% oxygen, 0.9% argon, and 0.04% carbon dioxide) (Bredenoord et al. 2004). Most of the gas in the stomach is eructated. The large quantity of nitrogen represented in atmospheric air is less represented further along the gastrointestinal tract. As swallowed air contains very little carbon dioxide, CO_2 diffuses from the blood into the stomach bubble (Tomlin et al. 1991). Much of the oxygen of swallowed air is absorbed from the stomach into the blood along its pressure gradient (Bredenoord et al. 2004).

In each segment of the intestine, the volume and composition of gas are determined by chemical reactions, bacterial fermentation, and consumption, diffusion between luminal and blood compartments all in the setting of swallowing and belching, gut motility, and anal evacuation (Wilkinson et al. 2019). In the healthy state, food substrate and bacterial populations contribute to individual variation; in disease states, both medical and surgical, enzyme deficiencies, malabsorption, bacterial overgrowth, and a host of other factors play a role as well (Rao 1997).

In the upper small intestine, bicarbonate and acid combine to produce CO_2. Bicarbonate is present in salivary, biliary, pancreatic, and small bowel secretions, and hydrochloric acid is secreted by the stomach (about 30 mEq/h after meals) (Rune 1972). Fatty acids are released from the digestion of triglycerides (about 100 mEq acid/ 30 gm fat). Although CO_2 diffuses rapidly into the blood, in the postprandial state, the high pCO_2 causes luminal pN_2 to fall below that of blood, and N_2 diffuses from the blood to the intestine (Levitt 1971). This results in both CO_2 and N_2 being propelled into the colon (Salvioli et al. 2006).

The gas formed in the colon is produced by colonic bacteria (endogenous) breaking down food residue resulting in the formation of hydrogen and methane (Azpiroz and Serra 2004). Approximately 100 ml of gas is present in the intestinal tract in the fasting state, distributed equally in the stomach, small intestine, ascending colon, transverse colon, descending colon, and pelvic colon (Tomlin et al. 1991). This volume, however, may increase postprandially by 65%, particularly in the pelvic colon (Stone-Dorshow and Levitt 1987). The average daily anal expulsion of gas is approximately 600–700 ml, of which greater than 50% is swallowed air (Azpiroz and Serra 2004; Bendezú et al. 2015). Nitrogen (N_2), oxygen (O_2), carbon dioxide (CO_2), hydrogen (H_2), and methane (CH_4) comprise over 99% of intraluminal gas. In the stomach, the principle gases found are N_2, O_2, and CO_2, whereas in flatus there is also H_2 and CH_4 (Pimentel et al. 2003a).

Colonic bacterial flora, currently termed gut microbiota, is the product of early environmental exposures, antibiotic usage, and dietary habits (Lee and Lee 2014). The gut microbiota is highly variable from one individual to another. Acting upon the delivered substrate, bacteria in the colon both produce and consume various gases. It is primarily here that the content of flatus is determined. Large numbers of bacteria, fermenting undigested carbohydrates and proteins, produce H_2 and CO_2 (Stephen and Cummings 1980). The substrate that is delivered to the colon is highly variable. The gas-producing components of the diet are usually the undigested carbohydrates (Perman and Modler 1982). Carbohydrate malabsorption may be from monosaccharides (glucose, galactose, fructose) and disaccharides (lactose, sucrose, maltose) (El-Salhy and Gundersen 2015). Undigested disaccharides in the colon cause an osmotic load attracting water and electrolytes into the colon, causing watery diarrhea (Nanayakkara et al. 2016). Bacterial fermentation of carbohydrates in the colon results in the accumulation of gases (hydrogen, carbon dioxide, and methane), resulting in excessive flatus, bloating and distention, and abdominal pain (Levitt et al. 1987; Perman and Modler 1982). The details of sugar malabsorption are provided later. Small quantities of starches present in wheat, oats, corn, and potatoes are resistant to digestion, a resistance enhanced by the refrigeration and reheating of food products. The fiber in a meal can decrease starch absorption, and the amylase inhibitors in the seeds of plants such as cereal (wheat, maize, rice, barley) and legumes (kidney beans, cowpea, adzuki beans) reduce carbohydrate digestion in the small intestine (Wilkinson et al. 2019; Bendezú et al. 2015; Manichanh et al. 2014).

Clinical Gas Syndromes

Belching and passing flatus are generally normal, not pathologic, events. Air swallowing is normal, and gas accumulates in the proximal stomach as a result of eating. To belch, the lower esophageal sphincter (LES) relaxes in response to distention, followed by relaxation of the upper esophageal sphincter (UES) (Rao 1997). Of interest, high-resolution manometry demonstrates that there are two different types of belching – supragastric and gastric – with the former executed by the descent of the diaphragm, decrease in intrathoracic pressure, and UES relaxation occurring before anterograde airflow.

Belching

The medical term for belching is *eructation*. Belching is defined as an audible escape of air from the esophagus or the stomach into the pharynx (Bredenoord et al. 2004). Aerophagia is a major cause of belching, based on the observation of the occurrence of excessive air swallowing (Bredenoord et al. 2004). Individuals with the problem of excessive aerophagia often develop repetitive belching. The topic has been defined and discussed at length recently by Stanghellini et al. under symptoms that can be attributed to the functional gastrointestinal disorders of the gastroduodenal region (Stanghellini et al. 2016). Belching is a physiological process and can be considered a disorder only when it is excessive and becomes troublesome (Rao 1997). Belching is classified into two types depending on the origin of the refluxed gas: the gastric belch and the supragastric belch (Wilkinson et al. 2019) (Fig. 2).

Intraluminal impedance measurement of air transport in the esophagus has demonstrated that different mechanisms of excessive belching occur (Kessing et al. 2014). Supragastric is a result of swallowed air that does not reach the stomach but returns orally, a brief period after swallowing (Stanghellini et al. 2016). The pathophysiology of supragastric belching can be studied using the impedance recording technique (Ooi et al. 2016). Excessive belching, gastric or supragastric, is described in the Rome IV criteria of functional GI disorders (Drossman 2016). Belching may occur as an atypical manifestation of dyspepsia or GERD, but is more often a manifestation of emotional stress (Schmulson and Drossman 2017). In a study by Hemmink et al., patients with GERD were seen to have a high frequency of both supragastric and gastric belching (Hemmink et al. 2009a, b). In 24 of the 50 patients with GERD, supragastric benching occurred more frequently in patients with GERD than in controls (Hemmink et al. 2009b). The authors concluded that the supragastric belches in GERD are secondary to the patient's response to an unpleasant esophageal sensation caused by excessive salivation, aerophobia, and belching (Hemmink et al. 2009a). A vicious cycle is initiated the belch promoting air swallowing, the aspirated air passes into the stomach, increasing the size of the gastric air bubble.

In gastric belching, a physiologic phenomenon occurs to help eliminate gas accumulated inside the upper gastrointestinal tract. There is an escape of swallowed intragastric air that enters the esophagus during a transient lower esophageal sphincter relaxation (TLESR) (Khalaf et al. 2017). TLESRs are referred to as the belch (Straathof et al. 2001). Normal healthy individuals have only occasional TLESR, but GERD patients have significantly more TLESRs. Distention of the proximal stomach triggers TLESR that permits the expulsion of air (Hemmink et al. 2009b; Straathof et al. 2001). This mechanism also prevents the entry of large volumes of air through the pylorus into the intestines (Khalaf et al. 2017). Gastric belches are involuntary, are controlled entirely by reflexes, occur 25 to 30 times per day, and are physiological (Hasler 2006).

Avoidance of carbonated beverages, slow eating, diaphragmatic breathing, and speech therapy to reduce air swallowing and baclofen are options (Hemmink et al. 2009a). Baclofen may decrease both gastric and supragastric belching events (Katzka 2013; Ryu et al. 2014). Symptomatic treatment with simethicone might prevent gas formation in the intestines and alleviate symptoms as well is appropriate although the success is variable (Azpiroz and Serra 2004). The management may require placing a nasogastric tube to relieve gastric air along with the use of sedatives. Anxiety, rapid eating, and chewing gum may cause excessive air swallowing (Ooi et al. 2016).

Supragastric Belching

The pathophysiology is just being elucidated with high sophisticated esophageal pH esophageal impedance monitoring that measures the resistance of a medium to an alternating electrical current and helps to measure the movement of air in the esophagus (Hemmink et al. 2009b). It is thus a very useful tool in the evaluation of belching and air swallowing (Ooi et al. 2016). An interesting recent observation is that supragastric belching is associated with globus, a sensation of a ball in the throat and GERD in a subgroup of proton-pump non-responders (Khalaf et al. 2017). A point of clinical importance is that supragastric belching is never observed during sleep. The Magenblase syndrome, often chronic and occurs mostly after an evening meal, is the fullness of the abdomen and bloating relieved by belching (Nigaglioni et al. 1963). Manometric studies of eructation show decreased lower esophageal sphincter tone followed by upper esophageal sphincter relaxation (Khalaf et al. 2017). Addressing psychiatric issues, diaphragmatic breathing therapy to "unlearn" abnormal behaviors, and cognitive therapy are recommended additional approaches to treatment (Kessing et al. 2014).

Bloating

The two words bloating and distention are terms that are used indiscriminately as a symptom and sign, occurring often together (Goldstein and Pitchumoni 2012; Bendezú et al. 2015; Lacy et al. 2011). These two terms are clinically different according to recent observers. Bloating is a subjective sensation of increased pressure within the abdomen, and the term "distention" should only be used when the sensation is accompanied by an actual increase in abdominal girth (Lasser et al. 1975). The terms bloating and distention have been interchangeably used by clinicians and patients as well. Bloating and distention are distinct entities and need not coexist (Lasser et al. 1975). Rome IV criteria explain the sensation of bloating as "a feeling of being puffed up in the abdomen" or as "wearing tight clothes" and can be felt after a full meal (Drossman 2016; Schmulson and Drossman 2017). We do not have adequate research on bloating and distention because of a lack of suitable methods of investigation (Simrén 2009; Lasser et al. 1975). To some extent, this has been improved by the gas challenge, which

suggests that the colon can physiologically accommodate moderate amounts of gas without symptoms unless large amounts of gas are produced (Chang et al. 1994; Major et al. 2017).

Functional abdominal bloating (FAB) is classified as a recurrent feeling of bloating or visible distention for at least 3 days per month over a period of at least 3 months (Schmulson and Drossman 2017; Tang et al. 2013; Sullivan 2012). FAB takes its place as a distinct syndrome among IBS and functional constipation and diarrhea in the Rome IV criteria of bowel disorders (Drossman 2016). FAB is also a component of the other disorders in up to 90% of functional gastrointestinal disorders, such as functional dyspepsia or characteristically as part of IBS (Drossman and Hasler 2016). FAB is more prevalent in women than men but is of similar prevalence in the young and old (Agrawal and Whorwell 2008). In geriatric patients bloating and abdominal distention may be manifestations of organic disease, and potential causes should be considered first in the differential diagnosis (Almario et al. 2017).

Bloating and distention are seen together more commonly in the setting of constipation with symptoms worsening as the day progresses (Tang et al. 2013). A short duration of bloating may occur secondary to any infectious diarrheal syndromes (Weinberg 1998). Dyspeptic bloating may be a key symptom in the postprandial symptom that a patient may classify as "indigestion." (Talley et al. 2001) Gastroparesis and gastric outlet obstruction may also cause bloating (Goetze et al. 2010). Gastroparesis is often caused by poorly controlled diabetes mellitus, whereas gastric outlet obstruction is often secondary to scarring peptic ulcer disease (Goetze et al. 2010).

The symptom of bloating may precede belching and may coexist with flatulence. The pathogenesis of bloating and flatulence is different; therefore, bloating can occur without flatulence (Bendezú et al. 2015). For example, the ingestion of low fermentable psyllium fiber may induce a bloating sensation without excess intestinal gas and increased flatulence (Mcrorie 2015). The pathogenesis of bloating varies among patients and includes a variety of etiologies: organic or functional, visceral hypersensitivity, digestive enzyme deficiencies, dysfunctional gut transit, impaired evacuation of rectal gas, small intestinal bacterial overgrowth (SIBO), colonic bacterial fermentation, and disorders of the colonic microbiome. The specifics regarding the pathogenesis of gas and bloating follow in this chapter.

Patients need not produce more gas to have gas-related symptoms. Many patients who complain of bloating have normal amounts of gas in the GI tract, as demonstrated by argon gas washout studies (Levitt 1971; Major et al. 2017). An abnormal abdominal-diaphragmatic reflex initially coined "splenic flexure syndrome" is a phenomenon in which patients exhibit excessive gas in anatomical bend between the transverse and descending colon resulting in bloating and abdominal pain (Osipenko et al. 2008; Lumsden et al. 1963). CT studies show increased lateral girth along with diaphragmatic descent, or dyssynergia, of diaphragm contraction with abdominal wall muscle relaxation (Osipenko et al. 2008). Many patients suffering from gas, bloating, and abdominal pain may benefit from exercise and biofeedback (Azpiroz and Serra 2004; Lacy et al. 2011; Sullivan 2012; Price et al. 1988; Barba et al. 2015).

Symptoms occurring within 30 min of eating or the inability to finish a meal are attributable to upper gastrointestinal disorders, usually functional dyspepsia (Weinberg 1998). However, the physician should also consider other symptoms that could attribute to early symptoms: gastroesophageal reflux disease (GERD), *Helicobacter pylori* infection, gastroparesis, impaired gastric accommodation, and gastric outlet obstruction (Talley et al. 2001). Definitive testing may be deferred in favor of empiric treatment (Rao 1997). Patients with malignant gastric belching often need to restrict carbonated beverages and other gassy foods; eliminate gum chewing, smoking, and the use of straws; and learn to eat more slowly (Drossman 2006; Barba et al. 2015; Azpiroz 2005).

Small bowel bloating is defined as abdominal distention occurring more than 30 min after eating (Weinberg 1998). Distention in the small bowel and proximal colon is caused by several small bowel disorders such as celiac disease, jejunal diverticulosis, Crohn's disease, and non-celiac gluten enteropathies (Salvioli et al. 2006). Other food sensitivities, functional abdominal bloating, and functional abdominal distention may also be related to abdominal wall muscle relaxation and not simply related to retained gas (El-Salhy and Gundersen 2015). Although functional disorders are as common in older people as in the young, more rigorous investigation of organic disease is appropriate in older patients before the treatment of functional bloating can safely ensue.

Thus far this chapter has focused on non-acute abdominal distention. In contrast, acute abdominal distention that is associated with pain is a clinical scenario that can have serious clinical implications if not recognized early. The differential diagnosis of pathologic abdominal distention associated with pain ranges from perforation, pneumoperitoneum, bowel obstruction, and volvulus (Weinberg 1998; Rami Reddy and Cappell 2017; Falch et al. 2014). The specifics regarding these diagnoses will not be discussed in detail in this chapter, but it is paramount to recognize the pathologic difference in the urgent versus nonurgent presentation in abdominal distention.

Flatulence

Flatulence is the sum of gas that is produced throughout the intestinal tract (Bendezú et al. 2015). There is an abundance of bacteria producing CO_2, H_2, and methane in the large bowel (Levitt 1971). Gas is also formed by a diet rich in fermentable substrate (Tomlin et al. 1991). Flatus also includes air that is swallowed (Ryu et al. 2014). CO_2 is formed in the upper intestine as a product of digestion (Suarez et al. 1997). In addition to CO_2, gases that diffuse along their concentration gradients from the bloodstream into the bowel lumen are also found in the intestinal tract (Price et al. 1988). The amount of gas in the intestinal lumen may be further increased by conditions of excessive mucous secretion interfering with CO_2 and H_2 diffusion, bacterial overgrowth conditions, rapid small intestinal transit, as well as conditions of maldigestion and malabsorption

(Levitt 1971; Azpiroz 2005). The aforementioned conditions lead to increased substrate availability for bacterial fermentation in the colon.

Passing gas through the anus is normal; however, when flatulence happens more often than expected, it can become an embarrassing problem. In extreme cases, flatulence can interfere with a person's ability to socialize. Although there is insufficient data, recent research has been gathered regarding the "normal" volume and component of flatus; an elegant study by Tomlin et al. noted that the volume of gas expelled by volunteers may range from 200 to 2400 ml/ 24 h. Interestingly, there was no consistent relationship between flatus volume and dietary fiber volume, likely reflecting bacterial adaptation to dietary intake (Tomlin et al. 1991). With the air passing through the intestine much more rapidly than liquids or solids, once introduced into the stomach, air can be passed as flatus in as little as 20–35 min, with postprandial flatus starting from approximately 1 hour after eating (Tomlin et al. 1991). The size of a single expulsion of flatus varies from 25 to 100 ml. Hydrogen and CO_2 were the predominant gases expelled, with 1/3 of participants expelling methane. One-third of expelled gas was unidentified, but it likely contains nitrogen of both swallowed air and air found in the gastrointestinal tract (Hemmink et al. 2009a). Men produce more aromatic flatus than women, and the utility of activated charcoal-lined undergarments to mask odor remains a matter of debate (Suarez et al. 1998). Finally, many types of colitidies and parasitic diseases, in particular, are associated with increased flatulence (Weinberg 1998).

At any given time, there is less than 200 mL of gas throughout the gastrointestinal tract (Goldstein and Pitchumoni 2012). On average, healthy men pass flatus about 14 times per day, especially after meals (Tomlin et al. 1991). Flatus rates up to 25 per day are normal. The average volume of flatus passage per hour is 100 ml, with volume per 24 h 400–2400 ml, and less than 25 times per day considered a normal number of passages (Suarez et al. 1997). Large volumes of flatus are expelled after a meal, illustrating both the greater interaction of substrate and bacteria after eating and the

impact of the well-known gastrocolic reflex (Price et al. 1988; Passos et al. 2005).

Although there is no good treatment for flatulence other than dietary manipulation, various remedies have been offered. Most interventions aimed at altering the normal colonic bacterial milieu with luminal probiotics or antibiotics have thus far not proved very successful (Ganiats et al. 1994). A recent randomized double-blind study, however, has reported the value of rifaximin therapy for abdominal bloating and flatulence (Sharara et al. 2006; Pimentel et al. 2006). On the other hand, flatus volume, as well as the degree of bloating, will improve by reducing the poorly digested simple sugars in the diet – lactose, fructose, and sorbitol (Nanayakkara et al. 2016). Similar benefit can be seen with reductions in dietary soluble fiber, legumes (beans, peas, soybeans), onions, celery, carrots, cruciferous vegetables (kale, collard greens, cabbage, Brussels sprouts, cauliflower, bok choy, radish, broccoli, arugula), raisins, apples, pears, grapes, and prune juice, and complex starches such as wheat and potato (Varney et al. 2017).

Dietary modifications form symptom amelioration, however, must be balanced by the broad health benefits of short-chain fatty acids (SCFA), the major metabolic product of bacterial fermentation in the colon (Scheppach 1994). These benefits include key roles in glucose and cholesterol regulation, colonocyte nutrition and blood flow, and gut immune function (Varney et al. 2017). In addition to being the fermentable substrates that yield H_2 and CO_2, most of these gas-forming foods contain sulfur moieties. In the presence of sulfur-reducing bacteria, these sulfate-containing foods will result in excessively odoriferous flatus (Suarez et al. 1998). Moreover, the sulfide ion itself inhibits carbonic anhydrase enzymes, active transporters for CO_2 across luminal membranes, and its presence, therefore, contributes to increased flatus volume (Tangerman and Winkel 2010; Serra et al. 1998).

Peppermint oil has intrinsic properties that have been hypothesized to treat the symptoms of bloating associated with IBS (Ford et al. 2008; Cappello et al. 2007). These properties are thought to be secondary to peppermint's antimicrobial, antiviral, antioxidant, antitumor, and some anti-allergenic activity. It has been used empirically with limited success (Masuy et al. 2018). In a meta-analysis of 12 randomized trials with 835 patients, Alammar et al. found that peppermint oil improved symptoms (Alammar et al. 2019).

SIBO

Small intestinal bacterial overgrowth (SIBO) is a clinical condition in which the proximal small bowel becomes colonized with a large (greater than 10 (Scaldaferri et al. 2013) per milliliter) number of gut microflora (Ford et al. 2009). SIBO can result from several pathophysiologic conditions and plays an important role in the prevalence of bloating. Female gender, older age, diarrhea-predominant IBS, bloating and flatulence, proton-pump inhibitor and narcotic intake, and low hemoglobin are associated with SIBO among IBS patients (Ford et al. 2009; Reddymasu et al. 2010; Sachdeva et al. 2011). SIBO can cause not only bloating but also abdominal pain, diarrhea, and macrocytic anemia.

Normally, the stomach and small intestine are relatively sterile when compared to the colon. Bacterial overgrowth can be seen in the setting of various types of obstructive processes and in cases of postoperative alterations in anatomy (Shah et al. 2010). Pernicious anemia, surgical vagotomy, and prolonged use of proton-pump inhibitors all result in a permissive environment of relative achlorhydria and are thought to increase SIBO (Reddymasu et al. 2010). Billroth II, gastric bypass surgeries, and small bowel diverticula create a static "blind-loop" environment where bacterial overgrowth can occur. Conditions such as diabetes mellitus, scleroderma, amyloidosis, and many degenerative neurologic disorders have their impact in altering the normal motor physiology of the GI tract, thereby altering gut transit and resulting in bacterial overgrowth (Tan et al. 2013). Obstructive conditions can also be seen in Crohn's disease, adhesions, radiation enteritis, and malignancy.

Validated guidelines for the evaluation of bloating do not exist, but many clinicians choose to empirically treat symptoms after studies to rule out SIBO, malabsorption, and other organic disorders have been carried out (Reddymasu et al. 2010). Theoretically, the definitive test for small bowel bacterial overgrowth is the culture of small bowel aspirate (Dukowicz et al. 2007). However, this test is invasive, time-consuming, and difficult to handle properly. The breath test (BT) with various substrates (e.g., glucose, lactulose, fructose, sorbitol, sucrose, and inulin) is useful in the diagnosis of lactose intolerance and small intestinal bacterial overgrowth (SIBO) and in evaluating fecal transit time (Gasbarrini et al. 2007). The results of the test are the measurement of breath for hydrogen (or other gases) in expired air as it relates to the time of administration of the substrates in question (Shah et al. 2010). The reliability of the results of breath tests can be improved by using standardized doses of the substrates. A consensus meeting of experts was convened to develop guidelines for clinicians and research (Dukowicz et al. 2007). The doses for various tests using lactulose, glucose, fructose, and lactose are 10, 75, 25, and 25 g. Fructose and lactose breath testing should be performed for at least 3 h. The results are interpreted as follows: A rise of ≥ 20 p.p.m. from the baseline in hydrogen during the test should be considered positive for fructose and lactose breath testing, whereas a rise of ≥ 20 p.p.m. from the baseline in hydrogen by 90 min should be considered a positive test for SIBO (Shah et al. 2010).

Pathogenesis of Gas and Bloating

The common denominator is a combination of diet-based factors, malabsorption, colonic fermentation, and excessive gas production (Tang et al. 2013). In this process, the substrate is a food item usually a carbohydrate (lactose, fructose, other components of dietary fiber), which is processed in the colon (Kerckhoffs et al. 2008). Some of the culprits of excessive gas production are referred to as being high in FODMAPs (fermentable oligo-, di-, monosaccharides and polyols) (Varney et al. 2017). The role of bacteria (gut microbiota) and dysbiosis is significant in the

Table 3 Examples of foods that can attribute to gas, belching, and bloating. These foods are also examples of FODMAPs

Molecule	Examples
Oligosaccharides (fructans)	Wheat (large amounts), rye (large amounts), onions, leeks, zucchini
Disaccharides (lactose)	Dairy products, cheese, milk, yogurt
Monosaccharides (excess fructose)	Honey, apples, pears, peaches, mangos, fruit juice, dried fruit
Polyols (sorbitol)	Apricots, peaches, artificial sweeteners, sugar-free gums
Galactose (raffinose)	Lentils, cabbage, Brussels sprouts, asparagus, green beans, legumes

genesis of fatty acids and gas as it relates to consumed food products (Fernández-Bañares et al. 2006). Maldigestion and malabsorption of both simple and complex carbohydrates and dietary fiber are a common cause of excess gas production (Stone-Dorshow and Levitt 1987) (Table 3).

The intestinal gas that is often a nuisance enough to seek medical attention is often a by-product of a high-fiber diet that is considered essential, deserving the title of a "functional food" and increasingly noted to be beneficial in preventing several metabolic and colonic disorders (Ganiats et al. 1994). The treatment of the functional symptoms thus is a delicate balance between choosing healthy food that causes IBD symptoms or to accept a less healthy fiber-poor diet. A qualified dietitian may be able to keep a healthy balance by choosing appropriate items (Mansueto et al. 2015).

Lactose Intolerance

Worldwide nearly 70% of adults are deficient in intestinal lactase, the enzyme required for the digestion of lactose (Fernández-Bañares et al. 2006). Lactose is a disaccharide consisting of galactose bound to glucose (Sieber et al. 1997). The consumption of lactose-containing milk and dairy products in these individuals can lead to the development of various gastrointestinal symptoms including abdominal pain, bloating, and diarrhea. In humans, the intestinal lactase activity is high at birth but starts to progressively decline during adolescence, curtailing the ability to digest dietary lactose and culminating in adult-type hypolactasia (Sieber et al. 1997). However, in some, a genetic trait enables intestinal lactase activity to persist into adulthood (Parker and Watson 2017).

The prevalence of lactase persistence varies between populations and ethnicities (Mattar et al. 2012). For example, over 90% of adults in Southeast Asia are lactase deficient, whereas, in Scandinavia, the prevalence of lactase deficiency is only ~10%. It is estimated that over 80% of individuals of African and Asian descent are considered to be lactase deficient as adults. Primary lactase insufficiency is estimated to be prevalent in 21% of Caucasians, 75% of African Americans, 51% of Hispanics, 79% of the Native American population, and 60% of Ashkenazi Jews (Lapides and Savaiano 2018).

The intestinal lactose, lactase-phlorizin hydrolase (LPH), or simply lactase, belongs to a group of intestinal disaccharidases located on the brush border of the small intestine. The concentration of LPH is highest in the duodenum and proximal jejunum and progressively declines towards the ileum (Parker and Watson 2017). The intestinal bacteria hydrolyze the unabsorbed lactose in the colon to glucose and galactose and subsequently ferment them to lactate, SCFAs, and gases, such as H_2, CO_2, and CH_4 contributing to the symptoms of bloating, pain, and diarrhea (Matthews et al. 2005). Lactase deficiency can also occur secondarily with many short duration gastrointestinal infections or in chronic disorders such as celiac disease inflammatory bowel disease, abdominal radiation, or bariatric surgery (Sieber et al. 1997; Mattar et al. 2012).

The symptoms of lactase deficiency are due to multiple pathophysiologic mechanisms. First, there is increased water content in the intestines due to the osmotic load (Parker and Watson 2017). This is followed by fermentation by the colonic microbiome leading to the production of short-chain fatty acids and gas, mainly hydrogen, CO_2, and CH_4 (Montalto et al. 2009). For every 5 g of

Table 4 List of some medications with lactose as an additive. (Data adapted from Drugs.com (2012))

Medications made with lactose
Alprazolam
Cetirizine
Cyclobenzaprine
Ethinyl estradiol/levonorgestrel
Hydromorphone
Lorazepam
Meloxicam
Nitrofurantoin
Penicillin V potassium
Promethazine
Viagra

unabsorbed carbohydrate reaching the colon, approximately 1 L of gas and 60 mmol of short-chain fatty acids are produced by fermentation (Miller and Wolin 1979; McRorie and Chey 2016). Half the amount is absorbed and excreted through the lungs, but the remaining half is passed through the gastrointestinal tract. Diarrhea is often mild and not typically high volume.

The diagnosis is often from history as well as by the result of a lactose elimination diet. In the lactose tolerance test (LTT) and the H_2-breath test, a subject is challenged with an oral dose of 20–50 g lactose after which blood glucose concentrations (LTT) or H_2 concentrations in expired air are measured for every 30 min for 2–3 h (Fernández-Bañares et al. 2006; Varney et al. 2017; Sieber et al. 1997). Different lactose feeding protocols have consistently produced negative findings suggesting that in humans, intestinal lactase is not an inducible enzyme (Miller and Wolin 1979). It is theorized that prolonged intake of lactose results in an adaptive mechanism of the gut microbiota relating to lactose processing. Individuals should practice looking at the contents of packed foods for lactose content if one is to avoid lactose-rich food. Lactose is found in many medications since lactose helps tablets highly compressible (see Table 4 for some lactose-containing medications) (Eadala et al. 2009).

Fructose Intolerance

Fructose is a six-carbon monosaccharide, present in a variety of foods. Fructose malabsorption was first described by Rumessen (Rumessen and Gudmand-Høyer 1987). The consumption of fructose from high-fructose corn syrup (HFCS) has increased over 1,000 percent from 1970 to 1990. Fructose is a monosaccharide that is found naturally in fruits. Fructose is consumed as sucrose (table sugar), which is a disaccharide composed of equal parts of fructose and glucose. Fructose is also consumed currently as a component of HFCS that is frequently added as sweeteners to many processed foods and beverages (Rumessen and Gudmand-Høyer 1987). HFCS is a preferred sweetening agent because it is less expensive and has additional beneficial properties, including sweetness, flavor enhancement, freezing point depression, and shelf-life extension (Stanhope and Havel 2010).

The third National Health and Nutrition Examination Survey reported that the mean intake of fructose was 37 g per day among all Americans. Fructose represents more than 10% of caloric intake for the total population, but older age groups (51 years and older) consumed a smaller percentage of their total fructose from sugar-sweetened beverages compared to their younger counterparts (Vos et al. 2008). An increasing number of functional disorders of the gastrointestinal tract are related to excessive fructose use. The daily recommended dosage for women should not exceed 20 g of fructose per day. Men should never consume more than 36 g per day, and children need no more than 12 g per day. On average, children, adults, and the elderly are consuming double to triple the recommended amount of fructose. The largest source of fructose was sugar-sweetened beverages (30%) followed by grains (22%) and fruit or fruit juice (19%).

Symptoms for fructose malabsorption and intolerance include nausea, bloating, gas, abdominal pain, diarrhea, and vomiting (Kyaw and Mayberry 2011). Excess dietary intake of fructose can quickly overwhelm the absorptive capacity of the small intestine, leading to incomplete absorption and resulting in fructose malabsorption (Stanhope and Havel 2010; Fedewa and Rao 2014; Rizkalla 2010). Abdominal bloating and diarrhea are the symptoms due to the inability to sufficiently absorb the ingested monosaccharide present in variable quantities in many fruits and vegetables.

The topic of fructose intolerance in Western and modern society was recently well discussed by Fedewa and Rao (Fedewa and Rao 2014). Human beings have a variable but only a limited capacity to digest and absorb fructose since glucose is much better absorbed through an active transport mechanism in the small intestine facilitated by GLUT 2 and GLUT 5 transporters. Fructose is mainly absorbed through carrier-mediated facilitated diffusion and GLUT 5. Malabsorption of fructose in the small intestine results in an osmotic force which increases the influx of water into the colonic lumen, rapid propulsion of fecal matter, and increased production of gas. The mechanism is this not different from that of lactose malabsorption (Rumessen and Gudmand-Høyer 1988; Stone-Dorshow and Levitt 1987).

Fructose is broken down by colon bacteria into short fatty acids, CO_2 and H_2, which can be measured in the expired air (Rizkalla 2010). Bloating, abdominal discomfort, and sometimes osmotic diarrhea are the consequences induced by the degradation products built by the colonic bacteria (Rumessen and Gudmand-Høyer 1988; Rumessen and Gudmand-Høyer 1987; Kyaw and Mayberry 2011). It is believed that about 36% of the European population suffers from fructose malabsorption in a more or less severe form, and about half of them are symptomatic.

Fructose malabsorption is a less well-understood disorder than that of lactose, as the absorptive capacity of fructose in "normal" individuals is not known. As with other carbohydrates, fructose fermentation by colonic bacteria can result in H_2, CO_2, methane, and short-chain fatty acids with resulting flatulence, bloating, and abdominal pain (Mansueto et al. 2015; Major et al. 2017). Patients with IBS appear to have more symptoms, but not more malabsorption by breath testing than normal controls (Skoog et al. 2008). Withdrawal of fructose from the diet results in high rates of symptom resolution (Fernández-Bañares et al. 2006; Fedewa and Rao 2014). Due to numerous false-positive and false-negative results, hydrogen breath testing has had limited usefulness. Therefore, the diagnosis of fructose malabsorption is often based upon history alone.

Sorbitol Intolerance

Sorbitol is a sugar alcohol rich in some fruits and plants and contains a laxative property. Sorbitol is a common sweetener used in "sugar-free" candy and other foods labeled "diabetic" (Gould and Sellin 2009). The use of sorbitol as a suitable substitute for sugar-containing foods is misunderstood by many, including diabetic individuals. Sorbitol is not well absorbed by 43% of Caucasians and 55% of non-Caucasians and causes a similar clinical syndrome (Jain et al. 1985; Fernández-Bañares et al. 2009). The pharmaceutical industry uses sorbitol in the production of several medications for protection against the loss of moisture. It is of great importance that the gastroenterologist takes into account hidden sources of sorbitol when evaluating a patient with functional symptoms (Johnston et al. 1994). See Table 5 for some sorbitol containing medications.

High-Fiber Diet

A high-fiber diet is considered to be the choice in maintaining good health and in preventing several metabolic disorders including obesity, diabetes

Table 5 List of some medications containing sorbitol as an additive. (Data adapted from Drugs.com (2012))

Medications made with sorbitol
Acetaminophen
Dextromethorphan
Alprazolam
Bexarotene
Calcitriol
Carbamazepine
Clonazepam
Didanosine
Didrex
Fasprin
Lithium
Multivitamins
Myambutol
Myorisan
Ondansetron hydrochloride
Phenylephrine
Staxyn
Simethicone
Vascepa
Xeljanz

mellitus, hyperlipidemia, and other related disorders (Després and Lemieux 2006). As discussed in detail in another chapter, dietary fiber is an essential component of our daily diet, and the Academy of Nutrition and Dietetics recommends 25 g of fiber per day for women and 38 g per day for men (Vos et al. 2008). In controlling functional symptoms, it was once a common practice to try a high-fiber diet which did not give consistent benefits (Jankovic et al. 2015; Owens et al. 1995). However, it is a common clinical observation that many individuals, especially in Western countries, are not accustomed to a high-fiber diet and often develop abdominal pain, bloating, and inconvenient flatulence when they consume foods that are high in fiber (Wilkinson et al. 2019).

Current research indicates that certain foods containing high FODMAPs (fermentable oligo-, di-, monosaccharides and polyols) exacerbate symptoms in some patients because of the fermentation and osmotic effects (El-Salhy and Gundersen 2015). The common properties of foods high in FODMAPs are that they are comprised of poorly absorbed short-chain carbohydrates and fatty acids: fructose, lactose, fructans, and galactans (Whelan et al. 2018). When administered in sufficient doses, they are fermented by gut microbiota and have a laxative effect by increasing the amount of fluid in the lumen and consequently intestinal motility (Mansueto et al. 2015; Major et al. 2017). In addition to the laxative effect, foods high in FODMAP are also gas-producing due to the fermentability of the fiber and short-chain carbohydrates that comprise fructose, FOS, and GOS (Macfarlane and Macfarlane 2012). These biologic processes are present also for other poorly absorbed, fermentable oligosaccharides, disaccharides, monosaccharides, and polyols. Excess intake of fructose overwhelms the absorptive capacity of the small intestine, leading to fructose malabsorption as mentioned earlier concerning fructose intolerance (Fedewa and Rao 2014).

Restriction of FODMAPs in the diet decreases symptoms of abdominal pain, bloating, and diarrhea associated with the production of short-chain fatty acids (Nanayakkara et al. 2016). It is clear that while a high-fiber diet is beneficial overall, there is a lot of overlap between foods that are high in fiber and foods that are high in FODMAPs (Staudacher et al. 2017). FODMAP foods are not necessarily unhealthy items in the diet. Indeed many of them are needed for the maintenance of health through healthy gut microbiota (Varney et al. 2017). Some of these foods contain fructans, inulin, and galacto-oligosaccharides (GOS), which are healthy prebiotics (Varney et al. 2017). It is a dilemma to choose a low-FODMAP diet, yet the diet is rich in fiber. Patients should meet with a qualified nutritionist before initiation of a food elimination diet (Kalantar-Zadeh et al. 2019; Linlawan et al. 2019). Following a low-FODMAP diet isn't a lifetime requirement since the offending item or items in the diet can be identified by careful elimination experiments by the patient. This enables the patient to avoid that particular item/items and consume other items in the list of FODMAPs (Owens et al. 1995; Whelan et al. 2018). For further details on the specifics of FODMPAs, please see the chapter by Haller et al.

Challenges Unique to the Older Adult

There are certain conditions associated with aging that result in increased intestinal gas. The condition of "lactase nonpersistence" is a well-known example of an age-related phenomenon and, in fact, may affect certain populations well before old age (Almario et al. 2017). In the majority of settings, however, it is the non-gastrointestinal medical conditions, seen more in the aging and aged populations, which secondarily cause belching, bloating, and flatus to be more exaggerated (Bharucha and Camilleri 2001).

There are several reasons why bloating may be more prevalent in older people. Bloating can be the result of both overproduction and defective transport of intestinal gas. Diabetes mellitus, more common in the elderly, is a disease in which both mechanisms can be operational (Azpiroz 2005). Decreased midgut motility may cause stasis and bacterial overgrowth, with the fermentation of substrate and gas production in the small intestine (Macfarlane and Macfarlane

2012). At the same time, increased motility may result in the delivery of partially digested, malabsorbed substrate to bacterial populations in the colon (Levitt 1969; Klaus et al. 2009).

Constipation is far more common in the older population (Gallegos-Orozco et al. 2012). Endocrine and neurologic diseases, medications, and poor nutrition all contribute to chronic constipation. Patients are often advised by mainstream media to take a daily soluble fiber product. This fermentable substrate is delivered to the large bowel, where H_2 and CO_2 are produced (Mcrorie 2015). If the patient is impacted, however, only bloating and discomfort result from ingestion fiber products (Gallegos-Orozco et al. 2012). Older patients should be advised to speak to their physician prior to initiating treatment for constipation as a detailed history, and evaluation of medications should be done prior.

A host of factors, cumulative with age, can cause relative obstructive processes in the bowel and may also contribute to bacterial overgrowth (Reddymasu et al. 2010). Adhesions form surgery or radiation, strictures following diverticulitis, and malignancy are a few examples. Any of these conditions which result in the increased delivery of fermentable substrate to colonic bacteria will cause flatus to be more prevalent (Keller and Layer 2009). In the battle to manage constipation, many old and young alike will increase their ingestion of cruciferous vegetables and other high-fiber foods and, in so doing, become quite flatulent (Ganiats et al. 1994).

An older individual with ill-fitting dentures might experience mouth pain, excessive salivation, and air swallowing (Ooi et al. 2016). Geriatric patients are more likely to have several medications to swallow, and with the swallowing of sequential pills, there may be significant swallowing of air as well (Hemmink et al. 2009a). Many older adults, for reasons of illness or diminished stamina, may spend proportionately more time in the supine rather than an upright position; and 2–3 times more air is swallowed in the supine position (Bredenoord et al. 2004; Hemmink et al. 2009a). The elderly are more likely to have encountered serious illness, such as post-laryngectomy, for example, and utilize a device that generates phonation by swallowing of air (Talley et al. 2001).

Older individuals undergo several metabolic changes associated with aging. One of these changes results in an increase of intestinal proteolytic bacteria and a decrease in saccharolytic bacteria (Bharucha and Camilleri 2001). This change results in a significant change in intestinal flora that can predispose the individual to bloating (Almario et al. 2017; Tang et al. 2013). There are some limited studies suggesting that the ingestion of prebiotic and probiotic formulations decrease these intestinal changes (Bischoff 2016; Duncan and Flint 2013).

Treatment of Intestinal Gas

Non-pharmacologic therapy is usually the appropriate first step in the intervention. Emotional factors and other underlying diseases should be identified and addressed. Habits and behavior patterns should be properly examined for their possible contribution to symptoms (gum chewing, rapid eating "on the run," consumption of large quantities of carbonated beverages or diet candies) with re-evaluation after a period of abstinence (Azpiroz and Serra 2004).

Diet must be thoroughly evaluated. To this end, it is helpful to have patients keep a daily record of what they are eating and when they are symptomatic. A trial of a targeted elimination diet can very quickly provide the diagnosis. Often, it is necessary to reduce lactose, fructose, complex carbohydrates, or fruits and vegetables in the diet. Malabsorption of complex carbohydrates is highly variable (Nanayakkara et al. 2016). Food preparation itself can affect digestion: soaking legumes increases oligosaccharide digestion by significantly decreasing concentrations of raffinose and stachyose (Fedewa and Rao 2014). Refrigeration and reheating of starches decrease digestion. Fiber and legumes in a meal can interfere with starch digestion. Although the concepts are basic, the subtleties of diet manipulation require an individualized approach. Success is reached by trial and with patience.

In addition to dietary modification, the physician should also consider additional lifestyle approaches to treatment. A meta-analysis explored the role of cognitive behavioral therapy (CBT) utilizing mindfulness and meditation in reducing functional symptoms and found an overall benefit (Hauser et al. 2014; Glasinovic et al. 2018; Shen and Nahas 2009). One of the barriers of CBT is access to qualified professionals to deliver treatment. In response to this barrier, one study evaluated the difference in using therapist-based versus web-based CBT in patients with IBS and found that there was no significant difference in the outcomes of either group (Everitt et al. 2015; Bonnert et al. 2017). CBT has been used in combination with diaphragmatic breathing techniques and found not only reduction in belching but also a reduction in dyspepsia (Katzka 2013; Ong et al. 2018; Punkkinen et al. 2016). In addition to CBT, there is some limited data on the usage of hypnotherapy to manage the symptoms of intestinal gas and IBS. The Cochrane Database of Systematic Review found that there is insufficient evidence to support the inclusion of hypnotherapy in the treatment of intestinal gas as there is a need for more high-quality studies on this subject (Webb et al. 2007).

Pharmacologic therapeutic intervention often begins by examining the side effect profile of medications being taken for other conditions, eliminating unnecessary drugs, and decreasing doses whenever possible (Weinberg 1998). Attention must be given to avoiding common pitfalls, such as gluten-containing drugs in the celiac patient and bicarbonate-based CO_2-generating antacids in the bloated patient.

Probiotics can be used in a pulsed fashion for achlorhydria, scleroderma, and blind-loop syndromes, where the concern for small intestinal bacterial overgrowth (SIBO) is ever-present (Dukowicz et al. 2007). Their use to alter microflora and achieve control of pain and bloating in the IBS patient is being studied in randomized trials. Antibiotics also provide benefit to individuals with bacterial overgrowth and IBS (Sharara et al. 2006; Pimentel et al. 2003b). Several studies have addressed the prevalence of SIBO in IBS patients and symptom improvement with "antibiotic decontamination." The role of antibiotics in the modification of small bowel and colonic microflora in the patient with IBS is an active area of investigation (Pimentel et al. 2006). Recent attention has turned to rifampin, a non-absorbable bactericidal antibiotic providing targeted results without entering the systemic circulation (Sharara et al. 2006).

Prokinetic agents such as metoclopramide and domperidone provide theoretical benefits in cases of gastroparesis and more generalized symptoms of nausea and bloating by targeting dopamine receptors (Caldarella et al. 2002). However, their use is limited by possible irreversible extrapyramidal sequelae. Since the disappearance of cisapride from the prokinetic arena, a safe and effective agent continues to be awaited. Neostigmine, a cholinesterase inhibitor used for myasthenia gravis, has short-term utility in the treatment of ileus (Jiang and Horvath 2010). Its poor oral absorption and short duration of action, along with undesirable side effects in patients with asthma, peptic ulcer disease, and bradycardia, narrow its real clinical utility. Prokinetic studies in functional bloating have demonstrated symptom improvement in the absence of changed gas volume, suggesting that motor stimulation alters symptom perception.

Anticholinergic, or antispasmodic, agents such as dicyclomine and glycopyrrolate are used to decrease bowel motility. In the elderly, however, their efficacy is limited by a myriad of side effects such as drowsiness, blurred vision, confusion, orthostatic hypotension, urinary retention, and constipation (Almario et al. 2017; Sprung 2014). One must also avoid this drug class in patients with narrow-angle glaucoma. Several categories of antidepressants – specifically, TCAs, SSRIs, and SNRIs – exert an antinociceptive effect on the efferent nerves of the intestine while generally decreasing bowel motility as well. These agents address gut hypersensitivity and have been a mainstay of treating irritable bowel syndrome for many years (Owens et al. 1995).

Gas and bloating may be decreased by using pancreatic enzymes for both primary and secondary pancreatic insufficiency states such as post-gastrectomy, short bowel syndrome, gastric bypass, and rapid transit states (Suarez et al. 1999). Their demonstrated efficacy in controlling symptoms in healthy subjects after a high-fat meal is in some fashion analogous to rapid transit states. Beta-galactosidases (lactase) is therapeutic in the setting of lactose intolerance. Alpha-glycosidase (Beano), harvested from aspergillus niger, decreases the flatulence resulting from ingesting legumes but not cruciferous vegetables and other poorly digestible fiber (Ganiats et al. 1994). Eight randomized controlled trials were located, and collectively they indicated that peppermint oil could be efficacious for symptom relief in IBS (Cappello et al. 2007). A meta-analysis of five placebo-controlled double-blind trials supports this notion of peppermint oil (Alammar et al. 2019). Agents such as simethicone and charcoal have a minor role in decreasing the volume of gas within the lumen of the intestine (Azpiroz and Serra 2004; Barba et al. 2016).

Modulating the gut microbiome is being evaluated in the treatment of many functional gastrointestinal symptoms (Hungin et al. 2018; Lee et al. 2017; Pimentel et al. 2013). Many observations contribute to the role of gut microbiota in the symptoms and the beneficial effects by altering the microbiota. One observation is the onset of IBS symptoms after an episode of infectious gastroenteritis (Gasbarrini et al. 2008). Another observation is the onset of symptoms beginning after a course of antibiotic therapy suggesting the dysbiosis of gut microbiota (Macfarlane and Macfarlane 2012). The final observation is the clinical improvement of symptoms after the use of a nonabsorbable antibiotic rifaximin and some probiotics and prebiotics (Sharara et al. 2006; Duncan and Flint 2013; Yoon et al. 2018). In added support of the above, a recent Asian data substantiate the research that places IBS as a disorder of gut-brain interaction, recognizing the key role of the intestinal microenvironment (Macfarlane and Macfarlane 2012; Duncan and Flint 2013). The research is in its early stages, but there is accumulating evidence that the combination of probiotics *Lactobacillus* and *Bifidobacterium* is a safe choice to improve the overall symptoms

for IBS patient (Lee and Lee 2014; Duncan and Flint 2013; Iovino et al. 2014).

Conclusions

Belching, bloating, and flatulence are ubiquitous. The underlying physiology of these symptoms involves a complex interplay of diet, bacterial gut flora, and basic metabolic pathways. Patterns of behavior and emotional factors play a role as well. The clinical gas syndromes intersect with the aging process to create issues that are unique to the older adult. Therapeutic intervention should be focused first on dietary modifications. Pharmacologic modalities are imperfect, and caution must be taken to avoid the untoward side effects to which the older population, by age and of polypharmacy, are particularly prone. When managing quality of life issues and non-life-threatening illness, caution and patience should be the cornerstone of care. Although belching, bloating, and abdominal distention are generally considered to be functional in origin, in the older adult, they may imply organic disorders that may require prompt attention. Future studies should evaluate the appropriate methods of assessing the severity of these symptoms in the geriatric population.

Key Points

1. Belching is defined as the audible escape of air from the esophagus into the pharynx. Belching is classified into two subtypes depending on the origin of the refluxed gas: the gastric belch and the supragastric belch.
2. Bloating is the manifestation of altered visceral sensation resulting in the subjective sensation of abdominal distention.
3. Abdominal pain with bloating is an alarm sign. Abdominal distention may be a sign of many disorders that may require prompt medical attention.
4. Flatulence is the sum of gas produced throughout the intestinal tract. Excessive

flatulence is a manifestation of consuming a diet rich in fiber and highly fermentable carbohydrates.

5. The composition of the belched gas is similar to atmospheric air; however, the composition of flatus includes additional gases produced by fermentation of undigested carbohydrates by bacteria.

6. Often, the symptoms of gaseousness are manifestations of disordered motility characteristic of irritable bowel syndrome (IBS).

7. Various food intolerances may be associated with bloating, abdominal distention, and diarrhea. The most common intolerances are lactose intolerance, fructose intolerance, and gluten intolerance.

8. The concept of intolerance to various components of food has contributed to the development of the low-FODMAP (fermentable oligosaccharides, disaccharides, monosaccharides, and polyols) diet.

9. Small intestinal bacterial overgrowth (SIBO) is to be recognized as a cause of abdominal distention, flatulence, and other IBS-like symptoms.

10. The role of gut microbiota is a new field in medicine with a wide clinical significance that includes the pathogenesis of functional symptoms of IBS.

11. Some of the symptoms considered to be functional in the younger adult may be indicative of significant pathology in the older adult.

References

Agrawal A, Whorwell PJ. Review article: abdominal bloating and distension in functional gastrointestinal disorders - epidemiology and exploration of possible mechanisms. Aliment Pharmacol Ther. 2008; https://doi.org/10.1111/j.1365-2036.2007.03549.x.

Alammar N, Wang L, Saberi B, et al. The impact of peppermint oil on the irritable bowel syndrome: a meta-analysis of the pooled clinical data. BMC Complement Altern Med. 2019; https://doi.org/10.1186/s12906-018-2409-0.

Almario CV, Almario AA, Cunningham ME, Fouladian J, Spiegel BMR. Old farts – fact or fiction? Results from a population-based survey of 16,000 Americans examining the association between age and flatus. Clin Gastroenterol Hepatol. 2017; https://doi.org/10.1016/j.cgh.2017.03.023.

Avgerinos A, Kalantzis N, Rekoumis G, Pallikaris G, Arapakis G, Kanaghinis T. Bowel preparation and the risk of explosion during colonoscopic polypectomy. Gut. 1984; https://doi.org/10.1136/gut.25.4.361.

Azpiroz F. Intestinal gas dynamics: mechanisms and clinical relevance. Gut. 2005; https://doi.org/10.1136/gut.2004.048868.

Azpiroz F, Levitt MD. Intestinal gas. In: Feldman M, Friedman L, Brandt L, editors. Schlesinger and Fortran's gastrointestinal and liver disease. 9th ed. Philadelphia: Elsevier; 2010. p. 233–40.

Azpiroz F, Serra J. Treatment of excessive intestinal gas. Curr Treat Options Gastroenterol. 2004; https://doi.org/10.1007/s11938-004-0016-2.

Barba E, Burri E, Accarino A, et al. Abdominothoracic mechanisms of functional abdominal distension and correction by biofeedback. Gastroenterology. 2015; https://doi.org/10.1053/j.gastro.2014.12.006.

Barba E, Accarino A, Soldevilla A, Malagelada JR, Azpiroz F. Randomized, placebo-controlled trial of biofeedback for the treatment of rumination. Am J Gastroenterol. 2016; https://doi.org/10.1038/ajg.2016.197.

Bendezú RA, Barba E, Burri E, et al. Intestinal gas content and distribution in health and in patients with functional gut symptoms. Neurogastroenterol Motil. 2015; https://doi.org/10.1111/nmo.12618.

Bharucha AE, Camilleri M. Functional abdominal pain in the elderly. Gastroenterol Clin N Am. 2001; https://doi.org/10.1016/S0889-8553(05)70193-X.

Bischoff SC. Microbiota and aging. Curr Opin Clin Nutr Metab Care. 2016; https://doi.org/10.1097/MCO.0000000000000242.

Bonnert M, Olén O, Lalouni M, et al. Internet-delivered cognitive behavior therapy for adolescents with irritable bowel syndrome: a randomized controlled trial. Am J Gastroenterol. 2017; https://doi.org/10.1038/ajg.2016.503.

Bredenoord AJ, Weusten BLAM, Sifrim D, Timmer R, Smout AJPM. Aerophagia, gastric, and supragastric belching: a study using intraluminal electrical impedance monitoring. Gut. 2004; https://doi.org/10.1136/gut.2004.042945.

Caldarella MP, Serra J, Azpiroz F, Malagelada JR. Prokinetic effects in patients with intestinal gas retention. Gastroenterology. 2002; https://doi.org/10.1053/gast.2002.33658.

Cappello G, Spezzaferro M, Grossi L, Manzoli L, Marzio L. Peppermint oil (Mintoil®) in the treatment of irritable bowel syndrome: a prospective double blind - placebo-controlled randomized trial. Dig Liver Dis. 2007; https://doi.org/10.1016/j.dld.2007.02.006.

Chang J, Chadwick RW, Allison JC, Hayes YO, Talley DL, Autry CE. Microbial succession and intestinal enzyme activities in the developing rat. J Appl Bacteriol. 1994; https://doi.org/10.1111/j.1365-2672.1994.tb02823.x.

Collins SM. A role for the gut microbiota in IBS. Nat Rev Gastroenterol Hepatol. 2014; https://doi.org/10.1038/nrgastro.2014.40.

Després JP, Lemieux I. Abdominal obesity and metabolic syndrome. Nature. 2006; https://doi.org/10.1038/nature05488.

Drossman DA. The functional gastrointestinal disorders and the Rome III process. Gastroenterology. 2006; https://doi.org/10.1053/j.gastro.2006.03.008.

Drossman DA. Functional gastrointestinal disorders: history, pathophysiology, clinical features, and Rome IV. Gastroenterology. 2016; https://doi.org/10.1053/j.gastro.2016.02.032.

Drossman DA, Hasler WL. Rome IV – functional GI disorders: disorders of gut-brain interaction. Gastroenterology. 2016; https://doi.org/10.1053/j.gastro.2016.03.035.

Drugs.com. Choice Rev Online. 2012; https://doi.org/10.5860/choice.49-5697.

Dukowicz AC, Lacy BE, Levine GM. Small intestinal bacterial overgrowth: a comprehensive review. Gastroenterol Hepatol. 2007;3(2):112–22.

Duncan SH, Flint HJ. Probiotics and prebiotics and health in ageing populations. Maturitas. 2013; https://doi.org/10.1016/j.maturitas.2013.02.004.

Eadala P, Waud JP, Matthews SB, Green JT, Campbell AK. Quantifying the "hidden" lactose in drugs used for the treatment of gastrointestinal conditions. Aliment Pharmacol Ther. 2009; https://doi.org/10.1111/j.1365-2036.2008.03889.x.

El-Salhy M, Gundersen D. Diet in irritable bowel syndrome. Nutr J. 2015; https://doi.org/10.1186/s12937-015-0022-3.

Everitt H, Landau S, Little P, et al. Assessing cognitive behavioural therapy in irritable bowel (ACTIB): protocol for a randomised controlled trial of clinical-effectiveness and cost-effectiveness of therapist delivered cognitive behavioural therapy and web-based self-management in irritable. BMJ Open. 2015; https://doi.org/10.1136/bmjopen-2015-008622.

Falch C, Vicente D, Häberle H, et al. Treatment of acute abdominal pain in the emergency room: a systematic review of the literature. Eur J Pain (United Kingdom). 2014; https://doi.org/10.1002/j.1532-2149.2014.00456.x.

Fedewa A, Rao SSC. Dietary fructose intolerance, fructan intolerance and FODMAPs. Curr Gastroenterol Rep. 2014; https://doi.org/10.1007/s11894-013-0370-0.

Fernández-Bañares F, Rosinach M, Esteve M, Forné M, Espinós JC, Maria Viver J. Sugar malabsorption in functional abdominal bloating: a pilot study on the long-term effect of dietary treatment. Clin Nutr. 2006; https://doi.org/10.1016/j.clnu.2005.11.010.

Fernández-Bañares F, Esteve M, Viver JM. Fructose-sorbitol malabsorption. Curr Gastroenterol Rep. 2009; https://doi.org/10.1007/s11894-009-0056-9.

Ford AC, Talley NJ, Spiegel BMR, et al. Effect of fibre, antispasmodics, and peppermint oil in the treatment of irritable bowel syndrome: systematic review and meta-analysis. BMJ. 2008; https://doi.org/10.1136/bmj.a2313.

Ford AC, Spiegel BMR, Talley NJ, Moayyedi P. Small intestinal bacterial overgrowth in irritable bowel syndrome: systematic review and meta-analysis. Clin Gastroenterol Hepatol. 2009; https://doi.org/10.1016/j.cgh.2009.06.031.

Gallegos-Orozco JF, Foxx-Orenstein AE, Sterler SM, Stoa JM. Chronic constipation in the elderly. Am J Gastroenterol. 2012; https://doi.org/10.1038/ajg.2011.349.

Ganiats TG, Norcross WA, Halverson AL, Burford PA, Palinkas LA. Does beano prevent gas? A double-blind crossover study of oral ??- galactosidase to treat dietary oligosaccharide intolerance. J Fam Pract. 1994;39:441–5.

Gasbarrini A, Lauritano EC, Gabrielli M, et al. Small intestinal bacterial overgrowth: diagnosis and treatment. Dig Dis. 2007; https://doi.org/10.1159/000103892.

Gasbarrini A, Lauritano EC, Garcovich M, Sparano L, Gasbarrini G. New insights into the pathophysiology of IBS: intestinal microflora, gas production and gut motility. Eur Rev Med Pharmacol Sci. 2008;12 (Suppl 1):111–7.

Glasinovic E, Wynter E, Arguero J, et al. Treatment of supragastric belching with cognitive behavioral therapy improves quality of life and reduces acid gastroesophageal reflux. Am J Gastroenterol. 2018; https://doi.org/10.1038/ajg.2018.15.

Goetze O, Fox MR, Erb A, et al. Gastric emptying, dyspeptic symptoms and eating behavior in healthy mountaineers after rapid ascent to 4559 M (14957 Ft). Gastroenterology. 2010;138:S-467.

Goldstein DR, Pitchumoni CS. Intestinal gas. Geriatr Gastroenterol. 2012; https://doi.org/10.1007/978-1-4419-1623-5_33.

Gould M, Sellin JH. Diabetic diarrhea. Curr Gastroenterol Rep. 2009; https://doi.org/10.1007/s11894-009-0054-y.

Hasler WL. Gas and bloating. Gastroenterol Hepatol. 2006.

Hauser G, Pletikosic S, Tkalcic M. Cognitive behavioral approach to understanding irritable bowel syndrome. World J Gastroenterol. 2014; https://doi.org/10.3748/wjg.v20.i22.6744.

Hemmink GJM, Weusten BLAM, Bredenoord AJ, Timmer R, Smout AJPM. Aerophagia: excessive air swallowing demonstrated by esophageal impedance monitoring. Clin Gastroenterol Hepatol. 2009a; https://doi.org/10.1016/j.cgh.2009.06.029.

Hemmink GJM, Bredenoord AJ, Weusten BLAM, Timmer R, Smout AJPM. Supragastric belching in patients with reflux symptoms. Am J Gastroenterol. 2009b; https://doi.org/10.1038/ajg.2009.203.

Hungin APS, Mitchell CR, Whorwell P, et al. Systematic review: probiotics in the management of lower gastrointestinal symptoms – an updated evidence-based international consensus. Aliment Pharmacol Ther. 2018; https://doi.org/10.1111/apt.14539.

Iovino P, Bucci C, Tremolaterra F, Santonicola A, Chiarioni G. Bloating and functional gastro-intestinal disorders: where are we and where are we going? World J Gastroenterol. 2014; https://doi.org/10.3748/wjg.v20.i39.14407.

Jain NK, Rosenberg DB, Ulahannan MJ, Glasser MJ, Pitchumoni CS. Sorbitol intolerance in adults. Am J Gastroenterol. 1985; https://doi.org/10.1111/j.1572-0241.1985.tb02206.x.

Jankovic N, Geelen A, Streppel MT, et al. WHO guidelines for a healthy diet and mortality from cardiovascular disease in European and American elderly: the CHANCES project. Am J Clin Nutr. 2015; https://doi.org/10.3945/ajcn.114.095117.

Jiang R, Horvath B. Neostigmine. In: The essence of analgesia and analgesics; 2010. https://doi.org/10.1017/CBO9780511841378.120.

Johnston KR, Govel LA, Andritz MH. Gastrointestinal effects of sorbitol as an additive in liquid medications. Am J Med. 1994; https://doi.org/10.1016/0002-9343(94)90029-9.

Kalantar-Zadeh K, Berean KJ, Burgell RE, Muir JG, Gibson PR. Intestinal gases: influence on gut disorders and the role of dietary manipulations. Nat Rev Gastroenterol Hepatol. 2019; https://doi.org/10.1038/s41575-019-0193-z.

Katzka DA. Simple office-based behavioral approach to patients with chronic belching. Dis Esophagus. 2013; https://doi.org/10.1111/dote.12006.

Keller J, Layer P. Intestinal and anorectal motility and functional disorders. Best Pract Res Clin Gastroenterol. 2009; https://doi.org/10.1016/j.bpg.2009.02.012.

Kerckhoffs APM, Visser MR, Samsom M, et al. Critical evaluation of diagnosing bacterial overgrowth in the proximal small intestine. J Clin Gastroenterol. 2008; https://doi.org/10.1097/MCG.0b013e31818474d7.

Kessing BF, Bredenoord AJ, Smout AJPM. The pathophysiology, diagnosis and treatment of excessive belching symptoms. Am J Gastroenterol. 2014; https://doi.org/10.1038/ajg.2014.165.

Khalaf, Mohamed MD; Schatz, Richard MD; Elias, Puja MD; Castell, Donald MD, MACG, AGAF Pathogenesis of GERD: Don't Forget the Resting LES Pressure! American Journal of Gastroenterology. 2017;112: S191–S192. https://journals.lww.com/ajg/fulltext/2017/10001/pathogenesis_of_gerd__don_t_forget_the_resting_les.355.aspx.

Klaus J, Spaniol U, Adler G, Mason RA, Reinshagen M, von Tirpitz CC. Small intestinal bacterial overgrowth mimicking acute flare as a pitfall in patients with Crohn's disease. BMC Gastroenterol. 2009; https://doi.org/10.1186/1471-230X-9-61.

Kunkel D, Basseri RJ, Makhani MD, Chong K, Chang C, Pimentel M. Methane on breath testing is associated with constipation: a systematic review and meta-analysis. Dig Dis Sci. 2011; https://doi.org/10.1007/s10620-011-1590-5.

Kyaw MH, Mayberry JF. Fructose malabsorption: true condition or a variance from normality. J Clin Gastroenterol. 2011; https://doi.org/10.1097/MCG.0b013e3181eed6bf.

Lacy BE, Gabbard SL, Crowell MD. Pathophysiology, evaluation, and treatment of bloating: hope, hype, or hot air? Gastroenterol Hepatol. 2011;7(11):729–39.

Lapides RA, Savaiano DA. Gender, age, race and lactose intolerance: is there evidence to support a differential symptom response? A scoping review. Nutrients. 2018; https://doi.org/10.3390/nu10121956.

Lasser RB, Bond JH, Levitt MD. The role of intestinal gas in Functional Abdominal Pain. N Engl J Med. 1975; https://doi.org/10.1056/NEJM197509112931103.

Lee KN, Lee OY. Intestinal microbiota in pathophysiology and management of irritable bowel syndrome. World J Gastroenterol. 2014; https://doi.org/10.3748/wjg.v20.i27.8886.

Lee HJ, Choi JK, Ryu HS, et al. Therapeutic modulation of gut microbiota in functional bowel disorders. J Neurogastroenterol Motil. 2017; https://doi.org/10.5056/jnm16124.

Levitt MD. Production and excretion of hydrogen gas in man. N Engl J Med. 1969; https://doi.org/10.1056/NEJM196907172810303.

Levitt MD. Volume and composition of human intestinal gas determined by means of an intestinal washout technic. N Engl J Med. 1971; https://doi.org/10.1056/NEJM197106242842502.

Levitt MD, Ingelfinger FJ. Hydrogen and methane production in man. Ann N Y Acad Sci. 1968; https://doi.org/10.1111/j.1749-6632.1968.tb19033.x.

Levitt MD, Hirsh P, Fetzer CA, Sheahan M, Levine AS. H2 excretion after ingestion of complex carbohydrates. Gastroenterology. 1987; https://doi.org/10.1016/0016-5085(87)90132-6.

Linlawan S, Patcharatrakul T, Somlaw N, Gonlachanvit S. Effect of Rice, wheat, and mung bean ingestion on intestinal gas production and postprandial gastrointestinal symptoms in non-constipation irritable bowel syndrome patients. Nutrients. 2019; https://doi.org/10.3390/nu11092061.

Lumsden K, Chaudhary NA, Truelove SC. The irritable colon syndrome. Clin Radiol. 1963; https://doi.org/10.1016/S0009-9260(63)80010-0.

Macfarlane GT, Macfarlane S. Bacteria, colonic fermentation, and gastrointestinal health. J AOAC Int. 2012; https://doi.org/10.5740/jaoacint.SGE_Macfarlane.

Major G, Pritchard S, Murray K, et al. Colon hypersensitivity to distension, rather than excessive gas production, produces carbohydrate-related symptoms in individuals with irritable bowel syndrome. Gastroenterology. 2017; https://doi.org/10.1053/j.gastro.2016.09.062.

Manichanh C, Eck A, Varela E, et al. Anal gas evacuation and colonic microbiota in patients with flatulence: effect of diet. Gut. 2014; https://doi.org/10.1136/gutjnl-2012-303013.

Mansueto P, Seidita A, D'alcamo A, Carroccio A. Role of FODMAPs in patients with irritable bowel syndrome. Nutr Clin Pract. 2015; https://doi.org/10.1177/0884533615569886.

Masuy I, Tackoen J, Deloose E, Van Oudenhove L, Tack J. The combination of peppermint oil and caraway oil does not affect gastric function, but increases hunger ratings and decreases satiation in healthy subjects. United Eur Gastroenterol J. 2018; https://doi.org/10.1177/2050640618792819.

Mattar R, Mazo DF de C, Carrilho FJ. Lactose intolerance: diagnosis, genetic, and clinical factors. Clin Exp Gastroenterol. 2012; https://doi.org/10.2147/CEG.S32368.

Matthews SB, Waud JP, Roberts AG, Campbell AK. Systemic lactose intolerance: a new perspective on an old problem. Postgrad Med J. 2005; https://doi.org/10.1136/pgmj.2004.025551.

Mcrorie JW. Psyllium is not fermented in the human gut. Neurogastroenterol Motil. 2015; https://doi.org/10.1111/nmo.12649.

McRorie JW, Chey WD. Fermented Fiber supplements are no better than placebo for a laxative effect. Dig Dis Sci. 2016; https://doi.org/10.1007/s10620-016-4304-1.

Miller TL, Wolin MJ. Fermentations by saccharolytic intestinal bacteria. Am J Clin Nutr. 1979;

Montalto M, Di Stefano M, Gasbarrini A, Corazza GR. Intestinal gas metabolism. Dig Liver Dis Suppl. 2009; https://doi.org/10.1016/S1594-5804(09)60015-2.

Nanayakkara WS, Skidmore PM, O'Brien L, Wilkinson TJ, Gearry RB. Efficacy of the low FODMAP diet for treating irritable bowel syndrome: the evidence to date. Clin Exp Gastroenterol. 2016; https://doi.org/10.2147/CEG.S86798.

Nigaglioni A, Finkelstein D, Bockus HL. Role of gastric distention in angina pectoris. Intractable angina pectoris with cascade stomach and magenblase syndrome treated with gastric resection. Am J Cardiol. 1963; https://doi.org/10.1016/0002-9149(63)90067-5.

Ong AML, Chua LTT, Khor CJL, Asokkumar R, s/o Namasivayam V, Wang YT. Diaphragmatic breathing reduces belching and proton pump inhibitor refractory gastroesophageal reflux symptoms. Clin Gastroenterol Hepatol. 2018. https://doi.org/10.1016/j.cgh.2017.10.038.

Onyenekwe PC, Njoku GC, Ameh DA. Effect of cowpea (Vigna unguiculata) processing methods on flatus causing oligosaccharides. Nutr Res. 2000; https://doi.org/10.1016/S0271-5317(00)00128-7.

Ooi JLS, Vardar R, Sifrim D. Supragastric belching. Curr Opin Gastroenterol. 2016; https://doi.org/10.1097/MOG.0000000000000276.

Osipenko MF, Bikbulatova EA, But-Gusaim VI. Splenic flexure and irritable colon syndromes: conjugate conditions. Ter Arkh. 2008;80(2):48–52.

Owens DM, Nelson DK, Talley NJ. The irritable bowel syndrome: long-term prognosis and the physician-patient interaction. Ann Intern Med. 1995; https://doi.org/10.7326/0003-4819-122-2-199501150-00005.

Parker AM, Watson RR. Lactose intolerance. In: Nutrients in dairy and their implications for health and disease; 2017. https://doi.org/10.1016/B978-0-12-809762-5.00016-4.

Passos MC, Serra J, Azpiroz F, Tremolaterra F, Malagelada JR. Impaired reflex control of intestinal gas transit in patients with abdominal bloating. Gut. 2005; https://doi.org/10.1136/gut.2003.038158.

Perman JA, Modler S. Glycoproteins as substrates for production of hydrogen and methane by colonic bacterial flora. Gastroenterology. 1982; https://doi.org/10.1016/S0016-5085(82)80333-8.

Pimentel M, Mayer AG, Park S, Chow EJ, Hasan A, Kong Y. Methane production during lactulose breath test is associated with gastrointestinal disease presentation. Dig Dis Sci. 2003a; https://doi.org/10.1023/A:1021738515885.

Pimentel M, Chow EJ, Lin HC. Normalization of lactulose breath testing correlates with symptom improvement in irritable bowel syndrome: a double-blind, randomized, placebo-controlled study. Am J Gastroenterol. 2003b; https://doi.org/10.1016/S0002-9270(02)05902-6.

Pimentel M, Park S, Mirocha J, Kane SV, Kong Y. The effect of a nonabsorbed oral antibiotic (Rifaximin) on the symptoms of the irritable bowel syndrome: a randomized trial. Ann Intern Med. 2006; https://doi.org/10.7326/0003-4819-145-8-200610170-00004.

Pimentel M, Mathur R, Chang C. Gas and the microbiome. Curr Gastroenterol Rep. 2013; https://doi.org/10.1007/s11894-013-0356-y.

Price KR, Lewis J, Wyatt GM, Fenwick GR. Review article flatulence – causes, relation to diet and remedies. Food Nahrung. 1988; https://doi.org/10.1002/food.19880320626.

Punkkinen J, Haak R, Kaartinen M, Walamies M. Help from habit reversal for supragastric belching. Duodecim. 2016;132(22):2073–9.

Rami Reddy SR, Cappell MS. A systematic review of the clinical presentation, diagnosis, and treatment of small bowel obstruction. Curr Gastroenterol Rep. 2017; https://doi.org/10.1007/s11894-017-0566-9.

Rao SSC. Belching, bloating, and flatulence: how to help patients who have troublesome abdominal gas. Postgrad Med. 1997; https://doi.org/10.3810/pgm.1997.04.208.

Reddymasu SC, Sostarich S, McCallum RW. Small intestinal bacterial overgrowth in irritable bowel syndrome: are there any predictors? BMC Gastroenterol. 2010; https://doi.org/10.1186/1471-230X-10-23.

Rizkalla SW. Health implications of fructose consumption: a review of recent data. Nutr Metab. 2010; https://doi.org/10.1186/1743-7075-7-82.

Roccarina D, Lauritano EC, Gabrielli M, Franceschi F, Ojetti V, Gasbarrini A. The role of methane in intestinal diseases. Am J Gastroenterol. 2010; https://doi.org/10.1038/ajg.2009.744.

Rumessen JJ, Gudmand-Høyer E. Malabsorption of fructose-sorbitol mixtures interactions causing abdominal distress. Scand J Gastroenterol. 1987; https://doi.org/10.3109/00365528708991486.

Rumessen JJ, Gudmand-Høyer E. Functional bowel disease: malabsorption and abdominal distress after ingestion of fructose, sorbitol, and fructose- sorbitol mixtures. Gastroenterology. 1988; https://doi.org/10.1016/S0016-5085(88)80016-7.

Rune SJ. Acid-Base parameters of duodenal contents in man. Gastroenterology. 1972; https://doi.org/10.1016/S0016-5085(72)80035-0.

Ryu HS e, Choi SC h, Lee JS e. Belching (eructation). Korean J Gastroenterol. 2014; https://doi.org/10.4166/kjg.2014.64.1.4.

Sachdeva S, Rawat AK, Reddy RS, Puri AS. Small intestinal bacterial overgrowth (SIBO) in irritable bowel syndrome: frequency and predictors. J Gastroenterol Hepatol. 2011; https://doi.org/10.1111/j.1440-1746.2011.06654.x.

Salvioli B, Serra J, Azpiroz F, Malagelada JR. Impaired small bowel gas propulsion in patients with bloating during intestinal lipid infusion. Am J Gastroenterol. 2006; https://doi.org/10.1111/j.1572-0241.2006.00702.x.

Scaldaferri F, Nardone O, Lopetuso LR, et al. Intestinal gas production and gastrointestinal symptoms: from pathogenesis to clinical implication. Eur Rev Med Pharmacol Sci. 2013;17(Suppl 2):2–10.

Scheppach W. Effects of short chain fatty acids on gut morphology and function. Gut. 1994;35(1 Suppl):35–8.

Schmulson MJ, Drossman DA. What is new in Rome IV. J Neurogastroenterol Motil. 2017; https://doi.org/10.5056/jnm16214.

Serra J, Azpiroz F, Malagelada JR. Intestinal gas dynamics and tolerance in humans. Gastroenterology. 1998; https://doi.org/10.1016/S0016-5085(98)70133-7.

Serra J, Azpiroz F, Malagelada JR. Mechanisms of intestinal gas retention in humans: impaired propulsion versus obstructed evacuation. Am J Physiol Gastrointest Liver Physiol. 2001;

Shah ED, Basseri RJ, Chong K, Pimentel M. Abnormal breath testing in IBS: a meta-analysis. Dig Dis Sci. 2010; https://doi.org/10.1007/s10620-010-1276-4.

Sharara AI, Aoun E, Abdul-Baki H, Mounzer R, Sidani S, Elhajj I. A randomized double-blind placebo-controlled trial of rifaximin in patients with abdominal bloating and flatulence. Am J Gastroenterol. 2006; https://doi.org/10.1111/j.1572-0241.2006.00458.x.

Shen Y-HA, Nahas R. Clinical review treatment of irritable bowel syndrome. Can Fam Physician. 2009;

Sieber R, Stransky M, de Vrese MZ. Lactose intolerance and consumption of milk and milk products. Ernahrungswiss. 1997;36(4):375–93. https://doi.org/10.1007/BF01617834.

Simrén M. Bloating and abdominal distention: not so poorly understood anymore! Gastroenterology. 2009; https://doi.org/10.1053/j.gastro.2009.03.023.

Skoog SM, Bharucha AE, Zinsmeister AR. Comparison of breath testing with fructose and high fructose corn syrups in health and IBS. Neurogastroenterol Motil. 2008; https://doi.org/10.1111/j.1365-2982.2007.01074.x.

Sprung, Douglas MD. FACG Is Treating Elderly Irritable Bowel Syndrome Patients With Anticholinergics Really Dangerous? Results of a Community-Based Study. American Journal of Gastroenterology. 2014;109:S531. https://journals.lww.com/ajg/Fulltext/2014/10002/Is_Treating_Elderly_Irritable_Bowel_Syndrome.1795.aspx.

Stanghellini V, Chan FKL, Hasler WL, et al. Gastroduodenal disorders. Gastroenterology. 2016; https://doi.org/10.1053/j.gastro.2016.02.011.

Stanhope KL, Havel PJ. Fructose consumption: recent results and their potential implications. Ann N Y Acad Sci. 2010; https://doi.org/10.1111/j.1749-6632.2009.05266.x.

Staudacher HM, Lomer MCE, Farquharson FM, et al. A diet low in FODMAPs reduces symptoms in patients with irritable bowel syndrome and a probiotic restores Bifidobacterium species: a randomized controlled trial. Gastroenterology. 2017; https://doi.org/10.1053/j.gastro.2017.06.010.

Stephen AM, Cummings JH. Mechanism of action of dietary fibre in the human colon. Nature. 1980; https://doi.org/10.1038/284283a0.

Stone-Dorshow T, Levitt MD. Gaseous response to ingestion of a poorly absorbed fructo-oligosaccharide sweetener. Am J Clin Nutr. 1987; https://doi.org/10.1093/ajcn/46.1.61.

Straathof JWA, Ringers J, Lamers CBHW, Masclee AAM. Provocation of transient lower esophageal sphincter relaxations by gastric distension with air. Am J Gastroenterol. 2001; https://doi.org/10.1016/S0002-9270(01)02498-4.

Suarez F, Furne J, Springfield J, Levitt M. Insights into human colonic physiology obtained from the study of flatus composition. Am J Physiol Gastrointest Liver Physiol. 1997;272:G1028.

Suarez FL, Springfield J, Levitt MD. Identification of gases responsible for the odour of human flatus and evaluation of a device purported to reduce this odour. Gut. 1998;48:100–4.

Suarez F, Levitt MD, Adshead J, Barkin JS. Pancreatic supplements reduce symptomatic response of healthy subjects to a high fat meal. Dig Dis Sci. 1999; https://doi.org/10.1023/A:1026675012864.

Sullivan SN. Functional abdominal bloating with distention. ISRN Gastroenterol. 2012; https://doi.org/10.5402/2012/721820.

Talley NJ, Phung N, Kalantar JS. ABC of the upper gastrointestinal tract: indigestion: when is it functional? Br Med J. 2001;323:1294.

Tan AH, Mahadeva S, Thalha AM, et al. Helicobacter pylori and small intestinal bacterial overgrowth in Parkinson'/INS;s disease: prevalence and clinical significance. J Neurol Sci. 2013; https://doi.org/10.1016/j.jns.2013.07.528.

Tang YR, Wang P, Yin R, Ge JX, Wang GP, Lin L. Five-year follow-up of 263 cases of functional bowel disorder. World J Gastroenterol. 2013; https://doi.org/10.3748/wjg.v19.i9.1466.

Tangerman A, Winkel EG. Extra-oral halitosis: an overview. J Breath Res. 2010; https://doi.org/10.1088/1752-7155/4/1/017003.

Tomlin J, Lowis C, Read NW. Investigation of normal flatus production in healthy volunteers. Gut. 1991; https://doi.org/10.1136/gut.32.6.665.

Varney J, Barrett J, Scarlata K, Catsos P, Gibson PR, Muir JG. FODMAPs: food composition, defining cutoff values and international application. J Gastroenterol Hepatol. 2017; https://doi.org/10.1111/jgh.13698.

Vos MB, Kimmons JE, Gillespie C, Welsh J, Blank HM. Dietary fructose consumption among US children and adults: the third National Health and nutrition examination survey CME. MedGenMed Medscape Gen Med. 2008;

Webb AN, Kukuruzovic RH, Catto-Smith AG, Sawyer SM. Hypnotherapy for treatment of irritable bowel syndrome. Cochrane Database Syst Rev. 2007; https://doi.org/10.1002/14651858.CD005110.pub2.

Weinberg DS. Handbook of gastroenterology. Ann Intern Med. 1998; https://doi.org/10.7326/0003-4819-129-8-199810150-00041.

Whelan K, Martin LD, Staudacher HM, Lomer MCE. The low FODMAP diet in the management of irritable bowel syndrome: an evidence-based review of FODMAP restriction, reintroduction and personalisation in clinical practice. J Hum Nutr Diet. 2018; https://doi.org/10.1111/jhn.12530.

Wilkinson JM, Cozine EW, Loftus CG. Gas, bloating, and belching: approach to evaluation and management. Am Fam Physician. 2019;

Yoon K, Kim N, Lee JY, et al. Clinical response of Rifaximin treatment in patients with abdominal bloating. Korean J Gastroenterol. 2018; https://doi.org/10.4166/kjg.2018.72.3.121.

Constipation

53

T. S. Dharmarajan, David Widjaja, and C. S. Pitchumoni

Contents

T. S. Dharmarajan (✉)
Department of Medicine, Division of Geriatrics,
Montefiore Medical Center, Wakefield Campus, Bronx,
NY, USA

Department of Medicine, Albert Einstein College of
Medicine, Bronx, NY, USA

Department of Medicine, New York Medical College,
Valhalla, NY, USA
e-mail: dharmarajants@yahoo.com

D. Widjaja
Bogor Senior Hospital, Bogor, Indonesia
e-mail: medicine.nyc@gmail.com

C. S. Pitchumoni
Department of Medicine, Robert Wood Johnson School of
Medicine, Rutgers University, New Brunswick, NJ, USA

Department of Medicine, New York Medical College,
Valhalla, NY, USA

Division of Gastroenterology, Hepatology and Clinical
Nutrition, Saint Peters University Hospital, New
Brunswick, NJ, USA
e-mail: pitchumoni@hotmail.com

© Springer Nature Switzerland AG 2021
C. S. Pitchumoni, T. S. Dharmarajan (eds.), *Geriatric Gastroenterology*,
https://doi.org/10.1007/978-3-030-30192-7_45

Abstract

Constipation is a common syndrome in older individuals. Constipation is defined as a frequency of defecation fewer than three times per week in association with additional manifestations as defined in the Rome criteria. Deviations from baseline habits deserve attention and perhaps evaluation. Motility and structural abnormalities are two important factors contributing to pathogenesis of constipation. Colonic motor dysfunction is associated with several factors, predominantly dietary, activity, medications, and disease. A thorough medical history helps identify the etiology, including the presence of systemic disorders that will need to be addressed to manage constipation. Acute development of constipation is likely to be on a different basis. More specialized tests of colonic transit or pelvic floor function are considered in older adults in selected cases and in settings where the findings are likely to influence management decisions. Management strategy includes primarily addressing lifestyle modification including the use of adequate fiber, sufficient fluid intake, optimizing defecation posture, and promoting activity; when the strategy is ineffective, pharmacological measures are utilized. Miscellaneous modalities are available as a last resort. Laxatives used long term to manage constipation are invariably associated with adverse drug effects.

Keywords

Constipation · Definition of constipation · Medication-induced constipation · Laxatives · Laxative misuse · Stool softeners · Bisacodyl · Senna · Lactulose · Polyethylene glycol · Docusate · Fecal impaction · Fecal incontinence · Dietary fiber · Fiber supplements · Rome criteria for constipation · Evaluation for constipation · Pelvic floor dysfunction · Pelvic dyssynergia · Slow transit constipation · Fecal impaction · Bristol Stool Form Scale · Defecatory disorders · Anorectal manometry · Balloon expulsion test · Colonic transit time · Enema · Rectal examination

Introduction

Constipation is a common syndrome in the geriatric age group in all settings and often poses a management enigma. The topic has been reviewed in several position papers (American College of Gastroenterology Chronic Constipation Task Force 2005; Bouras and Tangalos 2009; Camilleri 2011; Foxx-Orenstein et al. 2008; Ghoshal et al. 2018; Locke et al. 2000; Tariq 2008; Lindberg et al. 2011). The prevalence of constipation is significantly higher in the geriatric age group, compared to those younger, regardless of the methodology of data collection, self-reporting or utilizing the Rome criteria (Drossman et al. 1993; Harari et al. 1996; Pare et al. 2001; Sandler et al. 1990; Talley et al. 1996; Talley et al. 1993). The disorder is more common in older women than men (Bouras and Tangalos 2009). The prevalence of census-adjusted Rome IV functional bowel disorders were similar in the United States, Canada, and United Kingdom, with 7.9% to 8.6% for functional constipation (Palsson et al. 2020).

Constipation is more prevalent in nursing home residents compared to community adults (Rao and Go 2010), a finding perhaps relating to differences in comorbidity and medication use (Fosnes et al. 2010; Gage et al. 2010; van Dijk et al. 1998). In nursing homes, the prevalence of constipation increased between 2007 and 2013, from 36% to 40%; after controlling for age, sex, function and cognition, and medication use, the difference was statistically significant (Gustafsson et al. 2019). In particular, this calls to attention the need for awareness, especially in those prescribed with opioids and rated as constipated when not treated with laxatives. Residents on opioids and anticholinergics were at higher risk, and those with a higher activities of daily living (ADL) score were at lower risk (Gustafsson et al. 2019).

The association between constipation and cognitive impairment was studied in a cohort of 2806 patients over 60 years of age; score for constipation in total, directive force, calculating ability, delayed memory, writing, reading comprehension, and visual-spatial ability was lower than that in non-constipation subjects; cognitive impairment risk tended to increase with increasing severity of constipation in males and females (Wan et al. 2019).

The direct Medicare costs for constipation are significant. In 2001, of 5.7 million ambulatory visits that carried a diagnosis of constipation, 2.7 million listed constipation as the primary diagnosis; of these >1.8 million were outpatients, and >0.5 million were in those visiting the emergency department (ED) (Martin et al. 2006). Of the total cost incurred at $235 million/year, 55% was for inpatient care, 23% was in the ED, and 16% involved outpatient physicians (Martin et al.

2006). The in-hospital constipation-related complications such as intestinal obstruction, anal fissures, impaction, volvulus, and stercoral ulcers entailed much Medicare and Medicaid costs (Tuteja and Biskupiak 2007). The criteria used to identify constipation impact the prevalence of the disorder. In an Australian study involving a large national sample of community-dwelling adults, five simple definitions of constipation were compared with Rome III criteria. Simple definitions, commonly used in research, performed poorly with the Rome III criteria; self-reported criteria had the highest sensitivity and negative predictive value compared to the Rome III criteria, but had low specificity and positive predictive value (Werth et al. 2019). The authors suggest using the Rome criteria where possible for better estimates in prevalence studies. Similar findings were also reported in India. In a pan-Indian multicentric study of 2656 patients, 1404 reported experiencing constipation, although only 507(36%) of them had a stool frequency <3 per week (Ghoshal et al. 2018). In another multicentric irritable bowel syndrome study from India, involving 1618 patients with chronic lower GI symptoms, in 463 patients who had self-perceived constipation, only 319 patients were diagnosed as chronic constipation if the stool frequency criteria had been applied (Ghoshal et al. 2018).

Of interest and highlighted in an article highlighting "teaching primary care of frail older adults," the Frailty 5 Checklist included feelings, flow (constipation and urinary incontinence), function and falls, farmacy, and future and family; these are the five domains that affect frail seniors and should be evaluated (Freedman and McDougall 2019). Rates of constipation approach 50% in adults over age 80 years and may even be associated with syncope, coronary or cerebral ischemia, anorexia, nausea, discomfort, and poor quality of life (Freedman and McDougall 2019).

Definitions

Because clinicians and patients differ in their views on constipation, consensus criteria have helped in defining and categorizing the diagnosis of constipation. The American Gastroenterological Association criteria utilized colonic transit and anorectal tests to classify constipated patients into one of three groups: normal transit constipation, slow transit constipation, and pelvic floor dysfunction or defecatory disorders (Bharucha et al. 2013). On the other hand, Rome IV criteria incorporate symptoms and anorectal assessments of rectal evacuation in defining and categorizing constipation (Mearin et al. 2016; Rao et al. 2016). Based on the Rome criteria, defecatory disorders are defined by bowel symptoms and anorectal test results indicative of impaired rectal evacuation. However, functional constipation and constipation-predominant irritable bowel syndrome are defined only by symptoms (Bharucha and Wald 2019). Bowel symptoms are used for defining functional constipation. Abdominal pain that is temporally related to bowel disturbances is used for defining the constipation-predominant irritable bowel syndrome. Upper gastrointestinal tract symptoms (e.g., heartburn, dyspepsia), anxiety, depression, urinary symptoms, and the prevalence of increased rectal sensation are more common in constipation-predominant irritable bowel syndrome than functional constipation (Bharucha and Wald 2019). The symptoms of functional constipation and constipation-predominant irritable bowel syndrome based on Rome IV criteria are depicted in Table 1 (Mearin et al. 2016). Unlike the Rome III criteria, it is now specified in Rome IV criteria that abdominal pain and bloating may be present but are not predominant symptoms (i.e., the patient does not meet criteria for IBS). Although constipation-predominant irritable bowel syndrome and functional constipation both improve with dietary fiber supplementation and/or simple laxatives, an assessment of the phenotype of constipation guides and predicts the response to therapy (Bharucha and Wald 2019). For example, pelvic floor biofeedback therapy, not laxatives, is the cornerstone of managing defecatory disorder. The dose and response to treatment with secretagogues (e.g., lubiprostone) differs between functional constipation and constipation-predominant irritable bowel syndrome. Medically refractory isolated slow transit constipation is an indication for colectomy.

Table 1 Rome IV criteria for functional constipation (Mearin et al. 2016)

1. Must include two or more of the following:
(a) Straining during more than 25% of defecations
(b) Lumpy or hard stools (Bristol Stool Form Scale 1–2) more than 25% of defecations
(c) Sensation of incomplete evacuation more than 25% of defecations
(d) Sensation of anorectal obstruction/blockage more than 25% of defecations
(e) Manual maneuvers to facilitate more than 25% of defecations (e.g., digital evacuation, support of the pelvic floor)
(f) Fewer than three spontaneous bowel movements per week
2. Loose stools are rarely present without the use of laxatives
3. Insufficient criteria for irritable bowel syndrome

[a]Criteria fulfilled for the last 3 months with symptom onset at least 6 months prior to diagnosis

Rather than a disease entity, constipation is a term to describe difficulties experienced by a patient in moving the bowels (McCrea et al. 2008). In practice, clinicians use the frequency of defecation episodes, stool weight, colonic transit time, and anorectal manometry as proxy measures for constipation (Ashraf et al. 1996). Frequency of defecation fewer than three times per week is considered as constipation (Walter et al. 2010); however, this may be normal if it does not represent a deviation from baseline defecation practice and there is no associated discomfort (Abyad and Mourad 1996). Furthermore, patients often perceive constipation differently from the physician, with many defining constipation as just the presence of hard stools, infrequent evacuation, excessive straining, a sense of incomplete evacuation, excessive time spent on the toilet, and unsuccessful evacuation (Koch et al. 1997).

In a review of gastrointestinal disorders in older age, constipation was believed to affect 50% of nursing home residents; predispositions included decreased mobility, cognitive impairment, comorbidities, and polypharmacy; the disorder differs from IBS in that there is a lack of abdominal pain and discomfort; and stool impaction is a significant complication (Dumic et al. 2019).

Relevant Age-Related Physiological Changes

The daily input of water into the gastrointestinal (GI) tract is about 9.0 L per day (Pandol et al. 2009) About 1.5–2.0 liters of water enter the colon, with only 100–200 mL in feces (Pandol et al. 2009); higher water content makes stool softer (Danjo et al. 2008). Aging does not significantly reduce saliva production and pancreatic and gastric juice secretion (Bhutto and Morley 2008; Laugier et al. 1991). However, it is common for older adults to consume less water and poorly appreciate and respond to thirst. Data from the National Health and Nutrition Examination Survey (NHANES) evaluated water intake in different age groups, totaling 15,702 adults from the period 2005 through 2010; 83% of women and 95% of men over the age of 71 years failed to meet the Institute of Medicine average intake (AI) of water and stated it was a cause for concern in the old (Drewnowski et al. 2013).

Colonic motility plays a role in formation of stool. Aging is associated with enteric neurodegeneration and significant decline in cell number and density throughout the GI tract (Bernard et al. 2009; Peck et al. 2009; Phillips et al. 2007; Phillips and Powley 2007; Sprenger et al. 2009). Smooth muscle relaxation remains normal, but cholinergic neurons are reduced in number (Bernard et al. 2009). The functional consequence is delayed transit in the large bowel because there is less contraction with the bolus, leading to inefficient peristalsis (Bernard et al. 2009; Wiskur and Greenwood-Van Meerveld 2010). Extrinsic colonic nerves in rodents have shown a dramatic age-related degeneration of sympathetic motor neurons of the myenteric plexus and decline in colonic transit (Phillips et al. 2006), but there is paucity of data on age-related changes of the extrinsic innervation of the human colon and regarding degenerative process of interstitial cells of Cajal (intestinal pace maker) as a potential cause of constipation with age (Wiskur and Greenwood-Van Meerveld 2010).

Gastric distension and chemical stimulation by nutrients can stimulate peristaltic contractions in the colon to propel material toward the rectum via a neural reflex arc, commonly termed the gastrocolic reflex (Wiskur and Greenwood-Van Meerveld 2010). The reflex also stimulates colonic motility. The efficiency of gastrocolic reflex with age is not clear.

Endogenous opioids inhibit enteric nerve activity and inhibit both propulsive motor and secretory activities (Holzer 2007; Mehendale and Yuan 2006). Three major, distinct classes of opioid receptors are located in the enteric nervous system: delta, kappa, and mu (De Schepper et al. 2004; Holzer 2004). The enteric mu-opioid receptor is the principal mediator of opioid agonist effects on the GI tract (De Schepper et al. 2004). When opioid agonists bind to these receptors, the release of excitatory and inhibitory neurotransmitters is inhibited, interrupting coordinated rhythmic contractions required for intestinal motility, along with a reduction in mucosal secretions (Wood and Galligan 2004).

Aging in asymptomatic women is associated with reduced anal resting and squeeze pressures, reduced rectal compliance, reduced rectal sensation, and perineal laxity (Fox et al. 2006). Reduced rectal sensation may lead to stool impaction in the rectum (Wilson 1999). In addition, sarcopenia of aging (Glass and Roubenoff 2010) leads to weak abdominal musculature, which in turn decreases intra-abdominal pressure during straining, creating difficulty in evacuation.

Pathogenesis

Motility and structural abnormalities are two factors contributing to pathogenesis of constipation. Motility abnormalities include colonic and pelvic floor dysfunction. Colonic motor dysfunction is associated with dietary, medication, and disease factors (McCrea et al. 2008). Contributing diseases are listed in Table 2. In Parkinson's disease, constipation may be evident for a mean of 10 years (range 5 months to 19 years) prior to the onset of motor symptoms (Abbott et al. 2001). There is a high prevalence of constipation in patients with Parkinson's disease and

Table 2 Common disorders with colonic dysfunction constipation (Chinn and Schuffler 1988; Condom et al. 1993; Drukker et al. 2009; Gallagher and O'Mahony 2009; Viallard et al. 2005)

Endocrine or metabolic disorders	Neoplasms with paraneoplastic syndromes
Diabetes mellitus	Small cell lung cancers
Hypothyroidism	Pulmonary carcinoid
Hypercalcemia	**Musculoskeletal or connective tissue disorders**
Hypocalcemia	Amyloidosis
Hypokalemia	Dermatomyositis
Hypermagnesemia	Systemic sclerosis
Hyperparathyroidism	Psychogenic disorders
Hypoparathyroidism	Anxiety
Neurological disorders	Depression
Parkinson's disease	Somatization
Cerebrovascular disease, stroke	
Dementia	
Spinal cord lesions	
Autonomic neuropathy	

Table 3 Constipation-related presentations in older people

Behavioral: agitation, depression
Delirium
Megacolon
Overflow or spurious diarrhea
Quality of life impairment
Urinary retention

parkinsonism; a reduction of motor performance appears to be the primary basis for severe constipation and suggests that a good quality of gait and endurance may be helpful in reducing the risk of constipation (Frazzitta et al. 2019). A distinct category may be "Lewy body constipation," a cause for geriatric constipation; the disorder is characterized by the presence of dementia and parkinsonism features and is typical in older adults (Sakakibara et al. 2019).

Constipation is prevalent in those who suffer a stroke, although the pathophysiology of post-stroke constipation is not clear. A study of post-stroke patients suggested elevated thresholds for rectal sensation in those who developed a stroke followed by constipation, rather than an alteration in anorectal motility; in particular those with brainstem strokes develop constipation because the afferent pathways from the rectum to the brain are disrupted; elevated rectal sensation defecation threshold and decreased activity levels may be additionally contributory (Cheng et al. 2020). A complex neurohormonal mechanism

involving the dorsal vagal nucleus in the brain, vasoactive intestinal peptide (VIP) and gut appear involved (Braak et al. 2003). Data from subjects in the 2009–2010 National Health and Nutrition Examination Survey dataset who completed the Bowel Health Questionnaire suggested that there was an association between chronic constipation and poor kidney function in diabetes (Sommers et al. 2018).

Many medications lower colonic motility and are associated with constipation; a partial list is shown in Table 3. Opioid-induced constipation occurs in 40% of patients on opioids, through interference with GI motility by delaying transit, stimulating non-propulsive motility, segmentation tone and inhibition of colonic transit, intestinal and colonic secretion (Camilleri 2011); inhibition of acetylcholine release from the myenteric plexus and binding to opioid receptors in the intestine decreases intestinal motility and fluid secretion (Clemens and Klaschik 2008; Thomas et al. 2008). In patients with Parkinson's disease, the use of beta-blockers is associated with a lower risk of constipation, while dopaminergic treatments appear to increase risk of constipation (Pagano et al. 2015). Numerous drugs with anticholinergic effects decrease intestinal tone and motility (Lat et al. 2010); iron and calcium slow intestinal transit (Gartlehner et al. 2007); dehydration may be the basis with furosemide (Fosnes et al. 2010); inhibition of prostaglandins occurs with ibuprofen (prostaglandin analogues cause diarrhea) (Chang et al. 2007). With thalidomide, cisplatin, and vinca alkaloids, the mechanism is unclear (Gibson and Keefe 2006).

The term idiopathic slow transit constipation applies to a clinical syndrome characterized by intractable constipation and delayed colonic transit (Bharucha and Phillips 2001). The diagnosis is made after excluding colonic obstruction, metabolic disorders (e.g., hypothyroidism, hypercalcemia), drug-induced constipation, and pelvic floor dysfunction (Bharucha and Phillips 2001). In addition, in vitro and in vivo studies have shown that methane, a gas produced by gut bacteria, inhibits gastrointestinal motility (Chatterjee et al. 2007; Pimentel et al. 2006). The methane level in the gut may inversely correlate with stool form and stool frequency (Chatterjee et al. 2007; Pimentel et al. 2006). The level of the gas also appeared to correlate with the severity of constipation (Pimentel et al. 2006). The pathophysiology of ineffective colonic propulsion is incompletely understood, with potential mechanisms including reduced colonic contractile response to a meal, fewer colonic high amplitude propagated contractions, and disturbed visceral perception (Mertz et al. 1999; O'Brien et al. 1996). As the result of abnormal colonic activity, the bowel content remains in the ascending or transverse colon, without advancing to the rectosigmoid colon.

Pelvic floor dysfunction or disorders of the anorectum and pelvic floor create outlet dysfunction and inability to adequately evacuate rectal contents (McCrea et al. 2008). Terms used to describe these disorders include anismus, pelvic floor dyssynergia, paradoxical pelvic floor contraction, obstructed defecation, and functional rectosigmoid obstruction (Pezim et al. 1993). Pelvic floor dysfunction is most commonly due to dysfunction of the pelvic floor muscles or anal sphincters (Thompson et al. 2002). In the majority, it results from faulty toilet habits, painful defecation, obstetric or back injury, and brain-gut dysfunction (Rao 2008; Remes-Troche and Rao 2008). Damage to pelvic connective tissue, nerves, and muscles during childbirth may be contributory to the pathogenesis of pelvic floor dysfunction (Ryhammer et al. 1996). Patients with pelvic floor dysfunction are unable to coordinate abdominal, rectoanal, and pelvic floor muscles during defecation (Bharucha et al. 2006; Rao et al. 1998). The failure of rectoanal coordination may be impaired rectal contraction (61%), paradoxical anal contraction (78%), or inadequate anal relaxation (Rao 2008). Thus, incoordination or

dyssynergia of involved muscles is primarily responsible (Rao 2008). Further, up to half the patients may have rectal hyposensitivity (Rao et al. 1998; Scott and Gladman 2008).

Structural abnormalities causing constipation include nonobstructive and obstructive lesions. Anal fissure, a cut or split in the epithelial lining of the anal canal distal to the dentate line, is a nonobstructive cause of constipation. Anal fissure creates tearing pain and spasms with defecation for hours after defecation (Schubert et al. 2009; Talley 2008). The pain results in fear of the defecation process, resulting in constipation and even fecal impaction. Other painful anorectal lesions include abscess, hemorrhoids, proctalgia fugax, fistula, and levator ani syndrome (McCallum et al. 2009). Rectal prolapse, rectocele, and prolapsed hemorrhoids create obstructed defecation syndrome (Cruz et al. 2011; Scarlett 2004). With colon cancer, the location and depth of lesions determine the presentation of obstructive symptoms; the sites for greatest risk for obstruction are the splenic flexure and descending colon (Kaufman et al. 1989). Patients with obstructed defecation have a significant reduction in the amplitude of propagating pressure waves throughout the entire colon (McCrea et al. 2008).

Risk factors implicated in pathogenesis include aging, depression, inactivity, low caloric intake, low income, low education, number of medications taken (independent of adverse effect profile), physical and sexual abuse, and female gender (Lindberg et al. 2011).

Evaluation

History

A thorough medical history helps in identifying the etiology and in management of constipation. History should elicit the patient's perceptions of normal bowel habits; onset and duration of symptoms; defecation frequency; color, size, and volume of stool; rectal bleeding or pain; weight loss; straining with passage of stool; abdominal pain or bloating; fecal soiling or diarrhea; and need for digital manipulation during defecation (Gallagher and O'Mahony 2009). In addition, older adults should be encouraged to describe ability to sense complete evacuation and stool size using the Bristol Stool Form Scale and provide information about their cultural beliefs and expectations (Rao and Meduri 2010). Stool diaries and questionnaires help explore the bowel movement history, and minimize patient embarrassment (Ashraf et al. 1996; Rao et al. 2004).

Patient perception of normal bowel habits is a relevant initial question. Studies suggest that patient perception, which relates not only to the pathophysiology but also to sociocultural factors, determines symptom reporting and may increase the diagnostic sensitivity of symptom-based criteria (Ghoshal et al. 2013; Ghoshal et al. 2016; Sperber et al. 2014). Among persons without apparent GI motility disorders and not on relevant medications, 98% had frequency of movement between three stools per day and three per week (Walter et al. 2010). Using Rome criteria, those with fewer than three bowel movements per week may not have constipation if there is no straining, lumpy or hard stool, or sensation of incomplete evacuation. Some degree of urgency, straining, and incomplete evacuation should be considered normal (Walter et al. 2010). Excessive straining, feeling of incomplete evacuation, and abdominal bloating were reported by the majority with dyssynergic defecation (Rao et al. 2004). Patients with obstetric trauma-related pelvic floor dysfunction may manifest severe constipation, obstructed defecation, rectocele, hemorrhoids, rectal prolapse, or incontinence (Rikard-Bell et al. 2014).

Onset and duration of symptoms determine the chronicity in relation to etiologies and complications. Recent alarm symptoms or signs like rectal bleeding, anemia, guaiac-positive stool, or presence of an abdominal mass are red flags prompting evaluation to exclude organic illness and neoplastic disease; recurring problems of a long duration, poorly relieved with dietary measures or laxatives suggests a functional colorectal disorder (Rao and Meduri 2010). About 45% of patients with functional constipation report abdominal pain (Wong et al. 2010).

Constipation can be both a manifestation or symptom and a disorder, seen in both functional constipation and irritable bowel syndrome with constipation predominance, with common therapeutic approaches; while laxatives offer relief of discomfort in constipation, laxative response in IBS-C is just a small part of the puzzle (Wong et al. 2020).

At time, the older individual may present to the provider in the office or at the emergency room or long-term care institution with unusual manifestations pertinent to constipation; a lack of bowel movement may never be mentioned. A person with dementia may manifest new-onset agitation without expressing an abdominal complaint; the presentation may be accompanied by urinary retention or spurious diarrhea, calling for vigilance on the part of the provider to enable a diagnosis (Table 3).

Stool form is commonly recorded by using Bristol Stool Form Scale (Lewis and Heaton 1997) (Fig. 1). In clinical practice, stool form and frequency are often used as surrogate markers of intestinal and colonic transit (Heaton and O'Donnell 1994). Stool form and shape correlate better than stool frequency with whole gut transit time (Heaton and O'Donnell 1994; Lewis and Heaton 1997; Saad et al. 2010). Furthermore, fecal incontinence in older adults may be a presenting feature of severe constipation (Leung and Rao 2009).

Careful attention must be paid to the identification of prescriptions and over-the-counter preparations (Table 4). In general, older adults use opioids for cancer-related or back pain (Reid et al. 2010), and many develop constipation (Papaleontiou et al. 2010).

Lifestyle, especially diet and physical activity, is associated with bowel movements. A food diary helps assess fiber and fluid intake, frequency of meals, and nutrient content (Rao and Meduri 2010). Difficulties with chewing, swallowing, diet, and mobility are common in the old (Gallagher and O'Mahony 2009). In addition, screening for cognitive function, depression, anxiety, and systemic disease may uncover contributing factors (Gallagher and O'Mahony 2009).

Fig. 1 Bristol Stool Form Scale. Reproduced from Adv Therap. 2011; 28(4), pg 285 Fig. 2; a Springer Publication

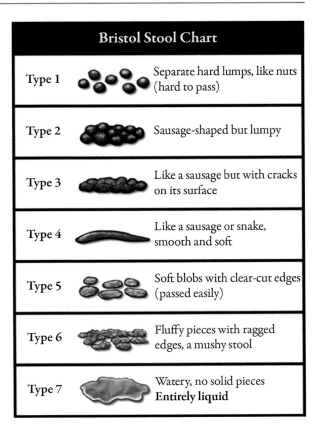

Physical Examination

Physical examination should be focused toward systemic disorders associated with constipation (Table 5). Neurological examination uncovers common disorders such as spinal cord lesions, prior stroke, and Parkinson's disease or parkinsonism. Testing for cognitive impairment may be helpful based on earlier discussion (Wan et al. 2019). Poor dentition or oral lesions should be identified (Gallagher and O'Mahony 2009). Gait and mobility must be assessed for two reasons: older adults may need to increase activity as part of lifestyle management and also require the essential mobility to access convenient sites for evacuation of bowels.

Abdominal examination evaluates distention, presence or absence of mass, and bowel sounds. Intestinal dilatation above an obstruction, with no peristalsis below the obstruction, suggests fecal impaction (Schlange's sign) (Williams 2008). A mass in the left lower quadrant suggests a colonic lesion or stool in the left colon (Rao and Meduri 2010; Williams 2008). Discomfort in the left lower quadrant on palpation suggests constipation or diverticular disease (Williams 2008). Pelvic examination in women may help detect internal prolapse or rectocele.

An adequate perianal and digital rectal examination may be the most revealing part of clinical evaluation and dictates subsequent investigation (Rao and Meduri 2010; Talley 2008; Tantiphlachiva et al. 2010). Digital rectal exam is reliable in detecting normal, but not abnormal, sphincter tone (Tantiphlachiva et al. 2010). A simple ten-step approach on performing a rectal examination has been well outlined by Talley (2008); the basics are provided in Table 6.

Table 4 Medications associated with constipation (Fosnes et al. 2010; Gallagher and O'Mahony 2009; Gibson and Keefe 2006; Hallberg et al. 1966; Lat et al. 2010; Ness et al. 2006; Opie 1988; Panchal et al. 2007; Talley et al. 2003; Trindade et al. 1998)

Analgesics	Clonidine
Alendronate	Disopyramide
Aluminum antacids	Diuretics
Anticholinergics	Fiber (with inadequate fluid intake)
Anticonvulsants	Furosemide
Anti-diarrheal preparations	Iron supplements
Anti-histamine-1 receptor antagonist	Nonsteroidal anti-inflammatory drugs
Antiparkinsonian drugs	Ondansetron
Antipsychotics	Opioid analgesics
Antispasmodics	Polystyrene resins
β-Adrenergic blockers	Selective serotonin reuptake inhibitors
Calcium channel blockers	Sucralfate
Calcium supplements	Sympathomimetics (e.g., ephedrine)
Cisplatin	Tricyclic antidepressants

Table 5 Valuable signs and clues from the physical examination

General inspection
Prior stroke
Parkinsonism
Myxedema
Poor dentition, oral lesions
Abdominal distention
Abdominal examination
Palpable abdominal mass
Abdominal distension
Abdominal tenderness
Abnormal bowel sounds (absent, high-pitched)
Distended bladder
Pelvic examination in women
Internal prolapse
Rectocele
Perianal and digital rectal examination
Sphincter tone
Pelvic floor contraction
Palpable rectal mass
Color of stool

Diagnostic Tests

Following the history and examination, several tests may be considered; the basics include a complete blood cell count, serum glucose, creatinine, and calcium, and all are inexpensive and serve a screening function (Locke et al. 2000). Hypothyroidism is a rare cause; we believe thyroid function testing is useful in the initial evaluation of constipation, particularly in older people. In those chronically constipated, without alarm symptoms or signs, there is inadequate data to make recommendations on routine blood or other diagnostic tests including flexible sigmoidoscopy, colonoscopy, and barium enema (Bharucha et al. 2013; Rao and Meduri 2011). Diagnostic studies are indicated in patients with alarm symptoms and signs (Bharucha et al. 2013; Rao and Meduri 2011). Plain abdominal radiography is often helpful, although controversial (Gallagher and O'Mahony 2009; Moylan et al. 2010). A recent study (Reber et al. 2018) reveals that clinicians somewhat agree that radiographs are helpful in determining management and find quantitation of stool burden

within the radiology report helpful. Radiologists tend to find radiographs inaccurate at quantifying stool burden. Figure 2 illustrates the diagnostic landmarks of an abdominal radiograph in a patient with constipation (Dharmarajan et al. 2004). Routine screening colonoscopy is recommended for all patients with chronic, uncomplicated constipation in the over 50-year-old age group who have not undergone screening for colorectal cancer (American College of Gastroenterology Chronic Constipation Task Force 2005; Locke et al. 2000). Abdominal sonogram or preferably a computed tomography scan of abdomen is indicated when a space-occupying lesion is suspected (Dharmarajan et al. 2004).

Specialized tests of colonic transit or pelvic floor function are considered only with severe, intractable constipation with no secondary cause apparent and in whom an adequate trial of high-fiber diet and laxatives is unsuccessful (Gallagher and O'Mahony 2009). In older patients with a defecatory disorder, anorectal manometry and balloon expulsion tests are considered only if they will affect management decisions (Gallagher and O'Mahony 2009).

Fig. 2 Diagnostic landmarks on abdominal radiograph in patient with constipation

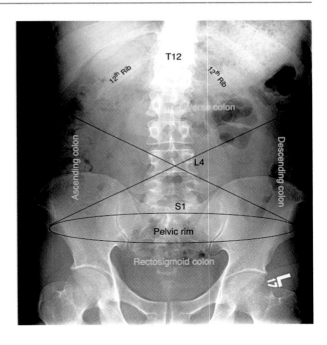

Table 6 The basics of rectal examination (Dobben et al. 2007; Talley 2008; Williams 2008)

Prepare the patient by providing an understanding of the procedure and reasons to undergo the examination

The left lateral decubitus position is most suitable, with the knees pulled up (Williams 2008)

Inspect the perineum; request the patient to strain; observe the perianal region for warts, fecal soiling, prolapsed hemorrhoids, or fistulae (Dobben et al. 2007)

The anal wink is tested by stroking a cotton swab around the anus: its absence indicates disrupted sacral nerve pathways

Digital examination using lubrication: check anal sphincter pressure; pain on examination may indicate anal fissure, inflamed hemorrhoids, or ischiorectal abscess; palpate the rectal walls to assess the prostate in men and cervix in women; the examination helps exclude a rectal mass and impacted stool

The finger in the rectum gauges resting tone of the internal anal sphincter, which correlates with absent, decreased, or normal resting and squeeze pressures (Dobben et al. 2007)

Evaluate for pelvic floor dysfunction by asking the patient to strain. Normally, the anal sphincter and puborectalis relax, with the perineum descending by 1–3.5 cm. Absence of a descent along with tight muscles supports the diagnosis of paradoxical external anal sphincter and puborectalis contraction (pelvic floor dysfunction or dyssynergia)

Examine the gloved finger for features of the stool and blood, mucus, or pus

Modified from Talley (2008)

Transit studies enable a distinction between patients with slow and normal colonic transit times. Presently, colonic transit studies can be performed at every unit with X-ray or fluoroscopy devices; they require a short time and are relatively inexpensive. The study can be a preliminary test to evaluate constipation, although over half of those with dyssynergic defecation have excessive retention of markers. The radiopaque marker test is performed by administering a single capsule containing 24 plastic markers on day 1 and by obtaining plain abdominal radiographs on day 6 (120 h later) (Rao and Meduri 2010). Retention of at least 20% of markers (more than six markers) on day 6 (120 h) is considered abnormal and is indicative of slow transit constipation (Rao and Meduri 2010). The median colonic transit time is 1.5 (1.0–3.7) days for women and 1.3 (0.8–1.9) days for men (Sadik et al. 2003).

Other modalities for colonic transit study are colonic transit scintigraphy and the use of a wireless motility capsule. Colonic transit scintigraphy is a noninvasive and quantitative method of evaluation of total and regional colonic transit by using an isotope (111In or 99Tc) (Rao and Meduri 2010). A wireless motility capsule has been reported to be useful and safe in older people (Rao and Go 2010).

Sixty percent of patients with dyssynergic defecation have an abnormal radiopaque marker test with excessive retention of markers (Rao et al. 1998). It is important to exclude dyssynergic defecation before making a diagnosis of slow transit constipation (Rao 2001; Rao et al. 2005). In older adults, the presence of dyssynergic defecation can be detected by anorectal manometry and balloon expulsion tests. Anorectal manometry is performed by inserting pressure-sensitive catheters to provide an assessment of pressure activity in the anorectum and to provide comprehensive information regarding rectal sensation, rectoanal reflexes, and anal sphincter function, at rest and during defecatory maneuvers (Diamant et al. 1999; Karlbom et al. 2004; Sun and Rao 2001). Normally when healthy subjects attempt to defecate, they generate an adequate propulsive force synchronized with relaxation of the puborectalis and the external anal sphincter. The inability to perform this coordinated maneuver represents the chief pathophysiological abnormality in dyssynergic defecation (Rao 2001; Rao et al. 1998).

The balloon expulsion test is a simple, physiologic assessment of simulated defecation dynamics, by assessing a participant's ability to expel an artificial stool, and is often conducted together with anorectal manometry (Rao and Singh 2011). This test is performed by inserting an empty 10-cm-long latex condom covered with lubricating jelly and tied to a catheter into the rectum of a patient lying in the left lateral position (Minguez et al. 2004). Water at a temperature of 36 °C is instilled into the balloon through the catheter with a 60-mL syringe. The total volume introduced is the minimum to induce a sustained desire to defecate (Minguez et al. 2004). Patients are asked to sit on a toilet and expel the balloon. Asymptomatic persons can expel the balloon in a median 50 s (range 10–90 s) and always within 5 min (Rao and Singh 2011). In a large study, the balloon expulsion test had a sensitivity of 88%, with a positive predictive value of 64% for diagnosing pelvic floor dysfunction; the specificity was 89%, with a negative predictive value of 97% for excluding pelvic floor dysfunction, suggesting that this may be a useful screening test for dyssynergic defecation (Minguez et al. 2004). Although the failure to expel a balloon strongly suggests dyssynergic defecation, a normal test does not exclude this possibility (Rao and Singh 2011).

Defecography or pelvic magnetic resonance imaging is indicated if the results of anal manometry or balloon expulsion tests are equivocal, or if there is a clinical suspicion of a structural rectal abnormality that hinders defecation (Diamant et al. 1999; Fletcher et al. 2003). Because pathological structural abnormalities and functional abnormalities are common in patients with chronic constipation and the structural abnormalities cannot be evaluated using non-imaging test modalities (balloon expulsion and anorectal manometry), defecography could be considered the first-line diagnostic test if resources allow (Grossi et al. 2018). Defecography involves filling the rectum with contrast media and observing the act of defecation with fluoroscopy or magnetic resonance imaging. Currently, magnetic resonance imaging is the only imaging modality that simultaneously can evaluate global pelvic floor anatomy and dynamic motion (Savoye-Collet et al. 2008). Magnetic resonance imaging defecography of the pelvic floor may detect rectoceles, cystoceles, enteroceles, intussusceptions, a dyskinetic puborectalis muscle (in males), changes in the anorectal angle, presence of paradoxical sphincter contraction, and additional pelvic floor abnormalities (Reiner et al. 2011; Rentsch et al. 2001). A study showed that the sensitivity of magnetic resonance defecography for the diagnosis of dyssynergic defecation is 100%, but a specificity of only 23% (Reiner et al. 2011). The limitations of MRI defecography include its high cost, lack of standardization, and availability (Rao 2010).

Management

Prevention of constipation involves primarily lifestyle measures, with medications utilized when non-pharmacological approaches fail. The

Table 7 Non-pharmacological management (Anti et al. 1998; Dharmarajan et al. 2004; Gallagher and O'Mahony 2009; Goldstein et al. 2009; Ostaszkiewicz et al. 2010; Romero et al. 1996; Schnelle et al. 2010)

| **Counseling** |
| On the range of variations in bowel habits that are accepted as normal |
| The need for regular bowel habits |
| **Diet** |
| Adequate meals, including recommended fiber content |
| Adequate fluids daily |
| Prune juice or prunes may be a helpful measure |
| **Habits** |
| Scheduled toileting around the same time daily, responding to the urge to defecate |
| Utilization of gastrocolic reflex 15–20 min following a beverage or food intake prior to scheduled toileting daily |
| Optimal sitting position on toilet during defecation |
| Avoid distractions (such as reading) while defecating |
| **Fluids** |
| Encourage adequate fluid intake especially with fiber intake or when at risk for dehydration |
| **Activity** |
| Mild or moderate physical activity daily, ideally 30–60 min after a meal |
| **Medications** |
| Review medications regularly; be aware of adverse drug effects on the GI tract and interactions |
| Revise drug regimens or limit use of those that tend to cause constipation |
| Special caution required for patients initiated on opioids |
| Discourage routine and excessive use of laxatives |
| **Fiber** |
| Encourage intake of fresh vegetables and fruits daily |
| Utilize fiber-rich food with a combination of soluble and insoluble fiber regularly |
| Commercial fiber formulas are an option when dietary fiber intake is inadequate |

prophylactic use of stool softeners and/or laxatives is appropriate in patients with opioid use (Camilleri 2011; Romero et al. 1996). The goals of treatment of constipation are to relieve symptoms, to restore normal bowel habits (i.e., passage of soft, formed stools at least thrice weekly without straining), and to improve quality of life (Gallagher and O'Mahony 2009). The management strategy includes lifestyle modification, the use of fiber, pharmacological measures, and miscellaneous modalities such as surgery. Non-pharmacological approaches are outlined in Table 7.

Lifestyle Modification

Bowel Training and Education

Regular habits go a long way in the management of constipation. Bowel evacuation is best attempted at a regular time daily. Utility of the gastrocolic reflex is recommended, typically attempted from 5 to 30 min after breakfast, or consumption of warm liquids (Dharmarajan et al. 2004). Sitting position on toilet must be an optimal condition of defecation. The older person should be educated to sit on the toilet seat with legs apart and lean forward with elbows (Ostaszkiewicz et al. 2010). Sensation of satisfactory bowel emptying in sitting defecation posture necessitates excessive expulsive effort compared to the squatting posture (Sikirov 2003). Bedbound older adults may experience position-related pelvic dyssynergia and difficulty in evacuating stool (Rao et al. 2006). Prolonged straining is discouraged, as is distractive behavior such as reading, while attempting to defecate (Dharmarajan et al. 2004; Goldstein et al. 2009). In the event of failure, the gastrocolic reflex may be attempted for a few days prior to discontinuation.

The Role for Squatting

The possible influence for body position to address defecation and avoid constipation has been studied. Squatting is widely practiced in Asia and Africa, whereas sitting is the typical custom in Western countries (Wald 2019). Squatting posture helps straighten the anorectal angle to help reduce straining and facilitate defecation; accordingly, toilets can be tailored to promote the squatting or semi-squatting position; such devices may be helpful to some older adults with musculoskeletal disorders with no ill effects (Wald 2019).

Exercise and Diet

Low physical activity is associated with constipation (Huang et al. 2014). It is hence logical to include physical training as a treatment measure; multicomponent interventions, including exercise in older nursing home residents, significantly helped increase bowel movements (Schnelle et al. 2010). Where possible, walking is the ideal exercise in older adults, for 30 min most days a week; abdominal and pelvic floor exercises during biofeedback therapy may be additive in effect, especially in those with pelvic floor dyssynergia (Chiarioni et al. 2005). The effect of exercise on bowel transit time is probably through stimulation of colonic transit (Song et al. 2018).

A minimum of 1.5 liters of fluid daily, perhaps more, is recommended especially with high-fiber intake (Anti et al. 1998); in dehydrated, febrile states, heavy exertion, and excessively hot weather and for frequent flyer seniors prior to long-distance air flights, large quantities of fluid intake are essential (Morley 2000). The National Academies of Sciences, Engineering, and Medicine recommended a minimum daily fluid intake of as much as 3.7 L for men and 2.7 L for women (Institute of Medicine 2005). However, in the healthy, encouraging fluids above usual recommendations does not serve additional benefit to relieve constipation (Lindeman et al. 2000); caffeinated beverages (coffee, tea, colas) are not considered as part of this quota of fluid consumption (Dharmarajan et al. 2004). Recent data analysis of the National Health and Nutrition Examination Survey (NHANES) 2005–2010 also showed that a lower dietary fiber intake, but not poor water consumption, was associated with a greater risk of constipation in US adults (Shen et al. 2019). Even so, it is worth emphasizing that the preached trio of diet (fiber), fluid intake, and exercise is not supported adequately by science and awaits more data (Annells and Koch 2003).

New insights on the intraluminal impact of food have been provided by magnetic resonance imaging, which allows analysis of the processing of complex multiphase meals, including viscosity, fat, and fiber content in controlling motility; intestinal secretions are shown to be stimulated by a range of fruits and vegetables; the modes of action of bran and psyllium are brought to light, enabling the serial evaluation of the impact of nutrients and drugs (Spiller and Marciani 2019). Dietary therapy for functional therapy should include a variety of specific foods, with a focus on dietary fiber; misconceptions about their physical effects have led to misconceptions and misunderstandings, although evidence of their clinical efficacy is present (Okawa et al. 2019).

Fiber

A low-fiber diet should not be assumed to be the cause of constipation. In general, dietary fiber plays a role in management of constipation by increasing stool mass, decreasing intestinal transit time, and increasing gastrointestinal motility (Tucker et al. 1981; Wrick et al. 1983). Based on an average from several studies, bulk laxatives and fiber increase bowel movement frequency by an overall weighted average of 1.4 bowel movements per week (Tramonte et al. 1997). Fiber and bulk laxatives decreased abdominal pain and improved stool consistency compared with placebo (Tramonte et al. 1997). However, many patients with slow colonic transit and dyssynergic defecation do not respond well to dietary fiber intake of 30 g/day (Voderholzer et al. 1997). In contrast, most constipated patients without an underlying motility disorder improve or became symptom-free with this amount of supplemental fiber (Voderholzer et al. 1997). A systematic review, which included six RCTs, suggested the benefits of dietary soluble fiber (e.g., psyllium or ispaghula) in chronic idiopathic constipation, while data for insoluble dietary fiber (e.g., wheat bran) was conflicting (Suares and Ford 2011).

Dietary Reference Intakes recommend consumption of 14 g dietary fiber per 1,000 kcal, or 25 g for adult women and 38 g for adult men, preferably as dietary form, with adequate water (Slavin 2008), with subtle and gradual changes to foods rich in residual fiber (Gallagher and O'Mahony 2009). A recent RCT demonstrated dried plums (prunes) to be more effective than psyllium in the management of mild to moderate constipation (Attaluri et al. 2011).

Less than 10% of most Western populations consume adequate dietary fiber in the form of fruits, most consuming half the recommended levels (Dreher 2018). The benefit of consuming adequate fruits is becoming clearer; the bioactive prebiotic effects of fruits help in many additional ways beyond protecting gastrointestinal health and constipation; they promote weight management and reduce risk of cardiovascular disease, type 2 diabetes, and colorectal cancer and odds of successful aging (Dreher 2018). A meta-analysis involving 1322 articles and retrieving 19 studies, 5 included, the findings suggested that dietary fiber intake can obviously increase stool frequency in those with constipation; but it does not improve stood consistency, treatment success, and laxative use (Yang et al. 2012). A study of dietary fiber intake and reduction in functional constipation among Canadian adults suggested an economic value of increasing dietary fiber intake beyond its well-known health benefits; with each 1 g/day increase in fiber intake, there was a 1.8% reduction in constipation rates and a substantial reduction in healthcare cost savings (Abdullah et al. 2015).

The effect of increasing dietary fiber is not immediate; patients should observe a gradual increase in bowel movement frequency over weeks. Bloating and flatulence may be an adverse effect, but usually resolve with continued use. To minimize this problem, fiber supplementation is commenced in small doses of 5 to 10 g/day and gradually titrated to the full dose of 20–35 g/day (Dharmarajan et al. 2004; Slavin 2008). Fecal impaction should be treated before increasing

dietary fiber (Gallagher and O'Mahony 2009). Importantly, fiber intake should not be increased during a period of severe constipation, fecal impaction, or ileus. Fiber supplementation should be avoided in patients with idiopathic megacolon and megarectum or bowel obstruction and in the hospitalized ill; these patients require a fiber-restricted diet with laxatives or enemas to prevent fecal retention and impaction (Gattuso and Kamm 1997). Fiber supplements interfere with drug absorption and hence are best not administered with medications.

Kiwifruit (*Actinidia*) is a fruit available in most international markets and is consumed in several forms such as juice, dry fruits, and jam and as the fruit. The nutritional biological properties of kiwifruit are many, including vitamins and polyphenols (Ma et al. 2019). Kiwi is rich in dietary fiber. Clinical evidence for the efficacy of green-fleshed kiwifruit regarding gastrointestinal health, comfort, and laxation is growing; the effect of a different gold-fleshed kiwifruit (Zesy002 kiwifruit, *Actinidia chinensis* var. *chinensis*) on gut was compared to Metamucil in a randomized crossover clinical trial (Eady et al. 2019). The number of complete, spontaneous bowel movements was significantly greater during daily consumption of three kiwifruit versus baseline and Metamucil treatment; stool consistency improved and was softer, and less straining was required (Eady et al. 2019). In mice experiments, ultramicro kiwifruit powder increased gut transit (intestinal propulsion) and decreased whole gut transit time (Zhuang et al. 2019). While the value of prunes is well-known, the benefits of kiwi for gut health are less recognized.

Prunes (dried plums, *Prunus domestica*) are traditionally used as a remedy for constipation. Besides its high dietary fiber content, prunes and their extracted juice also contain other components that may contribute to GI function, including the sugar alcohol sorbitol and phenolic compounds, predominantly chlorogenic and neochlorogenic acids, (Stacewicz-Sapuntzakis et al. 2001) all of which are poorly absorbed by the small intestine and pass undigested into the colon. In a systematic review of randomized controlled trials, 3 weeks of prune consumption

(100 g/day) improved stool frequency and stool consistency compared with psyllium (22 g/day) in subjects with constipation (Lever et al. 2014). However, the evidence for the outcomes and the effects in non-constipated subjects is weak (Lever et al. 2014). In a recent randomized controlled trial in 120 healthy adults with low-fiber intakes and low stool frequency of 3–6 stools/week, supplementation of prunes 80–120 g/day (plus water 300 ml/day) significantly increased stool weight and frequency (Lever et al. 2019). Although the incidence of flatulence was significantly higher after prune consumption, the subjects could tolerate the dried plums (Lever et al. 2019).

Besides kiwifruit and prunes, other fruits have been studied for relieving constipation. In a non-randomized trial of papaya (*Carica papaya* L.), volunteers who took 20 ml daily of papaya preparation/extract for 40 days had significant improvement of constipation compared to those who received placebo (Muss et al. 2013). A study involving the common fig (*F. carica*) showed that fig paste supplementation for 8 weeks was associated with a significant reduction in colonic transit time and a significant improvement in stool type and abdominal discomfort compared with placebo (Baek et al. 2016).

Pharmacotherapy of Constipation

Unfortunately, prescribing of medications has increasingly replaced non-pharmacological approaches for outpatient management of constipation in the United States, with hyperosmolar agents used most frequently and increasingly (Trinkley et al. 2010). Examples, mechanism of actions, and side effects of available pharmacological agents are listed in Table 8. Lactulose, sorbitol, senna compound, and bisacodyl may be the initial choices in older adults (Rao and Go 2010), with polyethylene glycol an option for those unresponsive (Rao and Go 2010; Siegel and Di Palma 2005). Newer agents are a consideration when conventional laxatives are ineffective. In general, the effectiveness of treatment remained similar when RCTs at low risk of bias were analyzed (Ford and Suares 2011), but modes of action of the medications differ. Costs vary, with senna and bisacodyl least expensive, while

secretory drugs and serotonin agonists incur costs (see Table 9). Based on data, a standardized fiber supplement should be considered as the first-line agent for constipated patients, particularly in the primary care setting (Bharucha and Wald 2019). In constipated patients with bloating, initial laxative choice could be polyethylene glycol (PEG)-based solution, administered daily and supplemented, when necessary, with stimulant laxatives (Bharucha and Wald 2019). Studies have shown that treatment of constipation with PEG is safe and effective for up to 24 months (Dipalma et al. 2007; Migeon-Duballet et al. 2006). PEG also appeared better than lactulose for improving stool frequency, stool consistency, and abdominal pain (Lee-Robichaud et al. 2010). The use of lactulose is associated with nausea (Lederle et al. 1990) as bacterial metabolism of these unabsorbed carbohydrates leads to gas production (Bharucha and Wald 2019). Despite laxatives being freely available over the counter in most countries, evidence for their safety and efficacy are still lacking. Age-related changes increase the likelihood for adverse effects in older people. Caution must be used when extrapolating laxative-related kinetics and dynamics in older persons, and their prescription must be tailored to comorbidity and concomitant medication use to reduce adverse drug events (Pont et al. 2019).

Stool Softeners and Emollients

Data on the effectiveness of stool softeners in chronic constipation are limited. A study on 170 patients revealed that docusate was less effective than psyllium, a bulk laxative, in increasing stool water content and overall laxative efficacy (McRorie et al. 1998). Stool softeners do not have a laxative effect.

Similar to stool softeners, there is insufficient evidence for the use of paraffin oil, also known as mineral oil, to treat chronic constipation (Pare et al. 2007). Mineral oil decreases water absorption and softens the stool, thereby allowing easier passage (Xing and Soffer 2001). It is no longer recommended in the old, as it may cause anal

Table 8 Pharmacological management (American College of Gastroenterology Chronic Constipation Task Force 2005; Bharucha and Wald 2019; Castle et al. 1991; Dharmarajan et al. 2004; Gallagher and O'Mahony 2009; Siegel and Di Palma 2005; Tack 2011; Wald 2019; Xing and Soffer 2001)

Bulk-forming laxatives	
Examples	Psyllium (natural fiber), methylcellulose (modified cellulose), calcium polycarbophil (synthetic)
Actions	Increase water content and stool bulk, with better stool consistency. In the colon, they are fermented by bacteria to produce short-chain fatty acids that increase luminal osmolarity and water retention, potentiating laxative effect
Dose	Psyllium: start 3.4 gram PO daily, increase dose gradually to 3.4 gram PO three times a day Methylcellulose: 1 gram PO daily, increase gradually to three times a day.
Adverse effects	Bloating, flatulence, and abdominal discomfort; fecal impaction with inadequate fluid intake. Esophageal obstruction in those with dysphagia
Stool softeners	
Examples	Docusate, mineral oil
Actions	Softens the stool as a surfactant and causes stool wetting Mineral oil acts as an emollient
Dose	Docusate: 100–600 mg PO daily, divided in 1–3 doses Mineral oil: 15–45 mL/day PO divided in 1–2 doses daily or 118 mL per rectal daily PRN
Adverse effects	Mineral oil causes lipid pneumonia, malabsorption of fat-soluble vitamins, anal seepage. Docusate may impair liver function
Saline laxatives	
Examples	Magnesium salts, sodium phosphate, sodium sulfate
Actions	Through osmotically mediated water retention and stimulation of peristalsis. Magnesium salts release cholecystokinin and activate constitutive nitric oxide synthase causing fluid secretion
Dose	Magnesium citrate: 8.725–17.45 grams/day PO divided in 1–2 doses
Adverse effects	Magnesium salts cause hypermagnesemia, especially impaired renal function. Sodium phosphate causes hypocalcemia, hyperphosphatemia, hypernatremia. Sodium and potassium losses may result via stool
Osmotic laxatives	
Examples	Lactulose, sorbitol, polyethylene glycol, glycerin rectal suppository
Action	Neither digested nor absorbed in the small intestine; act through osmotic properties. Lactulose is broken down by bacteria in the colon to lactic and acetic acids to lower colonic pH, favoring formation of less absorbable NH_4^+ from NH_3, effectively trapping ammonia in the colon
Dose	Lactulose:10–20 grams PO daily, 1–2/day, maximum 60 grams/day Polyethylene glycol 3350: 17 grams (1 capful) PO daily PRN; need to dissolve in 4–8 oz of liquid Glycerin: 5.6 grams (1 unit) rectal suppository daily PRN
Adverse effects	Lactulose and sorbitol cause flatulence, abdominal cramps, and diarrhea
Stimulant laxatives	
Examples	Bisacodyl, anthraquinone derivatives (senna, cascara)
Action	Stimulate intestinal motility and reduce absorption of water and electrolytes in the colon. Anthraquinone becomes active on being metabolized by colonic bacteria
Dose	Bisacodyl: 5–15 mg PO daily, oral or suppository. Maximum 30 mg/day. Senna: 17.2–34.4 mg PO at night PRN
Adverse effects	Bisacodyl causes rectal irritation, abdominal cramps, and colitis Anthraquinones may cause melanosis coli and urine discoloration
Secretory drugs	
Examples	Lubiprostone, linaclotide, plecanatide
Actions	Target guanylate cyclase-C receptors on the intestinal epithelium to increase intestinal chloride and bicarbonate secretion into the gut lumen to enhance gastrointestinal transit
Dose	Lubiprostone: 24 ug/day (chronic constipation), 8 ug (IBS-C) Linaclotide: 72 or 145 ug (chronic constipation), 290 ug (IBS-C) Plecanatide: 3 mg or 6 mg (chronic constipation), 3 mg or 6 mg (IBS-C)

(continued)

Table 8 (continued)

Adverse effects	Diarrhea for all secretory drugs. The common side effects of lubiprostone and linaclotide are flatulence, abdominal distention, headache, and abdominal pain
Serotonin agonists	
Example	Prucalopride
Actions	Agonist to serotonin 4 receptor that increases intracellular cyclic adenosine monophosphate to enhance release of acetylcholine, a major excitatory neurotransmitter in the gastrointestinal tract
Dose	Prucalopride 2 mg daily
Adverse effects	Headache, abdominal pain, nausea, diarrhea, abdominal distention, flatulence
Peripherally acting μ-opioid receptor antagonists (PAMORAs)	
Examples	Naldemedine, naloxegol, methylnaltrexone
Actions	Inhibit μ-opioid receptors in the gastrointestinal tract. PAMORAs counteract the effects of opioids to gastrointestinal tract such as delay GI transit, stimulate non-propulsive motor activity, increase intestinal segmentation, and decrease electrolyte and water secretion into the gut
Dose	Naldemedine: 0.2 mg daily Naloxegol: 12.5–25 mg daily Methylnaltrexone: 12 mg every other day (subcutaneous), 450 mg daily (oral)
Adverse effects	Gastrointestinal perforation, diarrhea, nausea, vomiting, abdominal pain

Table 9 The spectrum of laxative costs

Agents and daily doses	Cost category[a]
Bisacodyl, 10 mg	Low
Senna, 17 mg	Low
Psyllium 10 g	Low
Polyethylene glycol 3350, 17 g packet	Medium
Naldemedine, 0.2 mg	High
Naloxegol, 12.5–25 mg	High
Lubiprostone, 8–24 ug	High
Plecanatide, 3–6 mg	High
Prucalopride, 1–2 mg	High
Linaclotide, 72–290 ug	High
Methylnaltrexone 450 mg	High

[a]Low: less than US $ 10/month; medium: US $ 10–100/month; high: over US$ 100/month (Wald 2019)

seepage, reduces absorption of fat-soluble vitamins, and predisposes to aspiration lipoid pneumonia (Ramkumar and Rao 2005; Xing and Soffer 2001).

Bulk Laxatives

Bulk laxatives may help manifestations, such as abdominal pain, defecation effort, and painful defecation (Pare et al. 2007). Bulk laxatives are most effective in normal transit constipation;

the majority of patients with slow transit constipation or disordered defecation will have a poor response (Voderholzer et al. 1997). Effect takes several days (Gallagher and O'Mahony 2009). Bulk laxatives are generally not to be prescribed unless fiber cannot be increased in diet (Gallagher and O'Mahony 2009; Pampati and Fogel 2004). The American College of Gastroenterology Chronic Constipation Task Force (ACG-CCTF) found that psyllium was the only bulking agent with sufficient data for an evidence-based recommendation (American College of Gastroenterology Chronic Constipation Task Force 2005). The frail old should maintain adequate fluid intake while on bulk laxatives to avoid worsening of constipation due to mechanical obstruction. Compared to natural fiber, synthetic compounds undergo less bacterial fermentation and cause less bloating and flatulence (Romero et al. 1996). Bulk laxatives must be taken separately from medications, as they can interfere with absorption of drugs through an adsorbent effect. Bulk agents should be started on a small dose and titrated upward gradually; they are contraindicated at the time of fecal impaction or acute development of constipation, typically in hospitalized patients.

Saline Laxatives

Saline laxatives are not recommended for treatment of chronic constipation as data is inadequate for these agents in any age. Magnesium, sodium, and phosphate containing laxatives are usually well tolerated, but are risky in presence of renal and cardiac disease, both common in the old. Excessive absorption of sodium, phosphorus, or magnesium may lead to electrolyte and volume overload; saline laxatives cause dehydration when excessively used (Lembo and Camilleri 2003). Magnesium oxide is widely used as a laxative and easily available over the counter. Typically, magnesium levels are not checked and the alterations in concentrations are seldom recognized. In a study of 193 patients taking daily magnesium oxide, 16% had high magnesium concentrations and 5% had hypermagnesemia; factors predisposing were chronic kidney disease stage 4 or worse and dosage of magnesium oxide in excess of 1 g/day (Mori et al. 2019). Interestingly, age was not an association.

Stimulant Laxatives

In general, stimulant laxatives do not produce electrolyte disturbance when used in appropriate dosage (Kienzle-Horn et al. 2007). The development of tolerance to stimulant laxatives may occur in slow colonic transit constipation (Muller-Lissner et al. 2005). Sodium picosulfate should be used with caution in those with renal impairment or cardiac failure, for fear of electrolyte disturbance (Xing and Soffer 2001). Castor oil should no longer be used as it causes significant abdominal cramping and nutrient malabsorption (Pare et al. 2007; Wald 2006). Interestingly, a study involving institutionalized older individuals with chronic constipation showed application of topical castor oil to abdominal wall (castor oil pack) helped fecal consistency and minimized straining and incomplete evacuation (Arslan and Eser 2011). Oral bisacodyl is typically administered at bedtime because its time of onset is about 6 h later, in the morning; however, the suppository bisacodyl acts within 30–60 min and is generally best avoided at bedtime (Dharmarajan et al. 2004). Stimulant suppositories (i.e., bisacodyl and glycerin) should be given about 30 min after breakfast in order to synchronize their effects with the gastrocolic response (Bharucha and Wald 2019). Phenolphthalein, no longer marketed in the United States, has been associated with fixed drug eruption, protein-losing enteropathy, Stevens-Johnson syndrome, lupus reactions, and possible carcinogenicity (Corazziari et al. 2000; Murphy 2009). Phosphate preparations, formerly used for bowel preparation, are no longer used for laxation today.

Osmotic Laxatives

High-molecular-weight polyethylene glycol (PEG) is a large polymer with substantial osmotic activity that obligates intraluminal water (Schiller et al. 1988). There are several types of PEG, including polyethylene glycol electrolyte lavage solution (PEG-ELS), sulfate-free electrolyte lavage solution (SF-ELS), and PEG 3350 (MiraLAX, Braintree Laboratories, Braintree, MA) (Siegel and Di Palma 2005). PEG-ELS and SF-ELS, commonly used for preparation prior to colonoscopy, reach a steady-state equilibrium when given in large volumes at high infusion rates (1.5 L/h) and pass through the gastrointestinal tract with a claim of no net water or electrolyte absorption or secretion (DiPalma 2004). However, this is not necessarily the case when they are given in small amounts or ingested at slow rates (Siegel and Di Palma 2005). PEG-ELS is also effective for fecal impaction at a dose of 100 g in 1 L of water per day for up to 3 days (Culbert et al. 1998); however, manual fragmentation and extraction of impacted stool are required prior to use of oral laxatives (Wrenn 1989). PEG 3350 laxative is a chemically inert polymer that does not contain absorbable salts. For overnight treatment of constipation, 68 g of PEG 3350 provided reliable and safe relief within 24 h (DiPalma et al. 2000) without incontinence, cramps, diarrhea, or changes in electrolytes or serum osmolality.

Lactulose, sorbitol, mannitol, and glycerin are poorly absorbed sugars with osmotic action. A meta-analysis revealed polyethylene glycol to be better than lactulose in outcomes of stool frequency per week, form of stool, relief of abdominal pain, and the need for additional products (Lee-Robichaud et al. 2010). Glycerin is significantly absorbed in the small bowel to prevent its regular use to treat chronic constipation (Siegel and Di Palma 2005). Those who are lactose intolerant may simply adjust their consumption of lactose-containing foods to regulate their bowel habits (Siegel and Di Palma 2005).

Enemas

Enemas play an important role in the management and prevention of fecal impaction in those at risk (Wrenn 1989). Lubricant suppositories (glycerin) can help to initiate defecation in fecal impaction. In a study, administration of daily lactulose with a glycerin suppository and a once-weekly tap water enema achieved complete rectal emptying and prevented incontinence related to impaction in institutionalized older patients (Chassagne et al. 2000). Phosphate enemas should be used with extreme caution in patients with impaired renal dysfunction and preexisting electrolyte imbalance and are generally avoided today (Farah 2005; Hsu and Wu 2008; Pare et al. 2007). Soapsuds enemas are also not used currently, as they cause irritation and possible severe colitis (Harish et al. 2006; Pare et al. 2007).

The risks of enema use include perforation of intestinal wall, rectal mucosal damage, and bacteremia. Patients who take anticoagulants and those who have coagulation or bleeding disorders are at risk of bleeding complications or intramural hematoma (Niv et al. 2013; Rentea and Fehring 2017). Contraindications to enemas include neutropenia, thrombocytopenia, paralytic ileus, intestinal obstruction, recent colorectal or gynecological surgery, recent anal or rectal trauma, severe colitis, inflammation or infection of the abdomen, toxic megacolon, undiagnosed abdominal pain, and recent radiotherapy to the pelvic area (Larkin et al. 2018). Perforation,

hyperphosphatemia (after Fleet Enema), and sepsis may cause death in up to 4% of cases (Niv et al. 2013). Therefore, enemas for the treatment of constipation in older people elderly should be recommended with caution.

Serotonin Agonists

Tegaserod has been removed from the market because of its association with risk of cardiovascular events (Al-Judaibi et al. 2010). Prucalopride, unlike other drugs in its class, such as tegaserod, mosapride, and renzapride, has a lower affinity for the human Ether-a-go-go Related Gene protein (hERG) (Camilleri et al. 2008). It is believed that the effects on the hERG channel may have led to the unfavorable cardiovascular profile seen with tegaserod. In a RCT involving 84 elderly nursing home residents with chronic constipation, 2 mg prucalopride once daily for 4 weeks was safe and well tolerated (Camilleri et al. 2009). Prucalopride is a serotonin 4 receptor agonist that increases intracellular cyclic adenosine monophosphate to enhance the release of acetylcholine, a major excitatory neurotransmitter in the gastrointestinal tract (Omer and Quigley 2017). The usual recommended dose of prucalopride is 2 mg daily in individuals 65 years or younger and 1 mg daily in individuals older than 65 years (Wald 2019). Lower dose is recommended in older adults as the medication is exclusively excreted through the kidneys; renal function often declines in aging individuals. Prucalopride and also intestinal secretagogues should be used only if standard laxatives fail as they are more expensive compared to standard laxatives (e.g., bisacodyl, senna, or PEG-based solution), and there is no evidence that the newer medications are more effective than the standard laxatives (Wald 2019). Unlike intestinal secretagogues, prucalopride has not been approved by US FDA for the management of IBS-C (Bharucha and Wald 2019). A systematic review of randomized controlled trials assessing the efficacy of drugs (osmotic or stimulant laxatives, elobixibat, linaclotide, lubiprostone, mizagliflozin, naronapride, plecanatide, prucalopride, tegaserod, tenapanor, or velusetrag) in adults with chronic idiopathic constipation reveals that prucalopride ranked first at 12 weeks, suggesting that this drug is likely to be the most efficacious for patients with chronic idiopathic constipation (Luthra et al. 2019). As many of the included trials in this systematic review recruited patients who previously did not respond to laxatives, prucalopride seems beneficial in those who failed treatment with other laxatives. Additionally, prucalopride has demonstrated promise in the treatment of gastroparesis, postoperative ileus, and opioid-induced constipation (Vijayvargiya and Camilleri 2019).

Intestinal Secretagogues

Lubiprostone, linaclotide, and plecanatide are approved by the US FDA for treating chronic constipation and IBS-C (Schey and Rao 2011; Shah et al. 2018). These agents increase intestinal chloride secretion by activating channels on the apical (luminal) enterocyte surface to enhance gastrointestinal transit (Bharucha and Wald 2019; Schey and Rao 2011; Shah et al. 2018). To maintain electroneutrality, sodium is also secreted into the intestinal lumen, followed by water secretion to preserve isosmolality. By increasing intestinal secretion, these medications accelerate transit and facilitate ease of defecation (Bharucha and Wald 2019).

Lubiprostone, a bicyclic fatty acid derivative of prostaglandin E1, primarily activates the apical type 2 chloride channels (Schey and Rao 2011). Besides its action on colonic transit, lubiprostone also accelerates small intestine transit in healthy individuals (Camilleri et al. 2006). Lubiprostone, compared to placebo, has consistently increased complete and spontaneous bowel movements per week, as well as improved stool consistency, straining, constipation severity, and patient-reported treatment effectiveness (Johanson et al. 2008). The US FDA approves lubiprostone at a dose of 24 micrograms twice daily for the treatment of chronic idiopathic constipation in adults and at a dose of 8 micrograms twice daily for IBS-C in adult women (Tuteja and Rao 2008).

Systematic reviews of articles evaluating the treatment of chronic constipation in older individuals showed that lubiprostone was associated with 5.69 spontaneous bowel movements per week versus 3.46 per week for placebo (P = 0.001) (Fleming and Wade 2010). Common side effects of lubiprostone include nausea, diarrhea, abdominal pain and bloating, and the rare side effect dyspnea (Chamberlain and Rao 2012). Likely mechanisms for these side effects may be related to lubiprostone's primary action on small bowel secretion and the associated intestinal distension, as well as smooth muscle contraction (Chamberlain and Rao 2012).

Linaclotide is another intestinal secretagogue with its structure similar to the heat-stable enterotoxins that cause diarrhea (Bharucha and Waldman 2010; Shah et al. 2018). These heat-stable toxins act on guanylyl cyclase C which is expressed in brush border membranes of intestinal mucosal cells from the duodenum to the rectum that open the cystic fibrosis transmembrane conductance regulator chloride channel and produce a net efflux of ions and water into the intestinal lumen (Bharucha and Waldman 2010; Shah et al. 2018). Linaclotide increases spontaneous bowel movements and is effective in improving secondary endpoints, such as stool consistency, straining, abdominal discomfort, bloating, global assessments, and quality of life (Lembo et al. 2010). Linaclotide was first approved for IBS-C (290 micrograms daily) and chronic idiopathic constipation (145 micrograms daily) in 2012. The US FDA approved 72 micrograms daily dose for the management of chronic idiopathic constipation (Wald 2019).

Similar to linaclotide, plecanatide is an intestinal secretagogue for the treatment of both chronic constipation and IBS-C. Plecanatide demonstrated efficacy and safety in a randomized placebo-controlled trial of over 1300 patients with chronic constipation (DeMicco et al. 2017). Over the 12-week trial, 3 mg or 6 mg daily plecanatide significantly improved stool consistency and stool frequency. Significant increases in mean weekly spontaneous bowel movements and complete spontaneous bowel movements began in week 1 and were maintained through week 12 in plecanatide-treated patients. Plecanatide was approved by the US FDA for CIC (3 mg daily) and for IBS-C (3 mg or 6 mg daily) in January 2018 (Wald 2019).

A meta-analysis of 8 linaclotide trials (5 examining CIC and 3 examining IBS-C) and 7 plecanatide trials (4 examining CIC and 3 - examining IBS-C) encompassing over 10,000 patients concluded that there were no significant differences between the drugs concerning efficacy or adverse events, such as diarrhea (or diarrhea-related study withdrawals) (Bharucha and Wald 2019). Similar findings of the efficacy of the intestinal secretagogues (linaclotide, lubiprostone, plecanatide, and tenapanor) were also reported in a network meta-analysis of individuals with IBS-C (Black et al. 2018). In this systematic review, linaclotide (290 micrograms once daily) was ranked first in efficacy for decreasing abdominal pain and achieving complete spontaneous bowel movements. Tenapanor (50 mg twice daily) was ranked first for decreasing bloating. Total numbers of adverse events were significantly larger with linaclotide (290 and 500 micrograms once daily) and plecanatide (3 mg once daily) compared with placebo. However, plecanatide 6 mg once daily ranked first for safety. Diarrhea was significantly more common with all drugs, except lubiprostone (8 micrograms twice daily). Nausea was significantly more common in patients who received lubiprostone.

Peripherally Acting μ-Opioid Receptor Antagonists (PAMORAs)

Opioid-induced constipation (OIC) is entity by itself; opioids are commonly prescribed for those with advanced cancer, and adverse effects follow, particularly constipation. Constipation is a burdensome problem, and timely institution of prophylactic laxatives such as methylnaltrexone, a mu-opioid receptor antagonist, will help prevent the disorder; further intensification of a laxative when opioid dosage is increased will prevent OIC (Neefjes et al. 2019). Naldemedine and naloxegol, also known as peripherally acting μ-opioid receptor antagonists (PAMORAs) drugs, are

recommended in the American Gastroenterological Association (AGA) guideline for pharmacological treatment of opioid-induced constipation (OIC) if an adequate trial of traditional laxatives results in suboptimal symptom control (Crockett et al. 2019). The AGA also conditionally recommends use of methylnaltrexone in OIC as there is low quality of evidence for the use of methylnaltrexone (Crockett et al. 2019). The 2019 AGA guideline reduced the strength of supportive evidence to weak or nonexistent for alvimopan and methylnaltrexone. On the other hand, the guideline strongly recommends the use of naloxegol and naldemedine and the presence of moderately strong to strong quality of evidence for the use of these two medications. PAMORAs have shown to improve bowel symptoms without compromise to pain relief, although there can be associated side effects, including diarrhea and abdominal pain. PAMORAs do not enter the central nervous system but inhibit only μ-opioid receptors in the gastrointestinal tract (Wald 2019). Two randomized, placebo-controlled trials involving 1352 patients found that naloxegol in doses of 12.5 mg or 25 mg daily was superior to placebo over a 12-week trial (Chey et al. 2014). In these trials, adverse events (primarily gastrointestinal) occurred most frequently in the groups treated with 25 mg of naloxegol.

Currently, there is insufficient evidence to support the use of lubiprostone and prucalopride for the management of OIC (Crockett et al. 2019). In addition, more data related to the use of PAMORAs in older adults are needed (Moore et al. 2008). In spite of the perceived efficacy of these drugs in PIC, de-prescribing of combination controlled release oxycodone-naloxone in palliative/hospice care settings has been a consideration because of poor pain control or impaired hepatic function, with beneficial effects (Clark et al. 2020).

Other Agents

Colchicine, a gout medication, is known to induce diarrhea in higher doses.

In slow transit constipation, colchicine in a dose of 1 mg daily effectively reduces symptoms of constipation, although it is seldom used for the management of constipation (Abbott et al. 2001).

Prebiotics and probiotics are being evaluated as potential treatments for constipation. Several factors are vital to normal gut motility, including gastrointestinal microbiota; an imbalance or dysfunction in any of its components may contribute to aberrant gut motility and, consequently, symptoms of constipation (Dimidi et al. 2017). Studies that investigated the gastrointestinal microbiota in constipation consistently demonstrate decreased bifidobacteria and lactobacilli and increased *Bacteroidetes* compared with controls (Chassard et al. 2012; Khalif et al. 2005; Kim et al. 2015; Parthasarathy et al. 2016). On the other hand, the abundance of *Actinobacteria*, *Bacteroides*, *Lactococcus*, and *Roseburia* were correlated with faster gut transit time, whereas *Faecalibacterium* was directly correlated to slower gut transit time (Parthasarathy et al. 2016). Based on these facts, modifying the gut luminal environment with certain probiotic species and strains may affect gut motility and secretion and provide benefit for patients with constipation (Dimidi et al. 2017). However, much of the current evidence is derived from animal studies; their effect in humans is unclear due to a paucity of human studies (Dimidi et al. 2017).

A take-home point from a review on constipation by Wald (2016) suggests that polyethylene glycol (PEG 3350) was shown to be non-inferior to a high-affinity serotonin agonist and requires comparison to inexpensive laxatives such as bisacodyl; novel secretory drugs and high-affinity serotonin agonists remain a second-tier choice for the management of chronic idiopathic constipation. Choice of treatment for chronic constipation must take into account the cost and efficacy (Wald 2016).

Laxative Abuse or Misuse

Laxatives have been in use for centuries and have been abused or misused in 10–60% of situations (Roerig et al. 2010). Some users suffer from eating disorders, while others use laxatives for weight loss or to cause factitious diarrhea. Another group is constipated but believe that frequent bowel movements are required for good health. Use among older groups in care homes varies and is often not based on rational criteria (Gage et al. 2010). The most misused group is the stimulant class, perhaps because of their onset of action; electrolyte imbalance is often the result. Addressing the problem involves a high degree of suspicion, education, stopping the laxative and replacing with fiber supplements, along with nursing and psychiatrist involvement where appropriate (Gage et al. 2010; Roerig et al. 2010).

Miscellaneous Modalities

Manual Fragmentation

Manual fragmentation and extraction of the fecal mass are almost always initially indicated for fecal impaction (Wrenn 1989). The procedure usually requires local anesthesia and lubrication with lidocaine jelly, followed by gentle, progressive anal dilation with first one and then two fingers (Klein 1982). A scissoring action is used to fragment the impaction. In women, applying transvaginal pressure with the other hand may aid fragmentation and expulsion (Erdman 1985). A pudendal block or spinal or general anesthesia is rarely required (Klein 1982). Colonic perforation after manual disimpaction has been reported in a patient with stercoral ulceration (Lim et al. 2018). Therefore, manual disimpaction should be performed carefully in patients with long-standing fecal impaction in the rectum.

Endoscopy Intervention

When stool impaction is beyond the reach of the fingers, a lavage directed by sigmoidoscopic visualization can be effective to relieve transient bowel obstruction, abdominal pain, and distention (Wrenn 1989).

Surgical Therapy

In select patients with slow colonic transit, subtotal colectomy and ileorectal anastomoses are options when other measures have failed to relieve constipation, provided that defecation dysfunction disorder has been excluded (Hassan et al. 2006; Nyam et al. 1997). In the past, segmental colonic resection in constipation is disappointing (Bouras and Tangalos 2009; Rotholtz and Wexner 2001). Reported side effects of surgery include diarrhea, incontinence, infection, and bowel obstruction. Furthermore, older people may be unfit for surgery due to advanced age and comorbidities (Rao and Go 2010). However, a recent report (Yang et al. 2018) reveals that laparoscopic subtotal colonic bypass plus colostomy with antiperistaltic cecoproctostomy (SCBCAC) is an effective and safe procedure for the treatment of slow transit constipation in an aged population and can significantly improve the prognosis. The clinical efficacy of SCBCAC is more favorable compared with that of subtotal colonic bypass with antiperistaltic cecoproctostomy.

Surgical management may also be considered in constipated older adults with symptomatic grade 3–4 rectal prolapse (Patcharatrakul and Rao 2018) and large rectocele (>3 cm) who fail conservative treatment or those with coexisting symptomatic pelvic organ prolapse (Schey et al. 2012).

Biofeedback Therapy

Biofeedback is an effective treatment for pelvic floor dyssynergia but not slow transit constipation (Chiarioni et al. 2005). In addition, biofeedback therapy can be useful in constipation-related excessive perineal descent and solitary rectal ulcer syndrome (Patcharatrakul and Rao 2018). Biofeedback involves the use of pressure measurements or averaged electromyographic activity within the anal canal to teach patients to relax pelvic floor muscles when straining to defecate (Chiarioni et al. 2006). This is combined with use of appropriate techniques for straining (increasing intra-abdominal pressure) and having the patient practice defecation of a water-filled balloon (Chiarioni et al. 2006). Audiovisual feedback is provided to the patients as they attempt defecation (Rao and Go 2010); sensory defects in older adults must be initially corrected.

Indications for Referral

Physicians should not hesitate to seek consultation to address the presence of alarm signs such as weight loss, melena, recent change in bowel habits, and refractory constipation (Foxx-Orenstein et al. 2008); consultants in the category include gastroenterologist, geriatrician,

psychiatrist, surgeon, pharmacist, nutritionist, or others to meet individual needs (Table 10). A collaborative effort between the primary provider and the consultant offers the best chance for success (Dharmarajan et al. 2004).

Approach to Constipation: AGA Medical Position Statement

The American Gastroenterological Association (AGA) panel (released 2013) suggests a simple algorithmic approach. Discontinue medications that may be causative prior to further evaluation. Perform a digital rectal examination before referral. Only a blood count is needed, further testing only if indicated. Colonoscopy is not recommended in the absence of alarm features; anorectal manometry, rectal balloon expulsion test, and defecography are considered only when there is no response to laxatives. The treatment begins by addressing medications that may be causative, performing only clinically indicated tests, and followed by a therapeutic trial of fiber, osmotic, or stimulant laxatives before anorectal testing. Pelvic floor training by biofeedback is preferred to laxatives for defecatory disorders (Stern and Davis 2016).

Key Points

- Constipation is common in the geriatric population and often a management problem.
- Age-related physiological changes may contribute to development of chronic constipation, but it often is a result of a variable combination of improper personal habits involving lifestyle, comorbidity, and adverse drug effect or drug interaction.
- Evaluation of constipation should address the aforementioned areas. Suggested algorithms for the approach and management are provided in Figs. 3 and 4.
- A focused history on the patient's complaints and perception of normal bowel habits will be helpful.
- The presence of red flags such as anemia, prior history of cancer, weight loss,

Table 10 Indications for consultation in refractory constipation (Dharmarajan et al. 2004; Gallagher and O'Mahony 2009; Lacy and Brunton 2005; Locke et al. 2000; Pare et al. 2007; Rao and Singh 2011)

1. Gastroenterologist

Constipation with alarm signs, e.g., recent onset, weight loss, anemia, pain, constipation alternating with diarrhea, gastrointestinal bleeding

Chronic constipation requiring excessive use of laxatives or stool softeners

Fecal incontinence of recent onset

High stool impaction which is beyond the reach of finger

To identify colonic neuropathy, myopathy, or normal colonic motor function before consideration of colectomy in patients with severe constipation

To assess colonic involvement in patients with colonic pseudo-obstruction and/or megacolon syndromes and to assess tone/compliance changes

Clinical suggestion of pelvic floor dysfunction

2. Geriatrician

Chronic constipation not alleviated despite compliance with high-fiber diet, exercise regimen, and bowel training program

Coexisting cognitive impairment, e.g., dementia, Parkinson's disease

For the diagnosis of one or more coexisting conditions, requiring expertise in management, e.g., hypothyroidism, diabetes, and heart disease

Where coexisting pain and its management are contributory

Polypharmacy, requiring revision of drug regimen, where constipation may result from drug-drug, drug-nutrient, or drug-disease interaction

3. Surgeon

Constipation associated with vomiting and/or abdominal distension, where volvulus, obstruction, and ischemia are considerations

Complications of constipation, e.g., hemorrhoids, fissures, perirectal abscess

Refractory constipation, including presence of rectocele and rectal prolapse

Severe intractable constipation not due to anorectal dysfunction, suggesting slow colonic transit constipation

4. Psychiatrist/psychologist

Patients with depression and psychological distress

Following medical evaluation and maximal attempts at therapy, when investigations including bowel transit studies are futile

In those who fail to cooperate with conventional approaches

Patients with irritable bowel syndrome and laxative abuse

5. Nutritionist, nurse, pharmacist

As indicated, to counsel regarding diet, habits, review of medications, etc.

new-onset constipation, and fever call for evaluation, including specialists where indicated.

- Treatment of chronic constipation is tailored primarily to non-pharmacological approaches including dietary fiber, fluids, and activity.
- Revision of medication regimen is among the initial approaches; discontinue medications that may be causative, prior to resorting to use of stool softeners and laxatives.
- Opioid-induced constipation is a common entity in older adults; this is one area where laxatives are administered at the outset along with opioid administration.
- The recommendations are to use traditional laxatives as first-line agents for managing OIC, since many patients respond to them; PAMORAs are considered when traditional laxatives fail.
- Laxative misuse and adverse effects should be recognized and addressed.
- Laxative use must be tailored to individual based on their comorbidity and concomitant medication use.

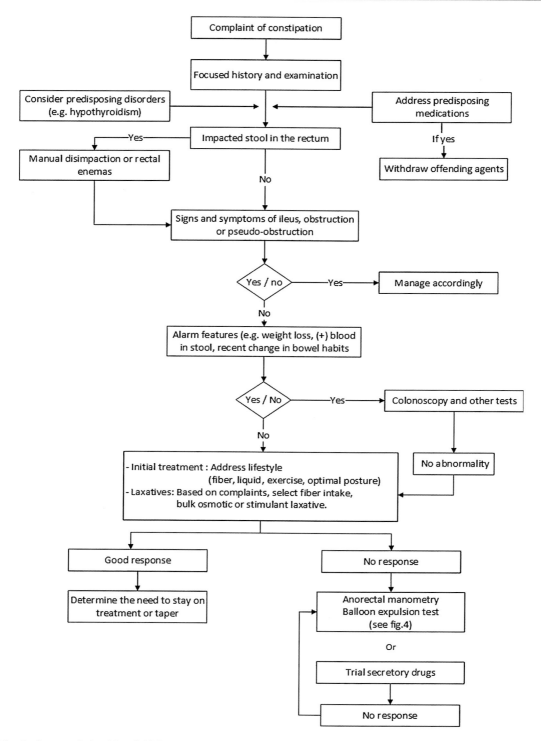

Fig. 3 Suggested algorithm: initial approach of constipation. Modified from Bharucha and Wald 2019; Ghoshal et al. 2018

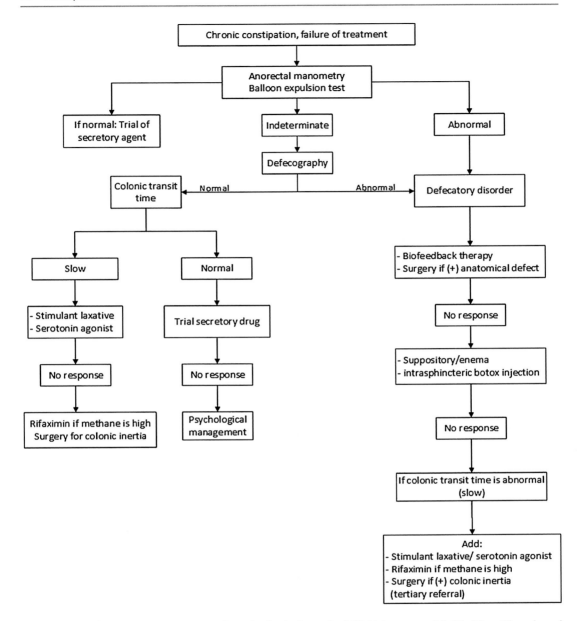

Fig. 4 Suggested algorithm: management of constipation in those who fail initial measures. Modified from Bharucha and Wald 2019; Ghoshal et al. 2018

References

Abbott RD, et al. Frequency of bowel movements and the future risk of Parkinson's disease. Neurology. 2001;57:456–62.

Abdullah MM, Gyles CL, Marinangeli CP, Carlberg JG, Jones PJ. Dietary fibre intakes and reduction in functional constipation rates among Canadian adults: a cost-of-illness analysis. Food Nutr Res. 2015;59:28646. https://doi.org/10.3402/fnr.v59.28646.

Abyad A, Mourad F. Constipation: common-sense care of the older patient. Geriatrics. 1996;51:28–34, 36.

Al-Judaibi B, Chande N, Gregor J. Safety and efficacy of tegaserod therapy in patients with irritable bowel syndrome or chronic constipation. Can J Clin Pharmacol. 2010;17:e194–200.

American College of Gastroenterology Chronic Constipation Task Force. An evidence-based approach to the management of chronic constipation in North America. Am J Gastroenterol. 2005;100(Suppl 1):S1–4. https://doi.org/10.1111/j.1572-0241.2005.50613_1.x. AJG50613_1 [pii].

Annells M, Koch T. Constipation and the preached trio: diet, fluid intake, exercise. Int J Nurs Stud. 2003;40:843–52.

Anti M, et al. Water supplementation enhances the effect of high-fiber diet on stool frequency and laxative consumption in adult patients with functional constipation. Hepato-Gastroenterology. 1998;45:727–32.

Arslan GG, Eser I. An examination of the effect of castor oil packs on constipation in the elderly. Complement Ther Clin Pract. 2011;17:58–62. https://doi.org/10.1016/j.ctcp.2010.04.004. S1744-3881(10)00032-0 [pii].

Ashraf W, Park F, Lof J, Quigley EM. An examination of the reliability of reported stool frequency in the diagnosis of idiopathic constipation. Am J Gastroenterol. 1996;91:26–32.

Attaluri A, Donahoe R, Valestin J, Brown K, Rao SS. Randomised clinical trial: dried plums (prunes) vs. psyllium for constipation. Aliment Pharmacol Ther. 2011;33:822–8. https://doi.org/10.1111/j.1365-2036.2011.04594.x.

Baek HI, et al. Randomized, double-blind, placebo-controlled trial of Ficus carica paste for the management of functional constipation. Asia Pac J Clin Nutr. 2016;25:487–96. https://doi.org/10.6133/apjcn.092015.06.

Bernard CE, et al. Effect of age on the enteric nervous system of the human colon. Neurogastroenterol Motil. 2009;21:746–e746. https://doi.org/10.1111/j.1365-2982.2008.01245.x. NMO1245 [pii].

Bharucha AE, Phillips SF. Slow transit constipation. Gastroenterol Clin N Am. 2001;30:77–95.

Bharucha AE, Wald A. Chronic constipation. Mayo Clin Proc. 2019;94:2340–57. https://doi.org/10.1016/j.mayocp.2019.01.031.

Bharucha AE, Waldman SA. Taking a lesson from microbial diarrheagenesis in the management of chronic constipation. Gastroenterology. 2010;138:813–7. https://doi.org/10.1053/j.gastro.2010.01.022.

Bharucha AE, Croak AJ, Gebhart JB, Berglund LJ, Seide BM, Zinsmeister AR, An KN. Comparison of rectoanal axial forces in health and functional defecatory disorders. Am J Physiol Gastrointest Liver Physiol. 2006;290: G1164–9. https://doi.org/10.1152/ajpgi.00487.2005.

Bharucha AE, Pemberton JH, Locke GR 3rd. American Gastroenterological Association technical review on constipation. Gastroenterology. 2013;144:218–38. https://doi.org/10.1053/j.gastro.2012.10.028.

Bhutto A, Morley JE. The clinical significance of gastrointestinal changes with aging. Curr Opin Clin Nutr Metab Care. 2008;11:651–60. https://doi.org/10.1097/MCO.0b013e32830b5d37. 00075197-200809000-00016 [pii].

Black CJ, Burr NE, Quigley EMM, Moayyedi P, Houghton LA, Ford AC. Efficacy of Secretagogues in patients with irritable bowel syndrome with constipation: systematic review and network meta-analysis. Gastroenterology. 2018;155:1753–63. https://doi.org/10.1053/j.gastro.2018.08.021.

Bouras EP, Tangalos EG. Chronic constipation in the elderly. Gastroenterol Clin N Am. 2009;38:463–80. https://doi.org/10.1016/j.gtc.2009.06.001. S0889-8553(09)00057-0 [pii].

Braak H, Rub U, Gai WP, Del Tredici K. Idiopathic Parkinson's disease: possible routes by which vulnerable neuronal types may be subject to neuroinvasion by an unknown pathogen. J Neural Transm. 2003;110:517–36. https://doi.org/10.1007/s00702-002-0808-2.

Camilleri M. Opioid-induced constipation: challenges and therapeutic opportunities. Am J Gastroenterol. 2011;106:835–42. https://doi.org/10.1038/ajg.2011.30. quiz. 843ajg201130 [pii].

Camilleri M, et al. Effect of a selective chloride channel activator, lubiprostone, on gastrointestinal transit, gastric sensory, and motor functions in healthy volunteers. Am J Physiol Gastrointest Liver Physiol. 2006;290: G942–7. https://doi.org/10.1152/ajpgi.00264.2005.

Camilleri M, Kerstens R, Rykx A, Vandeplassche L. A placebo-controlled trial of prucalopride for severe chronic constipation. N Engl J Med. 2008;358:2344–54. https://doi.org/10.1056/NEJMoa0800670. 358/22/2344 [pii].

Camilleri M, Beyens G, Kerstens R, Robinson P, Vandeplassche L. Safety assessment of prucalopride in elderly patients with constipation: a double-blind, placebo-controlled study. Neurogastroenterol Motil. 2009;21:1256–e1117. https://doi.org/10.1111/j.1365-2982.2009.01398.x. NMO1398 [pii].

Castle SC, Cantrell M, Israel DS, Samuelson MJ. Constipation prevention: empiric use of stool softeners questioned. Geriatrics. 1991;46:84–6.

Chamberlain SM, Rao SS. Safety evaluation of lubiprostone in the treatment of constipation and irritable bowel syndrome. Expert Opin Drug Saf. 2012;11:841–50. https://doi.org/10.1517/14740338.2012.708732.

Chang JY, Locke GR, Schleck CD, Zinsmeister AR, Talley NJ. Risk factors for chronic constipation and a possible role of analgesics. Neurogastroenterol Motil. 2007;19:905–11. https://doi.org/10.1111/j.1365-2982.2007.00974.x. NMO974 [pii].

Chassagne P, et al. Does treatment of constipation improve faecal incontinence in institutionalized elderly patients? Age Ageing. 2000;29:159–64.

Chassard C, et al. Functional dysbiosis within the gut microbiota of patients with constipated-irritable bowel syndrome. Aliment Pharmacol Ther. 2012; 35:828–38. https://doi.org/10.1111/j.1365-2036.2012.05007.x.

Chatterjee S, Park S, Low K, Kong Y, Pimentel M. The degree of breath methane production in IBS correlates with the severity of constipation. Am J Gastroenterol. 2007;102:837–41. https://doi.org/10.1111/j.1572-0241.2007.01072.x.

Cheng J, Li L, Xu F, Xu Y, Lin L, Chen JDZ. Poststroke constipation is associated with impaired rectal sensation. Am J Gastroenterol. 2020;115:105–14. https://doi.org/10.14309/ajg.0000000000000479.

Chey WD, Webster L, Sostek M, Lappalainen J, Barker PN, Tack J. Naloxegol for opioid-induced constipation in patients with noncancer pain. N Engl J Med. 2014;370:2387–96. https://doi.org/10.1056/NEJMoa1310246.

Chiarioni G, Salandini L, Whitehead WE. Biofeedback benefits only patients with outlet dysfunction, not patients with isolated slow transit constipation. Gastroenterology. 2005;129:86–97. https://doi.org/10.1053/j.gastro.2005.05.015.

Chiarioni G, Heymen S, Whitehead WE. Biofeedback therapy for dyssynergic defecation. World J Gastroenterol. 2006;12:7069–74.

Chinn JS, Schuffler MD. Paraneoplastic visceral neuropathy as a cause of severe gastrointestinal motor dysfunction. Gastroenterology. 1988;95:1279–86.

Clark K, et al. Pharmacovigilance in hospice/palliative care: de-prescribing combination controlled release oxycodone-naloxone. J Palliat Med. 2020; https://doi.org/10.1089/jpm.2019.0226.

Clemens KE, Klaschik E. Management of constipation in palliative care patients. Curr Opin Support Palliat Care. 2008;2:22–7. https://doi.org/10.1097/SPC.0b013e3282f53146. 01263393-200803000-00006 [pii].

Condom E, Vidal A, Rota R, Graus F, Dalmau J, Ferrer I. Paraneoplastic intestinal pseudo-obstruction associated with high titres of Hu autoantibodies. Virchows Arch A Pathol Anat Histopathol. 1993;423:507–11.

Corazziari E, et al. Long term efficacy, safety, and tolerability of low daily doses of isosmotic polyethylene glycol electrolyte balanced solution (PMF-100) in the treatment of functional chronic constipation. Gut. 2000;46:522–6.

Crockett SD, Greer KB, Heidelbaugh JJ, Falck-Ytter Y, Hanson BJ, Sultan S, American Gastroenterological Association Institute Clinical Guidelines C. American Gastroenterological Association Institute guideline on the medical management of opioid-induced constipation. Gastroenterology. 2019;156:218–26. https://doi.org/10.1053/j.gastro.2018.07.016.

Cruz JV, et al. TRREMS procedure (transanal repair of rectocele and rectal mucosectomy with one circular stapler): a prospective multicenter trial. Arq Gastroenterol. 2011;48:3–7.

Culbert P, Gillett H, Ferguson A. Highly effective new oral therapy for faecal impaction. Br J Gen Pract. 1998;48:1599–600.

Danjo K, et al. Effects of cellulose supplementation on fecal consistency and fecal weight. Dig Dis Sci. 2008;53:712–8. https://doi.org/10.1007/s10620-007-9938-6.

De Schepper HU, Cremonini F, Park MI, Camilleri M. Opioids and the gut: pharmacology and current clinical experience. Neurogastroenterol Motil. 2004;16:383–94. https://doi.org/10.1111/j.1365-2982.2004.00513.x. NMO513 [pii].

DeMicco M, Barrow L, Hickey B, Shailubhai K, Griffin P. Randomized clinical trial: efficacy and safety of plecanatide in the treatment of chronic idiopathic constipation. Ther Adv Gastroenterol. 2017;10:837–51. https://doi.org/10.1177/1756283X17734697.

Dharmarajan TS, Rao VSR, Pitchumoni CS. Constipation in older adults: an ancient malady, remains a management enigma. Pract Gastroenterol. 2004;28:40–65.

Diamant NE, Kamm MA, Wald A, Whitehead WE. AGA technical review on anorectal testing techniques. Gastroenterology. 1999;116:735–60.

Dimidi E, Christodoulides S, Scott SM, Whelan K. Mechanisms of action of probiotics and the gastrointestinal microbiota on gut motility and constipation. Adv Nutr. 2017;8:484–94. https://doi.org/10.3945/an.116.014407.

DiPalma JA. Current treatment options for chronic constipation. Rev Gastroenterol Disord. 2004;4(Suppl 2):S34–42.

DiPalma JA, DeRidder PH, Orlando RC, Kolts BE, Cleveland MB. A randomized, placebo-controlled, multicenter study of the safety and efficacy of a new polyethylene glycol laxative. Am J Gastroenterol. 2000;95:446–50. https://doi.org/10.1111/j.1572-0241.2000.01765.x. S0002927099008242 [pii].

Dipalma JA, Cleveland MV, McGowan J, Herrera JL. A randomized, multicenter, placebo-controlled trial of polyethylene glycol laxative for chronic treatment of chronic constipation. Am J Gastroenterol. 2007;102:1436–41. https://doi.org/10.1111/j.1572-0241.2007.01199.x.

Dobben AC, et al. Anal inspection and digital rectal examination compared to anorectal physiology tests and endoanal ultrasonography in evaluating fecal incontinence. Int J Color Dis. 2007;22:783–90. https://doi.org/10.1007/s00384-006-0217-3.

Dreher ML. Whole fruits and fruit fiber emerging health effects. Nutrients. 2018;10 https://doi.org/10.3390/nu10121833.

Drewnowski A, Rehm CD, Constant F. Water and beverage consumption among adults in the United States: cross-sectional study using data from NHANES 2005–2010. BMC Public Health. 2013;13:1068. https://doi.org/10.1186/1471-2458-13-1068.

Drossman DA, et al. U.S. householder survey of functional gastrointestinal disorders. Prevalence, sociodemography, and health impact. Dig Dis Sci. 1993;38:1569–80.

Drukker CA, Heij HA, Wijnaendts LC, Verbeke JI, Kaspers GJ. Paraneoplastic gastro-intestinal anti-Hu syndrome in neuroblastoma. Pediatr Blood Cancer. 2009;52:396–8. https://doi.org/10.1002/pbc.21807.

Dumic I, Nordin T, Jecmenica M, Stojkovic Lalosevic M, Milosavljevic T, Milovanovic T. Gastrointestinal tract disorders in older age. Can J Gastroenterol Hepatol. 2019;2019:6757524. https://doi.org/10.1155/2019/6757524.

Eady SL, Wallace AJ, Butts CA, Hedderley D, Drummond L, Ansell J, Gearry RB. The effect of

'Zesy002' kiwifruit (Actinidia chinensis var. chinensis) on gut health function: a randomised cross-over clinical trial. J Nutr Sci. 2019;8:e18. https://doi.org/10.1017/jns.2019.14.

Erdman LH. Fecal impaction. J S C Med Assoc. 1985; 81:404–5.

Farah R. Fatal acute sodium phosphate enemas intoxication. Acta Gastroenterol Belg. 2005;68:392–3.

Fleming V, Wade WE. A review of laxative therapies for treatment of chronic constipation in older adults. Am J Geriatr Pharmacother. 2010;8:514–50. https://doi.org/10.1016/S1543-5946(10)80003-0.

Fletcher JG, Busse RF, Riederer SJ, Hough D, Gluecker T, Harper CM, Bharucha AE. Magnetic resonance imaging of anatomic and dynamic defects of the pelvic floor in defecatory disorders. Am J Gastroenterol. 2003;98:399–411. https://doi.org/10.1111/j.1572-0241.2003.07235.x. S0002927002059038 [pii].

Ford AC, Suares NC. Effect of laxatives and pharmacological therapies in chronic idiopathic constipation: systematic review and meta-analysis. Gut. 2011;60: 209–18. https://doi.org/10.1136/gut.2010.227132. 60/2/209 [pii].

Fosnes GS, Lydersen S, Farup PG. Constipation and diarrhoea – common adverse drug reactions? A cross sectional study in the general population. BMC Clin Pharmacol. 2010;11:2. https://doi.org/10.1186/1472-6904-11-2. 1472-6904-11-2 [pii].

Fox JC, Fletcher JG, Zinsmeister AR, Seide B, Riederer SJ, Bharucha AE. Effect of aging on anorectal and pelvic floor functions in females. Dis Colon Rectum. 2006;49:1726–35. https://doi.org/10.1007/s10350-006-0657-4.

Foxx-Orenstein AE, McNally MA, Odunsi ST. Update on constipation: one treatment does not fit all. Cleve Clin J Med. 2008;75:813–24.

Frazzitta G, Ferrazzoli D, Folini A, Palamara G, Maestri R. Severe constipation in Parkinson's disease and in Parkinsonisms: prevalence and affecting factors. Front Neurol. 2019;10:621. https://doi.org/10.3389/fneur.2019.00621.

Freedman A, McDougall L. Frailty 5 checklist: teaching primary care of frail older adults. Can Fam Physician. 2019;65:74–6.

Gage H, et al. Laxative use in care homes. J Adv Nurs. 2010;66:1266–72. https://doi.org/10.1111/j.1365-2648.2010.05297.x. JAN5297 [pii].

Gallagher P, O'Mahony D. Constipation in old age. Best Pract Res Clin Gastroenterol. 2009;23:875–87. https://doi.org/10.1016/j.bpg.2009.09.001. S1521-6918(09)00129-2 [pii].

Gartlehner G, Jonas DE, Morgan LC, Ringel Y, Hansen RA, Bryant CM, Carey T. Drug class review on constipation drug: final report [internet]; 2007. NBK10503 [bookaccession].

Gattuso JM, Kamm MA. Clinical features of idiopathic megarectum and idiopathic megacolon. Gut. 1997;41:93–9.

Ghoshal UC, et al. Comparison of manning, Rome I, II, and III, and Asian diagnostic criteria: report of the multicentric Indian irritable bowel syndrome (MIIBS) study. Indian J Gastroenterol. 2013;32:369–75. https://doi.org/10.1007/s12664-013-0365-7.

Ghoshal UC, Verma A, Misra A. Frequency, spectrum, and factors associated with fecal evacuation disorders among patients with chronic constipation referred to a tertiary care center in northern India. Indian J Gastroenterol. 2016;35:83–90. https://doi.org/10.1007/s12664-016-0631-6.

Ghoshal UC, et al. Indian consensus on chronic constipation in adults: a joint position statement of the Indian motility and functional diseases association and the Indian Society of Gastroenterology. Indian J Gastroenterol. 2018;37:526–44. https://doi.org/10.1007/s12664-018-0894-1.

Gibson RJ, Keefe DM. Cancer chemotherapy-induced diarrhoea and constipation: mechanisms of damage and prevention strategies. Support Care Cancer. 2006;14:890–900. https://doi.org/10.1007/s00520-006-0040-y.

Glass D, Roubenoff R. Recent advances in the biology and therapy of muscle wasting. Ann N Y Acad Sci. 2010;1211:25–36. https://doi.org/10.1111/j.1749-6632.2010.05809.x.

Goldstein O, Shaham Y, Naftali T, Konikoff F, Lavy A, Shaoul R. Toilet reading habits in Israeli adults. Neurogastroenterol Motil. 2009;21:291–5. https://doi.org/10.1111/j.1365-2982.2008.01204.x.

Grossi U, Di Tanna GL, Heinrich H, Taylor SA, Knowles CH, Scott SM. Systematic review and meta-analysis: defecography should be a first-line diagnostic modality in patients with refractory constipation. Aliment Pharmacol Ther. 2018; https://doi.org/10.1111/apt.15039.

Gustafsson M, Lamas K, Isaksson U, Sandman PO, Lovheim H. Constipation and laxative use among people living in nursing homes in 2007 and 2013. BMC Geriatr. 2019;19:38. https://doi.org/10.1186/s12877-019-1054-x.

Hallberg L, Ryttinger L, Solvell L. Side-effects of oral iron therapy. A double-blind study of different iron compounds in tablet form. Acta Med Scand Suppl. 1966;459:3–10.

Harari D, Gurwitz JH, Avorn J, Bohn R, Minaker KL. Bowel habit in relation to age and gender. Findings from the National Health Interview Survey and clinical implications. Arch Intern Med. 1996;156:315–20.

Harish K, Tony J, Sunilkumar R, Thomas V. Severe colitis induced by soap enemas. Indian J Gastroenterol. 2006;25:99–100.

Hassan I, et al. Ileorectal anastomosis for slow transit constipation: long-term functional and quality of life results. J Gastrointest Surg. 2006;10:1330–6. https://doi.org/10.1016/j.gassur.2006.09.006. discussion 1336-1337. S1091-255X(06)00395-7 [pii].

Heaton KW, O'Donnell LJ. An office guide to whole-gut transit time. Patients' recollection of their stool form. J Clin Gastroenterol. 1994;19:28–30.

Holzer P. Opioids and opioid receptors in the enteric nervous system: from a problem in opioid analgesia to a possible new prokinetic therapy in humans. Neurosci Lett. 2004;361:192–5. https://doi.org/10.1016/j.neulet.2003.12.004. S0304394003013843 [pii].

Holzer P. Treatment of opioid-induced gut dysfunction. Expert Opin Investig Drugs. 2007;16:181–94. https://doi.org/10.1517/13543784.16.2.181.

Hsu HJ, Wu MS. Extreme hyperphosphatemia and hypocalcemic coma associated with phosphate enema. Intern Med. 2008;47:643–6. https://doi.org/10.2169/internalmedicine/47.0704. [pii].

Huang R, Ho SY, Lo WS, Lam TH. Physical activity and constipation in Hong Kong adolescents. PLoS One. 2014;9:e90193. https://doi.org/10.1371/journal.pone.0090193.

Institute of Medicine. Dietary reference intakes for water, potassium, sodium, chloride, and sulfate. Washington, DC: The National Academies Press; 2005. https://doi.org/10.17226/10925.

Johanson JF, Morton D, Geenen J, Ueno R. Multicenter, 4-week, double-blind, randomized, placebo-controlled trial of lubiprostone, a locally-acting type-2 chloride channel activator, in patients with chronic constipation. Am J Gastroenterol. 2008;103:170–7. https://doi.org/10.1111/j.1572-0241.2007.01524.x. AJG1524 [pii].

Karlbom U, Lundin E, Graf W, Pahlman L. Anorectal physiology in relation to clinical subgroups of patients with severe constipation. Color Dis. 2004;6:343–9. https://doi.org/10.1111/j.1463-1318.2004.00632.x. CDI632 [pii].

Kaufman Z, Eiltch E, Dinbar A. Completely obstructive colorectal cancer. J Surg Oncol. 1989;41:230–5.

Khalif IL, Quigley EM, Konovitch EA, Maximova ID. Alterations in the colonic flora and intestinal permeability and evidence of immune activation in chronic constipation. Dig Liver Dis. 2005;37:838–49. https://doi.org/10.1016/j.dld.2005.06.008.

Kienzle-Horn S, Vix JM, Schuijt C, Peil H, Jordan CC, Kamm MA. Comparison of bisacodyl and sodium picosulphate in the treatment of chronic constipation. Curr Med Res Opin. 2007;23:691–9. https://doi.org/10.1185/030079907X178865.

Kim SE, et al. Change of fecal flora and effectiveness of the short-term VSL#3 probiotic treatment in patients with functional constipation. J Neurogastroenterol Motil. 2015;21:111–20. https://doi.org/10.5056/jnm14048.

Klein H. Constipation and fecal impaction. Med Clin North Am. 1982;66:1135–41.

Koch A, Voderholzer WA, Klauser AG, Muller-Lissner S. Symptoms in chronic constipation. Dis Colon Rectum. 1997;40:902–6.

Lacy BE, Brunton SA. Partnering with gastroenterologists to evaluate patients with chronic constipation. MedGenMed. 2005;7:19.

Larkin PJ, et al. Diagnosis, assessment and management of constipation in advanced cancer: ESMO clinical practice guidelines. Ann Oncol. 2018;29:iv111–25. https://doi.org/10.1093/annonc/mdy148.

Lat I, Foster DR, Erstad B. Drug-induced acute liver failure and gastrointestinal complications. Crit Care Med. 2010;38:S175–87. https://doi.org/10.1097/CCM.0b013e3181de0db2. 00003246-201006001-00012 [pii].

Laugier R, Bernard JP, Berthezene P, Dupuy P. Changes in pancreatic exocrine secretion with age: pancreatic exocrine secretion does decrease in the elderly. Digestion. 1991;50:202–11.

Lederle FA, Busch DL, Mattox KM, West MJ, Aske DM. Cost-effective treatment of constipation in the elderly: a randomized double-blind comparison of sorbitol and lactulose. Am J Med. 1990;89:597–601. https://doi.org/10.1016/0002-9343(90)90177-f.

Lee-Robichaud H, Thomas K, Morgan J, Nelson RL. Lactulose versus polyethylene glycol for chronic constipation. Cochrane Database Syst Rev. 2010:CD007570. https://doi.org/10.1002/14651858.CD007570.pub2.

Lembo A, Camilleri M. Chronic constipation. N Engl J Med. 2003;349:1360–8. https://doi.org/10.1056/NEJMra020995. 349/14/1360 [pii].

Lembo AJ, et al. Efficacy of linaclotide for patients with chronic constipation. Gastroenterology. 2010;138:886–95. https://doi.org/10.1053/j.gastro.2009.12.050. e881. S0016-5085(09)02247-1 [pii].

Leung FW, Rao SS. Fecal incontinence in the elderly. Gastroenterol Clin N Am. 2009;38:503–11. https://doi.org/10.1016/j.gtc.2009.06.007. S0889-8553(09)00063-6 [pii].

Lever E, Cole J, Scott SM, Emery PW, Whelan K. Systematic review: the effect of prunes on gastrointestinal function. Aliment Pharmacol Ther. 2014;40:750–8. https://doi.org/10.1111/apt.12913.

Lever E, Scott SM, Louis P, Emery PW, Whelan K. The effect of prunes on stool output, gut transit time and gastrointestinal microbiota: a randomised controlled trial. Clin Nutr. 2019;38:165–73. https://doi.org/10.1016/j.clnu.2018.01.003.

Lewis SJ, Heaton KW. Stool form scale as a useful guide to intestinal transit time. Scand J Gastroenterol. 1997;32:920–4. https://doi.org/10.3109/00365529709011203.

Lim D, Liu S, Ferzli G. Management of sigmoid perforation from chronic constipation and manual disimpaction. BMJ Case Rep. 2018; https://doi.org/10.1136/bcr-2018-226886.

Lindberg G, Hamid SS, Malfertheiner P, et al. World Gastroenterology Organisation global guideline: constipation-a global perspective. J Clin Gastroenterol, 45. 2011:483–7. https://doi.org/10.1097/MCG.0b013e31820fb914. 00004836-201107000-00004 [pii].

Lindeman RD, Romero LJ, Liang HC, Baumgartner RN, Koehler KM, Garry PJ. Do elderly persons need to be encouraged to drink more fluids? J Gerontol A Biol Sci Med Sci. 2000;55:M361–5.

Locke GR 3rd, Pemberton JH, Phillips SF. American Gastroenterological Association medical position statement: guidelines on constipation. Gastroenterology. 2000;119:1761–6.

Luthra P, Camilleri M, Burr NE, Quigley EMM, Black CJ, Ford AC. Efficacy of drugs in chronic idiopathic constipation: a systematic review and network meta-analysis. Lancet Gastroenterol Hepatol. 2019; 4:831–44. https://doi.org/10.1016/S2468-1253(19) 30246-8.

Ma T, Lan T, Geng T et al. Nutritional properties and biological proeprties of kiwifruit (Actinidia) and kiwi-fruit products under simulated gastrointestinal in vitro digestion. Food and Nutrition. 2019;63:1674. https://doi.org/10.29219/fncv63.1674.

Martin BC, Barghout V, Cerulli A. Direct medical costs of constipation in the United States. Manag Care Interface. 2006;19:43–9.

McCallum IJ, Ong S, Mercer-Jones M. Chronic constipation in adults. BMJ. 2009;338:b831.

McCrea GL, Miaskowski C, Stotts NA, Macera L, Varma MG. Pathophysiology of constipation in the older adult. World J Gastroenterol. 2008;14:2631–8.

McRorie JW, Daggy BP, Morel JG, Diersing PS, Miner PB, Robinson M. Psyllium is superior to docusate sodium for treatment of chronic constipation. Aliment Pharmacol Ther. 1998;12:491–7.

Mearin F, Lacy BE, Chang L, Chey WD, Lembo AJ, Simren M, Spiller R. Bowel disorders. Gastroenterology. 2016; https://doi.org/10.1053/j.gastro.2016.02.031.

Mehendale SR, Yuan CS. Opioid-induced gastrointestinal dysfunction. Dig Dis. 2006;24:105–12. https://doi.org/10.1159/000090314. 90314 [pii].

Mertz H, Naliboff B, Mayer E. Physiology of refractory chronic constipation. Am J Gastroenterol. 1999; 94:609–15. https://doi.org/10.1111/j.1572-0241.1999.922_a.x. S000292709800803X [pii].

Migeon-Duballet I, Chabin M, Gautier A, Mistouflet T, Bonnet M, Aubert JM, Halphen M. Long-term efficacy and cost-effectiveness of polyethylene glycol 3350 plus electrolytes in chronic constipation: a retrospective study in a disabled population. Curr Med Res Opin. 2006;22:1227–35. https://doi.org/10.1185/030079906X112543.

Minguez M, et al. Predictive value of the balloon expulsion test for excluding the diagnosis of pelvic floor dyssynergia in constipation. Gastroenterology. 2004;126:57–62.

Moore J, Firoozan S, Martinez N. Advancements in the treatment of constipation in hospitalized older adults: utilizing Secretagogues and peripherally acting mu-opioid receptor antagonists. Am J Ther. 2008;25: e15–27.

Mori H, et al. Clinical features of hypermagnesemia in patients with functional constipation taking daily magnesium oxide. J Clin Biochem Nutr. 2019;65:76–81. https://doi.org/10.3164/jcbn.18-117.

Morley J. Water, water everywhere and not a drop to drink. J Gerontol A Biol Sci Med Sci. 2000;55:M359–60.

Moylan S, Armstrong J, Diaz-Saldano D, Saker M, Yerkes EB, Lindgren BW. Are abdominal x-rays a reliable way to assess for constipation? J Urol. 2010;184:1692–8.

https://doi.org/10.1016/j.juro.2010.05.054. S0022-5347(10)03595-0 [pii].

Muller-Lissner SA, Kamm MA, Scarpignato C, Wald A. Myths and misconceptions about chronic constipation. Am J Gastroenterol. 2005;100:232–42. https://doi.org/10.1111/j.1572-0241.2005.40885.x. AJG40885 [pii].

Murphy J. Movement away from phenolphthalein in laxatives. JAMA. 2009;301:1770. https://doi.org/10.1001/jama.2009.585. 301/17/1770-a [pii].

Muss C, Mosgoeller W, Endler T. Papaya preparation (Caricol(R)) in digestive disorders. Neuro Endocrinol Lett. 2013;34:38–46.

Neefjes ECW, et al. Optimal treatment of opioid induced constipation in daily clinical practice – an observational study. BMC Palliat Care. 2019;18:31. https://doi.org/10.1186/s12904-019-0416-7.

Ness J, Hoth A, Barnett MJ, Shorr RI, Kaboli PJ. Anticholinergic medications in community-dwelling-older veterans: prevalence of anticholinergic symptoms, symptom burden, and adverse drug events. Am J Geriatr Pharmacother. 2006;4:42–51. https://doi.org/10.1016/j.amjopharm.2006.03.008. S1543-5946(06)00009-2 [pii].

Niv G, Grinberg T, Dickman R, Wasserberg N, Niv Y. Perforation and mortality after cleansing enema for acute constipation are not rare but are preventable. Int J Gen Med. 2013;6:323–8. https://doi.org/10.2147/IJGM.S44417.

Nyam DC, Pemberton JH, Ilstrup DM, Rath DM. Long-term results of surgery for chronic constipation. Dis Colon Rectum. 1997;40:273–9.

O'Brien MD, et al. Motility and tone of the left colon in constipation: a role in clinical practice? Am J Gastroenterol. 1996;91:2532–8.

Okawa Y, Fukudo S, Sanada H. Specific foods can reduce symptoms of irritable bowel syndrome and functional constipation: a review. Biopsychosoc Med. 2019;13:10. https://doi.org/10.1186/s13030-019-0152-5.

Omer A, Quigley EMM. An update on prucalopride in the treatment of chronic constipation. Ther Adv Gastroenterol. 2017;10:877–87. https://doi.org/10.1177/1756283X17734809.

Opie LH. Calcium channel antagonists. Part IV: side effects and contraindications drug interactions and combinations. Cardiovasc Drugs Ther. 1988;2:177–89.

Ostaszkiewicz J, Hornby L, Millar L, Ockerby C. The effects of conservative treatment for constipation on symptom severity and quality of life in community-dwelling adults. J Wound Ostomy Continence Nurs. 2010;37:193–8. https://doi.org/10.1097/WON.0b013e3181cf7206.

Pagano G, Tan EE, Haider JM, Bautista A, Tagliati M. Constipation is reduced by beta-blockers and increased by dopaminergic medications in Parkinson's disease. Parkinsonism Relat Disord. 2015;21:120–5. https://doi.org/10.1016/j.parkreldis.2014.11.015.

Palsson OS, Whitehead W, Tornblom H, Sperber AD, Simren M. Prevalence of Rome IV functional Bowel disorders among adults in the United States, Canada, and the United Kingdom. Gastroenterology. 2020; https://doi.org/10.1053/j.gastro.2019.12.021.

Pampati V, Fogel R. Treatment options for primary constipation. Curr Treat Options Gastroenterol. 2004;7:225–33.

Panchal SJ, Muller-Schwefe P, Wurzelmann JI. Opioid-induced bowel dysfunction: prevalence, pathophysiology and burden. Int J Clin Pract. 2007;61:1181–7. https://doi.org/10.1111/j.1742-1241.2007.01415.x. IJCP1415 [pii].

Pandol SJ, Raybould HE, Yee HF. Integrative response of the gastrointestinal tract and liver to a meal. In: Yamada T, Alpers DH, Kalloo AN, Kaplowitz N, Owyang C, Powell DW, editors. Textbook of gastroenterology, vol. 1. 5th ed. Chichester: Blackwell Publishing; 2009. p. 3–14.

Papaleontiou M, Henderson CR Jr, Turner BJ, Moore AA, Olkhovskaya Y, Amanfo L, Reid MC. Outcomes associated with opioid use in the treatment of chronic noncancer pain in older adults: a systematic review and meta-analysis. J Am Geriatr Soc. 2010;58: 1353–69. https://doi.org/10.1111/j.1532-5415.2010.02 920.x. JGS2920 [pii].

Pare P, Ferrazzi S, Thompson WG, Irvine EJ, Rance L. An epidemiological survey of constipation in Canada: definitions, rates, demographics, and predictors of health care seeking. Am J Gastroenterol. 2001;96: 3130–7. https://doi.org/10.1111/j.1572-0241.2001. 05259.x. S0002-9270(01)03821-7 [pii].

Pare P, et al. Recommendations on chronic constipation (including constipation associated with irritable bowel syndrome) treatment. Can J Gastroenterol. 2007;21 (Suppl B):3B–22B.

Parthasarathy G, et al. Relationship between microbiota of the colonic mucosa vs feces and symptoms, colonic transit, and methane production in female patients with chronic constipation. Gastroenterology. 2016;150:367–79. https://doi.org/10.1053/j.gastro.2015.10.005. e361.

Patcharatrakul T, Rao SSC. Update on the pathophysiology and management of anorectal disorders. Gut Liver. 2018;12:375–84. https://doi.org/10.5009/gnl17172.

Peck CJ, Samsuria SD, Harrington AM, King SK, Hutson JM, Southwell BR. Fall in density, but not number of myenteric neurons and circular muscle nerve fibres in Guinea-pig colon with ageing. Neurogastroenterol Motil. 2009;21:1075–e1090. https://doi.org/10.1111/j.1365-2982.2009.01349.x. NMO1349 [pii].

Pezim ME, Pemberton JH, Levin KE, Litchy WJ, Phillips SF. Parameters of anorectal and colonic motility in health and in severe constipation. Dis Colon Rectum. 1993;36:484–91.

Phillips RJ, Powley TL. Innervation of the gastrointestinal tract: patterns of aging. Auton Neurosci. 2007;136:1–19. https://doi.org/10.1016/j.autneu.2007.04.005. S1566-0702(07)00108-7 [pii].

Phillips RJ, Rhodes BS, Powley TL. Effects of age on sympathetic innervation of the myenteric plexus and gastrointestinal smooth muscle of Fischer 344 rats.

Anat Embryol (Berl). 2006;211:673–83. https://doi.org/10.1007/s00429-006-0123-z.

Phillips RJ, Pairitz JC, Powley TL. Age-related neuronal loss in the submucosal plexus of the colon of Fischer 344 rats. Neurobiol Aging. 2007;28:1124–37. https://doi.org/10.1016/j.neurobiolaging.2006.05.019. S0197 -4580(06)00178-3 [pii].

Pimentel M, et al. Methane, a gas produced by enteric bacteria, slows intestinal transit and augments small intestinal contractile activity. Am J Physiol Gastrointest Liver Physiol. 2006;290:G1089–95. https://doi.org/ 10.1152/ajpgi.00574.2004.

Pont LG, Fisher M, Williams K. Appropriate use of laxatives in the older person. Drugs Aging. 2019;36:999–1005. https://doi.org/10.1007/s40266-019-00701-9.

Ramkumar D, Rao SS. Efficacy and safety of traditional medical therapies for chronic constipation: systematic review. Am J Gastroenterol. 2005;100:936–71. https://doi.org/10.1111/j.1572-0241.2005.40925.x. AJG40925 [pii].

Rao SS. Dyssynergic defecation. Gastroenterol Clin N Am. 2001;30:97–114.

Rao SS. Dyssynergic defecation and biofeedback therapy. Gastroenterol Clin North Am. 2008;37:569–86. https://doi.org/10.1016/j.gtc.2008.06.011. viii. S0889-8553 (08)00051-4 [pii].

Rao SS. Advances in diagnostic assessment of fecal incontinence and dyssynergic defecation. Clin Gastroenterol Hepatol. 2010;8:910–9. https://doi.org/10.1016/j.cgh. 2010.06.004. S1542-3565(10)00601-4 [pii].

Rao SS, Go JT. Update on the management of constipation in the elderly: new treatment options. Clin Interv Aging. 2010;5:163–71.

Rao SS, Meduri K. What is necessary to diagnose constipation? Best Pract Res Clin Gastroenterol. 2010;25:127–40. https://doi.org/10.1016/j.bpg.2010.11.001. S1521-6918 (10)00156-3 [pii].

Rao SS, Meduri K. What is necessary to diagnose constipation? Best Pract Res Clin Gastroenterol. 2011;25:127–40. https://doi.org/10.1016/j.bpg.2010.11.001.

Rao SS, Singh S. Clinical utility of colonic and anorectal manometry in chronic constipation. J Clin Gastroenterol. 2011;44:597–609. https://doi.org/10.1097/MCG.0b01 3e3181e88532.

Rao SS, Welcher KD, Leistikow JS. Obstructive defecation: a failure of rectoanal coordination. Am J Gastroenterol. 1998;93:1042–50. https://doi.org/10.1111/j.1572-0241. 1998.00326.x. S0002-9270(98)00207-X [pii].

Rao SS, Tuteja AK, Vellema T, Kempf J, Stessman M. Dyssynergic defecation: demographics, symptoms, stool patterns, and quality of life. J Clin Gastroenterol. 2004;38:680–5. https://doi.org/10.10 97/01.mcg.0000135929.78074.8c. 00004836-20040 9000-00012 [pii].

Rao SS, Ozturk R, Laine L. Clinical utility of diagnostic tests for constipation in adults: a systematic review. Am J Gastroenterol. 2005;100:1605–15. https://doi.org/ 10.1111/j.1572-0241.2005.41845.x. AJG41845 [pii].

Rao SS, Kavlock R, Rao S. Influence of body position and stool characteristics on defecation in humans. Am J Gastroenterol. 2006;101:2790–6. https://doi.org/10.1111/j.1572-0241.2006.00827.x. AJG827 [pii].

Rao SS, Bharucha AE, Chiarioni G, Felt-Bersma R, Knowles C, Malcolm A, Wald A. Functional anorectal disorders. Gastroenterology. 2016; https://doi.org/10.1053/j.gastro.2016.02.009.

Reber J, McGauvran A, Froemming A. Abdominal radiograph usage trends in the setting of constipation: a 10-year experience. Abdom Radiol (NY). 2018;43:2231–8. https://doi.org/10.1007/s00261-018-1466-7.

Reid MC, et al. Characteristics of older adults receiving opioids in primary care: treatment duration and outcomes. Pain Med. 2010;11:1063–71. https://doi.org/10.1111/j.1526-4637.2010.00883.x. PME883 [pii].

Reiner CS, Tutuian R, Solopova AE, Pohl D, Marincek B, Weishaupt D. MR defecography in patients with dyssynergic defecation: spectrum of imaging findings and diagnostic value. Br J Radiol. 2011;84:136–44. https://doi.org/10.1259/bjr/28989463. 84/998/136 [pii].

Remes-Troche JM, Rao SS. Neurophysiological testing in anorectal disorders. Expert Rev Gastroenterol Hepatol. 2008;2:323–35. https://doi.org/10.1586/17474124.2.3.323.

Rentea RM, Fehring CH. Rectal colonic mural hematoma following enema for constipation while on therapeutic anticoagulation. J Surg Case Rep. 2017; https://doi.org/10.1093/jscr/rjx001.

Rentsch M, Paetzel C, Lenhart M, Feuerbach S, Jauch KW, Furst A. Dynamic magnetic resonance imaging defecography: a diagnostic alternative in the assessment of pelvic floor disorders in proctology. Dis Colon Rectum. 2001;44:999–1007.

Rikard-Bell J, Iyer J, Rane A. Perineal outcome and the risk of pelvic floor dysfunction: a cohort study of primiparous women. Aust N Z J Obstet Gynaecol. 2014;54:371–6. https://doi.org/10.1111/ajo.12222.

Roerig JL, Steffen KJ, Mitchell JE, Zunker C. Laxative abuse: epidemiology, diagnosis and management. Drugs. 2010;70:1487–503. https://doi.org/10.2165/11898640-000000000-00000. 2 [pii].

Romero Y, Evans JM, Fleming KC, Phillips SF. Constipation and fecal incontinence in the elderly population. Mayo Clin Proc. 1996;71:81–92.

Rotholtz NA, Wexner SD. Surgical treatment of constipation and fecal incontinence. Gastroenterol Clin N Am. 2001;30:131–66.

Ryhammer AM, Laurberg S, Hermann AP. Long-term effect of vaginal deliveries on anorectal function in normal perimenopausal women. Dis Colon Rectum. 1996;39:852–9. https://doi.org/10.1007/bf02053982.

Saad RJ, et al. Do stool form and frequency correlate with whole-gut and colonic transit? Results from a multicenter study in constipated individuals and healthy controls. Am J Gastroenterol. 2010;105:403–11. https://doi.org/10.1038/ajg.2009.612. ajg2009612 [pii].

Sadik R, Abrahamsson H, Stotzer PO. Gender differences in gut transit shown with a newly developed radiological procedure. Scand J Gastroenterol. 2003;38:36–42.

Sakakibara R, Doi H, Fukudo S. Lewy body constipation. J Anus Rectum Colon. 2019;3:10–7. https://doi.org/10.23922/jarc.2018-022.

Sandler RS, Jordan MC, Shelton BJ. Demographic and dietary determinants of constipation in the US population. Am J Public Health. 1990;80:185–9.

Savoye-Collet C, Koning E, Dacher JN. Radiologic evaluation of pelvic floor disorders. Gastroenterol Clin North Am. 2008;37:553–67. https://doi.org/10.1016/j.gtc.2008.06.004. viii. S0889-8553(08)00048-4 [pii].

Scarlett Y. Medical management of fecal incontinence. Gastroenterology. 2004;126:S55–63. https://doi.org/10.1053/j.gastro.2003.10.007.

Schey R, Rao SS. Lubiprostone for the treatment of adults with constipation and irritable bowel syndrome. Dig Dis Sci. 2011;56:1619–25. https://doi.org/10.1007/s10620-011-1702-2.

Schey R, Cromwell J, Rao SS. Medical and surgical management of pelvic floor disorders affecting defecation. Am J Gastroenterol. 2012;107:1624–33. https://doi.org/10.1038/ajg.2012.247. quiz p 1634.

Schiller LR, Emmett M, Santa Ana CA, Fordtran JS. Osmotic effects of polyethylene glycol. Gastroenterology. 1988;94:933–41.

Schnelle JF, Leung FW, Rao SS, Beuscher L, Keeler E, Clift JW, Simmons S. A controlled trial of an intervention to improve urinary and fecal incontinence and constipation. J Am Geriatr Soc. 2010;58:1504–11. https://doi.org/10.1111/j.1532-5415.2010.02978.x. JGS2978 [pii].

Schubert MC, Sridhar S, Schade RR, Wexner SD. What every gastroenterologist needs to know about common anorectal disorders. World J Gastroenterol. 2009;15:3201–9.

Scott SM, Gladman MA. Manometric, sensorimotor, and neurophysiologic evaluation of anorectal function. Gastroenterol Clin N Am. 2008;37:511–38. https://doi.org/10.1016/j.gtc.2008.06.010. vii. S0889-8553(08)00052-6 [pii].

Shah ED, Kim HM, Schoenfeld P. Efficacy and tolerability of guanylate cyclase-C agonists for irritable Bowel syndrome with constipation and chronic idiopathic constipation: a systematic review and meta-analysis. Am J Gastroenterol. 2018;113:329–38. https://doi.org/10.1038/ajg.2017.495.

Shen L, Huang C, Lu X, Xu X, Jiang Z, Zhu C. Lower dietary fibre intake, but not total water consumption, is associated with constipation: a population-based analysis. J Hum Nutr Diet. 2019;32:422–31. https://doi.org/10.1111/jhn.12589.

Siegel JD, Di Palma JA. Medical treatment of constipation. Clin Colon Rectal Surg. 2005;18:76–80. https://doi.org/10.1055/s-2005-870887.

Sikirov D. Comparison of straining during defecation in three positions: results and implications for human health. Dig Dis Sci. 2003;48:1201–5.

Slavin JL. Position of the American dietetic association: health implications of dietary fiber. J Am Diet Assoc. 2008;108:1716–31.

Sommers T, et al. Prevalence of chronic constipation and chronic Diarrhea in diabetic individuals in the United States. Am J Gastroenterol. 2018; https://doi.org/10.1038/s41395-018-0418-8.

Song BK, Kim YS, Kim HS, Oh JW, Lee O, Kim JS. Combined exercise improves gastrointestinal motility in psychiatric in patients. World J Clin Cases. 2018;6:207–13. https://doi.org/10.12998/wjcc.v6.i8.207.

Sperber AD, et al. Conducting multinational, cross-cultural research in the functional gastrointestinal disorders: issues and recommendations. A Rome foundation working team report. Aliment Pharmacol Ther. 2014;40:1094–102. https://doi.org/10.1111/apt.12942.

Spiller R, Marciani L. Intraluminal impact of food: new insights from MRI. Nutrients. 2019;11 https://doi.org/10.3390/nu11051147.

Sprenger N, Julita M, Donnicola D, Jann A. Sialic acid feeding aged rats rejuvenates stimulated salivation and colon enteric neuron chemotypes. Glycobiology. 2009;19:1492–502. https://doi.org/10.1093/glycob/cwp124. cwp124 [pii].

Stacewicz-Sapuntzakis M, Bowen PE, Hussain EA, Damayanti-Wood BI, Farnsworth NR. Chemical composition and potential health effects of prunes: a functional food? Crit Rev Food Sci Nutr. 2001;41:251–86. https://doi.org/10.1080/20014091091814.

Stern T, Davis AM. Evaluation and treatment of patients with constipation. JAMA. 2016;315:192–3. https://doi.org/10.1001/jama.2015.16995.

Suares NC, Ford AC. Systematic review: the effects of fibre in the management of chronic idiopathic constipation. Aliment Pharmacol Ther. 2011;33:895–901. https://doi.org/10.1111/j.1365-2036.2011.04602.x.

Sun WM, Rao SS. Manometric assessment of anorectal function. Gastroenterol Clin N Am. 2001;30:15–32.

Tack J. Current and future therapies for chronic constipation. Best Pract Res Clin Gastroenterol. 2011;25:151–8. https://doi.org/10.1016/j.bpg.2011.01.005. S1521-6918 (11)00006-0 [pii].

Talley NJ. How to do and interpret a rectal examination in gastroenterology. Am J Gastroenterol. 2008;103:820–2. https://doi.org/10.1111/j.1572-0241.2008.01832.x.

Talley NJ, Weaver AL, Zinsmeister AR, Melton LJ 3rd. Functional constipation and outlet delay: a population-based study. Gastroenterology. 1993;105:781–90.

Talley NJ, Fleming KC, Evans JM, O'Keefe EA, Weaver AL, Zinsmeister AR, Melton LJ 3rd. Constipation in an elderly community: a study of prevalence and potential risk factors. Am J Gastroenterol. 1996;91:19–25.

Talley NJ, Jones M, Nuyts G, Dubois D. Risk factors for chronic constipation based on a general practice sample. Am J Gastroenterol. 2003;98:1107–11. https://doi.org/10.1111/j.1572-0241.2003.07465.x. S0002927003002399 [pii].

Tantiphlachiva K, Rao P, Attaluri A, Rao SS. Digital rectal examination is a useful tool for identifying patients with dyssynergia. Clin Gastroenterol Hepatol. 2010;8:955–60. https://doi.org/10.1016/j.cgh.2010.06.031. S1542-3565 (10)00678-6 [pii].

Tariq S. Constipation in long-term care. Ann Long Term Care. 2008;16:1–45.

Thomas JR, Cooney GA, Slatkin NE. Palliative care and pain: new strategies for managing opioid bowel dysfunction. J Palliat Med. 2008;11(Suppl 1): S1–19. https://doi.org/10.1089/jpm.2008.9839.supp. quiz S21-12.

Thompson WG, Irvine EJ, Pare P, Ferrazzi S, Rance L. Functional gastrointestinal disorders in Canada: first population-based survey using Rome II criteria with suggestions for improving the questionnaire. Dig Dis Sci. 2002;47:225–35.

Tramonte SM, Brand MB, Mulrow CD, Amato MG, O'Keefe ME, Ramirez G. The treatment of chronic constipation in adults. A systematic review. J Gen Intern Med. 1997;12:15–24.

Trindade E, Menon D, Topfer LA, Coloma C. Adverse effects associated with selective serotonin reuptake inhibitors and tricyclic antidepressants: a meta-analysis. CMAJ. 1998;159:1245–52.

Trinkley KE, Porter K, Nahata MC. Prescribing patterns for the outpatient treatment of constipation in the United States. Dig Dis Sci. 2010;55:3514–20. https://doi.org/10.1007/s10620-010-1196-3.

Tucker DM, et al. Dietary fiber and personality factors as determinants of stool output. Gastroenterology. 1981;81:879–83.

Tuteja AK, Biskupiak JE. Chronic constipation: overview and treatment options. PT. 2007;32:91–105.

Tuteja AK, Rao SS. Lubiprostone for constipation and irritable bowel syndrome with constipation. Expert Rev Gastroenterol Hepatol. 2008;2:727–33. https://doi.org/10.1586/17474124.2.6.727.

van Dijk KN, de Vries CS, van den Berg PB, Dijkema AM, Brouwers JR, de Jong-van den Berg LT. Constipation as an adverse effect of drug use in nursing home patients: an overestimated risk. Br J Clin Pharmacol. 1998;46:255–61.

Viallard JF, Vincent A, Moreau JF, Parrens M, Pellegrin JL, Ellie E. Thymoma-associated neuromyotonia with antibodies against voltage-gated potassium channels presenting as chronic intestinal pseudo-obstruction. Eur Neurol. 2005;53:60–3. https://doi.org/10.1159/000084300.

Vijayvargiya P, Camilleri M. Use of prucalopride in adults with chronic idiopathic constipation. Expert Rev Clin Pharmacol. 2019;12:579–89. https://doi.org/10.1080/17512433.2019.1620104.

Voderholzer WA, Schatke W, Muhldorfer BE, Klauser AG, Birkner B, Muller-Lissner SA. Clinical response to dietary fiber treatment of chronic constipation. Am J Gastroenterol. 1997;92:95–8.

Wald A. Pathophysiology, diagnosis and current management of chronic constipation. Nat Clin Pract Gastroenterol Hepatol. 2006;3:90–100. https://doi.org/10.1038/ncpgasthep0406. ncpgasthep0406 [pii].

Wald A. Constipation: advances in diagnosis and treatment. JAMA. 2016;315:185–91. https://doi.org/10.1001/jama.2015.16994.

Wald A. Update on the Management of Constipation. JAMA. 2019; https://doi.org/10.1001/jama.2019.16029.

Walter SA, Kjellstrom L, Nyhlin H, Talley NJ, Agreus L. Assessment of normal bowel habits in the general adult population: the Popcol study. Scand J Gastroenterol. 2010;45:556–66. https://doi.org/10.3109/00365520903551332.

Wan Y, Zhang D, Qian Y, Chang S, Qian H. Association between constipation and cognitive impairment among adults aged 60 years and older: a cohort study; 2019. Available at SSRN: https://ssrn.com/abstract=3463266 or https://doi.org/10.2139/ssrn.3463266.

Werth BL, Williams KA, Fisher MJ, Pont LG. Defining constipation to estimate its prevalence in the community: results from a national survey. BMC Gastroenterol. 2019;19:75. https://doi.org/10.1186/s12876-019-0994-0.

Williams ME. Geriatric physical diagnosis: a guide to observation and assessment. Jefferson: McFarland Company, Inc.; 2008.

Wilson JA. Constipation in the elderly. Clin Geriatr Med. 1999;15:499–510.

Wiskur B, Greenwood-Van Meerveld B. The aging colon: the role of enteric neurodegeneration in constipation. Curr Gastroenterol Rep. 2010;12:507–12. https://doi.org/10.1007/s11894-010-0139-7.

Wong RK, Palsson OS, Turner MJ, Levy RL, Feld AD, von Korff M, Whitehead WE. Inability of the Rome III criteria to distinguish functional constipation from constipation-subtype irritable Bowel syndrome. Am J Gastroenterol. 2010;105:2228–34. https://doi.org/10.1038/ajg.2010.200. ajg2010200 [pii].

Wong MYW, Hebbard G, Gibson PR, Burgell RE. Chronic constipation and abdominal pain: independent or closely-interrelated symptoms? J Gastroenterol Hepatol. 2020; https://doi.org/10.1111/jgh.14970.

Wood JD, Galligan JJ. Function of opioids in the enteric nervous system. Neurogastroenterol Motil. 2004;16 (Suppl 2):17–28. https://doi.org/10.1111/j.1743-3150.2004.00554.x. NMO554 [pii].

Wrenn K. Fecal impaction. N Engl J Med. 1989;321:658–62. https://doi.org/10.1056/NEJM198909073211007.

Wrick KL, Robertson JB, Van Soest PJ, Lewis BA, Rivers JM, Roe DA, Hackler LR. The influence of dietary fiber source on human intestinal transit and stool output. J Nutr. 1983;113:1464–79.

Xing JH, Soffer EE. Adverse effects of laxatives. Dis Colon Rectum. 2001;44:1201–9.

Yang J, Wang HP, Zhou L, Xu CF. Effect of dietary fiber on constipation: a meta analysis. World J Gastroenterol. 2012;18:7378–83. https://doi.org/10.3748/wjg.v18.i48.7378.

Yang Y, Cao YL, Wang WH, Zhang YY, Zhao N, Wei D. Subtotal colonic bypass plus colostomy with antiperistaltic cecoproctostomy for the treatment of slow transit constipation in an aged population: a retrospective control study. World J Gastroenterol. 2018;24:2491–500. https://doi.org/10.3748/wjg.v24.i23.2491.

Zhuang Z, et al. The manufacturing process of kiwifruit fruit powder with high dietary Fiber and its laxative effect. Molecules. 2019;24 https://doi.org/10.3390/molecules24213813.

Chronic Diarrhea in the Older Adult

54

Lawrence R. Schiller

Contents

Abstract

Diarrhea is a common problem in all age groups. It can be particularly troubling in older individuals, especially those who are frail, because of secondary problems such as fecal incontinence or fluid and electrolyte disorders. Physiologic fitness may be impaired in older individuals due to senescence of the immune system, decreased renal function, abnormal nutritional status, and the accumulation of chronic diseases. Some conditions appear to be more common in elders, and it is important to realize that the presentation of illnesses in older individuals may be different than in younger patients. Diarrhea may be more or less severe and its response to treatment may be different than in younger individuals. Quality of life may be impacted more intensely in the old, and diarrhea may lead to institutionalization, especially individuals affected by fecal incontinence. This chapter will review some of the changes in intestinal structure and function that occur with normal aging, common conditions that may cause

L. R. Schiller (✉)
Baylor University Medical Center, Dallas, TX, USA

Texas A&M College of Medicine, Dallas Campus,
Dallas, TX, USA
e-mail: LRSMD@aol.com

© Springer Nature Switzerland AG 2021
C. S. Pitchumoni, T. S. Dharmarajan (eds.), *Geriatric Gastroenterology*,
https://doi.org/10.1007/978-3-030-30192-7_46

diarrhea in the geriatric population, and rational approaches to evaluation and management of chronic diarrhea.

Keywords

Diarrhea · Fecal incontinence · Intestinal fluid and electrolyte absorption · Malabsorption · Infectious diarrhea · Chronic diarrhea · Diagnosis and management · Antidiarrheal drugs

Introduction

Diarrhea is a symptom that most individuals have had at one time or another. Acute gastroenteritis attributed to food poisoning occurs in millions each year, and it has been estimated that the average American has a transient episode of diarrhea every few years (Hall et al. 2013). Chronic diarrhea (lasting more than 4 weeks) occurs up to 6% of the population (Singh et al. 2018). For most individuals, diarrhea is defined as the passage of loose stools, often associated with increased stool frequency (>2 bowel movements per day).

The prevalence of diarrhea in the old is uncertain, but its impact can be severe. Because of decreased mobility and impaired anal sphincter function, fecal incontinence may complicate the course of chronic diarrhea in many elders and may result in the need for increased assistance by caregivers or even admission to a nursing facility. Impaired physiologic fitness also may make diarrhea more of a problem than in younger individuals. For example, aging often is accompanied by decreased renal function, which may make it difficult to compensate for dehydration and electrolyte loss. Another problem that can make diarrhea catastrophic for frail elders is impaired nutritional status; decreased food intake due to diarrhea may make marginal nutritional status even worse. Senescence of the immune system may make it difficult to clear infections causing diarrhea, thus prolonging episodes of infectious diarrhea.

Institutionalization of older people may increase the chances of developing infectious

diarrhea, particularly if satisfactory sanitation is not maintained. Common-source food-borne infections or person-to-person infections may affect residents in institutions (White et al. 2019). Many elders are at risk for contracting *Clostridioides difficile* infection from spores contaminating hospital and nursing home environments. In addition, *Clostridioides difficile* infection may be more likely to relapse in older patients who are less capable than more youthful persons of mounting an effective immune response (Asempa and Nicolau 2017; Donskey 2017).

Some concomitant diseases that predispose to diarrhea, such as diabetes, occur more frequently in the old. Geriatric patients also may have been treated for various diseases and have residuals from that treatment that may predispose to diarrhea. For example, patients may have had bowel resections or radiation therapy that have left them with short bowel syndrome or radiation enteritis. Many elders may be on drugs that have diarrhea as a side effect (Philip et al. 2017). This must be recognized promptly to avoid unneeded and extensive evaluation.

Another complicating feature or management of diarrhea in older adults is that some diarrheal diseases may present differently in elders than in younger patients. For example, celiac disease which typically produces diarrhea and weight loss in the young may present with fatigue, reduced appetite, cognitive decline, or neuropathy rather than diarrhea (Collin et al. 2018). Physicians dealing with the elderly need to consider diseases that primarily present with diarrhea or malabsorption in younger adults, when seeing older patients with a variety of symptoms.

Changes in Intestinal Structure and Function with Normal Aging

The intestinal epithelium abuts a harsh luminal environment and is bathed with raw nutrients, powerful digestive enzymes, and multiple microorganisms. Because of this, the epithelial cells may be damaged; they are replaced every 5 or 6 days by fresh cells produced by stem cells in the crypts. This means that the intestinal epithelial cells are always "young." Except for rare patients in whom the stem cells are damaged, mucosal function is well maintained into old age. Direct tests of mucosal absorption with d-xylose tests remain normal to age 80 and decline only slightly thereafter (Webster and Leeming 1975).

The regulatory systems controlling intestinal physiology are not as robust. Extrinsic autonomic nerves and the enteric nervous system may suffer attrition over time. It has been estimated that 40–60% of nerves innervating the gut are lost over a lifetime (Wade 2002). Loss of cholinergic nerves may account for some of the motility changes observed in older individuals. Hormone-secreting cells in the epithelium are more fortunate in that they are replaced along with the intestinal epithelial cells and generally are well maintained as we age. The immune system plays an important role in regulating gut activities but becomes less capable in old age, so-called "immunosenescence" (Sadighi Akha 2018). This may alter the composition of the microbiome. Multiple studies suggest that the microbiome of older people has fewer bifidobacteria and more bacteroides than in younger individuals, but age is only one factor that may be responsible for alterations in the flora (O'Toole and Jeffery 2015; An et al. 2018). How much impact this has on gut function or susceptibility to pathogenic infection is uncertain.

Some gut functions tend to diminish with age, but these may be secondary to factors that accompany aging, and not just aging itself. For example, calcium absorption may decrease in older individuals, but this is probably due to lower intake, lower plasma vitamin D levels that relate to decreased sun exposure, less vitamin D intake, and impaired renal processing of this vitamin (Gallagher and Vitamin 2013; Sanders et al. 2014; ter Borg et al. 2015). Similarly, gastric acid secretion and intrinsic factor secretion may diminish with age, but much of this may relate to previous *Helicobacter pylori* infection, not necessarily aging itself (Salles 2007).

Differential Diagnosis of Diarrhea in the Elderly

Chronic diarrhea is arbitrarily defined (and differentiated from acute diarrhea) as production of loose stools for more than 4 weeks (Schiller et al. 2014). This criterion eliminates most acute infectious diarrheas that typically last less than 1 week and focuses the physician's attention on conditions that have a longer time course. For purposes of thinking about the causes of diarrhea and getting to a specific diagnosis, it is useful to characterize diarrhea into four pathophysiological categories: secretory diarrhea, osmotic diarrhea, inflammatory diarrhea, and fatty diarrhea.

Secretory Diarrhea

Secretory diarrhea is the most common mechanism of diarrhea and is due to reduced rates of absorption of fluid and electrolytes from the lumen. (Despite the name, net secretion of fluid and electrolytes is rarely present.) This can have many different causes (Table 1). Most of these disorders occur in people of all ages; some occur more often in older individuals. When assessing any patient with diarrhea, the physician must consider all of them.

Infections. Most acute diarrhea is due to transient infection with pathogenic bacteria, viruses, or protozoa. Chronic diarrhea is less likely to be due to microbes, but can be due to longer-lasting infections, particularly with protozoa, or due to recurrent infection (DuPont 2016). Published epidemiological studies disagree about the incidence of acute diarrhea in the elderly. A population survey study using random telephone calls by the Foodborne Diseases Active Surveillance Network (FoodNet) suggested that the risk of having diarrhea in the 4 weeks preceding the survey in patients 65 years of age or older was half that of the general population (0.32 episodes per person-year versus 0.72 episodes per person-year) (Imhoff et al. 2004). In another study, the risk of hospitalization for gastroenteritis was higher for older patients than for younger persons (White

Table 1 Causes of secretory diarrhea

Infections
Bacteria
Protozoa
Viruses
Iatrogenic diarrhea
Drugs
Tube feeding
Postsurgical
Radiation therapy
Stimulant laxative abuse
Ileal bile acid malabsorption
Microscopic colitis syndrome
Lymphocytic colitis
Collagenous colitis
Disordered motility/regulation
Diabetic neuropathy
Idiopathic neuropathy
Irritable bowel syndrome
Colorectal disease
Systemic diseases
Addison's disease
Hyperthyroidism
Hormone-secreting tumors (e.g., gastrinoma, VIPoma)
Autoimmune diseases/vasculitis
Idiopathic secretory diarrhea
Sporadic
Epidemic (Brainerd diarrhea)

et al. 2019). The easiest way to reconcile these studies is to conclude that the risk of contracting infection may be lower in the elderly, but once infected, the risk of being hospitalized is greater. Most of these infections are acute, but some become chronic or recurrent, possibly due to an aging immune system. The prevalence of chronic infectious diarrhea in older persons is not well-defined.

The spectrum of organisms causing infectious diarrhea probably is no different in older as compared to younger adults, although the frequency and presentations of specific infections may vary (White et al. 2019). Commonly identified organisms include *Salmonella*, *Shigella*, *Campylobacter*, *Clostridioides difficile*, *Escherichia coli*, Norovirus, Rotavirus, *Giardia*, *Cryptosporidium*, and *Entamoeba histolytica*. Immunosuppressed patients may have cytomegalovirus or herpesvirus. It is important to realize that many able older persons travel the world and so traveler's diarrhea (some of which can present as chronic diarrhea) should be considered as well. In most cases, the diagnosis and management of these infections are similar to that in younger adults.

One exception to this rule is infection with *Clostridioides difficile* (Asempa and Nicolau 2017; Donskey 2017). Epidemiological studies suggest that two-thirds of healthcare-associated *Clostridioides difficile* infections occur in patients aged 65 years or older. This may relate to frequent exposure to healthcare environments, greater use of antibiotics, altered intestinal microbiome, or immunosenescence. Moreover, older individuals seem to be more likely to have a severe clinical course and to develop recurrent *Clostridioides difficile* infection. Colonization with *Clostridioides difficile* may be ten times higher in nursing home residents than in the general population, making nursing homes fertile soil for this infection. Any institutionalized patient with diarrhea should be regarded as having *Clostridioides difficile* infection and placed in contact isolation until proven otherwise.

Diagnosis of infectious diarrhea depends on recognition of the possibility and selection of microbiological tests to make a specific diagnosis (Jump et al. 2018; Sell and Dolan 2018). Traditional testing regimens have included stool tests, such as bacterial culture for enteric pathogens, microscopy for ova and parasites, and antigen detection tests for giardiasis, cryptosporidiosis, and *Clostridioides difficile* toxin. Limitations of this approach include the time it takes to get results back, expertise needed to do the tests, and expense. This has led to the development of culture-independent testing with PCR multiplex technology (Zboromyrska and Vila 2016; Liesman and Binnicker 2016). This allows for rapid reporting of the presence of bacteria, protozoa, and viruses associated with acute diarrhea. Test results are available in as little as 4 h and permit directed antibiotic therapy when necessary and avoidance of antibiotic therapy when not needed. The main limitation of this technique is its high sensitivity. Organisms that are merely being carried by the patient may be identified but may not be responsible for the diarrheal disease. Also, multiplex tests may be positive for weeks after the clinical diarrheal disorder has resolved. Multiplex testing should only be done when stools are liquid, and results need to be interpreted with care.

The same is true for standard testing for *Clostridioides difficile* (Asempa and Nicolau 2017; Donskey 2017). Because rates of carriage are so high, particularly in hospitalized elders, the use of sensitive testing for *Clostridioides difficile* toxin will overestimate the number of people in whom the organism is responsible for diarrhea. Patients developing diarrhea while hospitalized should first be screened for laxative use, drug-associated diarrhea, and diarrhea associated with enteral feeding before sending off tests for *Clostridioides difficile*. Even then, only liquid stools should be sent for testing.

Antibiotic therapy for identified causes of infectious diarrhea is no different for older patients versus the young. Empiric antibiotic therapy used while awaiting the results of stool testing should be discouraged except in two circumstances. The first is when patients present with dysentery (fever with blood or pus in the stool) and the other is when patients have clear-cut travelers' diarrhea. In most other circumstances, antibiotics should be held pending identification of the responsible pathogen.

Clostridioides difficile demands particular attention in the old (Asempa and Nicolau 2017; Donskey 2017). Risk factors for development of *Clostridioides difficile* infection include previous use of antibiotics, particularly high-risk antibiotics such as clindamycin and fluoroquinolones. Use of proton pump inhibitors, poor functional status, prior hospitalization, and residency in a long-term care facility also contribute to the development of *Clostridioides difficile*. Development of *Clostridioides difficile* in a resident of a long-term care facility should be a stimulus to review antibiotic stewardship, isolation procedures, and disinfection protocols in the facility (Jump et al. 2018). Elders are at particular risk for severe or recurrent infection due to impaired host immunity (e.g., poor

antibody response to *Clostridioides difficile* toxin) and comorbidities.

Antibiotic therapy with oral vancomycin (125 mg QID for 10 days) is appropriate for most older individuals with *Clostridioides difficile*, especially those with more severe disease (Daniels and Kufel 2018). Metronidazole (500 mg TID) is now second-line therapy and should be limited to those with mild disease who cannot receive vancomycin. Fidaxomicin (200 mg BID) is equally effective to vancomycin in leading to resolution of acute episodes, but may be associated with fewer recurrences – a major concern in the elderly. A high acquisition cost has limited its use. Another expensive adjunctive therapy is bezlotoxumab (Deeks 2017). This monoclonal antibody to *Clostridioides difficile* toxin B is administered intravenously to patients receiving standard-of-care anti-*C. difficile* therapy; with this additive therapy, the recurrence rate in patients 65 years and older was 51% lower than that with placebo. This drug should be considered in patients who are at a high risk for recurrence and should be used with care in patients with a history of congestive heart failure since there is a risk of exacerbating that condition.

Recurrence is common in *Clostridioides difficile* infection, occurring in 10–25% of patients. Patients who have had at least three infections have a 50–60% chance of relapse. Recurrences are treated with repeat rounds of antibiotics and some physicians have recommended protocols emphasizing tapering doses over long periods of time or use of probiotics to minimize the chance of another recurrence. Evidence for these approaches is mixed. Many gastroenterologists have turned to fecal microbial transplant (FMT) as an alternative for treating recurrent *Clostridioides difficile* infection. Multiple studies have suggested that FMT can result in a durable cure rate of over 90%, but a recent meta-analysis of observational studies suggests that older patients fare less well (87.0% vs. 99.4% in those 65 years of age or older as compared to younger patients) (Li et al. 2016).

Iatrogenic diarrhea. Older individuals take many different medicines for their multiple ailments. Diarrhea is a frequent side effect of

Table 2 Medications associated with diarrhea

Acid-reducing agents (e.g., histamine H_2-receptor antagonists, proton pump inhibitors)
Antacids (e.g., those that contain magnesium)
Antiarrhythmics (e.g., quinidine)
Antibiotics (most)
Anti-inflammatory agents (e.g., NSAIDs, gold salts, 5-aminosalicylates)
Antihypertensives (e.g., beta-adrenergic receptor blocking drugs, olmesartan)
Antineoplastic agents (many)
Antiretroviral agents
Colchicine
Herbal products
Heavy metals
Metformin
Prostaglandin (e.g., misoprostol)
Theophylline
Vitamin and mineral supplements (e.g., vitamin C, magnesium)

NSAIDs nonsteroidal anti-inflammatory drugs

drugs, and drugs represent an important cause of diarrhea that needs to be recognized to avoid unnecessary diagnostic evaluations (Philip et al. 2017; Abraham and Sellin 2012). A careful review of the patient's drug list, including any over-the-counter and herbal remedies, is essential. A list of medications commonly associated with diarrhea is provided in Table 2. Usually, drug-induced diarrhea begins shortly after introduction of a new drug, but this is not always recognized in a timely way. Delayed onset due to changes in drug metabolism or drug interactions may make the temporal association of the onset of diarrhea and the initiation of drug therapy obscure.

Identification of the responsible drug and replacement with a drug less likely to cause diarrhea often will solve the problem. If the drug producing diarrhea cannot be discontinued, use of antidiarrheal drugs may mitigate diarrhea. It is important to note that many institutionalized patients are given standing orders for laxatives in case they develop constipation; in that case, the offending medications should be discontinued if the patient complains of diarrhea.

Another cause of iatrogenic diarrhea is enteral feeding (Mobarhan and DeMeo 1995; Eisenberg 2002). Tube feeding is used to support individuals

who can no longer consume enough by mouth to maintain good nutritional status. Many of these patients have neurologic problems that limit their ability to swallow. Others may have primary gastrointestinal problems, such as gastroparesis, which limit their ability to eat. When nutrients are introduced directly into the gut, normal regulatory mechanisms are bypassed and diarrhea may ensue. For example, jejunal tube feeding bypasses the duodenal feedback mechanisms that regulate gastric emptying and nutrient presentation to the absorptive surface. This creates a situation in which hypertonicity-induced increases in intraluminal volume and motility, abnormal stimulation of gastrointestinal peptide release, and bacterial overgrowth can produce diarrhea. Carbohydrate malabsorption may produce osmotic diarrhea in some patients (see below). Diarrhea can develop with other routes of enteral nutrition as well. Modification of the rate of infusion, alteration of the formula to increase fiber, and administration of antidiarrheal drugs, such as loperamide or diphenoxylate, can mitigate this problem.

Older patients are more likely to have had illnesses requiring surgery or radiation therapy than younger patients, and these therapies sometimes can cause diarrhea (Buchman 2018; Teo et al. 2015). Diarrhea can complicate gastrointestinal surgeries or radiation therapy decades after the therapy was provided. For example, diarrhea may not occur in a patient with gastrectomy until bacterial overgrowth has developed years later. A thorough past history is essential when evaluating patients with chronic diarrhea. Antidiarrheal drugs have a role in controlling postsurgical or postradiation diarrhea when more specific therapy (e.g., antibiotics or bile acid sequestrants) is not effective.

Laxative abuse. Factitious diarrhea due to stimulant laxative abuse occurs in four groups of patients: (1) those with eating disorders who use laxatives to purge, (2) those with secondary gains from feigned illness (e.g., disability payments, attention from relatives), (3) patients with Munchausen syndrome, and (4) dependent patients poisoned by a caregiver (Polle syndrome) (Roerig et al. 2010). The prevalence of laxative abuse in older individuals has not been well studied. Some older individuals may take or be given laxatives as part of their "routine" medications and may not be aware that these drugs may be causing diarrhea. This sort of situation is probably best considered as a drug side effect and not an attempt to create a factitious illness. On the other hand, deliberate ingestion or administration of laxatives to produce diarrhea represents laxative abuse and indicates psychopathology in the patient or caregiver. Chemical tests can detect laxatives in stool samples from patients suspected of having surreptitious laxative abuse. Management of these patients is difficult and often requires psychiatric consultation if laxatives are being abused by the patient or criminal investigation if being given inappropriately by caregivers.

Ileal bile acid malabsorption. Each day the liver secretes bile acids to assist with solubilizing dietary fat. When bile acids reach the ileum, they are reabsorbed and recycled back to the liver. This process is ordinarily very efficient with 90–95% of the bile acids being recycled. If ileal bile acid absorption is abnormally low, bile acids enter the colon. If the concentration of conjugated dihydroxy bile acid in the colon reaches 3–5 mM, sodium absorption by the mucosa is reduced, chloride secretion is increased, and colonic motility is stimulated, resulting in watery diarrhea. This situation can occur after ileal resection or disease, several gastrointestinal diseases, such as small bowel bacterial overgrowth, cholecystectomy, and celiac disease, and if the feedback regulation of bile acid synthesis is disordered, resulting in overproduction of bile acids by the liver (Camilleri 2015; Vijayvargiya and Camilleri 2018). This last mechanism is surprisingly common, occurring in up to one-third of patients with otherwise undiagnosed chronic secretory diarrhea.

The diagnosis of bile acid malabsorption can be made by measuring excess fecal bile acid excretion in a timed stool collection, whole-body retention of radiolabeled bile acid (SeHCAT test – not available in the USA), increased serum levels of the bile acid synthesis intermediate C4 (7α-hydroxyl-4-cholesten-3-one), or low serum levels of fibroblast growth factor 19 (FGF19). These

tests are not that good at predicting responses to therapy (in one retrospective study, only 50% of patients with abnormal SeHCAT tests responded (Damsgaard et al. 2018)), and so the diagnosis usually depends on an empiric trial of a bile acid sequestrant, such as cholestyramine, colestipol, or colesevelam.

Microscopic colitis syndrome. Although its name suggests that diarrhea in microscopic colitis syndrome should be inflammatory, the colonic mucosa does not ulcerate in this condition, and so blood and pus are not frequently found. This syndrome includes two disorders, lymphocytic colitis and collagenous colitis (Pardi 2017). Both conditions are characterized by increased intraepithelial lymphocytes and inflammatory changes in the lamina propria that are evident on histologic study. The inflammation reduces the ability of the mucosa to absorb water and salt. The distinction between lymphocytic colitis and collagenous colitis is the finding of a thickened subepithelial collagen layer in the latter condition. The cause for microscopic colitis is unknown, but it is thought to be an immunologic disorder, perhaps pathophysiologically similar to celiac disease (but not due to gluten ingestion).

Microscopic colitis syndrome is a common problem that is frequently seen in older patients (Gentile and Yen 2018). In the general population, it is as common as Crohn's disease, but the age distribution of microscopic colitis skews older, with a median age of onset of 68 years. In older individuals, microscopic colitis often is complicated by fecal incontinence; older patients presenting with watery diarrhea and fecal incontinence should have microscopic colitis excluded.

The diagnosis of microscopic colitis syndrome depends on finding a normal or near normal gross appearance of the colonic mucosa and identifying the characteristic histologic changes on mucosal biopsy specimens taken from the colon. It is recommended that multiple specimens be obtained from above the rectum to give the pathologist the best opportunity to make the diagnosis. Once a diagnosis of microscopic colitis is made, several therapies can be employed. Budesonide has the best evidence supporting its use, but recurrence is common and re-treatment is needed frequently. Mesalamine and prednisone have been recommended by some, but are frequently disappointing. Azathioprine has been recommended for refractory cases (Pardi 2017; Gentile and Yen 2018).

Disordered motility/regulation. Secretory diarrhea complicates the course of about 20% of those with type 2 diabetes. (Steatorrhea also may occur in people with diabetes but usually is due to coexisting celiac disease, pancreatic exocrine insufficiency, or small intestinal bacterial overgrowth.) Watery diabetic diarrhea usually is attributed to coexisting autonomic neuropathy (Azpiroz and Malagelada 2016), but also may be due to metformin treatment. Idiopathic neuropathy also may cause chronic diarrhea. Presumably neuropathy produces diarrhea by altering intestinal fluid and electrolyte absorption or motility. A similar mechanism may explain diarrhea after sympathectomy or vagotomy. Neuropathy is also associated with impairment of continence mechanisms and may result in fecal incontinence, magnifying the disruption due to diarrhea. Clonidine has been suggested as therapy for diabetic diarrhea. Opiate antidiarrheal drugs also have a role.

Irritable bowel syndrome. IBS is the most common diagnosis made in patients with chronic diarrhea, but it often is not the correct or final diagnosis. According to the Rome committee, IBS is a chronic disorder in which abdominal pain is associated temporally with a change in stool frequency or form (Lacy et al. 2016). By definition, painless diarrhea is not IBS. In addition, with proper testing, most patients with IBS and diarrhea can be shown to have an underlying problem (Schiller 2018). The three most likely final diagnoses in patients with IBS with diarrhea are food intolerances, bile acid malabsorption, and small intestinal bacterial overgrowth or dysbiosis. IBS typically starts in adolescence or young adulthood, and it is unusual (but not impossible) for IBS to present in the elderly. Clinicians should search for other causes of diarrhea before settling on IBS as a diagnosis in an older patient, especially if published criteria are not met.

Colorectal disease. Conditions such as diverticulitis, left-sided colon cancer or lymphoma, and villous adenoma sometimes present with watery diarrhea. This may be due to partial obstruction or local irritation. More often neoplasia will present with an inflammatory pattern (blood or pus in stools).

Systemic diseases. Endocrinopathies, such as Addison's disease or hyperthyroidism, may present with chronic diarrhea. Addison's disease is less common than diabetes and can be difficult to diagnose in the elderly because of its subtle presentation. The weight loss, fatigue, and lassitude that are common in Addison's disease may be passed off as symptoms related to "old age." The typical electrolyte changes seen in Addison's disease may be masked by concurrent use of diuretics. It is important to consider a cosyntropin stimulation test in the second tier of investigations of older patients with chronic diarrhea. The presentation of hyperthyroidism also may be atypical in older people. Adrenergic symptoms, such as tachycardia and tremor, may be absent and so it makes sense to check thyroid hormone and thyroid-stimulating hormone levels in elders with chronic diarrhea. Hormone-secreting tumors (e. g., gastrinoma, VIPoma) are unlikely causes of diarrhea at any age and should only be considered when patients present with characteristic clinical syndromes or findings of possible endocrine tumor on imaging studies (Fabian et al. 2012).

Several autoimmune diseases, especially those that produce vasculitis, may be complicated by chronic diarrhea (Geboes and Dalle 2002). This is most often secretory diarrhea unless the condition is associated with ulceration in which case diarrhea will be more inflammatory in nature.

Idiopathic secretory diarrhea. Some patients with secretory diarrhea have no diagnosis after a detailed evaluation and empiric trials of antibiotics and cholestyramine. These patients have a characteristic clinical presentation with the sudden onset of watery diarrhea (often accompanied by modest acute weight loss) that persists for months or years and then subsides gradually (Afzalpurkar et al. 1992). This has been seen in isolated individuals and in outbreaks epidemiologically associated with common sources of food or drink (so-called "Brainerd diarrhea") (Kimura et al. 2006). While this would seem to be an infectious disease, no pathogen has been identified, even when sought while the outbreaks were ongoing. Nonspecific antidiarrheal agents may be useful until the disease subsides on its own.

Osmotic Diarrhea

Osmotic diarrhea is due to ingestion of a poorly absorbed substances that result in retention of water within the intestinal lumen (Schiller et al. 2014). These poorly absorbed substances are either nutrients, such as disaccharides, ions with limited absorptive capacity, such as magnesium, or poorly absorbed polymers, such as polyethylene glycol.

Dietary carbohydrates and lactulose. The archetype for poorly absorbed nutrients is lactose. Lactose is a disaccharide that must be cleaved into its constituent monosaccharides, glucose and galactose, to be absorbed. Most young mammals have abundant lactose phlorizin hydrolase (LPH, "lactase") in the brush border of the intestine which allows complete digestion of lactose in breast milk during infancy and childhood. Most mammals repress expression of the LPH gene after weaning, and in most human populations, its activity decreases substantially by age 20, making most adults lactase deficient (Bayless et al. 2017; Storhaug et al. 2017). Mutations that developed independently in Northwestern Europe and in several locations in Africa and Asia allow some adults to maintain LPH activity and digest lactose successfully. This leads to the expectation in many individuals that they can ingest milk and dairy products throughout life. The level of lactase expression tends to decrease through adulthood, however, even in those who have the mutations favoring LPH persistence. At some point, LPH activity may decline sufficiently to produce diarrhea if too much lactose is ingested. Patients presenting with diarrhea will not suspect dairy products as the cause of their symptoms since they have not had problems tolerating lactose-containing foods before.

Investigations in the last 10 years have identified a family of poorly absorbed dietary carbohydrates that may produce symptoms, the so-called FODMAPs (fermentable oligosaccharides, disaccharides, monosaccharides, and polyols) (Vakil 2018). These occur in a variety of foods and include not only lactose, but fructose and fructans, galacto-oligosaccharides (GOS, stachyose and raffinose), and sugar alcohols (mannitol and sorbitol). Studies using dietitian-directed low FODMAPs diets suggest that irritable bowel symptoms can be substantially reduced by eliminating these chemicals from the diet (Schumann et al. 2018). As many as 40% of patients with IBS-D may benefit by reducing FODMAPs, making carbohydrate malabsorption a leading identifiable cause for this syndrome.

Lactulose, a synthetic disaccharide composed of fructose and galactose, is not able to be hydrolyzed by LPH and therefore is poorly absorbable. It is used therapeutically as a laxative and as a treatment for hepatic encephalopathy. It is readily fermented by colonic bacteria and can produce diarrhea if consumed in excess. The pathophysiology of diarrhea produced by lactulose is identical to that of other forms of carbohydrate malabsorption (Hammer et al. 1989).

In patients with carbohydrate malabsorption, symptoms are dose dependent and may be intermittent, depending on the amount of the poorly absorbed substance ingested and the residual capacity to digest the offending carbohydrate. Malabsorbed carbohydrate passes into the colon where the bacterial flora ferments it. For every 5 g of carbohydrate reaching the colon approximately, 1 L of gas and 60 mmol of short-chain fatty acids are produced by fermentation (Miller and Wolin 1979). About half of the gas is absorbed into the blood and excreted by the lungs; the remaining amount is passed as flatus or is consumed by other bacteria. Short-chain fatty acids are partially absorbed by the colonic mucosa; those remaining in the lumen along with unfermented carbohydrate have an osmotic effect and obligate water retention. This may produce watery diarrhea depending on the amount of poorly absorbed carbohydrates entering the colon.

Clues to the diagnosis of carbohydrate malabsorption as a cause of chronic diarrhea include intermittency of symptoms, variability of stool volume day-to-day (depending on the amount of poorly absorbed carbohydrates ingested), and the presence of bloating and increased flatus. Stool analysis can help confirm the diagnosis by showing an acid pH ($<$6) due to the presence of short-chain fatty acids and a large osmotic gap (Hammer et al. 1990). The osmotic gap represents unmeasured osmoles in stool water and is calculated by subtracting twice the sum of the sodium and potassium concentrations (to account for the anions accompanying these cations) from 290, the osmolality of luminal contents within the colon. Because there is no problem with absorbing electrolytes in patients with osmotic diarrhea, the concentrations of sodium and potassium will be low, and the calculated osmotic gap will be high ($>$50 mosm/kg).

Review of a diet and symptom diary can help identify carbohydrate malabsorption as a factor driving chronic diarrhea. Intake of high FODMAPs foods followed several hours later by bloating, gas, increased flatus, or loose stools is consistent with carbohydrate malabsorption. The time gap is critical since it allows time for transit of the meal through the small intestine and metabolism of carbohydrate by the colonic flora. Some physicians have advocated use of breath hydrogen testing to confirm the presence of specific carbohydrate malabsorption by giving the specific substrate in a test meal and looking for a spike in hydrogen concentration in expired air (Rezaie et al. 2017). Test protocols vary widely as to the dose of substrate, timing of breath sampling, and criteria for a positive test. The sensitivity and specificity of breath hydrogen testing for carbohydrate malabsorption is not good enough to recommend routine use of these tests before trial of a low FODMAPs or specific carbohydrate exclusion diet in patients suspected of having carbohydrate-induced diarrhea.

Treatment of osmotic diarrhea due to carbohydrate malabsorption is straightforward: the offending carbohydrate needs to be removed from the diet. Alternatively, patients with lactase insufficiency can be given exogenous lactase with meals to improve lactose hydrolysis. This approach is limited by incomplete mixing of the enzyme with substrate but may reduce the severity of symptoms when lactose ingestion cannot be avoided.

Poorly absorbed ions and polyethylene glycol. The other major cause of osmotic diarrhea is ingestion of poorly absorbed ions, such as magnesium, sulfate, or phosphate, or the poorly absorbed polymer, polyethylene glycol. Ingestion and absorption of these poorly absorbed ions is essential for health, but absorption is limited. For instance, although there is an element of active absorption of magnesium at low luminal magnesium concentrations, passive absorption is limited to 7% of the load (Fine et al. 1991). Thus, for any substantial magnesium dose, over 90% will remain in the lumen, obligating retention of anions and water to maintain electrical neutrality and osmotic equilibrium with body fluids. This accounts for magnesium's effectiveness as a laxative. Sulfate and phosphate salts also are poorly absorbed and obligate retention of water and electrolytes in the lumen. Polyethylene glycol is a large polymer (MW 3350) that is poorly absorbable and exerts an anomalous osmotic activity due to complexing with water (Schiller et al. 1988); it is used as a laxative and in colonic lavage solutions.

Patients may take magnesium purposely to induce factitious diarrhea or may take it inadvertently in the form of an antacid or calcium – magnesium supplement and produce diarrhea as a drug side effect. The diagnosis of magnesium-induced diarrhea can be made by finding a high concentration of magnesium in stool water and a high osmotic gap (Fine et al. 1991). Patients with osmotic diarrhea due to ingestion of the multivalent anions, sulfate, or phosphate retain sodium within the lumen to maintain electrical neutrality and may have a negative osmotic gap. They will have high concentrations of the offending anion in stool water. Patients who take polyethylene glycol as a laxative produce stools with a substantial osmotic gap and a high concentration of polyethylene glycol.

Identification of the cause of osmotic diarrhea can lead to measures to reduce intake of the offending agent which should mitigate diarrhea.

Inflammatory Diarrhea

Diseases that produce inflammation and ulceration of the wall of the intestine result in blood or pus in the stools, the key features of inflammatory diarrhea. Causes of inflammatory diarrhea are outlined in Table 3. The differential diagnosis of inflammatory diarrhea in older patients includes conditions that are not seen as often in younger patients, such as *Clostridioides difficile* colitis, NSAID-induced colitis, ischemic colitis, segmental colitis associated with diverticular disease, radiation colitis, diversion colitis, colon cancer, and solitary rectal ulcer syndrome.

Idiopathic inflammatory bowel disease. While ulcerative colitis and Crohn's disease are typically viewed as diseases of young and middle-aged adults, epidemiologic studies suggest that they also may present initially in older patients. These sorts of studies are complicated by the occurrence of other causes of inflammatory diarrhea in the elderly that may be mistaken for IBD, such as ischemic or infectious colitis (van Walree et al. 2015; Butter et al. 2018). However, studies suggest that the incidence and prevalence of true idiopathic inflammatory bowel disease in older patients is increasing. Some patients have had IBD for years and continue to have problems as they age, but roughly 10–15% of IBD patients are diagnosed for the first time after age 60 (van Walree et al. 2015). Ulcerative colitis seems to

be more common than Crohn's disease in this group. The presentations of ulcerative colitis and Crohn's disease in the older age group may be atypical and more subtle than in younger people. For example, older ulcerative colitis patients are less likely to have abdominal pain and rectal bleeding than younger patients. Also, isolated proctitis is less often seen in the elderly. Crohn's disease in older patients is associated more with colonic and perianal disease than with small bowel disease. Older patients with Crohn's disease are more likely to have rectal bleeding and less likely to have diarrhea, abdominal pain, or weight loss than younger patients. Crohn's disease tends to be more inflammatory in the elderly and progression to stricturing or penetrating disease seems to occur less often (Butter et al. 2018).

Chronic ulcerating infections. Infectious diseases that produce ulceration in the intestine may present with inflammatory diarrhea. These include pseudomembranous colitis due to *Clostridioides difficile*, bacterial infections such as tuberculosis and yersiniosis, protozoal diseases such as amebiasis, and ulcerating viral infections such as cytomegalovirus and *Herpes simplex*.

Diverticular disease and diverticular colitis. Up to 65% of people who are 65 years or older have diverticulosis. Most are asymptomatic, but 5–10% may develop symptoms of diverticulitis or diverticular hemorrhage in their lifetime (Young-Fadok 2018; John et al. 2016). A small percentage of patients develop abdominal pain and diarrhea and are found to have a segmental colitis in the diverticula-bearing part of the colon (SCAD, "segmental colitis associated with diverticulosis"). It is unclear whether this is a unique entity or represents an overlap between IBD and diverticular disease. Diagnosis is based on colonoscopic inspection and biopsy with histologic findings of inflammation. Treatment remains undefined; some physicians recommend antibiotics, such as metronidazole, and others use aminosalicylates, such as mesalamine, but evidence suggests little effect on the course of this condition.

Ischemia. Ischemic colitis produces bloody diarrhea and abdominal pain. It is often seen

Table 3 Causes of inflammatory diarrhea in the elderly

Inflammatory bowel disease
Crohn's disease
Ulcerative colitis
Chronic ulcerating infections
Pseudomembranous colitis
Tuberculosis, yersiniosis
Amebiasis
Cytomegalovirus, herpes simplex virus
Diverticular disease and diverticular colitis
Ischemia
Radiation colitis
Neoplasia
Colon cancer
Lymphoma

with low-flow conditions affecting the inferior mesenteric artery, drugs, and vasculitis. In older patients, constipation seems to be a frequent predisposing factor (Sherid et al. 2016). Unlike small intestinal ischemia, it has a self-limited course and is not associated with transmural necrosis and death. Diagnosis is made on the basis of the clinical syndrome and supporting colonoscopic findings. Management is focused on reversing the underlying cardiovascular problem. Most patients recover with supportive care.

Neoplasia. Colon cancer and lymphoma sometimes present with diarrhea which may contain blood or pus if mucosal ulceration is present. Large villous adenomas of the rectum produce large amounts of mucus which may be confused with diarrhea.

Any evaluation of inflammatory diarrhea must consider all of these conditions. Accordingly, most patients with inflammatory diarrhea require colonoscopy with biopsies, cross-sectional imaging, and a detailed evaluation for infection.

Fatty Diarrhea

The presence of excess fat in the stool implies a problem with fat digestion or absorption. In order to be digested, fat must be solubilized so that it can interact with digestive enzymes in the aqueous environment. Solubilization is accomplished by bile acids and therefore conditions which limit bile acid secretion, such as primary biliary cholangitis or bile duct obstruction, can produce steatorrhea. Classical small intestinal bacterial overgrowth deconjugates bile acids which also may lead to impaired fat solubilization. Pancreatic exocrine insufficiency also impedes fat digestion and can produce fatty diarrhea. Fat absorption can be limited by mucosal diseases, such as celiac disease or Whipple's disease, reduction in absorptive surface area as seen in short bowel syndrome, and impaired circulation as seen with chronic mesenteric ischemia.

Older individuals may be at more risk for several of these problems (Holt 2007; Thomson 2009). For example, it is thought that small intestinal bacterial overgrowth is more likely to occur in older people due to a greater prevalence of hypochlorhydria related to late effects of *Helicobacter pylori* infection or use of proton pump inhibitors, or due to a greater prevalence of gastrointestinal motility disorders associated with aging or diabetes. There may be some age-related pancreatic atrophy evident on cross-sectional imaging in older patients, but it is uncertain as to whether this ever becomes severe enough to produce pancreatic exocrine insufficiency (Löhr et al. 2018). Patients with chronic pancreatitis may have progressive reduction of pancreatic exocrine secretion that first may become clinically evident as steatorrhea as age advances.

Mucosal diseases. Historically, celiac disease has been viewed as a disease of childhood, but it is clear now that the diagnosis may first come to light in adults. Roughly 25% of patients with classic celiac disease are first diagnosed at age 65 or greater (Collin et al. 2018). Older individuals may present with other forms of enteropathy, such as autoimmune enteropathy or drug-related enteropathy, which need to be included in the differential diagnosis. Autoimmune enteropathy is a rare condition that presents with intractable diarrhea, villous atrophy, and absence of typical serologic markers for celiac disease (Ahmed et al. 2018). It does not respond to a gluten-free diet and treatment with immunosuppressive drugs is often needed to control symptoms. Some drugs, most prominently olmesartan, are associated with villous atrophy and steatorrhea (Philip et al. 2017; Ebrahim et al. 2017). These patients do not have serologic markers for celiac disease and do not respond to a gluten-free diet. The mechanisms causing drug-associated enteropathy are unknown. Withdrawal of the offending drug allows for reconstitution of the intestinal mucosa and resolution of steatorrhea.

The presentation of mucosal disease in the elderly is often different than that in younger patients: weight loss and diarrhea may not be as prominent, and osteopenia, hypoprothrombinemia, and neurological symptoms, such as neuropathy and mental fogginess, may be more evident (Holt 2007; Thomson 2009). All patients presenting with steatorrhea should have biopsies obtained from the small intestine and reviewed by pathologists knowledgeable in the diagnosis of enteropathy.

Whipple's disease is a rare infection with *Tropheryma whipplei* that can be associated with steatorrhea (Marth 2015). Diarrhea may not be the presenting symptom. Systemic infection may produce arthritis, neurological symptoms, and endocarditis which may produce more prominent symptoms. Elderly patients with progressive decline of mental function and evidence of steatorrhea should be screened for this condition.

Pancreatic exocrine insufficiency. The prevalence of pancreatic exocrine insufficiency as a cause of steatorrhea in the elderly is not been well defined (Löhr et al. 2018). It is clear that pancreatic exocrine insufficiency can occur, but whether it can occur independently as a result of aging or only as a consequence of chronic pancreatitis is unknown. Chronic pancreatitis presents most often in middle-aged adults, in whom it may be due to heavy alcohol abuse, autoimmune disease, genetic mutations, or anatomic problems with pancreatic duct drainage. Cigarette smoking appears to enhance the chances of developing chronic pancreatitis. When chronic pancreatitis occurs in older individuals, it may produce less pain and may progress more rapidly to both exocrine and endocrine pancreatic insufficiency (Hirth et al. 2019). Because pancreatic cancer is increasingly common in older individuals and may present with exocrine pancreatic insufficiency due to pancreatic duct obstruction, older patients presenting with steatorrhea should have cross-sectional imaging of the upper abdomen to assess pancreatic anatomy.

Bile acid deficiency. Bile acid deficiency is often overlooked as a potential cause for steatorrhea. Unlike mucosal diseases or pancreatic exocrine insufficiency which produce malabsorption of all categories of nutrients, bile acid deficiency produces fat malabsorption exclusively. Bile acid concentrations in the duodenum are critical to fat solubilization and digestion; if duodenal bile acid concentration is inadequate, fat solubilization will not occur. This occurs when adequate amounts of bile acid are not secreted by the liver as in primary biliary cholangitis or if bile acid is not released into the duodenum as with bile duct obstruction.

Bile acid deficiency may also exist if the enterohepatic circulation of bile acids is disrupted by ileal resection or disease and the liver cannot increase bile acid synthesis enough to compensate for losses.

If bile acid deficiency is recognized as the cause of steatorrhea, it can be remedied by providing supplemental exogenous conjugated bile acids (Little et al. 1992). This can be accomplished by giving ox bile (300 mg with meals) and titrating the dose up. Dose titration should be gradual, since any malabsorbed bile acid may reach the colon in sufficiently high concentrations to cause secretory diarrhea.

Small intestinal bacterial overgrowth (SIBO). Ordinarily, the small intestine maintains a relatively sparse microbiome. This is accomplished by gastric acid secretion which works to inhibit microbial proliferation, active motility which moves material rapidly through the small intestine, and by secretion of specific and nonspecific antimicrobial substances, such as secretory immunoglobulin, defensins, and cathelicidins. These mechanisms work together to keep the bacterial population in luminal fluid less than 10^5/mL. If bacterial counts increase beyond this threshold, bile acids may become deconjugated and can be absorbed from the lumen, lowering the concentration of bile acid available to solubilize fat. In addition, bacterial overgrowth may disrupt the absorption of other nutrients, such as vitamin B_{12}, and lead to the fermentation of dietary carbohydrates. The net results of these changes are symptoms of bloating, pain, diarrhea, and weight loss (Holt 2007; Quigley 2019). In addition, several extraintestinal symptoms, such as fatigue and brain fogginess, have been attributed to SIBO. It is thought (without much good evidence) that the density of SIBO determines the type of symptoms produced, with lower bacterial counts associated with IBS and higher bacterial counts associated with more classic malabsorption syndrome.

SIBO may develop as a result of structural changes in the intestine that produce stasis, such as jejunal diverticulosis or strictures, gastrocolic fistula, or upper gastrointestinal tract surgeries, including gastric bypass. SIBO can also be seen with intestinal motility disorders, such as scleroderma, and with hypochlorhydria due to chronic gastritis or prolonged proton pump inhibitor therapy. There is some evidence that SIBO may develop as a result of preceding gastroenteritis leading to development of autoantibodies to vinculin, a molecule involved with mucosal and enteric nervous system function (Pimentel et al. 2015). This has been alleged to be a mechanism for development of SIBO in postinfectious IBS.

The prevalence of SIBO and its contribution to the development of diarrhea in older individuals is not well defined. Testing for SIBO is controversial (Rezaie et al. 2016). Quantitative culture of intestinal contents has been considered to be the "gold standard" for diagnosis, with a threshold of 10^5/mL considered to be abnormal on the basis of studies in patients with steatorrhea well-established to be due to SIBO. More recent studies suggest that the upper limit of normal is much lower than this and that colony counts of 10^3–10^4 may be abnormal. Hydrogen breath testing using fermentable carbohydrate substrates, such as glucose or lactulose, is often used in the clinic to try to confirm a diagnosis of SIBO. Performance characteristics for breath tests are not that good, with sensitivities of ~80% and specificities of ~75%. This means that the tests may be inaccurate in 20–25% of patients tested, making them confirmatory tests at best. Nevertheless, when these have been used in older patients, there seems to be a higher prevalence of SIBO than in younger individuals, making the pretest probability of a diagnosis of SIBO higher in elderly patients with diarrhea. It should be a consideration in any older patient with chronic diarrhea, particularly those with steatorrhea.

When a diagnosis of SIBO seems likely due to clinical circumstances or positive testing, a trial of antibiotic therapy is in order. Many different antibiotics have been advocated over the years, and therapy is almost always empirical (i.e., not guided by sensitivity testing). Commonly used antibiotics include trimethoprim/sulfamethoxazole, tetracyclines, metronidazole, fluoroquinolones, and rifaximin. There is little reliable evidence to guide therapy since treatment trials used varying diagnostic criteria, medications, doses, and duration of therapy. If steatorrhea is present, antibiotics that are effective against the anaerobic bacteria that deconjugate bile acids (such as metronidazole) are recommended, either alone or with another antibiotic. Initially, patients should receive a short course of therapy (10–14 days) and the effectiveness should be judged at the end of the treatment period. If results are favorable, the antibiotic should be stopped until relapse occurs. Relapse is a likely outcome since the fundamental causes for SIBO are not addressed by antibiotic therapy. Long-term suppressive therapy is only indicated in patients with frequent relapses. If there is no response to therapy, trial of an alternative antibiotic should be considered.

Mesenteric vascular insufficiency. Acute loss of blood flow to the small intestine is a life-threatening medical emergency. Chronic progressive loss of blood flow leads to a syndrome of abdominal pain, reduced food intake, and weight loss, known as "intestinal angina" (Cardin et al. 2012). This may be associated with steatorrhea, but most of the weight loss is attributed to sitophobia triggered by meal-induced abdominal pain. Many of these patients have advanced peripheral vascular disease due to atherosclerosis, and almost all of them are cigarette smokers. Diagnosis of this syndrome depends on recognizing the classic history and obtaining Doppler sonography, magnetic resonance or CT angiography, or standard mesenteric angiography (Zacho and Abrahamsen 2008). Revascularization or stenting is used to treat this syndrome.

Diabetic steatorrhea. Long-standing diabetes can be associated with watery diarrhea attributed to neuropathy (see discussion above) or with fatty diarrhea. Diabetics are more likely to have celiac disease, SIBO, and pancreatic exocrine insufficiency than nondiabetic patients; studies should be done to look for these conditions in diabetics presenting with steatorrhea (Zsóri et al. 2018).

Postsurgical steatorrhea. Gastric surgery for peptic ulcer disease is sometimes complicated by steatorrhea, especially when the operation includes vagotomy or gastroenterostomy. Vagotomy has multiple adverse effects, including disruption of orderly emptying by the stomach leading to "dumping syndrome" and reduction of pancreatic exocrine secretion. Gastroenterostomy also disrupts gastric emptying and may be associated with anatomic changes that predispose to SIBO. Ulcer surgery is less frequently done nowadays, but bariatric surgery is done very frequently. While some bariatric operations are designed mainly to limit food intake, some are deliberately designed to promote malabsorption by excluding food from a large part of the absorptive surface of the small intestine (Borbély and Osterwalder 2017). This also occurs after extensive small bowel resection for other indications. In both of these situations, steatorrhea will occur as a matter of course. Sometimes the onset of steatorrhea is delayed because it depends on additional factors such as development of SIBO. Patients with postsurgical malabsorption should be evaluated for these complicating factors, since they may provide a target for therapy. Otherwise, nonspecific antidiarrheal therapy is all that can be offered.

Other Situations Presenting as "Diarrhea"

Patients sometimes report "diarrhea" when problems that may be causing the passage of loose stools cannot be described adequately. Two disorders of particular importance in older adults are fecal impaction and fecal incontinence. It is important to identify these processes, since their management is very different than the management of chronic diarrhea. Both of these situations can be identified with digital rectal examination; hence it is important to perform a digital rectal examination to look for these conditions whenever patients complain of "diarrhea."

Fecal impaction. Fecal impaction occurs in constipated patients when a mass of stool too large to be passed through the anus accumulates in the rectum (Serrano Falcón et al. 2016). Rectal distention causes relaxation of the internal anal sphincter. Leakage of liquid stools occurs when secretions that form above the obstructing bolus pass around the impaction and through the relaxed anal canal. This may be reported as diarrhea or fecal incontinence, but a careful digital rectal examination should identify the true cause of the problem. Once the impaction is removed, loose stools should subside. A bowel program to prevent recurrence (usually use of laxatives or enemas to prevent the accumulation of stool in the rectum) should be put in place.

Fecal incontinence. Another condition that can be mistaken for chronic diarrhea is fecal incontinence. Patients usually do not distinguish incontinence and diarrhea, and often describe incontinence as "bad" diarrhea. Fecal incontinence is not due to passage of voluminous stools. Instead, it indicates that there is a compromise of the nerves and muscles that preserve continence which may be age-related (Yu and Rao 2014). Digital rectal examination will find evidence of sphincter weakness or impaired sensation. Anorectal manometry can confirm the physiologic impairments that may be present. Sentient patients with some level of sensory and muscle function may be able to participate in biofeedback training to manage this problem. Others may benefit from an anticipatory bowel program emphasizing regular toileting to prevent incontinence. Patients who have both chronic diarrhea and fecal incontinence usually need to have the diarrhea controlled to have any hope of controlling incontinence.

Evaluation and Management of Chronic Diarrhea in Older Adults

The evaluation and management of chronic diarrhea in older adults is conceptually no different than in the young. Because some conditions are more common in the elderly and others are less common, the pretest probabilities of specific diagnoses are different than in younger adults, but the diagnostic framework is the same (Schiller et al. 2014; Schiller 2018).

Initial Evaluation

When diarrhea has lasted for 4 weeks or more, the physician's first duty is to obtain a comprehensive and thoughtful history. It is absolutely essential to review previous evaluations, including the primary data (test results and images) and not just reports of what was done. This should be complemented by a thorough physical examination, including a digital rectal examination to exclude fecal impaction and sphincter defects that might predispose to fecal incontinence. Sometimes the likelihood of a specific diagnosis will be so high after this initial encounter that specific diagnostic tests or an empiric therapeutic trial can be instituted to confirm the tentative diagnosis. An example of this would be someone who developed diarrhea after starting a new drug; the drug could be discontinued, and the patient observed for improvement before doing anything else. In other cases, a specific diagnosis may not

be overwhelmingly likely and so a stepwise approach to diagnosis is key.

The initial diagnostic evaluation should focus on four groups of entities: fecal impaction management or fecal incontinence, iatrogenic conditions, infection, and irritable bowel syndrome or functional diarrhea (Fig. 1). Fecal impaction and fecal incontinence can be evaluated by history and digital rectal examination. Iatrogenic conditions can be excluded by review of the patient's drug therapy (including over the counter medications), previous surgeries, or previous radiation therapy. Infections should be sought in most patients with chronic diarrhea and testing for *Clostridioides difficile* toxin should be routine if there is no compelling alternative diagnosis. Irritable bowel

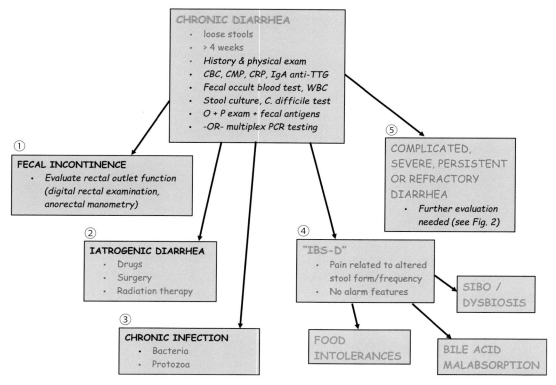

Fig. 1 Initial diagnostic considerations and approaches for patients with chronic diarrhea. Following a thorough history and physical examination, assess the likelihood of any of four possibilities: fecal incontinence or impaction, infection, iatrogenic diarrhea, and irritable bowel syndrome with diarrhea (IBS-D). Incontinence and impaction can be assessed by history and digital rectal examination. Infection should be excluded by appropriate microbiological testing. Iatrogenic diarrhea can be suggested by the patient's history of medications, surgery, or radiation therapy. IBS-D can be diagnosed by published criteria; food intolerances, bile acid malabsorption, and small intestinal bacterial overgrowth should be considered in patients with IBS-D. Patients not fitting into any of these categories with complicated, severe, persistent, or refractory diarrhea need further evaluation. (From Schiller 2019)

syndrome and functional diarrhea are best diagnosed by reviewing published criteria. If the patient does not meet criteria for these conditions, a diagnosis of IBS or functional diarrhea should not be made.

In patients who *do* meet criteria for IBS, the physician should consider three likely diagnoses that may cause IBS: (1) food intolerances, most likely related to poorly absorbed carbohydrates; (2) bile acid-induced diarrhea; and (3) small intestinal bacterial overgrowth. Surveys mainly in younger patients with IBS suggest that these diagnoses might account for the majority of IBS patients (Schiller 2018). They can be sorted out by assessing a diet and symptom diary, an empiric trial of a bile acid sequestering resin, and an empiric trial of antibiotic therapy for SIBO. In most settings, diagnostic testing for these entities is not accurate enough to define their presence, but

this is likely to change as better diagnostic tests are developed (Fig. 1).

Further Evaluation

Patients who have reached this point without a diagnosis are candidates for further diagnostic testing (Fig. 2). In most individuals, imaging of the intestine and associated organs with CT enteroscopy and colonoscopy is appropriate. When colonoscopy is done, multiple biopsies of the mucosa above the rectum should be obtained for histologic assessment, even if the mucosa appears grossly normal. Patients who are found to have steatorrhea by either qualitative Sudan staining of a fecal smear or quantitative analysis of a timed stool sample also should be candidates for upper gastrointestinal endoscopy with small

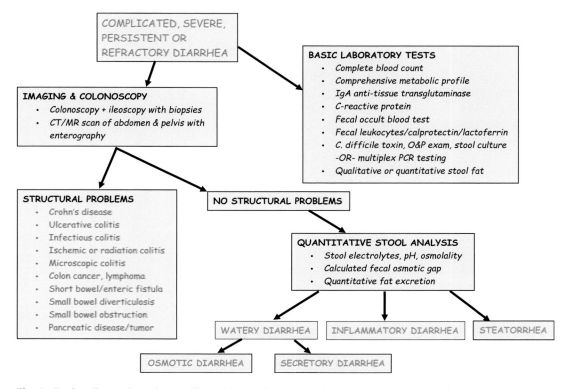

Fig. 2 Further diagnostic testing. Radiographic imaging and colonoscopy/endoscopy with biopsies reasonably can be used next to look for structural problems that might be causing diarrhea. If no diagnosis is forthcoming, stool analysis can help to categorize diarrhea as watery (with subtypes of secretory and osmotic), inflammatory or fatty. This information can help direct the next steps toward diagnosis (From Schiller 2019)

Table 4 Components of a complete stool analysis

Stool weight
Stool fat content
Stool electrolytes
Na, K
Cl, HCO$_3$
Stool pH
Stool lactoferrin (or calprotectin)
Reducing substances
Stool osmolality
Laxative screening
Mg, P
PEG
Senna
Bisacodyl

bowel biopsy to exclude mucosal disease as the cause of fat malabsorption.

If the diagnosis is still in doubt, patients should have a complete stool analysis done on either a spot or a timed stool collection (Fig. 2). In most patients, a 48-h timed collection is sufficient, if diarrhea is present. A timed stool collection allows calculation of quantitative fat excretion which can be of use as a baseline for follow-up in most patients. Analysis of a spot collection may yield valuable data, if a timed collection is not possible. For example, the finding of white blood cells in stool by microscopy or by abnormal concentrations of the neutrophil markers, lactoferrin, or calprotectin can point the way to diagnosis of an inflammatory process. The components of a complete stool analysis are listed in Table 4. A retrospective study concluded that the results of a complete stool analysis could be used to categorize diarrhea as shown in Table 5 and provide diagnostic clues that could allow for a more directed evaluation (Steffer et al. 2012). The key outcome from stool analysis is the ability to categorize the diarrhea as watery (with subtypes of secretory and osmotic diarrhea), inflammatory, or fatty. This serves to limit the differential diagnosis that needs to be explored and the tests that need to be ordered (Fig. 3).

Therapy

Supportive care trials with hydration and electrolyte replacement are critically important in elderly

Table 5 Patterns of stool composition in chronic diarrhea

Category/findings	Implications
Stool weight <200 g/24 h	
No objective evidence of diarrhea	Change in stool frequency, intermittent diarrhea, fecal incontinence, treatment with antidiarrheal drugs during collection
Hyperdefecation (increased frequency without excess volume)	Possible IBS, proctitis, abnormal rectal reservoir function
Abnormal consistency (unformed – runny stools)	Possible IBS
Elevated fecal osmotic gap	Presumed mild carbohydrate malabsorption or excess Mg intake from supplements
Steatorrhea	Malabsorption or maldigestion
Stool weight >200 g/24 h	
Secretory diarrhea without steatorrhea	Microscopic colitis or other cause of secretory diarrhea
	Carbohydrate malabsorption without steatorrhea
High fecal osmotic gap	Ingestion of poorly absorbed carbohydrates, malabsorption
Steatorrhea with or without carbohydrate malabsorption	Small bowel mucosal disease, small intestinal bacterial overgrowth, pancreatic exocrine insufficiency, bile acid deficiency
Osmotic diarrhea	Ingestion of poorly absorbed ions (e.g., magnesium, phosphate, sulfate) or osmotically active polymers (e.g., polyethylene glycol)
Unclassified	Blood or pus suggests inflammatory causes of diarrhea

patients with diarrhea. Older patients are much more likely to have physiologic compromise and the rate of rehydration needs to be customized to their cardiovascular and renal status. If hydration is too rapid, preexisting heart failure may be exacerbated. If hydration is too slow, azotemia may persist. Serum creatinine, electrolytes, hematocrit, and urine output should be followed closely

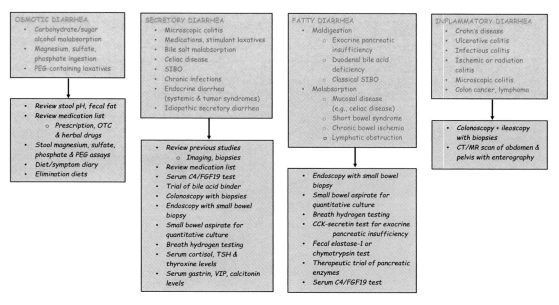

Fig. 3 Classification by stool characteristics limits differential diagnosis and directs further diagnostic testing. In most cases, this allows establishment of a likely diagnosis and initiation of therapy (Modified, from Schiller 2019)

during rehydration in frail patients. Nutritional status may be compromised by diarrhea: many older patients reduce or stop eating when they are ill. Diseases causing diarrhea may limit the tolerance of patients for feeding and consultation with a dietitian should be routine in patients hospitalized with chronic diarrhea.

If a specific diagnosis can be reached, therapy for that condition can be instituted. In most situations, a response should be seen within 1–2 weeks.

Therapeutic trials. When therapeutic trials are part of the diagnostic strategy (e.g., antibiotic therapy for SIBO or pancreatic enzyme replacement therapy for exocrine pancreatic insufficiency), a sufficient dose of medicine should be given to produce an effect and treatment should be assessed by both symptom response and quantitative testing after the medication has had a chance to work, if possible. For example, a patient with steatorrhea receiving a clinical trial of pancreatic enzyme replacement therapy should receive a large dose of enzymes with each meal and have symptoms assessed and fecal fat excretion measured before and after a few days of treatment to document its effectiveness.

Nonspecific antidiarrheal drug therapy. While waiting for diagnostic testing to be completed or when no specific treatment is available for the patient's diagnosis, nonspecific antidiarrheal drug therapy may be considered (Table 6). The most effective drugs for this purpose are μ-opioid agonists (Schiller 2017). Loperamide works well enough in most patients with chronic diarrhea, but the dose is limited to 4 mg four times a day, because it is not more effective above this dose. Potent opioid drugs with a higher ceiling effect, such as morphine or deodorized tincture of opium, sometimes need to be used. These potent agents may be less well tolerated in older patients due to sedation, and so initial doses should be low and titrated up more slowly than in younger patients. Unlike the brain, the gut does not manifest tolerance to opiates, and so once an effective dose is reached, it should not need to be increased. Patients should be warned that their use of opioids will be monitored and that use of more than the prescribed dose will result in the drug being stopped. In my experience, use of potent opiates in very low doses is generally well tolerated and does not lead to serious drug abuse in these patients.

Table 6 Therapies for chronic diarrhea

Drug class	Agent	Typical doses
Opiates (μ-opiate receptor selective)		
	Diphenoxylate	2.5–5 mg four times a day
	Loperamide	2–4 mg four times a day
	Codeine	15–60 mg four times a day
	Opium tincture	2–20 drops four times a day
	Morphine	2–20 mg four times a day
Adrenergic agonists		
	Clonidine	0.1–0.3 mg three times a day
Somatostatin analogue		
	Octreotide	50–250 μg three times a day (subcutaneously)
Bile acid-binding resins		
	Cholestyramine	4 g daily up to four times a day
	Colestipol	4 g daily up to four times a day
	Colesevelam	1875 mg up to twice a day
Fiber supplements		
	Calcium polycarbophil	5–10 g daily
	Psyllium	10–20 g daily

In addition to opiates, several other drugs have nonspecific antidiarrheal effects that may help to mitigate diarrhea (Table 6).

Key Points

- Chronic diarrhea – loose stools for more than 4 weeks – is a common problem in older patients.
- It has an extensive differential diagnosis that is similar to that in younger individuals, but individual diagnoses may have different likelihoods in older individuals.
- Conditions that seem to be more likely in older patients with chronic diarrhea include *Clostridioides difficile*, iatrogenic diarrhea, small intestinal bacterial overgrowth, ischemia, microscopic colitis, and systematic diseases, such as diabetes mellitus.
- Conditions that may be less likely in older patients include new-onset idiopathic inflammatory bowel disease and irritable bowel syndrome.
- Initial evaluation of older individuals with chronic diarrhea includes a thoughtful history and physical examination, and a detailed review of available medical records.
- Initial laboratory testing should include a complete blood count, comprehensive metabolic profile to assess electrolyte status and renal function, serum C-reactive protein to look for inflammation, and analysis of stool for blood, pus, and infectious agents.
- Imaging of the colon and small intestine by enterography, and colonoscopy and endoscopy with biopsies can evaluate possible structural causes of diarrhea.
- If no diagnosis is apparent, detailed chemical analysis of stool for electrolytes (sodium and potassium with calculation of fecal osmotic gap), qualitative or quantitative fat content, and white blood cell markers (lactoferrin or calprotectin) can be used to categorize diarrhea as secretory, osmotic, inflammatory, or fatty. This can help direct further testing.
- Initial therapy consists of rehydration with electrolyte repletion and symptomatic management with nonspecific antidiarrheal drugs. If a specific diagnosis can be made, specific therapy often can be employed.

References

Abraham BP, Sellin JH. Drug-induced, factitious, & idiopathic diarrhoea. Best Pract Res Clin Gastroenterol. 2012;26(5):633–48.

Afzalpurkar RG, Schiller LR, Little KH, et al. The self-limited nature of chronic idiopathic diarrhea. N Engl J Med. 1992;327(26):1849–52.

Ahmed Z, Imdad A, Connelly JA, Acra S. Autoimmune enteropathy: an updated review with special focus on stem cell transplant therapy. Dig Dis Sci. 2018; https://doi.org/10.1007/s10620-018-5364-1.

An R, Wilms E, Masclee AAM, et al. Age-dependent changes in GI physiology and microbiota: time to reconsider? Gut. 2018;67:2213–22.

Asempa TE, Nicolau DP. *Clostridium difficile* infection in the elderly: an update on management. Clin Interv Aging. 2017;12:1799–809.

Azpiroz F, Malagelada C. Diabetic neuropathy in the gut: pathogenesis and diagnosis. Diabetologia. 2016;59 (3):404–8.

Bayless TM, Brown E, Paige DM. Lactase non-persistence and lactose intolerance. Curr Gastroenterol Rep. 2017; 19(5):23. https://doi.org/10.1007/s11894-017-0558-9.

Borbély YM, Osterwalder A, Kröll D, et al. Diarrhea after bariatric procedures: diagnosis and therapy. World J Gastroenterol. 2017;23(26):4689–700.

Buchman AL. Intestinal failure and rehabilitation. Gastroenterol Clin N Am. 2018;47(2):327–40.

Butter M, Weiler S, Biedermann L, et al. Clinical manifestations, pathophysiology, treatment and outcome of inflammatory bowel diseases in older people. Maturitas. 2018;110:71–8.

Camilleri M. Bile acid diarrhea: prevalence, pathogenesis, and therapy. Gut Liver. 2015;9(3):332–9.

Cardin F, Fratta S, Inelmen EM, et al. Diagnosis of chronic mesenteric ischemia in older patients: a structured review. Aging Clin Exp Res. 2012;24(6):635–9.

Collin P, Vilppula A, Luostarinen L, et al. Review article: coeliac disease in later life must not be missed. Aliment Pharmacol Ther. 2018;47:563–72.

Damsgaard B, Dalby HR, Krogh K, et al. Long-term effect of medical treatment of diarrhoea in 377 patients with SeHCAT scan diagnosed bile acid malabsorption from 2003 to 2016: a retrospective study. Aliment Pharmacol Ther. 2018;47:951–7.

Daniels LM, Kufel WD. Clinical review of *Clostridium difficile* infection: an update on treatment and prevention. Expert Opin Pharmacother. 2018;19(16): 1759–69.

Deeks ED. Bezlotoxumab: a review in preventing *Clostridium difficile* infection recurrence. Drugs. 2017;77(15):1657–63.

Donskey CJ. *Clostridium difficile* in older adults. Infect Dis Clin N Am. 2017;31(4):743–56.

DuPont HL. Persistent diarrhea: a clinical review. JAMA. 2016;315(24):2712–23.

Ebrahim VS, Martin J, Murthy S, et al. Olmesartan-associated enteropathy. Proc (Bayl Univ Med Cent). 2017;30(3):348–50.

Eisenberg P. An overview of diarrhea in the patient receiving enteral nutrition. Gastroenterol Nurs. 2002;25(3):95–104.

Fabian E, Kump P, Krejs GJ. Diarrhea caused by circulating agents. Gastroenterol Clin N Am. 2012;41(3): 603–10.

Fine KD, Santa Ana CA, Fordtran JS. Diagnosis of magnesium-induced diarrhea. N Engl J Med. 1991;324 (15):1012–7.

Gallagher JC, Vitamin D. aging. Endocrinol Metab Clin N Am. 2013;42(2):319–32.

Geboes K, Dalle I. Vasculitis and the gastrointestinal tract. Acta Gastroenterol Belg. 2002;65(4):204–12.

Gentile N, Yen EF. Prevalence, pathogenesis, diagnosis, and management of microscopic colitis. Gut Liver. 2018;12(3):227–35.

Hall AJ, Wikswo ME, Karunya Manikonda K, et al. Acute gastroenteritis surveillance through the National Outbreak Reporting System. US Emerg Infect Dis. 2013;19(8):1305–9.

Hammer HF, Santa Ana CA, Schiller LR, Fordtran JS. Studies of osmotic diarrhea induced in normal subjects by ingestion of polyethylene glycol and lactulose. J Clin Invest. 1989;84(4):1056–62.

Hammer HF, Fine KD, Santa Ana CA, et al. Carbohydrate malabsorption. Its measurement and its contribution to diarrhea. J Clin Invest. 1990;86(6):1936–44.

Hirth M, Härtel N, Weiss C, et al. Clinical course of chronic pancreatitis in elderly patients. Digestion. 2019;10:1–8. https://doi.org/10.1159/000494349.

Holt PR. Intestinal malabsorption in the elderly. Dig Dis. 2007;25(2):144–50.

Imhoff B, Morse D, Shiferaw B, et al. Burden of self-reported acute diarrheal illness in FoodNet surveillance areas, 1998–1999. Clin Infect Dis. 2004;38(Suppl 3): S219–26.

John ES, Katz K, Saxena M, et al. Management of inflammatory bowel disease in the elderly. Curr Treat Options Gastroenterol. 2016;14(3):285–304.

Jump RLP, Crnich CJ, Mody L, et al. Infectious diseases in older adults of long-term care facilities: update on approach to diagnosis and management. J Am Geriatr Soc. 2018;66(4):789–803.

Kimura AC, Mead P, Walsh B, et al. A large outbreak of Brainerd diarrhea associated with a restaurant in the Red River Valley. Texas Clin Infect Dis. 2006;43(1): 55–61.

Lacy BE, Mearin F, Chang L, et al. Bowel disorders. Gastroenterology. 2016;150:1393–407.

Li Y-T, Cai H-F, Wang Z-H, et al. Systematic review with meta-analysis: long-term outcomes of faecal microbiota transplantation for *Clostridium difficile* infection. Aliment Pharmacol Ther. 2016;43:445–57.

Liesman RM, Binnicker MJ. The role of multiplex molecular panels for the diagnosis of gastrointestinal infections in immunocompromised patients. Curr Opin Infect Dis. 2016;29(4):359–65.

Little KH, Schiller LR, Bilhartz LE, Fordtran JS. Treatment of severe steatorrhea with ox bile in an ileectomy patient with residual colon. Dig Dis Sci. 1992;37(6): 929–33.

Löhr JM, Panic N, Vujasinovic M, Verbeke CS. The ageing pancreas: a systematic review of the evidence and analysis of the consequences. J Intern Med. 2018;283(5): 446–60.

Marth T. *Tropheryma whipplei*, immunosuppression and Whipple's disease: from a low-pathogenic, environmental infectious organism to a rare, multifaceted inflammatory complex. Dig Dis. 2015;33(2): 190–9.

Miller TL, Wolin MJ. Fermentations by saccharolytic intestinal bacteria. Am J Clin Nutr. 1979;32(1):164–72.

Mobarhan S, DeMeo M. Diarrhea induced by enteral feeding. Nutr Rev. 1995;53(3):67–70.

O'Toole PW, Jeffery IB. Gut microbiota and aging. Science. 2015;350(6265):1214–5.

Pardi DS. Diagnosis and management of microscopic colitis. Am J Gastroenterol. 2017;112(1):78–85.

Philip NA, Ahmed N, Pitchumoni CS. Spectrum of drug-induced chronic diarrhea. J Clin Gastroenterol. 2017;51(2):111–7.

Pimentel M, Morales W, Rezaie A, et al. Development and validation of a biomarker for diarrhea-predominant irritable bowel syndrome in human subjects. PLoS One. 2015;10(5):e0126438. https://doi.org/10.1371/journal.pone.0126438.

Quigley EMM. The spectrum of small intestinal bacterial overgrowth (SIBO). Curr Gastroenterol Rep. 2019;21(1):3. https://doi.org/10.1007/s11894-019-0671-z.69.

Rezaie A, Pimentel M, Rao SS. How to test and treat small intestinal bacterial overgrowth: an evidence-based approach. Curr Gastroenterol Rep. 2016;18(2):8. https://doi.org/10.1007/s11894-015-0482-9.

Rezaie A, Buresi M, Lembo A, et al. Hydrogen and methane-based breath testing in gastrointestinal disorders: the north American consensus. Am J Gastroenterol. 2017;112(5):775–84.

Roerig JL, Steffen KJ, Mitchell JE, Zunker C. Laxative abuse: epidemiology, diagnosis and management. Drugs. 2010;70(12):1487–503.

Sadighi Akha AA. Aging and the immune system: an overview. J Immunol Methods. 2018;463:21–6.

Salles N. Basic mechanisms of the aging gastrointestinal tract. Dig Dis. 2007;25:112–7.

Sanders KM, Scott D, Ebeling PR. Vitamin D deficiency and its role in muscle-bone interactions in the elderly. Curr Osteoporos Rep. 2014;12(1):74–81.

Schiller LR. Antidiarrheal drug therapy. Curr Gastroenterol Rep. 2017;19(5):18. https://doi.org/10.1007/s11894-017-0557-x.

Schiller LR. Evaluation of chronic diarrhea and irritable bowel syndrome with diarrhea in adults in the era of precision medicine. Am J Gastroenterol. 2018;113(5):660–9.

Schiller LR. Diarrhea and constipation. In: Berg CL, Teitelman MG, Marino DE, (eds.) Digestive Diseases Self-Education Program 9, Chap. 9. American Gastroenterological Association, Bethesda (MD). 2019: 275–305.

Schiller LR, Emmett M, Santa Ana CA, Fordtran JS. Osmotic effects of polyethylene glycol. Gastroenterology. 1988;94(4):933–41.

Schiller LR, Pardi DS, Spiller R, et al. Gastro 2013 APDW/WCOG Shanghai working party report: diarrhea: definition, classification, diagnosis. J Gastroenterol Hepatol. 2014;29:6–25.

Schumann D, Klose P, Lauche R, et al. Low fermentable, oligo-, di-, mono-saccharides and polyol diet in the treatment of irritable bowel syndrome: a systematic review and meta-analysis. Nutrition. 2018;45:24–31.

Sell J, Dolan B. Common gastrointestinal infections. Prim Care. 2018;45(3):519–32.

Serrano Falcón B, Barceló López M, Mateos Muñoz B, et al. Fecal impaction: a systematic review of its medical complications. BMC Geriatr. 2016;16:4. https://doi.org/10.1186/s12877-015-0162-5.

Sherid M, Samo S, Sulaiman S, et al. Comparison of ischemic colitis in the young and the elderly. WMJ. 2016;115(4):196–202.

Singh P, Mitsuhashi S, Ballou S, et al. Demographic and dietary associations of chronic diarrhea in a representative sample of adults in the United States. Am J Gastroenterol. 2018;113(4):593–600.

Steffer KJ, Santa Ana CA, Cole JA, Fordtran JS. The practical value of comprehensive stool analysis in detecting the cause of idiopathic chronic diarrhea. Gastroenterol Clin N Am. 2012;41(3):539–60.

Storhaug CL, Fosse SK, Fadnes LT. Country, regional, and global estimates for lactose malabsorption in adults: a systematic review and meta-analysis. Lancet Gastroenterol Hepatol. 2017;2(10):738–46.

Teo MTW, Sebag-Montefiore D, Donnellan CF. Prevention and management of radiation-induced late gastrointestinal toxicity. Clin Oncol. 2015;27:656–67.

ter Borg S, Verlaan S, Hemsworth J, et al. Micronutrient intakes and potential inadequacies of community-dwelling older adults: a systematic review. Br J Nutr. 2015;113(8):1195–206.

Thomson AB. Small intestinal disorders in the elderly. Best Pract Res Clin Gastroenterol. 2009;23(6):861–74.

Vakil N. Dietary fermentable oligosaccharides, disaccharides, monosaccharides, and polyols (FODMAPs) and gastrointestinal disease. Nutr Clin Pract. 2018;33(4):468–75.

van Walree IC, van Tuyl SA, Hamaker ME. Late-onset inflammatory bowel disease in the very elderly. Neth J Med. 2015;73(1):4–9.

Vijayvargiya P, Camilleri M. Update on bile acid malabsorption: finally ready for prime time? Curr Gastroenterol Rep. 2018;20(3):10. https://doi.org/10.1007/s11894-018-0615-z.

Wade PR. Aging and neural control of the GI tract. I. Age-related changes in the enteric nervous system. Am J Physiol Gastrointest Liver Physiol. 2002;283: G489–95.

Webster SG, Leeming JT. Assessment of small bowel function in the elderly using a modified xylose tolerance test. Gut. 1975;16:109–13.

White AE, Ciampa N, Chen Y, et al. Characteristics of campylobacter, Salmonella infections and acute gastroenteritis in older adults in Australia, Canada, and the United States. Clin Infect Dis. 2019; https://doi.org/10.1093/cid/ciy1142.

Young-Fadok TM. Diverticulitis. N Engl J Med. 2018;379(17):1635–42.

Yu SW, Rao SS. Anorectal physiology and pathophysiology in the elderly. Clin Geriatr Med. 2014;30(1):95–106.

Zacho HD, Abrahamsen J. Chronic intestinal ischaemia: diagnosis. Clin Physiol Funct Imaging. 2008;28(2): 71–5.

Zboromyrska Y, Vila J. Advanced PCR-based molecular diagnosis of gastrointestinal infections: challenges and opportunities. Expert Rev Mol Diagn. 2016;16(6): 631–40.

Zsóri G, Illés D, Terzin V, et al. Exocrine pancreatic insufficiency in type 1 and type 2 diabetes mellitus: do we need to treat it? A systematic review. Pancreatology. 2018. pii: S1424-3903(18)30111-X; https://doi.org/10. 1016/j.pan.2018.05.006.

Upper Gastrointestinal Bleeding

55

Nicholas J. Costable and David A. Greenwald

Contents

Abstract

Upper gastrointestinal bleeding is a common reason for hospital admission in older adult patients and carries a high morbidity and mortality if not properly managed. Risk factors for developing upper GI bleeding include advanced age, H pylori infection, medication use (NSAIDs, Aspirin, $P2Y_{12}$ inhibitors, anticoagulants, and steroids), smoking, and history of liver disease. Providers caring for older adults should try to minimize all modifiable risk factors for upper GI bleeding including reducing use of aspirin and NSAIDs (whenever possible) as well as coprescribing PPIs in patients who will be initiated on long-term NSAID therapy. The most common etiology of upper GI bleeding is peptic ulcer disease, followed by erosive gastroesophagitis, gastroesophageal varices, Mallory-Weiss tears, Dieulafoy's lesions, gastric antral vascular ectasia (GAVE), portal hypertensive gastropathy (PHG), aortoenteric fistula, malignancy, and other rare conditions.

N. J. Costable
Department of Internal Medicine, Icahn School of Medicine at Mount Sinai, New York, NY, USA
e-mail: Nicholas.costable@mountsinai.org

D. A. Greenwald (✉)
Department of Internal Medicine, Division of Gastroenterology, Icahn School of Medicine at Mount Sinai, New York, NY, USA
e-mail: David.greenwald@mountsinai.org

© Springer Nature Switzerland AG 2021
C. S. Pitchumoni, T. S. Dharmarajan (eds.), *Geriatric Gastroenterology*,
https://doi.org/10.1007/978-3-030-30192-7_47

Early recognition and management of upper GI bleeding in adult patients is imperative and can potentially be lifesaving. A detailed history regarding prior history of upper GI bleeding, peptic ulcer disease, NSAIDs or anticoagulant use, and liver disease is vital. Common symptoms of upper GI bleeding include melena, hematemesis, nausea, and abdominal pain. Management begins with assessment of airway protection (and intubation if indicated), placement of two large bore IVs, administration of isotonic crystalloid solution and/or blood products, and administration of IV PPI. Patients with known or suspected liver disease and suspected variceal bleeding should also receive IV antibiotics and IV somatostatin analogs. Risk stratification scores should be used to determine patients at highest risk for further decompensation. Upper endoscopy is both a diagnostic and therapeutic tool used in the management of upper GI bleeding. Endoscopy should be performed within 24 h of presentation after appropriate resuscitation. Management of anticoagulation in upper GI bleeding largely depends on the indication for anticoagulation, the risk of continued bleeding with continuing the medication, and the risk of thrombosis with discontinuing the medication. A multidisciplinary approach to the decision of anticoagulation continuation is preferred when possible.

Keywords

Gastrointestinal bleeding · Ligament of Treitz · Hematemesis · Melena · Hematochezia · NSAIDs · Aspirin · Warfarin · Direct-acting oral anticoagulants (DOACs) · Peptic ulcer disease · *H. pylori* · Esophageal varices · Erosive esophagitis · AV malformations · Mallory-Weiss Tear · Dieulafoy's lesion · Gastric antral vascular ectasia (GAVE) · Portal hypertensive gastropathy (PHG) · Aortoenteric fistula · PPI · Urease breath testing · Esophagogastroduodenoscopy (EGD) · Endoscopic management · Glasgow-Blatchford score

Introduction

Upper gastrointestinal tract hemorrhage is defined as gastrointestinal bleeding that arises proximal to the Ligament of Treitz, the anatomical division between the duodenum and jejunum. The annual incidence of hospitalization for acute upper GI bleeding is approximately 100 per 100,000 individuals (Longstreth 1995), and the incidence of upper GI bleeding is about six-fold higher compared to lower GI bleeding. Approximately 70% of cases of upper GI bleeding occur in patients over the age of 60 (Van Leerdam et al. 2003), and the incidence, morbidity, and mortality all increase with age, making it an important disease to understand in this patient demographic (Rockall et al. 1995).

Risk Factors for Upper GI Bleeding

Age, smoking, alcohol intake, history of peptic ulcer disease, portal hypertension, and certain medications have all been associated with a greater risk of upper GI hemorrhage. Several studies have shown age to be an independent risk factor for upper GI hemorrhage (Kaplan et al. 2001). This is likely due in concert to physiologic alterations of the aging gastrointestinal tract, as well as the development of other medical comorbidities that predispose one to GI bleeding.

The parietal cells of the stomach produce about two liters of hydrochloric acid per day, creating an intragastric pH of around 1–2 (Leung 2014). This acidic environment is imperative for digestion, as well as providing an antimicrobial barrier from the outside world. The epithelial lining of the stomach would not be able to tolerate the high acidity of the stomach were it not for the production of a bicarbonate rich mucosal layer that serves as a protective barrier. These protective and destructive factors normally exist in equilibrium and prevent mucosal destruction while permitting the initial stages of digestion. In elderly patients, this equilibrium tends to be disrupted primarily by decreased gastric mucus production due to the use of nonspecific cyclooxygenase (COX) inhibitors such as aspirin and other nonsteroidal anti-inflammatory medications (NSAIDs). Cyclo-oxygenases are enzymes involved in the production of prostaglandins, a group of lipid compounds that are involved in both inflammatory response (primarily via COX-2) and vasodilation to promote blood flow to splanchnic organs (primarily via COX-1). Medications that inhibit the synthesis of these prostaglandins lead to decreased submucosal blood flow and mucous production, thus disrupting the delicate acid-mucous equilibrium, and leaving the mucosa prone to injury.

Aspirin is one of the most prescribed medications among elderly adults. Its main utility is for secondary prophylaxis of coronary artery disease, peripheral vascular disease, and nonembolic stroke. However, it is estimated that approximately 25% of all adults in the United States over the age of 40 without known cardiovascular disease, around 29 million people, take a daily aspirin without the recommendation of a physician (O'Brien et al. 2019). Recent data have shown that aspirin as primary prophylaxis in low-risk patients without known cardiovascular disease may be more harmful than beneficial. A multicenter, double-blinded, placebo controlled trial of nearly 20,000 patients investigated the effect of low-dose aspirin for primary cardiovascular disease prophylaxis in adults age 70 or older. At five years, the trial found that use of aspirin did not significantly improve rates of disability-free survival, but patients taking aspirin had a 38% increased risk of major hemorrhage compared to placebo (McNeil et al. 2018). Additionally, a large multicenter trial showed that in patients with moderate cardiovascular disease risk with no prior history of coronary artery disease, aspirin was not shown to decrease the rate of cardiovascular ischemic events, but was associated with a higher rate of gastrointestinal bleeding (Gaziano et al. 2018).

Similar to aspirin, NSAIDs are also a class of COX inhibitors that are among the most prescribed medications in the United States. They are frequently prescribed as analgesics and anti-inflammatory agents for conditions commonly associated with older age, such as osteoarthritis, making them an important risk factor for upper GI

bleeding in these patients. An estimated 1.2% of the population reports taking an NSAID at least once daily, and about 7.3% of patients over the age of 60 report filling at least one NSAID prescription within the past year (Wongrakpanich et al. 2018). Approximately 2–4% of chronic NSAID users will experience at least one major GI complication related to their NSAID use, including development of peptic ulcer disease (Straus and Ofman 2001). In the late 1990s, specific COX-2 inhibitors were introduced as potential GI sparing anti-inflammatory agents owing to the lack of COX-1 inhibition. Use of these agents, however, has been shown to be associated with increased risk of myocardial infarction as compared to nonselective COX inhibitors in patients with preexisting cardiovascular disease (Bombardier et al. 2000), and therefore their use warrants careful consideration in this patient population.

Patients who will be prescribed long-term NSAIDs should be evaluated for other risk factors for the development of peptic ulcer disease such as the presence of *Helicobacter pylori* to minimize risk of GI bleeding. A 2005 meta-analysis looking at *H. pylori* eradication prior to starting chronic NSAID therapy showed a 57% risk reduction in the development of peptic ulcer disease (Leontiadis et al. 2005a). The effect on patients who are already on NSAID therapy is less well-defined. Guidelines suggest patients, at high risk for peptic ulcer disease who will be initiated on chronic NSAID therapy (age > 64, corticosteroid use, antiplatelet agent use, and previous history of peptic ulcer disease), should be coprescribed prophylactic agents to prevent NSAID-induced GI toxicity (Bhatt et al. 2008). Randomized trials have demonstrated that coadministration of either a proton pump inhibitor (PPIs) (Cullen et al. 1998) or misoprostol (Raskin et al. 1995) (a prostaglandin E analog) reduces rates of symptomatic peptic ulcer development. Histamine-2 receptor blockers (H2 antagonists) use has not been demonstrated to be beneficial in the prevention of peptic ulcer disease in these patients; however, their use can be considered in patients who are intolerant or have contraindications to PPIs or misoprostol (Hooper et al. 2004).

P2Y$_{12}$ inhibitors, such as clopidogrel, prasugrel, and ticagrelor, directly inhibit platelet aggregation and thus pose an increased risk of GI bleeding. Inhibition of the P2Y$_{12}$ ADP receptor expressed on the surface of platelets leads to impaired clot formation. P2Y$_{12}$ inhibitors are commonly prescribed for conditions that increase in prevalence with advancing age, such as secondary stroke prevention, acute coronary syndrome, and peripheral vascular disease. While the increased risk for GI bleeding is a class effect of these medications, it should be noted that the rates of bleeding differ between the agents (Guo et al. 2019). A meta-analysis of over 60,000 patients showed that prasugrel, one of the third generation P2Y$_{12}$ inhibitors, had a significantly higher rate of GI bleeding compared to clopidogrel (Hooper et al. 2004).

Warfarin is a commonly used anticoagulant that inhibits the vitamin K-dependent synthesis of factors II, VII, IX, and X as well as protein C and S. It is primarily used for embolic stroke prevention in patients with atrial fibrillation, a condition affecting approximately 9% of patients over age 65, venous thromboembolism (VTE) prophylaxis, and anticoagulation after heart valve replacement (January et al. 2014). It is well established that warfarin use is associated with an increased risk of GI hemorrhage (Chen et al. 2014). Recently, warfarin use has declined due to the development of newer anticoagulants that do not require coagulation monitoring and have much less drug-drug interaction.

Direct acting oral anticoagulants (DOACs) are a class of relatively new anticoagulants that include dabigatran, rivaroxaban, apixaban, and edoxaban. These agents exert their effect by inhibiting different stages of the coagulation cascade. Like warfarin, they are primarily used in the prevention of stroke in atrial fibrillation and VTE prophylaxis, but unlike warfarin they are not approved for anticoagulation after heart valve replacement. The landmark trials investigating the efficacy of these agents showed that the rates of GI bleeding were comparable to rates seen with warfarin (Connolly et al. 2009; Granger et al. 2011; Patel et al. 2011). However, dabigatran was shown to have a 50% relative risk increase

in the rates of GI bleeding as compared to warfarin (Connolly et al. 2009). A large population-based study investigating the risk of GI bleeding among patients using these agents found that apixaban had the most favorable GI safety profile while Rivaroxaban had the most unfavorable profile (Abraham et al. 2017). The study also demonstrated that regardless of agents, the rates of GI bleeding in patients of age 75 or older were significantly increased (Abraham et al. 2017).

Presentation

Upper gastrointestinal bleeding can manifest anywhere on a spectrum from occult bleeding to life-threatening hemorrhage. The most important step in the evaluation of a patient with suspected upper gastrointestinal bleeding is a careful history and thorough physical examination. Special attention should be paid to the onset of symptoms, prior history of peptic ulcer disease or gastrointestinal bleeding, prior endoscopy, use of high-risk medications (NSAIDs, aspirin, DOACs, P2Y$_{12}$ inhibitors, and corticosteroids), alcohol use, and known diagnosis of cirrhosis.

The most common presenting symptoms for an upper GI bleed are melena (black, tarry stool) and hematemesis. Melena occurs when the iron in hemoglobin is oxidized to Fe^{3+}, from which melena derives its distinct color. It infers that the blood has spent a considerable amount of time in the GI tract (typically greater than 4–6 h) and therefore implies a more proximal source of bleeding. About 90% of cases of melena are due to a GI bleed proximal to the ligament of Treitz, though it may also originate from the nasopharynx, small bowel, or right colon depending on gut transit time (Cappell and Friedel 2008). Large volume upper GI bleeding may also present as hematochezia (bright red blood per rectum) due to the more rapid transit of blood and less iron oxidation, and this is usually accompanied by hemodynamic instability.

Hematemesis refers to the presence of bright red blood in vomited material. Hematin colored material in vomit is sometimes referred to as "coffee ground emesis" for its resemblance to ground coffee. Coffee ground emesis generally implies blood in the stomach has been acted upon by acid over time, while hematemesis can suggest a larger volume bleed. Other symptoms that are less specific for upper GI bleeding that may be present include nausea, abdominal pain (primarily epigastric), lightheadedness, syncope, dyspnea, and fatigue.

Etiologies

Differential diagnosis of upper GI hemorrhage may be categorized as etiologies due to portal hypertension and cirrhosis vs. etiologies not associated with portal hypertension. Among etiologies not due to portal hypertension, the most common causes are peptic ulcer disease and erosive gastritis/esophagitis. Peptic ulcer disease is the most common etiology of upper gastrointestinal bleeding and will be discussed in its own section. Erosive esophagitis and gastritis typically arise as a result of chronic acid reflux, adverse effects of medications (including NSAIDs, bisphosphonates, and tetracyclines), or infection (ex. candida species, CMV, and HSV). Long-standing acid reflux tends to affect elderly patients more commonly, and they are more likely to suffer consequences such as erosive esophagitis compared to younger patients (Chait 2010). Medication-induced esophagitis is also particularly important in geriatric patients as the associated medications are more commonly prescribed in the elderly. Bisphosphonates are a class of medications well recognized as causing erosive esophagitis, perhaps in as many as 26% of patients (De Groen et al. 1996). Patients taking bisphosphonates should be advised to take the pill with 6–8 oz. of water and remain upright for at least 30 min after swallowing to minimize the likelihood of esophageal injury (De Groen et al. 1996). Patients with erosive gastritis/esophagitis tend to present with hematemesis more commonly than melena, and the overall clinical course is generally more benign compared to bleeding from other etiologies (Chait 2010; Guntipalli et al. 2014).

Mallory-Weiss tears are longitudinal mucosal lacerations at the gastroesophageal junction (GEJ) that occur with repeated episodes of retching or vomiting (Mallory 1929). These lacerations can lead to bleeding from submucosal blood vessels. Classically, these tears will present in patients who have repeated episodes of emesis that are initially clear and progress to hematemesis (Harris and DiPalma 1993). Arteriovenous malformations (AVMs) are the most common vascular abnormalities associated with upper GI bleeding and are more common with increasing age (Foutch 1993). The abnormal blood vessels dilate and erode through the overlying mucosa and lead to occult venous bleeding. They typically are present in the small bowel, but rarely, also can be seen in the stomach. Patients with renal dysfunction are at increased risk of developing AVMs. GI bleeding from AVMs also can be seen in patients with aortic stenosis in a triad known as Heyde Syndrome. Dieulafoy's lesions, in contrast, are abnormally dilated submucosal arteries that erode overlying mucosa and can cause brisk arterial bleeding. Due to the arterial nature of the bleeding, they have a greater propensity to cause significant hemodynamic compromise as compared to AVMs. Aortoenteric fistulas are a rare, but potentially devastating cause of upper GI bleeding. They may either arise as de novo fistulas (primary) or as a result of aortic reconstruction (secondary), most commonly between the aorta and the duodenum (O'Mara and Imbembo 1977). They typically present first with a sentinel bleed that may occur hours or days prior to a later massive hemorrhage. Due to the high mortality associated with aortoenteric fistulas, patients with known history of aortic disease who are being evaluated for GI bleeding should undergo radiographic and endoscopic evaluation for fistulization. If an aortoenteric fistula is detected, emergent surgical repair of the fistula is indicated.

Esophageal variceal rupture is the most feared manifestation of upper GI bleeding due to portal hypertension. Portal hypertension is most often caused by cirrhosis, but it also can be due to portal venous thrombus, hepatic vein thrombus (Budd-Chiari Syndrome), or heart disease. Cirrhosis leads to portal hypertension via two distinct mechanisms: increased resistance to portal vein outflow due to the fibrozed liver and increased production of splanchnic vasodilators such as nitric oxide and endothelial-like growth factor (García-Pagán et al. 2012). This leads to shunting of portal blood into tributary veins and formation of thin-walled varices which are susceptible to rupture. The most common site of variceal formation is the distal esophagus, but they can be found in the stomach and other points of the GI tract as well. The annual rate of bleeding from varices is 5% and 15% among small and large varices, respectively (North Italian Endoscopic Club for the Study and Treatment of Esophageal Varices 1988). Portal hypertensive gastropathy (PHG) is another, usually less severe, cause of upper GI bleeding due to portal hypertension. PHG refers to increased mucosal friability and edema as a result of portal hypertension. Gastric antral vascular ectasia (GAVE) may occur in patients with portal hypertension as a result of ectatic (dilated) gastric mucosal veins. Due to its appearance on endoscopy, GAVE is sometimes referred to as "watermelon stomach."

Peptic Ulcer Disease and *H. pylori*

Peptic ulcer disease is by far the most common cause of upper GI bleeding, accounting for approximately 60% of all presentations of upper GI bleeding (Longstreth 1995). A peptic ulcer refers to a defect in the gastric or duodenal mucosa that extends beyond the muscularis mucosa into the deeper layers of the gastrointestinal wall (Vakil et al. 2016). These ulcers can manifest anywhere on a spectrum from asymptomatic to life-threatening gastrointestinal perforation. The most common causes of peptic ulcer disease are *Helicobacter pylori (H. pylori)* infection and chronic NSAID use (as described earlier).

Helicobacter pylori is a spiral shaped, urease producing, and gram negative bacterium that is among the most common bacterial infections in the world (Cave 1996). The worldwide prevalence of *H. pylori* infection is estimated to be around 50%, and the prevalence increases with age. Studies have shown that *H. pylori* is found in over 50% of people over the age of 60 in developed countries, such as the United States, and as high as 80% in underdeveloped countries

(Pounder and Ng 1995). The exact method of transmission is still unknown; however, studies have shown that children of *H. pylori* infected parents have higher rates of *H. pylori* detection than children of uninfected parents, suggesting person-to-person and fecal-oral transmission.

Upon entry into the GI tract, *H. pylori* will use its flagella to travel toward the mucosal epithelium and move toward areas of high urea using chemotaxis (Yoshiyama and Nakazawa 2000). The bacterium is able to adhere to foveolar cells in the mucosa and secrete virulence factors important for bacterial survival and proliferation. Urease is one of the most important virulence factors for *H. pylori* survival as it cleaves urea into ammonia, which is used to buffer the highly acidic gastric environment. *H. pylori* secretes other virulence factors that induce mucosal epithelial cell damage and weaken mucosal integrity leading to the development of gastroduodenitis and peptic ulcers. Chronic gastritis as a result of *H. pylori* infection leads to an increased risk of developing gastric adenocarcinoma or mucosal associated lymphoid tissue (MALT) lymphoma.

In most patients, *H. pylori* infection is asymptomatic. However, in those with symptoms, disease may range from mild gastritis to severe peptic ulcer disease leading to gastroduodenal perforations. Common presenting complaints include postprandial epigastric pain or discomfort, usually starting within a few hours of eating, which may radiate toward the back (Barkun and Leontiadis 2010). Patients who develop ulcers along the gastric antrum may present with symptoms of gastric outlet obstruction including early satiety, bloating, nausea, or vomiting.

Diagnosis of *H. pylori* infection can be performed either through endoscopic biopsy, stool antigen testing, or urease breath testing (Chey et al. 2017). Endoscopic biopsy with urease staining is one of the most sensitive and specific means of diagnosing *H. pylori* with a sensitivity and specificity of 90% and 95%, respectively; however, it is also the most invasive and most expensive of all of the diagnostic tests. Urea breath testing (UBT) is a noninvasive test that may be used to detect *H. pylori* presence. Patients are given a solution containing urea with a labeled carbon isotope (either C^{13} or C^{14}), which in the presence of *H. pylori* is metabolized to ammonia and radiolabeled CO_2. The radiolabeled CO_2 is detected by machine, and high levels of radiolabeled CO_2 imply the presence of *H. pylori*. The sensitivity and specificity of UBT ranges 88–95% and 95–100%, respectively (Crowe et al. 2010). There is, however, a high false negative rate in patients using PPIs, bismuth, or antibiotics. One study looking at false negative rates in patients taking PPIs showed a 33% false negative rate in subsequent breath tests in patients who were taking PPIs (Laine et al. 1998). Patients should be instructed to stop taking their PPI at least 14 days prior to UBT as studies have shown that detection rates return to those of non-PPI users (Laine et al. 1998). Stool antigen testing is another noninvasive diagnostic option that carries a sensitivity and specificity of 94–97% respectively (Crowe et al. 2010). As with UBT, stool antigen sensitivity is decreased in patients taking PPIs, bismuth, and antibiotic use. Serologic tests for *H. pylori* exist, however, they do not reliably predict active infection from previous exposure, limiting their use.

First-line treatment of *H. pylori* infection is treatment with clarithromycin-based triple therapy consisting of 14 days of clarithromycin, amoxicillin, and PPI (Chey et al. 2017). In patients who are allergic to penicillins, metronidazole can be substituted for amoxicillin. However, it should be noted that eradication rates with triple therapy are below 80%, mainly due to increasing clarithromycin resistance (Chey et al. 2017). Guidelines suggest that patients with any prior macrolide exposure or patients in areas with known high rates of clarithromycin resistance should be given bismuth-based quadruple therapy consisting of bismuth sulfate, metronidazole, tetracycline, and a PPI for 10–14 days (Chey et al. 2017). All patients who undergo treatment for *H. pylori* should be tested for cure, usually with UBT or stool antigen testing (Chey et al. 2017). Patients should be off antibiotics for 4 weeks prior to stool-antigen testing and PPI for at least 2 weeks to decrease rates of false negative results (Chey et al. 2017).

Initial Evaluation

Initial diagnostic evaluation should always begin with a thorough history and physical exam. Careful attention should be paid to the patient's mental status as well as for any signs of respiratory distress or difficulty protecting the airway. Patients should be evaluated for stigmata of chronic liver disease including scleral icterus, jaundice, splenomegaly, ascites, spider angiomata, and palmar erythema. Every patient presenting with concern for upper GI bleeding should undergo digital rectal examination to evaluate for melanotic stool. A meta-analysis comparing presentation of upper vs. lower GI bleeding found that patient-reported melena was associated with a likelihood ratio (LR) of 5.1–5.9 in favor of upper GI bleeding while the presence of melena on digital rectal exam was associated with a LR of 25 demonstrating the diagnostic importance of a rectal exam in suspected upper GI bleeding (Srygley et al. 2012). Nasogastric lavage is no longer recommended as part of the initial evaluation, as it has not been shown to reduce mortality (Huang et al. 2011).

Labs including complete blood count, comprehensive metabolic panel, coagulation factors, and a type and screen should be done in all patients as part of the initial evaluation. BUN/creatinine ratio of >30 can suggest an upper GI source of bleeding and has been associated with a LR of 7.5 (Srygley et al. 2012). Liver test abnormalities, thrombocytopenia, and coagulopathy without obvious cause can suggest undiagnosed cirrhosis and prompt consideration of variceal hemorrhage as a possible etiology.

Several predictive models using demographic information as well as lab values have been developed to help stratify those with higher risk bleeding from those with less high-risk bleeding. Among these predictive models, two of the most commonly used are the AIM65 score and the Glasgow-Blatchford score. The AIMS65 score uses preendoscopy data to predict in hospital mortality for patients presenting with upper GI bleeding (Saltzman et al. 2011). The score was derived from a large, multicenter database of over 22,000 patients hospitalized for upper GI bleed. The study found that the following factors were associated with increased inpatient mortality: albumin <3.0, INR >1.5, altered mental status, systolic blood pressure <90 mmHg at presentation, and age >65. Mortality ranged from 0.3% in patients with 0 of these risk factors, to 25% in patients with all 5 risk factors present (Saltzman et al. 2011). The Glasgow-Blatchford score was developed to help predict patients who are at high risk for requiring urgent endoscopic intervention for the management of upper GI bleeding. The score is based on BUN, hemoglobin, systolic blood pressure, heart rate, and the presence of melena, syncope, liver disease, and/or heart failure (Blatchford et al. 2000). The score ranges from 0 to 23 and the risk of urgent endoscopy increases with increasing score. Scores ≤1 have been associated with a low risk for needing urgent endoscopic intervention, and these patients can be considered for outpatient evaluation (Stanley et al. 2017).

Management

Management of upper GI bleeding can be considered in terms of management of nonvariceal hemorrhage vs. management of variceal hemorrhage. Regardless of etiology, care of all patients with suspected upper GI bleeding should always begin with assessing the patient's ABCs (airway, breathing, and circulation) and vital signs. Patients who are unable to protect their airway due to ongoing large volume emesis or altered mental status should be intubated. All patients should have two large bore IVs placed for volume resuscitation and possible transfusion of blood products. It is not recommended to use central venous catheters for volume resuscitation as the longer catheter length increases resistance and therefore hinders flow of IV fluids and blood products (Reddick et al. 2011).

With regard to nonvariceal hemorrhage, all patients should be made nil per os (NPO) and immediately started on intravenous PPI therapy. PPIs help raise gastric pH, which in turn stabilizes blood clots and helps reduce rates of rebleeding (Leontiadis et al. 2005b; Kaviani et al. 2003; Green et al. 1978). A meta-analysis of

13 randomized trials published in 2014 comparing intermittent PPI therapy twice daily to continuous PPI infusion sought to compare rates of rebleeding. The trial showed that intermittent PPI dosing was associated with a 28% relative risk reduction of rebleeding and was noninferior to continuous PPI dosing (Sachar et al. 2014). The use of intermittent PPI dosing also allows increased accessibility to intravenous access, often needed for the administration of fluids and/or blood products. Administration of prokinetic agents such as IV metoclopramide or erythromycin given 30–90 min prior to endoscopy may help with visualization of bleeding lesions during endoscopy and has been shown to reduce the rate of second-look endoscopy (Rahman et al. 2016).

Patients with known or suspected cirrhosis and upper GI bleeding should be administered high dose PPI, a vasoactive somatostatin analog, and initiated on antibiotic prophylaxis for prevention of spontaneous bacterial peritonitis (SBP). Somatostatin analogs promote splanchnic vasoconstriction, which in turn helps to counteract the overproduction of vasodilatory compounds due to cirrhosis (Wells et al. 2012). This helps to decrease forward flow into the portal venous system, thereby decreasing blood loss through bleeding varices. The use of vasoactive medications has been shown to improve rates of hemostasis and decreases mortality in patients with variceal hemorrhage (Wells et al. 2012; Garcia-Tsao et al. 2017). Octreotide is the only available somatostatin analog in the United States and should be administered as a 50mcg IV bolus, followed by a continuous 50mcg/h. infusion for 3–5 days. Antibiotic prophylaxis (with either norfloxacin or ceftriaxone) should be administered to all patients with suspected or known cirrhosis admitted for upper GI bleeding. A meta-analysis published in 2012 showed that antibiotic prophylaxis reduces the rate of bacterial infection (including SBP) and decreases mortality (Chavez-Tapia et al. 2011). A trial comparing norfloxacin with ceftriaxone showed that ceftriaxone was superior to norfloxacin in prophylaxis of bacterial infections, making it the antibiotic of choice (Fernández et al. 2006).

Patients should be treated for a total of 7 days and can be transitioned to oral antibiotics once the patient is able to tolerate liquids and solids by mouth (Garcia-Tsao et al. 2017).

Patients should be transfused with packed red blood cells when the hemoglobin is <7.0, with a goal hemoglobin of ≥7.0. A trial comparing restrictive (goal Hgb ≥7.0) vs. liberal (Hgb ≥10.0) transfusion in patients hospitalized for acute upper GI bleeding found that the restrictive transfusion protocol was associated with a lower 45-day mortality (Villanueva et al. 2013). Patients with thrombocytopenia, found to have platelets less than 50,000/microliter, should be transfused with the goal being above 50,000. Patients with an INR >2.0 not secondary to cirrhosis should be transfused with fresh frozen plasma. The management of coagulopathy in patients with cirrhosis is more challenging as the INR is not a reliable indication of coagulation status in cirrhosis (Garcia-Tsao et al. 2017).

Endoscopic management is the mainstay of treatment both for patients with nonvariceal upper GI bleeding as well as patients with variceal hemorrhage. Current guidelines suggest that early endoscopy (defined as endoscopy within 24 h of presentation) should be performed on patients presenting with nonvariceal GI bleeding, as it has been shown to reduce hospital length of stay and inhospital mortality (Garg et al. 2017). Urgent endoscopy (earlier than 12 h of presentation) in patients with nonvariceal bleeding has been associated with higher risks of rebleeding and inhospital mortality, likely due to inadequate initial resuscitation (Kumar et al. 2017). Patients presenting with suspected variceal bleeding should undergo urgent endoscopy (Garcia-Tsao et al. 2017). For peptic ulcers with visible bleeding or stigmata of recent bleeding, endoscopic therapy usually entails injection of the bleeding site with epinephrine along with a second means of obtaining hemostasis (such as placement of hemostatic clips, thermal coaptive coagulation, argon plasma coagulation, or fibrin sealant) (Laine and Jensen 2012). AVMs with visible bleeding can be treated with thermic therapy, such as argon plasma coagulation (APC) (Gerson et al. 2015).

Esophageal varices typically are managed with esophageal variceal ligation (i.e., banding), which has been proven superior to endoscopic sclerotherapy in terms of rebleeding and eradication of varices (Dai et al. 2015). All patients who undergo esophageal variceal ligation should have a follow-up endoscopy within two weeks to ensure obliteration of varices (Garcia-Tsao et al. 2017). Those with persistent varices at 2 weeks should undergo biweekly endoscopy until complete variceal eradication is achieved (Garcia-Tsao et al. 2017). For variceal bleeding that cannot be controlled with endoscopic therapy, treatment options include emergent placement of a transjugular intrahepatic portosystemic shunt (TIPS) or surgery. TIPS is generally preferred to surgery as it has a high success rate and a much lower mortality rate compared to surgery (Sanyal 2014). Patients hospitalized with esophageal variceal bleeding should be started on a nonselective beta blocker prior to discharge, as the combination of endoscopic therapy and nonselective beta blockade has been shown superior to either therapy alone in secondary prevention of variceal bleeding (Thiele et al. 2012).

Management of Anticoagulation in Acute Upper GI Bleeding

The decision regarding the management of anticoagulation in the setting of acute upper GI bleeding largely depends on the amount of bleeding, the risk of thrombosis while discontinuing anticoagulation, and the indication for anticoagulation in the first place (Acosta et al. 2016). Patients taking antiplatelet agents who are at especially high risk for thrombotic events with cessation of these antithrombotic agents include patients within 90 days of acute coronary syndrome (ACS), recent coronary stent placement (<1 year for drug eluting stents or < 1 month for bare metal stents), patients with multiple stents, and those with a prior history of stent occlusion. The most significant complication of cessation of antiplatelet agent for these patients is stent thrombosis. Up to 6% of patients who have had a stent occlusion in the past will develop a second stent occlusion within 1 year and have a much higher rate of cardiovascular death (Acosta et al. 2016). In addition, approximately 2.3% of patients hospitalized with ACS will develop GI bleeding during the index hospitalization (Abbas et al. 2005), and these patients have a significantly higher inhospital mortality compared to patients hospitalized with ACS who do not develop GI bleeding (Al-Mallah et al. 2007). Guidelines recommend a multidisciplinary approach with the cardiology consultation prior to discontinuing antiplatelet agents in these high-risk patients as the risk of adverse cardiac events may exceed the risk of bleeding (Acosta et al. 2016).

Management of patients on warfarin presenting with upper GI bleeding depends on the severity of the bleeding and the indication for warfarin use. Patients with relatively minor bleeding sometimes can be observed off Warfarin without the administration of reversal agents (Acosta et al. 2016). Patients with supratherapeutic INR and life-threatening hemorrhage should be given either prothrombin complex concentrates (PCC) or fresh frozen plasma (FFP) to correct the coagulopathy (Acosta et al. 2016). Patients should be transfused to a goal INR of ≤2.5, as studies have shown comparable rates of successful hemostasis between patients with INRs of 1.5–2.5 and nonanticoagulated patients (Acosta et al. 2016). Therefore, it is recommended that endoscopic therapy should not be delayed in patients with serious GI bleeding and an INR <2.5. Vitamin K is less useful in the acute setting of hemorrhage as production of vitamin K-dependent factor can take several days. One study showed an absolute risk of embolism of about 1% in patients who had warfarin held for 4–7 days (Garcia et al. 2008). Patients with mechanical heart valves (especially patients with mitral valve replacement) are at particularly high risk of developing thrombotic complications from cessation of warfarin and INR reversal (Roudaut et al. 2007). One should strongly consider cardiology consultation prior to reversal or cessation of warfarin in patients with mechanical valve replacement given the high mortality of prosthetic valve thrombus (Roudaut et al. 2007). Reinitiation of warfarin

after procedure depends on the thromboembolic risk of the patient as well as risk of rebleeding (Acosta et al. 2016). A randomized trial published in 2015 showed that bridging with heparin in low-risk patients with atrial fibrillation during the periprocedural period did not decrease the risk of thromboembolic events, but did result in a statistically increased risk of bleeding (Douketis 2015). It is therefore recommended that low-risk patients start warfarin once adequate hemostasis is achieved, and not be bridged with heparin (Doherty 2017). Patients with high thromboembolic risk, however, do benefit from bridging with heparin while awaiting a therapeutic INR after restarting warfarin (Doherty 2017).

Few guidelines exist for the management of patients taking DOACs who present with upper GI bleeding. The most important principle is that DOACs have rapid onset of action (most between 1 and 4 h of onset) and relatively rapid offset (usually within 12–24 h). Drug clearance is dependent on the patient's creatinine clearance, which declines with age, and therefore, patients with decreased renal function will have impaired clearance of the drug (Lutz et al. 2017). Patients taking DOACs presenting with minor upper GI bleeding should have their next dose of DOAC held if the benefit of hemostasis is outweighed by the risk of thrombosis. For patients with moderate to severe GI bleeding who are hemodynamically stable, anticoagulation should be held and endoscopic evaluation should be deferred for 12–24 h to allow for normal coagulation to return (Acosta et al. 2016). It is reasonable to consider administration of PCC or FFP along with urgent endoscopy in patients who have hemodynamically compromising bleeds. Additionally, there are two available FDA approved reversal agents: Idarucizumab (for dabigatran) and Andexanet Alpha (for rivaroxaban, apixaban, and edoxaban) that can be used in life-threatening hemorrhage (Acosta et al. 2016; Pollack Charles Jr. et al. 2017; Connolly et al. 2019). Reinitiation of DOACs should be deferred until adequate hemostasis is ensured given the rapidity of onset of these agents (Acosta et al. 2016). (Images 1, 2, 3, 4, 5, Fig. 1, Tables 1, 2, and 3).

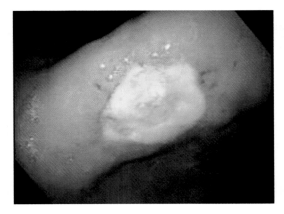

Image 1 Peptic ulcer

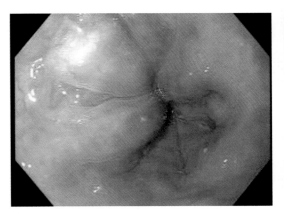

Image 2 Esophageal varices

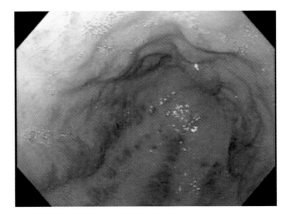

Image 3 Gastric antral vascular ectasia

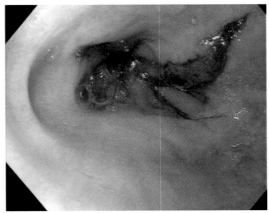

Image 4 Mallory-Weiss tear

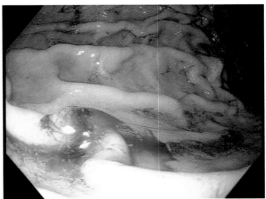

Image 5 Dieulafoy's lesion

Key Points

- It is prudent that providers caring for geriatric patients have a sound understanding of upper GI bleeding, as several age-related processes contribute to the increased incidence, morbidity, and mortality in this population.
- Risk factors for upper GI bleeding include advanced age, H pylori infection, medication use (NSAIDs, Aspirin, P2Y$_{12}$ inhibitors, anticoagulants, and steroids), smoking, and history of liver disease.
- High clinical suspicion is imperative as prompt evaluation and treatment of older patients with suspected upper GI bleeding may help minimize the risk of poor outcomes.

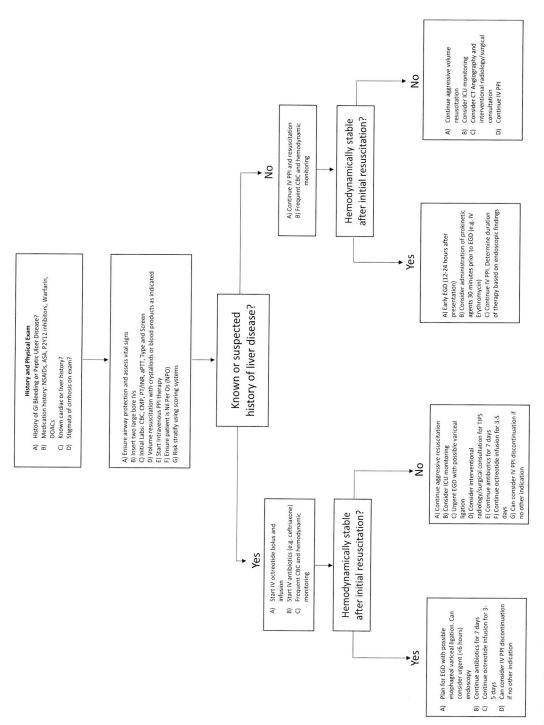

Fig. 1 Approach to patients with suspected upper GI bleeding

Table 1 Glasgow-Blatchford bleeding score table

	Score value
Blood urea (mmol/L)	
6.5–7.9	2
8.0–9.9	3
10.0–25.0	4
>25.0	6
Hemoglobin for men (g/dL)	
12.0–12.9	1
10.0–11.9	3
<10.0	6
Hemoglobin for women (g/dL)	
10.0–11.9	1
<10.0	6
Other markers	
Pulse ≥100 BPM	1
Melena	1
Syncope	2
Liver disease	2
Heart failure	2

Table 2 Etiologies of upper GI bleeding

Causes of upper gastrointestinal bleeding	Comments
Peptic ulcer disease	Most common cause of upper gastrointestinal bleeding in hospitalized patients. Risk factors include *H. pylori* infection and NSAID use.
Erosive gastroesophagitis	Occurs as a part of long-standing gastroesophageal reflux and/or NSAID use. Rarely causes major bleeding.
Esophageal/gastric varices	Can occur with diseases that cause increased risk of portal venous pressure including cirrhosis, portal venous thrombosis, and others.
Mallory-Weiss tear	Mucosal tear near esophagogastric junction usually as a result of repetitive vomiting/retching. Predominant symptom is hematemesis.
Dieulafoy lesion	Abnormally dilated submucosal arterial bleed. Can cause severe hemodynamic compromise given arterial nature
Arteriovenous malformations (AVMs)	Abnormal connection between arteries and veins. Mainly seen in distal small bowel, but may be present in upper GI tract.
Gastric antral vascular ectasia (GAVE)	Abnormal dilation of gastric veins associated with cirrhosis and chronic kidney disease
Portal hypertensive gastropathy (PHG)	Result of submucosal congestion in diseases that increase portal pressure.
Malignancy	Rare cause of overt upper GI bleeding.
Aortoenteric fistula	Rare, but potentially fatal cause of upper GI bleeding. Should be considered in patients with aortic disease or recent aortic surgery

- Providers caring for older adults should address modifiable risk factors for upper GI bleeding including reducing the use of aspirin and NSAIDs (whenever possible) as well as coprescribing PPIs in patients who will be initiated on long-term NSAID therapy.
- The most common etiology of upper GI bleeding is peptic ulcer disease, followed by erosive gastroesophagitis, gastroesophageal varices, Mallory-Weiss tears, Dieulafoy's lesions, gastric antral vascular ectasia (GAVE), portal hypertensive gastropathy (PHG), aortoenteric fistula, malignancy, and other rare conditions.
- Early recognition and management of upper GI bleeding in adult patients is imperative and can potentially be lifesaving. A detailed history regarding prior history of upper GI bleeding, peptic ulcer disease, NSAIDs or anticoagulant use, and liver disease is vital.
- Management begins with assessment of airway protection (and intubation if indicated), placement of large bore IVs, administration of isotonic crystalloid solution and/or blood products, and administration of IV PPI.
- Management of anticoagulation in upper GI bleeding largely depends on the indication for anticoagulation, the risk of continued bleeding with continuing the medication, and the risk of thrombosis with discontinuing the medication.

Table 3 Forrest classification of peptic ulcer bleeding

Forrest grade	Endoscopic findings	Rate of rebleeding*
I	Active hemorrhage	
Ia	Active pulsatile bleeding	55%
Ib	Active nonpulsatile (oozing) bleeding	
II	Stigmata of recent bleeding	
IIa	Visible, nonbleeding vessel	50%
IIb	Adherent clot	22%
IIc	Hematin coated lesion	10%
III	Clean based ulcer	5%

Source: Laine L, Peterson WL. Bleeding peptic ulcer. New Engl J Med. 1994;331 (Bombardier et al. 2000):717–27
[a]Rate of rebleeding when endoscopic therapy is not performed

References

Abbas AE, et al. Incidence and prognostic impact of gastrointestinal bleeding after percutaneous coronary intervention for acute myocardial infarction. Am J Cardiol. 2005;96(2):173–6.

Abraham NS, et al. Gastrointestinal safety of direct oral anticoagulants: a large population-based study. Gastroenterology. 2017;152(5):1014–22.

Acosta RD, et al. The management of antithrombotic agents for patients undergoing GI endoscopy. Gastrointest Endosc. 2016;83(1):3–16.

Al-Mallah M, et al. Predictors and outcomes associated with gastrointestinal bleeding in patients with acute coronary syndromes. J Thromb Thrombolysis. 2007;23(1):51–5.

Barkun A, Leontiadis G. Systematic review of the symptom burden, quality of life impairment and costs associated with peptic ulcer disease. Am J Med. 2010;123(4):358–66.

Bhatt DL, et al. ACCF/ACG/AHA 2008 expert consensus document on reducing the gastrointestinal risks of antiplatelet therapy and NSAID use: a report of the American College of Cardiology Foundation task force on clinical expert consensus documents. J Am Coll Cardiol. 2008;52(18):1502–17.

Blatchford O, Murray WR, Blatchford M. A risk score to predict need for treatment for upper gastrointestinal haemorrhage. Lancet. 2000;356(9238):1318–21.

Bombardier C, et al. Comparison of upper gastrointestinal toxicity of rofecoxib and naproxen in patients with rheumatoid arthritis. N Engl J Med. 2000;343(21):1520–8.

Cappell MS, Friedel D. Initial management of acute upper gastrointestinal bleeding: from initial evaluation up to gastrointestinal endoscopy. Med Clin N Am. 2008; 92(3):491–509.

Cave DR. Transmission and epidemiology of helicobacter pylori. Am J Med. 1996;100:12S–8S.

Chait MM. Gastroesophageal reflux disease: important considerations for the older patients. World J Gastrointest Endosc. 2010;2(12):388.

Chavez-Tapia NC, et al. Meta-analysis: antibiotic prophylaxis for cirrhotic patients with upper gastrointestinal bleeding–an updated Cochrane review. Aliment Pharmacol Ther. 2011;34(5):509–18.

Chen W-C, et al. Gastrointestinal hemorrhage in warfarin anticoagulated patients: incidence, risk factor, management, and outcome. Bio Med Res Int. 2014;2014

Chey WD, et al. ACG clinical guideline: treatment of helicobacter pylori infection. Am J Gastroenterol. 2017;112(2):212–39.

Connolly SJ, et al. Dabigatran versus warfarin in patients with atrial fibrillation. N Engl J Med. 2009;361(12):1139–51.

Connolly SJ, et al. Full study report of andexanet alfa for bleeding associated with factor Xa inhibitors. N Engl J Med. 2019;380(14):1326–35.

Crowe, S. E., M. Feldman, and C. H. Ginsburg. Indications and diagnostic tests for Helicobacter pylori infection. *Uptodate. Wellesley* (2010);17(3).

Cullen D, et al. Primary gastroduodenal prophylaxis with omeprazole for non-steroidal anti-inflammatory drug users. Aliment Pharmacol Ther. 1998;12(2):135–40.

Dai C, et al. Endoscopic variceal ligation compared with endoscopic injection sclerotherapy for treatment of esophageal variceal hemorrhage: a meta-analysis. World J Gastroenterol: WJG. 2015;21(8):2534.

De Groen PC, et al. Esophagitis associated with the use of alendronate. N Engl J Med. 1996;335(14):1016–21.

Doherty, John U., et al. 2017 ACC expert consensus decision pathway for periprocedural management of anticoagulation in patients with nonvalvular atrial fibrillation: a report of the American College of Cardiology Clinical Expert Consensus Document Task Force. J Am Coll Cardiol 69(7): 2017 871–898.

Douketis JD, et al. Perioperative bridging anticoagulation in patients with atrial fibrillation. New Engl J Med. 2015;373(9):823–33.

Fernández J, et al. Norfloxacin vs ceftriaxone in the prophylaxis of infections in patients with advanced cirrhosis and hemorrhage. Gastroenterology. 2006;131(4):1049–56.

Foutch PG. Angiodysplasia of the gastrointestinal tract. Am J Gastroenterol. 1993;88:6.

Garcia DA, et al. Risk of thromboembolism with short-term interruption of warfarin therapy. Arch Intern Med. 2008;168(1):63–9.

García-Pagán J-C, Gracia-Sancho J, Bosch J. Functional aspects on the pathophysiology of portal hypertension in cirrhosis. J Hepatol. 2012;57(2):458–61.

Garcia-Tsao G, et al. Portal hypertensive bleeding in cirrhosis: risk stratification, diagnosis, and management: 2016 practice guidance by the American association for the study of liver diseases. Hepatology. 2017;65(1):310–35.

Garg SK, et al. Early esophagogastroduodenoscopy is associated with better outcomes in upper gastrointestinal bleeding: a nationwide study. Endosc Int Open. 2017;5(05):E376–86.

Gaziano JM, et al. Use of aspirin to reduce risk of initial vascular events in patients at moderate risk of cardiovascular disease (ARRIVE): a randomised, double-blind, placebo-controlled trial. Lancet. 2018;392(10152):1036–46.

Gerson LB, et al. ACG clinical guideline: diagnosis and management of small bowel bleeding. Am J Gastroenterol. 2015;110(9):1265–87.

Granger CB, et al. Apixaban versus warfarin in patients with atrial fibrillation. N Engl J Med. 2011;365(11):981–92.

Green FW, et al. Effect of acid and pepsin on blood coagulation and platelet aggregation: a possible contributor to prolonged gastroduodenal mucosal hemorrhage. Gastroenterology. 1978;74(1):38–43.

Guntipalli P, et al. Upper gastrointestinal bleeding caused by severe esophagitis: a unique clinical syndrome. Dig Dis Sci. 2014;59(12):2997–3003.

Guo C-G, et al. Systematic review with meta-analysis: the risk of gastrointestinal bleeding in patients taking third-generation P2Y12 inhibitors compared with clopidogrel. Aliment Pharmacol Ther. 2019;49(1):7–19.

Harris JM, DiPalma JA. Clinical significance of Mallory-Weiss tears. Am J Gastroenterol. 1993;88:12.

Hooper L, et al. The effectiveness of five strategies for the prevention of gastrointestinal toxicity induced by non-steroidal anti-inflammatory drugs: systematic review. BMJ. 2004;329(7472):948.

Huang ES, et al. Impact of nasogastric lavage on outcomes in acute GI bleeding. Gastrointest Endosc. 2011;74(5):971–80.

January CT, et al. 2014 AHA/ACC/HRS guideline for the management of patients with atrial fibrillation: a report of the American College of Cardiology/American Heart Association task force on practice guidelines and the Heart Rhythm Society. J Am Coll Cardiol. 2014;64(21):e1–e76.

Kaplan RC, Heckbert SR, Koepsell TD, Furberg CD, Polak JF. Risk factors for gastrointestinal bleeding among older patients. Cardiovascular health study investigators. J Am Geriatr Soc. 2001;49(2):126–33.

Kaviani MJ, et al. Effect of oral omeprazole in reducing re-bleeding in bleeding peptic ulcers: a prospective, double-blind, randomized, clinical trial. Aliment Pharmacol Ther. 2003;17(2):211–6.

Kumar NL, et al. Timing of upper endoscopy influences outcomes in patients with acute nonvariceal upper GI bleeding. Gastrointest Endosc. 2017;85(5):945–52.

Laine L, Jensen DM. Management of patients with ulcer bleeding. Am J Gastroenterol. 2012;107(3):345–60.

Laine L, et al. Effect of proton-pump inhibitor therapy on diagnostic testing for helicobacter pylori. Ann Intern Med. 1998;129(7):547–50.

Leontiadis GI, Sharma VK, Howden CW. Systematic review and meta-analysis of proton pump inhibitor therapy in peptic ulcer bleeding. BMJ. 2005a;330(7491):568.

Leontiadis GI, Sharma VK, Howden CW. Systematic review and meta-analysis of proton pump inhibitor therapy in peptic ulcer bleeding. BMJ. 2005b;330(7491):568.

Leung PS, editor. The gastrointestinal system: gastrointestinal, nutritional and hepatobiliary physiology: Springer Science & Business; 2014.

Longstreth GF. Epidemiology of hospitalization for acute upper gastrointestinal hemorrhage: a population–based study. Am J Gastroenterol. 1995;90:2.

Lutz J, Jurk K, Schinzel H. Direct oral anticoagulants in patients with chronic kidney disease: patient selection and special considerations. Int J Nephrol Renov Dis. 2017;10:135.

Mallory GK. Hemorrhages from lacerations of the cardiac orifice of stomach due to vomiting. Am J Med Sci. 1929;178:506–15.

McNeil JJ, et al. Effect of aspirin on disability-free survival in the healthy elderly. N Engl J Med. 2018;379(16):1499–508.

North Italian Endoscopic Club for the Study and Treatment of Esophageal Varices. Prediction of the first variceal hemorrhage in patients with cirrhosis of the liver and esophageal varices. N Engl J Med. 1988;319(15):983–9.

O'Brien CW, Juraschek SP, Wee CC. Prevalence of aspirin use for primary prevention of cardiovascular disease in the United States: results from the 2017 National Health Interview Survey. Ann Intern Med. 2019;

O'Mara C, Imbembo AL. Paraprosthetic-enteric fistula. Surgery. 1977;81(5):556–66.

Patel MR, et al. Rivaroxaban versus warfarin in non-valvular atrial fibrillation. N Engl J Med. 2011;365(10):883–91.

Pollack Charles V Jr, et al. Idarucizumab for dabigatran reversal – full cohort analysis. N Engl J Med. 2017;377(5):431–41.

Pounder RE, Ng D. The prevalence of helicobacter pylori infection in different countries. Aliment Pharmacol Ther. 1995;9:33–9.

Rahman R, et al. Pre-endoscopic erythromycin administration in upper gastrointestinal bleeding: an updated meta-analysis and systematic review. Ann Gastroenterol. 2016;29(3):312.

Raskin JB, et al. Misoprostol dosage in the prevention of nonsteroidal anti-inflammatory drug-induced gastric and duodenal ulcers: a comparison of three regimens. Ann Intern Med. 1995;123(5):344–50.

Reddick AD, Ronald J, Morrison WG. Intravenous fluid resuscitation: was Poiseuille right? Emerg Med J. 2011;28(3):201–2.

Rockall TA, et al. Incidence of and mortality from acute upper gastrointestinal haemorrhage in the United Kingdom. BMJ. 1995;311(6999):222–6.

Roudaut R, Serri K, Lafitte S. Thrombosis of prosthetic heart valves: diagnosis and therapeutic considerations. Heart. 2007;93(1):137–42.

Sachar H, Vaidya K, Laine L. Intermittent vs continuous proton pump inhibitor therapy for high-risk bleeding ulcers: a systematic review and meta-analysis. JAMA Intern Med. 2014;174(11):1755–62.

Saltzman JR, et al. A simple risk score accurately predicts in-hospital mortality, length of stay, and cost in acute upper GI bleeding. Gastrointest Endosc. 2011;74(6): 1215–24.

Sanyal B. Methods to achieve hemostasis in patients with acute variceal hemorrhage: UpToDate; 2014.

Srygley FD, et al. Does this patient have a severe upper gastrointestinal bleed? JAMA. 2012;307(10):1072–9.

Stanley AJ, et al. Comparison of risk scoring systems for patients presenting with upper gastrointestinal bleeding: international multicentre prospective study. BMJ. 2017;356:i6432.

Straus WL, Ofman JJ. Gastrointestinal toxicity associated with nonsteroidal anti-inflammatory drugs: epidemiologic and economic issues. Gastroenterol Clin. 2001;30(4):895–920.

Thiele M, et al. Meta-analysis: banding ligation and medical interventions for the prevention of rebleeding from oesophageal varices. Aliment Pharmacol Ther. 2012;35(10):1155–65.

Vakil NB, Feldman M, Grover S. Peptic ulcer disease: clinical manifestations and diagnosis. UpToDate. 2016;2016

Van Leerdam ME, et al. Acute upper GI bleeding: did anything change?: time trend analysis of incidence and outcome of acute upper GI bleeding between 1993/1994 and 2000. Am J Gastroenterol. 2003;98(7):1494–9.

Villanueva C, et al. Transfusion strategies for acute upper gastrointestinal bleeding. N Engl J Med. 2013;368(1):11–21.

Wells M, et al. Meta-analysis: vasoactive medications for the management of acute variceal bleeds. Aliment Pharmacol Ther. 2012;35(11):1267–78.

Wongrakpanich S, Wongrakpanich A, Melhado K, Rangaswami J. A comprehensive review of non-steroidal anti-inflammatory drug use in the elderly. Aging Dis. 2018;9(1):143.

Yoshiyama H, Nakazawa T. Unique mechanism of helicobacter pylori for colonizing the gastric mucus. Microbes Infect. 2000;2(1):55–60.

Lower Gastrointestinal Bleeding

56

Edward Sheen, Jennifer Pan, Andrew Ho, and George Triadafilopoulos

Contents

E. Sheen (✉) · G. Triadafilopoulos
Division of Gastroenterology and Hepatology, Stanford University School of Medicine, Stanford, CA, USA
e-mail: esheen@stanford.edu; vagt@stanford.edu

J. Pan
Division of Gastroenterology and Hepatology, Stanford University School of Medicine, Stanford, CA, USA

Division of Gastroenterology and Hepatology, Veterans Affairs Palo Alto Medical Center, Palo Alto, CA, USA
e-mail: jenpan@stanford.edu

A. Ho
Division of Gastroenterology and Hepatology, Stanford University School of Medicine, Stanford, CA, USA

Division of Gastroenterology and Hepatology, Santa Clara Valley Medical Center, San Jose, CA, USA
e-mail: Andrew.Ho@hhs.sccgov.org

© Springer Nature Switzerland AG 2021
C. S. Pitchumoni, T. S. Dharmarajan (eds.), *Geriatric Gastroenterology*,
https://doi.org/10.1007/978-3-030-30192-7_48

Abstract

Lower gastrointestinal bleeding is a frequent clinical challenge that appears to be increasing in incidence among older adults. Bleeding episodes are associated with a higher mortality rate, longer hospitalization, and higher resource utilization, compared to that associated with upper gastrointestinal bleeding. The increase in incidence is attributed to the high prevalence of age-related disorders such as diverticulosis, ischemic colitis, colorectal neoplasms, and angiodysplasia. Additional associated contributors include the prevalent use of aspirin, nonsteroidal anti-inflammatory drugs, anticoagulants, and anti-platelet medications.

The guidelines of two major professional organizations, the American College of Gastroenterology and American Society for Gastrointestinal Endoscopy, can help inform the management of lower gastrointestinal bleeding and anticoagulant therapy in the setting of bleeding. Management principles include the proper triage of patients, timely resuscitation, and identification of the source of bleeding by endoscopic and/or imaging procedures such as angiography, which can be both diagnostic and therapeutic. Emergency surgery is seldom needed.

Keywords

Angiodysplasia · Angiography · Colitis · Colon cancer · Colonoscopy · Diverticular bleeding · Endoscopy safety · Hematochezia · Hemostasis · Lower gastrointestinal bleeding · Post-polypectomy bleeding · Rectal bleeding · Upper endoscopy

Introduction

Gastrointestinal bleeding is a common and growing challenge in the older population. The estimated incidence of lower gastrointestinal bleeding requiring hospitalization ranges from 20.5 to 27 cases per 100,000 individuals per year, with a greater than 200-fold increase with advancing age between the third and ninth decades of life, and higher prevalence among males (Longstreth 1997; Tariq and Mekhjian 2007; Wilcox and Clark 1999). This incidence appears to be increasing. A population-based study from Spain suggested that hospitalization rates for lower gastrointestinal complications, mostly for hematochezia, increased by more than 50% from 20/100,000 in 1996 to 33/100,000 individuals in 2005 (Lanas et al. 2009). Lower gastrointestinal events were also associated with a higher mortality rate, longer hospitalization, and higher resource utilization, compared to upper gastrointestinal events, particularly among older adults. Acute lower gastrointestinal bleeding is associated with longer length of stay and higher direct medical costs, especially among the elderly (Comay and Marshall 2002). Peery et al. reported more than 885,000 ambulatory and emergency room presentations nationwide for rectal bleeding in 2010 (Peery et al. 2015). They also estimated that there were more than 342,000 emergency department visits for lower gastrointestinal bleeding in 2012 (109 visits per 100,000 individuals), a 17% increase since 2006. An observational, prospective study performed in 2013 across the 110 emergency departments comprising the French Emergency Medicine Research network found an estimated lower gastrointestinal bleeding incidence of 93/100,000, which the authors noted was generally higher than that reported in prior studies. The authors believed their finding might be related to all types of bleeding being counted in their study, including "weak bleeding due to anorectal lesions," as well as aging of the population and increased utilization of antithrombotic medications (Thiebaud et al. 2019).

The increased incidence of lower gastrointestinal bleeding in older adults is attributed to the higher rate of diverticulosis, cardiopulmonary disease, ischemic colitis, colorectal neoplasms, and angiodysplasia, as well as more prevalent use of aspirin, nonsteroidal anti-inflammatory drugs, and anticoagulants in this population (Lanas et al. 2009; Farrell and Friedman 2000).

Most patients with lower gastrointestinal bleeding have a favorable outcome despite the frequency of advanced age and other comorbid conditions among these patients (Boley et al. 1979; Bokhari et al. 1996). The estimated mortality rate is 4–10% or greater; mortality is associated with severe hemorrhage and emergent surgery (Browder et al. 1986; Richter et al. 1995; Schiller et al. 1970; Leitman et al. 1989; Levy et al. 2003). The mortality rate has been reported to be higher (23%) among patients admitted for other causes and who experience lower gastrointestinal bleeding during their hospitalization, compared to patients admitted for lower gastrointestinal

bleeding (2.4%, Tariq and Mekhjian 2007). Reported independent predictors of all-cause mortality include increasing age, length of hospitalization, and the number of comorbid conditions (Longstreth 1997).

The economic burden of lower gastrointestinal bleeding is not fully known but is substantial, given the prevalence of this problem in the geriatric population. Thomas et al. estimated that diverticular bleeding alone cost $1.3 billion in 2001 (Thomas et al. 2004). With the growing elderly population, both the clinical burden and health-care expenditures from lower gastrointestinal bleeding are expected to increase significantly in the years ahead (Comay and Marshall 2002).

Definitions and Clinical Presentation

Lower gastrointestinal bleeding has traditionally been defined as bleeding that occurs from a source distal to the ligament of Treitz, though since the advent of small bowel enteroscopy techniques, small bowel bleeding sources are now considered midgut bleeding. A newly proposed definition of lower gastrointestinal bleeding is therefore bleeding distal to the ileocecal valve (Eisen et al. 2001; Raju et al. 2007; Ell and May 2006). Endoscopy is usually the first-line method for both diagnosis and management of gastrointestinal bleeding.

To best differentiate upper gastrointestinal bleeding – which is bleeding proximal to the ligament of Treitz – from lower gastrointestinal bleeding sources and to expedite appropriate procedures, as well as minimize unnecessary interventions, a focused history, physical examination, and laboratory evaluation should be performed. The classical presentation of patients with acute (bleeding duration <3 days) upper gastrointestinal bleeding includes hematemesis and melena, which is the passage of black, tarry, and foul-smelling stools from degradation of blood to hematin. In contrast, overt lower gastrointestinal bleeding usually presents with hematochezia, defined as the rectal passage of bright red blood with or without stool. Brisk upper gastrointestinal bleeding can also present with hematochezia if bleeding is rapid enough to avoid degradation to hematin and melena before blood completes transit through the gastrointestinal tract (Trivedi and Pitchumoni 2006). Patients with slow or chronic lower gastrointestinal bleeding can present with occult fecal blood, intermittent melena, maroon stools, or small amounts of bright-red blood per rectum.

When gastrointestinal bleeding is suspected without overt symptoms, occult bleeding sources should be considered. Older references may utilize the term "obscure" gastrointestinal bleeding, which the American College of Gastroenterology proposes using only for patients in whom a source of bleeding cannot be identified anywhere in the digestive tract. Therefore, small bowel evaluation with video capsule endoscopy should be considered a first-line procedure if both upper and lower endoscopic examinations are unrevealing (Gerson et al. 2015). Table 1 summarizes key terms and their significance.

Aggravating Factors in Older Adults

Medical Comorbidities

In older adults, there is an increased prevalence of comorbidity from cardiopulmonary disease, renal disease, diabetes, and cancer. These comorbidities are associated with increased incidence risk of clinically significant bleeding (Comay and Marshall 2002). For example, as will be discussed further, patients with atherosclerosis and atrial fibrillation are at higher risk of ischemic colitis, while aortic stenosis may be associated with vascular ectasias, which can be found throughout the body and digestive tract (Brandt et al. 1982). Given the increased incidence of prostate cancer with age, radiation proctopathy is another common cause of lower gastrointestinal bleeding, though this tends to be more chronic in nature and presents as intermittent scant hematochezia. In patients who develop lower gastrointestinal bleeding after intensive care unit admission for critical illness, 32% of cases are found to be due to rectal ulcers, which can have early rebleeding

Table 1 Terms and their significance. (From Pitchumoni and Dharmarajan 2012)

Hematemesis: Vomiting of blood. It indicates an upper GI source of bleeding proximal to the ligament of Treitz. It may consist of bright red blood indicative of active bleeding or coffee ground material

Melena: Passage of black, tarry, foul smelling stool as a result of degradation of hemoglobin to hematin. At least 50 cc of blood in the upper GI tract is required to cause melena. The source of bleeding is almost always in the upper GI tract, but may be in the distal small bowel or right colon (early and slow bleeding)

Hematochezia: Passage of bright red blood through the rectum with or without stool. The source is often the lower GI tract, but brisk UGIB can cause hematochezia

Obscure bleeding: Can have two forms
  Obscure – occult bleeding which is not visible to the patient and is manifested by recurrent iron deficiency anemia and/or repeated positive fecal occult blood test results
  Obscure – overt bleeding as manifested by recurrent passage of visible blood

Upper gastrointestinal bleeding: Bleeding site proximal to the ligament of Treitz

Middle gastrointestinal bleeding: Bleeding from the small bowel not visible by EGD or colonoscopy

Lower gastrointestinal bleeding: Bleeding site is usually in the colon
  Acute lower gastrointestinal bleeding: Bleeding of recent duration (arbitrarily defined as <3 days) and may result in the need for blood transfusion, instability of vital signs, and/or anemia
  Chronic lower gastrointestinal bleeding: Bleeding associated with intermittent or slow blood loss over a period of several days or longer

rates of 44–48% after endoscopic therapy, as well as a mortality rate of 33–48% in patients with multiple comorbidities and high-risk stigmata (Kanwal et al. 2003; Lin et al. 2011).

Medications

Use of medications for the management of comorbid disorders alongside additional risks from polypharmacy can also aggravate bleeding and contribute to greater morbidity and mortality (Farrell and Friedman 2000). While nonsteroidal anti-inflammatory drugs (NSAIDs) are well-known to be associated with upper gastrointestinal bleeding, the lower gastrointestinal tract can also experience NSAID-induced toxicity, though the mechanisms involved are not yet well-understood. It is thought that NSAIDs may cause local mucosal trauma and platelet inhibition (Patrono 1994). The prevalence of NSAID use has been reported to be as high as 86% among patients with lower gastrointestinal bleeding (Lanas et al. 1992). Studies have shown that oral and/or parenteral nonselective NSAIDs are associated with a two- to fivefold increase in risk for lower gastrointestinal bleeding and development of anemia, including diverticular bleeding (Laine et al. 2003). In addition, NSAID use can contribute to exacerbation of inflammatory bowel disease (Matuk et al. 2004). NSAID-associated colopathy can also cause colonic ulcerations and diaphragm-like strictures (predominantly in the terminal ileum and right colon), as well as present with lower gastrointestinal bleeding and perforation (Bjarnason et al. 1993).

Anticoagulant and antiplatelet use are also more prevalent in the elderly and in susceptible individuals has been associated with an increased risk of gastrointestinal bleeding. While warfarin had traditionally been the mainstay of anticoagulant therapy for patients with atrial fibrillation and other pro-coagulable states, new target-specific direct-acting/novel oral anticoagulants (DOACs/NOACs) are now widely used. Though all-cause bleeding rates for DOACs were reportedly similar when compared with warfarin, the rate of gastrointestinal bleeding for patients treated with dabigatran, rivaroxaban, and edoxaban was higher (Feagins and Weideman 2018). In contrast, the rates of gastrointestinal bleeding in patients treated with apixaban were similar – if not lower – than that in patients treated with warfarin (1.2% vs 1.3%) (Granger et al. 2011). While the incidence rates (per 1000 person-years) of lower gastrointestinal bleeding (LGIB) have been found to be higher than the incidence of upper gastrointestinal bleeding (UGIB) among new low-dose aspirin users (1.68 vs. 0.97), incidence rates of gastrointestinal bleeds requiring hospitalization (0.45 vs. 0.57) and 30-day mortality rates (0.01 vs. 0.06) were lower for LGIB than for UGIB (Cea Soriano et al. 2019). In addition, prior studies have found that among aspirin users with a history of lower gastrointestinal bleeding, while there is an

Table 2 Drugs that may contribute to lower gastrointestinal bleeding in the elderly. (Adapted from Triadafilopoulos 2012)

Drug or drug class	Type(s) of injury
Nonsteroidal anti-inflammatory drugs (NSAIDs)	Intestinal/colonic ulcers; colitis; exacerbation of underlying inflammatory bowel disease (IBD); ischemic colitis, diverticular bleeding
Amphetamines	Ischemic colitis
Cocaine	Ischemic colitis
Imipramine	Ischemic colitis
Vasopressin	Ischemic colitis
Aspirin	Exacerbation of underlying IBD; allergic colitis
Methyldopa	Allergic colitis
Gold salts	Allergic colitis
Anticoagulants	Intestinal intramural hematomas
Chemotherapeutic agents	Neutropenic enterocolitis
Neuroleptics	Hemorrhagic diarrhea

increased risk of recurrent LGIB bleeding with continuation of aspirin, there was a concurrent reduced risk of serious cardiovascular events and death (Chan et al. 2016). A multidisciplinary management approach is recommended for patients on anticoagulant medications in order to balance the risk of thromboembolic events with the risk of bleeding. Periprocedural anticoagulation management recommendations are discussed below. Other drugs that may contribute to lower gastrointestinal bleeding in older adults are summarized in Table 2.

Evaluation, Assessment, and Management

A general approach for the management of lower gastrointestinal bleeding is summarized in Fig. 1.

History

Alongside resuscitation, evaluation of all patients with suspected lower gastrointestinal bleeding

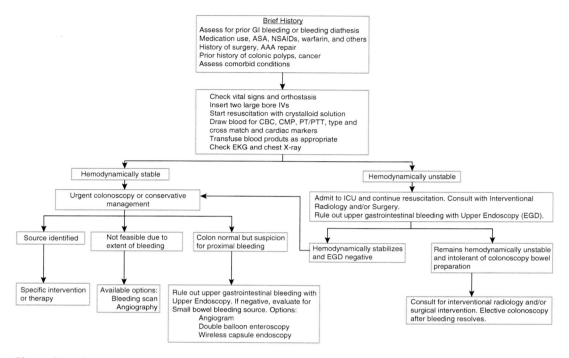

Fig. 1 General management of lower gastrointestinal bleeding. (Adapted from Pitchumoni and Dharmarajan 2012)

should begin with a thorough history and physical examination to guide subsequent diagnostic and management steps. This can be challenging with elderly patients, a significant proportion of whom may be poor historians, have difficulty communicating, or live in a nursing home setting. In these situations, it is especially important to obtain additional corroborating information from family members, primary care physicians, and other care team members to help ensure an accurate and thorough medical history. Important components of the history include timing, duration, and characteristics of bleeding; prior history of gastrointestinal bleeding; recent endoscopic instrumentation or relevant surgeries; comorbid conditions; and use of NSAIDs, anticoagulants, antiplatelet agents, selective serotonin reuptake inhibitors, or other medications that may increase bleeding risk. It is also important to evaluate for evidence of comorbidities which may increase bleeding risk including prior history of vascular, connective tissue, and inflammatory bowel disease; cirrhosis of the liver; radiation therapy; and anemia; as well

as conditions such as cardiopulmonary disease that may impact tolerance for endoscopy. Table 3 summarizes important clinical questions for assessment of lower gastrointestinal bleeding.

Physical Examination and Initial Laboratory Studies

The initial evaluation should include measurement of vital signs and examination for orthostatic changes, which suggest at least a 10–20% loss of circulatory volume. Hypotension with a systolic blood pressure less than 100 mmHg or baseline tachycardia suggests significant hemodynamic compromise requiring urgent volume resuscitation. A proper digital rectal examination can help to evaluate for a rectal mass and confirm the reported description of stool color. Initial laboratory testing should include a complete blood count, coagulation profile, electrolytes, renal and liver function tests, as well as typing and cross matching of blood for potential transfusions. An

Table 3 Important clinical questions for assessing a patient with lower gastrointestinal bleeding. (Adapted from Triadafilopoulos 2012)

When did the bleeding start?
What is the duration?
Is this the first episode of bleeding or a recurrent event?
What is the stool color? Red (fresh blood), maroon (partly digested blood), or black (melena)?
Is blood coating the stool or mixed in it?
Is blood dripping after passing stools?
Are blood clots being passed?
Is there any tenesmus, perianal pain, or spasm?
Is the bleeding painless?
Is there any associated abdominal pain?
Has there been any vomiting of blood?
Has there been any chest pain, shortness of breath, loss of consciousness, or altered mental status?
Was there any colonic instrumentation (e.g., colonoscopy with polypectomy) within the past 30 days?
Are there any relevant previous surgeries (e.g., peptic ulcer surgery or abdominal aneurysm repair)?
Is the patient on NSAIDs, aspirin, anticoagulants, or antiplatelet agents?
Is there a history of chronic liver disease?
Is there a history of inflammatory bowel disease?
Is there a history of cardiovascular disease?

electrocardiogram should be performed to help evaluate for preexisting coronary artery disease and evidence of active ischemia.

Resuscitation

Volume resuscitation should include fluid administration via large-bore intravenous catheters. Blood transfusion is also frequently required. Age, bleeding rate, and the presence of comorbid conditions should inform the target hemoglobin concentration. Red blood cell transfusion is recommended for a hemoglobin level less than 7.0 g/dL (Barkun et al. 2010). Hemoglobin level should be maintained at or around 10 g/dL (hematocrit 30%) in elderly patients with coronary artery disease (Barnert and Messmann 2009). Maintaining an international normalized ratio (INR) below 1.8 is associated with lower mortality and fewer myocardial infarctions (Baradarian et al. 2004; Barkun et al. 2004).

Discontinuation of anticoagulants and vitamin K administration may also be required. All patients with significant bleeding should be considered for admission to the intensive care unit.

Assessment and Diagnostic Approach

Severe bleeding has been defined as bleeding requiring transfusion of two units of packed red blood cells and/or hematocrit decreasing by greater than 20% within 24 h of presentation (Strate and Syngal 2005). Strate and Syngal evaluated seven predictors of severity in acute lower gastrointestinal bleeding, including hypotension, tachycardia, syncope, nontender abdominal examination, bleeding within 4 h of presentation, aspirin use, and more than two comorbid diseases. Patients with more than three, one to three, and no risk factors were reported to have 84%, 43%, and 9% risk for severe bleeding, respectively (Strate et al. 2005). Velayos et al. prospectively evaluated patients admitted for acute lower gastrointestinal bleeding and reported that abnormal vital signs, gross blood on rectal examination, and initial hematocrit less than 35% were each predictors of severity (Velayos et al. 2004). The first UK national guidelines for acute lower gastrointestinal bleeding were recently released, and they represent the largest prospective study to date on this topic (Oakland et al. 2019). The guidelines include recommendations for diagnosis and management, including risk assessment. Patients with an Oakland score ≤8 without other indications for hospital admission were found to have a 95% probability for safe discharge with outpatient follow-up. The Oakland score was reportedly better able to predict safe discharge, blood transfusion, and readmission than were six other gastrointestinal bleeding scores, including the Rockall and Blatchford scores (Oakland et al. 2019; Rockall et al. 1996; Blatchford et al. 2000). However, it was not intended to predict the requirement for urgent intervention such as emergent colonoscopy and angiography, which is a major decision point in management.

There are several potential reasons why current prediction tools still have significant limitations

(Kosowicz and Strate 2019). Among them, lower gastrointestinal bleeding includes a range of conditions with variable potential for "severe bleeding," and bleeding itself may be intermittent. Clinical outcomes also have not been clearly and consistently defined across studies. A number of outcome measures are impacted by the process of care, which can vary significantly across institutions. Additionally, outcome measures such as length of stay and mortality can be influenced by comorbid conditions in addition to bleeding itself. Most predictive models were derived from small populations or large administrative datasets lacking generalizability and detailed patient level data, respectively. Kosowicz and Strate envision the optimal predictive model as being able to identify high-risk patients who would benefit from urgent intervention such as emergent colonoscopy and angiography versus those who can be safely managed in the outpatient setting (Kosowicz and Strate 2019). In addition, such a model would be easy to use, based on data available at the time of patient presentation, and able to predict clinically meaningful outcomes not significantly influenced by processes of care. Rather than developing numerous predictive models, they advocate focusing future studies on validating and fine-tuning the best existing models.

The 2016 American College of Gastroenterology (ACG) Clinical Guideline for Management of Patients with Acute Lower Gastrointestinal Bleeding provides recommendations for evaluation and management (Strate and Gralnek 2016). High-risk patients with alarming clinical features, hemodynamic instability, signs and symptoms of ongoing bleeding, or serious comorbid disease should be considered for intensive care unit admission. Hemodynamically unstable patients with hematochezia – especially those with history of cirrhosis – should be considered for urgent upper endoscopy to rule out upper gastrointestinal tract hemorrhage. Indeed, in one study, 15% of patients with hematochezia were found to have an upper gastrointestinal source of bleeding, a sizable proportion (Zuccaro 1998). While nasogastric lavage was previously recommended to support the identification of an upper gastrointestinal source of bleeding, more recent studies have

suggested that nasogastric lavage does not change primary outcomes and may not be as useful as previously believed (Rockey et al. 2017; Kessel et al. 2016; Huang et al. 2011).

Colonoscopy is the initial evaluation of choice for most high-risk patients and should be performed within 24 h of presentation following resuscitation, including blood product transfusion as indicated, and restoration of hemodynamic stability. High-risk patients with continued active bleeding and hemodynamic instability despite aggressive resuscitation may be unable to safely undergo colonoscopy and should be considered for radiographic localization of the bleeding source, followed by angiography or surgical consultation, which will be further discussed below. Low-risk patients with no or few high-risk clinical features, no serious comorbidities, hemodynamic stability, and no ongoing bleeding can often be monitored on a regular hospital floor. Colonoscopy remains the initial evaluation of choice for these patients.

Colonoscopy is able to examine the entire colon and terminal ileum to help localize and confirm the bleeding source. It can detect a definite source of bleeding in up to 90% of lower gastrointestinal bleeding cases and guide therapeutic intervention (Richter et al. 1995). Table 4 summarizes criteria for diagnosing a colonic source of bleeding.

In non-hemodynamically significant cases of small volume hematochezia, where history and physical examination suggest a distal colonic or anorectal source of bleeding, flexible sigmoidoscopy can be considered as opposed to a colonoscopy. Sigmoidoscopy may also be considered for evaluation of frail elderly patients if there is a need to avoid large-volume, oral colonic preparation, or

Table 4 Colonoscopic criteria for diagnosis of colonic hemorrhage. (Adapted from Triadafilopoulos 2012)

Active bleeding
Non-bleeding visible vessel
Sentinel clot overlying a lesion
Fresh bleeding localized in one colonic segment
Diverticular inflammation with surrounding fresh blood
Absence of blood in the terminal ileum with fresh blood in the colon

if colonoscopy is considered too risky. This can be an acceptable option if sigmoidoscopy is able to provide adequate endoscopic evaluation of the colonic mucosa proximal to the source of bleeding and there is no evidence for an alternative source of bleeding.

Endoscopic Therapy

There are multiple endoscopic options available to achieve hemostasis, including mechanical clips, bipolar circumactive probe (BICAP), heater probe, argon plasma coagulation, band ligation, acryl glue injection, epinephrine, and sclerosant injection. Table 5 summarizes these options.

Table 5 Available options for endoscopic control of bleeding. (Adapted from Pitchumoni and Dharmarajan 2012)

Procedure[a]	Comments
Injection of epinephrine/ sclerosing agents	Sclerosant agents such as polidocanol or ethanol are popularly used in the USA
Argon plasma coagulation	For noncontact coagulation. Ideal for lesions with large surface areas, i.e., watermelon stomach and portal hypertensive gastropathy
Clips	Provide mechanical hemostasis. Better than epinephrine injection or heater probe. Desirable in patients with coagulopathy, cirrhosis, and multi-system disease. Useful for ulcers, Dieulafoy's lesions, and post-polypectomy bleeds
Thermal coagulation Bipolar/heater probe	Applied directly to bleeding point
Band ligation	Effective for varices
Histoacryl glue injection	For acute bleeding and fundal varices; it is available in certain countries outside USA
TC-325 (Hemospray)	Inorganic powder, after contact with blood, forms a protecting gel providing adhesive mechanical barrier

[a]Option is chosen based on the lesion and *expertise of the endoscopist*. Procedures may be combined for better hemostasis

Special Considerations in Geriatric Patients

Upon deciding to pursue endoscopic evaluation of an older adult, special considerations are required to optimize safety.

Bowel Preparation

Thorough cleansing of the colon enables adequate endoscopic evaluation. Polyethylene glycol-based preparations are preferred because they do not induce significant absorption or excretion of ions across the intestinal mucosa and do not cause significant fluid and electrolyte shifts (Mamula et al. 2009; Pelham et al. 2008; Rothfuss et al. 2006). In contrast, magnesium and sodium phosphate-based products raise particular safety concerns because their hypertonicity can shift fluid and electrolyte balance, worsen renal function, and impair cardiac function, and many older adults are already vulnerable to such disturbances. These cleansing agents can cause hyperphosphatemia and hypermagnesemia in the setting of decreased glomerular filtrate rates, as well as medications altering intestinal phosphate absorption, water, or electrolyte balance, both of which are relatively common in the elderly. They may predispose to the development of acute phosphate nephropathy (Carl and Sica 2007). Careful attention should be directed toward reducing the risk of dehydration by maintaining adequate hydration.

Older adults experience higher rates of poor colonic preparations (between 16% and 21%), which is the single most important impediment to adequate colonoscopy (Lukens et al. 2002). This is often due to poor tolerance of high-volume oral preparations. Depending on procedural urgency, split dose preparation or placement of a nasogastric tube for expedited bowel cleansing may improve preparation quality. Given the higher rates of cognitive and functional limitations in the elderly, aspiration precautions should be taken during the preparation process. Tables 6 and 7 summarize potential adverse effects of osmotically active cleansing solutions as well as risk factors for acute phosphate nephropathy.

Table 6 Adverse effects of osmotically active cathartics. (From Pitchumoni and Dharmarajan 2012)

	Sodium phosphate	Magnesium citrate	Polyethylene glycol lavage
Hyponatremia	+	+	+
Hypokalemia	+		+
Hypocalcemia	+		
Hypernatremia	+		+
Hyperphosphatemia	+		
Hypermagnesemia		+	+
Other	Acute phosphate nephropathy, Aphthous ulcers (rectosigmoidal)		Allergic reactions, Aspiration

Table 7 Acute phosphate nephropathy risk factors. (Adapted from Pitchumoni and Dharmarajan 2012)

Age >60
Female
Medications
Angiotensin-converting-enzyme inhibitors
Angiotensin receptor blockers
Diuretics
NSAIDs
Comorbidities
Congestive heart failure
Chronic renal disease
Diabetes mellitus
Hypertension
Low body weight

Sedation Safety and Complications

While monitoring equipment during endoscopy is the same for all patients, sedation safety in the elderly requires awareness of increased sedation risks (Muravchick 2002). Physiologic responses to hypoxia or hypercarbia tend to be blunted and delayed in the geriatric population (Shaker et al. 2003). Reduced hepatic and renal clearance functions alongside expansion of distribution volume for lipid-soluble sedatives from age-related increase in lipid fraction of body mass can produce deeper respiratory depression, increased risk of aspiration, and need for prolonged recovery after sedation. Closer and continuous monitoring as well as administration of sedation at a slower rate with lower initial and total doses is therefore recommended (Darling 1997). Most colonoscopy cases are performed under moderate sedation, but

patients considered high-risk should undergo evaluation for anesthesia support.

Although colonoscopy is generally considered safe in the elderly, advanced age (>80 years of age) is a risk factor for serious procedure-related adverse events, including perforation, gastrointestinal bleeding, and need for blood transfusion (Warren et al. 2009; Arora et al. 2009). Patients of advanced age experience higher rates of cumulative gastrointestinal adverse events (34.9 per 1000 colonoscopies, incidence rate ratio 1.7) and higher risk of perforation (1.5 per 1000 colonoscopies, incidence rate ratio 1.6), when compared with younger patients (Day et al. 2011). Altogether, the risks associated with colonoscopy in elderly patients should be discussed and considered in partnership with patients, family members, and other care team members to determine whether they outweigh the potential benefits of a procedure.

Anticoagulation Management

As discussed above, the use of anticoagulant and antiplatelet (APA) therapy is more prevalent in the elderly. The use of these medications can be associated with postprocedural bleeding, though these risks vary depending on the procedure performed (Anderson et al. 2009). When deciding how to manage antithrombotic agents, the patient's risk for a thromboembolic event (VTE) should be weighed alongside the urgency of the planned procedure. Upper endoscopy, colonoscopy, and flexible sigmoidoscopy performed for diagnosing and treating gastrointestinal bleeding are considered low-risk procedures, even with mucosal biopsy samples taken, and thus when these procedures are performed in an elective setting, anticoagulants and APAs can generally be continued up to the procedure.

In the setting of urgent and emergent endoscopic procedures, especially for patients presenting with serious acute gastrointestinal bleeding, however, American Society for Gastrointestinal Endoscopy Guidelines recommend holding anticoagulant therapy to facilitate hemostasis (Acosta et al. 2016). While reversal agents for warfarin anticoagulant therapy including four-factor prothrombin complex concentrate and vitamin K or fresh-frozen plasma can be given for life-threatening bleeding, endoscopic therapy should not be delayed for serious bleeding in patients on antithrombotic therapy with an INR <2.5. Most endoscopic interventions for hemostasis can still be performed in the setting of ongoing antiplatelet agent use, and current multidisciplinary consensus statements recommend reinitiating APAs as soon as hemostasis is achieved (Becker et al. 2009; Bhatt et al. 2008). In patients with life-threatening bleeding, multidisciplinary discussions should be conducted to consider how to balance the risks of rebleeding with those from thrombotic events. In cases in which incidental lesions (such as larger polyps) are discovered during endoscopy, and a follow-up elective procedure such as colonoscopy with polypectomy with higher-risk for bleeding is recommended, the procedure can be deferred until the patient is able to undergo safe cessation of the antithrombotic agent. For patients on APAs, consultation with the prescribing specialists should be performed before discontinuing these agents to confirm the risk of adverse cardiac events, especially in patients with drug-eluting stents placed within the past year, bare- metal stents placed within 30 days, or acute coronary syndrome within 90 days. The recommendations for management of antithrombotic agents in the elective endoscopic setting should be made in consultation with the prescribing physician and endoscopist.

Non-endoscopic Management

When the source of lower gastrointestinal bleeding cannot be diagnosed and/or treated with endoscopic interventions or if a patient is too hemodynamically unstable to prepare for and undergo a colonoscopic evaluation, alternative diagnostic and therapeutic options must be considered.

Angiography

Angiography can localize a bleeding site with an arterial bleeding rate of at least 0.5 ml/min (Scheffel et al. 2007). In this small subset of patients, angiography can localize a lower gastrointestinal bleeding source in 25–70% of exams and also provide immediate hemostasis in 40–100% of cases of diverticular bleeding (Yi et al. 2013; Khanna et al. 2005). Major adverse events typically involve vascular injuries and include bowel infarction, transient ischemic attacks, and hematomas, as well as contrast reactions, and nephrotoxicity, which may occur in up to 17% of patients who undergo angiography (Strate and Naumann 2010).

If a diagnostic test for localization is desired prior to angiography, multidetector row CT scanning is now recommended as first-line imaging over nuclear red blood cell scintigraphy, which involves the injection of technetium into the patient's bloodstream, due to decreased scanning time and more accurate arterial images with contrast material extravasation (Zink et al. 2008; Strate and Gralnek 2016). Red blood cell scintigraphy can be helpful, however, in identifying slower-bleeding lesions, such as angioectasias which are more difficult to treat with angiography and embolization, as these scans are able to detect arterial bleeding rates as low as 0.04 mL/min (Zuckier 2003).

Surgery

Surgery is now rarely required and is reserved for the minority of patients experiencing persistent or refractory gastrointestinal bleeding or those in which other diagnostic and therapeutic options have failed. Surgical consultation should be considered in patients experiencing persistent bleeding with transfusion of six or more units of packed red blood cells (Bokhari et al. 1996). It is important, however, to carefully localize the source of bleeding whenever possible before surgical resection, because while the rebleeding rate is higher in patients after segmental resection compared with total colectomy (18% vs 4%), limited colonic resection is associated with a lower mortality rate (Farner et al. 1999; Vernava et al. 1997).

Balloon Tamponade

Balloon tamponade has rarely been utilized for lower gastrointestinal hemorrhage, but there are a few cases in the literature, including a recent case report by emergency medicine physicians in which an elderly man presented late in the evening with profuse rectal bleeding of unclear source (Neeki et al. 2019). Gastroenterology and interventional radiology teams were not available in-house. Anoscopy was not feasible due to heavy bleeding. Manual application of intrarectal pressure and Foley balloon application were not successful. With other options exhausted, a Minnesota tube was subsequently deployed transrectally and able to achieve adequate hemostasis. Flexible sigmoidoscopy the next morning revealed a circumferential, ulcerated mucosa at the dentate line that was subsequently cauterized. In summary, in emergent cases of acute onset lower gastrointestinal hemorrhage for which access to specialty intervention is not available, balloon tamponade may provide another option to control bleeding until definitive therapy can be delivered.

Causes of Lower Gastrointestinal Bleeding

Diverticulosis

Diverticulosis is an age-related disease. The prevalence increases by age, from less than 5% at age 40–65% by age 85 (Painter and Burkitt 1975).

Most patients with diverticulosis are asymptomatic, but an estimated 3–5% of patients develop acute bleeding (Painter and Burkitt 1975). Even though bleeding is relatively uncommon, the high prevalence of diverticulosis in the geriatric population explains why it is the single most common cause of lower gastrointestinal bleeding in this population, accounting for 33% of episodes (Strate et al. 2008). Risk factors for bleeding include a low fiber diet, regular aspirin or NSAID use, and constipation (Bjarnason and Macpherson 1994; Wilcox et al. 1997). Approximately 50–90% of cases originate from the right colon and occur without associated diverticulitis (Meyers et al. 1976).

Other than potential mild abdominal cramping from intraluminal blood-induced colonic spasm, bleeding is usually painless and stops spontaneously more than 80% of the time. It has been estimated that less than 1% of patients require more than four units of blood transfusion (McGuire 1994). However, because the bleeding source is arterial, some episodes can involve large volume blood loss and hemodynamic compromise. The mortality rate among older patients is approximately 4% (Alvarez et al. 2007). Rebleeding is relatively common and estimated to occur in 18–38% of cases after spontaneous cessation (Jensen 2005; Elta 2004) (Fig. 2).

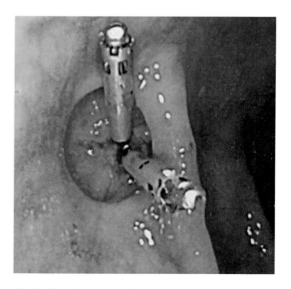

Fig. 2 Diverticular bleeding post clipping

Rapid bowel purge followed by timely colonoscopy can enable identification of the culprit bleeding diverticulum. Hemostasis can be achieved utilizing epinephrine injection, hemostatic clips, bipolar probe coagulation, band ligation, and fibrous glue (Jensen et al. 2000; Farrell et al. 2003). A recently published study from Japan suggested that use of a new hemostasis technique with endoscopic detachable snare ligation (EDSL) might be superior to conventional endoscopic clipping for colonic diverticular hemorrhage, but the study was small and performed at a single center (Kobayashi et al. 2019). Further research is required.

If the diverticular bleeding source cannot be identified or if bleeding is persistent, angiographic intervention with bleeding vessel embolization usually achieves hemostasis (Kuo et al. 2003; Funaki et al. 2001; Defreyne et al. 2001). However, given the risk of post-embolization infarction, angiographic intervention generally is not considered the first choice therapy for patients who are clinically stable.

Vascular Ectasias

Vascular ectasias (or angiodysplasia) are dilated, distorted, and tortuous veins, venules, and capillaries, mostly lined only by endothelium and occasionally a small amount of smooth muscle (Boley et al. 1977; Reinus and Brandt 1994). Endoscopically, they appear as peripherally expanding capillaries with a central origin, single or multiple, and of variable diameter, usually between 0.1 and 1.0 cm. They may develop anywhere in the gastrointestinal tract including throughout the colon. Bleeding colonic vascular ectasias are typically cecal or right colonic lesions (Diggs et al. 2011).

Because bleeding is from a venous origin, it is usually less severe than diverticular bleeding, though significant hemorrhage has been reported to occur in 15% of patients (Trivedi and Pitchumoni 2006). Overt bleeding can present as painless, recurrent, self-limited melena, or hematochezia but is more often chronic and occult, with consequent stool occult blood

positivity and iron deficiency anemia. As with diverticular disease, the incidence and bleeding risk increase with age. Additional conditions that have been associated with vascular ectasias include aortic stenosis, chronic renal failure, and von Willebrand disease (Boley et al. 1977).

Colonoscopic evaluation should thoroughly and carefully examine the colonic mucosa without causing traumatic suction injury which may be confused for culprit ectasias. Endoscopists can also miss vascular ectasias if they are small in size or if patients are volume depleted. Hemostasis can be achieved with argon laser coagulation, heater or bipolar probe, and injection sclerotherapy, but rebleeding can occur. Embolization or partial colectomy may be considered in cases of emergent hemorrhage.

Colitis

Colitis is the common response to acute mucosal injury and subsequent activation of the inflammatory cascade. The initial clinical presentation and clinical findings of ischemic, infectious, and inflammatory colitis may not be distinguishable, but ischemic and infectious etiologies are more common among older adults. Presentation may include bloody stools, diarrhea, abdominal pain, fever, dehydration, and hemodynamic compromise. Severe hemorrhage is unusual. Endoscopically, the mucosal appearance may be nonspecific, appearing edematous, pale, dark, or erythematous, friable, and ulcerated, in either a segmental or focal distribution. The clinical context should therefore be carefully interpreted, and biopsies should be obtained for histopathologic diagnosis.

Ischemic Colitis

Ischemic colitis accounts for an estimated 3–9% of lower gastrointestinal bleeding cases (Longstreth 1997; Bramley et al. 1996). Elderly patients are at higher risk for ischemic colitis due to atherosclerotic disease, heart failure, arrhythmias, blood pressure fluctuations, embolic events,

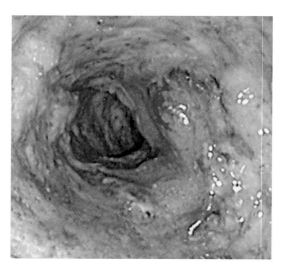

Fig. 3 Segmental ischemic colitis

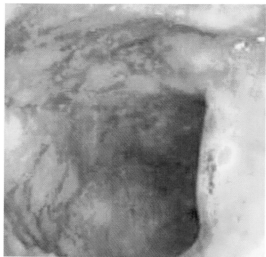

Fig. 4 *Clostridium difficile* pseudomembranous colitis

and treatment with digoxin or aspirin (Cubiella Fernández et al. 2010). Patients often experience crampy abdominal pain followed by passage of bloody stools. The watershed areas of the splenic flexure, right colon, and rectosigmoid junction are commonly involved. Colonoscopy often reveals continuous and segmental involvement and may include a clear demarcation between normal and involved mucosa, consistent with compromise of a specific vascular territory. Biopsies typically reveal necrosis without significant acute or chronic inflammation. Management usually consists of supportive care and underlying risk factor modification. Most cases self-resolve, but some severe cases can be complicated by perforation or stricture formation (Fig. 3).

Infectious Colitis

Common sources of infectious colitis include *Campylobacter*, *Salmonella*, *Shigella*, *Escherichia coli O157:H7*, and *Clostridium difficile*. *Clostridium difficile* infection causes hematochezia in less than 10% of cases (Slotwiner-Nie and Brandt 2001). Older patients are at higher risk for infectious colitis, particularly *Clostridium difficile* infection in the setting of recent antibiotic therapy, hospitalization, intensive care unit admission, tube feeding, or

residence in a long-term care facility. They are also at higher risk for complications such as thrombocytopenic purpura from *E. Coli O157: H7*, and mortality increases with age (Slotwiner-Nie and Brandt 2001; Lew et al. 1991; Garthright et al. 1988) (Fig. 4).

Most causative organisms can be identified by stool culture or polymerase chain reaction (PCR), while *Clostridium difficile* infection is typically diagnosed via a specialized stool test for *Clostridium difficile* toxins or genes. Treatment consists of supportive care including volume repletion and electrolyte replacement, alongside specific antimicrobial therapy. Treatment options for *Clostridium difficile* infection include vancomycin, metronidazole, fidaxomicin, and fecal microbiota transplantation. It should be noted that metronidazole may interfere with warfarin metabolism and increase bleeding risk (further details provided in chapter on *C. difficile* colitis).

Inflammatory Bowel Disease

Approximately 15% of patients with inflammatory bowel disease experience onset of symptoms after age 65 (Robertson and Grimm 2001). Crohn's disease and ulcerative colitis may each present with bleeding, but hematochezia is a more

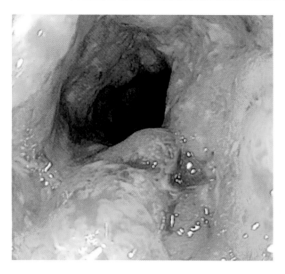

Fig. 5 Crohn's colitis

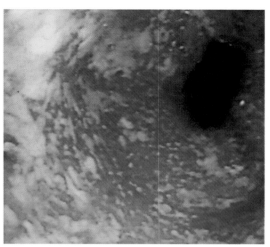

Fig. 6 Ulcerative colitis

common initial presentation in the latter, and severe bleeding is uncommon. Both conditions are typically accompanied by further evidence of active inflammation such as leukocytosis and elevated erythrocyte sedimentation rate as well as C-reactive protein. Endoscopic differentiation between inflammatory bowel disease and ischemic colitis may be a challenge, but imperative, given the distinct management required. Features more consistent with ischemia include history of the risk factors reviewed earlier such as cardiovascular disease, arrhythmias, hypotensive episodes, and embolic events, accompanying segmental colitis – possibly involving a watershed area – and dark mucosal discoloration. Biopsies should be obtained to help confirm the diagnosis. The general management principles for Crohn's disease and ulcerative colitis still apply to the older population (Figs. 5 and 6).

Neoplasms

Bleeding from colon cancer or colonic polyps is relatively uncommon, accounting for 5–11% and 2–8% of acute lower gastrointestinal bleeding cases, respectively (Zuckerman and Prakash 1999; Farrell and Friedman 2005). Bleeding is the presenting symptom of approximately 2–26% of neoplasms (Richter et al. 1995; Peura et al. 1997). Bleeding is more frequently occult but can also present as recurrent slow overt bleeding. The source may be an erosion or ulceration of the neoplasm, which can be further aggravated by antiplatelet or anticoagulant medications. Left-sided malignancies classically present with bright red blood per rectum, while more proximal lesions present with maroon colored blood or even melena. Colonoscopy with biopsy should be performed to confirm the presence of malignancy, and to rule out synchronous lesions, and ensure there are no additional sources of bleeding (Fig. 7).

Endoscopic interventions are limited due to the friability and frequently diffuse distribution of lesions, as well as risk of perforation. Endoscopic application of TC-325 (Hemospray), an inorganic powder for diffuse bleeding sources such as colon cancer, has been described and is currently the only such spray available for use in the USA, though it is not yet widely available (Soulellis et al. 2013; Saltzman 2019). After contact with blood, the powder absorbs water and forms a protecting gel serving as an adhesive mechanical barrier covering the bleeding site. The mineral material within the spray is able to absorb fluid 30–40 times its dry weight, leading to hemostasis (Saltzman 2019). A recent study also reported that TC-325 was safe and effective at achieving

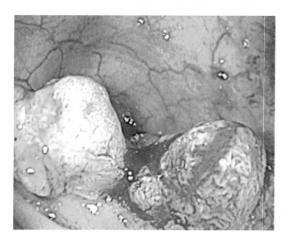

Fig. 7 Sigmoid colon cancer

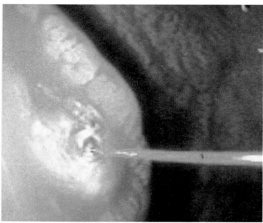

Fig. 8 Actively bleeding rectal ulcer

hemostasis of nonvariceal lower gastrointestinal bleeding from a variety sources, particularly post-polypectomy hemorrhage (Hookey et al. 2019). The powder was effective as monotherapy, part of combination therapy, or as a rescue approach.

Anorectal Sources

Hemorrhoids are frequently asymptomatic but are the second most common cause of hematochezia, accounting for 10–20% of lower gastrointestinal bleeding episodes (Strate et al. 2008; Jensen 2005). Hemorrhoidal bleeding classically presents as painless, intermittent passage of low-volume bright red blood-coated stools, dripping into the toilet, or staining toilet paper but can also present with pruritis or thrombosis. Bleeding is rarely significant. Though common, the source of bleeding in elderly patients should generally be confirmed with endoscopic examination to rule out bleeding from malignancy or other serious pathology. Treatment with fiber supplementation, stool softeners, sitz baths, and suppositories is usually sufficient. Persistent, significant bleeding can be treated with endoscopic or surgical intervention (Fig. 8).

Stercoral and solitary rectal ulcers are typically found in patients with a history of chronic constipation. Anal fissures may cause episodic rectal bleeding but present with severe, sharp anal pain during defecation. Treatment may consist of stool softeners, topical calcium channel blockers, fiber supplementation, and sitz baths.

Post-polypectomy Bleeding

Delayed, painless bleeding following polypectomy may occur up to 3 weeks following polyp removal, possibly due to sloughing of the coagulated eschar. It is typically self-limited, but some cases of active arterial bleeding can present acutely with life-threatening large volume hemorrhage. Patients experiencing significant blood loss after a recent colonoscopy with polypectomy should be hospitalized and undergo rapid colonic lavage followed by urgent colonoscopy to confirm the bleeding site and achieve hemostasis (Fig. 9).

Radiation Proctitis

Radiation therapy is commonly part of the treatment regimen for urologic, gynecologic, and anorectal malignancies. Radiation proctitis can present with rectal bleeding that is rarely hemodynamically significant, as well as urgency, tenesmus, and diarrhea. Acute radiation injury occurs within 6 weeks of radiation exposure. Chronic

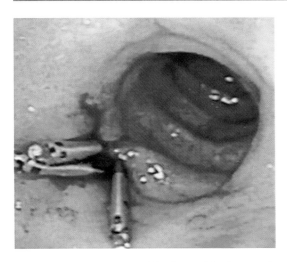

Fig. 9 Post-polypectomy bleeding with hemostasis achieved by clipping

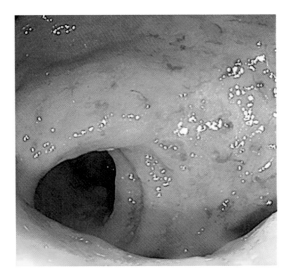

Fig. 10 Radiation proctitis

radiation proctitis affects an estimated 5–20% of patients (Vanneste et al. 2015), often occurring 9–14 months after radiation therapy. In some patients, onset may occur a few years after initial radiation exposure and rarely up to 30 years afterward. Treatment usually consists of medical therapies including sucralfate enemas and endoscopic thermal interventions such as application of argon plasma coagulation to the affected area, which may require multiple treatments (Fig. 10).

Key Points

- Lower gastrointestinal bleeding is a common and growing challenge in the older population. The clinical and economic burden appears to be increasing.
- Multiple comorbidities among older patients as well as use of NSAIDs, anticoagulant, and antiplatelet medications increase the risk of clinically significant bleeding.
- Colonoscopy is the initial evaluation of choice for most patients who are hemodynamically stable and able to tolerate bowel preparation.
- Although colonoscopy is generally considered safe in the older age group, advanced age is a risk factor for sedation and endoscopic-related adverse events. The potential risks and benefits associated with colonoscopy should be discussed and considered in partnership with patients, family members, and other care providers.
- Lower gastrointestinal bleeding in geriatric patients is most commonly caused by diverticular disease, vascular ectasias, colitis, anorectal sources, and malignancies.

References

Acosta RD, Abraham NS, Chandrasekhara V, Chathadi KV, Early DS, Eloubeidi MA, Evans JA, Faulx AL, Fisher DA, Fonkalsrud L, Hwang JH, Khashab MA, Lightdale JR, Muthusamy VR, Pasha SF, Saltzman JR, Shaukat A, Shergill AK, Wang A, Cash BD, Dewitt JM, Committee, A. S. O. P. The management of antithrombotic agents for patients undergoing GI endoscopy. Gastrointest Endosc. 2016;83:3–16.

Alvarez JA, Baldonedo RF, Bear IG, Otero J, Pire G, Alvarez P, Jorge JI. Presentation, management and outcome of acute sigmoid diverticulitis requiring hospitalization. Dig Surg. 2007;24:471–6.

Anderson MA, Ben-Menachem T, Gan SI, Appalaneni V, Banerjee S, Cash BD, Fisher L, Harrison ME, Fanelli RD, Fukami N, Ikenberry SO, Jain R, Khan K, Krinsky ML, Lichtenstein DR, Maple JT, Shen B, Strohmeyer L, Baron T, Dominitz JA, Committee, A. S. O. P. Management of antithrombotic agents for endoscopic procedures. Gastrointest Endosc. 2009;70: 1060–70.

Arora G, Mannalithara A, Singh G, Gerson LB, Triadafilopoulos G. Risk of perforation from a colonoscopy in adults: a large population-based study. Gastrointest Endosc. 2009;69:654–64.

Baradarian R, Ramdhaney S, Chapalamadugu R, Skoczylas L, Wang K, Rivilis S, Remus K, Mayer I, Iswara K, Tenner S. Early intensive resuscitation of patients with upper gastrointestinal bleeding decreases mortality. Am J Gastroenterol. 2004;99:619–22.

Barkun A, Sabbah S, Enns R, Armstrong D, Gregor J, Fedorak RN, Rahme E, Toubouti Y, Martel M, Chiba N, Fallone CA, Investigators, R. The Canadian registry on nonvariceal upper gastrointestinal bleeding and endoscopy (RUGBE): endoscopic hemostasis and proton pump inhibition are associated with improved outcomes in a real-life setting. Am J Gastroenterol. 2004;99:1238–46.

Barkun AN, Bardou M, Kuipers EJ, Sung J, Hunt RH, Martel M, Sinclair P, Group, I. C. U. G. B. C. International consensus recommendations on the management of patients with nonvariceal upper gastrointestinal bleeding. Ann Intern Med. 2010;152:101–13.

Barnert J, Messmann H. Diagnosis and management of lower gastrointestinal bleeding. Nat Rev Gastroenterol Hepatol. 2009;6:637–46.

Becker RC, Scheiman J, Dauerman HL, Spencer F, Rao S, Sabatine M, Johnson DA, Chan F, Abraham NS, Quigley EM, Gastroenterology, A. C. O. C. A. T. A. C. O. Management of platelet-directed pharmacotherapy in patients with atherosclerotic coronary artery disease undergoing elective endoscopic gastrointestinal procedures. Am J Gastroenterol. 2009;104:2903–17.

Bhatt DL, Scheiman J, Abraham NS, Antman EM, Chan FK, Furberg CD, Johnson DA, Mahaffey KW, Quigley EM, Harrington RA, Bates ER, Bridges CR, Eisenberg MJ, Ferrari VA, Hlatky MA, Kaul S, Lindner JR, Moliterno DJ, Mukherjee D, Schofield RS, Rosenson RS, Stein JH, Weitz HH, Wesley DJ, Foundation, A. C. O. C, Gastroenterology, A. C. O, Association, A. H. ACCF/ACG/AHA 2008 expert consensus document on reducing the gastrointestinal risks of antiplatelet therapy and NSAID use. Am J Gastroenterol. 2008;103:2890–907.

Bjarnason I, Macpherson AJ. Intestinal toxicity of nonsteroidal anti-inflammatory drugs. Pharmacol Ther. 1994;62:145–57.

Bjarnason I, Hayllar J, Macpherson AJ, Russell AS. Side effects of nonsteroidal anti- inflammatory drugs on the small and large intestine in humans. Gastroenterology. 1993;104:1832–47.

Blatchford O, Murray WR, Blatchford M. A risk score to predict need for treatment for upper gastrointestinal haemorrhage. Lancet. 2000;356:1318–21.

Bokhari M, Vernava AM, Ure T, Longo WE. Diverticular hemorrhage in the elderly–is it well tolerated? Dis Colon Rectum. 1996;39:191–5.

Boley SJ, Sprayregen S, Sammartano RJ, Adams A, Kleinhaus S. The pathophysiologic basis for the angiographic signs of vascular ectasias of the colon. Radiology. 1977;125:615–21.

Boley SJ, Dibiase A, Brandt LJ, Sammartano RJ. Lower intestinal bleeding in the elderly. Am J Surg. 1979;137:57–64.

Bramley PN, Masson JW, McKnight G, Herd K, Fraser A, Park K, Brunt PW, Mckinlay A, Sinclair TS, Mowat NA. The role of an open-access bleeding unit in the management of colonic haemorrhage. A 2-year prospective study. Scand J Gastroenterol. 1996;31:764–9.

Brandt LJ, Boley SJ, Mitsudo S. Clinical characteristics and natural history of colitis in the elderly. Am J Gastroenterol. 1982;77:382–6.

Browder W, Cerise EJ, Litwin MS. Impact of emergency angiography in massive lower gastrointestinal bleeding. Ann Surg. 1986;204:530–6.

Carl DE, Sica DA. Acute phosphate nephropathy following colonoscopy preparation. Am J Med Sci. 2007;334: 151–4.

Cea Soriano L, Lanas A, Soriano-Gabarró M, García Rodríguez LA. Incidence of upper and lower gastrointestinal bleeding in new users of low-dose aspirin. Clin Gastroenterol Hepatol. 2019;17(5):887–95.

Chan FK, Leung Ki EL, Wong GL, Ching JY, Tse YK, Au KW, Wu JC, Ng SC. Risks of bleeding recurrence and cardiovascular events with continued aspirin use after lower gastrointestinal hemorrhage. Gastroenterology. 2016;151:271–7.

Comay D, Marshall JK. Resource utilization for acute lower gastrointestinal hemorrhage: the Ontario GI Bleed study. Can J Gastroenterol. 2002;16:677–82.

Cubiella Fernández J, Núñez Calvo L, González Vázquez E, García García MJ, Alves Pérez MT, Martínez Silva I, Fernández Seara J. Risk factors associated with the development of ischemic colitis. World J Gastroenterol. 2010;16:4564–9.

Darling E. Practical considerations in sedating the elderly. Crit Care Nurs Clin N Am. 1997;9:371–80.

Day LW, Kwon A, Inadomi JM, Walter LC, Somsouk M. Adverse events in older patients undergoing colonoscopy: a systematic review and meta-analysis. Gastrointest Endosc. 2011;74:885–96.

Defreyne L, Vanlangenhove P, De Vos M, Pattyn P, Van Maele G, Decruyenaere J, Troisi R, Kunnen M. Embolization as a first approach with endoscopically unmanageable acute nonvariceal gastrointestinal hemorrhage. Radiology. 2001;218:739–48.

Diggs NG, Holub JL, Lieberman DA, Eisen GM, Strate LL. Factors that contribute to blood loss in patients with colonic angiodysplasia from a population-based study. Clin Gastroenterol Hepatol. 2011;9:415–20; quiz e49.

Eisen GM, Dominitz JA, Faigel DO, Goldstein JL, Kalloo AN, Petersen BT, Raddawi HM, Ryan ME, Vargo JJ, Young HS, Fanelli RD, Hyman NH, Wheeler-Harbaugh J, Committee, A. S. F. G. E. S. O. P. An annotated algorithmic approach to acute lower gastrointestinal bleeding. Gastrointest Endosc. 2001;53:859–63.

Ell C, May A. Mid-gastrointestinal bleeding: capsule endoscopy and push-and-pull enteroscopy give rise to a new medical term. Endoscopy. 2006;38:73–5.

Elta GH. Urgent colonoscopy for acute lower-GI bleeding. Gastrointest Endosc. 2004;59:402–8.

Farner R, Lichliter W, Kuhn J, Fisher T. Total colectomy versus limited colonic resection for acute lower gastrointestinal bleeding. Am J Surg. 1999;178:587–91.

Farrell JJ, Friedman LS. Gastrointestinal bleeding in older people. Gastroenterol Clin North Am. 2000;29:1–36, v.

Farrell JJ, Friedman LS. Review article: the management of lower gastrointestinal bleeding. Aliment Pharmacol Ther. 2005;21:1281–98.

Farrell JJ, Graeme-Cook F, Kelsey PB. Treatment of bleeding colonic diverticula by endoscopic band ligation: an in-vivo and ex-vivo pilot study. Endoscopy. 2003;35:823–9.

Feagins LA, Weideman RA. GI bleeding risk of DOACs versus warfarin: is newer better? Dig Dis Sci. 2018;63:1675–7.

Funaki B, Kostelic JK, Lorenz J, Ha TV, Yip DL, Rosenblum JD, Leef JA, Straus C, Zaleski GX. Superselective microcoil embolization of colonic hemorrhage. AJR Am J Roentgenol. 2001;177:829–36.

Garthright WE, Archer DL, Kvenberg JE. Estimates of incidence and costs of intestinal infectious diseases in the United States. Public Health Rep. 1988;103:107–15.

Gerson LB, Fidler JL, Cave DR, Leighton JA. ACG clinical guideline: diagnosis and management of small bowel bleeding. Am J Gastroenterol. 2015;110:1265–87; quiz 1288.

Granger CB, Alexander JH, McMurray JJ, Lopes RD, Hylek EM, Hanna M, Al-Khalidi HR, Ansell J, Atar D, Avezum A, Bahit MC, Diaz R, Easton JD, Ezekowitz JA, Flaker G, GarcIA D, Geraldes M, Gersh BJ, Golitsyn S, Goto S, Hermosillo AG, Hohnloser SH, Horowitz J, Mohan P, Jansky P, Lewis BS, Lopez-Sendon JL, Pais P, Parkhomenko A, Verheugt FW, Zhu J, Wallentin L, Investigators, A. C. A. Apixaban versus warfarin in patients with atrial fibrillation. N Engl J Med. 2011;365:981–92.

Hookey L, Barkun A, Sultanian R, Bailey R. Successful hemostasis of active lower GI bleeding using a hemostatic powder as monotherapy, combination therapy, or rescue therapy. Gastrointest Endosc. 2019;89:865–71.

Huang ES, Karsan S, Kanwal F, Singh I, Makhani M, Spiegel BM. Impact of asogastric lavage on outcomes in acute GI bleeding. Gastrointest Endosc. 2011;74:971–80.

Jensen DM. Management of patients with severe hematochezia–with all current evidence available. Am J Gastroenterol. 2005;100:2403–6.

Jensen DM, Machicado GA, Jutabha R, Kovacs TO. Urgent colonoscopy for the diagnosis and treatment of severe diverticular hemorrhage. N Engl J Med. 2000;342:78–82.

Kanwal F, Dulai G, Jensen DM, Gralnek IM, Kovacs TO, Machicado GA, Jutabha R. Major stigmata of recent hemorrhage on rectal ulcers in patients with severe hematochezia: endoscopic diagnosis, treatment, and outcomes. Gastrointest Endosc. 2003;57:462–8.

Kessel B, Olsha O, Younis A, Daskal Y, Granovsky E, Alfici R. Evaluation of nasogastric tubes to enable differentiation between upper and lower gastrointestinal bleeding in unselected patients with melena. Eur J Emerg Med. 2016;23:71–3.

Khanna A, Ognibene SJ, Koniaris LG. Embolization as first-line therapy for diverticulosis-related massive lower gastrointestinal bleeding: evidence from a meta-analysis. J Gastrointest Surg. 2005;9:343–52.

Kobayashi K, Furumoto Y, Akutsu D, Matsuoka M, Nozaka T, Asano T, Fujiki K, Gosho M, Narasaka T, Mizokami Y. Endoscopic detachable snare ligation improves the treatment for colonic diverticular hemorrhage. Digestion. 2019;6:1–9.

Kosowicz RL, Strate LL. Predicting outcomes in lower gastrointestinal bleeding: more work ahead. Gastrointest Endosc. 2019;89(5):1014–6.

Kuo WT, Lee DE, Saad WE, Patel N, Sahler LG, Waldman DL. Superselective microcoil embolization for the treatment of lower gastrointestinal hemorrhage. J Vasc Interv Radiol. 2003;14:1503–9.

Laine L, Connors LG, Reicin A, Hawkey CJ, Burgos-Vargas R, Schnitzer TJ, Yu Q, Bombardier C. Serious lower gastrointestinal clinical events with nonselective Nsaid or coxib use. Gastroenterology. 2003;124:288–92.

Lanas A, Sekar MC, Hirschowitz BI. Objective evidence of aspirin use in both ulcer and nonulcer upper and lower gastrointestinal bleeding. Gastroenterology. 1992;103:862–9.

Lanas A, García-Rodríguez LA, Polo-Tomás M, Ponce M, Alonso-Abreu I, Perez-Aisa MA, Perez-Gisbert J, Bujanda L, Castro M, Muñoz M, Rodrigo L, Calvet X, Del-Pino D, Garcia S. Time trends and impact of upper and lower gastrointestinal bleeding and perforation in clinical practice. Am J Gastroenterol. 2009;104:1633–41.

Leitman IM, Paull DE, Shires GT. Evaluation and management of massive lower gastrointestinal hemorrhage. Ann Surg. 1989;209:175–80.

Levy R, Barto W, Gani J. Retrospective study of the utility of nuclear scintigraphic-labelled red cell scanning for lower gastrointestinal bleeding. ANZ J Surg. 2003;73:205–9.

Lew JF, Glass RI, Gangarosa RE, Cohen IP, Bern C, Moe CL. Diarrheal deaths in the United States, 1979 through 1987. A special problem for the elderly. JAMA. 1991;265:3280–4.

Lin CK, Liang CC, Chang HT, Hung FM, Lee TH. Acute hemorrhagic rectal ulcer: an important cause of lower gastrointestinal bleeding in the critically ill patients. Dig Dis Sci. 2011;56:3631–7.

Longstreth GF. Epidemiology and outcome of patients hospitalized with acute lower gastrointestinal hemorrhage: a population-based study. Am J Gastroenterol. 1997;92:419–24.

Lukens FJ, Loeb DS, Machicao VI, Achem SR, Picco MF. Colonoscopy in octogenarians: a prospective outpatient study. Am J Gastroenterol. 2002;97:1722–5.

Mamula P, Adler DG, Conway JD, Diehl DL, Farraye FA, Kantsevoy SV, Kaul V, Kethu SR, Kwon RS, Rodriguez SA, Tierney WM, Committee, A. T.

Colonoscopy preparation. Gastrointest Endosc. 2009;69:1201–9.

Matuk R, Crawford J, Abreu MT, Targan SR, Vasiliauskas EA, Papadakis KA. The spectrum of gastrointestinal toxicity and effect on disease activity of selective cyclooxygenase-2 inhibitors in patients with inflammatory bowel disease. Inflamm Bowel Dis. 2004;10:352–6.

McGuire HH. Bleeding colonic diverticula. A reappraisal of natural history and management. Ann Surg. 1994;220:653–6.

Meyers MA, Alonso DR, Gray GF, Baer JW. Pathogenesis of bleeding colonic diverticulosis. Gastroenterology. 1976;71:577–83.

Muravchick S. The elderly outpatient: current anesthetic implications. Curr Opin Anaesthesiol. 2002;15: 621–5.

Neeki MM, Raj V, Archambeau B, Arabian S, Hussain F. Novel application of balloon tamponade in management of acute lower gastrointestinal hemorrhage. Clin Pract Cases Emerg Med. 2019;3:243–7.

Oakland K, Chadwick G, East JE, Guy R, Humphries A, Jairath V, Mcpherson S, Metzner M, Morris AJ, Murphy MF, Tham T, Uberoi R, Veitch AM, Wheeler J, Regan C, Hoare J. Diagnosis and management of acute lower gastrointestinal bleeding: guidelines from the British Society of Gastroenterology. Gut. 2019;68:776–89.

Painter NS, Burkitt DP. Diverticular disease of the colon, a 20th century problem. Clin Gastroenterol. 1975;4: 3–21.

Patrono C. Aspirin as an antiplatelet drug. N Engl J Med. 1994;330:1287–94.

Peery AF, Crockett SD, Barritt AS, Dellon ES, Eluri S, Gangarosa LM, Jensen ET, Lund JL, Pasricha S, Runge T, Schmidt M, Shaheen NJ, Sandler RS. Burden of gastrointestinal, liver, and pancreatic diseases in the United States. Gastroenterology. 2015;149: 1731–1741.e3.

Pelham RW, Nix LC, Chavira RE, Cleveland MV, Stetson P. Clinical trial: single- and multiple-dose pharmacokinetics of polyethylene glycol (Peg-3350) in healthy young and elderly subjects. Aliment Pharmacol Ther. 2008;28:256–65.

Peura DA, Lanza FL, Gostout CJ, Foutch PG. The American College of Gastroenterology bleeding registry: preliminary findings. Am J Gastroenterol. 1997;92: 924–8.

Pitchumoni CS, Dharmarajan TS, editors. Geriatric gastroenterology. New York: Springer; 2012.

Raju GS, Gerson L, Das A, Lewis B, Association, A. G. American Gastroenterological Association (Aga) Institute technical review on obscure gastrointestinal bleeding. Gastroenterology. 2007;133:1697–717.

Reinus JF, Brandt LJ. Vascular ectasias and diverticulosis. Common causes of lower intestinal bleeding. Gastroenterol Clin N Am. 1994;23:1–20.

Richter JM, Christensen MR, Kaplan LM, Nishioka NS. Effectiveness of current technology in the diagnosis

and management of lower gastrointestinal hemorrhage. Gastrointest Endosc. 1995;41:93–8.

Robertson DJ, Grimm IS. Inflammatory bowel disease in the elderly. Gastroenterol Clin N Am. 2001;30:409–26.

Rockall T, Logan RF, Devlin HB, Northfield TC. Selection of patients for early discharge or outpatient care after acute upper gastrointestinal haemorrhage. National audit of acute upper gastrointestinal haemorrhage. Lancet. 1996;347:1138–40.

Rockey DC, Ahn C, De Melo SW. Randomized pragmatic trial of nasogastric tube placement in patients with upper gastrointestinal tract bleeding. J Investig Med. 2017;65:759–64.

Rothfuss KS, Bode JC, Stange EF, Parlesak A. Urinary excretion of polyethylene glycol 3350 during colonoscopy preparation. Z Gastroenterol. 2006;44:167–72.

Saltzman J. Hemostatic spray for the management of gastrointestinal bleeding. Gastroenterol Hepatol. 2019;15:4.

Scheffel H, Pfammatter T, Wildi S, Bauerfeind P, Marincek B, Alkadhi H. Acute gastrointestinal bleeding: detection of source and etiology with multi-detector-row Ct. Eur Radiol. 2007;17:1555–65.

Schiller KF, Truelove SC, Williams DG. Haematemesis and melaena, with special reference to factors influencing the outcome. Br Med J. 1970;2:7–14.

Shaker R, Ren J, Bardan E, Easterling C, Dua K, Xie P, Kern M. Pharyngoglottal closure reflex: characterization in healthy young, elderly and dysphagic patients with predeglutitive aspiration. Gerontology. 2003;49: 12–20.

Slotwiner-Nie PK, Brandt LJ. Infectious diarrhea in the elderly. Gastroenterol Clin N Am. 2001;30:625–35.

Soulellis CA, Carpentier S, Chen YI, Fallone CA, Barkun AN. Lower GI hemorrhage controlled with endoscopically applied Tc-325 (with videos). Gastrointest Endosc. 2013;77:504–7.

Strate LL, Gralnek IM. ACG clinical guideline: management of patients with acute lower gastrointestinal bleeding. Am J Gastroenterol. 2016;111:755.

Strate LL, Naumann CR. The role of colonoscopy and radiological procedures in the management of acute lower intestinal bleeding. Clin Gastroenterol Hepatol. 2010;8:333–43; quiz e44.

Strate LL, Syngal S. Predictors of utilization of early colonoscopy vs. radiography for severe lower intestinal bleeding. Gastrointest Endosc. 2005;61:46–52.

Strate LL, Saltzman JR, Ookubo R, Mutinga ML, Syngal S. Validation of a clinical prediction rule for severe acute lower intestinal bleeding. Am J Gastroenterol. 2005;100:1821–7.

Strate LL, Ayanian JZ, Kotler G, Syngal S. Risk factors for mortality in lower intestinal bleeding. Clin Gastroenterol Hepatol. 2008;6:1004–10; quiz 955.

Tariq SH, Mekhjian G. Gastrointestinal bleeding in older adults. Clin Geriatr Med. 2007;23:769–84, vi.

Thiebaud PC, Yordanov Y, Galimard JE, Naouri D, Brigant F, Truchot J, Moustafa F, Pateron D. Suspected lower gastrointestinal bleeding in emergency departments, from bleeding symptoms to diagnosis. Am J Emerg Med. 2019;37(4):772–4.

Thomas S, Wong R, Das A. Economic burden of acute diverticular hemorrhage in the U.S.: a nationwide estimate [abstract W1290]. Presented at the 105th annual meeting of the American Gastroenterological Association, New Orleans, May 15–20, 2004.

Triadafilopoulos G. Management of lower gastrointestinal bleeding in older adults. Drugs Aging. 2012;29: 707–15.

Trivedi CD, Pitchumoni CS. Gastrointestinal bleeding in older adults. Pract Gastroenterol. 2006;30:15–42.

Vanneste BG, Van De Voorde L, De Ridder RJ, Van Limbergen EJ, Lambin P, Van Lin EN. Chronic radiation proctitis: tricks to prevent and treat. Int J Color Dis. 2015;30:1293–303.

Velayos FS, Williamson A, Sousa KH, Lung E, Bostrom A, Weber EJ, Ostroff JW, Terdiman JP. Early predictors of severe lower gastrointestinal bleeding and adverse outcomes: a prospective study. Clin Gastroenterol Hepatol. 2004;2:485–90.

Vernava AM, Moore BA, Longo WE, Johnson FE. Lower gastrointestinal bleeding. Dis Colon Rectum. 1997;40:846–58.

Warren JL, Klabunde CN, Mariotto AB, Meekins A, Topor M, Brown ML, Ransohoff DF. Adverse events after outpatient colonoscopy in the Medicare population. Ann Intern Med. 2009;150:849–57, W152.

Wilcox CM, Clark WS. Causes and outcome of upper and lower gastrointestinal bleeding: the Grady Hospital experience. South Med J. 1999;92:44–50.

Wilcox CM, Alexander LN, Cotsonis GA, Clark WS. Nonsteroidal antiinflammatory drugs are associated with both upper and lower gastrointestinal bleeding. Dig Dis Sci. 1997;42:990–7.

Yi WS, Garg G, Sava JA. Localization and definitive control of lower gastrointestinal bleeding with angiography and embolization. Am Surg. 2013;79:375–80.

Zink SI, Ohki SK, Stein B, Zambuto DA, Rosenberg RJ, Choi JJ, Tubbs DS. Noninvasive evaluation of active lower gastrointestinal bleeding: comparison between contrast-enhanced Mdct and 99mTc-labeled RBC scintigraphy. AJR Am J Roentgenol. 2008;191:1107–14.

Zuccaro G. Management of the adult patient with acute lower gastrointestinal bleeding. American College of Gastroenterology. Practice Parameters Committee. Am J Gastroenterol. 1998;93:1202–8.

Zuckerman GR, Prakash C. Acute lower intestinal bleeding. Part II: etiology, therapy, and outcomes. Gastrointest Endosc. 1999;49:228–38.

Zuckier LS. Acute gastrointestinal bleeding. Semin Nucl Med. 2003;33:297–311.

Part X

Hepatobiliary System and Pancreas

Aging Liver and Interpretation of Liver Tests

Ritu Agarwal

Contents

Abstract

Older adults exhibit various alterations in morphology, blood flow, cellular activity, and functions of the liver. Decreases are seen in the liver volume, liver blood flow, phagocytotic activity, immune responses, and ability to regenerate. Simultaneously, there is increased cellular senescence, oxidative stress, inflammatory response, and vulnerability to injury. The cumulative effects result in an increased prevalence of liver diseases and pose an additional risk factor for older adults with underlying comorbidities. However, liver function remains remarkably resilient during aging. Therefore, an abnormal liver chemistry in an older patient needs to be fully investigated in the context of coexisting medical conditions.

An extensive detailed medical history, including a probing history of all medications, prescription as well as over the counter, vitamins and minerals and herbals, serologic tests, and imaging help determine a clinical diagnosis without a liver biopsy. Other studies including vibration controlled transient elastography and liver biopsy may be performed to confirm the diagnosis.

R. Agarwal (✉)
Division of Liver Diseases, The Mount Sinai Hospital, Icahn School of Medicine, New York, NY, USA
e-mail: ritu.agarwal@mssm.edu

© Springer Nature Switzerland AG 2021
C. S. Pitchumoni, T. S. Dharmarajan (eds.), *Geriatric Gastroenterology*,
https://doi.org/10.1007/978-3-030-30192-7_49

Keywords

Older adults · Elderly · Aging and liver · Liver morphology · Liver functions · Liver diseases · Liver chemistry test · Alanine aminotransferase (ALT) · Aspartate aminotransferase (AST) · Gamma-glutamyl-transferase (GGT) · Alkaline phosphatase (ALP) · Bilirubin · Albumin · Globulins · Acute phase proteins (APP) · Hepcidin · Prothrombin time (PT) · International normalized ratio (INR) · Serology tests · Abdominal ultrasound · CT · MRI · Vibration controlled transient elastography (FibroScan) · Liver biopsy · Drug induced liver disease (DILI) · Surgery · Anesthesia · Critical illness · Ischemia · Cholestasis · Sepsis

Introduction

The prevalence and economic burden of chronic liver disease is rapidly changing in the United States (Hirode et al. 2020; Paik et al. 2020; Volk 2020; Younossi et al. 2020). Worldwide liver disease has become a major cause of mortality (12th leading cause worldwide). Over the last decade, while deaths in United States from chronic hepatitis C have plateaued, those from alcoholic liver disease and nonalcoholic fatty liver disease (NAFLD) have increased (Paik et al. 2020). From 2012 to 2016, the rate of hospitalizations from chronic liver disease in USA increased by approximately 21%. While the proportion of hospitalizations for patients aged 45–64 years decreased (55.5% to 50.3%), that for adults 65 and greater increased (27.4–32.2%). In 2016, older adults (=>65 years) also experienced the highest in mortality (10.7%) compared to 2.8% for patients <25 years. In terms of economic burden, from 2012 to 2016 there was a 26% increase in total hospitalization costs resulting in an expenditure of $18.8 billion in 2016 (Hirode et al. 2020). Liver disease develops insidiously without symptoms. The liver can sustain considerable damage before hepatic dysfunctions become clinically manifest. Signs and symptoms develop only when the complications of liver failure or portal hypertension develop.

Liver tests are among the most frequently ordered laboratory tests during routine physical checkup. These include alanine aminotransferase (ALT), aspartate aminotransferase (AST), gamma-glutamyl transferase (GGT), alkaline phosphatase (ALP), bilirubin, albumin, prothrombin time (PT), and international normalized ratio (INR). A minimal change in liver tests is common with aging. Older adults over 60 years of age, especially women, may have a mildly elevated alkaline phosphatase. Serum ALT levels decrease with age independent of gender or metabolic factors (Dong et al. 2012). Bilirubin may slightly decline with age due to reductions in muscle mass and hemoglobin concentrations. A slight decrease in serum albumin is also encountered (Tietz et al. 1992). Prothrombin time is normal unless affected by vitamin K deficiency. Abnormalities of liver tests in routine evaluations at least one are not uncommon (Fleming et al. 2011). In a cohort study on 13,276 people aged 75 years and above, registered with general practices, with a valid measurement of one or more liver test, calculating the prevalence of abnormal aspartate transaminase (AST), alkaline phosphatase (ALP) or bilirubin, Fleming and associates stress the importance of abnormal liver tests in the older adults. In their study, the prevalence of a single abnormal liver test was 16.1% (95% CI [15.4%, 16.7%]). The findings are not to be dismissed, as they signify overall poor prognosis, a modest increase in overall mortality. The prevalence for the tests and their prognostic significance were 3.3% (95% CI [3.0%, 3.7%]) for AST, 9.2% (95% CI [8.8%, 9.7%]) for ALP and 5.4% (95% CI [5.1%, 5.9%]) for bilirubin (Fleming et al. 2011). Abnormal AST, ALP, and bilirubin were associated with increased risks of all-cause mortality; adjusted HRs, 1.27(95% CI [1.09, 1.47]), 1.47(95% CI [1.35, 1.61]), and 1.15(95% CI [1.02, 1.30]), respectively. Abnormal AST and ALP were associated with sevenfold and sixfold increased risk of death from liver disease, respectively. Two or more abnormal tests were associated with two-fold and 17-fold increased risk of death from cancer and liver disease.

As the aging population rapidly grows worldwide, a frequent cause of referral to the hepatology clinic is the observation of an abnormal liver test in an older adult. There is no liver disease specific for older age. Evaluation of an older adult even with mild abnormalities is important (Newsome et al. 2018). This warrants initiation of necessary tests without resorting to over evaluation. However, to do this we need to understand the natural history associated with the abnormalities found.

Aging and Liver

Various changes both in structure and function (Table 1) are seen in the liver with aging that have a significant impact on systemic aging and increases the risk of various liver diseases.

Anatomy: While the liver weighs only up to 2.5% of body weight, it receives approximately 25% of cardiac output. The blood supply from the liver is mainly from the portal vein (70%) with the rest from the hepatic arteries. Each one of them meets approximately half of the liver's oxygen demand. The hepatic veins return the blood back to the heart. The functional unit of the liver is the hepatic lobule: a building block of liver tissue that consisting of portal triad, hepatocytes arranged in linear cords between the capillary network and central vein. The sinusoids are low pressure channels that receive blood from the terminal branches of the hepatic artery and portal vein at the periphery of the lobules and deliver it into the central veins. Sinusoids are lined with endothelial cells known as liver sinusoidal endothelial cells (LSEC) and Kupffer cells (KC). LSEC make up half of the nonparenchymal cells of the liver. Hepatocytes are separated from the sinusoids by the space of Disse. Hepatic stellate cells (HSC) are present in the space of Disse and are involved in scar formation in response to liver damage. LSEC are perforated with pores called "fenestrations" which allows size selective filtration of blood borne molecules. Moreover, there is no underlying basement membrane in the extracellular space of Disse. This unique microvasculature enables the bidirectional exchange of substrate between

Table 1 Morphological and functional changes in the liver with aging

Morphological changes	Functional changes
Hepatocyte	
Decreased number	Accelerated cellular senescence
Decreased volume	Decreased metabolism
Decreased smooth endoplasmic reticulum	Decreased function
Decreased mitochondria	Increased oxidative stress
Increased polyploidy	Increased inflammatory response
Increased lipofuscin	Increased insulin resistance
Increased vacuolation	Decreased regeneration
Increased chromosomal abnormalities	Suppression of autophagy
	Increased vulnerability to injury
Liver sinusoidal endothelial cells	
Defenestration pseudocapillarization	Impaired transfer of substrates
	Hyperlipidemia
	Impaired insulin clearance
	Decreased endocytic activity
Kupffer cells and NK cells	
Increase in number	Increased cytokine production
Increased activation	Increased inflammatory response
	Decreased autophagy
Stellate cells	
Increase in number	Increased activation
	Increased fibrogenesis

the blood originating from both the gut and systemic circulation and hepatocytes (Hunt et al. 2019).

Morphological and functional changes. Aging has a direct impact on all the different cell types: hepatocytes, LSECs, KCs, and HSCs. There is one third loss of hepatic volume and perfusion between the ages 30 and 100 years (Wynne et al. 1989). The aging liver has been described macroscopically as "brown atrophy." This is caused by the accumulation of a brown pigment called lipofuscin within the lysosomes of hepatocytes (Schmucker and Sachs 2002). Lipofuscin accumulation is associated with chronic oxidative stress and a failure to degrade denatured proteins. The volume of the hepatocytes gradually increases as they approach maturity and then decrease with aging. There are increases in the number of abnormal nuclei (polyploidy nuclei) and chromosomal abnormalities. Mitochondria within hepatocytes have an increase in volume, a decrease in number, and dysfunction of mitochondria resulting in decline of ATP levels. Also, there is decreased generation of smooth endoplasmic reticulum and synthesis of microsomal proteins in the liver (Schmucker 2005; Kim et al. 2015). Impairment of metabolic pathways also is related to increased hepatocyte senescence and suppression of autophagy (Hunt et al. 2019). The sinusoidal endothelial cells undergo defenestration. The sinusoids undergo "pseudo-capillarization." This refers to age related changes: thickening and defenestration of LSEC, sporadic deposition of collagen and basal lamina in the extracellular space of Disse, and increased number of fat engorged nonactivated stellate cells resulting in marked reduced porosity or impaired transfer of substances (such as dissolved or the albumin bound drugs, proteins, lipoproteins, etc.). There is also an increase in Von Willebrand factor expression, a decrease in caveolin-1 expression, and increased intracellular adhesive molecule-1 expression. Defenestration also leads to hyperlipidemia and hepatic insulin resistance by impairing the uptake of lipoproteins and insulin (Mohamad et al. 2016). In addition, endocytic activity is diminished. KCs increase in number, reveal reduced phagocytosis and autophagy. Their activation is increased resulting in increased production of cytokines that results in inflammatory changes. Hepatic stellate cells increase in number with increased size of lipid droplets and when activated produce collagen, a key initiating process in development of fibrosis. Therefore, with aging there are multiple structural changes in all types of liver cells resulting in impairment of their function (Kim et al. 2015; Hunt et al. 2018, 2019; Shetty et al. 2018).

Physiology: As a vital organ the liver has a central role in various functions: (a) storage of blood, iron and vitamins such as A, D, E, K, B 6, B 9, and B12, (b) metabolism of carbohydrate, protein, fat and drugs, (c) synthesis of coagulation factors, (d) synthesis and excretion of bile, and (e) clearance of pathogens and immunity.

Storage of blood. The liver can store 450ml of bold (10% of the blood volume) in the hepatic veins and sinusoids. It is clinically important to note that the liver is expandable and increase in pressure in the right atrium as in congestive cardiac failure or constrictive pericarditis is reflected in simultaneous increase in hepatic pressure expanding the storing capacity to 0.5–1 L (see liver test abnormalities in cardiac diseases) . The liver also has a high lymph flow. Fluid leak (sweating from the surface of the liver) in hepatic disorders is attributed to the rapid and high inflow of arterial blood into the splanchnic microcirculation increasing hydrostatic pressure in the splanchnic capillaries. Lymph leakage from the liver and other splanchnic organs is also one of the mechanism of ascites.

Storage of iron. The liver stores iron as ferritin. About 27% of total blood iron is stored in the liver and the rest 68% is present as hemoglobin in the red blood cells. Hepatocytes are a major site of ferritin (an acute phase protein) synthesis with high iron content stimulating and lower content decreasing ferritin synthesis. Serum ferritin levels as well as serum iron and iron binding capacity are often performed to evaluate the cause of anemia in the older adult but care is needed in interpretation (Cullis et al. 2018). Low ferritin levels are only found in patients with reduced body iron stores. But every case of raised ferritin even in a diabetic, a frequent co-morbidity in the older adult is not hemochromatosis. Many older adults are subjected to tests to exclude hemochromatosis unnecessarily. Reactive causes of raised serum ferritin levels, including malignancy, inflammatory disorders, renal failure, liver disease, and metabolic syndrome, should always be considered first as they are all considerably more common than true iron overload (Cullis et al. 2018). Transferrin (a glycoprotein) also synthesized by the hepatocytes functions as the major transport protein for iron in plasma.

Storage of vitamins. In general, vitamin deficiencies in liver disease are related to disorders of hepatic function and diminished reserves. Liver stores fat soluble vitamins (A, D, E, K) as well as vitamins pyridoxine (B6), folate (B9), and cobalamin (B12). Vitamin A is principally stored in the hepatic stellate cells. Activation of quiescent stellate cells results in loss of vitamin A stores enabling production of collagen and subsequent fibrosis. Vitamin D undergoes 25 hydroxylation in the liver rendering the liver critical to the metabolic activation of this vitamin. Furthermore, inadequate dietary intake and/or malabsorption can contribute to deficiencies (Bemeur and Butterworth 2014).

Metabolism of carbohydrate. The liver regulates blood sugar levels via several ways: glycolysis, glucose uptake, glycogenolysis, and gluconeogenesis. The two major sites of glycogen storage are the liver and skeletal muscle. In the liver, glycogen can make up 5–6% of the weight and can store roughly 100–120 grams of glycogen. As a storage organ the liver has glucose buffer action; it can remove excess glucose from blood and deliver glucose when needed. The aging liver has reduced insulin sensitivity and contributes to impaired insulin clearance in part secondary to age related change in the liver sinusoidal epithelium (Hunt et al. 2019). This may be a major factor for type 2 diabetes and hepatic steatosis in the elderly (Petersen et al. 2003). Gluconeogenesis refers to the ability of the liver to produce glucose from amino acids and glycerol. Although not considered to be a liver test, hypoglycemia is a known complication of acute liver failure and easily and repeatedly tested in the management of patients with fulminant liver failure.

Protein metabolism. Hepatocytes synthesize most (hundreds) of the plasma proteins (i.e., albumin, globulin, acute phase proteins, enzymes, hormones) except immunoglobulins which are produced by plasma cells (Devi and Kumar 2012). The normal serum protein level is 6–8 g/dL.

Albumin. The normal serum albumin level is 3.5–5.0 g/dL. Normally the liver synthesizes approximately 150–250 mg/kg/day of albumin, less than half of the capacity (Busher 1990). Factors stimulating protein synthesis are protein intake, decrease in colloid oncotic pressure and hormones: thyroid, corticosteroids, growth hormone, and insulin (Devi and Kumar 2012). Conversely, chronic (but not acute acidosis) and proinflammatory cytokines such as tumor necrosis factor (TNF) and interleukin (IL)-6 and -1B inhibit albumin synthesis (Carvalho and Machado 2018). It has a long circulating half-life of 3 weeks. This makes it difficult to interpret in setting of acute hepatic injury. Decreased albumin synthesis in liver disease accounts for the hypoalbuminemia and often indicates liver disease of >3 weeks in duration. The acute development of hypoalbuminemia with sepsis, severe acute pancreatitis, or trauma results from increased albumin capillary permeability leading to redistribution of albumin from the vascular to interstitial space and increased catabolism. In older adults, other comorbidities should be considered to explain a low albumin. This may be due to either decrease in synthesis (protein malnutrition) or increased albumin loss in the urine (nephrosis), intestine (protein losing enteropathy), or wounds (decubitus ulcers and severe burns) (Levitt and Levitt 2016).

Albumin accounts for the majority (70%) of the colloid osmotic pressure. A decrease in albumin results in shift of fluid from the intravascular space to interstitial space resulting in intravascular volume depletion and edema formation. Another important function is its binding capacity. It can bind to a variety of substances such as bilirubin, hormones (e.g., thyroxine), metals (e.g., copper, zinc), vitamins (e.g., A, D), and drugs (e.g., warfarin, phenytoin, lorazepam). The binding of the drug to albumin influences its distribution, metabolism, biologic half-life, and pharmacologic effect. A decrease in protein binding seen in hypoalbuminemia increases the free fraction of the drug available for clearance resulting in an increase in volume of distribution and shorter elimination half-life (Keller et al. 1984). Similarly, it binds fatty acids, a possible explanation of why hyperlipidemia is seen with hypoalbuminemia. It has a negative charge and retains cations: a reason why calcium is corrected for albumin levels. Hypoalbuminemia is also a prognostic predictor of mortality in elderly people irrespective whether they are independently living in a community, hospitalized or institutionalized (Cabrerizo et al. 2015).

Table 2 Globulins and their levels in various disorders (Busher 1990; Zhao et al. 2020)

Type	Major component	Decreased	Increased
Alpha-1	Alpha-1 antitrypsin	Alpha-1 antitrypsin deficiency	Acute inflammation
Alpha-2	Alpha-2 macroglobulin		Nephrotic syndrome
	Haptoglobin	Hemolytic reaction	Stress, inflammation
Beta	Transferrin	Iron deficiency	
	C 3, C4, C5		
Gamma	Polyclonal	Congenital immunodeficiency Nephrotic syndrome Corticosteroids	Liver diseases Autoimmune conditions Chronic infections Malignancies
	Monoclonal		Plasma cell myeloma B cell lymphoma Amyloidosis Chronic Lymphocytic leukemia Lymphoplasmacytic lymphoma

Globulins. The normal globulin level is 2.6–3.6 g/dL and consists of several proteins: carrier proteins, enzymes, compliments, and immunoglobulins. They fall into four categories by electrophoresis: alpha-1, alpha-2, beta, and gamma. The gamma-globulins are classified according to their heavy chain type: IgG, IgA, IgM, IgE, and IgG. IgG accounts for nearly 75% of total immunoglobulins and is either polyclonal or monoclonal. Table 2 lists the various globulins and their clinical significance (Busher 1990; Zhao et al. 2020). Liver diseases account for majority (61%) of polyclonal hypergammaglobulinemia followed by autoimmune conditions (22%), chronic infections (6%), hematologic disorders (5%), and in nonhematologic malignancies (3%) (Dispenzieri et al. 2001). Maximum immunoglobins levels are seen in the third decade. Both IgM and IgG levels decreased significantly in the elderly while IgA levels are maintained (Buckley and Dorsey 1970; Lock and Unsworth 2003).

Acute phase proteins (APP) are a group of proteins primarily synthesized in hepatocytes. Their production increases in response to infection, inflammation, or trauma by proinflammatory cytokines. Maximum serum concentrations is typically reached within 24–48 h after the infection and decline coincides with recovery. Their main functions include optimization and trapping of microorganisms and their products, activation of complement system, binding cellular remnants like nuclear fractions, neutralizing enzymes, scavenging (free hemoglobin, radicals), and modulating the immune response of the host (Jain et al. 2011). Levels of APP which are overexpressed are known as "positive" APP (C reactive protein, D-dimer protein, mannose-binding protein, alpha 1 antitrypsin, alpha1 antichymotrypsin, alpha 2 macroglobulin, fibrinogen, prothrombin, factor VIII, von-Willebrand factor, plasminogen, complement factors, ceruloplasmin, ferritin, haptoglobin, serum amyloid A, fibrinogen, alpha-1 acid glycoprotein, etc.). Those proteins whose synthesis is reduced are known as "negative" APP (albumin, transferrin, and transthyretin) (Jain et al. 2011; Khalil and Al-Humadi 2020).

Hepcidin is also synthesized predominantly in hepatocytes. It is the main regulator of systemic iron homeostasis. It influences intestinal iron absorption, plasma iron concentration, and tissue iron distribution, through its receptor, the cellular iron exporter ferroportin. Hepcidin deficiency results in iron overload; the liver is most frequently affected due to avid uptake of nontransferrin bound iron by hepatocytes. Common disorders associated with deficiency are hereditary hemochromatosis, iron loading anemias (B- thalassemia and congenital dyserythropoietic anemias), and chronic hepatitis C. Hepcidin excess is pathogenic in anemias of inflammation (infection and inflammation rapidly increase hepcidin synthesis), chronic kidney disease (renal excretion is a route of hepcidin clearance), and iron refractory iron deficiency anemia (Nemeth and Ganz 2009; Sangkhae and Nemeth 2017). When hepcidin is elevated, iron absorption is hindered.

Alpha fretoprotein (AFP). AFP is a serum glycoprotein, a marker for HCC, is not considered as a traditional liver test. In many countries, and until recently in the US estimation of serum AFP levels in outpatients is considered a tool to evaluate hepatic malignancy although abdominal ultrasound is a preferred test. It is pertinent to mention the utility of the test since the older adult has a high risk for hepatic neoplasms. The test has lost its importance. AFP >400–500 ng/ml is considered diagnostic for HCC. However, AFP levels are normal in as many as 30% of patients with hepatocellular cancer, at time of diagnosis and usually remains low, even with advanced HCC. With very high values, the specificity of AFP is close to 100% but at a cost to the sensitivity which falls below 45% (Bialecki and Bisceglie 2005). The interpretation of this test in the older adult is critical.

Liver forms urea from ammonia, deamination of amino acids, synthesis of plasma proteins, and synthesis of various compounds from amino acids. A hallmark of protein and amino acid metabolism in liver disease is the decrease in circulating branched-chain and increased concentrations of circulating aromatic amino acids with concomitantly altered amino acid kinetics (Charlton 2006). In the management of patients with hepatic encephalopathy, the latter function is considered. However, it is not a liver test in clinical situations.

Fat metabolism. The liver plays a role in oxidation of fatty acids, synthesis of cholesterol, phospholipids, and lipoproteins. Peterson et al. have demonstrated that there is an age associated decline in mitochondrial oxidative and phosphorylation activity by nearly 40% resulting in increased fat accumulation in liver (Petersen et al. 2003). Overall, the neutral fat and cholesterol volumes in the liver gradually expand with aging. The blood cholesterol, high density lipoprotein cholesterol, and neutral fat levels also increase overtime (Alves-Bezerra and Cohen 2017). Meanwhile, the metabolism of low-density lipoprotein cholesterol decreases by 35% (Kim et al. 2015). All can be easily measured. Although not considered liver tests, one has to be aware of the laboratory abnormalities.

Drug metabolism and detoxifications. The cytochrome P450 group of enzymes are responsible in detoxification in the first phase of drug metabolism. Cytochrome P-450 activity decreases by 32% in adults older than 70 years compared to adults 20–29 years old. This may account for the reduction of drug metabolism by up to 30% after 70 years of age (Sotaniemi et al. 1997).

Synthesis of coagulation factors. The liver synthesizes most of the coagulation factors (FI, FII, FV, FVII, FVIII, FIX, FX, FXI, FXII, FXIII). Although in milder cases the synthesis is not evident, a reduction of activities of the coagulation factors is notable in end stage liver disease. Von Willebrand factor, synthesized in endothelial cells, plays an important role in hemostatic processes and exhibits increased activity in liver disease (Hartman et al. 2016). The four procoagulant vitamin K–dependent factors of the clotting system are factors II, VII, IX, and X. The above four and the two anticoagulant factors (protein C and protein S) and protein Z require postribosomal modification after synthesis for proper physiologic function. Measurement of these factors is not routine. But the decrease in procoagulants results initially in a slightly prolonged PT and ultimately in a markedly abnormal PT and APTT (the standard tests).

Synthesis and excretion of bile. Bile synthesized and excreted by the liver consists mainly of bile salts, phospholipids, cholesterol, conjugated bilirubin, electrolytes, and water. Of the total bile flow of approximately 600 ml/day, 75% is derived from the hepatocytes and the rest 25% from the cholangiocytes. The majority of bile acids are reabsorbed from the ilium and transported to the liver by the portal venous system (enterohepatic circulation) and only 5% is eventually excreted (Hundt et al. 2020). With aging there is an increment in the lithogenic index of gallbladder bile without significant change in bile acid metabolism suggesting that the canicular secretion of cholesterol increases with age. This may partly account for the increased frequency of gallstones in the elderly (Valdivieso et al. 1978).

Clearance of pathogens from blood and immunity. Liver also serves as a vital organ for immunity and clearing pathogens. Non-hepatocytes cells of the liver (LSEC, Kupffer cells, stellate cells, and natural killer cells) are involved in both inmate and adaptive immunity. KCs constitute 80–90% of the tissue macrophages in the body. With nearly one third to one half of lymphocytes being natural killer (NK) cells, the liver contains the largest population of NK cells in the body. In combination LSEC and KC constitute the most powerful scavenger system in the body. The first exposure of food and microbial antigens to the hepatic sinusoids via portal vein enables them to be important players in endotoxin removal, pathogen recognition, antigen presentation, recruitment of leukocytes, and meditating the liver immune response during infection or injury. The overall balance determines whether the injury or infection resolves, persists, or progresses (Kubes and Jenne 2018; Shetty et al. 2018; Ortega-Rivera et al. 2020).

Aging and Liver Function

Liver function remains remarkably resilient during aging (Tietz et al. 1992). Recent experience with orthotopic transplants of liver from aged donors when compared to younger donors have demonstrated comparable function and duration (Morsiani et al. 2019). Hepatic grafts from older donors (=>80 years) are being successfully used in transplantation (Salizzoni et al. 2017).

Cieslak et al. have suggested that the currently used tests bilirubin, AST, ALT, ALP, and GGT do not represent real liver function but are surrogate parameters. Using a quantitative dynamic liver function test that measured the uptake of an isotope by the hepatocyte in 203 patients with healthy liver, a negative correlation was observed between age and isotope uptake suggesting that liver function declines with age (Cieslak et al. 2016). Nevertheless, the liver does show relatively modest physiological alterations during aging. Several molecular changes appear to be

relevant: an increase of micro-RNA expression after 60 years of age, a remodeling of genome-wide DNA methylation profile evident until 60 years of age, and then plateauing and changes in transcriptome including the metabolic zone of hepatocyte lobules (Morsiani et al. 2019). These contribute to dysregulation of mitochondrial function and nutrient sensing pathways, leading to cellular senescence, low grade inflammatory changes, and impairment of function in all liver cells: hepatocytes, LSEC, KC, and stellate cells (Hunt et al. 2019).

Aging, Inflammation, and Liver

Inflammation has a critical role in the aging process of the liver that contributes to "inflammaging" of old age. It accelerates the aging process as a continuum largely as a result of lifestyles and exposure to noxious agents. Individual "immunobiography" of every individual depends largely on their lifestyle and environment (i.e., diet, alcohol consumption, gut microbiome, viral or bacterial infections, drugs, etc.). It can either accelerate or decelerate the liver aging process (Morsiani et al. 2019). The biologic age of the liver can differ substantially from the chronologic age of the liver. For example, liver fibrosis is a consequence of excess healing response; the biological mechanisms are not well understood (Hunt et al. 2019). Hopefully, ongoing research involving dietary manipulations, drugs, nanoparticles, antibodies, etc., will lead to future therapies (Hunt et al. 2018; Shetty et al. 2018).

Liver Regeneration or Recovery

The liver has a remarkable regenerating capacity, better than any other organ. As little as 25% of a liver can regenerate into a whole liver (Sheedfar et al. 2013). The ability for the liver to regenerate or recover after injury declines with age (Tajiri and Shimizu 2013; Zhu et al. 2014; Kim et al. 2015; Xu et al. 2020). The change in liver volume at 6 months after hepatectomy in older adults >65 years was lower when compared to young <65 years (23.3% versus 45.6%, respectively)

(Xu et al. 2020). Hepatocytes remain quiescent under normal physiologic conditions.

Routine Biochemical Tests of Liver

Liver chemistries are included in commonly ordered comprehensive metabolic profiles during routine evaluations. These include alanine aminotransferase (ALT), aspartate aminotransferase (AST), gamma-glutamyl-transferase (GGT), alkaline phosphatase (ALP), bilirubin, albumin (mentioned earlier), and prothrombin time (PT or INR) (Table 3).

Alanine and aspartate aminotransferases (ALT and AST) are enzymes involved in transfer amino groups of alanine and aspartate to ketoglutaric acid. Both are sensitive indicators of liver cell injury. ALT is present primarily in liver cells and is therefore a more specific marker of hepatic injury than AST. The ACG clinical guidelines recommend a normal ALT without risk factors for liver disease is 29–33 IU/l for males and 19–25 IU/l for females (Kwo et al. 2017). This upper limit of normal (ULN) is notably lower than that has been previously accepted (men 35–79 IU/l and 31–55 IU/l for women). The latter recommendation was based upon reference populations without consideration of features including BMI (higher BMI is linearly related with higher ALT) and the use of different values by the laboratories for defining ULN. An elevated ALT is associated with increased liver-related mortality. A higher ULN thereby excludes a significant number of patients, specifically with obesity and possible

Table 3 Liver chemistry tests

Test	Origin
AST	Liver, skeletal and cardiac muscle, pancreas, lungs
ALT	Liver, kidney, skeletal muscle, lung
ALP	Liver, bone, placenta, kidneys, intestines
GGT	Liver, kidney, pancreas, heart, brain
Bilirubin	Hemolysis, biliary obstruction
Albumin	Liver
Prothrombin time	Liver

NAFLD. Furthermore, a normal ALT does not exclude significant liver disease (Kwo et al. 2017).

AST is present in liver, cardiac muscle, skeletal muscle, kidney, brain, pancreas, lungs, leukocytes, and red cells. It is therefore less sensitive and specific for the liver. Isolated AST elevation can be suggestive of cardiac or muscle or thyroid disorders, celiac sprue, and hemolysis (Oh et al. 2017).

Alkaline Phosphatase: The single serum test that causes considerable diagnostic dilemma in geriatric practice is the interpretation of isolated elevated alkaline phosphatase. Estimation of ALP is a component of all evaluations in inpatients as well as outpatients. The incidental detection of an "isolated" elevation of alkaline phosphatase in the presence of normal ALT, AST, and bilirubin creates dilemmas in diagnosis; the value cannot be ignored since a large number of benign and malignant bone diseases, liver diseases, and even few cancers outside the liver (e.g., lung); most of them, if not all, are age related and create a major diagnostic dilemma. Along with many liver diseases, a major concern is bone disease, since this metalloenzyme is expressed on osteoblasts and elevated serum levels of the enzyme correlate with increased osteoblastic activity. Many recent clinical publications and professional societies have addressed the problem. Unless a careful diagnostic approach is followed, one is likely to exhaust a large number of easily expensive imaging studies and unnecessary interventional endoscopic procedures.

Elevated alkaline phosphatase (ALP) is a marker for cholestasis. Cholestatic liver disease can be categorized as intrahepatic (functional impairment of bile formation by hepatocytes) or extrahepatic (anatomic obstruction to bile flow) (Table 4).

Alkaline phosphatase is found in the liver, bone, placenta, intestine, and the kidney. In normal serum, ALP comprises mostly the liver and bone portions. For this reason, an elevated alkaline phosphatase must be determined to be hepatic or nonhepatic in origin. A combined increase of ALP and other liver chemistries is suggestive of hepatic origin. As ALP is synthesized by the

Table 4 Elevated alkaline phosphatase

Hepatic	Nonhepatic
Intrahepatic	Bone disease
Primary biliary cholangitis	Hyperthyroidism
Primary sclerosing cholangitis	Infection
Medications	Congestive heart failure
Hepatic metastasis	Blood type O and B
Extra hepatic	Increasing age (women)
Bile duct obstruction	Lymphoma
Bile duct stricture	
Ductopenia	
Neoplasms	

canalicular epithelium, it is raised in biliary obstruction (intrahepatic or extrahepatic) and is usually normal or marginally elevated in hepatocellular injury. Elevations can be seen in the absence of raised bilirubin when the degree of obstruction is minor. An elevated alkaline phosphatase can be complemented by GGT. GGT is normal in bone disease. A simultaneous GGT and alkaline phosphatase elevation supports a hepatic source for the elevated alkaline phosphatase. If alkaline phosphatase is elevated and confirmed to be hepatic in origin, abdominal ultrasound imaging is the initial study; the findings will identify the need for a subsequent MRCP. Serology including autoimmune markers is indicated depending on the clinical diagnosis. A liver biopsy may be considered for further evaluation, to evaluate for infiltrative disorders such as granulomatous liver disease (Fig. 1).

In older adults, alkaline phosphatase is normal in osteoporosis and osteopenia but does go up in vitamin D deficiency (osteomalacia). The increased bone turnover is especially the case in older women (Mukaiyama et al. 2015). Osteomalacia while less common, characterized by marked softening of bones, raises ALP. Besides inadequate intake of vitamin D, osteomalacia also occurs after certain surgeries (gastric resection and intestinal bypass), celiac disease, chronic kidney disease, hepatobiliary disease, and use of phenytoin and phenobarbital (Noh et al. 2013). Liver has a significant role in vitamin D metabolism; not surprisingly, liver disease is strongly linked to vitamin D deficiency (Keane et al. 2018). The prevalence of osteoporosis in patients with chronic liver diseases particularly liver cirrhosis and cholestatic liver disease is 12–55% (Jeong and Kim 2019). ALP can also be mildly elevated after a fatty meal due to influx of intestinal alkaline phosphatase into the circulation (Kasarala and Tillmann 2016). It is an interesting observation.

Low levels of serum alkaline phosphatase can occur in hypothyroidism, pernicious anemia, zinc deficiency, and Wilsons disease (Poynard and Imbert-Bismut 2012).

Gamma-glutamyl-transferase (GGT) is present in highest concentration in the liver and is a well-established serum marker for liver dysfunction, biliary disorders, and alcoholism. Since it is also present in kidneys, pancreas, and other tissues, the predictive utility of GGT as a sole marker for liver disease is low (Koenig and Seneff 2015). It is most useful in confirming whether an elevated ALP is of hepatic origin (Newsome et al. 2018). Similarly, a GGT level of two hundred or more in patients with AST/ALT ratio >2 also supports the diagnosis of alcoholic liver disease (Pratt and Kaplan 2000). Normal values range from 0 to 30 IU/l. Maximal values 5–30 times normal are seen in cases of intra- or posthepatic biliary obstruction. Alcohol related cirrhosis, heavy alcohol consumption, primary and metastatic malignancy are associated with high elevations while only modest rises 2–5 times normal occur in infectious hepatitis. Because it is not specific for liver, it is not recommended as a screening test for liver disease in the absence of other abnormal liver enzymes (Kwo et al. 2017).

Bilirubin is a breakdown product of hemoglobin, released from aging red blood cells. Bilirubin is conjugated in the liver to water soluble form. Conjugated bilirubin is then secreted into bile. An elevated unconjugated or indirect bilirubin is due to over production of bilirubin from hemolysis, resorption of hematoma, muscle injury rarely, decreased hepatic uptake, or decreased hepatic conjugation. Gilberts syndrome affects 3–7% of the US population and is due to a genetic defect of UDP-glucuronosyltransferase resulting in

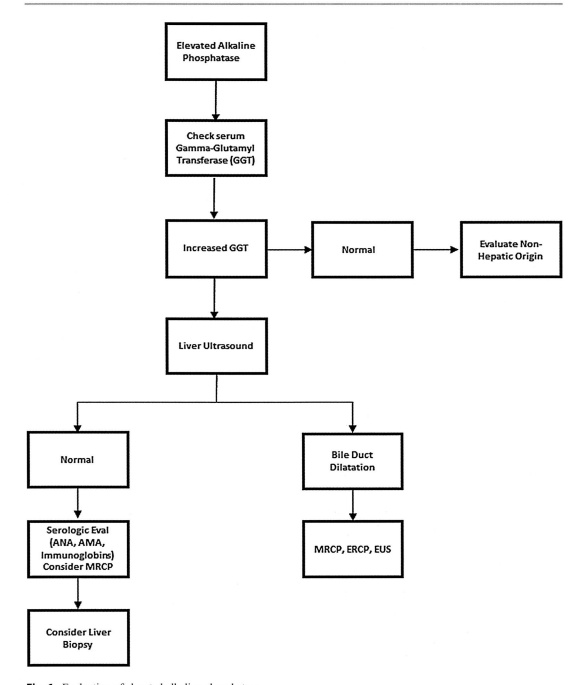

Fig. 1 Evaluation of elevated alkaline phosphatase

impaired conjugation of bilirubin with glucuronic acid with other normal liver enzymes that increases with fasting (as it happens in hospitalized patients requiring various tests). Unnecessary evaluations are initiated in the older adult who demonstrates a modest elevation of total bilirubin often following an "NPO" status which is only a reflection of Gilberts. The levels also increase with sepsis. Diagnosis can be confirmed by fractionating the amount of conjugated bilirubin that is less than 20–30% of the total bilirubin level, in the absence of hemolysis (Palmer et al. 2020). In most cases, total bilirubin levels are minimally elevated and rarely greater than 4–5 mg/dL. Conjugated hyperbilirubinemia signifies presence of either biliary obstruction (stones, strictures, or neoplasm) or a parenchymal liver disorder. Very rarely, two inherited disorders associated with conjugated hyperbilirubinemia that can be encountered in the elderly are Dubin-Johnson syndrome and Rotor syndrome. In both, ALP and GGT are normal (Kwo et al. 2017) (Fig. 2).

Prothrombin Time (PT) and International Normalized Ratio (INR): Commonly used tests for identifying and monitoring coagulopathy are partial thromboplastin time (PTT), prothrombin time (PT), and international normalized ratio (INR). PTT and PT are measures of intrinsic and extrinsic pathways, respectively, of the coagulations system. INR is a ratio of patient's PT as compared to a laboratory normative PT. It is usually measured simultaneously to standardize the reporting of PT. INR avoids interlaboratory variability in PT, while its interpretation is similar to that of PT (Limdi and Hyde 2003; Harrison 2018).

As a function test, PT is more sensitive than albumin for acute liver injury because it measures liver disease of <24 h duration. It is a marker of hepatic synthesis of coagulation factors I, II, V, VII, IX, and X. Prolonged PT elevation may also reflect malnutrition or vitamin K deficiency that is needed for synthesis of the clotting factors II, VII, IX, and X. Reduction of prolonged PT by intravenous vitamin K administration differentiates nutritional causes from intrinsic liver disease (Limdi and Hyde 2003).

Several limitations exist with estimations of PT and INR. First, elevations in PT and INR do not occur until loss of >70% synthetic function. Second, PT and INR measure only one clotting pathway while in vivo clotting homeostasis is dependent on multiple factors. Third, the value of PT and INR depends on the assay or available reagents and can differ significantly for the same individual. Fourth, the commonly held and widely practiced myth that an elevated PT or INR is associated with increased risk of a hemorrhagic event is unproven (Segal et al. 2005). It leads to inappropriate interventions, exposing the patient to increased risk of adverse events. Fifth, the accuracy of an abnormal PT in predicting bleeding after invasive procedures is minimal. Indeed, the incidence of bleeding after bedside procedures in the presence of abnormal PT is <3% for minor and <1% for a major bleed, respectively, with a mortality of approximately 0.016% after a major hemorrhagic complication (Harrison 2018). Lastly, PT and INR when used in Child-Pugh or Model for End Stage Liver Disease (MELD), scores correlate well with mortality but not hemorrhagic events. Therefore, currently in patients with suspected coagulopathy, newer tests such as thromboelastography (TEG) are superior. TEG allows rapid bed-side representation of the various components of clot formation and fibrinolysis allowing targeted intervention (e.g., platelets, fresh frozen plasma, cryoprecipitate, or medications like tranexamic acid) (Harrison 2018; O'Leary et al. 2019). Other tests of coagulation abnormalities in liver diseases are occasionally performed in acute and chronic liver diseases and it is justifiable because the liver is the primary source of numerous proteins that are critical for normal function of the blood coagulation cascade requiring an individualized approach (Pant et al. 2018).

Evaluation of an Abnormal Liver Chemistry Test

Evaluation of the older adult even with mild abnormalities is important (Newsome et al. 2018). Just repeating liver tests are inefficient (Lilford et al. 2013). An extensive history should include: alcohol and herbal consumption,

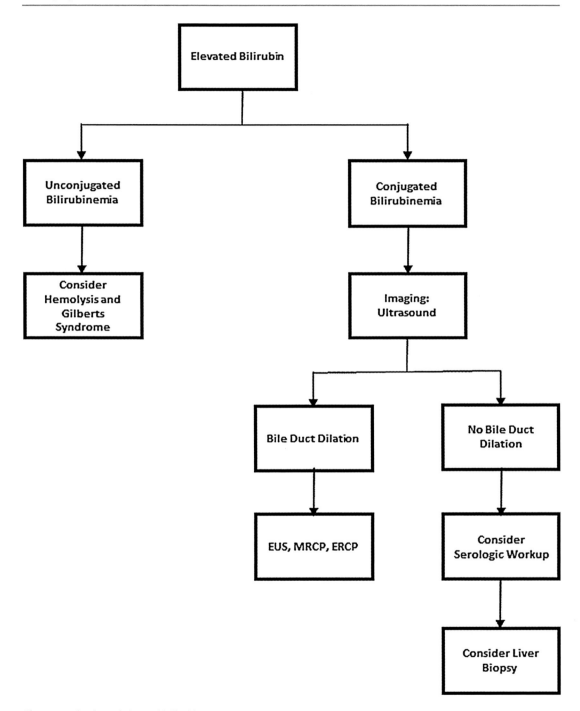

Fig. 2 Evaluation of elevated bilirubin

medication use in the past and present (prescription and nonprescription), family history of chronic liver disease, personal history of autoimmune disease and possible exposure to viral hepatitis, risk assessment for metabolic profile (hyperlipidemia, obesity, diabetes, and hypertension). Immunosuppression can raise possibility for Hepatitis B reactivation or CMV or HSV infection. A hypercoagulable state can put a patient at risk for developing thrombosis or Budd Chiari syndrome. Cardiovascular disease (heart failure or relative hypotension) can be concerning for ischemic hepatitis.

In addition to the liver test, a complete blood count with platelets is significant. Thrombocytopenia is the most common hematological abnormality found in patients with chronic liver diseases as a result of decreased production, splenic sequestration, and increased destruction. Factors that can contribute to bone marrow suppression resulting in decreased production are alcohol, iron overload, drugs, and reduction of thrombopoietin levels in chronic liver disease. Splenic sequestration results from hypersplenism due to portal hypertension. Increased destruction occurs due to immunologically mediated antiplatelet immunoglobulins in autoimmune liver diseases (Newsome et al. 2018). Therefore, if thrombocytopenia is noted, further testing for a liver disease is appropriate.

Pattern of Liver Enzyme Elevation. Liver enzyme elevations typically present in either of two patterns: hepatocellular or cholestatic. The predominant pattern can help in determining the clinical diagnosis (Table 5). Hepatocellular pattern is associated with a disproportionate increase in AST/ALT relative to ALP reflective of hepatocyte injury. Cholestatic pattern has a disproportionately elevated alkaline phosphatase relative to AST/ALT. This can be reflective of obstruction of bile ducts or infiltrative disease. Bilirubin can be elevated in both patterns. Conjugated bilirubin is typically predominantly elevated in cholestatic injury. The distinction between hepatocellular and cholestatic patterns is sometimes not definitive as overlap can occur (Sanchez and Corey 2016).

Table 5 Patterns of liver injury, enzyme elevations, and liver diseases

Type	Elevations	Disease
Hepatocellular	AST and ALT	DILI, viral hepatitis, alcohol hepatitis, autoimmune hepatitis, ischemic hepatitis
Cholestatic	ALP and GGT	DILI, bile duct obstruction (biliary strictures, choledocholithiasis, PSC, PBC, neoplasms
Mixed pattern	AST, ALT, ALP, and GGT	Overlap of both type

The degree of increase of ALT and AST helps to guide the evaluation in the clinical setting. Increase of ALT and/or AST < 5 upper limit of normal (ULN) is suggestive of viral hepatitis B and C, alcoholic and NAFLD, hemochromatosis, Wilson's disease, A1 antitrypsin deficiency, autoimmune hepatitis, and drug induced liver injury. In patients with increase ALT and/or AST of 5–15x ULN acute hepatitis A, B, and C is a possibility in addition to the above conditions. Furthermore, ALT and/or AST >15xULN or massive elevations of ALT >10,000 IU/l is suggestive of acetaminophen toxicity and ischemic hepatopathy (shock liver) (Kwo et al. 2017). An AST/ALT ratio >2:1 is typically seen in alcoholic hepatitis. This is thought to be related to pyridoxal 5-phosphatase deficiency. In contrast, nonalcoholic steatohepatitis is associated with AST/ALT ratio <1 (Pratt and Kaplan 2000). As the liver fibrosis progresses towards advanced fibrosis/cirrhosis serum ALT levels tend to fall, whereas AST levels remain stable or increase leading to an increase in AST/ALT (Younossi et al. 2018). However, it needs to be stressed that elevations in levels of aminotransferases correlate poorly with the degree of liver cell damage. There exists considerable overlap and any increase needs to be determined on the clinical context.

Additional tests. Serologic test (Table 6), ultrasound, ultrasound elastography, CT MRI, and a liver biopsy should be performed as necessary to confirm the diagnosis.

Table 6 Serologic evaluation of liver injury

Serologic test	Clinical disease
Hepatitis-A IgM	Acute hepatitis A
Hepatitis-A IgG	Hepatitis A past exposure and immunity
Hepatitis B s Ag	Hepatitis B infection
Hepatitis B core Ab	Hepatitis B prior exposure
Hepatitis B surface Ab	Hepatitis B immunity
Hepatitis C Ab	Hepatitis C
Hepatitis E IgG, IgM	Hepatitis E
Antimitochondrial antibody (AMA)	Primary biliary cholangitis
Smooth muscle antibody (SMA)	Autoimmune Hepatitis
Transferrin saturation	Hemochromatosis
Alpha-antitrypsin	Alpha antitrypsin deficiency
Immunoglobin G quantitative	Autoimmune hepatitis
Immunoglobin M	Primary biliary cholangitis

Ultrasound (US): Transabdominal ultrasound is used as initial imaging for evaluation on elevated liver enzymes. It is widely available, safe, well tolerated, cheap, and noninvasive. It provides information regarding biliary tree, liver size and texture, and focal liver lesions. Doppler studies facilitate portal vein flow, presence of clot, and development of collateral vessels. Presence of obesity and ascites reduces the accuracy. It is helpful in diagnosing hepatic steatosis and the degree of steatosis can be subjectively graded as mild, moderate, and severe. In a meta-analysis of 34 studies (2815 patients) comparing ultrasound to liver biopsy as the gold standard, Hernaez et al. found a sensitivity of 85% and specificity of 93% for ultrasound to distinguish moderate-to-severe fatty liver from the absence of steatosis (Hernaez et al. 2011). Usually steatosis is detected by ultrasound when the liver fat content approaches 20%. In contrast, the presence of fat greater than 5% is considered abnormal. Therefore, a significant number of patients with steatosis starting at 5% of liver fat can be missed. Furthermore, it is unable to differentiate nonalcoholic fatty liver disease (NAFLD) from nonalcoholic steatohepatitis (NASH) (Castera et al. 2019; Younossi et al. 2018). Nevertheless, the British Society of Gastroentrology guidelines on the

management of abnormal liver blood tests recommend using abdominal ultrasound as the initial standard screening radiologic test (Newsome et al. 2018).

US is also best and initial diagnostic study for gallstones. In contrast, it has poor sensitivity (22–55%) for detecting common bile duct (CBD) stones. Despite this it is superior for detecting dilation of CBD (sensitivity 77–87%) (ASGE 2010). Choledocholithiasis, a leading cause of obstructive jaundice, present in 10–20% of patients with symptomatic cholelithiasis is associated with dilatation of biliary tree (Frossard and Morel 2010). These patients should then undergo ERCP if they have high risk criteria while in those with intermediate risk criteria MRCP, endoscopic ultrasound, intraoperative cholangiogram, or intraoperative ultrasound is the next recommended modality based on available resources and expertise (Table 7) (ASGE 2019).

CT: CT can be utilized for better characterization of liver size and texture. Multiphase and contrast enhanced CT can further differentiate focal liver lesions and better characterize vasculature. Intravenous contrast should be administered with caution in the elderly because of possible decline in renal function.

MRI: Multiphase and gadolinium contrast enhanced MRI with T1 and T2 weighted images can help to characterize liver diseases and masses better than CT. Among the various benefits are identification of active liver disease, quantification of fatty liver, hepatic fibrosis that correlates with the histologic stage of fibrosis, regenerative nodules seen in setting of chronic liver disease and hepatocellular carcinoma (Chundru et al. 2014). As an example, the characteristic magnetic resonance cholangiography findings of multiple structure and dilatation of bile ducts when associated with raised ALP establish the diagnosis of sclerosing cholangitis and avoid the need for liver biopsy (Palmer et al. 2020). Table 8 lists the indications for MRI of liver (ACR 2020) and MRCP (Griffin et al. 2012).

While MRI avoids ionizing radiation, there are several concerns relating to the safety or toxicity of gadolinium contrast agents even in patients with normal renal function. Gadolinium is filtered

Table 7 Proposed investigations for abnormal liver test in symptomatic cholelithiasis based on predictors of choledocholithiasis (ASGE guidelines 2019)

Probability	Predictors of choledocholithiasis	Proposed investigation
High (>50%)	Choledocholithiasis on US/CT or Clinical ascending cholangitis or Total bilirubin >4 mg/dL and dilated CBD on US/CT (>6 mm or 8 mm postcholecystectomy)	ERCP
Intermediate (10–50%)	Abnormal liver test or Dilated CBD (6 mm or 8 mm postcholecystectomy)	MRCP, EUS, laparoscopic IOC, or intra operative US

Table 8 Indications for MRI of liver (ACR 2020) and MRCP (Griffin et al. 2012)

MRI of liver
Detection of focal hepatic lesions
Characterization of focal hepatic lesions
Evaluation of vascular patency
Evaluation and noninvasive quantification of iron, fat, fibrosis in chronic liver disease such as hemochromatosis, hemosiderosis, NASH, and hepatitis
Evaluation of cirrhotic liver and HCC surveillance
Evaluation of infection
Clarification of findings from laboratory anomalies and other imaging studies
Alternative imaging for contraindication to CT scan
MRCP
Congenital anomalies of cystic and hepatic ducts
Choledochal cyst
Choledocholithiasis
Biliary strictures (benign and malignant)
Pancreas division
Chronic pancreatitis
Pancreatic tumors
Postsurgical biliary anatomy and complications

by the kidney, but deposits can occur in the brain, bone, and skin. A variety of conditions (neurological, musculoskeletal, dermal, pancreatitis, hepatotoxicity, and nephrotoxicity) have been reported (Rogosnitzky and Branch 2016). Other drawbacks of MRI are cost of procedure, patient size, availability, claustrophobia, and presence of metal implants.

Fibrosis Evaluation. While most NAFLD patients have simple steatosis, only a minority (10–20%) have NASH that can progress to severe fibrosis and complications of chronic liver disease. A critical issue is to identify those with NASH and to differentiate those with advanced hepatic fibrosis (Castera et al. 2019; Younossi et al. 2018). Numerous scores that utilize commonly checked tests including aminotransferases, GGT, bilirubin, INR, and platelets have been proposed to indirectly assess fibrosis. Most studied are AST to platelet ratio index (APRI), AST to ALT ratio, Fibrosis-4 score (FIB-4), FibroTest, and NAFLD fibrosis score. Among these, the FIB-4 (uses age, AST, ALT, platelets) and NAFLD fibrosis score (uses age, ALT, AST, albumin, platelets, BMI, and diabetes) are the most accurate with a high negative predictive value of >90% for ruling out advanced fibrosis and thereby identify patients who do not need further assessment. Only in case of a positive test, further diagnostic workup is required for confirming advanced fibrosis (Castera et al. 2019). The scores have been developed and validated in patients aged 35–65 years old. The specificity for detecting advanced fibrosis in patients >65 years old with the NAFLD fibrosis score and FIB4 has been shown to be low resulting in high false positive rates. This is not surprising as age is utilized in the calculation. It has been suggested to modify cutoffs for patients >65 years, in order to reduce the false positive rate (McPherson et al. 2017).

Direct serum biomarkers measure components of the fibrosis pathway: procollagen peptides I/III, type IV collagen, cytokines interleukin-10, and transforming growth factor alpha. ELF (Enhanced

Liver Fibrosis Test uses hyaluronic acid, PIIINP, and TIMP-1) has been recommended as the next testing for those patients with intermediate FIB-4 or NAFLD fibrosis score (Newsome et al. 2018) as they are limited in distinguishing intermediate stages of fibrosis (Castera 2020). The ELF test does not utilize age in the calculation model. However, a study suggested that the test has a reduced accuracy in patients >45 years old (Fagan et al. 2015).

Vibration Controlled Transient Elastography: Vibration Controlled Transient Elastography (FibroScan; Echosens, Paris, France) is an ultrasound-based technique that permits rapid, painless, noninvasive measurement of liver fibrosis with high accuracy and no potential complications. It has been validated with high intra- and interobserver reproducibility and can be performed quickly at bedside. An ultrasound transducer probe is placed between two ribs in the intercostal space and measures the generated elastic shear wave and velocity. This gives a liver stiffness measurement expressed in kilopascals that correlates with fibrosis stage. To improve reliability, a minimum of ten valid readings are taken. The limiting factors are that it is operator dependent (<500 examinations) and may be difficult to interpret in obese patients (BMI > 30). Older age (>50 years) has also been identified as a possible limiting factor for reliable results (Castera et al. 2010). It has an accuracy of approximately 80% and 90% for diagnosing advanced fibrosis and cirrhosis, respectively (Castera et al. 2019, Younossi et al. 2018). While there is considerable overlap in distinguishing mild and moderate degree of fibrosis, its greatest value is the negative predictive value of 90% whereby it can exclude both advanced fibrosis/cirrhosis in approximately 90% of the patients and avoid the need for a liver biopsy. It is therefore recommended as the second line radiologic test in the American (Chalasani et al. 2018), British (Newsome et al. 2018), and European (EASL 2016) guidelines for management of patients with NAFLD.

Liver Biopsy. Despite availability of extensive serologic workup and noninvasive measurements

Table 9 Liver biopsy (Pandey et al. 2020; Neuberger et al. 2020)

Purpose	Indications
Diagnosis	Differentiate complex conditions Autoimmune hepatitis (AIH) from NASH AIH/primary biliary cholangitis overlap Drug induced liver injury Posttransplant rejection from underlying Pathology Determine etiology and grade of mass lesions
Prognosis	Determine severity of damage NASH: advanced fibrosis from cirrhosis Hemochromatosis: presence of cirrhosis
Management	Treatment decisions Monitor treatment efficacy

of fibrosis, liver biopsy is the gold standard in the management of several complex liver conditions for diagnosis, prognosis, and management (Table 9). Liver biopsy is relatively safe. The few relative contraindications are the uncooperative patient, increased risk of bleeding, vascular tumors of the liver, ascites, morbid obesity, extrahepatic biliary obstruction, bacterial cholangitis, and amyloidosis (Neuberger et al. 2020; Pandey et al. 2020). Percutaneous liver biopsy is usually performed with or without or under ultrasound guidance; image guidance increases the safety and yield. Transvenous (trans-jugular or trans-femoral) liver biopsy is another option for the high-risk patients (ascites, obesity, and coagulopathy). Endoscopic ultrasound guided (EUS) or laparoscopic liver biopsy are other options. The most frequent complication is pain in 84% (Pandey et al. 2020). The incidence of serious complication is approximately 1% with a mortality of only 0.2%. Bleeding occurs in <10% with major bleed in <2% (Neuberger et al. 2020). Rarely bile peritonitis from puncture of gallbladder or a dilated intrahepatic bile duct is seen (Pandey et al. 2020). However, risks can be greater in older age because of decreased liver size. Patient's age >50 has been identified as having higher likelihood for postbiopsy bleeding (Midia et al. 2019). Mortality is not increased with advancing age (Gilmore et al. 1995).

Liver Tests and Disorders

Drug induced liver injury (DILI). Medications whether prescribed, over the counter or complimentary alternative medications are common causes for drug induced liver injury (DILI) (Table 10). Spectrum of DILI can range from asymptomatic elevations of liver enzymes to acute liver failure. Diagnosis of DILI is challenging and is based on a comprehensive history of drug exposure and exclusion of other causes (Hoofnagle and Bjornsson 2019). Medications can cause injury in hepatocellular, cholestatic of mixed patterns (Table 11). Injury can be caused in a predictable time-dose dependent pattern or unpredictably (idiosyncratic) (Hoofnagle and Bjornsson 2019). This risk is believed to be multifactorial: drug dose, drug clearance, drug distribution, and polypharmacy (Leise et al. 2014).

Drugs that have high first pass hepatic uptake, such as propranolol, have declined hepatic clearance in the elderly because of reduced liver volume and hepatic blood flow. A reduction in liver cytochrome P450 may also contribute to decreased drug clearance in elderly patients.

Cytochrome P450 activity has been shown to be 32% lower in patients >70 years than patients 20–29 years (Sotaniemi et al. 1997). The distribution of medications is also altered because of decreased albumin levels. Water soluble drug distribution can be altered because of change in ratio of body fat to water in older patients. Polypharmacy also impacts risk of drug-drug interactions. Elderly patients are more likely to take multiple medications because of multiple comorbidities. In a prospective study from Netherlands, 94.2% of elderly patients, mean age 82.3 years, were taking more than one medication and 73.3% were prescribed four or more medications (Tulner et al. 2009).

Older patients are more likely to present with cholestatic pattern of drug induced liver injury, whereas younger patients are more prone to hepatocellular injury. (Lucena et al. 2009; Chalasani et al. 2015). It is unclear if there is a biological explanation for this or simply a reflection that older patients may be more likely to be prescribed medications such as antibiotics, cardiovascular medications, and analgesics/antipyretics medications that are more prone to cholestatic injury.

Table 10 Drugs commonly related to Drug Induced Liver Injury in Older Adults (Leise et al. 2014; Hoofnagle and Bjornsson 2019)

Class	Drug
Analgesics	Acetaminophen, allopurinol, aspirin, NSAIDs
Antimicrobial	Amoxicillin-clavulanate, azithromycin, cephalosporins floxacillin
Antineoplastic	Methotrexate, tyrosine kinase inhibitors
Cardiac	Amiodarone, statins, diltiazem, hydralazine
CNS agents	Phenytoin, carbamazepine
Dietary	Green tea extracts (high dose)
Endocrine	Acarbose, glucocorticoids
Herbal	Hydroxycut, OxyELITE Pro
Gastrointestinal	Omeprazole
Psychiatric	Bupropion, haloperidol, risperidone, selective serotonin reuptake inhibitors, trazodone, valproic acid
Rheumatologic	Azathioprine, methotrexate, Tumor necrosis factor alpha inhibitors

Table 11 Most frequent medications and type of drug-induced liver injury (Adapted from Chalasani et al. 2015)

Medication	Phenotype
Amoxicillin-Clavulanate	Cholestatic or mixed Hepatitis
Isoniazid	Acute hepatocellular hepatitis
Nitrofurantoin	Acute or chronic hepatocellular hepatitis
TMP-SMZ	Mixed hepatitis
Minocycline	Acute or chronic hepatocellular hepatitis
Cefazolin	Cholestatic Hepatitis
Azithromycin	Hepatocellular, mixed or cholestatic hepatitis
Ciprofloxacin	Hepatocellular, mixed or cholestatic hepatitis
Levofloxacin	Hepatocellular, mixed or cholestatic hepatitis
Diclofenac	Acute or chronic hepatocellular hepatitis
Phenytoin	Hepatocellular or mixed hepatitis
Methyldopa	Hepatocellular or mixed hepatitis
Azathioprine	Cholestatic hepatitis

Patients >75 years old require significantly longer hospitalization for DILI (Onji et al. 2009). However, the prospective study of DILI in the USA did not observe older patients (=>65 years) to have higher frequency of liver transplant or death (Chalasani et al. 2015).

Cirrhosis in the Elderly. There is increasing prevalence of cirrhosis in older adults. The etiology of cirrhosis due to NAFLD is increasing while that due to chronic viral hepatitis is decreasing. Other causes in the elderly are autoimmune hepatitis, primary biliary cholangitis, primary sclerosing cholangitis, and idiopathic (Carrier et al. 2019). However, cirrhosis is often underdiagnosed in older persons. Possible explanations are fewer clinical signs on presentation and infrequent use of diagnostic modalities (Carrier et al. 2019). An autopsy study revealed that 23.7% of elderly with liver cirrhosis had not been diagnosed as having cirrhosis before death (Fujimoto et al. 2008). Similarly, in a study of 135 patients aged 80 years or above with chronic liver disease, 54.1% were found to have cirrhosis. Cirrhosis was a major risk factor affecting the prognosis in this study (Hoshida et al. 1999).

Cirrhosis increases risk of perioperative morbidity and mortality depending on the severity of liver dysfunction. Perioperative mortality is 2–10 times higher in patients with cirrhosis compared to patients without cirrhosis (Newman et al. 2020). The two commonly used predictors of perioperative mortality in patients with cirrhosis are the Child-Turcotte-Pugh (CTP) score and Model for End Stage Liver Disease (MELD) score. The components of CTP score are serum albumin, bilirubin, PT-INR, encephalopathy, and ascites. Patients are categorized as class A (5–6 points), class B (7–9 points), and Class C (10–15 points). Overall surgical mortality for various nonhepatic abdominal surgeries is <5–10% for Class A, 10–40% for Class B and 22–100% for Class C (Newman et al. 2020). The major drawbacks of CPT score are that it has fixed cut off values and uses two subjective parameters (ascites and encephalopathy). In contrast, MELD is a linear regression model that is calculated by using three serum tests: bilirubin, PT-INR, and creatinine. The risk of postoperative mortality increases linearly especially for values of eight and above (Newman et al. 2020). Northrup and associates have demonstrated that mortality increases by 1% for each rise of MELD point up to score of 20 and then by 2% for each point above 20 (Northup et al. 2005).

Postsurgical Liver Enzyme Elevations. Postsurgical liver enzyme elevations can occur in older adults without underlying liver disease. The abnormalities can range from mild enzyme elevations to fulminant hepatic failure (Patel 1999). Risk factors for postsurgical abnormalities can be classified as: prehepatic, hepatocellular, and posthepatic (Labori and Raeder 2004) (Table 12).

The changes are secondary to the duration of surgery, type and technique of surgery, and type of anesthesia utilized. Minor surgical procedures under anesthesia lasting for short duration less than 1 h reveal no abnormalities in liver enzymes. In contrast, surgical procedures involving large body surface area (hernia repair, total mastectomy) demonstrated transient elevations that were more marked after intrabdominal (gastric or biliary) procedures. Transaminases increased within an hour of starting surgery and peaked at the end of surgery. All values decreased to near normal levels at 96 h (Clarke et al. 1976).

Laparoscopic abdominal procedures may impair hepatic function more in older patients. The increase in intraabdominal pressure (IAP) produced by insufflation of carbon-dioxide results in direct and indirect effects on the splanchnic circulation (Hatipoglu et al. 2014). The targeted mean IAP during laparoscopic surgery is 12–15 mm Hg. Even with a modest increase of IAP up to 15 mm Hg, hepatic portal venous flow decreases significantly compared to those undergoing conventional open surgery (Liu et al. 2017). The decrease in portal blood flow is more pronounced in older adults (Sato et al. 2000). Elevations in serum bilirubin, AST and ALT are more pronounced after laparoscopic compared to open cholecystectomy (Singal et al. 2015).

Anesthesia and liver function tests. Hepatic blood flow normally decreases by approximately 40% during the initial 30 min of anesthesia induction (Rahimzadeh et al. 2014). The hepatotoxic

Table 12 Risk factors for abnormal liver function tests in surgery

Prehepatic	Hemolysis
	Hematoma resorption
	Transfusions
Hepatocellular	Hypoxia
	Hypotension
	Type of surgery
	Type of anesthesia
	Infection
	Hepatotoxic drugs
	Total parenteral nutrition
Posthepatic	Compression of liver
	Bile duct injury
	Choledocholithiasis
	Neoplasms

effect of different inhalation anesthetics is halothane > enflurane > isoflurane > desflurane > sevoflurane (Rajan et al. 2019). Regional anesthesia (spinal or epidural anesthesia and nerve blocks) and total intravenous anesthesia are safer alternatives to inhalation anesthetics. Fentanyl is considered the opioid drug of choice as it does not decrease hepatic oxygen and blood supply (Rahimzadeh et al. 2014). Wang et al. (2013) in their randomized control study of older patients undergoing laparoscopic colon or rectal resections have demonstrated that combined general and regional anesthesia is more conducive to the protection of perioperative liver function than general anesthesia alone.

Liver Enzymes in Critical Illness. The liver has a critical role in the systemic response during critical illness (Bernal 2016). It serves a role in clearance of pathogenic microorganisms and toxins from circulation. In response to systemic inflammation, the liver releases cytokines, inflammatory mediators, and coagulation cascade components. Hepatic dysfunction occurs in approximately 11–31% of critically ill patients (Kluge and Tacke 2019) and up to 41% in patients with intraabdominal infections (Guo et al. 2015) is associated with worst outcomes (Kramer et al. 2007; Jager et al. 2012; Kluge and Tacke 2019; Yang 2020). Kramer and associates in their prospective multicenter study of 4146 critically ill patients observed that early hepatic dysfunction

was associated with a twofold increase in mortality (30.4% versus 16.4%) (Kramer et al. 2007). Similarly, one-year survival rate was significantly lower (8% vs 25%) in patients with hypoxic hepatitis (Jager et al. 2012). Hepatic dysfunction in critical illness can be classified into ischemic hepatitis and cholestasis of sepsis.

Ischemic hepatitis seen in 5–10% occurs because of decreased hepatic blood flow in the setting of cardiac, respiratory, or circulatory failure (Kluge and Tacke 2019). It often impacts older patients with underlying cardiac disease. It clinically presents as an acute rise in serum transaminases with the exclusion of other causes of acute liver injury such as viral or drug induced liver injury. Transaminase elevation is rapid and profound (often in thousands) and peaks in 48–72 h after a drop in cardiac output or blood pressure. It is typically accompanied by rise in bilirubin, which may have a delayed peak. Mild coagulopathy can also be present which is reflective of compromised hepatic synthetic function. Liver enzymes improve after hemodynamic status has been restored.

Cholestasis of sepsis seen in approximately 20% presents with progressive rise in bilirubin, ALP, and GGT (Kluge and Tacke 2019; Jenniskens et al. 2016). It is usually not due to obstruction but is thought to be secondary to inflammation induced alterations in the transport of bile acids which appear to drive bile acids and bilirubin towards the systemic circulation. This is usually defined as total bilirubin >2 mg/dl (Guo et al. 2015). Management entails treating underlying infection, minimizing inflammation, and hypoxia in the liver, preventing hyperglycemia, avoiding early use of parenteral nutrition and reducing the administration of avoidable drugs (Jenniskens et al. 2018).

Hepatocellular carcinoma (HCC). The incidence of HCC increases with age. Elderly patients with HCC are more likely to be women, suffer from hepatitis C virus infection and NAFLD (Brunot et al. 2016). Although prognosis is poor, surveillance in high risk patients is associated with early detection and improved survival. Surveillance for HCC in 363 elderly Italian patients >=70 years of age with cirrhosis using both ultrasound and AFP determinations every 6–12 months reduced risk of dealing with an advanced cancer and improved survival as the cancers were amenable to effective treatments (Trevisani et al. 2004). In a single center study of 1530 patients diagnosed with HCC, older patients =>65 years (n = 318, 21%) were compared to younger patients <65 years (n = 1212, 79%). Elderly patients when stratified by stage or treatment showed comparable long-term outcome. In multivariate analysis, age was not an independent risk factor for prognosis, whereas performance status, stage, and effective treatments were independent predictors of long-term survival (Guo et al. 2017). Hence, surveillance and aggressive treatments options are indicated in select elderly (including extremely old) patients with good liver function and good performance status (Brunot et al. 2016; Carrier et al. 2019; Guo et al. 2017).

Key Points

- The prevalence of liver disease with abnormal liver tests is rapidly increasing in older people.
- Nonalcoholic fatty liver disease (NAFLD) is a common disorder in older people.
- Various alterations in morphology, blood flow, cellular activity, and functions of the liver are seen in the older adults.
- Routinely requested liver tests include ALT, AST, GGT, ALP, bilirubin, albumin, and PT or INR; incidental abnormalities are common.
- Liver function remains remarkably resilient during aging.
- ALT and AST assess hepatocellular injury; ALP and bilirubin represent excretion while albumin and PT are markers of protein synthesis.
- An extensive history and identification of predominant patterns of liver blood test helps in determining the clinical diagnosis and further investigations to confirm it.
- Abnormal liver enzymes in older adults, even when mild, should be fully investigated in the context of co-existing medical conditions and risk factors for liver disease.

References

Alves-Bezerra M, Cohen D. Triglyceride metabolism in the liver. Compr Physiol. 2017;8:1–8.

American College of Radiology. ACR-SAR-SPR practice parameter for the performance of magnetic resonance imaging (MRI) of the liver; 2020. Available at https://www.acr.org. Revised 2020 (Resolution 27).

ASGE Standards of Practice Committee, Maple J, Ben-Menachem T, Anderson M, et al. The role of endoscopy in the evaluation of suspected choledocholithiasis. Gastrointest Endosc. 2010;71:1–9.

ASGE Standards of Practice Committee, Buxbaum J, Fehmi S, Sultan S, et al. ASGE guideline on the role of endoscopy in the evaluation and management of choledocholithiasis. Gastrointest Endosc. 2019;89: 1075–105.

Bemeur C, Butterworth R. Nutrition in the management of cirrhosis and its neurological complications. J Clin Exp Hepatol. 2014;4:141–50.

Bernal W. The liver in systemic disease: sepsis and critical Illness. Clin Liver Dis. 2016;7:88–91.

Bialecki E, Bisceglie A. Diagnosis of hepatocellular carcinoma. HPB (Oxford). 2005;7:26–34.

Brunot A, Le Sourd S, Pracht M, Edeline J. Hepatocellular carcinoma in elderly patients: challenges and solutions. J Hepatocellular Carcinoma. 2016;3:9–18.

Buckley C, Dorsey F. The effect of aging on human serum immunoglobulin concentrations. J Immunol. 1970;105: 964–72.

Busher JT. Serum albumin and globulin. In: Walker HK, Hall WD, Hurst JW, editors. Clinical methods: the history, physical, and laboratory examinations. 3rd ed. Boston: Butterworts; 1990.

Cabrerizo S, Cuadras D, Gomez-Busto F, et al. Serum albumin and health in older people: review and meta-analysis. Maturitas. 2015;81:17–27.

Carrier P, Debette-Gratien M, Jacques J, Loustaud-Ratti V. Cirrhotic patients and older people. World J Hepatol. 2019;11:663–77.

Carvalho J, Machado M. New insights about albumin and liver disease. Ann Hepatol. 2018;17:547–60.

Castera L. Noninvasive markers of fibrosis: how reliable are they? In: Foster GR, Reddy RR, editors. Clinical dilemmas in viral liver disease. 2nd ed; 2020. Chapter 1, p. 1–8. https://doi.org/10.1002/97811195 33481ch1.

Castera L, Foucher J, Bernard PH, et al. Pitfalls of liver stiffness measurement: a 5-year prospective study of 13,369 examinations. Hepatology. 2010;51:828–35.

Castera L, Friedrich-Rust M, Loomba R. Noninvasive assessment of liver disease in patients with non-alcoholic fatty liver disease. Gastroenterology. 2019;156:1264–81.

Chalasani N, Bonkovsky H, Fontana R, et al. Features and outcomes of 899 patients with drug-induced liver injury: the DILIN prospective study. Gastroenterology. 2015;148:1340–52.

Chalasani N, Younossi Z, Lavine J, et al. The diagnosis and management of nonalcoholic fatty liver disease: practice guidance from the American Association for the Study of Liver Diseases. Hepatology. 2018;67:328–57.

Charlton M. Branched-chained amino acids enriched supplements as therapy for liver disease. J Nutr. 2006;136 (Suppl 1):295S–8S.

Chundru S, Kalb B, Arif-Tiwari H, et al. MRI of diffuse liver disease: characteristics of acute and chronic disease. Diagn Interv Radiol. 2014;20:200–8.

Cieslak K, Baur O, Verheij J, et al. Liver function declines with increased age. HPB. 2016;18:691–6.

Clarke RSJ, Doggart JR, Lavery T. Changes in liver function after different types of surgery. Br J Anaesth. 1976;48:119–28.

Cullis J, Fitzsimons E, Griffiths W, et al. Investigation and management of a raised serum ferritin. Br J Hematol. 2018;181:331–40.

Devi R, Kumar M. Effect of aging and sex on the caeruloplasmin (Cp) and the plasma protein levels. J Clin Diagn Res. 2012;6:577–80.

Dispenzieri A, Gertz M, Themeau T, Kyle R. Retrospective cohort study of 148 patients with polyclonal gammopathy. Mayo Clin Proc. 2001;76:476–87.

Dong M, Bettencourt R, Brenner D, et al. Serum levels of alanine aminotransferase decrease with age in longitudinal analysis. Clin Gastroenterol Hepatol. 2012;10:285–90.

EASL. EASL-EASD-EASO Clinical practice guidelines for the management of non-alcoholic fatty liver disease. J Hepatol. 2016;64:1388–402.

Fagan KJ, Pretorius CJ, Horsfall LU, et al. ELF score >9.8 indicates advanced hepatic fibrosis and is influenced by age, steatosis and histological activity. Liver Int. 2015;35:1673–81.

Fleming KM, et al. Abnormal liver tests in people aged 75 and above: prevalence and association with mortality. Aliment Pharmacol Ther. 2011;34:324–34.

Frossard JL, Morel PM. Detection and management of bile duct stones. Gastrointest Endosc. 2010;72:808–16.

Fujimoto K, Sawabe M, Sasaki M, et al. Undiagnosed cirrhosis occurs frequently in the elderly and requires periodic follow ups and medical treatments. Geriatr Gerontol Int. 2008;8(3) https://doi.org/10.1111/j.1447-0594.2008.00470.x.

Gilmore I, Burroughs A, Murray-Lyon I, et al. Indications, methods and outcomes of percutaneous liver biopsy in England and Wales: an audit by the British Society of Gastroenterology and the Royal College of Physicians of London. Gut. 1995;36:437–41.

Griffin N, Charles-Edwards G, Grant L. Magnetic resonance cholangiopancreatography: the ABC of MRCP. Insights Imaging. 2012;3:11–21.

Guo K, Ren J, Wang G, et al. Early liver dysfunction in patients with intra-abdominal infections. Medicine. 2015;94(42):e1782.

Guo H, Wu T, Lu Q, et al. Hepatocellular carcinoma in elderly: clinical characteristics, treatments and outcome compared with younger adults. PLoS One. 2017;12(9):

e 0184160. https://doi.org/10.1371/journal.phone.0184160.

Harrison MF. The misunderstood coagulopathy of liver disease: a review for the acute setting. West J Emerg Med. 2018;19:863–71.

Hartman M, Szalai C, Saner F. Hemostasis in liver transplantation: pathophysiology, monitoring and treatment. World J Gastroenterol. 2016;22:1541–50.

Hatipoglu S, Akbulut S, Hatipoglu F, Abdullayev R. Effect of laparoscopic abdominal surgery on splanchnic circulation: Historical developments. World J Gastroenterol. 2014;20:18165–76.

Hernaez R, Lazo M, Bonekamp S, et al. Diagnostic accuracy and reliability of ultrasonography for the detection of fatty liver : a meta-analysis. Hepatology. 2011;54:1082–90.

Hirode G, Saab S, Wong R. Trends in the burden of chronic liver disease among hospitalized US adults. JAMA Netw Open. 2020;3(4):e201997.

Hoofnagle J, Bjornsson E. Drug induced liver injury – types and phenotypes. N Engl J Med. 2019;381:264–73.

Hoshida Y, Ikeda K, Kobayashi M, et al. Chronic liver disease in the extremely elderly of 80 years or more: clinical characteristics, prognosis and patient survival analysis. J Hepatol. 1999;31:860–6.

Hundt M, Basit H, John S. Physiology, bile secretion. StatPearls [Internet]. Treasure Island: StatPearls Publishing; 2020. PMID: 29262229.

Hunt N, McCourt P, Le Couteur D, Cogger V. Novell targets for delaying aging: the importance of the liver and advances in drug delivery. Adv Drug Deliv Rev. 2018;135:39–49.

Hunt N, Kang S, Lockwood G, et al. Hallmarks of aging in the liver. Comput Struct Biotechnol J. 2019;17:1151–61.

Jager B, Drolz A, Michl B, et al. Jaundice increases the rate of complications and one-year mortality in patients with hypoxic hepatitis. Hepatology. 2012;56:2297–304.

Jain S, Gautam V, Naseem S. Acute-phase proteins: as diagnostic tool. J Pharm Bioallied Sci. 2011;3:118–27.

Jenniskens M, Langouche L, Vanmijngaerden Y, et al. Cholestatic liver dysfunction during sepsis and other critical illness. Intensive Care Med. 2016;42:16–27.

Jenniskens M, Langouche L, Van den Berghe G. Choleestatic alterations in the critically ill: some new light on an old problem. Chest. 2018;153:733–43.

Jeong H, Kim D. Bone diseases in patients with chronic liver disease. Int J Mol Sci. 2019;20:4270. https://doi.org/10.3390/ijms20174270.

Kasarala G, Tillmann H. Standard liver tests. Clin Liver Dis. 2016;8:13–8.

Keane J, Eleangovan H, Stokes R, Gunton J. Vitamin D and the liver – correlation or cause? Nutrients. 2018;10:496. https://doi.org/10.3390/nu10040496.

Keller F, Maiga M, Neumayer H, et al. Pharmacokinetic effect of altered plasma protein binding of drugs in renal disease. Eur J Drug Metab Pharmacokinet. 1984;9:275–82.

Khalil R, Al-Humadi N. Types of acute phase reactants and their importance in vaccination (review). Biomed Rep. 2020;12:143–52.

Kim H, Kisseleva T, Brenner D, et al. Aging and liver disease. Curr Opin Gastroenterol. 2015;31:184–91.

Kluge M, Tacke F. Liver impairment in critical illness and sepsis: the dawn of new biomarkers? Ann Transl Med. 2019;7(Suppl 8) https://doi.org/10.21037/atm2019.12.79.

Koenig G, Seneff S. Gama glutamyl transferase: a predictive biomarker of cellular antioxidant inadequacy and disease risk. Dis Markers. 2015:818570. https://doi.org/10.1155/2015/818570.

Kramer L, Jordan B, Drumi W, et al. Incidence and prognosis of early hepatic dysfunction in critically ill patients – a prospective multicenter study. Crit Care Med. 2007;35:1099–104.

Kubes P, Jenne C. Immune response in the liver. Annu Rev Immunol. 2018;36:247–77.

Kwo P, Cohen S, Lim J. ACG clinical guideline: evaluation of abnormal liver chemistries. Am J Gastroenterol. 2017;112:18–35.

Labori KJ, Raeder MG. Diagnostic approach to the patient with jaundice following trauma. Scand J Surg. 2004;93:176–83.

Leise M, Poterucha J, Talwalkar J. Drug-induced liver injury. Mayo Clin Proc. 2014;89:95–106.

Levitt D, Levitt M. Human serum albumin homeostasis: a new look at the role of synthesis, catabolism, renal and gastrointestinal excretion, and the clinical value of serum albumin measurements. Int J Gen Med. 2016;9:229–55.

Lilford R, Bentham L, Girling A, et al. Birmingham and Lambeth liver evaluation testing strategies (BALLETS): a prospective cohort study. Health Technol Assess. 2013;17:1–307.

Limdi JK, Hyde GM. Evaluation of abnormal liver function test. Postgrad Med J. 2003;79:307–12.

Liu Y, Cao W, Liu Y, et al. Changes in duration of action of rocuronium following decrease in hepatic blood flow during pneumoperitoneum for laparoscopic gynaecological surgery. BMC Anaesthesiol. 2017;17:45.

Lock RJ, Unsworth DJ. Immunoglobulins and immunoglobulin subclasses in the elderly. Ann Clin Biochem. 2003;40:143–8.

Lucena MI, Spanish Group for the Study of Drug Induced Liver Disease, et al. Phenotypic characterization of idiosyncratic drug induced liver injury: the influence of age and sex. Hepatology. 2009;49:2001–9.

McPherson S, Hardy T, Dufour J, et al. Age as a confounding factor for the accurate non-invasive diagnosis for advanced NAFLD fibrosis. Am J Gastroenterol. 2017;112:740–51.

Midia M, Odedra D, Shuster A, et al. Predictors of bleeding complications following percutaneous image-guided liver biopsy: a scoping review. Diagn Interv Radiol. 2019;25:71–80.

Mohamad M, Mitchell S, Wu L, et al. Ultrastructure of the liver microcirculation influences hepatic and systemic insulin activity and provides a mechanism for age related insulin resistance. Aging Cell. 2016;15:706–15.

Morsiani C, Bacalini M, Santoro A, et al. The peculiar aging of human liver: a geroscience perspective within transplant context. Aging Res Rev. 2019;51:24–34.

Mukaiyama K, Kamimura M, Uchiyama S, et al. Evaluation of serum alkaline phosphatase (alp) level in post-menopausal woman is caused by high bone turnover. Aging Clin Exp Res. 2015;27:413.

Nemeth E, Ganz T. The role of hepcidin in iron metabolism. Acta Haematol. 2009;122:78–86.

Neuberger J, Patel J, Caldwell H, et al. Guidelines on the use of liver biopsy in clinical practice from the British Society of Gastroenterology, the Royal College of Radiologists and the Royal College of Pathology. Gut. 2020;69:1382–403.

Newman K, Johnson K, Cornia P, et al. Perioperative evaluation and management of patients with cirrhosis: risk assessment, surgical outcomes and future directions. Clin Gastroenterol Hepatol. 2020;18:2398–414.

Newsome P, Cramb R, Davison S, et al. Guidelines on the management of abnormal liver blood tests. Gut. 2018;67:6–19.

Noh C, Lee M, Kim B, Chung Y. A case of nutritional osteomalacia in young adult male. J Bone Metab. 2013;20:51–5.

Northup PG, Wanamaker RC, Lee VD, et al. Model for End Stage Liver Disease (MELD) predicts non-transplant surgical mortality in patients with cirrhosis. Ann Surg. 2005;242:244–51.

O'Leary J, Greenberg C, Patton H, Caldwell S. AGA clinical practice update: coagulation in cirrhosis. Gastroenterology. 2019;157:34–43.

Oh R, Hustead T, Ali S, Pantsari M. Mildly elevated liver transaminase levels: causes and evaluation. Am Fam Physician. 2017;96:709–15.

Onji M, et al. Clinical characteristics of drug induced liver injury in the elderly. Hepatol Res. 2009;39:546–52.

Ortega-Rivera M, Hunt N, Garcia-Sancho J, Cogger V. The hepatic sinusoid in aging and disease: update and advances from the 20th liver sinusoid meeting. Hepatol Commun. 2020;4:1087–98.

Paik J, Golabi P, Biswas R, et al. Nonalcoholic fatty liver disease and alcoholic liver disease are major drivers of liver mortality in the United States. Hepatol Commun. 2020;4:890–903.

Palmer M, Regev A, Lindor K, et al. Consensus guidelines: best practices for detection, assessment and management of suspected acute drug-induced liver injury occurring during clinical trials in adults with chronic cholestatic liver disease. Aliment Pharmacol Ther. 2020;51:90–109.

Pandey N, Hoilat G, John S. Liver biopsy. StatPearls Intranet. Treasure Island: StatPearls Publishing; 2020.

Pant A, Kopec A, Luyendyk J, et al. Role of blood coagulation cascade in hepatic fibrosis. Am J Physiol Gastrointest Liver Physiol. 2018;315:G171–6.

Patel T. Surgery in patients with liver disease. Mayo Clin Proc. 1999;74:593–9.

Petersen K, Befroy D, Shulman G. Mitochondrial dysfunction in the elderly: possible role of insulin resistance. Science. 2003;300:1140–2.

Poynard T, Imbert-Bismut F. Laboratory testing for liver disease. In: Thomas D Boyer, Michael P Manns and Arun J Sanyal, editors. Zakim and Boyer's Hepatology. 6th ed. Science Direct, 2012;201–215. https://doi.org/10.1016/B978-1-4377-0881-3.00072-3.

Pratt D, Kaplan M. Evaluation of abnormal liver-enzyme results in asymptomatic patients. N Engl J Med. 2000;342:1266–71.

Rahimzadeh P, Safari S, Faiz SHR, Alavian M. Anesthesia for patients with liver disease. Hepat Mon. 2014;14(7):e19881.

Rajan S, Garg D, Cummings K III, Krishnaney A. Hepatotoxity after sevoflurane anaesthesia: a new twist to an old story. Br J Anaesth. 2019;122(4):e63–71.

Rogosnitzky M, Branch S. Gadolinium-based contrast agent toxicity: a review of known and proposed mechanisms. Biometals. 2016;29:365–76.

Salizzoni M, Amoroso A, Lupo F, et al. Centenarian livers: very long-term outcomes of old grafts. Transplantation. 2017;101:e292.

Sanchez J, Corey K. Interpretation of abnormal liver chemistries in the hospitalized patient. Clin Liv Dis. 2016;7:132–4.

Sangkhae V, Nemeth E. Regulation of the iron homeostatic hormone hepcidin. Adv Nutr. 2017;8:126–36.

Sato K, Kawamura T, Wakusawa R. Hepatic blood flow and function in elderly patients undergoing laparoscopic cholecystectomy. Anesth Analg. 2000;90:1198–202.

Schmucker D. Age related changes in liver structure and function: implications for disease? Exp Gerontol. 2005;40:650–9.

Schmucker D, Sachs H. Quantifying dense bodies and a lipofuscin during aging: a morphologist's perspective. Arch Gerontol Geriatr. 2002;34:249–61.

Segal J, Dzik W, Transfusion medicine/ Hemostasis Clinical Trials network. Paucity of studies to support that abnormal coagulation test results predict bleeding in the setting of invasive procedures: an evidence based review. Transfusion. 2005;45:1413–25.

Sheedfar F, Di Biase S, Koonen D, Vinciguerra M. Liver diseases and aging: friends or foe? Aging Cell. 2013;12:950–4.

Shetty S, Lalor P, Adams D. Liver sinusoidal endothelial cells – gatekeepers of hepatic immunity. Nature Rev: Gastroenterol Hepatol. 2018;15:555–67.

Singal RS, Singal RP, Sandhu K, et al. Evaluation and comparison of post-operative levels of serum bilirubin, serum transaminases and alkaline phosphatase in laparoscopic cholecystectomy versus open cholecystectomy. J Gastrointest Oncol. 2015;6:479–86.

Sotaniemi EA, et al. Age and cytochrome P450-linked drug metabolism in humans: an analysis of 226 subjects with equal histopathologic conditions. Clin Pharmacol Ther. 1997;61:331–9.

Tajiri K, Shimizu Y. Liver physiology and liver disease in the elderly. World J Gastroenterol 2013; 19: 8459-8467.

Tietz N, Shuey D, Wekstein D. Laboratory values in fit and aging individuals – sexagenarians through centenarians. Clin Chem. 1992;38:1167–85.

Trevisani F, Cantarini M, Labate A, et al. Surveillance of hepatocellular carcinoma in elderly Italian patients with cirrhosis: effects of cancer staging and patient survival. Am J Gastroenterol. 2004;99:1470–6.

Tulner LR, et al. Discrepancies in reported drug use in geriatric outpatients: relevance to adverse events and drug-drug interactions. Am J Geriatr Pharmacother. 2009;7:93–104.

Valdivieso V, Palam R, Wunkhaus R, et al. Effect of aging on biliary lipid composition and bile acid metabolism in normal Chilean women. Gastroenterology. 1978;74:871–4.

Volk ML. Burden of cirrhosis on patients and caregivers. Hepatol Commun. 2020;4:1107–11.

Wang P, Wang H, Zhong T. Influence of different anesthesia on liver and renal function in elderly patients undergoing laparoscopic colon or rectal resection. Hepato-Gastroenterology. 2013;60:79–82.

Wynne H, Cope L, Mutch E, et al. The effect of age upon the liver volume and apparent liver blood flow in healthy man. Hepatology. 1989;9:297–301.

Xu F, Hua C, Tautenhahn H, et al. The role of autophagy for the regeneration of the aging liver. Int J Mol Sci. 2020;21:3606.

Yang JH. Hepatic dysfunction in critically ill patients. Acute Crit Care. 2020;35:44.

Younossi Z, Loomba R, Anstee Q, et al. Diagnostic modalities for nonalcoholic fatty liver disease, nonalcoholic steatohepatitis and associated fibrosis. Hepatology. 2018;68:349–60.

Younossi Z, Stepanova M, Younossi Y, et al. Epidemiology of chronic liver diseases in the USA in the past three decades. Gut. 2020;69:564–8.

Zhao E, Carruthers M, Li C, et al. Conditions associated with polyclonal hypergammaglobulinemia in the IgG-4 related disease era: a retrospective study from a hematology tertiary care center. Hema. 2020;105(3):e121–3.

Zhu C, Ikemoto T, Utsunomiya T, et al. Senescence related genes possibly responsible for poor liver regeneration after hepatectomy in elderly patients. J Gastroenterol Hepatol. 2014;29:1102–8.

Viral Liver Diseases

58

Satheesh Nair and Rajanshu Verma

Contents

S. Nair (✉)
Medical Director of Liver Transplantation, Endowed Chair of Excellence in Transplant Medicine, University of Tennessee Health Science Center, Memphis, TN, USA
e-mail: snair@uthsc.edu

R. Verma
Division of Transplant Hepatology, University of Tennessee Health Science Center, Memphis, TN, USA
e-mail: rverma@uthsc.edu

Abstract

Hepatitis A, hepatitis B, and hepatitis C are the most common types of viral hepatitis. Other types include hepatitis E and hepatitis D. Hepatitis A virus (HAV) infection can produce a significant illness in adults with severity increasing with advancing age. Once acute HAV infection resolves, patients develop lifelong immunity. Hepatitis E virus (HEV) is

© Springer Nature Switzerland AG 2021
C. S. Pitchumoni, T. S. Dharmarajan (eds.), *Geriatric Gastroenterology*,
https://doi.org/10.1007/978-3-030-30192-7_50

similar to HAV, but acute infection causes higher mortality in older adults. Hepatitis B virus (HBV) is one of the most common infections in the world and a leading cause of liver cancer. Majority of adult patients with acute HBV spontaneously clear the infection. Five percent of patients, however, progress into chronic hepatitis B. Chronic HBV is a dynamic disease with four phases: *HBe antigen positive* immune tolerance and immune clearance phases; and *HBe antigen negative* inactive and reactivation phases. Most chronic HBV encountered in older patients are "E antigen" negative/E antibody positive chronic HBV. Treatment of chronic HBV is indicated when there is evidence of liver injury based on elevated ALT and advanced fibrosis on liver biopsy. Entecavir or tenofovir are the currently approved treatments and both have excellent safety and efficacy. HCV is the one of the leading indications for liver transplant in the United States and Europe. Most patients, who get infected with HCV, develop chronic HCV with many eventually progressing to cirrhosis. Screening is recommended for people born between 1945 and 1965 irrespective of risk factors; this screening recommendation may be expanded further to all adults in the near future. Specific drugs targeting HCV replication can cure most patients and hence treatment is recommended if there is detectable HCV RNA.

Keywords

Hepatitis A · HBV · HCV · Cirrhosis · Liver transplantation · HEV · HDV · Hepatocellular carcinoma · Interferon · Hepatitis B · Hepatitis C · Hepatitis E · Viral liver diseases · Viral hepatitis

Abbreviations

HAV	Hepatitis A virus
HBV	Hepatitis B virus
HCC	Hepatocellular carcinoma
HCV	Hepatitis C virus
HDV	Hepatitis D virus
HEV	Hepatitis E virus
HIV	Human immunodeficiency virus
IgG	Immunoglobulin G
IgM	Immunoglobulin M
NS3A/4	Nucleoside 3A/4
NS5A	Nucleoside 5A
NS5B	Nucleoside 5B
PCR	Polymerase chain reaction
RAS	Resistance-associated substitutions
RNA	Ribonucleic acid
SVR	Sustained virologic response

Introduction

Viral hepatitis (hepatitis A–E) affect millions of people in the world. The World Health Organization estimates that in 2015, 257 million people were living with chronic hepatitis B infection (defined as hepatitis B surface antigen positive). Acute liver failure, end-stage liver disease, and hepatocellular carcinoma from viral hepatitis are leading causes of mortality in the world. Hepatitis A and E cause acute infection, while hepatitis B and C mostly present as chronic infections (Fig. 1). Tremendous progress has been made in the treatment of viral hepatitis, especially with hepatitis C over the last few years. This chapter highlights the recent advances in the field of viral hepatitis. The key diagnosis criteria and treatment recommendations based on the current data and practice guidelines are summarized with easy to read tables (Table 1).

Hepatitis A

According to the World Health Organization, approximately 1.5 million clinical cases of hepatitis A occur worldwide annually (Daniels et al. 2009), but seroprevalence data indicate that tens of millions of hepatitis A virus (HAV) infections occur each year. Even though the prevalence of anti-HAV antibody is high among the older population (75%) (Bell et al. 2005), those who are not immune and acquire the infection are at increased risk of complications and higher likelihood of hospitalization.

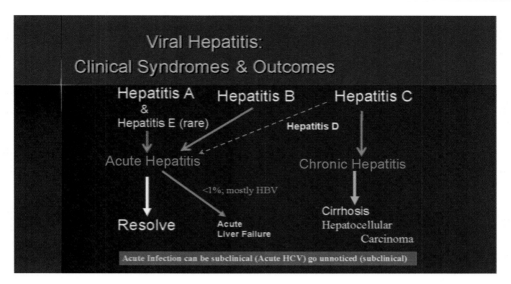

Fig. 1 Viral hepatitis: clinical presentations and outcomes

Table 1 Viral hepatitis serology and interpretation

IgM anti HAV antibody	Acute hepatitis A
IgG anti HAV antibody	Previous exposure; immunity
IgM HEV antibody	Acute hepatitis E infection
Ig G HEV	Prior infection
HCV antibody	Chronic hepatitis C or prior infection – no immunity
HCV RNA	Active HCV infection
HB surface antigen(HBsAg)	Active HBV infection (>6 months indicates chronic HBV infection)
Anti HB surface antibody (HBsAb)	No active HBV and Immunity
IgM Anti HB core Ab	Acute HBV (rarely seen in reactivation phase)
IgG HB core Ab	Prior exposure to HBV
Anti HBs Ab (+) and IgG HBcore Ab (+)	Resolved HBV infection
Anti HBs Ab (+) and IgG HBcore Ab (−)	Vaccination
Anti HBs Ab (−) IgG HBcore (+) HBsAg (−)	Prior infection (small % can have DNA in serum/liver-occult infection- risk of reactivation with immunosuppression)
HBe antigen	Active replication (early phases of infection)
Anti-HBe antibody	Late phases of infection or resolved HBV
HBV DNA	Active infection and for treatment monitoring
HDV antibody	Infection/exposure
HDV PCR	Active infection

Clinical Features and Diagnosis

Clinical illness varies from a mild flu-like sickness to fulminant hepatic failure. The average incubation period is 28 days (range: 15–50 days), after which symptoms include nausea, abdominal pain, fatigue, fever, dark urine, and jaundice along with abnormal liver function including high transaminases and bilirubin. The illness is usually self-limited with most symptoms resolving within 2–4 weeks (Fig. 2).

Rarely, HAV infection can cause a relapsing or cholestatic form of hepatitis lasting several

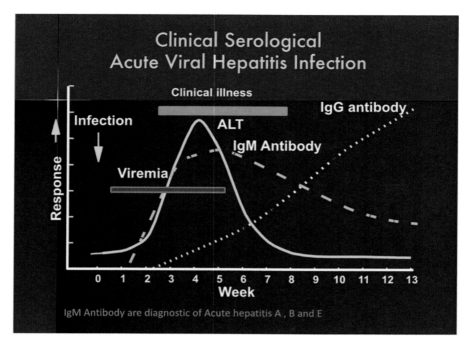

Fig. 2 Clinical and serological features of acute viral hepatitis A and E. (Modified from CDC website)

months before eventual recovery. However, unlike hepatitis B and C, hepatitis A does not cause chronic infection and only rarely leads to fulminant hepatic failure. Acute liver failure from HAV is seen more commonly in patients with chronic liver disease, particularly when it is secondary to chronic hepatitis C virus infection (Vento et al. 1998).

The diagnosis of acute HAV infection is established by the detection of IgM antibodies to HAV (IgM anti-HAV). Following resolution, IgM antibody is replaced by immunoglobulin G (IgG) anti-HAV, which remains detectable for life, and affords lifelong immunity (Fig. 2). People who have received hepatitis A vaccine will also have detectable total anti-HAV antibodies (Table 2).

Treatment

HAV infection is usually self-limited and treatment is therefore supportive. The majority recover without sequelae. However, fatalities associated with the infection and the rate of hospitalization are more common with advancing age (Daniels

et al. 2009; Vento et al. 1998; Forbes and Williams 1988). Thus, special care is indicated for the elderly with acute infection.

Prevention

There are two kinds of vaccine available in the United States (HARVIX, VAQTA). Two doses of the vaccine elicit good immune response in almost 100% of recipients (antibody titer of >20 mIU/ml). HAV vaccination is recommended for everyone with chronic liver disease including those with fatty liver disease and those with persistently elevated ALT (more than two times upper limit of normal). However, the older population and immunocompromised patients may have a suboptimal immune response to vaccination. International travel remains the most commonly identified risk factor for acquiring HAV for US citizens. Travel to endemic areas is common among older adults who now have increased life expectancy and mobility. Therefore, all older travelers lacking naturally acquired immunity should be vaccinated as soon as travel is planned. The

Table 2 Treatment for viral hepatitis

Hepatitis A	Supportive
Acute HBV supportive	Entecavir or tenofovir in prolonged acute HBV
chronic hepatitis B[a]	Entecavir, tenofovir (TDF/TAF[a])
	PEGylated interferon α (contraindicated in cirrhosis)
Hepatitis D	Pegylated interferon α
HBV cirrhosis with liver failure or HCC	Liver transplantation is the best treatment (treat HBV before transplant to prevent recurrence in the allograft)
Acute liver failure (HBV, HEV, HAV)	Liver transplant/supportive
HCV	Glecaprevir/pibrentasvir (Mavyret) or
	Sofosbuvir/velpatasvir, (Epclusa)
HCV cirrhosis with no liver failure	Treat with antiviral agents as above
HCV cirrhosis with liver failure or HCC	Liver transplantation is the best treatment; treat Epclusa if patient is not a candidate for transplant

[a]treat only if advanced fibrosis, high ALT, and high DNA; tenofovir alafenamide has less bone and renal toxicity than TDF

HAV prophylaxis guidelines depend on the underlying health condition of the traveler, endemicity of the area one is traveling to, and the timing of the travel. If travelling to an area with high or intermediate risk of HAV endemicity within 2 weeks, administration of immunoglobulin is also recommended in addition to the vaccine. Detailed guidelines can be accessed on the CDC site (https://www.cdc.gov/mmwr/volumes/67/wr/mm6743a5.htm).

Hepatitis E

Hepatitis E resembles HAV in mode of transmission, clinical presentation, and natural history. HEV causes approximately 20 million infections worldwide each year; however, it is rare in the United States, although sporadic cases have been reported (Rein et al. 2012). HEV in endemic areas of the world is caused by genotype 1 and 2 and results in maternal mortality by affecting pregnant women. In the industrial world, HEV infection is caused by genotypes 3 and 4, possibly acquired as a zoonotic infection. There are several reports of HEV evolving into a chronic infection in severely immunocompromised patients and solid organ recipients.

Acute hepatitis due to HEV is a self-limited disease but is known to be more serious in the older people. There are no FDA approved tests for

diagnosing HEV, but IgM anti-HEV antibody testing is available commercially. Like HAV, detection of IgM anti-HEV indicates acute infection and IgG anti-HEV becomes positive when the infection resolves. HEV PCR assays are also available and usually positive during the acute illness. These commercial assays are not well standardized and false positive results are possible. Vaccine against HEV (HEV 239, Hecolin®) has been developed and licensed in China with limited availability outside Chinese mainland (Li et al. 2015; World Health Organization).

Hepatitis C

It is estimated that more than 170 million persons are infected with hepatitis C worldwide with an incidence of 3–4 million new cases annually. According to the US National Health and Nutrition Examination Survey (NHANES) 2003–2010 data, 1.3% of US population (3.6 million individuals) have anti-HCV antibodies (Denniston et al. 2014). The prevalence of HCV in the geriatric population is projected to increase in the next two to three decades. Because of the longer duration of infection, older adults with hepatitis C are more likely to have advanced disease. HCV is one of the leading indications for liver transplant in the United States and Europe. Twenty-five to 30% of those chronically infected will progress to cirrhosis in 20–25 years after acquiring the infection. The rate of progression depends on the age at which infection was acquired; when contracted at an older age, the disease progression is more rapid (Thabut et al. 2006). Once cirrhosis is established, the risk of liver failure is 5% every year and the risk of hepatocellular carcinoma is 1–3% per year. Several other factors have been linked with higher rate of disease progression (Poynard et al. 1997, 2001).

Mode of Transmission and Risk Factors

HCV is transmitted primarily through exposure to infected blood and blood products. Most patients with HCV in a geriatric practice probably acquired the infection from the use of unsterilized syringes and needles or from blood transfusion prior to 1992 (Thabut et al. 2006).

Clinical Features and Diagnosis

Majority of patients (80%) infected with HCV evolve into chronic hepatitis C, without presenting with an acute phase, with the remaining 20% spontaneously clearing the virus. Hence acute HCV is rarely encountered in clinical practice. Factors including younger age, female gender, certain major histocompatibility complex genes, white race, and interleukin 28 gene polymorphism (IL 28 CC genotype) are associated with spontaneous clearance of HCV infection. Chronic HCV infection is asymptomatic and is routinely diagnosed during evaluation for elevated transaminases or by birth cohort-based screening. In many instances, however, the initial presentation can be with symptoms and signs of liver failure, especially in geriatric patients, who may have acquired the infection 30–40 years earlier. Serum ALT and AST are typically elevated up to five times the upper limit of normal. Serum ALT is higher than AST in the milder stages of HCV, but as the disease evolves into cirrhosis, AST/ALT ratio is reversed (serum AST > ALT). The diagnosis is established by HCV RNA assay in the serum using polymerase chain reaction

assay. The presence of HCV antibody indicates exposure but testing for HCV RNA is required to diagnose active infection. The HCV RNA levels are reported as IU/ml.

Since the degree of fibrosis determines the prognosis and risk of hepatocellular carcinoma, assessment of fibrosis is an important part of evaluation of the patients with chronic hepatitis C (and HBV). Fibrosis is typically classified from I–IV (METAVIR system, stage IV = cirrhosis). Several noninvasive tests (FIB-4, APRI from online calculators) and imaging modalities (transient elastography FibroScan®, shear wave elastography, MR elastography) are now available to estimate the degree of fibrosis. Hence, liver biopsy is no longer indicated in most patients with HCV infection. However, liver biopsy is useful if concomitant diseases such as hemochromatosis, alcoholic hepatitis, and hepatic sarcoidosis are suspected.

HCV Genotypes

HCV viral genome exhibits substantial genetic variations; six major types of HCV, called genotypes, are identified worldwide. About 75% of patients in the United States have genotype 1 and 25% have genotype 2 and 3. Within these genotypes, there are several subtypes and quasispecies. The current treatment of HCV is effective for all genotypes.

Extrahepatic Manifestations

HCV infection is well known to be associated with membranous glomerulonephritis, porphyria cutanea tarda, and mixed cryoglobulinemia, whereas its association with B cell lymphoma is not proven. There are reports of higher incidence of diabetes and increased insulin resistance in patients with HCV, even in the absence of cirrhosis. It is not unreasonable to screen patients with diabetes for HCV and cirrhosis (Eslam et al. 2011). Insulin resistance is also associated with higher rate of progression of fibrosis and is known to improve with HCV

Table 3 Extrahepatic manifestation of viral hepatitis[a]

Condition	Comments
1. **Polyarteritis nodosa**	HBV, HBV treatment may be indicated
2. **Membranous nephropathy**	HBV (Rx effect not known)
3. **Membranoproliferative nephropathy**	HBV (Rx effect not known) and HCV
4. **Essential mixed cryoglobulinemia**	90% have HCV; HCV cure may not decrease Cryoglobulin levels or its manifestation
5. **B-cell non-Hodgkin's lymphoma**	Treatment is similar to other lymphoma All lymphoma patients be tested for HCV HCV treatment may cause regression
6. **Elevated gamma globulin**	Reported with HCV but not very conclusive Elevated IG levels are seen in chronic liver disease
7. **Porphyria cutanea tarda**	50% patients have HCV HCV treatment may not affect skin lesions HIV and hemochromatosis need to be ruled out
8. **Lichen planus**	Test for HCV in patients with lichen planus
9. **Thyroid disorder**	HCV patients are at risk of hypothyroidism TSH and T4 should be checked at diagnosis of HCV
10. **Diabetes mellitus**	HCV increases insulin resistance HCV cure may improve glycemic control
11. **Autoantibodies**	Rheumatoid factor antinuclear antibodies are seen in HCV-may lead to false diagnosis

[a]Lower mortality from cardiovascular and neurological diseases has been observed in HCV patients who achieved SVR compared to those without SVR

treatment (Conjeevaram et al. 2011; Patel et al. 2011). HCV antibody is frequently seen in patients with rheumatoid arthritis, and HCV PCR is required to confirm the diagnosis of active infection. Conversely, rheumatoid factor is present in many patients with HCV, but without any other evidence of rheumatoid arthritis. A detailed review of extrahepatic manifestations of HCV was recently published (Jacobson et al. 2010) (Table 3).

Treatment

Treatment of chronic hepatitis C is truly one of the miracles of modern medicine. Within the last decade, its treatment has transformed from, year-long treatment with multiple injections with interferon with suboptimal response, multiple side effects to simple tablet-based treatment that effectively cures nearly 100% of patients.

The end point of HCV therapy is defined as sustained virologic response (SVR), meaning undetectable HCV RNA by a sensitive assay,

12 weeks after stopping the treatment. Once SVR is achieved, HCV RNA remains undetectable (durability of response), and hence clinicians use the term "cure" in patients who achieve SVR (Swain et al. 2010). In addition to reducing liver complications, in achieving SVR in HCV-infected patients, there is a decrease in non-liver-related mortality. Moreover, several studies have shown that fibrosis is reversible in those who achieve sustained viral suppression in both HCV and HBV. However, patients with cirrhosis need hepatocellular carcinoma screening every 6 months even after achieving SVR (Morgan et al. 2010).

HCV was first discovered in 1989. Interferon-alpha was the first drug used to treat HCV which resulted in treatment response in up to a third of patients; however, it led to significantly high relapse rates and thus a low true SVR of 6% (Davis et al. 1989). Addition of ribavirin to interferon helped increase SVR rates to 34–42% (McHutchison et al. 1998). Subsequently, it was found that use of pegylated form of interferon when used with ribavirin helped achieve higher

SVR rates (Zeuzem et al. 2000). The development of HCV replicon in 2006 has made it possible to develop many direct acting agents that target the key enzymes (NS3, NS 5B, and NS 5A) involved in the HCV replication. A NS5B polymerase inhibitor, sofosbuvir (Sovaldi®, Gilead Sciences), was approved in 2013 (FDA approves Sovaldi for chronic hepatitis C). *Sofosbuvir* in combination of N5A inhibitors (Ledipasvir (Harvoni) and *velpatasvir* (Epclusa) have led the way in HCV treatment during the last few years (Feld et al. 2015; Foster et al. 2015). In 2017, another combination regimen with NS5a inhibitor, *pibrentasvir* and NS3 inhibitor, *glecaprevir* (Mavyret, Abbvie Inc.) was approved to treat HCV (Forns et al. 2017).

The two recommended regimens for HCV patients, who have not failed previous treatment, are either *sofosbuvir + velpatasvir* (Epclusa), 1 tablet/per day with or without food for 12 weeks, or *pibrentasvir* and *glecaprevir* (Mavyret), 3 tablets/day with food for 8 weeks. Both regimens are highly effective with near 100% cure rate and are effective for all genotypes (Zeuzem et al. 2018; FDA approves Mavyret). Cirrhosis, genotype 3, and baseline NS5A *resistance-associated substitutions* (RAS) may lower the response by 5–10%. Age, race, gender, BMI, and baseline viral RNA levels do not affect response to treatment. The safety of both regimens is well established in patients with decreased renal function and those with ESRD on hemodialysis. There is no need for dose adjustment.

The current simplified treatment regimen encourages primary care physicians and physician extenders to treat HCV. Liver biopsy is not required before treatment. There is no need for follow-up or laboratory testing during treatment in majority of patients. However, SVR need to be documented. Cirrhosis can be diagnosed with reasonable accuracy by using APRI (https://www.mdcalc.com/ast-platelet-ratio-index-apri) or FIB-4 score (https://www.mdcalc.com/fibrosis-4-fib-4-index-liver-fibrosis). If cirrhosis is suspected or patient had failed treatment in the past or has coinfection with HBV, closer follow-up and a referral to a specialist are indicated. The most updated guidelines for treatment of HCV are jointly published by Infectious Diseases Society of America (IDSA) and American Association for the Study of Liver Diseases (AASLD) on https://www.hcvguidelines.org.

The HCV treatment regimen is safe and effective in patients over 65 years. The phase 3 clinical trials included several patients over 65 years and the SVR rate is similar to younger patients. These regimens were also equally well tolerated. Age by itself should not be consideration for eligibility of HCV treatment but treatment should not be offered to patents with life expectancy of less than 1 year. Protease inhibitor (NS3 inhibitor) containing regimens such as pibrentasvir and glecaprevir (Mavyret) are contraindicated in patients with decompensated liver disease (Child-Pugh score 7 or more) or in patients who had a decompensating event in the past. An FDA update in September 2019 reported several deaths in patients taking protease inhibitor drugs. Hence patients with cirrhosis need careful assessment before protease inhibitors are prescribed.

Since patients over 65 are likely to be on multiple cardiovascular drugs for metabolic syndrome, *drug–drug interaction* (DDI) is an important consideration. For example, sofosbuvir (Epclusa) is contraindicated in patients taking amiodarone due to life-threatening brady-arrhythmias. Statins also have significant drug interactions with these drugs; dose adjustment or discontinuation may be required. *Epclusa* has lower efficacy when used in patients taking high dose of proton pump inhibitors as the absorption of velpatasvir is reduced at higher pH. Interactions with warfarin and hypoglycemic agents may require closer monitoring. All drugs have lower efficacy in patients taking CYP3A inducers such as phenytoin sodium and carbamazepine. There are app-based services one can use to verify DDI (Liverpool HEP1Chart: http://www.hep-druginteraction.org).

It is very rare for HCV treatment to fail; failure is often due to inadequate exposure to the drugs either because of nonadherence or drug interactions as mentioned above. Rarely treatment emergent *resistance-associated substitutions* (RAS) lead to virologic failure. Sofosbuvir, velpatasvir, and voxilaprevir combination (Vosevi) is effective in treating most patients who have failed treatment (Jacobson et al. 2017). Resistance testing is not indicated for HCV.

On basis of these highly effective treatments, World Health Organization (WHO) has set a goal to eliminate hepatitis C by 2030 (WHO 2016). Effective HCV treatment has also helped expand the donor pool by allowing use of HCV positive organs in solid organ transplantation where there is always a scarcity of suitable donors and demand outstrips the supply of available organs by many-fold (WHO 2016).

Hepatitis B (HBV)

The incidence of hepatitis B infection in the United States is increasing due to immigration from endemic areas. The Center for Disease Control recommends screening for all individuals from endemic countries (Far East, sub-Saharan Africa). HBV is parenterally transmitted and hence screening is recommended for individuals with high risk behavior or those with exposure to blood products or contaminated needles.

Clinical Features and Diagnosis

HBV can present as acute HBV, with a clinical presentation very similar to acute HAV (Fig. 3). Almost 90–95% patients with acute HBV sponta-neously clear the infection and develop immunity. Five percent of patients, however, progress into chronic hepatitis B as evidenced by persistence of HBV surface antigen (HBsAg) beyond 6 months. Once chronic infection is established, HBV infec-tion evolves through different stages based on the interaction with the immune system of the host (Fig. 2). Most chronic HBV encountered in adults over 65 years will be "e antigen" negative chronic HBV and have "pre-core mutant HBV" (HBV loses the ability to produce HBV e antigen) and hence the typical serological pattern will be HBsAg antigen positive, HBV e antibody positive (anti-HBe), and HBV e antigen negative (HBeAg). The HBV DNA and the serum ALT levels will depend on whether the patient is in the inactive phase or the reactivation phase of chronic HBV disease (Fig. 3).

It is important to note that unlike hepatitis C, HBV can cause hepatocellular carcinoma (HCC)

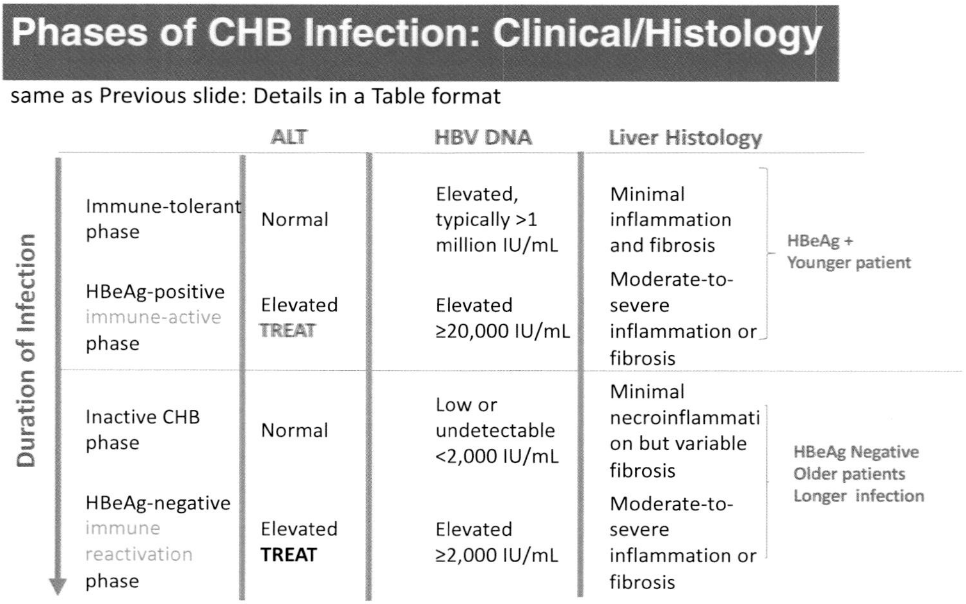

Phases of CHB Infection: Clinical/Histology

same as Previous slide: Details in a Table format

Duration of Infection		ALT	HBV DNA	Liver Histology	
	Immune-tolerant phase	Normal	Elevated, typically >1 million IU/mL	Minimal inflammation and fibrosis	HBeAg + Younger patient
	HBeAg-positive immune-active phase	Elevated **TREAT**	Elevated ≥20,000 IU/mL	Moderate-to-severe inflammation or fibrosis	
	Inactive CHB phase	Normal	Low or undetectable <2,000 IU/mL	Minimal necroinflammati on but variable fibrosis	HBeAg Negative Older patients Longer infection
	HBeAg-negative immune reactivation phase	Elevated **TREAT**	Elevated ≥2,000 IU/mL	Moderate-to-severe inflammation or fibrosis	

Fig. 3 Chronic HBV stages and treatment indications

even in the absence of cirrhosis. Age is an important risk factor for HCC in hepatitis B, and hence older adults need close surveillance for HCC irrespective of the severity of liver disease. Other factors that increase the risk of HCC in patients with chronic HBV include male gender, family history of HCC, presence of cirrhosis, higher level of HBV DNA, and coinfection with HIV, HDV

HBV Genotypes

Several genotypes of HBV are identified named A to F. Some genotypes are responsive to interferon (genotype A), while others are associated with higher risk of cancer (genotype C) (Lin and Kao 2011). But unlike HCV, there are no definitive treatment guidelines based on the genotype.

Reactivation of HBV

Since hepatitis B can be clinically silent in many patients, it is important to screen for HBV markers (HBsAg) in patients scheduled for immunosuppressive treatments such as prolonged course of steroids, chemotherapy, anti B cell treatment, or anti-TNF alfa agents (Gisbert et al. 2011). This risk of reactivation also depends on the agent used with the highest risk reported with rituximab. This is particularly relevant in patients over 65 who may have inactive HBV and is at higher risk of malignancy due to age. If a patient is HBsAg positive and does not meet the criteria for HBV treatment, prophylaxis is recommended for the entire duration therapy and 6–12 months following completion of immunosuppressive therapy. Even in patients with resolved prior infection (negative HBsAg, positive HB core antibody, Table 1), a small amount of HBV DNA may be present in the hepatocytes and reactivation is possible. Prophylaxis may be indicated in these patients also if they are receiving rituximab. Any of the oral antiviral agents can be used for prophylaxis but entecavir or tenofovir is preferred. HBV reactivation can lead to rapid onset of liver failure. Many of these patients may not qualify for

transplant due to underlying medical conditions such as malignancy that led to immunosuppressive therapy. Generally liver transplantation is not offered to patients over 70 years and many centers consider age over 75 years as an absolute contraindication.

HBV reactivation can also occur in coinfected patients with HCV who are undergoing treatment for HCV (Chen et al. 2017). If they have active HBV, treatment of HBV needs to be instituted before HCV is treated. In patients with no active HBV (i.e., HBs Ag negative, but HBcore Ab positive), HBV DNA levels may need to be checked if there are abnormal liver function tests.

Treatment of HBV

HBV treatment guidelines have been recently revised and decision to treat is based on presence of liver injury and advanced fibrosis. Primary goal of HBV treatment is to limit progression of liver injury; hence treatment is reserved for patients with evidence of liver injury on liver biopsy or elevated ALT (Yuen and Lai 2011). HBV infection is not curable in most individuals even though viral suppression to undetectable levels of HBV DNA is possible in most patients. Patients in the "inactive stage" of liver disease, i.e., those with normal ALT and no fibrosis, should not be treated. Similarly, patients in the immune tolerant phase require no treatment, unless there is concern for higher risk of cancer or liver injury (Fig. 3).

HBV treatment has evolved over the last 10 years with advent of potent antiviral agents. Earlier antiviral agents such as lamivudine (Epivir™), adefovir (Hepsera™), and telbivudine (Tyzeka®) are no longer used as first-line therapy for HBV because of unacceptably high rate of resistance. As per recent AASLD guidelines, the first line of treatment is tenofovir disoproxil fumarate (TDF) (Viread™; Gilead Sciences) 300 mg PO/day, tenofovir alafenamide (TAF) (Vemlidy®; Gilead Sciences) 25 mg daily, entecavir (Baraclude™; Bristol-Myers Squibb) 0.5 mg/day PO, or pegylated interferon-α-2a (PEGASYS 180 mcg/week) (Terrault et al. 2018). Unlike

HCV, HBV is treated with a single drug. Both entecavir and tenofovir are well tolerated, while PEG interferon has myriad of side effects. The only indication to use two drugs is following documented resistance to one of the drugs. Tenofovir resistance is not seen in clinical studies with long-term follow-up, while entecavir resistance can be rarely seen particularly in patients who have taken lamivudine in the past. Tenofovir alafenamide (TAF) has the advantage over tenofovir disoproxil fumarate (TDF) as it has lower toxicity regarding bone density and renal function (Liaw et al. 2011). Interferon is contraindicated in patients with cirrhosis due to risk of liver failure with treatment-associated flares. On the other hand, both entecavir and tenofovir are well tolerated even in decompensated cirrhotic patients (Liaw et al. 2011). It is worth noting that the current HBV treatment will not cure HBV infection (defined as HBsAg loss) in most patients even with prolonged treatment. In HBeAg negative individuals, the clearance of HBsAg is only 5%. This is in contrast to HCV, where the majority can be "cured." Hepatitis B "cure" is now the focus of intense research.

Since HBV infection cannot be cured, surrogate goals of treatment are often used. These include: (1) seroconversion of HBe antigen to anti-HBe antibody positivity in HBeAg positive patients and (2) decrease in HBV DNA to undetectable levels in HBeAg negative patients with the eventual improvement/stabilization of the liver histology.

HIV and HBV coinfection also demands special attention; the choice of agents depends on whether HIV needs treatment. If HIV is to be treated, tenofovir is the agent of choice as it has excellent activity against both HIV and HBV.

Most patients over 65 are likely to have HBe antigen negative chronic infection as they have likely acquired infection in the remote past (Fig. 3). In addition, many may have significant fibrosis because of long duration of infection even in the presence of normal transaminases. The treatment is usually lifelong unless there is clearance of hepatitis B surface antigen. Many

hepatologists believe that these patients should be on treatment to decrease HBV replication and minimize the risk of hepatocellular carcinoma. There is no age limit to treat HBV as the treatment is well tolerated. There are some preliminary data that tenofovir may be superior to entecavir in reducing the risk of HCC. Renal and bone toxicity from long-term exposure to tenofovir disoproxil fumarate (Viread) is a concern in older adults and those patients should be switched to tenofovir alafenamide.

Hepatitis Delta (HDV)

Hepatitis D, being an incomplete virus, will only infect patients who have hepatitis B surface antigen. It is a coinfection, i.e., infection along with HBV or as super infection (in other words, infection of a patient with already established HBV). HDV increases the severity of HBV infection or can cause acute exacerbation of chronic HBV. HDV is difficult to treat; about 25% response can be achieved with pegylated interferon (Wedemeyer et al. 2011). Recent data suggest that long-term HBV viral suppression may also suppress HDV RNA levels even in the absence of HBsAg loss. Newer drugs such as Lonafarnib (a farnesyltransferase inhibitor), Myrcludex B (HBV/HDV entry inhibitor), and REP 2139 (inhibitor of virion release) hold promise in treating HDV

Key Points

- Hepatitis A presents as acute hepatitis and, in most patients, resolves without complications.
- Hepatitis E is rare and clinically resembles hepatitis A.
- Hepatitis E infection carries a higher mortality in older adults.
- Most cases of acute HBV resolve but rarely develop fulminant hepatic failure.
- About 5% of HBV develop chronic infection; most chronic HBV infections in the older population is either inactive carrier state or reactivation phase.

- Chronic hepatitis B can be effectively controlled by antiviral agents, but HBV infection cannot be eradicated.
- Tenofovir alafenamide has a better renal and bone safety profile and hence the preferred regimen in patients over 65 years.
- HBV can cause liver cancer even in the absence of cirrhosis; hence surveillance is indicated in high-risk patients https://www.aasld.org; Practice Guidelines Hepatocellular Carcinoma: Hepatology 2018; 68:723–750.
- HCV is the most common viral hepatitis in the United States and the leading cause of cirrhosis and liver cancer.
- Acute HCV is rarely seen in clinical practice; most cases are chronic HCV.
- All patients with HCV RNA should be treated (acute or chronic).
- Hepatitis C can be cured by Epclusa or Mavyret in most patients (99%).
- HCV drugs are safe and well tolerated, but drug–drug interaction requires attention.

References

Bell BP, Kruszon-Moran D, Shapiro CN, Lambert SB, McQuillan GM, Margolis HS. Hepatitis A virus infection in the United States: serologic results from the Third National Health and Nutrition Examination Survey. Vaccine. 2005;23(50):5798–806.

Chen G, Wang C, Chen J, Ji D, Wang Y, Wu V, Karlberg J, Lau G. Hepatitis B reactivation in hepatitis B and C coinfected patients treated with antiviral agents: a systematic review and meta-analysis. Hepatology. 2017;66(1):13–26.

Conjeevaram HS, Wahed AS, Afdhal N, Howell CD, Everhart JE, Hoofnagle JH, Virahep CSG. Changes in insulin sensitivity and body weight during and after peginterferon and ribavirin therapy for hepatitis C. Gastroenterology. 2011;140(2):469–77.

Daniels D, Grytdal S, Wasley A. Centers for disease C, prevention: surveillance for acute viral hepatitis – United States, 2007. MMWR Surveill Summ. 2009;58(3):1–27.

Davis GL, Balart LA, Schiff ER, Lindsay K, Bodenheimer HC Jr, Perrillo RP, Carey W, Jacobson IM, Payne J, Dienstag JL, et al. Treatment of chronic hepatitis C with recombinant interferon alfa. A multicenter randomized, controlled trial. N Engl J Med. 1989;321(22):1501–6.

Denniston MM, Jiles RB, Drobeniuc J, Klevens RM, Ward JW, McQuillan GM, Holmberg SD. Chronic hepatitis C virus infection in the United States, National Health and Nutrition Examination Survey 2003 to 2010. Ann Intern Med. 2014;160(5):293–300.

Eslam M, Khattab MA, Harrison SA. Insulin resistance and hepatitis C: an evolving story. Gut. 2011;60(8):1139–51.

FDA approves Mavyret for Hepatitis C. In

FDA approves Sovaldi for chronic hepatitis C. https://www.hhs.gov/hepatitis/blog/2013/12/09/fda-approves-sovaldi-for-chronic-hepatitis-c.html

Feld JJ, Jacobson IM, Hezode C, Asselah T, Ruane PJ, Gruener N, Abergel A, Mangia A, Lai CL, Chan HL, et al. Sofosbuvir and velpatasvir for HCV genotype 1, 2, 4, 5, and 6 infection. N Engl J Med. 2015;373(27):2599–607.

Forbes A, Williams R. Increasing age – an important adverse prognostic factor in hepatitis A virus infection. J R Coll Physicians Lond. 1988;22(4):237–9.

Forns X, Lee SS, Valdes J, Lens S, Ghalib R, Aguilar H, Felizarta F, Hassanein T, Hinrichsen H, Rincon D, et al. Glecaprevir plus pibrentasvir for chronic hepatitis C virus genotype 1, 2, 4, 5, or 6 infection in adults with compensated cirrhosis (EXPEDITION-1): a single-arm, open-label, multicentre phase 3 trial. Lancet Infect Dis. 2017;17(10):1062–8.

Foster GR, Afdhal N, Roberts SK, Brau N, Gane EJ, Pianko S, Lawitz E, Thompson A, Shiffman ML, Cooper C, et al. Sofosbuvir and velpatasvir for HCV genotype 2 and 3 infection. N Engl J Med. 2015;373(27):2608–17.

Gisbert JP, Chaparro M, Esteve M. Review article: prevention and management of hepatitis B and C infection in patients with inflammatory bowel disease. Aliment Pharmacol Ther. 2011;33(6):619–33.

Jacobson IM, Cacoub P, Dal Maso L, Harrison SA, Younossi ZM. Manifestations of chronic hepatitis C virus infection beyond the liver. Clin Gastroenterol Hepatol. 2010;8(12):1017–29.

Jacobson IM, Lawitz E, Gane EJ, Willems BE, Ruane PJ, Nahass RG, Borgia SM, Shafran SD, Workowski KA, Pearlman B, et al. Efficacy of 8 weeks of sofosbuvir, velpatasvir, and voxilaprevir in patients with chronic HCV infection: 2 phase 3 randomized trials. Gastroenterology. 2017;153(1):113–22.

Li SW, Zhao Q, Wu T, Chen S, Zhang J, Xia NS. The development of a recombinant hepatitis E vaccine HEV 239. Hum Vaccin Immunother. 2015;11(4):908–14.

Liaw YF, Sheen IS, Lee CM, Akarca US, Papatheodoridis GV, Suet-Hing Wong F, Chang TT, Horban A, Wang C, Kwan P, et al. Tenofovir disoproxil fumarate (TDF), emtricitabine/TDF, and entecavir in patients with decompensated chronic hepatitis B liver disease. Hepatology. 2011;53(1):62–72.

Lin CL, Kao JH. The clinical implications of hepatitis B virus genotype: recent advances. J Gastroenterol Hepatol. 2011;26(Suppl 1):123–30.

McHutchison JG, Gordon SC, Schiff ER, Shiffman ML, Lee WM, Rustgi VK, Goodman ZD, Ling MH, Cort S, Albrecht JK. Interferon alfa-2b alone or in combination with ribavirin as initial treatment for chronic hepatitis C. Hepatitis Interventional Therapy Group. N Engl J Med. 1998;339(21):1485–92.

Morgan TR, Ghany MG, Kim HY, Snow KK, Shiffman ML, De Santo JL, Lee WM, Di Bisceglie AM, Bonkovsky HL, Dienstag JL, et al. Outcome of sustained virological responders with histologically advanced chronic hepatitis C. Hepatology. 2010;52(3):833–44.

Patel K, Thompson AJ, Chuang WL, Lee CM, Peng CY, Shanmuganathan G, Thongsawat S, Tanwandee T, Mahachai V, Pramoolsinsap C, et al. Insulin resistance is independently associated with significant hepatic fibrosis in Asian chronic hepatitis C genotype 2 or 3 patients. J Gastroenterol Hepatol. 2011;26(7):1182–8.

Poynard T, Bedossa P, Opolon P. Natural history of liver fibrosis progression in patients with chronic hepatitis C. The OBSVIRC, METAVIR, CLINIVIR, and DOSVIRC groups. Lancet. 1997;349(9055):825–32.

Poynard T, Ratziu V, Charlotte F, Goodman Z, McHutchison J, Albrecht J. Rates and risk factors of liver fibrosis progression in patients with chronic hepatitis c. J Hepatol. 2001;34(5):730–9.

Rein DB, Stevens GA, Theaker J, Wittenborn JS, Wiersma ST. The global burden of hepatitis E virus genotypes 1 and 2 in 2005. Hepatology. 2012;55(4):988–97.

Swain MG, Lai MY, Shiffman ML, Cooksley WG, Zeuzem S, Dieterich DT, Abergel A, Pessoa MG, Lin A, Tietz A, et al. A sustained virologic response is durable in patients with chronic hepatitis C treated with peginterferon alfa-2a and ribavirin. Gastroenterology. 2010;139(5):1593–601.

Terrault NA, Lok ASF, McMahon BJ, Chang KM, Hwang JP, Jonas MM, Brown RS Jr, Bzowej NH, Wong JB. Update on prevention, diagnosis, and treatment of chronic hepatitis B: AASLD 2018 hepatitis B guidance. Hepatology. 2018;67(4):1560–99.

Thabut D, Le Calvez S, Thibault V, Massard J, Munteanu M, Di Martino V, Ratziu V, Poynard T. Hepatitis C in 6,865 patients 65 yr or older: a severe and neglected curable disease? Am J Gastroenterol. 2006;101(6):1260–7.

Vento S, Garofano T, Renzini C, Cainelli F, Casali F, Ghironzi G, Ferraro T, Concia E. Fulminant hepatitis associated with hepatitis A virus superinfection in patients with chronic hepatitis C. N Engl J Med. 1998;338(5):286–90.

Wedemeyer H, Yurdaydin C, Dalekos GN, Erhardt A, Cakaloglu Y, Degertekin H, Gurel S, Zeuzem S, Zachou K, Bozkaya H, et al. Peginterferon plus adefovir versus either drug alone for hepatitis delta. N Engl J Med. 2011;364(4):322–31.

WHO. Combating hepatitis B and C to reach elimination by 2030. Advocacy brief. 2016. https://www.who.int/hepatitis/publications/hep-elimination-by-2030-brief/en/

World Health Organization. Hepatitis E fact sheet. http://www.who.int/news-room/fact-sheets/detail/hepatitis-e

Yuen MF, Lai CL. Treatment of chronic hepatitis B: evolution over two decades. J Gastroenterol Hepatol. 2011;26(Suppl 1):138–43.

Zeuzem S, Feinman SV, Rasenack J, Heathcote EJ, Lai MY, Gane E, O'Grady J, Reichen J, Diago M, Lin A, et al. Peginterferon alfa-2a in patients with chronic hepatitis C. N Engl J Med. 2000;343(23):1666–72.

Zeuzem S, Foster GR, Wang S, Asatryan A, Gane E, Feld JJ, Asselah T, Bourliere M, Ruane PJ, Wedemeyer H, et al. Glecaprevir-pibrentasvir for 8 or 12 weeks in HCV genotype 1 or 3 infection. N Engl J Med. 2018;378(4):354–69.

Tumors of the Liver

59

Mumtaz Niazi, Pratik A. Shukla, and Nikolaos Pyrsopoulos

Contents

M. Niazi
Department of Medicine, Division of Gastroenterology
and Hepatology, Rutgers University, New Jersey Medical
School, Newark, NJ, USA
e-mail: man202@njms.rutgers.edu

P. A. Shukla
Department of Radiology, Division of Interventional
Radiology, Rutgers University, New Jersey Medical
School, Newark, NJ, USA
e-mail: pshukla@njms.rutgers.edu

N. Pyrsopoulos (✉)
Department of Medicine, Division of Gastroenterology
and Hepatology, Physiology, Pharmacology and
Neuroscience, Medical Director Liver Transplantation,
Rutgers – New Jersey Medical School, University
Hospital, Newark, NJ, USA
e-mail: pyrsopni@njms.rutgers.edu

© Springer Nature Switzerland AG 2021
C. S. Pitchumoni, T. S. Dharmarajan (eds.), *Geriatric Gastroenterology*,
https://doi.org/10.1007/978-3-030-30192-7_51

Abstract

Sensitivity of abdominal imaging studies is improving and use of radiologic modalities is getting more common, leading to diagnosis of incidental liver lesions. Some of the lesions need further investigations and some can be left alone. Hepatic hemagioma is the most common benign mesenchymal primary solid liver tumor. In patients with underlying cirrhosis and with chronic Hepatitis B, hepatocellular cancer (HCC) must be highly suspected. HCC is now the fifth most common cancer in the world and third most common cause of cancer-related mortality.

Keywords

Liver tumors · Hepatocellular cancer · Benign lesions · Malignant lesions · Focal nodular hyperplasia

Introduction

Due to the widespread and very common use of abdominal imaging studies, along with their continuous improvement in sensitivity, incidental liver lesions are now identified with increasing frequency either in solitary or multiple. The majority of these liver lesions, so-called incidentalomas, are benign and thus discovered in healthy and asymptomatic individuals. The major challenge is to establish an accurate diagnosis, so that further management recommendations can be provided. For hepatocellular lesions, a descriptive nomenclature was set and summarized by an international panel of experts sponsored by the World Congress of Gastroenterology in 1994 (International Working Party 1995). The combination of clinical history and appropriate radiological descriptions can help in the diagnosis of majority of the liver tumors. In patients with chronic liver disease, chronic hepatitis B, advanced age, previous history of cancer, or constitutional symptoms (anorexia, weight loss, asthenia, etc.), these incidentally discovered liver lesions have a high likelihood for malignant potential which require further investigation.

The liver tumors can be further divided into three categories: (i) benign lesions usually requiring no further investigations/treatment (ii); benign lesions requiring further investigation and may need therapy (iii); and malignant lesions requiring appropriate investigations and therapy (Table 1).

Benign Liver Tumors Requiring No Further Investigation

Hepatic Hemangiomas

Hepatic hemangioma is the most common benign mesenchymal primary solid liver tumor. The prevalence of hemangioma is estimated to be 5% as reported in imaging series (Horta et al. n.d.) and up to 20% in autopsy series (Bahirwani and Reddy 2008; Karhunen 1986). Hemangiomas can occur in all age groups but are more frequently diagnosed among women ranging between 30 and 50 years age. Hemangiomas are asymptomatic and are most commonly diagnosed incidentally with no major clinical implications. Hemangiomas range in size from a few millimeters to more than 20 cm in diameter. Even when they are large, most of the patients are asymptomatic (Bahirwani and Reddy 2008). In rare circumstances, large hepatic hemangioma can present with spontaneous or post-traumatic rupture resulting in symptomatic bleeding or mass effect on adjacent organs. Hemangiomas can be diagnosed radiologically by both dynamic contrast-enhanced computed tomography (CT) scan and magnetic resonance imaging (MRI) with a high degree of sensitivity and specificity (Fowler et al. n.d.). The classic appearance of a hepatic hemangioma on both imaging modalities is described as peripheral nodular, discontinuous enhancement with progressive centripital enhancement on delayed sequences (Mukundan et al. 2005). Although less sensitive, this imaging

Table 1 Categories of Liver Tumors

Benign lesions usually requiring no further investigations/treatment
Hepatic hemangiomas
Focal nodular hyperplasia
Simple hepatic cyst
Polycystic liver disease
Benign lesions requiring further investigation and may need therapy
Hepatocellular adenoma
Nodular regenerative hyperplasia
Malignant lesions requiring appropriate investigations and therapy
Hepatocellular carcinoma
Cholangiocarcinoma
Liver metastases

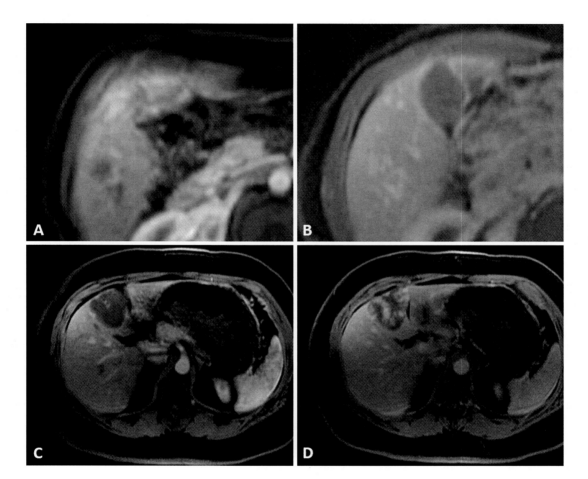

Fig. 1 (**a**) Post contrast MRI demonstrates a segment 6 hepatic lesion that demonstrates peripheral, discontinuous arterial enhancement which (**b**) progresses to coalesce and fill in on portal venous phase. (**c**) Second patient with a segment 4 lesion that demonstrates peripheral, nodular enhancement on arterial phase MRI with (**d**) progressive and more robust nodular enhancement on portal venous phase

appearance can also be seen on dynamic contrast-enhanced ultrasound. Small "flash-filling" hemangiomas (i.e., <2 cm) demonstrate prompt and robust arterial enhancement and subsequently blend in with liver parenchyma. Most hepatic hemangiomas remain stable over time (i.e., on follow-up imaging) and require no treatment (Figs. 1, 2, 3, and 4).

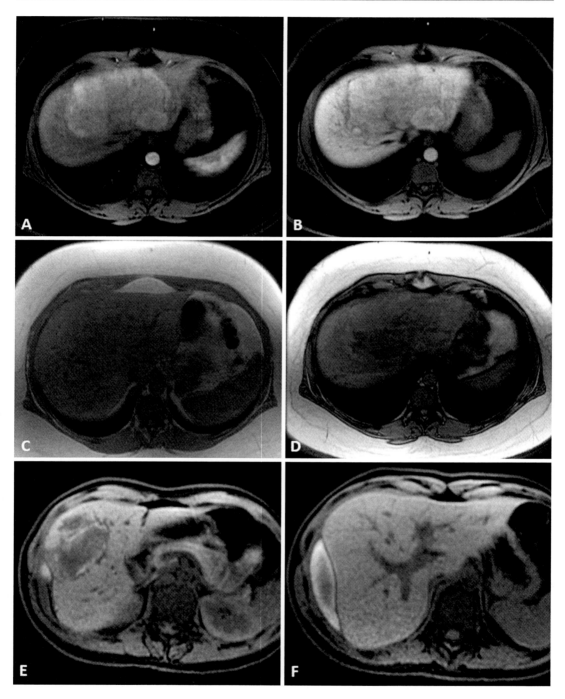

Fig. 2 (**a**) Arterial phase MRI demonstrates a large enhancing lesion that (**b**) appears to blend in on portal venous phase. (**c**) The mass is not clearly seen on "in-phase" imaging and (**d**) demonstrates "drop-out" of signal on "out-of-phase" or "opposed phase" imaging consistent with intralesional fat, seen in hepatic adenomas. (**e**) Hepatic adenoma in a different female patient on OCPs that demonstrates T1 hyperintensity compatible with intralesional blood. (**f**) Subcapsular hematoma seen in the same patient suggests rupture

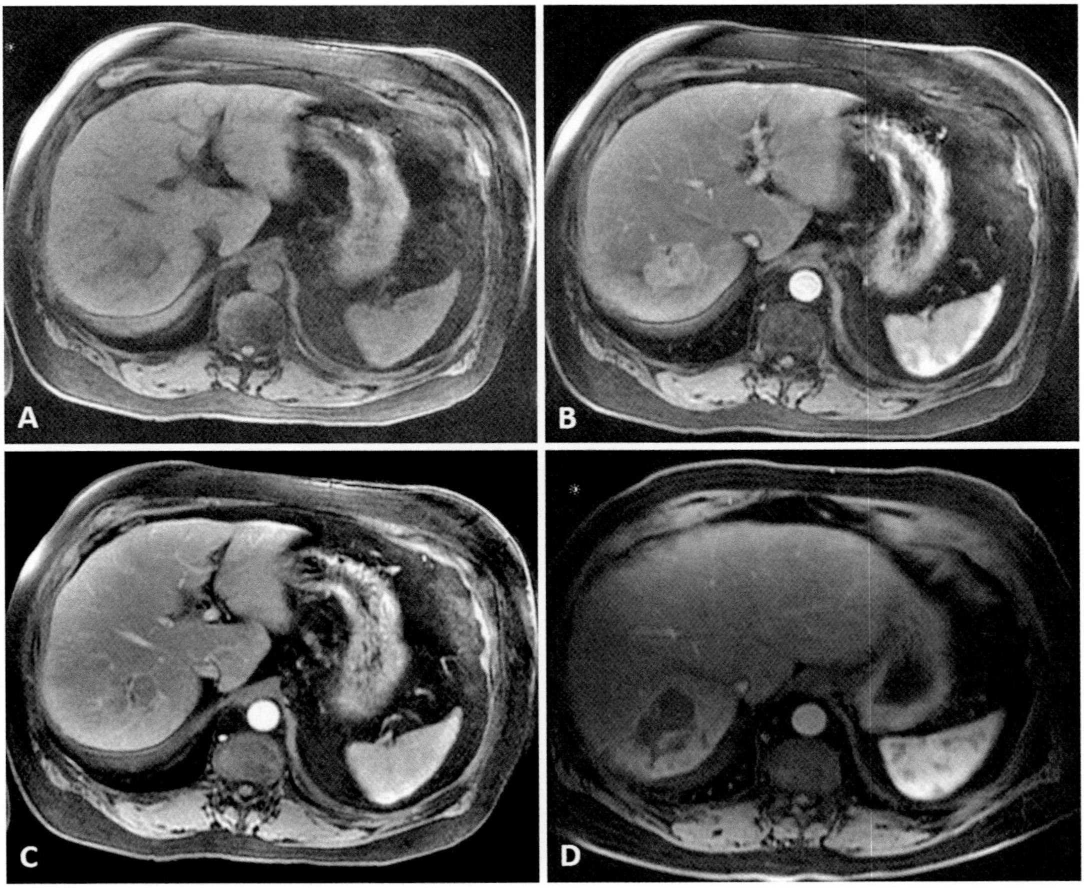

Fig. 3 (**a**) Non-contrast T1 weighted MRI demonstrates a hypodense lesion in segment 7 that (**b**). demonstrates enhancement on the arterial phase and (**c**) washes out on the portal venous phase with retained contrast in the capsule consistent with LI_RADS 5 diagnosis of HCC. (**d**) Post Yttrium-90 radio-embolization (TARE) scan demonstrates an ablative cavity in the region of the tumor with a surrounding area of hyper-intensity demonstrating the zone of treatment

Focal Nodular Hyperplasia

Focal nodular hyperplasia (FNH) is the second most common solid benign hepatic lesion. These lesions occur as a result of hyperplasia of normal hepatocytes without a well-differentiated vascular and biliary system. It has an estimated prevalence of 0.3–3% but clinically relevant prevalence is reduced to 0.03% (Marrero et al. 2014). FNH is seen in both sexes and throughout the age spectrum, although it occurs more commonly in females (up to 90%) between the ages of 20 and 50 years old (Wanless et al. 1985). Multiphasic abdominal CT or MRI can aid in the diagnosis.

In contrast to hemangiomas, these lesions demonstrate robust, homogeneous arterial enhancement and become isointense to liver parenchyma on delayed phase imaging. The classic "central scar" does not enhance on the arterial phase and retains the contrast on delayed phase imaging. This "central scar" also appears hyperintense on T2 weighted sequences (Silva et al. 2009). Furthermore, FNH lesions will uptake hepatobiliary secreted contrast agents (i.e., Eovist), which has the highest sensitivity as FNH cells are essentially maldeveloped hepatocytes (up to 90%) (Suh et al. 2015). Furthermore, if a diagnostic dilemma still exists, a Tc-99 m sulfur colloid test can be

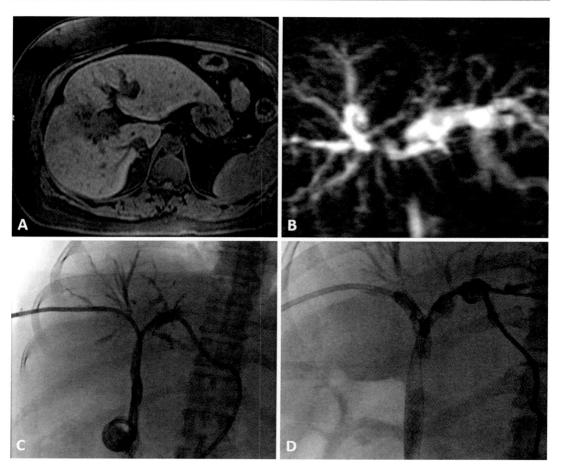

Fig. 4 (**a**) Non-contrast MRI demonstrates an irregular shaped central mass in the hilum resulting in biliary ductal dilation and capsular retraction, consistent with cholangiocarcinoma. (**b**). Severe biliary ductal dilation is demonstrated on MRCP. (**c**) Bilateral internal/external biliary drainage performed in this patient and cholangiography demonstrates persistent biliary ductal dilation. (**d**) Palliative double barrel CBD stent placement extending into the right and left hepatic ducts in this patient with unresectable disease

performed which will be taken up by hepatic Kupffer cells, present in FNH. A conservative approach is recommended for the management of FNH. Symptomatic lesions can be managed with partial hepatic resection, trans-arterial embolization, or percutaneous ablation (Mukundan et al. 2005; Silva et al. 2009).

Simple Hepatic Cyst

The prevalence of simple cysts has been reported 3% to 5% on ultrasonography (Rungsinaporn and Phaisakamas 2008) and 18% on cross-sectional imaging (Carrim and Murchison 2003). Hepatic cyst size can range from a few millimeters to massive lesions. Hepatic cysts are most commonly found incidentally and are asymptomatic. Large cysts tend to occur more frequently in women older than 50 years of age and can be symptomatic (abdominal pain, early satiety, and epigastric fullness). Cross-sectional imaging scans may confirm the diagnosis. Cysts typically measure fluid density on CT imaging and obey fluid characteristics on different MRI sequences. Along with that cyst do not enhance on either modality (Mortelé and Ros 2001). Asymptomatic cysts are best managed with observation. For symptomatic large liver cysts, therapeutic intervention could be ultrasound-guided aspiration which has high recurrence rates and more definite surgical treatment options are cyst fenestration (laparoscopic or open) and rarely hepatic resection (Reid-Lombardo et al. 2010). Sclerotherapy after aspiration has also been described as a treatment option for recurrent cysts (Wijnands et al. 2017).

Polycystic Liver Disease (PCLD)

PCLD are microscopically similar to simple hepatic cysts. PCLD is arbitrarily defined as a liver that contains >20 cysts (Gevers and Drenth 2013). It occurs in the setting of two distinct hereditary disorders, either as primary presentation of autosomal dominant polycystic liver disease (ADPLD) or associated with autosomal dominant polycystic kidney disease (ADPKD) (Gevers and Drenth 2013; van Aerts et al. 2018). PCLD tends to be asymptomatic, but due to increasing liver volume from cysts growth, the patient typically presents with hepatomegaly. They may have symptoms from mass effect such as abdominal pain, bloating, and fullness. Rare complications include portal hypertension with relatively preserved hepatic synthetic function (Chauveau et al. 2000; Marrero et al. 2014). The presence of multiple hepatic cysts on US, CT, or MRI supports the diagnosis of PCLD. Some cysts may have a complex fluid appearance on imaging modalities due to the presence of intracystic hemorrhage, uncommonly seen in patients with one or a few simple cysts. Treatment of PCLD is guided by the presence of symptoms. Surgical fenestration or CT-guided aspiration for a large dominant cyst can cause symptomatic relief, but reoccurrence is common. Liver transplantation with or without concomitant kidney transplantation has been considered in selected patients as well (Drenth et al. 2010; Garcea et al. 2013).

Benign Liver Tumors Requiring Further Investigation and Therapy

Hepatocellular Adenoma (HCA)

HCA is rare benign tumor of the liver with reported prevalence between 0.001% and 0.004%. It occurs predominantly in childbearing women (F: M prevalence 10:1). It has strong association with estrogen use (OCPs) and anabolic steroid use in men. HCA typically occurs in solitary (70%–80%), although patients with liver adenomatosis or glycogen storage disease (type 1 and 3) may have multiple lesions. HCAs range in size from <1 to 15 cm and are usually asymptomatic. Lesions greater than 5 cm in size are prone to complications such as spontaneous/traumatic rupture resulting in potentially life-threatening bleeding. In rare cases, malignant transformation in hepatocellular carcinoma (HCC) has been reported with larger lesions. HCA are now categorized into four subtypes based on genetic and pathologic criteria. Inflammatory HCAs are associated with the high risk of hemorrhage. Beta-catenin mutated adenomas are more often found in male patients and are more frequently associated with the development of hepatocellular carcinoma (Farges et al. 2011). CT scan can be used to diagnose HCA but MRI with gadobenate dimeglumine or gadoxetate disodium can be very effective in differentiating hepatocellular adenomas from FNH and other lesions (Laumonier et al. 2008). Distinguishing features on MRI include T1 hyperintensity due to intralesional hemorrhage or intracellular fat. The hyperintensity may be suppressed using an opposed phase imaging technique which indicates the presences of intralesional fat (Silva et al. 2009).

Small lesions (<5 cm) can be managed conservatively by repeated periodic imaging as well as discontinuing OCPs and anabolic steroids. Resection is recommended for symptomatic large lesion greater than 5 cm in size and particularly for HCAs with beta-catenin subtype as malignant transformation occurs most frequently in this subtype. Rarely liver transplantation is indicated in the case of glycogen storage disease or multiple adenomas (Thomeer et al. 2016; Bonder and Afdhal 2012; Grazioli et al. 2001).

Nodular Regenerative Hyperplasia (NRH)

NRH is a rare condition characterized by the widespread benign transformation of normal hepatic parenchyma into small regenerative nodules. The nodules are also separated by atrophic areas with little to no fibrosis. These nodules can vary in size from 1 mm to 1 cm. It affects men and women equally. NRH has a prevalence of over 5.3% in individuals greater than 80 years of age.

NRH is associated with medications and wide spectrum of systemic diseases such as myeloproliferative disorders, collagen vascular disorders, lymphoproliferative disorders, primary biliary cholangitis, bone marrow transplantation, Budd-Chiari syndrome, amyloidosis, and polyarteritis nodosa (Bonder and Afdhal 2012; Shastri et al. 2004). Imaging characteristics are nonspecific and are similar to cirrhosis thus definitive diagnosis is established by liver biopsy. The minimal to absence of fibrosis and unaltered architecture of the portal tract differentiate NRH from cirrhotic transformation. Hepatic biochemical tests are normal in these patients. Most patients with NRH are asymptomatic; however, patients may present with stigmata of portal hypertension. Treatment of NRH is directed at treating the underlying medical condition and preventing complications of portal hypertension. Liver transplantation may be required in patients with severely complicated portal hypertension or liver failure (Tateo et al. 2008).

Malignant Liver Lesions Requiring Appropriate Investigation and Therapy

Hepatocellular Carcinoma (HCC)

HCC is now the fifth most common cancer in the world and third most common cause of cancer-related mortality (The Global Cancer Observatory 2018). The age-specific incidence rate of HCC starts increasing in the mid-40s and reaches peak at approximately 70 years of age. It has a higher prevalence in males compared to females (El-Serag 2011). Major risk factors for hepatocellular carcinoma include infection with chronic hepatitis B (HBV) or chronic hepatitis C (HCV), alcoholic liver disease, and nonalcoholic fatty liver disease (NAFLD). The incidence of HCC in the United States has been rapidly rising secondary to HCV-related cirrhosis, particularly among the population born between 1945 and 1965, known as "baby boomers" (El-Serag 2013), and also cirrhosis secondary to non-alcoholic steatohepatitis (NASH). Obesity is a common and well-documented risk factor for nonalcoholic fatty liver disease (NAFLD). As the obesity epidemic progresses, the number of patients developing HCC on the background of NAFLD-related cirrhosis is projected to increase (White et al. 2012). Immigration to the United States from high endemic areas for hepatitis B (HBV) also reflects the increasing incidence of HBV-related HCC. HBV is unique in that patients with the disease can develop HCC even without cirrhosis. Not only that, active viral replication is also associated with high risk for HCC. Therefore, HCC screening is recommended in patients with HBV-related cirrhosis, family history of HCC in patients with chronic hepatitis B, and HBV carriers with ages higher than 40 (males) or 50 (females). Cirrhosis is the most important risk factor for HCC. More than 80% of the cases of HCC occurs in the setting of cirrhosis (Bruix et al. 2011). Any patient with a predisposing condition leading to chronic liver disease and cirrhosis should be screened for HCC.

Surveillance for hepatocellular carcinoma should be offered for patients with cirrhosis when the risk for HCC is 1.5% per year or greater. The American Association for the Study of Liver Diseases (AASLD) recommends surveillance of adults with cirrhosis using ultrasound, with or without alpha-fetoprotein (AFP) every 6 months as it has been shown to improve overall survival rates (Heimbach et al. 2018). Other tumor biomarkers such as AFP-L3%, which measures a subfraction of the AFP is shown to be more specific but less sensitive than AFP; des gamma carboxy prothrombin (DCP) is also specifically produced at high levels by a proportion of HCCs. However, no specific recommendations exist for their use as HCC surveillance. Despite high diagnostic performance of cross-sectional multiphasic imaging studies such as CT or MRI, their use as a primary modality for HCC surveillance has not been recommended secondary to lack of data on their efficacy and cost effectiveness.

Imaging studies play a critical role in the diagnosis of HCC. HCC is a unique tumor in which the diagnosis can be established, confirmed, and treated based on imaging characteristics, removing the necessity for subsequent histologic confirmation. Any solid liver lesion in the background of a cirrhotic liver or in a patient with chronic hepatitis B should be considered as HCC unless proven otherwise. If the lesion is seen on an abdominal ultrasound, further investigation with a multiphasic CT or MRI of the abdomen is warranted. The choice of MRI versus CT is controversial. The small studies have shown that a dynamic MRI has slightly better performance than CT scan for the diagnosis of HCC but further large studies are needed. Liver Imaging Reporting and Data System (LI-RADS) was initially published in 2011 by the American College of Radiology and is a comprehensive system for standardizing the terminology, technique, interpretation, reporting, and data collection of the liver imaging. The latest updated version was released in July 2018 (Mri and Core n.d.). LI-RADS can only be applied for lesions seen in patients with cirrhosis. It is consistent with and fully integrated into the AASLD HCC clinical practice guidelines and NCCN guidelines. In the LI-RADS classification system, any liver lesion visible on a multiphasic imaging studies is assigned category codes reflecting the relative probability of being benign, HCC or hepatic malignant neoplasm. LI-RADS 1 indicates definitely benign whereas LI-RADS 5 indicates definitely HCC. LI-RADS 5 criteria are consistent with the Organ procurement and Transplantation Network (OPTN) class 5 criteria. On a multiphasic MRI or CT scan, LI-RADS 5 category lesions are ≥1 cm and show arterial phase hyperenhancement on the arterial phase, and depending

on exact size, combination of additional features (hypodense "Washout" on a portal venous phase and enhancing capsule or maximum diameter increase ≥50% documented on previous multiphasic CT or MRI at least 6 months apart). In those who do not have these characteristics features on radiological examination, a directed biopsy of the mass may be considered especially for LI-RADS 4 (i.e., washout without capsule) and LI-RADS M. Diagnosis of HCC cannot be made by imaging criteria in patients without cirrhosis and a biopsy is therefore required in those cases.

The management of HCC requires a multidisciplinary approach and has been shown to be associated with the overall survival (Yopp et al. 2014). The first step in the treatment of HCC is to determine the stage of the HCC, the patient's functional status, the severity of liver synthetic dysfunction, and the degree of the portal hypertension. The Barcelona Clinic Liver Cancer (BCLC) staging system offers the most prognostic information as it comprehensively includes tumor burden, the patient's functional status, and the degree of liver dysfunction. The BCLC staging has been recently modified (Forner et al. 2018). Different criteria have been set to gauge the severity of liver function, the most commonly used being Child Pugh scoring system (and more recently the albumin-bilirubin scoring system). Functional status is determined using the Eastern Cooperative Oncology Group (ECOG) Performance Scoring system.

The therapeutic options can be curative such as surgical resection, orthotopic liver transplantation, and locoregional ablative techniques. Additional interventions including transarterial therapies (chemoembolization, radioembolization), systemic chemotherapy, or combination therapy (i.e., chemoembolization + ablation; systemic and locoregional chemoembolization, etc.). Generally, surgical resection is the treatment of choice for resectable HCC in patients without cirrhosis and also for smaller tumors with preserved liver synthetic function, in the absence of significant portal hypertension. Liver transplantation (LT) is the treatment of choice for the patient with clinically significant portal hypertension and with early stage HCC within Milan criteria, defined as one tumor measuring up to 5 cm or 2–3 tumors with the largest being less than 3 cm with no evidence of gross vascular invasion or regional/distant metastasis (Mazzaferro et al. 1996). LT for HCC within Milan criteria occurring in the setting of decompensated liver disease is highly effective therapy because it offers optimal treatment of both, the underlying liver disease and tumor, with excellent long-term survival rates. Liver transplantation in the elderly can be challenging, but in the absence of significant comorbidities, older recipient age is not a contraindication to liver transplant. Patients who meet "Milan criteria" get a high priority on the transplant waiting list and are automatically granted additional points on the Model for End Stage Liver Disease (MELD) score for organ allocation system in the United States. However, because the wait time for liver transplantation can be long (longer in some states than others) due to the allocation algorithm set forth by the United Network of Organ Sharing (UNOS), many patients undergo locoregional therapy (TACE, TARE, ablation, or combination treatment) to prevent the progression of disease while waiting for a donor liver, that is, "bridge" to transplantation. A waiting period is included in the UNOS criteria to ensure that the patient's disease stands the biologic test of time in order to prevent transplantation in a patient with an aggressive genotype, who poses a high risk of recurrence in the donor liver.

The patients who do not qualify for transplantation but are just outside of the Milan criteria may be treated by the aforementioned locoregional therapies including chemoembolization, radioembolization, or radiofrequency ablation/microwave ablation to "downstage" the patient to transplantation (Yao et al. 2015). Tumor ablation can be achieved by the injection of chemical substances such as ethanol or by creating heat with radiofrequency or microwaves. These techniques are best option for patients with BCLC stage A who are not a candidate for surgical resection for curative intent. Randomized controlled trials have confirmed the superiority of RFA over ethanol injection in terms of survival. There are no randomized controlled trials comparing

thermal ablative techniques. These techniques have the best results in tumors with a maximum diameter of less than 3 cm. Efficacy and outcomes have been shown to improve when used in conjunction with transarterial chemo-embolization.

The patients who are not candidate for curative therapies (resection, ablation, or LT) may be also considered for locoregional therapy (TACE or TARE) in Child-Pugh class A and highly selective Child-Pugh class B (i.e., good ECOG functional status). There is no data to support the use of locoregional therapy for patients with Child-Pugh class C. In fact, patients' liver function and performance status can worsen if treated with arterial therapies. Systemic chemotherapy should be considered for patients with Child class A and highly selective Child class B with advanced HCC and macrovascular invasion/metastatic disease. Multi-kinase inhibitor, Sorafenib, in a large phase 3 randomized placebo-controlled trial demonstrated a survival advantage (Llovet et al. 2008). Lenvatinib, multi-kinase inhibitor, has recently been approved also as a first-line therapy for advanced HCC (Kudo et al. 2018). Second-line therapy options are Regorafenib (multi-kinase inhibitor) (Bruix et al. 2017) and Nivolumab (programmed cell death protein 1 inhibitor) (El-Khoueiry et al. 2017) upon radiological progression to Sorafenib.

Cholangiocarcinoma (CCA)

CCA is the most common primary malignancy of the biliary tract and is best classified anatomically as intrahepatic (iCCA), perihilar (pCCA,) or distal (dCCA) (Blechacz et al. 2011). CCA is the second most common primary hepatic neoplasm in adults, with incidence increasing worldwide. The prognosis of CCA is dismal, 1-year survival for iCCA at 27.6% and 5-year survival is less than 10% because of the diagnosis is made at advanced stages. CCA arises from the epithelial cells of the intrahepatic bile ducts. The male-to-female ratio of CCA is 1:1.2–1.5. Globally, the average age at diagnosis is >50 years. In Western industrialized nations, the median age at presentation is 65 years. It is uncommon before age 40 except in patients with primary sclerosing cholangitis (PSC) (Blechacz 2017). ICCA may occur in patients with or without underlying chronic liver disease. It is usually classified pathologically as an adenocarcinoma but mixed hepatocellular-cholangiocarcinoma occurs especially in chronic liver disease. Other risk factors associated with CCA are smoking, alcohol use, liver fluke infestation, Caroli's disease, choledochal cysts, intrahepatic cholelithiasis, and cirrhosis (Endo et al. 2008).

The clinical presentation of CCA is nonspecific. CCA is often detected as an incidental liver lesion on imaging studies performed for other purposes. Laboratory tests are usually nonspecific. Patients with iCCA usually become symptomatic at the advanced stage of the disease with nonspecific symptoms such as abdominal pain, malaise, night sweats, and cachexia. Painless jaundice is the presenting symptom in about 90% of the patients with pCCA and acute cholangitis in about 10%. The most common used tumor marker for CCA is carbohydrate antigen 19-9 (CA 19-9), which can be measured to identify patients with iCCA, with 62% sensitivity and 63% specificity (Blechacz et al. 2011). However, CA 19-9 can also be elevated in other gastrointestinal, pancreatic, and benign cholangiopathies. Seven percent of the population are Lewis antigen negative and do not express CA 19-9 regardless of the tumor burden. Dynamic cross-sectional imaging (CT or MRI) can assist in the diagnosis of CCA, tumor size, the presence of satellite lesions, and the preoperative planning for CCA. Perihilar cholangiocarcinoma (i.e., Klatskin tumor) usually presents with diffuse biliary ductal dilatation due to compression/occlusion of the common bile duct. Intrahepatic cholangiocarcinoma can have a variety of imaging features including any combination of irregular mass with irregular enhancement and washout pattern, focal biliary dilations, capsular retraction, and/or hilar lymphadenopathy. Diagnosis of CCA cannot be confidently made with radiological imaging alone and a biopsy specimen is usually required to confirm the diagnosis. pCCA typically presents as a dominant stricture or filling defect. The patient may need endoscopic retrograde cholangiography (ERCP) percutaneous transhepatic cholangiography (PTC). ERCP or PTC allows sampling of the stricture and therapeutic biliary stent placement but unfortunately sensitivity of cytology of biliary brushing is only 20–43%, it can be increased up to 46–68% by using fluorescent in situ hybridization (FISH).

Surgical resection of CCA is the only potential curative option; however, the majority of CCA patients are diagnosed at late stage and are unresectable candidates. With surgical resection for iCCA, the median survival time is 36 months, and the reoccurrence rate is 62% after a median of 26-month follow-up (Endo et al. 2008). Contraindication to surgical resection includes bilateral disease, multifocal disease, and distant metastatic disease. For unresectable iCCA, systemic chemotherapy is the standard of care. Liver transplantation is contraindicated in iCCA because of its poor outcomes and prognosis. PSC patients with pCCA should preferentially be treated with liver transplantation (LT). Special protocols with neo-adjuvant chemoradiation therapy followed with LT are an effective treatment for pCCA with the recurrence 5-year survival of 68% (Murad et al. 2012). Locoregional therapies for CCA are currently being studied.

Liver Metastases

Metastases are the most common malignant liver tumors. The liver is a common metastatic site for large variety of primary tumors. Presumably because of hepatic portal venous drainage from gastrointestinal tract, metastatic liver disease is very common in most gastrointestinal malignancies. Most liver metastases typically manifest as multiple discrete lesions but may present as a solitary mass. Metastases isolated to the liver are a unique feature of colorectal carcinoma. On multiphasic CT of the liver, neuroendocrine tumors, renal cell carcinoma, breast carcinoma, melanoma, and thyroid carcinoma are hypervascular metastases whereas metastatic liver lesions from the colon, stomach, and pancreas usually are hypoattenuation in contrast to brighter surrounding liver parenchyma. Usually liver biopsy is required for the diagnosis unless the primary site is already known.

Liver metastases are one of the major causes of death in patient with colorectal cancer (CRC). Approximately 60% of CRC patients develop liver metastases during the course of the illness. About 85% of these patients have unresectable disease at the time of presentation. Surgery for colorectal metastases is increasingly being used as part of multimodality treatment as it considerably improved the overall survival. The 5-year survival for colorectal liver metastases patients receiving surgery and neoadjuvant therapy has increased up to 50% (Hof et al. 2016). Neuroendocrine tumors (NETs) are typically slow growing tumors, for metastatic NET, 5-year survival is between 19% and 38% and metastatic to liver having the worst prognosis. The liver is the most common site of metastases (82%) (Riihimäki et al. 2016). It does require a multidisciplinary team approach including surgical, ablative therapy, hepatic arterial chemoembolization/radio embolization, and somatostatin analogs. Liver transplantation may provide a survival benefit among patients with diffuse NETs metastases to liver in selected patients with 1, 3, and 5-year survival 89%, 69%, and 63%, respectively (Moris et al. 2017).

Key Points

- Most of the tumors of liver are identified incidentally and identified in asymptomatic patients.
- Majority of liver tumors are benign and very few needs further evaluation.
- Hepatic hemangioma is the most common solid tumor but benign in nature.
- MRI with EOVIST can help in differentiating FNH from hepatic adenoma.
- Hormonal contraceptives have been associated with hepatic adenoma.
- HCC is the fifth most common tumor in the world.
- Cirrhosis is the leading cause of HCC; hence, HCC screening should be done every 6 months with imaging modality such as US liver or contrast-induced imaging studies.

- BCLC staging system is the best way of managing the patients with HCC.
- Metastases are the most common malignant liver tumors.

References

Bahirwani R, Reddy KR. Review article: the evaluation of solitary liver masses. Aliment Pharmacol Ther. 2008. https://doi.org/10.1111/j.1365-2036.2008.03805.x.

Blechacz B. Cholangiocarcinoma: current knowledge and new developments. Gut Liver. 2017;11(1):13–26. https://doi.org/10.5009/gnl15568.

Blechacz B, et al. Clinical diagnosis and staging of cholangiocarcinoma. Nat Rev Gastroenterol Hepatol. 2011. https://doi.org/10.1038/nrgastro.2011.131.

Bonder A, Afdhal N. Evaluation of liver lesions. Clin Liver Dis. 2012;16(2):271–83. https://doi.org/10.1016/j.cld.2012.03.001. Elsevier Inc.

Bruix J, Sherman M, American Association for the Study of Liver Diseases. Management of hepatocellular carcinoma: an update. Hepatology (Baltimore). 2011. https://doi.org/10.1002/hep.24199.

Bruix J, et al. Regorafenib for patients with hepatocellular carcinoma who progressed on sorafenib treatment (RESORCE): a randomised, double-blind, placebo-controlled, phase 3 trial. Lancet. 2017;389 (10064):56–66. https://doi.org/10.1016/S0140-6736 (16)32453-9.

Carrim ZI, Murchison JT. The prevalence of simple renal and hepatic cysts detected by spiral computed tomography. Clin Radiol. 2003;58(8):626–9. https://doi.org/10.1016/S0009-9260(03)00165-X.

Chauveau D, Fakhouri F, Grünfeld JP. Liver involvement in autosomal-dominant polycystic kidney disease: therapeutic dilemma. J Am Soc Nephrol. 2000;11 (9):1767–75. https://doi.org/10.1109/ACCESS.2017. 2746838.

Drenth JPH, et al. Medical and surgical treatment options for polycystic liver disease. Hepatology. 2010;52(6): 2223–30. https://doi.org/10.1002/hep.24036.

El-Khoueiry AB, et al. Nivolumab in patients with advanced hepatocellular carcinoma (CheckMate 040): an open-label, non-comparative, phase 1/2 dose escalation and expansion trial. Lancet. 2017;389 (10088):2492–502. https://doi.org/10.1016/S0140-6736(17)31046-2. Elsevier Ltd.

El-Serag HB. Current concepts: hepatocellular carcinoma. NEJM. 2011. https://doi.org/10.1007/s10354-014-0296-7.

El-Serag HB. NIH public access. Gastroenterology. 2013;142(6):1264–73. https://doi.org/10.1053/j.gastro. 2011.12.061.Epidemiology.

Endo I, et al. Intrahepatic cholangiocarcinoma: rising frequency, improved survival, and determinants of outcome after resection. Ann Surg. 2008. https://doi.org/10.1097/SLA.0b013e318176c4d3.

European Association for Study of the Liver, E. EASL Clinical practice guidelines on the management of benign liver tumours. 2016. https://doi.org/10.1016/j.jhep.2016.04.001.

Farges O, et al. Changing trends in malignant transformation of hepatocellular adenoma. Gut. 2011;60(1):85–9. https://doi.org/10.1136/gut.2010.222109.

Forner A, Reig M, Bruix J. Hepatocellular carcinoma. Lancet. 2018;391(10127):1301–14. https://doi.org/10.1109/FCS.2017.8088863. Elsevier Ltd.

Fowler KJ, Brown JJ, Narra VR. Magnetic resonance imaging of focal liver lesions: approach to imaging diagnosis. n.d. https://doi.org/10.1002/hep.24679.

Garcea G, Rajesh A, Dennison AR. Surgical management of cystic lesions in the liver. ANZ J Surg. 2013;83(7–8):516–22. https://doi.org/10.1111/ans.12049.

Gevers TJG, Drenth JPH. Diagnosis and management of polycystic liver disease. Nat Rev Gastroenterol Hepatol. 2013. https://doi.org/10.1038/nrgastro.2012.254.

Grazioli L, et al. Hepatic adenomas: imaging and pathologic finding. Radiographics. 2001. https://doi.org/10.1148/radiographics.21.4.g01jl04877.

Heimbach JK, et al. AASLD guidelines for the treatment of hepatocellular carcinoma. Hepatology. 2018. https://doi.org/10.1002/hep.29086.

Hof J, et al. Outcomes after resection and/or radio-frequency ablation for recurrence after treatment of colorectal liver metastases. Br J Surg. 2016;103 (8):1055–62. https://doi.org/10.1002/bjs.10162.

Horta G, et al. Lesiones focales hepáticas benignas: un hallazgo frecuente a la tomografía computada. ARTíCULOS Rev. n.d.;143:197–202. Available at: http://repositorio.uchile.cl/bitstream/handle/2250/132 590/Benign-focal-liver-lesions-detected-by-computed.pdf?sequence=1&isAllowed=y. Accessed 9 June 2018.

International Working Party. Terminology of nodular hepatocellular lesions. Hepatology (Baltimore). 1995;22(3):983–93. Available at: http://www.ncbi.nlm.nih.gov/pubmed/7657307. Accessed 7 June 2018.

Karhunen P. Benign hepatic tumours and tumour like conditions in men. J Clin Pathol. 1986;39:183–8. Available at: https://www.ncbi.nlm.nih.gov/pmc/articles/PMC49 9674/pdf/jclinpath00197-0063.pdf. Accessed 9 June 2018.

Kudo M, et al. Lenvatinib versus sorafenib in first-line treatment of patients with unresectable hepatocellular carcinoma: a randomised phase 3 non-inferiority trial. Lancet. 2018;391(10126):1163–73. https://doi.org/10.1016/S0140-6736(18)30207-1. Elsevier Ltd.

Laumonier H, et al. Hepatocellular adenomas: magnetic resonance imaging features as a function of molecular pathological classification. Hepatology. 2008;48 (3):808–18. https://doi.org/10.1002/hep.22417.

Llovet JM, et al. Sorafenib in advanced hepatocellular carcinoma. N Engl J Med. 2008;359(4):378–90. https://doi.org/10.1056/NEJMoa0708857.

Marrero JA, et al. ACG clinical guideline: the diagnosis and management of focal liver lesions. Am J Gastroenterol. 2014. https://doi.org/10.1038/ajg.2014.213.

Mazzaferro V, et al. Liver transplantation for the treatment of small hepatocellular carcinomas in patients with cirrhosis. N Engl J Med. 1996. https://doi.org/10.1056/NEJM199603143341104.

Moris D, et al. Liver transplantation in patients with liver metastases from neuroendocrine tumors: a systematic review. Surgery (United States). 2017;162(3):525–36. https://doi.org/10.1016/j.surg.2017.05.006. Elsevier Inc.

Mortelé KJ, Ros PR. Cystic focal liver lesions in the adult: differential CT and MR imaging features. Radiographics. 2001. https://doi.org/10.1148/radiographics.21.4.g01jl16895.

Mri CT, Core L. CT/MRI LI-RADS® v2018 CORE, Acr. n.d.

Mukundan G, Lammle M, Brown JJ. Focal hepatic lesions: diagnostic value of enhancement pattern approach with contrast- enhanced 3D gradient- Echo MR imaging. Radiographics. 2005. https://doi.org/10.1148/rg.255045180.

Murad SD, et al. Predictors of pretransplant dropout and posttransplant recurrence in patients with perihilar cholangiocarcinoma. Hepatology. 2012;56(3):972–81. https://doi.org/10.1002/hep.25629.

Reid-Lombardo KM, Khan S, Sclabas G. Hepatic cysts and liver abscess. Surg Clin N Am. 2010;90(4):679–97. https://doi.org/10.1016/j.suc.2010.04.004. Elsevier Ltd.

Riihimäki M, et al. The epidemiology of metastases in neuroendocrine tumors. Int J Cancer. 2016;139(12):2679–86. https://doi.org/10.1002/ijc.30400.

Rungsinaporn K, Phaisakamas T. Frequency of abnormalities detected by upper abdominal ultrasound. J Med Assoc Thail. 2008;91(7):1072–5.

Shastri S, et al. Early nodular hyperplasia of the liver occurring with thioguanine therapy. Arch Pathol Lab Med. 2004;128:49–53.

Silva AC, et al. MR imaging of hypervascular liver masses: a review of current techniques. Radiographics. 2009. https://doi.org/10.1148/rg.292085123.

Suh CH, et al. The diagnostic value of Gd-EOB-DTPA-MRI for the diagnosis of focal nodular hyperplasia: a systematic review and meta-analysis. Eur Radiol. 2015;25(4):950–60. https://doi.org/10.1007/s00330-014-3499-9.

Tateo M, et al. A new indication for liver transplantation: nodular regenerative hyperplasia in human immunodeficiency virus-infected patients. Liver Transpl. 2008. https://doi.org/10.1002/lt.21493.

The Global Cancer Observatory. All cancers. Globocan. 2018;876:1–2. https://doi.org/10.1051/0004-6361/201016331.

Thomeer MG, et al. Hepatocellular adenoma: when and how to treat? Update of current evidence. Ther Adv

Gastroenterol. 2016;9(6):898–912. https://doi.org/10.1177/1756283X16663882.

van Aerts RMM, et al. Clinical management of polycystic liver disease. J Hepatol. 2018. https://doi.org/10.1016/j.jhep.2017.11.024.

Wanless IR, Mawdsley C, Adams R. On the pathogenesis of focal nodular hyperplasia of the liver. Hepatology. 1985. https://doi.org/10.1002/hep.1840050622.

White DL, Kanwal F, El–Serag HB. Association between nonalcoholic fatty liver disease and risk for hepatocellular cancer, based on systematic review. Clin Gastroenterol Hepatol. 2012. https://doi.org/10.1016/j.cgh.2012.10.001.

Wijnands TFM, et al. Efficacy and safety of aspiration sclerotherapy of simple hepatic cysts: a systematic review. Am J Roentgenol. 2017. https://doi.org/10.2214/AJR.16.16130.

Yao FY, et al. Downstaging of hepatocellular cancer before liver transplant: long-term outcome compared to tumors within Milan criteria. Hepatology. 2015;61(6):1968–77. https://doi.org/10.1002/hep.27752.

Yopp AC, et al. Establishment of a multidisciplinary hepatocellular carcinoma clinic is associated with improved clinical outcome. Ann Surg Oncol. 2014;21(4):1287–95. https://doi.org/10.1245/s10434-013-3413-8.

Nonalcoholic Fatty Liver Disease (NAFLD) and Nonalcoholic Steatohepatitis (NASH)

60

Steven Krawitz and Nikolaos Pyrsopoulos

Contents

Abstract

The exact prevalence of nonalcoholic fatty liver disease (NAFLD) is approximately 25% and is increasing globally. NAFLD is a component of metabolic syndrome and is becoming more prevalent among older adults. In the USA., Hispanics have been noted to have higher risks compared to African Americans.

Nonalcoholic steatohepatitis (NASH), a consequence of NAFLD, leads to progressive fibrosis, culminating in cirrhosis and rarely hepatocellular carcinoma (HCC). The majority of patients come to the clinician's attention usually because of elevated serum aspartate aminotransferase (AST) or alanine aminotransferase (ALT) levels noted in routine studies. Abdominal US, CT scan of abdomen, and MRI have different degrees of sensitivity in diagnosing NAFLD. Elastography uses imaging techniques to estimate liver stiffness and gauge fibrosis. Liver biopsy as an invasive test

S. Krawitz
VA New Jersey Health Care System, East Orange VA Medical Center, East Orange, NJ, USA
e-mail: Steven.Krawitz@va.gov

N. Pyrsopoulos (✉)
Department of Medicine, Division of Gastroenterology and Hepatology, Physiology, Pharmacology and Neuroscience, Medical Director Liver Transplantation, Rutgers – New Jersey Medical School, University Hospital, Newark, NJ, USA
e-mail: pyrsopni@njms.rutgers.edu

© Springer Nature Switzerland AG 2021
C. S. Pitchumoni, T. S. Dharmarajan (eds.), *Geriatric Gastroenterology*,
https://doi.org/10.1007/978-3-030-30192-7_52

is not practical, but is considered the gold standard. Control and avoidance of risk factors remain important in the management of NAFLD.

Keywords

Nonalcoholic fatty liver disease (NAFLD) · Metabolic syndrome · Nonalcoholic steatohepatitis (NASH) · Cirrhosis · Cryptogenic cirrhosis · Hepatoma · Cytokeratin 18 (CK18) · Fibroblast growth factor 21 (FGF21) · CK18-M65 (uncleaved CK18) · Abdominal ultrasound · Elastography · Vitamin E · Metformin · Obeticholic acid · Selonsertib

Introduction

The deposition of fat within the liver is a normal part of biosynthesis and physiology. However, when beyond the threshold of 5% hepatic steatosis, or when steatosis is visible on imaging, it is considered abnormal fat deposition and labeled nonalcoholic fatty liver disease (NAFLD). This definition requires no alternative etiology for the increased hepatic fat deposition or "steatosis" (Table 1). NAFLD is considered in the spectrum of metabolic syndrome, and therefore is becoming more prevalent among older adults as the population ages and the prevalence of metabolic diseases increases (for example diabetes, hypertension, obesity) (Chalasani et al. 2018). As the obesity epidemic worsens on a global stage, the incidence and therefore prevalence of NAFLD are also expected to rise (Angulo 2007). In a subset of individuals with NAFLD, steatosis induces an inflammatory cascade leading to injury within the hepatocyte. The term "nonalcoholic steatohepatitis" (NASH) is used to encapsulate this population and was first described as a clinical entity by Ludwig et al. describing liver biopsy findings resembling alcoholic hepatitis in patients who did not have a significant history of alcohol intake (Ludwig et al. 1980). Although there is some evidence that steatosis itself can lead to progressive liver injury and in rare cases

hepatocellular carcinoma (HCC), most of the risk for chronic liver disease and NAFLD is in the NASH subset of patients. NASH leads to progressive fibrosis, culminating in cirrhosis and possible hepatocellular carcinoma (HCC). Not all patients with NAFLD are obese, up to 20% of nonobese Americans and Asians develop NAFLD, sometimes labeled as "lean NAFLD." Given widely available antiviral treatment against the hepatitis C virus combined with the obesity epidemic, it is not surprising that NAFLD is the most prevalent etiology of chronic liver disease today and is commonly encountered in older adults. "Cryptogenic cirrhosis" is a term used in describing cirrhosis of the liver with no identifiable etiology; currently, it is evident that in older adults cryptogenic cirrhosis is likely previously unrecognized NASH from decades earlier.

Epidemiology and Prevalence of NAFLD and NASH

The exact prevalence of nonalcoholic fatty liver disease and NASH is elusive as the majority of those affected are unaware of their diagnosis. Moreover, only a fraction of those patients noted to have steatosis have undergone liver biopsy, technically the gold standard for diagnosing NASH. Prevalence varies among different populations, but NAFLD is a global disease with a worldwide distribution. Recently, the worldwide prevalence of NAFLD was projected at 25.24% (Younossi et al. 2016). The regions with the highest prevalence were South America and the Middle East, as opposed to Africa with a lower rate of NAFLD (Younossi et al. 2016). NAFLD also has massive impact in the USA. The condition is estimated to affect roughly one out of three Americans and is the most common liver condition in the Western world (Younossi et al. 2018). With an annual direct medical cost of 103 billion dollars, NAFLD also significantly impacts the American healthcare system (Younossi et al. 2018). Moreover, of large concern is the fact that the prevalence seems to be increasing. One study done in a cohort of US veterans showed a threefold increase in

Table 1 Causes of fatty liver disease (Chalasani et al. 2018)

Microvesicular steatosis	Macrovesicular steatosis
Excessive alcohol intake[a]	Reye's syndrome
Hepatitis C	Medications[c]
Wilson disease	Acute fatty liver of pregnancy
Lipodystrophy	HELLP syndrome
Starvation	Inborn errors of metabolism
Parental nutrition	
Medications[b]	

[a]>21 standard drinks per week in men and > 14 standard drinks per week in women over a 2-year period preceding baseline liver histology (Kleiner et al. 2005)
[b]Amiodarone, methotrexate, tamoxifen, corticosteroids
[c]Valproate, antiretroviral medications

prevalence between 2003 and 2011. Other studies corroborate this increase in prevalence in NAFLD between 1994 and 2008 (Younossi et al. 2011). Moreover, prevalence increased regardless of sex, age, or race (Kanwal et al. 2016). The prevalence of NAFLD after age 75 actually decreases, likely due to mortality from comorbid conditions (Clark 2006).

NAFLD affects all age groups, races, and both sexes. However, there are populations that have a higher prevalence of NAFLD and NASH. Higher risk demographics include: Latin Americans, patients with metabolic risk factors, and men (Saab et al. 2016; Chalasani et al. 2012). Hispanics have been demonstrated to have higher risks of NAFLD compared to Blacks (Rich et al. 2017). South Asians represent a growing population with NAFLD, although many do not have the traditional risk factor of elevated BMI (Chitturi et al. 2011). Any level of obesity increases the prevalence of NAFLD in patients with diabetes mellitus (Wanless and Lentz 1990; Silverman et al. 1990). It is estimated that in those individuals with both obesity and diabetes, the prevalence of NAFLD reaches 70% (Kim et al. 2018). Nonalcoholic steatohepatitis is estimated to affect 19% of the obese American population (Wanless and Lentz 1990; Silverman et al. 1990). In the morbidly obese, the prevalence of NAFLD is as high as 95%, with NASH

close to 25% (Dixon and Bhathal 2001). Moreover, the metabolic syndrome (Table 2) and all its components are widely known to be associated with the development of NAFLD and NASH. Clinically, its recognition is vital, as the all-cause mortality rate of patients with NAFLD is at least 34% higher than that of the general population (Marengo et al. 2016). NASH is a more aggressive condition that is associated with inflammation, hepatocyte injury with progressive fibrosis, and ultimately cirrhosis. Cirrhosis is largely irreversible resulting in multiple systemic sequelae and can lead to hepatocellular carcinoma and death. Even more concerning is growing evidence that HCC can even develop in the absence of cirrhosis in the NAFLD/NASH population (Mittal et al. 2016).

Diagnosis of NAFLD and NASH

Clinical Evaluation

The goals in diagnosis are to confirm the etiology of liver disease, to evaluate the specific type of fatty liver (Table 1), and to stage the disease (to establish clinical severity). The definition of nonalcoholic fatty liver disease (NAFLD) requires that (a) there is evidence of hepatic steatosis and (b) there are no causes for secondary hepatic fat accumulation such as significant alcohol consumption or use of steatogenic medication; and other liver diseases including hepatitis C (especially genotype 3), hemochromatosis, alpha-1 antitrypsin deficiency, and Wilson's disease are adequately ruled out (Chalasani et al. 2018). It is possible to have NALFD in conjunction with the abovementioned diseases.

Most people with NAFLD are asymptomatic. Fatigue, weight loss, weakness, and right upper quadrant abdominal pain are rare; and signs including jaundice, ascites, gynecomastia, and spider angiomata are noted only in advanced stages of the disease. This leads many individuals to present with more advanced disease at the time of diagnosis. In 15–50% of cases, liver fibrosis or cirrhosis is seen as the initial presentation (Falchuk et al. 1980).

Table 2 Components of metabolic syndrome

Criteria	Variable
Waist circumference	>102 cm men; >88 cm women
Fasting glucose	≥100 mg/dL
Triglycerides	≥150 mg/dL
HDL cholesterol	<40 mg/dL men; <50 mg/dL women
Blood pressure	Systolic ≥130 and/or diastolic ≥85 mm hg

The majority of patients come to the clinician's attention usually because of abnormal serum aspartate aminotransferase (AST) or alanine aminotransferase (ALT) levels noted often in routine serologic examination. No specific serologic markers for NAFLD are available. Testing is done to exclude other liver diseases such as hepatitis B, hepatitis C, autoimmune hepatitis, primary biliary cholangitis, hereditary hemochromatosis, Wilson's disease, or alpha-1 antitrypsin deficiency. Markers of metabolic syndrome (Table 2) including hemoglobin-A1c, increased total cholesterol, increased low density lipoproteins (LDL), and increased triglycerides in the setting of hypertension and obesity should alert clinicians to the possibility of concomitant NAFLD. Patients with NAFLD, and more commonly NASH, usually have mild (two to three-fold) fluctuating elevation of serum AST, ALT, or both and rarely more than three times the upper limit of normal (Harrison and Neuschwander-Tetri 2004). Autoantibodies may be positive in patients with NAFLD in the absence of autoimmune hepatitis (Vuppalanchi et al. 2012). The international normalized ratio (INR), serum bilirubin, and serum creatinine may be abnormal in advanced disease.

Given the massive number of people potentially affected by NAFLD, noninvasive tools to diagnose and stage the disease are paramount. Several panels have been developed to predict and diagnose hepatic steatosis and even fibrosis based on both biochemical measurements or patient characteristics/risk factors. The NAFLD fibrosis score is a noninvasive model used to predict which patients with NAFLD are more likely to have advanced fibrosis based on the following parameters: age, hyperglycemia, body mass index, platelet count, albumin, and AST/ALT ratio (Angula et al. 2007). Other models used to predict fibrosis, such as the Fibrosis-4 (FIB-4) and APRI score, were validated in the hepatitis C population and can be borrowed to be utilized in the NAFLD population.

There are several proprietary panels of biomarkers currently available in clinical practice. Biomarkers are pathway products and proteins associated with the pathophysiology of the transition from NAFLD to NASH (Tsai and Lee 2018). No one specific marker has been found to be reliably diagnostic. Some examples of NASH biomarkers include cytokeratin 18 (CK18), fibroblast growth factor 21 (FGF21), and CK18-M65 (uncleaved CK18) (Tsai and Lee 2018). Therefore, panels of biomarkers have been developed which utilize different breakdown products, proteins, and inflammatory markers in an effort to predict NASH and advanced fibrosis. Many of these models and panels still require external validation (Tsai and Lee 2018).

Imaging Studies

Imaging studies, including abdominal ultrasound, CT scan of the abdomen/pelvis, and magnetic resonance imaging (MRI), can detect fatty infiltration of the liver. Hepatic ultrasound is a simple, cost-effective, and noninvasive study to assess for hepatic steatosis. Hepatic steatosis induces an increase in echogenicity, and therefore the hepatic parenchyma appears brighter on imaging. This effect is largely due to increased reflection of ultrasound from the parenchyma and from intracellular accumulation of fat vacuoles (Lee and Park 2014). The sensitivity of US varies based on different reports and decreases in the presence of chronic liver disease and based on body habitus. Sensitivity for moderate steatosis (>33%) is estimated at 66–100% (McCullough 2004). The diagnostic performance of ultrasound in thin individuals is quite good, but even in mildly obese individuals (common in patients with fatty liver) the diagnostic accuracy of ultrasound declines (Mottin et al. 2004). Various techniques are used to assess the hepatic parenchyma, including comparison to the renal parenchyma to derive a ratio as well as assessing the visibility of specific structures such as the diaphragm and portal triads.

Cross-sectional imaging with CT scan can also assess for hepatic steatosis. Noncontrast CT scan of the abdomen gains accuracy in predicting steatosis only when the steatosis is greater than 30% (Park et al. 2006). Indeed, most studies assessing the accuracy of CT scan in diagnosing hepatic steatosis have only included populations with at least moderate steatosis, thus limiting knowledge regarding CT use to diagnosis steatosis in other populations. Iron deposition in the liver will increase its attenuation and can therefore confound diagnostic accuracy of CT scan for hepatic steatosis (Ma et al. 2009).

MRI has become the gold standard for hepatic steatosis quantification. Although costlier and historically not used solely for this purpose, with advances in technology, MRI has become superior to other modalities and is therefore becoming more utilized in clinical practice. Based on the phase of protons in water and fat, different signal strengths can be detected by most liver protocol MRI studies. By utilizing this principle in the so-called dual-echo chemical shift imaging, studies report 77–100% sensitivity and 87–91% specificity in detecting any degree of hepatic steatosis (Esterson and Grimaldi 2018). Even more advanced measurements like proton density fat fraction (PDFF) allow even more precise steatosis quantification, with some evidence even suggesting detection as precise as the gold standard of histology (Fischer et al. 2012). Moreover, since biopsy can assess only one fraction of the liver, and steatosis is known to have a heterogenous pattern, MR imaging might be superior as it allows global hepatic steatosis quantification. This global assessment can be followed over time and offers prognostic information as well as aid in following intervention efficacy. That said, MRI cannot be performed in those with implantable devices and is a difficult examination for individuals with claustrophobia. Both problems might be encountered in the older adult.

Elastography uses imaging techniques to estimate liver stiffness and gauge fibrosis. Since liver biopsy, an invasive test, is not always appropriate or practical, it may not be prudent to subject an older adult to liver biopsy in the absence of compelling indications. Elastography can be both non-image based (i.e., transient elastography) and image based (acoustic radiation force impulse {ARFI} elastography, MRE). A stepwise decrease in elasticity is seen in hepatic fibrosis (Yoneda et al. 2007). Ultrasound-based elastography can have disadvantages including a limited sample size and decreased reliability in obese patients. Use of a larger XL probe can help improve diagnostic accuracy in larger patients. Use of MR imaging to quantify fibrosis (MR elastography) is superior to ultrasound, and some studies report sensitivity and specificity above 98% (Yin et al. 2007).

Pathophysiology

The exact pathogenesis of NASH remains unknown. Initial theory revolved around the "two-hit" hypothesis developed in 1998 by Day et al. (Day and James 1998). This theory suggested that insulin resistance leads to hepatic steatosis and subsequent injury through oxidative stress. It has become clear that a more complicated multihit model is more comprehensive and representative of the true pathophysiology.

Hepatic steatosis remains the predisposing hepatic milieu from which to eventually develop NASH. Steatosis development is multifactorial, often growing out of obesity and metabolic syndrome with resultant adipose tissue dysfunction releasing excess free fatty acids (FFA) into the portal circulation leading to excess accumulation of triglycerides in hepatocytes. Adipose tissue dysfunction and increased levels of FFA can lead to increased lipid synthesis and gluconeogenesis and ultimately insulin resistance (Wang et al. 2005; Boden 1997). Moreover, FFA can directly lead to inflammation thus bridging steatosis to NASH (Shi et al. 2006; Suganami et al. 2005). It is becoming more evident that genetic predisposition also plays a large role by regulating insulin sensitivity, obesity and its distribution, degree of steatosis formation, and oxidative stress generation (Shepherd and Kahn 1999; Masuzaki et al. 2001; Barsh et al. 2000).

Excessive adiposity contributes to tissue damage that occurs in metabolic syndrome via fat-derived factors that regulate the inflammatory response. Several of these factors including fatty acids, adiponectin, leptin, and tumor necrosis factor-alpha (TNF-alpha) promote NAFLD by modulating the hepatic inflammatory response (Chitturi et al. 2002; Garg et al. 2003; Chaldakov et al. 2003). TNF-alpha is proinflammatory causing apoptosis, recruiting white blood cells (WBC), and promoting insulin resistance. Adiponectin is anti-inflammatory, inhibiting fatty acid uptake, stimulating fatty acid oxidation, and enhancing insulin sensitivity. Obesity can lead to the overproduction of TNF-alpha leading to reduced adiponectin activity. Interestingly, TNF-alpha and adiponectin inhibit each other's production and activity. In summary, the combination of high TNF-alpha and low adiponectin favors steatosis (NAFLD), cell death, inflammation (NASH), and insulin resistance (Stefan and Stuvoll 2002; Hotamisligil et al. 1993; Bruun et al. 2003).

Gut microbiota have shown increasing relevance to the development of NAFLD. Microbiota can influence several factors in the pathogenesis including absorption of dietary lipids promoting obesity, diabetes (type 1 and type 2), and generation of free fatty acids (Abu-Shanab and Quigley 2010). All these factors promote steatosis, leading to NAFLD and NASH. Medications such as antibiotics often used in the older adult can influence microbiota and contribute directly to fatty liver through adverse effects.

Pathology

Liver biopsy is the "gold standard" to confirm or exclude NASH (Tiniakos 2010), although biopsy is only done selectively in those suspected to have NAFLD. The diagnosis and differentiation between NAFLD and NASH can be determined only by liver histology and cannot be predicted by clinical or laboratory findings alone (Matteoni et al. 1999). The minimum histologic criteria for NAFLD is the presence of fat in more than 5% of hepatocytes, with or without lobular inflammation. NASH is differentiated from simple steatosis by hepatocellular injury, pathologically seen as hepatocyte ballooning. When there is sustained injury, the extracellular matrix accumulates along with fibrosis (Brunt 2010). Fibrosis, when present, has a typical pattern within the perisinusoidal/pericellular spaces of zone three, sometimes referenced as a "chicken wire" appearance. Other features of NASH include Mallory hyaline bodies, megamitochondria, glycogenated nuclei, and variable degrees of ductular reaction correlating with advance stages of fibrosis (Richardson et al. 2007). NASH and NAFLD may coexist with other diseases such as Wilson's disease, hemochromatosis, alpha-1-anti trypsin deficiency, and chronic hepatitis C infection.

A scoring system has been developed by the NIH for use in research and clinical grading known as the NAFLD Activity Score (NAS score) (Kleiner et al. 2005). The score grades the degree of steatosis, hepatocellular ballooning, and lobular inflammation. Although becoming more widely adapted, the score remains mostly a research tool at this time.

Management of NAFLD

Currently there are no FDA approved treatments specifically targeting NAFLD. General principles of treatment revolve around lifestyle modification and control of underlying metabolic risk factors. Although there are some medications utilized off label for NAFLD, the search is on for more targeted treatments. The number of NAFLD related registered phase two and three trials has been dramatically increasing (Gawrieh and Chalasani 2018). Goals of therapy have become focused on both stabilization of histology and liver disease, as well as improvement in fibrosis. The three major causes of NASH related mortality are cardiovascular disease, all-cause malignancy, and liver-related death (Ahmed et al. 2015).

Therefore, the scope of care needs to address all the concerns above.

- Lifestyle modification includes increased activity level and exercise in an attempt to lose weight, although even exercise alone can lead to steatosis reversal. A weight loss of 3–5% of body weight improves hepatic steatosis, and further loss to 7–10% can even improve NASH histology (Ahmed et al. 2015). Effective weight loss can improve steatohepatitis, inflammation, hepatic ballooning, and even possibly fibrosis (liver scarring) (Vilar-Gomez and Martinez-Perez 2015). Bariatric surgery intuitively seems like a possible effective intervention in NAFLD; however, more research is needed prior to its recommendation. Despite its effectiveness, sustained weight loss is difficult to sustain in the NAFLD patient population, and therefore medications are needed.
- Control and avoidance of risk factors remain important in the management of NAFLD. General principles of treatment involve weight reduction, control of underlying metabolic risk factors, and avoidance of excessive alcohol and hepatotoxic medications. Alcohol should be limited as much as possible (Ajmera and Belt 2018). Treatment should be directed at controlling and optimizing diabetes, hyperlipidemia, and hypertension.
- Current Pharmaceutical Treatments: Vitamin E is an antioxidant thought to counteract the oxidative stress underlying hepatocyte injury in nonalcoholic steatohepatitis. Vitamin E inhibits lipid peroxidation and inflammatory cytokines. A dose of 800 IU per day of vitamin E has been shown to decrease serum aminotransferase levels and improve steatosis and histology (Sanyal et al. 2010). Unfortunately, there was no benefit for fibrosis. Importantly, there may be risks associated with Vitamin E including increased risks of cardioembolic events, prostate cancer (Klein et al. 2011), and even mortality (Bjelakovic et al. 2007). Currently, some guidelines caution the use of vitamin E in patients with diabetes and men for these reasons (Chalasani et al. 2012). The use of insulin-sensitizing agents, even in individuals without diabetes, has been proposed to treat patients with NASH (Ratzui and Pienar 2011). Metformin (a biguanide) improves insulin sensitivity by suppressing hepatic gluconeogenesis, increasing peripheral glucose uptake, and increasing fatty acid oxidation. Metformin can lead to reductions of serum aminotransferases, insulin resistance, and liver volume but has minimal benefit for liver histology (Marchesini et al. 2001). Thiazolidinediones (TZD) improve insulin resistance in skeletal muscle, adipose tissue, and in the liver by increasing adiponectin levels and fatty acid oxidation and decreasing fatty acid synthesis. Pioglitazone is a ligand for the nuclear transcription peroxisome proliferator-activated receptor gamma (PPARγ). A large trial with pioglitazone showed significant improvement in histology with limited benefit on fibrosis (Sanyal et al. 2010). There was also significant weight gain seen with taking the medication subsequently lost after drug cessation.
- Future Pharmaceutical Treatments: Results with antioxidant and insulin-sensitizing agents have been underwhelming, therefore significant interest remains in developing new pharmaceuticals. Goals of therapy have become focused on both stabilization of histology and liver disease, as well as improvement in fibrosis. It is likely modern treatments will involve multiple agents aimed at different metabolic pathways. Obeticholic acid is a modified bile acid and FXR agonist that has been shown to decrease liver fat load and fibrosis in animal models. The FLINT trial demonstrated that obeticholic acid in a dose of 25 mg improved NASH histology without worsening of fibrosis (Neuschwander-Tetri et al. 2015). Selonsertib is a selective inhibitor of apoptosis signal-regulating kinase 1. This agent has been shown to decrease inflammation and fibrosis in animal models of NASH. A phase 2 trial in subjects with NASH showed improvement in fibrosis in both 6 mg and 18 mg doses of selonsertib (Loomba et al. 2018). Current drugs under investigation include: elafibranor (a peroxisome proliferator-activated receptor),

liraglutide (a glucagon-like peptide-1 analogue), and emricasan (a pan caspase inhibitor), with more to come.

Key Points

- NAFLD affects all age groups, races, and both sexes. There is higher prevalence of NAFLD and NASH in Hispanics and South Asians.
- Most people with NAFLD are asymptomatic, but it may lead to steatohepatitis, cirrhosis, and rarely hepatocellular carcinoma.
- The exact pathogenesis of NASH remains unknown. Initial theory revolved around the "two-hit" hypothesis but is now recognized as more complicated.
- Hepatic ultrasound is a simple, cost-effective, and noninvasive study to assess for hepatic steatosis.
- Other imaging studies, CT scan of the abdomen, and magnetic resonance imaging (MRI) can detect fatty infiltration of the liver.
- A scoring system was developed by the NIH for use in research and clinical grading known as the NAFLD Activity Score (NAS score).
- Liver biopsy is the "gold standard" to confirm or exclude NASH and for staging.
- Goals of therapy are focused on both stabilization of histology and liver disease, as well as improvement in fibrosis.
- Lifestyle modification and control of underlying metabolic risk factors are the basis of management.
- Obeticholic acid is a modified bile acid and FXR agonist that has been shown to decrease liver fat load and fibrosis in animal models.

References

Abu-Shanab A, Quigley E. The role of the gut microbiota in nonalcoholic fatty liver disease. Nat Rev Gastroenterol Hepatol. 2010;7:691–701.

Ahmed A, Wong RJ, Harrison SA. Nonalcoholic fatty liver disease review: diagnosis, treatment, and outcomes. Clin Gastroenterol Hepatol. 2015;13(12):2062–70. https://doi.org/10.1016/j.cgh.2015.07.029.

Ajmera V, Belt P. Among patients with nonalcoholic fatty liver disease, modest alcohol use is associated with less improvement in histologic steatosis and steatohepatitis. Clin Gastroenterol Hepatol. 2018;16(9):1511.

Angula P, Hui JM, Marchesini G. The NAFLD fibrosis score: a noninvasive system that identifies liver fibrosis in patients with NAFLD. Hepatology. 2007;45:846–54.

Angulo P. Obesity and nonalcoholic fatty liver disease. Nutr Rev. 2007;65(6 Pt 2):57–63. https://doi.org/10.1301/nr.2007.jun.S57.

Barsh G, Farooqi I, O'Rahilly S. Genetics of body-weight regulation. Nature. 2000;404:644–51.

Bjelakovic G, Nikolova D, Gluud L. Mortality in randomized trials of antioxidant supplements for primary and secondary prevention: systematic review and meta-analysis. JAMA. 2007;297(8):842–57.

Boden G. Role of fatty acids in the pathogenesis of insulin resistance and NIDDM. Diabetes. 1997;46:3–10.

Brunt E. Pathology of nonalcoholic fatty liver disease. Nat Rev Gastroenterol Hepatol. 2010;7:195–203.

Bruun J, Lihn A, Verdich C. Regulation of adiponectin by adipose tissue-derived cytokines: in vivo and in vitro investigations in humans. Am J Physiol Endocrinol Metab. 2003;285:E527–33.

Chalasani N, Younossi Z, Lavine JE, et al. The diagnosis and management of non-alcoholic fatty liver disease: practice guideline by the American Association for the Study of Liver Diseases, American College of Gastroenterology, and the American Gastroenterological Association. Hepatology. 2012;55(6):2005–23. https://doi.org/10.1002/hep.25762.

Chalasani N, Younossi Z, Lavine JE, et al. The diagnosis and management of nonalcoholic fatty liver disease: practice guidance from the American Association for the Study of Liver Diseases. Hepatology. 2018;67(1):328–57. https://doi.org/10.1002/hep.29367.

Chaldakov G, Stankulov I, Hristova M, Ghenev P. Adipobiology of diseases: adipokines and adipokine-targeted pharmacology. Curr Pharm Des. 2003;9:1023–31.

Chitturi S, Farrell G, Frost L. Serum leptin in NASH correlates with hepatic steatosis but not fibrosis: a manifestation of lipotoxicity? Hepatology. 2002;36:403–9.

Chitturi S, Wong VW, Farrell G. Nonalcoholic fatty liver in Asia: firmly entrenched and rapidly gaining ground. J Gastroenterol Hepatol. 2011;26:163–72. https://doi.org/10.1111/j.1440-1746.2010.06548.x.

Clark J. The epidemiology of nonalcoholic fatty liver disease in adults. J Clin Gastroenterol. 2006;40:S5.

Day C, James O. Steatohepatitis: a tale of the "hits"? Gastroenterology. 1998;114:842–5.

Dixon JB, Bhathal PS. Nonalcoholic fatty liver disease: predictors of nonalcoholic steatohepatitis and liver fibrosis in the severely obese. Gastroenterology. 2001;121:91–100. https://doi.org/10.1053/gast.2001.25540.

Esterson YB, Grimaldi GM. Radiologic imaging in nonalcoholic fatty liver disease and nonalcoholic steatohepatitis. Clin Liver Dis. 2018;22(1):93–108. https://doi.org/10.1016/j.cld.2017.08.005.

Falchuk K, Fiske S, Haggitt R. Pericentral hepatic fibrosis and intracellular hyalin in diabetes mellitus. Gastroenterology. 1980;78:535–41.

Fischer M, Raptis D, Montani M. Liver fat quantification by dual-echo MR imaging outperforms traditional histopathological analysis. Acad Radiol. 2012;19 (10):1208–14.

Garg R, Tripathy D, Dandona P. Insulin resistance as a proinflammatory state: mechanisms, mediators, and therapuetic interventions. Curr Drug Targets. 2003;4:487–92.

Gawrieh S, Chalasani N. Emerging treatments for non-alcoholic fatty liver disease and nonalcoholic steatohepatitis. Clin Liver Dis. 2018;22(1):189–99. https://doi.org/10.1016/j.cld.2017.08.013.

Harrison S, Neuschwander-Tetri BA. Nonalcoholic fatty liver disease and nonalcoholic steatohepatitis. Clin Liver Dis. 2004;8:861–79.

Hotamisligil G, Shargill N, Spiegelman B. Adipose expression of tumor necrosis factor-alpha: direct role in obesity-linked insulin resistance. Science (80–). 1993;259:87–91.

Kanwal F, Kramer JR, Duan Z, Yu X, White D, El-Serag HB. Trends in the burden of nonalcoholic fatty liver disease in a United States cohort of veterans. Clin Gastroenterol Hepatol. 2016;14(2):301–8. https://doi.org/10.1016/j.cgh.2015.08.010.

Kim D, Touros A, Kim WR. Nonalcoholic fatty liver disease and metabolic syndrome. Clin Liver Dis. 2018;22(1):133–40. https://doi.org/10.1016/j.cld.2017.08.010.

Klein E, Thompson I, Tangen C. Vitamin E and the risk of prostate cancer: the selenium and vitamin E cancer prevention trial (SELECT). JAMA. 2011;306(14):1549–56.

Kleiner DE, Brunt EM, Van Natta M, et al. Design and validation of a histological scoring system for nonalcoholic fatty liver disease. Hepatology. 2005;41(6):1313–21. https://doi.org/10.1002/hep.20701.

Lee SS, Park SH. Radiologic evaluation of nonalcoholic fatty liver disease. World J Gastroenterol. 2014;20(23):7392–402. https://doi.org/10.3748/wjg.v20.i23.7392.

Loomba R, Lawitz E, Mantry PS. The ASK1 inhibitor selonsertib in patients with nonalcoholic steatohepatitis: a randomized, phase 2 trial. Hepatology. 2018;67:549–59.

Ludwig J, Viggiano TR, McGill DB, Oh BJ. Nonalcoholic steatohepatitis: Mayo Clinic experiences with a hitherto unnamed disease. Mayo Clin Proc. 1980;55(7):434–8.. http://europepmc.org/abstract/MED/7382552

Ma X, Holalkere N-S, Kambadakone A. Imaging-based Quanti- fi cation of Hepatic Fat: methods and clinical. Radiographics. 2009;29:1253–80.

Marchesini G, Brizi M, Bianchi G. Metfomin in non-alcoholic steatohepatitis. Lancet. 2001;358:893–4.

Marengo A, Jouness R, Bugianesi E. Progression and natural history of nonalcoholic fatty liver disease in adults. Clin Liver Dis. 2016;20(2):313–24.

Masuzaki H, Paterson J, Shinyama H. A transgenic model of visceral obesity and the metabolic syndrome. Science (80–). 2001;294:166–70.

Matteoni C, Younossi Z, Gramlich T, Al E. Nonalcoholic fatty liver disease: a spectrum of clinical and pathological severity. Gastroenterology. 1999;116:1413–9.

McCullough A. The clinical features, diagnosis and natural history of nonalcoholic fatty liver disease. Clin Liver Dis. 2004;8:521–33.

Mittal S, El-Serag HB, Sada YH, et al. Hepatocellular Carcinoma in the Absence of Cirrhosis in United States Veterans Is Associated With Nonalcoholic Fatty Liver Disease. Clin Gastroenterol Hepatol. 2016;14(1):124–131.e1. https://doi.org/10.1016/j.cgh.2015.07.019.

Mottin CC, Moretto M, Padoin AV, et al. The Role of ultrasound in the diagnosis of hepatic steatosis in morbidly obese patients. Obes Surg. 2004;14:635–7.

Neuschwander-Tetri BA, Loomba R, Sanyal AJ. Farsenoid X nuclear receptor ligand obeticholic acid for non-cirrhotic, non-alcoholic steatohepatitis (FLINT): a multicentre, randomised, placebo-controlled trial. Lancet. 2015;385(9972):956–65.

Park S, Kim P, Kim K. Macrovesicular hepatic steatosis in living liver donors: use of CT for quantitative and qualitative assessment. Radiology. 2006;239(239):105–12.

Ratzui V, Pienar L. Pharmacological therapy for non-alcoholic steatohepatitis: how efficient are thiazolidinediones? Hepatol Res. 2011;41:687–95.

Rich NE, Oji S, Mufti AR, et al. Racial and ethnic disparities in nonalcoholic fatty liver disease prevalence, severity, and outcomes in the United States: a systematic review and meta-analysis. Clin Gastroenterol Hepatol. 2017;16(2):198–210.e2. https://doi.org/10.1016/j.cgh.2017.09.041.

Richardson M, Jonsson J, Powell E. Progressive fibrosis in nonalcoholic steatohepatitis: association with altered regeneration and a ductular reaction. Gastroenterology. 2007;133:80–90.

Saab S, Manne V, Nieto J, Schwimmer JB, Chalasani NP. Nonalcoholic fatty liver disease in Latinos. Clin Gastroenterol Hepatol. 2016;14(1):5–12. https://doi.org/10.1016/j.cgh.2015.05.001.

Sanyal AJ, Chalasani N, Kowdley KV, et al. Pioglitazone, vitamin E, or placebo for nonalcoholic steatohepatitis. N Engl J Med. 2010;362(18):1675–85. https://doi.org/10.1056/NEJMoa0907929.

Shepherd P, Kahn B. Glucose transporters and insulin action- implications for insulin resistance and diabetes mellitus. N Engl J Med. 1999;341:248–57.

Shi H, Kokoeva M, Inouye K. TLR4 links innate immunity and fatty acid- induced insulin resistance. J Clin Invest. 2006;116:3015–25.

Silverman J, O'brien K, Long S. Liver pathology in morbidly obese patients with and without diabetes. Am J Gastroenterol. 1990;85:1349–55.

Stefan N, Stuvoll M. Adiponectin- its role in metabolism and beyond. Horm Metab Res. 2002;34:469–74.

Suganami T, Nishida J, Ogawa Y. A paracrine loop between adipocytes and macrophages aggravates inflammatory changes: role of free fatty acid and tumor necrosis factor alpha. Arter Thromb Vasc Biol. 2005;25:2062–8.

Tiniakos D. Nonalcoholic fatty liver disease/nonalcoholic steatohepatitis:histological diagnostic criteria and scoring systems. Eur J Gastroenterol Hepatol. 2010;22:643–50.

Tsai E, Lee TP. Diagnosis and evaluation of nonalcoholic fatty liver disease/nonalcoholic steatohepatitis, including noninvasive biomarkers and transient Elastography. Clin Liver Dis. 2018;22(1):73–92. https://doi.org/10.1016/j.cld.2017.08.004.

Vilar-Gomez E, Martinez-Perez Y. Weight loss through lifestyle modification significantly reduces features of nonalcoholic steatohepatitis. Gastroenterology. 2015;149(2):367–78.

Vuppalanchi R, Gould R, Wilson L. Clinical significance of serum autoantibodies in patients with NAFLD: results from the nonalcoholic steatohepatitis clinical research network (NASH CRN). Hepatol Int. 2012;6(1):379–85.

Wang Y, Rimm EB, Stampfer MJ, Willett WC, Hu FB. Comparison of abdominal adiposity and overall obesity in predicting risk of type 2 diabetes among men. Am J Clin Nutr. 2005;81:1–3.

Wanless I, Lentz J. Fatty liver hepatitis (Steatohepatitis) and obesity: an autopsy study with analysis of risk factors. Hepatology. 1990;12:1106–10.

Yin M, Talwalkar J, Glaser K. Assessment of hepatic fibrosis with magnetic resonance elastography. Clin Gastroenterol Hepatol. 2007;5:1207–13.

Yoneda M, Fujita K, Inamori M. Transient elastography in patients with non-alcoholic fatty liver disease (NAFLD). Gut. 2007;56:1330–1.

Younossi ZM, Stepanova M, Afendy M, et al. Changes in the prevalence of the most common causes of chronic liver diseases in the United States from 1988 to 2008. YJCGH. 2011;9(6):524–530.e1. https://doi.org/10.1016/j.cgh.2011.03.020.

Younossi ZM, Koenig AB, Abdelatif D, Fazel Y, Henry L, Wymer M. Global epidemiology of nonalcoholic fatty liver disease – meta-analytic assessment of prevalence, incidence, and outcomes. Hepatology. 2016;64(1):73–84. https://doi.org/10.1002/hep.28431.

Younossi ZM, Henry L, Bush H, Mishra A. Clinical and economic burden of nonalcoholic fatty liver disease and nonalcoholic steatohepatitis. Clin Liver Dis. 2018;22(1):1–10. https://doi.org/10.1016/j.cld.2017.08.001.

Drug-Induced Liver Injury in Older Adults

61

Ethan D. Miller, Hamzah Abu-Sbeih, and Naga P. Chalasani

Contents

Abstract

The estimated incidence of idiosyncratic drug-induced liver injury (DILI) in the general population is 13.9 to 19.1 per 100,000 patients per year. Age itself is not a risk factor, but older adults appear to be at risk for DILI from a few, specific drugs, including several antibiotics. Older adults with DILI do not have a higher mortality compared to other age groups. The pathogenesis of idiosyncratic DILI remains poorly understood. Patients with suspected DILI may present with a variety of clinical signs and symptoms. DILI remains a diagnosis of exclusion, and its identification involves obtaining a careful history, select lab and imaging studies, and sometimes a liver biopsy. Older adults may exhibit a cholestatic biochemical profile compared to younger patients in response to the same offending agent. The suspected drug should be discontinued, followed by close monitoring. Spontaneous resolution occurs in most, but normalization of liver function may take days to months,

E. D. Miller · H. Abu-Sbeih
Department of Gastroenterology, Hepatology and Nutrition, The University of Texas MD Anderson Cancer Center, Houston, TX, USA
e-mail: emiller1@mdanderson.org; habusbeih@mdanderson.org

N. P. Chalasani (✉)
Division of Gastroenterology and Hepatology, Indiana University School of Medicine, Indianapolis, IN, USA
e-mail: nchalasa@iu.edu

© Springer Nature Switzerland AG 2021
C. S. Pitchumoni, T. S. Dharmarajan (eds.), *Geriatric Gastroenterology*,
https://doi.org/10.1007/978-3-030-30192-7_53

while some progress to cirrhosis. Drug re-challenge is not advisable but is on rare occasions unavoidable. Sometimes steroids are needed to treat DILI, especially when there is an autoimmune hepatitis-like reaction. Biomarkers to predict and monitor DILI are needed. There is under-reporting of DILI worldwide. More information regarding DILI in older adults is needed, including from clinical trials and case reports in registries.

Keywords

DILI · Hepatotoxicity · Hepatocellular · Cholestatic · Antibiotics · Diclofenac · Steroid therapy · Jaundice · Drug-induced hepatitis · Liver biopsy · Autoimmune liver disease · Idiosyncratic DILI · Supplement use · Liver injury

Introduction

The topic of drug-induced liver injury (DILI) in the elderly is important for several reasons. First, with increasing age come increasing comorbidities, medical visits, and testing, with the opportunity that test results concerning for liver injury may be identified. The clinician needs to have an approach to interpreting these tests and how to respond: when to be alert to certain medications which might pose a risk of liver injury and – just as important – when to be alert to knowing which medications might be a risk if discontinued. Indeed, it has been reported that older patients may be under-prescribed many medications, including statins (Barry et al. 2007). Second, "polypharmacy," the presence of more than five medications in a routine regimen, has also been cited as a risk factor for DILI in the elderly (Bell and Chalasani 2009; Onji et al. 2009; Stine et al. 2013). Although it has been questioned as to whether polypharmacy itself a risk factor for DILI (Chalasani and Bjornsson 2010; Chalasani et al. 2014), it is nevertheless a valid concern that with a longer list of medications, additional vigilance for the risk of hepatotoxicity is needed to ensure

hepatic issues do not overtake other medical conditions as a primary focus. Third, many patients, including the elderly, may take non-prescription medications and other supplements (Qato et al. 2016) that their providers may or may not have been informed about or consider as possibly hepatotoxic. It is important to be aware of this possibility since these compounds could be hepatotoxic and in fact have been cited as common causes of hepatotoxicity (Chalasani et al. 2015; Navarro et al. 2017). Finally, it is of paramount importance that registries around the world receive more cases of DILI in the elderly and that more studies include elderly patients, to improve our understanding of hepatotoxicity-related concerns in this important population.

DILI may be defined in several ways. Mainly it may be defined by the pattern of hepatic-related biochemistries observed after drug exposure (Danan and Benichou 1993). A hepatocellular pattern – in which the hepatocyte itself is injured – is characterized predominantly by elevated aminotransferases, whereas a cholestatic pattern, with disruption of flow within the biliary system, is characterized predominantly by an elevated alkaline phosphatase. A mixed pattern of injury reflects hepatocellular and biliary injury.

DILI is also defined in terms of the characteristics known to result from exposure to a particular drug. Drugs can cause intrinsic or idiosyncratic injury. Specific drugs may elicit injury in a predictable, dose-dependent fashion, usually at a fixed latency. This "intrinsic" type of injury is best typified by acetaminophen. While not toxic to the liver when taken as intended, acetaminophen can cause acute injury if taken in excess, particularly in the context of significant alcohol consumption.

By contrast, idiosyncratic DILI from a particular drug is not predictable with respect to dose, latency, or incidence. Idiosyncratic DILI tends to be what can limit drug development and, while rare, can cause significant morbidity and mortality (Chalasani et al. 2015) and is responsible for up to 17% of cases of acute liver failure (Nicoletti et al. 2017). Idiosyncratic DILI will be the focus of this chapter.

The estimated incidence of idiosyncratic DILI in the general population is 13.9 to 19.1 per 100,000 patients per year (Bjornsson et al. 2013; Sgro et al. 2002), although estimates from different parts of the world vary, and global data reporting is incomplete (Ahmad and Odin 2017). Because of its infrequency and also incomplete and under-reporting, including in clinical trials (Chalasani and Bjornsson 2010), it is especially difficult to estimate the incidence among the elderly as a distinct population. Moreover, the median age of DILI patients from a number of large studies ranges between 48 and 55 years (Fontana 2014), underscoring the paucity of data regarding the elderly.

It has long been an assumed that older patients are at higher risk for DILI compared to younger adults. Age greater than 50 years confers additional points to a historical and widely- used scale (RUCAM) for assessing for DILI (Danan and Benichou 1993), predicated on this belief. There is some evidence that the incidence of DILI increases with age, but for unclear reasons, possibly related to increased number of prescriptions with age (Bjornsson et al. 2013). But a risk of DILI in older patients, in general, has not been demonstrated on a consistent basis (Bell and Chalasani 2009; Chalasani et al. 2015; Andrade et al. 2019; Lucena et al. 2009; Suk et al. 2012). However, there is more consistent evidence that the biochemical pattern of DILI may shift with increasing age (Chalasani et al. 2015; Lucena et al. 2009) and that the elderly appear to be at risk for DILI not as a general rule, but from a few, specific drugs (Chalasani and Bjornsson 2010; de Lemos et al. 2016).

Pathophysiology

The pathogenesis of idiosyncratic DILI remains poorly understood and involves complex interactions among patient- and drug-related factors. Patient-related factors include genetic and non-genetic host susceptibility factors (Chalasani and Bjornsson 2010; Daly and Day 2009; Fontana 2014; Tujios and Fontana 2011; Wilke et al. 2007) and innate and adaptive immunity (Chen et al. 2015). In the future as the pathophysiology becomes clarified, this understanding will be the basis for clinically useful tools in the care of DILI patients (Vuppalanchi et al. 2014).

The liver plays an important role in the clearance and biotransformation of drugs and may be adversely affected due to the generation of toxic metabolites. Hepatic drug-metabolizing enzymes convert lipid-soluble molecules into a water-soluble form, thus permitting their entry into the plasma and excretion in the urine or elimination into the bile. Most drugs are transformed by hepatic phase I (reactive metabolite production) and phase II (reactive metabolite detoxification) metabolic reactions. Oxidation (e.g., hydroxylation and dealkylation) and reduction (e.g., nitroreduction) are phase I reactions, whereas phase II reactions include conjugation via an endogenous compound (via glucuronidation, sulfation, or acetylation) of the parent compound or a metabolite to make it more hydrophilic for eventual excretion into bile or urine (Fig. 1). The cytochrome P450 superfamily (CYP) is involved in the bioactivation and metabolism of drugs, mostly in phase I reactions. Factors that alter CYP activity increase toxicity by reducing drug conversion to nontoxic metabolites or by increasing conversion to toxic metabolites (Walgren et al. 2005). CYP is abundant in the centrilobular zone compared to the periportal area; centrilobular necrosis is characteristic of DILI, suggesting that drug-metabolizing enzymes play a role in DILI. Most hepatically cleared substrates are metabolized by CYP1, CYP2, and CYP3 families.

It has been proposed that due to various factors, including changes in liver mass, hepatic circulation and Phase I metabolism, the liver ages in clinically relevant ways (Tan et al. 2015). CYP3A is a prominent subfamily, and it has been postulated that age-related reductions in hepatic blood flow, and hepatic volume may have an impact on the clearance of some CYP3A substrates (Cotreau et al. 2005). Yet, in practice, there is a lack of evidence that these alterations are significant or can be used to anticipate or manage DILI (Onji et al. 2009; Stine et al. 2013). Also, it has been pointed out that such changes would,

PHASE I

- Redox reactions generate metabolically active polar groups

- Can generate toxic metabolites

PHASE II

- Conjugates highly polar moieties (i.e. glucuronide) to chemicals

- Mediated mainly by transferases

PHASE III

- Excretion into bile canaliculi or blood via transporters

- Transporters also involved in drug uptake into cells

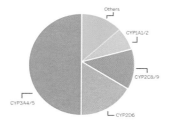
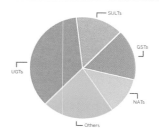

Fig. 1 Phases I, II, and III drug metabolism. (Abbreviations: **CYP1A1/2**: Cytochrome P450 1A1 and 1A2; **CYP2C8/9**: Cytochrome P450 2C8/2C9; **CYP2D6**: Cytochrome P450 2D6; and **CYP3A4/5**: Cytochrome P450 3A4/3A5)

if relevant to DILI, be expected to account for intrinsic rather than idiosyncratic DILI (Chalasani and Bjornsson 2010). In addition, it does not appear that older patients are at higher risk of worse outcomes compared to younger patients when DILI occurs. Rather, the presence of pre-existing liver disease is a risk factor for higher mortality from DILI (Chalasani et al. 2015).

In addition to Phase I and II reactions, other components of hepatic metabolism have been implicated in DILI. Hepatic transport systems maintain uptake and efflux processes in bile formation and play a role in drug clearance (Corsini and Bortolini 2013). Cholestatic DILI may result from drug-mediated inhibition of hepatobiliary transporter systems (Ho and Kim 2005; Pauli-Magnus and Meier 2006). Mutations and polymorphisms of the exporter proteins cause intracellular accumulation of toxic bile constituents with cholestatic liver injury (Lang et al. 2007; Noe et al. 2005). Some drugs (e.g., valproate, salicylate, antiretroviral agents) cause liver injury via mitochondrial toxicity; alteration of mitochondrial function in the liver may induce fat accumulation (microvesicular steatosis) (Begriche et al. 2011). Drugs can also cause damage to the endothelial cells, which may lead to nodular regenerative hyperplasia, sinusoidal injury, and accompanying manifestations of portal hypertension even in the absence of cirrhosis (Fontana 2014).

Genetic risk factors have been identified in association with idiosyncratic DILI, including related to specific Phase I CYP enzymes, Phase II enzymes, drug transporters, and mitochondrial DNA, as well as immunologic factors such as HLA alleles (Chalasani and Bjornsson 2010). Genome-wide association studies, which can be especially useful in screening the genome for possible genetic risk factors for a variety of conditions, have been done to identify DILI-related polymorphisms, which has led to the identification of HLA-related risk factor for DILI for several drugs, including amoxicillin-clavulanate (Lucena et al. 2011), flucloxacillin (Daly et al. 2009), and also for statins (Nicoletti et al. 2017), but not pertaining specifically to age-related DILI. There is also evidence for associations between the HLA haplotype and a cholestatic or mixed biochemistry pattern in response to injury from amoxicillin-clavulanic acid (Hautekeete et al. 1999). Such studies may reveal more polymorphisms related to specific drugs and help shed light on the mechanisms underlying DILI.

Specific immune pathways that may influence the occurrence of liver injury have also been investigated. For example, diclofenac, a non-steroidal anti-inflammatory drug (NSAID) that has been reported to cause hepatotoxicity including in the elderly, may suppress TNF-alpha, thereby leading to apoptosis (Fredriksson et al. 2011).

Various drug properties play a role in DILI. As one might expect, DILI is more likely to occur for drugs that are metabolized by the liver, although there are exceptions (Lammert et al. 2010). In one study, among a group of drugs that can cause DILI, ones that were reported more frequently among the elderly, as compared to a pediatric population, tended to have higher lipophilic indices (Hunt et al. 2014), possibly by causing increased metabolic demands on the liver (Fontana 2014). It has been observed that dose of an oral medication, regardless of its class or indication, is also a factor for causing liver injury, with higher oral dose presenting an increased risk of DILI, especially in daily doses exceeding 50 mg (Lammert et al. 2008). There also may be a connection between higher lipophilicity and higher drug dose in leading to DILI (Chen et al. 2013). When a variety of drug characteristics were assessed together, drug dose >50 mg was associated with a shorter latency to DILI, but drug properties were not helpful in determining outcomes (Vuppalanchi et al. 2014). While idiosyncratic DILI is not dose-related, there may be a threshold dose of 50–100 mg/day for DILI to be more likely (Andrade et al. 2019). However, it is not clear how to apply information about biochemical properties or dose, other than to note that idiosyncratic DILI can occur even when drugs are taken according to standard dosing.

Patterns of Liver Injury

DILI is a pattern of injury with characteristics that encompass a range of biochemical, histologic, and other clinical features (such as fever or rash, which may signal an allergic-based reaction). The "R" value (Table 1), the ratio of ALT/ULN to alkaline phosphatase/ULN, is used to categorize the pattern of presenting biochemistries as reflective of injury that is hepatocellular (R > 5), cholestatic (R < 2), or mixed (R = 2–5). Irrespective of what is "classically" expected in terms of a biochemical profile from a particular drug, older adults appear to be more likely to exhibit a cholestatic or mixed biochemical pattern of injury in response to a given drug, when compared to younger adults who may exhibit a hepatocellular pattern (Bjornsson et al. 2013; Chalasani et al. 2015; Onji et al. 2009) (Andrade et al. 2019; Hunt et al. 2014; Lucena et al. 2009) (Table 1).

There are a variety of histologic patterns that may be seen in the setting of DILI, including acute or chronic hepatocellular or cholestatic injury, granuloma formation, steatosis, macro- and micro-vesicular steatohepatitis, necrosis, vascular injury, and nodular regenerative hyperplasia. Regarding histologic patterns, in a large cohort, there were five patterns that were seen in the majority of cases: acute hepatitis, chronic hepatitis, acute cholestasis, chronic cholestasis, and cholestatic hepatitis. There was limited correlation between histologic and biochemical patterns at the time of injury when it came to classification into hepatocellular, cholestatic, or mixed patterns of injury based on the "R" value (Kleiner et al. 2014). Caution is urged in predicting the pattern of histologic changes based on the pattern of biochemistries.

Age may be a risk factor for the development of chronic DILI, but findings have not been consistent. Defining chronic DILI as persistently abnormal biochemistries, histology, or imaging lasting a year or more after drug withdrawal, older age was a risk factor in one study (Medina-Caliz et al. 2016). However, using abnormal biochemistries, imaging, or exam findings noted at least 6 months after drug withdrawal to define chronicity, a separate study found that older patients are actually less likely to have chronic DILI compared to other age groups (Chalasani et al. 2015).

Table 1 Patterns of liver injury in drug induced liver injury

R-value	Pattern	Key feature	Comment
<2	Cholestatic	Predominantly elevated alkaline phosphatase	Amoxicillin-clavulanate is the prototype. Elderly individuals are at higher risk for cholestatic DILI
>5	Hepatocellular	Predominantly elevated alkaline aminotransferase	Isoniazid is the prototype
2<R<5	Mixed	Equally elevated alkaline phosphatase and alkaline phosphatase	Interestingly, and for entirely unknown reasons, DILI with mixed pattern injury appears to be associated with lower mortality than other patterns of liver injury

The R-value is defined as serum ALT/ULN divided by serum alkaline phosphatase/ULN (ULN, upper limit of normal)

Medications in Older Adults

The majority of DILI cases are caused by a single prescription medication, and the rest are caused by multiple agents or dietary supplements (Bjornsson et al. 2013).

Medication, herbal preparation, and supplement use is common throughout the world. Most older adults in the US take prescription and over-the-counter medications and supplements (Qato et al. 2016). While older adults comprise less than 15% of the US population (Hunt et al. 2014), over 30% of serious medication-related adverse events are reported in adults >65 years old (Sonawane et al. 2018).

Several large, prospective, registry-based studies have consistently shown that by class, antibiotics are the most common cause of idiosyncratic DILI in the general population (Andrade et al. 2005; Bjornsson et al. 2013; Chalasani et al. 2015). Other common classes of medications causing DILI include herbal agents and dietary supplements, cardiovascular drugs (including some statins), antineoplastic agents, central nervous system medications, and NSAIDs (especially diclofenac) (Andrade et al. 2005; Bjornsson et al. 2013; Chalasani et al. 2015).

Safety and Risks of Common Drugs

The risk of DILI (Table 2) is higher for older adults for certain drugs, such as amoxicillin-clavulanate (Chalasani et al. 2014), but age itself is not a risk factor for DILI related to all drugs (Chalasani et al. 2015; Leise et al. 2014). For example, in one study comparing categories of drugs causing DILI in those under age 65 to those age 65 or older, the four of the five most common categories of drugs were the same (i.e, antimicrobials, cardiovascular drugs, herbals and dietary supplements, and antineoplastics). The two groups differed in that analgesics were listed for the older age group, whereas central nervous system agents were listed for the younger age group. Also, except for antimicrobials topping the lists in frequency in both groups, the relative frequencies of the other categories differed (Chalasani et al. 2015). Importantly, older adults do not have higher mortality compared to other age groups when DILI does happen (Chalasani et al. 2015).

Below are highlighted some common medications and categories of medications which are relevant to older adults. There are online resources available with information regarding liver toxicities associated with specific agents. In the USA, the Drug-Induced Liver Injury Network (DILIN) maintains LiverTox, a National Institutes of Health (NIH) online database that can be searched for information on hepatotoxicity for an expansive and increasing number of available medications, herbal preparations, and supplements. LiverTox searches include associated monographs and case reports, describing expected clinical, biochemical, and, when available, histologic patterns of injury, described treatments, with references (Hoofnagle et al. 2013). There are also instructions about submitting DILI cases to LiverTox and to the US Federal Drug Administration. The LiverTox website can be accessed at: https://livertox.nih.gov/.

Table 2 Drugs commonly associated with DILI in the elderly

Medication	Comment
Amoxicillin-clavulanate	Most common cause for DILI in the Western world. Elderly are more susceptible.
Erythromycin	Cholestatic pattern.
Flucloxacillin	Not available in the USA. HLA-B*57:01 is a very strong risk factor for DILI due to flucloxacillin.
Nitrofurantoin	Used chronically for prophylaxis against urosepsis, nitrofurantoin is associated with autoimmune like liver injury.
Isoniazid	Hepatocellular pattern liver injury. Elderly are more susceptible for liver injury from anti-TB medications.
Diclofenac	Diclofenac consumed systemically is associated with chronic hepatitis - like picture. Topical creams are not associated with liver injury.

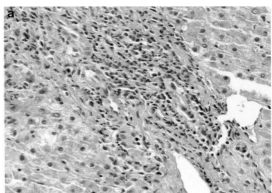 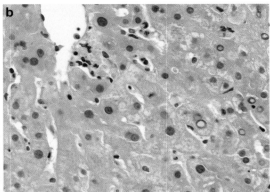

Fig. 2 Panel A: Liver injury due to amoxicillin-clavulanate. Portal area with inflammation and bile duct injury (arrow), 400x. **Panel B: Amoxicillin-clavulanate-induced liver injury**. Canalicular cholestasis (arrows) near central vein, 600x. (Courtesy of David E. Kleiner, MD, PhD at the Laboratory of Pathology/ National Cancer Institute, USA)

Antibiotics

Certain antibiotics are more likely to be hepatotoxic among elderly patients, compared to younger adults and children (Hunt et al. 2014; Medina-Caliz et al. 2016). Older age has been shown to be a risk factor for susceptibility to amoxicillin-clavulanate, which is more likely to cause a cholestatic pattern or mixed biochemistry pattern of injury in older patients, compared to the hepatocellular pattern seen in younger patients (Bjornsson et al. 2013; de Lemos et al. 2016; Hunt et al. 2014). Liver biopsy may show cholestasis and portal inflammation with duct injury (Figs. 2a and b).

Isoniazid also poses increased risk of DILI with age (Chalasani and Bjornsson 2010), as well as when it is used in the combination anti-tuberculosis regimen of isoniazid, rifampin, and pyrazinamide. Flucloxacillin, an antibiotic used in many parts of the world, may also cause DILI more frequently in elderly patients (Chalasani and Bjornsson 2010; Wing et al. 2017). Erythromycin and nitrofurantoin have also been cited as causing DILI more commonly in older patients (Chalasani and Bjornsson 2010). Nitrofurantoin has can cause a chronic, autoimmune hepatitis-like histologic pattern (Fig. 3) (Stricker et al. 1988) (Fig. 3).

Antineoplastics

DILI from antineoplastic agents can occur and can limit cancer therapy (Bjornsson et al. 2013). Age has been identified as one factor that can increase the risk of hepatotoxicity (Vincenzi et al. 2018), often when agents are used in

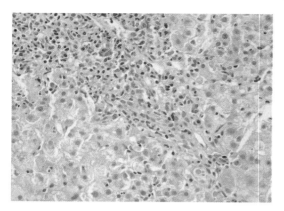

Fig. 3 Nitrofurantoin-induced liver injury. Portal inflammation with interface hepatitis and plasma cells (arrows) 400x. (Courtesy of David E. Kleiner, MD, PhD at the Laboratory of Pathology/ National Cancer Institute, USA)

combination (Bjornsson et al. 2013). The patterns of injury are widely variable. Immune checkpoint inhibitors, which are increasingly being used due to their impressive efficacy against a large and growing list of malignancies, are thought to cause injury through immune mechanisms and thus may cause an autoimmune-like form of liver injury (Postow et al. 2018), although histologic findings can vary widely (De Martin et al. 2018), as with all DILI. Typically, they can lead to elevated aminotransferases, with or without elevated alkaline phosphatase. Antineoplastics can also lead to chronic and progressive injury, not always apparent from routine biochemistries. For example, oxaliplatin, a drug used to treat colorectal cancer, may cause sinusoid injury and portal hypertension (Overman et al. 2018). Oxaliplatin injury can thus mimic clinical signs and symptoms of cirrhosis (varices, enlarges spleen, thrombocytopenia) in the absence of cirrhosis. Tamoxifen, a widely-used treatment for breast cancer, can cause or worsen fatty liver disease (Pan et al. 2016), can be superimposed upon non-alcohol-related steatohepatitis, and can even lead to cirrhosis. While vigilance for antineoplastic-related DILI is important, it is also important to not be overly cautious in limiting use of these drugs. Risk/benefit analysis is challenging, and further studies are needed.

Steroids

Steroids can cause liver injury, even acute liver failure in high doses (Sisti et al. 2015). Two steroids, cyproterone and danazol, have been reported as causing DILI in elderly, although it is not clear that the risk is actually higher among older patients (Hunt et al. 2014). However, steroids in general are the mainstay of treatment in a variety of conditions, including in the management of autoimmune hepatitis (Manns et al. 2010) or immune checkpoint inhibitor-related liver injury (Brahmer et al. 2018). Their use should always be carefully considered with a thorough discussion with the patient regarding the many risks. When possible, a liver biopsy should be considered before starting steroids to treat DILI.

Nonsteroidal Anti-inflammatory Drugs

NSAIDs may lead to liver injury. While the elderly are not always at higher risk of DILI from these medications, it has been reported that older patients, especially women, may be more susceptible (O'Connor et al. 2003). Diclofenac, a potent NSAID, may cause DILI more frequently in older adults (Banks et al. 1995), typically after chronic use rather than as a result of acute exposure (Medina-Caliz et al. 2016). Aspirin, widely used and often thought of as not hepatotoxic, occasionally causes elevated ALT levels and can (rarely) lead to hepatic failure with extremely high blood levels (O'Connor et al. 2003), but is not of higher risk for DILI specifically among older patients.

Alcohol and Drug Interactions

Alcohol consumption, especially heavy drinking (defined as consumption of over 2 drinks/day or 14 drinks/week for women or over 3 drinks/day or 21 drinks/week for men), is a risk factor for alcohol-related acute and chronic liver disease, including cirrhosis. Indeed, in the USA, the relative contribution of alcohol-related liver disease to cirrhosis-related death is anticipated to increase (Crabb et al. 2019). Heavy alcohol consumption increases the risk of acetaminophen hepatotoxicity (Schmidt et al. 2002).

Although acetaminophen is safe in usual therapeutic doses, hepatic and other organ damage occur with overdose. Acetaminophen overdose is responsible for nearly half of all cases of acute liver failure in the USA (Ramachandran and Jaeschke 2019). Older age has been shown to be an independent risk factor for developing hepatotoxicity from acetaminophen (Schmidt et al. 2002). In contrast to drugs that cause idiosyncratic DILI, liver damage from acetaminophen is dose-dependent. Overdose may be intentional, as in acute ingestion in suicide attempt. Or ingestion may be unintentional, as in consumption of excess dosage of a medication regimen, often through use of multiple acetaminophen-containing medications. Indeed, in early 2011, the US Food and Drug Administration asked manufacturers to limit the strength of acetaminophen to 325 mg in acetaminophen-containing medications, since acetaminophen is often a constituent of several drug combinations, especially opioids. In addition, the maximum daily dose of extra-strength acetaminophen (500 mg) is 3000 mg/day, also to reduce overuse, although most if not all physicians consider 4000 mg/day to be the maximum acetaminophen dose. Prognosis is better when acetaminophen liver injury is treated with *N*-acetylcysteine within hours of ingestion.

The role that alcohol consumption plays in the occurrence of idiosyncratic DILI is less clear than in acetaminophen toxicity but has been investigated. Alcohol use can increase the risk of DILI from isoniazid and halothane (two drugs also more likely to be hepatotoxic in older patients) (Dakhoul et al. 2018) as well as methotrexate (Malatjalian et al. 1996). In a recent study of heavy alcohol drinkers compared to non-alcohol drinkers, alcohol was not linked to worse outcomes when DILI was known or suspected. Interestingly, anabolic steroids were significantly linked to DILI among heavy drinkers, possibly because it was younger, male adults who were the heavy drinkers, although the causative role was not investigated (Dakhoul et al. 2018).

Cardiovascular Drugs

As a class, these agents have been implicated among the top causes of DILI in the elderly at a frequency higher than for younger adults (Chalasani et al. 2015). Many of these drugs have been reported to cause DILI, including common drugs such as amlodipine, atenolol, enalapril, labetalol, lisinopril, valsartan, and verapamil (Fontana et al. 2014). Amiodarone, a widely used antiarrhythmic drug, has long been known to pose a risk of DILI (Chalasani et al. 2008; Lewis et al. 1989). It causes elevated aminotransferases in a quarter of recipients, can cause injury long after drug withdrawal (Lewis et al. 1989), and has been linked to liver failure and cirrhosis (Bratton et al. 2019; Lewis et al. 1989). Cases of jaundice have been reported as well (Bratton et al. 2019). It also has a long latency (Chalasani et al. 2015), which means that a high index of suspicion for amiodarone-related toxicity is needed in the setting of elevated aminotransferases. A liver biopsy may show steatohepatitis, in a pattern similar to alcohol or non-alcoholic steatohepatitis (Fig. 4).

Hydralazine, an antihypertensive drug, is another cardiovascular drug that can cause a variety of liver injuries, including an autoimmune hepatitis-like pattern of serologic findings (de Boer et al. 2017), and can cause both cholestatic and hepatocellular patterns of injury.

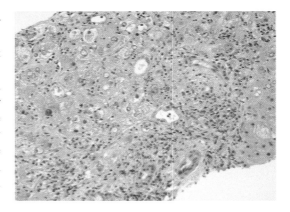

Fig. 4 Amiodarone-induced liver injury. Periportal ballooning with numerous Mallory-Denk bodies (arrows), 200x. (Courtesy of David E. Kleiner, MD, PhD at the Laboratory of Pathology/ National Cancer Institute, USA)

Statins

Among older adults in the USA, the most commonly prescribed medications include several statin medications (Qato et al. 2016). Medications in this class (atorvastatin, rosuvastatin, simvastatin, pravastatin, fluvastatin, and lovastatin) have been cited among the top 100 drugs responsible for DILI (Chalasani et al. 2015). Yet older adults do not appear to be at higher risk than other age groups for experiencing DILI from any of these statins. Because of the proven efficacy of these drugs, caution should be used in making a decision to discontinue a statin.

Other

It has been reported that older adults may be at increased risk from halothane use (Chalasani and Bjornsson 2010). This drug carries the risk of hepatotoxicity in the general population, and is often actively avoided for that reason.

Herbals and Dietary Supplements

This is a heterogeneous group of products that includes multivitamins, natural extracts, and other botanicals as well as weight loss and bodybuilding preparations. The use of herbals and dietary supplements is common worldwide. Hepatotoxicity may occur with their use (Bjornsson et al. 2013; Bunchorntavakul and Reddy 2013; Navarro et al. 2017), accounting for up to 20% of reported cases in the USA, with wide variations in rates reported in registries around the world (Navarro et al. 2017). Due to poor regulation and oversight of these products, there could be significant variations between the listed ingredients and contents of the supplement, including batch-to-batch differences. And given how available and common and potentially under-reported these products are, it is worthwhile to remain aware that supplements are not always safe and should not be considered so, despite the perception that they are harmless (Navarro et al. 2014). To this point, one study of emergency department visits identified that micronutrients, such as vitamins or multivitamins, calcium, iron, and potassium supplements accounted for two-thirds of ER visits among elderly patients (Geller et al.

2015). Common supplements taken among the elderly in the USA include vitamins, omega-3 fish oil, calcium, vitamin D, and saw palmetto (Qato et al. 2016). While none of these compounds in general has been linked to DILI in the elderly, it is important to maintain some degree of suspicion toward any compound when DILI is suspected.

Clinical Presentation and Diagnosis

DILI remains a diagnosis of exclusion. Identifying DILI involves taking a careful history and obtaining select lab and imaging studies and sometimes a liver biopsy. Patients with suspected DILI may present with a variety of clinical signs and symptoms, such as jaundice, fever, abdominal pain, nausea and vomiting, and also of liver failure (altered mental status/confusion), and a range of abnormal laboratory results. Obtaining a thorough history is essential (Table 3). It is particularly important to review the patient's medications with them. This involves confirming with them all the medications listed in their medical records and their own lists. If possible, patients should bring records of recent hospitalizations and have bottles with their own medications with them when a history is obtained. Do not rule out drugs they may not have taken for some time, as latencies can vary and may be as long as 12 months for certain medications (e.g., nitrofurantoin and statins). Include questions about any medications taken for a short time (e.g., analgesics and antibiotics) or that were stopped recently and why. It is also important to ask about herbal and dietary supplements. Even under the best of circumstances, lists and memories may be erroneous, and it can be valuable to enlist the assistance of a patient's family and friends – to help recall brief illnesses, treatments, and hospitalizations that may have involved drug exposure. Be sure to obtain information about comorbid illness that may cause liver injury. Physical exam may reveal signs of other causes of liver injury (Table 3).

It is helpful to review the pattern of abnormal hepatic biochemistry studies. The R value (Table 1) should be obtained if there is any question about

Table 3 Assessment for DILI in individuals presenting with acute or chronic liver injury

Obtain careful current and past medication history
Dose, duration, and timing of drug ingestion
Temporal relationship between exposure to known hepatotoxic agent and injury
Use of herbal medications, nutritional supplements, and over-the-counter medications
History of chronic liver diseases
Alternate causes of liver injury
Viral hepatitis (HAV, HBV, HCV, HEV, HSV, CMV, EBV)
Autoimmune hepatitis (separate from DILI)
Iron overload (hemochromatosis or transfusion-related)
Wilson disease
Primary biliary cholangitis
Wilson's disease
Gallstone-related diseases
Exclusion of other causes of abnormal biochemistries
Alcohol use
Ischemic liver injury, including congestive heart failure
Sepsis
Muscle disease/injury
Budd-Chiari syndrome
Hemolysis

whether the pattern of injury is hepatocellular (elevated ALT and/or AST) or cholestatic (elevated alkaline phosphatase) or a mix.

There are several caveats in assessing for DILI. It should be kept in mind that the R value can change with time, and also that, as mentioned above, older patients may present with a cholestatic pattern in the setting of DILI irrespective of the pattern expected by the inciting agent, based on the agent's listed side effect profile or published literature. Additionally, not all drugs fall neatly into one category or another, and it is often helpful to begin with a broad investigation into possible causes of liver injury rather than to focus on one pattern of injury alone.

When hepatocellular or mixed injury is suspected, assessment may be focused on ruling out other possible causes of such injury. This includes serology for viral hepatitis (HAV, HBV, HCV). If HEV PCR is available, it may be obtained. Other considerations include HSV, EBV, and CMV. (Ischemic hepatopathy and even

gallstone disease may present as hepatocellular or mixed injury as well, depending on the timing of injury). Serology for autoimmune hepatitis should be obtained (either to assess for possible autoimmune hepatitis or for a high titer of antinuclear antibody, which can be seen with nitrofurantoin and minocycline (Chalasani et al. 2015)). Assessment for Wilson's disease should be considered. Sometimes the markers do not reflect liver injury at all: skeletal muscle injury can cause elevated AST and even ALT. Consider creatine kinase and aldolase to assess for myositis.

To assess for cholestatic injury, imaging should be obtained to assess for biliary disease, including obstruction. Consider serology for primary biliary cholangitis.

The severity of DILI, generally for hepatocellular injury, should not be estimated by the degree of elevation of aminotransferases (which are not in general a good indicator of liver function, although there are exceptions, such as acute severe hepatitis with acetaminophen toxicity, Wilson's disease or HSV infection) but rather on whether there is evidence of impaired liver synthetic function associated with the injury. Biochemical clues to impaired synthetic function include acute changes such as elevated INR or total bilirubin and decline in albumin or platelets. Hy's law is a useful guideline, and postulates that those who develop bilirubin >2x ULN in the setting of AST or ALT >3x the upper limit of normal have an approximately 10–50% risk of DILI-related mortality or need for liver transplant (Temple 2006). This rule, in fact, is the basis for the model used by the US Federal Drug Administration in drug development, to determine whether a compound proceeds through the drug approval process (Senior 2014), highlighting its importance in considering DILI.

A liver biopsy is useful in certain circumstances but is by no means a required element in the evaluation of any possible DILI. Histologic findings of DILI, as mentioned, are diverse and not pathognomonic. However, a biopsy may be needed for one of several reasons. First, it can help diagnostically to identify a pattern of injury when one or more possible causes of liver injury are being considered, usually to rule out a cause.

Second, it can help to establish the severity of injury. This information is often needed, particularly to serve as a baseline if serial biopsies are being considered, or when the patient already has a known chronic liver disease, or if re-challenge with the suspected or known cause of DILI is being considered.

Management

When DILI is suspected, the first step is to discontinue the causative drug(s). Most cases improve upon withdrawal of the suspected medication(s) with no long-term sequelae (Hayashi et al. 2017). Normalization of liver function may take days to months, and some develop chronic DILI, with an incidence of 5–10% (Hayashi and Bjornsson 2018). Regular monitoring of labs and, when relevant, signs or symptoms of possible persistence or progression of DILI is advised (Bessone et al. 2019; Reuben et al. 2010; Andrade et al. 2019; European Association for the Study of the Liver 2016; Martin et al. 2014)

Sometimes steroids are needed, especially when there may be an autoimmune-like reaction (Stine and Chalasani 2015), including for immune checkpoint inhibitors which are increasingly being used for a variety of cancers (Brahmer et al. 2018). Steroid use should be limited to situations in which they are specifically indicated, and not as part of the general management of DILI.

N-acetylcysteine is a well-known treatment of acetaminophen-related DILI (Ramachandran and Jaeschke 2019). Its use for other causes of liver failure in DILI is controversial, largely due to lack of clear evidence of efficacy. There is some evidence that it can improve survival if administered to adults with acute liver failure not due to acetaminophen (Lee et al. 2009). USA and European guidelines recommend its use in ALF due to idiosyncratic DILI early on (e.g., coma grade I–II) (Chalasani et al. 2014; Andrade et al. 2019). With its low side-effect profile and lack of other definitive and safe treatments of DILI, its administration is encouraged when available.

Prior history of DILI increases the risk of injury on re-exposure to the same or structurally similar agents. Re-challenge is not advisable, since recurrent injury may be more severe than the initial insult, especially with immunologic injury. Ideally, re-challenge should be avoided. It is essential to closely monitor hepatic function in those with a prior history of DILI if re-exposure is necessary.

The presence of jaundice, coagulopathy, new-onset fluid retention, and encephalopathy or coma is evidence of DILI-related acute liver failure (Reuben et al. 2010). DILI can be associated with significant mortality, and is one of the most common causes of liver failure leading to death or liver transplant (Bessone et al. 2019). Compared to other causes of acute liver failure, it leads to a lower transplant-free survival (Andrade et al. 2019). When there are features concerning for liver failure, it is important to consider whether liver transplant is an option, based on patient factors and access to a transplant center. It is important to recognize that older age is not a contraindication to liver transplantation based on the most recent USA (Martin et al. 2014) and European guidelines (European Association for the Study of the Liver 2016), with liver transplants having been successfully performed in older adults. However, for this population, assessment of comorbidities is essential due to the risk of posttransplant cardiovascular complications.

Next Steps: Future Goals

The prediction and monitoring of the course of DILI remains a challenge. Novel biomarkers are needed and have been the subject of recent work (Barnhill et al. 2018; Church et al. 2018). There is also a computer-based modeling system, DILIsym, used to characterize the effects of drugs on a selected patient population by mathematically simulating its mechanism of injury (Church and Watkins 2018). Another model incorporates lab values and comorbidities to estimate 6-month mortality in DILI. The study that led to this model was also novel in providing insight into the context in which DILI occurs:

higher burden of comorbid illness (particularly for older males) was an independent risk factor for 6-month mortality in DILI (Ghabril et al. 2019). This observation merits additional investigation into the role comorbid diseases play in DILI, especially in older patients.

Finally, better data for elderly patients and inclusion in clinical trials are needed (Mitchell and Hilmer 2010). Older adults are often underrepresented in clinical trials (Stine et al. 2013; van Riet-Nales et al. 2016). There is an initiative by the NIH in the USA that trials include patients across the life span, with the goal of requiring expanded age criteria in new grants (https://grants.nih.gov/grants/guide/notice-files/NOT-OD-18-116.html). It is also essential for registries, worldwide, to include cases of DILI among older patients (Haugen et al. 2019).

Key Points

- Older adults are not, in general, at higher risk of drug-induced liver injury compared to other age groups.
- A few medications, including antibiotics (amoxicillin-clavulanate, erythromycin, flucloxacillin, isoniazid) and diclofenac, may be more likely to cause DILI in older adults.
- DILI may present more commonly with a cholestatic biochemical pattern in the elderly age group compared to younger adults or children.
- Although statins can cause DILI, they are not riskier to use as age increases.
- Cessation of the offending agent and clinical monitoring are needed when DILI is suspected.

References

Ahmad J, Odin JA. Epidemiology and genetic risk factors of drug hepatotoxicity. Clin Liver Dis. 2017;21:55–72. https://doi.org/10.1016/j.cld.2016.08.004.

Andrade RJ, et al. Drug-induced liver injury: an analysis of 461 incidences submitted to the Spanish registry over a 10-year period. Gastroenterology. 2005;129:512–21. https://doi.org/10.1016/j.gastro.2005.05.006.

Andrade RJ, et al. EASL clinical practice guidelines: drug-induced liver injury. J Hepatol. 2019;70:1222–61. https://doi.org/10.1016/j.jhep.2019.02.014.

Banks AT, Zimmerman HJ, Ishak KG, Harter JG. Diclofenac-associated hepatotoxicity: analysis of 180 cases reported to the Food and Drug Administration as adverse reactions. Hepatology. 1995;22:820–7.

Barnhill MS, Real M, Lewis JH. Latest advances in diagnosing and predicting DILI: what was new in 2017? Expert Rev Gastroenterol Hepatol. 2018;12:1–11. https://doi.org/10.1080/17474124.2018.1512854.

Barry PJ, Gallagher P, Ryan C, O'Mahony D. START (screening tool to alert doctors to the right treatment) – an evidence-based screening tool to detect prescribing omissions in elderly patients. Age Ageing. 2007;36:632–8. https://doi.org/10.1093/ageing/afm118.

Begriche K, Massart J, Robin MA, Borgne-Sanchez A, Fromenty B. Drug-induced toxicity on mitochondria and lipid metabolism: mechanistic diversity and deleterious consequences for the liver. J Hepatol. 2011;54:773–94. https://doi.org/10.1016/j.jhep.2010.11.006.

Bell LN, Chalasani N. Epidemiology of idiosyncratic drug-induced liver injury. Semin Liver Dis. 2009;29:337–47. https://doi.org/10.1055/s-0029-1240002.

Bessone F, Robles-Diaz M, Hernandez N, Medina-Caliz I, Lucena MI, Andrade RJ. Assessment of serious acute and chronic idiosyncratic drug-induced liver injury in clinical practice. Semin Liver Dis. 2019. https://doi.org/10.1055/s-0039-1685519.

Bjornsson ES, Bergmann OM, Bjornsson HK, Kvaran RB, Olafsson S. Incidence, presentation, and outcomes in patients with drug-induced liver injury in the general population of Iceland. Gastroenterology. 2013;144:1419–25, 1425.e1411–3; quiz e1419–20. https://doi.org/10.1053/j.gastro.2013.02.006.

Brahmer JR, et al. Management of immune-related adverse events in patients treated with immune checkpoint inhibitor therapy: American Society of Clinical Oncology Clinical Practice Guideline. J Clin Oncol. 2018;36:1714–68. https://doi.org/10.1200/jco.2017.77.6385.

Bratton H, Alomari M, Al Momani LA, Aasen T, Young M. Prolonged jaundice secondary to amiodarone use: a case report and literature review. Cureus. 2019;11:e3850. https://doi.org/10.7759/cureus.3850.

Bunchorntavakul C, Reddy KR. Review article: herbal and dietary supplement hepatotoxicity. Aliment Pharmacol Ther. 2013;37:3–17. https://doi.org/10.1111/apt.12109.

Chalasani N, Bjornsson E. Risk factors for idiosyncratic drug-induced liver injury. Gastroenterology. 2010;138:2246–59. https://doi.org/10.1053/j.gastro.2010.04.001.

Chalasani N, et al. Causes, clinical features, and outcomes from a prospective study of drug-induced liver injury in the United States. Gastroenterology. 2008;135:1924–34., 1934.e1921-1924. https://doi.org/10.1053/j.gastro.2008.09.011.

Chalasani NP, Hayashi PH, Bonkovsky HL, Navarro VJ, Lee WM, Fontana RJ. ACG clinical guideline: the diagnosis and management of idiosyncratic drug-induced liver injury. Am J Gastroenterol. 2014;109:950–66. https://doi.org/10.1038/ajg.2014.131.

Chalasani N, et al. Features and outcomes of 899 patients with drug-induced liver injury: the DILIN prospective study. Gastroenterology. 2015;148:1340–1352.e1347. https://doi.org/10.1053/j.gastro.2015.03.006.

Chen M, Borlak J, Tong W. High lipophilicity and high daily dose of oral medications are associated with significant risk for drug-induced liver injury. Hepatology. 2013;58:388–96. https://doi.org/10.1002/hep.26208.

Chen M, Suzuki A, Borlak J, Andrade RJ, Lucena MI. Drug-induced liver injury: interactions between drug properties and host factors. J Hepatol. 2015;63:503–14. https://doi.org/10.1016/j.jhep.2015.04.016.

Church RJ, Watkins PB. In silico modeling to optimize interpretation of liver safety biomarkers in clinical trials. Exp Biol Med. 2018;243:300–7. https://doi.org/10.1177/1535370217740853.

Church RJ, et al. Candidate biomarkers for the diagnosis and prognosis of drug-induced liver injury: an international collaborative effort. Hepatology. 2018. https://doi.org/10.1002/hep.29802.

Corsini A, Bortolini M. Drug-induced liver injury: the role of drug metabolism and transport. J Clin Pharmacol. 2013;53:463–74. https://doi.org/10.1002/jcph.23.

Cotreau MM, von Moltke LL, Greenblatt DJ. The influence of age and sex on the clearance of cytochrome P450 3A substrates. Clin Pharmacokinet. 2005;44:33–60. https://doi.org/10.2165/00003088-200544010-00002.

Crabb DW, Im GY, Szabo G, Mellinger JL, Lucey MR. Diagnosis and treatment of alcohol-related liver diseases: 2019 Practice Guidance from the American Association for the Study of Liver Diseases. Hepatology. 2019. https://doi.org/10.1002/hep.30866.

Dakhoul L, Ghabril M, Gu J, Navarro V, Chalasani N, Serrano J. Heavy consumption of alcohol is not associated with worse outcomes in patients with idiosyncratic drug-induced liver injury compared to non-drinkers. Clin Gastroenterol Hepatol. 2018;16:722–729.e722. https://doi.org/10.1016/j.cgh.2017.12.036.

Daly AK, Day CP. Genetic association studies in drug-induced liver injury. Semin Liver Dis. 2009;29:400–11. https://doi.org/10.1055/s-0029-1240009.

Daly AK, et al. HLA-B∗5701 genotype is a major determinant of drug-induced liver injury due to flucloxacillin. Nat Genet. 2009;41:816–9. https://doi.org/10.1038/ng.379.

Danan G, Benichou C. Causality assessment of adverse reactions to drugs – I. A novel method based on the conclusions of international consensus meetings: application to drug-induced liver injuries. J Clin Epidemiol. 1993;46:1323–30.

de Boer YS, et al. Features of autoimmune hepatitis in patients with drug-induced liver injury. Clin Gastroenterol Hepatol. 2017;15:103. https://doi.org/10.1016/j.cgh.2016.05.043.

de Lemos AS, et al. Amoxicillin-clavulanate-induced liver injury. Dig Dis Sci. 2016;61:2406–16. https://doi.org/10.1007/s10620-016-4121-6.

De Martin E, et al. Characterization of liver injury induced by cancer immunotherapy using immune checkpoint inhibitors. J Hepatol. 2018;68:1181–90. https://doi.org/10.1016/j.jhep.2018.01.033.

European Association for the Study of the Liver. EASL clinical practice guidelines: liver transplantation. J Hepatol. 2016;64:433–85. https://doi.org/10.1016/j.jhep.2015.10.006.

Fontana RJ. Pathogenesis of idiosyncratic drug-induced liver injury and clinical perspectives. Gastroenterology. 2014;146:914–28. https://doi.org/10.1053/j.gastro.2013.12.032.

Fontana RJ, et al. Idiosyncratic drug-induced liver injury is associated with substantial morbidity and mortality within 6 months from onset. Gastroenterology. 2014;147:96–108.e104. https://doi.org/10.1053/j.gastro.2014.03.045.

Fredriksson L, et al. Diclofenac inhibits tumor necrosis factor-alpha-induced nuclear factor-κB activation causing synergistic hepatocyte apoptosis. Hepatology. 2011;53:2027–41. https://doi.org/10.1002/hep.24314.

Geller AI, et al. Emergency department visits for adverse events related to dietary supplements. N Engl J Med. 2015;373:1531–40. https://doi.org/10.1056/NEJMsa1504267.

Ghabril M, et al. Development and validation of model consisting of comorbidity burden to calculate risk of death within 6 months for patients with suspected drug-induced liver injury. Gastroenterology. 2019. https://doi.org/10.1053/j.gastro.2019.07.006.

Haugen CE, et al. Assessment of trends in transplantation of liver grafts from older donors and outcomes in recipients of liver grafts from older donors, 2003–2016. JAMA Surg. 2019. https://doi.org/10.1001/jamasurg.2018.5568.

Hautekeete ML, et al. HLA association of amoxicillin-clavulanate–induced hepatitis. Gastroenterology. 1999;117:1181–6.

Hayashi PH, Bjornsson ES. Long-term outcomes after drug-induced liver injury. Curr Hepatol Rep. 2018;17:292–9. https://doi.org/10.1007/s11901-018-0411-0.

Hayashi PH, et al. Death and liver transplantation within 2 years of onset of drug-induced liver injury. Hepatology. 2017;66:1275–85. https://doi.org/10.1002/hep.29283.

Ho RH, Kim RB. Transporters and drug therapy: implications for drug disposition and disease. Clin Pharmacol Ther. 2005;78:260–77. https://doi.org/10.1016/j.clpt.2005.05.011.

Hoofnagle JH, Serrano J, Knoben JE, Navarro VJ. LiverTox: a website on drug-induced liver injury. Hepatology. 2013;57:873–4. https://doi.org/10.1002/hep.26175.

Hunt CM, Yuen NA, Stirnadel-Farrant HA, Suzuki A. Age-related differences in reporting of drug-associated liver injury: data-mining of WHO safety report database. Regul Toxicol Pharmacol. 2014;70:519–26. https://doi.org/10.1016/j.yrtph.2014.09.007.

Kleiner DE, et al. Hepatic histological findings in suspected drug-induced liver injury: systematic evaluation and clinical associations. Hepatology. 2014;59:661–70. https://doi.org/10.1002/hep.26709.

Lammert C, Einarsson S, Saha C, Niklasson A, Bjornsson E, Chalasani N. Relationship between daily dose of oral medications and idiosyncratic drug-induced liver injury: search for signals. Hepatology. 2008;47:2003–9. https://doi.org/10.1002/hep.22272.

Lammert C, Bjornsson E, Niklasson A, Chalasani N. Oral medications with significant hepatic metabolism at higher risk for hepatic adverse events. Hepatology. 2010;51:615–20. https://doi.org/10.1002/hep.23317.

Lang C, et al. Mutations and polymorphisms in the bile salt export pump and the multidrug resistance protein 3 associated with drug-induced liver injury. Pharmacogenet Genomics. 2007;17:47–60. https://doi.org/10.1097/01.fpc.0000230418.28091.76.

Lee WM, et al. Intravenous *N*-acetylcysteine improves transplant-free survival in early stage non-acetaminophen acute liver failure. Gastroenterology. 2009;137:856–64, 864.e851. https://doi.org/10.1053/j.gastro.2009.06.006.

Leise MD, Poterucha JJ, Talwalkar JA. Drug-induced liver injury. Mayo Clin Proc. 2014;89:95–106. https://doi.org/10.1016/j.mayocp.2013.09.016.

Lewis JH, et al. Amiodarone hepatotoxicity: prevalence and clinicopathologic correlations among 104 patients. Hepatology. 1989;9:679–85.

Lucena MI, et al. Phenotypic characterization of idiosyncratic drug-induced liver injury: the influence of age and sex. Hepatology. 2009;49:2001–9. https://doi.org/10.1002/hep.22895.

Lucena MI, et al. Susceptibility to amoxicillin-clavulanate-induced liver injury is influenced by multiple HLA class I and II alleles. Gastroenterology. 2011;141:338–47. https://doi.org/10.1053/j.gastro.2011.04.001.

Malatjalian DA, Ross JB, Williams CN, Colwell SJ, Eastwood BJ. Methotrexate hepatotoxicity in psoriatics: report of 104 patients from Nova Scotia, with analysis of risks from obesity, diabetes and alcohol consumption during long term follow-up. Can J Gastroenterol. 1996;10:369–75. https://doi.org/10.1155/1996/213596.

Manns MP, Czaja AJ, Gorham JD, Krawitt EL, Mieli-Vergani G, Vergani D, Vierling JM. Diagnosis and management of autoimmune hepatitis. Hepatology. 2010;51:2193–213. https://doi.org/10.1002/hep.23584.

Martin P, DiMartini A, Feng S, Brown R Jr, Fallon M. Evaluation for liver transplantation in adults: 2013 practice guideline by the American Association for the Study of Liver Diseases and the American Society of Transplantation. Hepatology. 2014;59:1144–65.

Medina-Caliz I, et al. Definition and risk factors for chronicity following acute idiosyncratic drug-induced liver injury. J Hepatol. 2016;65:532–42. https://doi.org/10.1016/j.jhep.2016.05.003.

Mitchell SJ, Hilmer SN. Drug-induced liver injury in older adults. Ther Adv Drug Saf. 2010;1:65–77. https://doi.org/10.1177/2042098610386281.

Navarro VJ, et al. Liver injury from herbals and dietary supplements in the U.S. Drug-Induced Liver Injury Network. Hepatology. 2014;60:1399–408. https://doi.org/10.1002/hep.27317.

Navarro VJ, Khan I, Bjornsson E, Seeff LB, Serrano J, Hoofnagle JH. Liver injury from herbal and dietary supplements. Hepatology. 2017;65:363–73. https://doi.org/10.1002/hep.28813.

Nicoletti P, et al. Association of liver injury from specific drugs, or groups of drugs, with polymorphisms in HLA and other genes in a genome-Wide Association Study. Gastroenterology. 2017;152:1078–89. https://doi.org/10.1053/j.gastro.2016.12.016.

Noe J, et al. Impaired expression and function of the bile salt export pump due to three novel ABCB11 mutations in intrahepatic cholestasis. J Hepatol. 2005;43:536–43. https://doi.org/10.1016/j.jhep.2005.05.020.

O'Connor N, Dargan PI, Jones AL. Hepatocellular damage from non-steroidal anti-inflammatory drugs QJM: monthly. J Assoc Physicians. 2003;96:787–91.

Onji M, Fujioka S, Takeuchi Y, Takaki T, Osawa T, Yamamoto K, Itoshima T. Clinical characteristics of drug-induced liver injury in the elderly. Hepatol Res. 2009;39:546–52. https://doi.org/10.1111/j.1872-034X.2009.00492.x.

Overman MJ, et al. The addition of bevacizumab to oxaliplatin-based chemotherapy: impact upon hepatic sinusoidal injury and thrombocytopenia. J Natl Cancer Inst. 2018;110:888–94. https://doi.org/10.1093/jnci/djx288.

Pan HJ, Chang HT, Lee CH. Association between tamoxifen treatment and the development of different stages of nonalcoholic fatty liver disease among breast cancer patients. J Formos Med Assoc. 2016;115:411–7. https://doi.org/10.1016/j.jfma.2015.05.006.

Pauli-Magnus C, Meier PJ. Hepatobiliary transporters and drug-induced cholestasis. Hepatology. 2006;44:778–87. https://doi.org/10.1002/hep.21359.

Postow MA, Sidlow R, Hellmann MD. Immune-related adverse events associated with immune checkpoint blockade. N Engl J Med. 2018;378:158–68. https://doi.org/10.1056/NEJMra1703481.

Qato DM, Wilder J, Schumm LP, Gillet V, Alexander GC. Changes in prescription and over-the-counter medication and dietary supplement use among older adults in the United States, 2005 vs 2011. JAMA Intern Med. 2016;176:473–82. https://doi.org/10.1001/jamainternmed.2015.8581.

Ramachandran A, Jaeschke H. Acetaminophen hepatotoxicity. Semin Liver Dis. 2019;39:221–34. https://doi.org/10.1055/s-0039-1679919.

Reuben A, Koch DG, Lee WM, Acute Liver Failure Study Group. Drug-induced acute liver failure: results of a U.S. multicenter, prospective study. Hepatology. 2010;52:2065–76. https://doi.org/10.1002/hep.23937.

Schmidt LE, Dalhoff K, Poulsen HE. Acute versus chronic alcohol consumption in acetaminophen-induced hepatotoxicity. Hepatology. 2002;35:876–82. https://doi.org/10.1053/jhep.2002.32148.

Senior JR. Evolution of the Food and Drug Administration approach to liver safety assessment for new drugs: current status and challenges. Drug Saf. 2014;37(Suppl 1): S9–17. https://doi.org/10.1007/s40264-014-0182-7.

Sgro C, et al. Incidence of drug-induced hepatic injuries: a French population-based study. Hepatology. 2002;36:451–5. https://doi.org/10.1053/jhep.2002. 34857.

Sisti E, et al. Age and dose are major risk factors for liver damage associated with intravenous glucocorticoid pulse therapy for graves' orbitopathy. Thyroid. 2015;25:846–50. https://doi.org/10.1089/thy.2015.0061.

Sonawane KB, Cheng N, Hansen RA. Serious adverse drug events reported to the FDA: analysis of the FDA adverse event reporting system 2006–2014 database. J Manag Care Spec Pharm. 2018;24:682–90. https://doi.org/10.18553/jmcp.2018.24.7.682.

Stine JG, Chalasani N. Chronic liver injury induced by drugs: a systematic review. Liver Int. 2015;35:2343–53. https://doi.org/10.1111/liv.12958.

Stine JG, Sateesh P, Lewis JH. Drug-induced liver injury in the elderly. Curr Gastroenterol Rep. 2013;15:299. https://doi.org/10.1007/s11894-012-0299-8.

Stricker BH, Blok AP, Claas FH, Van Parys GE, Desmet VJ. Hepatic injury associated with the use of nitrofurans: a clinicopathological study of 52 reported cases. Hepatology. 1988;8:599–606.

Suk KT, et al. A prospective nationwide study of drug-induced liver injury in Korea. Am J Gastroenterol. 2012;107:1380–7. https://doi.org/10.1038/ajg.2012.138.

Tan JL, Eastment JG, Poudel A, Hubbard RE. Age-related changes in hepatic function: an update on implications for drug therapy. Drugs Aging. 2015;32:999–1008. https://doi.org/10.1007/s40266-015-0318-1.

Temple R. Hy's law: predicting serious hepatotoxicity. Pharmacoepidemiol Drug Saf. 2006;15:241–3. https://doi.org/10.1002/pds.1211.

Tujios S, Fontana RJ. Mechanisms of drug-induced liver injury: from bedside to bench. Nat Rev Gastroenterol Hepatol. 2011;8:202–11. https://doi.org/10.1038/nrgastro.2011.22.

van Riet-Nales DA, Hussain N, Sundberg KA, Eggenschwyler D, Ferris C, Robert JL, Cerreta F. Regulatory incentives to ensure better medicines for older people: From ICH E7 to the EMA reflection paper on quality aspects. Int J Pharm. 2016;512:343–51. https://doi.org/10.1016/j.ijpharm.2016.05.001.

Vincenzi B, et al. The use of SAMe in chemotherapy-induced liver injury. Crit Rev Oncol Hematol. 2018;130:70–7. https://doi.org/10.1016/j.critrevonc.2018.06.019.

Vuppalanchi R, et al. Relationship between characteristics of medications and drug-induced liver disease phenotype and outcome. Clin Gastroenterol Hepatol. 2014;12:1550–5. https://doi.org/10.1016/j.cgh.2013.12.016.

Walgren JL, Mitchell MD, Thompson DC. Role of metabolism in drug-induced idiosyncratic hepatotoxicity. Crit Rev Toxicol. 2005;35:325–61.

Wilke RA, et al. Identifying genetic risk factors for serious adverse drug reactions: current progress and challenges. Nat Rev Drug Discov. 2007;6:904–16. https://doi.org/10.1038/nrd2423.

Wing K, et al. Quantification of the risk of liver injury associated with flucloxacillin: a UK population-based cohort study. J Antimicrob Chemother. 2017;72:2636–46. https://doi.org/10.1093/jac/dkx183.

Gallstones and Benign Gallbladder Disease

62

C. S. Pitchumoni and Nishal Ravindran

Contents

C. S. Pitchumoni (✉)
Department of Medicine, Robert Wood Johnson School of
Medicine, Rutgers University, New Brunswick, NJ, USA

Department of Medicine, New York Medical College,
Valhalla, NY, USA

Division of Gastroenterology, Hepatology and Clinical
Nutrition, Saint Peters University Hospital, New
Brunswick, NJ, USA
e-mail: pitchumoni@hotmail.com

N. Ravindran
Robert Wood Johnson School of Medicine, Rutgers
University, New Brunswick, NY, USA

Saint Peters University Hospital, New Brunswick, NY,
USA

© Springer Nature Switzerland AG 2021
C. S. Pitchumoni, T. S. Dharmarajan (eds.), *Geriatric Gastroenterology*,
https://doi.org/10.1007/978-3-030-30192-7_54

Abstract

The prevalence of gallstones progressively increases as age advances. Although asymptomatic in most, the clinical manifestations depend on the location of the stone in the biliary system. Gallstones, when in the gallbladder, may be painless or cause a postprandial biliary type of pain in the right upper quadrant related to a meal. When a stone migrates to the cystic duct and causes obstruction, it results in acute cholecystitis. Between 5% and 30% of cholelithiasis patients have concurrent choledocholithiasis. Gallstones obstructing the common bile duct (CBD) cause ascending cholangitis and acute biliary pancreatitis when the stone blocks the ampulla of Vater. Other complications include cholecystoduodenal or choledocho-duodenal fistula and gallstone ileus. Older adults are more likely to present with complications such as acute cholecystitis, gallstone pancreatitis, and common bile-duct stones than the young.

Tokyo guidelines are useful. There is an increase in the number of emergency and elective surgical cases involving older patients. Elective instead of emergency and a laparoscopic approach is the preferred method of surgery. In the management of CBD stones, endoscopic retrograde cholangiography, and stone extraction and stent placement are safe and effective in advanced age groups.

Keywords

Cholelithiasis · Gallstone disease · Gallbladder disease · Cholesterol stones · Pigment stones · Acute cholecystitis · Chronic cholecystitis · Common bile duct stones · Ascending cholangitis · Mirizzi's syndrome · Bouveret's syndrome · Gallstone ileus · Biliary fistulas · Magnetic resonance cholangiopancreatography · Endoscopic retrograde chloangiopancreatography · Stent placements · Laparoscopic cholecystectomy · Post cholecystectomy pain · Biliary drainage · Biliary fistula · Functional gallbladder disorder

Introduction

Among the biliary diseases, gallstones and gallbladder cancer increase with age, with gallstones affecting 33% of older adults (McSherry et al. 1985; Sugiyama and Atomi 1997). Other biliary disorders are polyps, biliary dyskinesia, and biliary cancers.

Gallstones (GS) have been found in Chinese and Egyptian mummies from more than 3500 years ago. The modern history of GS perhaps began in the eighteenth century with Morgagni, who made a number of observations based on autopsy studies, the findings being still relevant today (Moore 1937). He noted that the prevalence of gallstone disease increased with age and hypothesized that obesity could be a risk factor and that gallstones can remain asymptomatic for a lifetime.

GS form in the biliary system and may be cholesterol, the more common type, or pigment stones, the less common form. Along with diverticulitis, cholecystitis is also a principal gastrointestinal diagnosis for inpatients in the United States. The frequency of hospital admissions and surgery for cholelithiasis is steadily increasing in Western countries since the 1950s and more rapidly since the advent of minimally invasive laparoscopic cholecystectomy (Lam et al. 1996; Shaffer 2005).

About 20–25 million Americans have gallstones, predominantly of cholesterol, (see Fig. 1) with more than 700,000 cholecystectomies done annually in the United States (Shaffer 2006).

Symptomatic gall stone disease has a low mortality rate of 0.6%, which has fallen dramatically since 1979 but can be still significant in older people (Everhart and Ruhl 2009a). With the advent of laparoscopic cholecystectomy, there has been an increase in surgery in the United States by 28% (Nenner et al. 1994). The cost of biliary tract disease in the United States in 2015 was $10.3 billion (Peery et al. 2019). Epidemiological data suggests higher risk of cardiovascular disease and mortality associated with gallstones (Zheng et al. 2018; Upala et al. 2017). The Society of American Gastrointestinal and Endoscopic Surgeons (SAGES) recommended cholecystectomy in most symptomatic patients. Despite this recommendation, older adults are often excluded from cholecystectomy. The low rate of surgery reflects concerns and uncertainty about the risk and benefits of cholecystectomy in the elderly (Overby et al. 2010).

Recent demographic changes of increasing older population, coupled with the fact that the prevalence of gallstones progressively increases with age, predict a dramatic increase in the incidence of all types of gallstone disease – asymptomatic, symptomatic, and complicated.

Epidemiology

Risk factors for cholesterol gallstones include non-modifiable factors like ethnicity, family history, female sex, increasing age, and modifiable

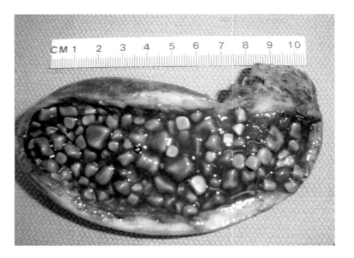

Fig. 1 Gallbladder specimen with cholesterol gallstones

Table 1 Risk factors for cholesterol stones

Modifiable	Comment
High-calorie diet/ high-carbohydrate diet	High-carb diets noted to increase risk (Tsai et al. 2005)
Low-fiber diet ("Western diet")	Cholesterol stones now are majority of stones in East Asia (Shaffer 2005)
Sedentary lifestyle	Exercise reduces lithogenic risk (Banim et al. 2010)
Obesity/metabolic syndrome (MS)	BMI more than 45 increases risk sevenfold (Stampfer et al. 1992)
Diabetes mellitus/insulin resistance	T2DM (Nervi et al. 2006), insulin resistance (Chapman et al. 1996), increased risk
Low HDL, high TG	Increased risk (Petitti et al. 1981; Ahlberg 1979)
NAFLD	Insulin resistance and MS (Loria et al. 2005)
Rapid weight loss /weight cycling	Weight loss > 1.5 kg/week increased risk (Erlinger 2000)
Bariatric surgery/gastrectomy	Most likely in first 6 weeks (Melmer et al. 2015; Liang et al. 2017)
Pregnancy and parity	Increased sludge, gallstones in 5% (Maringhini et al. 1993)
Total parenteral nutrition	Sludge formation after 4 weeks (Roslyn et al. 1983)
Drugs	Ceftriaxone, octreotide, thiazides, estrogen, progesterone (Stinton and Shaffer 2012)
Crohn's disease	Two- to threefold increase (Whorwell et al. 1984)
Spinal cord injury	Threefold increase (Apstein and Dalecki-Chipperfield 1987)
Solid organ transplant	Increased in the first 2 years (Spes et al. 1990) (Except liver transplant as cholecystectomy done)
Liver cirrhosis	Mostly pigment but also cholesterol stones
	Higher in child B C (Conte et al. 1999)
Chronic hepatitis C	More in hepatitis C (Acalovschi et al. 2009)
Non-modifiable	
Increasing age	4–10 times more after 40 (Everhart and Ruhl 2009b)
	In 80 year old risk 40–50%
Female sex	2:1
	Difference in risk disappears in elderly (Everhart et al. 1999)
Family history	Higher in twins
	5 times higher in families (Sarin et al. 1995)
	Lith genes
Ethnicity	Lith genes include ABC cholesterol transporter (Krawczyk et al. 2013)
	Highest in Pima Indians, south and Central America parts of North India
	Lowest in Sub-Saharan Africa (Shaffer 2005)

Adapted from "The Growing Global Burden of Gallstone disease" **Acalovschi and Lammert**

factors like diet, drugs, rapid weight loss, low physical activity, total parenteral nutrition, and spinal cord injury (Shaffer 2006). Solid organ transplantation, except liver transplant (as gallbladder is removed) is associated with increased risk of gallstones in the first 2 years (Kao et al. 2003). In 1999, Everhart JE et al. published a landmark paper which was the first large US population-based estimate of the prevalence of gallstones and gallbladder disease. It included 14,000 participants who underwent screening ultrasonography, as part of the Third National Health and Nutrition Examination Survey (NHANES III) (Everhart et al. 1999). Risk factors for gallstones, cholesterol, and pigment stones are tabulated in Tables 1 and 2.

Age and Gender

Prevalence of gallstones increases with age. The risk of gallstones after 40 years rises by

Table 2 Risk factors for pigment stones

Modifiable	Comment
Chronic hemolysis – sickle cell disease Thalassemia	Black pigment stones (Haley 2017)
	Consider prophylactic cholecystectomy
Crohn's disease	Both cholesterol and black stones (Brink et al. 1999)
Extensive ileal resection	Black pigment stones (Pitt et al. 1984)
Cystic fibrosis	Mostly black pigment stones (Angelico et al. 1991)
Liver cirrhosis	Mostly black pigment stones (Alvaro et al. 1990)
Biliary infection	Brown stones (Maki 1966)
	Form in bile ducts
	More common in East Asia
	Infestation with Clonorchis *Opisthorchis*
Non-modifiable	
Increasing age	Increase in black pigment stones in the elderly (Everhart and Ruhl 2009b)
Asian ethnicity	Brown pigment stones (Shoda et al. 2003)

Adapted from "The Growing Global Burden of Gallstone disease" **Acalovschi and Lammert**

4–10 times (Stinton and Shaffer 2012). The prevalence of gallstones in women at age 70 was 24% in the MICOL study and about 40% in the 80-year-old and near 50% in the above 90 group in a study from Dundee (Festi et al. 2008; Bateson 2000). Women are twice as likely as men to form gallstones, related to the effect of female sex hormones on cholesterol. Multiparous women have increased likelihood for gallstones. The female and male prevalence rates are nearly similar in the older age groups.

Ethnicity

There is a wide variation in occurrence of gallstones in relation to ethnicity. Gallstone disease affects at least 10–15% of the Caucasian population but is a disease of epidemic proportions in Native Americans with a prevalence of 60–70% in Pima Indians of North America (Comess et al. 1967; Sampliner et al. 1970). Gallstones affect over 35–50% of the Hispanic population in Central and South America. A higher incidence is seen among Northern Europeans, 4–25% compared to Southern Europeans, 6–14% (Barbara et al. 1987; Aerts and Penninckx 2003). In Northern India, the rate is 6–21% (Singh et al. 2001). Frequency is lower in African Americans, East

Asia, and Sub-Saharan Africa, 5–13% (Everhart et al. 1999; Nomura et al. 1988). The propensity of North American Indians to develop obesity and diabetes, the two risk factors associated with cholelithiasis is a growing trend in most population groups. Familial incidence of gallstones is seen in nearly 1/3 of all patients (Hemminki et al. 2017).

Obesity

Obesity is a risk factor for the formation of cholesterol gallstones (Amaral and Thompson 1985; Maclure et al. 1989). Stampfer et al. evaluated the effect of obesity in 90,000 women in the Nurses Health Study which showed a sevenfold rise in gallstones in those with a BMI more than 45 (Stampfer et al. 1992). Metabolic syndrome and diabetes mellitus are risk factors for gall stone formation. Complex metabolic pathways are thought to link gallstones to metabolic syndrome. Insulin resistance leads to altered cholesterol and bile salt metabolism (Ruhl and Everhart 2000). There are also more stone-related complications in the obese (Ata et al. 2011). Metabolic obesity associated with insulin resistance is being recognized as a risk factor in addition to insulin resistance in the non-obese non-diabetic in the prevalence of gallstone disease (Chang et al. 2008). The alarming rise in attempts to lose weight rapidly by medical treatment or by bariatric surgery increases the risk. Women who had a rapid weight loss of more than 4 kg had 44% increased risk of gallstones compared to an equal weight loss of 4 kg over a 2 year period. Women who lost more than 10 kg had more than 94% risk for gallstones when other risk factors were controlled (Everhart 1993). Ehrlinger observed that the prevalence of new gallstones increases by 10–12% after 8–16 weeks of a low-calorie diet and more than 30% about 12–18 months after gastric bypass, with 1/3 of stones becoming symptomatic. Risk factors that were identified were a relative loss of weight greater than 24% of the initial body weight, rate of weight loss more than 1.5 kg per week, a very low-calorie diet without fat, long overnight fasting period, and high serum triglycerides. Ursodeoxycholic acid (UDCA) decreases lithogenicity by lowering cholesterol saturation of bile (Erlinger 2000).

TPN is a rare risk factor for microlithiasis and gallstones (Guglielmi et al. 2006; Roslyn et al. 1983). Drugs known to increase the risk of gallstones are octreotide, cephalosporins, and thiazides (Trendle et al. 1997; Lopez et al. 1991; Angelin 1989). Octreotide reduces motility and leads to biliary stasis. Ceftriaxone is secreted in high concentrations and crystallizes in bile, resulting in sludge.

Pathogenesis

Gallstones are divided based on chemical composition into cholesterol, pigment, and mixed stones, depending on location as intrahepatic, gallbladder stones or choledocholithiasis.

Most stones are cholesterol stones comprising 37–68%, pigment stones account for 2–27%, mixed stones 4–16%, and calcium stones 1–17%. Mixed stones are a combination of cholesterol and pigment stones (Tazuma 2006; Johnston and Kaplan 1993; Gurusamy and Davidson 2014). This classification is not of much practical use since composition can be determined only after surgery and chemical analysis of stones.

Cholesterol stones form in the gallbladder mostly, but about 10% may form in the bile ducts.

Pigment stones are seen in patients with chronic hemolytic anemias such as sickle cell disease and thalassemia. Hemolysis leads to increased bilirubin and stone formation. These are black pigment stones consisting of calcium bilirubinate and form in the gallbladder or sometimes in the common bile duct (Trotman 1991). They contain less than 20% cholesterol. Sickle cell disease, although not a major problem in older people, frequently requires prophylactic cholecystectomy, in order to distinguish clinical features of sickle cell crisis from infarction of viscera (Bonatsos et al. 2001). Brown pigment stones are composed of unconjugated bilirubin, calcium salts and cholesterol and are intrahepatic. In East Asians brown pigment stones develop secondary to biliary infections due to bacteria or parasites or inflammation. There is changing epidemiology in that currently cholesterol stones are now more common than pigment stones in East Asia. Pigment stones can be seen in older adults as well (Van Erpecum et al. 1988).

Although the discussion on the pathogenesis that follows here pertains to cholesterol stones, the clinical manifestations are the same.

The pathogenesis of gallstones represents a failure of biliary cholesterol homeostasis (Wang et al. 2017). In bile, cholesterol, phospholipids, and bile acids are three major lipids, and bile pigments are minor lipids. Five primary defects in the pathogenesis are (i) genetic factors and *Lith* genes; (ii) hypersecretion of biliary cholesterol leading to supersaturated bile; (iii) rapid phase transitions of cholesterol in bile; (iv) impaired gallbladder motility associated with hypersecretion of mucins; and (v) increased amounts of cholesterol of intestinal origin (Dowling 2000; Wang et al. 2010, 2018). Bile salts are important to keep cholesterol in solution. Bile salts in critical micellar concentration aggregate to form simple micelles which can solubilize cholesterol (Somjen and Gilat 1985). Bile salts incorporate phospholipids to form mixed micelles that can solubilize triple the amount of cholesterol in simple micelles. The relative proportion of these three main components plays a critical role in determining the maximal solubility of cholesterol. Cholesterol gallstones are a polygenic disorder with several underlying mechanisms, but the main factor is excess biliary cholesterol (Venneman and van Erpecum 2010). Genes that contribute to cholesterol gallstones are those that encode for membrane transporters, regulatory enzymes, transcription factors, lipoprotein receptors, hormone receptors, and biliary mucins (Wang et al. 2018; Wang and Afdhal 2004). The complex genetic relationship to gallstone disease is still evolving.

Gallstones form as microcrystals in the biliary system. Sludge is an intermediate stage in stone formation (Lee et al. 1988; Carey and Cahalane 1988). Sludge is a particulate matter composed of cholesterol, calcium bilirubinate, and mucin. Sludge may contain larger particles seen under microscopy called microliths (1–3 mm in size) which may lead to gallstones. Biliary sludge is reversible in most situations but may persist in 12–20% and cause complications like acute cholecystitis, cholangitis, or acute pancreatitis (Lee et al. 2015).

Clinical Features of Gallstone Disease (Table 3)

Gallstones are asymptomatic in most people and only about 20% develop symptoms, necessitating removal of the gallbladder in 1–2% yearly (Gibney 1990; Portincasa et al. 2016).

Table 3 Summarizes the clinical presentations

Clinical presentation of gallstones
Asymptomatic gallstones
Biliary pain
Acute cholecystitis
Empyema of gallbladder
Choloenteric fistula
Gallstone Ileus
Mirizzi's syndrome
Bouveret's syndrome
Chronic cholecystitis
Asymptomatic choledocholithiasis
Obstructive jaundice
Acute cholangitis
Acute pancreatitis
Pyogenic liver abscess

Because of the high prevalence of gallstones in older adults, cause of pain may falsely be attributed to the presence of gallstones, and although we call this entity symptomatic disease, the source of pain is not biliary in etiology.

When symptomatic, the classic symptoms are sudden and rapidly intensifying pain in the right upper quadrant, radiating to the right scapula or shoulder, lasts several minutes to a few hours, associated with nausea and vomiting. In the geriatric population, however, similar to many other conditions, biliary disease may also present atypically, with atypical pain or no pain, associated with a confused state of mind and without leukocytosis. The clinical presentations depend on the site in the biliary system where the stone has lodged.

Biliary Pain

Biliary pain is a consequence of transient obstruction of the cystic duct by a stone and is often erroneously called biliary colic. The term is a misnomer as the pain is steady and not colicky. Abdominal pain occurs in epigastrium or RUQ and may last for 1–5 h. The pain starts, gradually progresses to plateau, and stays constant for several hours prior to gradual resolution. It may be associated with dyspepsia. Right upper quadrant tenderness may be present. Laboratory tests are usually normal.

Acute Calculous Cholecystitis and its Complications

Gallstones cause more than 90% of acute cholecystitis. Acalculous cholecystitis accounts for the remaining 5–10% of acute cholecystitis. Acute calculous cholecystitis (ACC) occurs when a gallstone gets impacted in the cystic duct leading to acute inflammation of the gallbladder (Gurusamy and Davidson 2014). In 75% of patients, this is preceded by biliary pain. Initially there is epigastric pain that lasts more than 6 h, followed by right upper quadrant (RUQ) pain, which may be accompanied by nausea and vomiting. Patients

Table 4 Tokyo guidelines TG18/TG13 diagnostic criteria for acute cholecystitis (Yokoe et al. 2018)

A. Local signs of inflammation, etc.
(1) Murphy's sign, (2) RUQ mass/pain/tenderness
B. Systemic signs of inflammation, etc.
(1) Fever, (2) elevated CRP, (3) elevated WBC count
C. Imaging findings Imaging findings characteristic of acute cholecystitis
Suspected diagnosis: one item in A + one item in B
Definite diagnosis: one item in A + one item in B + C

may have RUQ tenderness on palpation (Murphy's sign) which is highly sensitive and specific (Trowbridge et al. 2003). Serum bilirubin may be mildly elevated; serum alkaline phosphatase and aminotransferases may be elevated as well. These classic findings may be obscure in the elderly, and clinical findings may not always be reliable. Complications like empyema or gallbladder perforation can occur if untreated in about 10% (Morris et al. 2007). Gangrenous cholecystitis is a rare but severe condition associated with intramural hemorrhage, mucosal ulcers, intraluminal purulent debris, hemorrhage, and fibrinous exudate (Bennett and Balthazar 2003; Morfin et al. 1968).

Emphysematous cholecystitis (EC), also rare, is a rapidly progressive condition due to bacteria like Clostridia and *E. coli* with gas formation within the gallbladder. EC is seen more in men, in those with diabetes and bowel ischemia, with a fivefold increase in perforation and may be fatal (Gill et al. 1997).

Tokyo guidelines 2013/2018 suggest guidelines for management of acute cholangitis and acute cholecystitis (see Tables 4 and 5).

"Grade I" acute cholecystitis does not meet the criteria of "Grade III" or "Grade II" acute cholecystitis. It can also be defined as acute cholecystitis in a healthy patient with no organ dysfunction and mild inflammatory changes in the gallbladder, making cholecystectomy a safe and low-risk operative procedure.

Gallbladder perforation is a rare complication occurring in 2–5% of acute cholecystitis (Jansen et al. 2018; Roslyn et al. 1987). It is more common in the elderly and can be associated with increased morbidity and mortality. Gallbladder

Table 5 Tokyo guidelines TG18/13 severity of acute cholecystitis (Yokoe et al. 2018)

Grade III acute cholecystitis
"Grade III" acute cholecystitis is associated with dysfunction of any one of the following organs/systems:
1. Cardiovascular dysfunction: hypotension requiring treatment with dopamine ≥ 5 µg/kg per min, or any dose of norepinephrine
2. Neurological dysfunction: decreased level of consciousness
3. Respiratory dysfunction: PaO_2/FiO_2 ratio < 30
4. Renal dysfunction: oliguria, creatinine >2.0 mg/dl
5. Hepatic dysfunction: PT-INR >1.5
6. Hematological dysfunction: platelet count $<100,000/mm^3$
Grade II (moderate) acute cholecystitis
"Grade II" acute cholecystitis is associated with any one of the following conditions:
1. Elevated WBC count ($>18,000/mm^3$)
2. Palpable tender mass in the right upper abdominal quadrant
3. Duration of complaints >72 h
4. Marked local inflammation (gangrenous cholecystitis, pericholecystic abscess, hepatic abscess biliary peritonitis, emphysematous cholecystitis
Grade I acute cholecystitis

perforation may be of three types: type 1 into the peritoneal cavity, type 2 localized perforation, and type 3 cholecystoenteric fistula (Roslyn et al. 1987).

Biliary fistulas are a rare complication of gallstone disease (Crespi et al. 2016). The primary fistulas are spontaneous complication, while the secondary ones are related to surgical complications. The incidence of primary biliary fistulas range from 1% to 2% and may be as high as 5% in endemic areas. The types of fistulas may be cholecystoduodenal, cholecystogastric, or cholecystocolic. Large stones, recurrent cholangitis, female sex, and in particular old age are risk factors for bilio-enteric fistulas.

Gallbladder wall erosion and fistula formation can occur with gallstones causing obstruction when lodged in narrow parts of the GI tract, the ileocecal valve being the commonest area (gallstone ileus). Proximal migration or direct invasion to the stomach can result in the stone, usually of more than 2.5 cm size, causing gastric outlet obstruction (Bouveret syndrome).

Table 6 Cesendes classification of Mirizzi's syndrome (Csendes et al. 1989)

Type of Mirizzi's	Description
Type I	External compression of the common bile duct by stone impacted in the gallbladder or cystic duct
Type II	Cholecystobiliary fistula present with erosion of less than one-third of the circumference of the bile duct
Type III	Cholecystobiliary fistula involves up to two-thirds of the bile duct circumference
Type IV	Cholecystobiliary fistula with complete destruction of the bile duct

When a gallstone in the cystic duct causes compression on the bile duct or fistulizes into the bile duct and is associated with jaundice, it is termed Mirizzi's syndrome (Zaliekas and Munson 2008).

There are four types of Mirizzi's syndrome as classified by Cesendes depending on the location (Table 6).

Pathology in Mirizzi's syndrome is due to impaction of stone and obstruction by direct mass effect or development of stricture due to inflammation and pressure necrosis which leads to fistula formation (Clemente et al. 2018). ERCP and MRCP help in diagnosis, but often this is only recognized during surgery (Alemi et al. 2019). A few authors include cholecystoenteric fistulas in the types of Mirizzi's syndrome (Beltran et al. 2008). A discussion on secondary fistulas is discussed in major surgical textbooks.

Common Bile Duct (CBD) Stones

The incidence/prevalence of choledocholithiasis is not known but estimated to be 10–20% in patients with gallstones and the incidence increases with age (Chen et al. 2015). Recent studies have demonstrated that the clinical presentation of CBD stones may vary with age (Hu et al. 2016). Unlike in younger adults who present with classic biliary colic symptoms, older adults may be asymptomatic with no apparent clinical features or present with biliary colic and jaundice (Rosseland and Glomsaker 2000). There are

reports of cases of CBD stones impacted in the CBD that were asymptomatic for years.

CBD stones may be classified as primary, secondary, residual, or recurrent.

Primary CBD stones form in the bile ducts in setting of biliary ductal dilatation.

Secondary stones form in the gallbladder and escape into the CBD. Residual stones are those stones in the CBD that are missed at the time of cholecystectomy but present within 2 years of cholecystectomy. Recurrent stones develop in the biliary ducts and occur longer than 2 years after cholecystectomy.

CBD stones can cause intermittent obstruction of the bile duct, with transient increase in bilirubin, alkaline phosphatase, aminotransferases, and pancreatic enzymes.

Younger adults with CBD stones were significantly more likely to have abnormal liver function tests than those without. The sensitivity and accuracy of transabdominal ultrasound scans in screening for CBD stones increases with age (Hu et al. 2016). Unless removed, CBD stones can cause acute pancreatitis, obstructive jaundice, acute ascending cholangitis, and hepatic abscess.

ASGE criteria that stratify the risk of having choledocholithiasis are used in patients with intact gallbladder (Maple et al. 2010). Although CBD dilatation is not a predictive factor for choledocholithiasis post cholecystectomy, ASGE criteria are applicable similar to non-cholecystomized patients based on a retrospective study of 327 patients by Sousa et al. (2019). ASGE criteria have been shown to have a sensitivity varying from 55% to 89% (Gouveia et al. 2018; Suarez et al. 2016; Magalhaes et al. 2015). The criteria suggests high probability for CBD stones requiring further evaluation with ERCP.

ASGE criteria for risk stratification for CBD stones suggest: Very strong predictors are the presence of a CBD stone on transabdominal US, clinical features of acute cholangitis, and serum bilirubin greater than 4 mg/dL. Dilated CBD was defined as > 6 mm in adults and > 8 mm post cholecystectomy. Intermediate risk (10–50%) patients had abnormal liver biochemical tests or age more than 55 or dilated CBD on imaging. Low-risk patients (< 10%) had no predictors.

Ascending Cholangitis

Ascending cholangitis can occur with distal CBD obstruction (see Tables 7 and 8). This presents as Charcot's triad with RUQ abdominal pain, fever, and jaundice (Attasaranya et al. 2008; Kimura et al. 2007). Charcot's triad has high specificity but low sensitivity as older adults with cholangitis may not manifest all the findings. More than 1/3 of patients, in particular older people, may not present with Charcot's triad. In a prospective study assessing the diagnostic power of Charcot's triad only 22% of patients documenting suppurative bile on surgical choledochotomy demonstrated all three criteria, indicating the suboptimal utility of the triad. However the triad has high specificity. Reynold's pentad (Charcot's triad with septic shock and altered mental status) is present only in 30–45% adults with cholangitis but with elderly patients, delirium, or dementia may confound the clinical picture.

Bile cultures are positive in 80–100% of patients and blood cultures in 70% (Tanaka et al. 2007). Bacteria most frequently cultured are *E. coli*, *Klebsiella*, and *Enterococcus* (Gomi et al. 2013). Anaerobes and Clostridia may also occur. Staphylococcal infections are rare. Resistance to quinolones, ceftriaxone, ampicillin-sulbactam, and piperacillin-tazobactam has been reported from 30% to 52% (Reuken et al. 2017).

"Grade I" acute cholangitis does not meet the criteria of "Grade III" or "Grade II (moderate)" acute cholangitis at initial diagnosis.

Biliary Pancreatitis

Acute biliary pancreatitis occurs as a result of CBD obstruction by gallstones at the ampullary region. Additional details on biliary pancreatitis are discussed in another chapter.

Chronic Cholecystitis (See Fig. 2)

Chronic cholecystitis occurs with recurrent attacks of biliary pain associated with gallstones (Nesland 2004). Chronic cholecystitis is seen in the setting of cholelithiasis.

Table 7 Tokyo guidelines 2018 TG18/13 criteria cholangitis (Kiriyama et al. 2018)

A. Systemic inflammation
A-1. Fever and/or shaking chills
A-2. Laboratory data: evidence of inflammatory response
B. Cholestasis
B-1. Jaundice
B-2. Laboratory data: abnormal liver function tests
C. Imaging
C-1. Biliary dilatation
C-2. Evidence of the etiology on imaging (stricture, stone, stent, etc.)
Suspected diagnosis: one item in A + one item in either B or C
Definite diagnosis: one item in A, one item in B and one item in C

Table 8 Tokyo 2018 TG18/13 severity of acute cholangitis (Kiriyama et al. 2018)

Grade III acute cholangitis
"Grade III" acute cholangitis is defined as acute cholangitis that is associated with the onset of dysfunction at least in any one of the following organs/systems:
1. Cardiovascular dysfunction: hypotension requiring dopamine $\geq$5 μg/kg per min, or any dose of norepinephrine
2. Neurological dysfunction: disturbance of consciousness
3. Respiratory dysfunction: PaO_2/FiO_2 ratio < 300
4. Renal dysfunction: oliguria, serum creatinine >2.0 mg/dl
5. Hepatic dysfunction: PT-INR >1.5
6. Hematological dysfunction: platelet count $<100,000/mm^3$
Grade II (moderate) acute cholangitis
"Grade II" acute cholangitis is associated with any two of the following conditions:
1. Abnormal WBC count ($>12,000/mm^3$, $<4000/mm^3$)
2. High fever (≥39 °C)
3. Age (≥75 years old)
4. Hyperbilirubinemia (total bilirubin ≥5 mg/dl)
5. Hypoalbuminemia ($<$STD $\times$ 0.7)
Grade I acute cholangitis

There is no correlation to size of gallstones or severity of inflammation. Patients present with pain as in acute cholecystitis and the two conditions form a spectrum which can coexist. Histologically

Fig. 2 Chronic cholecystitis (Thickened gallbladder wall with mononuclear inflammatory infiltrates involving the mucosa and wall, smooth muscle hypertrophy, and Rokitansky-Aschoff sinuses)

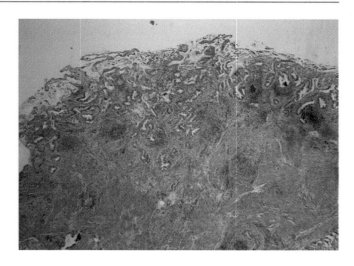

this is seen as subepithelial and subserosal fibrosis. US abdomen is the test of choice, and treatment is elective cholecystectomy (Knab et al. 2014). Chronic acalculous cholecystitis is a functional biliary disorder discussed below.

Porcelain Gallbladder

The presence of gallstones increases the risk of gallbladder carcinoma but is less than 0.1%. In contrast, earlier it was thought that all patients with gallbladder calcification had high risk for gallbladder cancer (Khan et al. 2011; Stephen and Berger 2001). Porcelain gallbladder (PGB), in which there is mural calcification of the gallbladder, seen with chronic cholecystitis has higher risk of gallbladder carcinoma (6–33%) when the calcification is incomplete (patchy) (Schnelldorfer 2013). It is seen more in women in the 50–70 year age group. Porcelain gallbladder is a rare finding seen in 0.05–0.08% cholecystectomy patients (Thakrar et al. 2019). Modern imaging techniques have led to earlier and more frequent detection of PGB. Current opinion is that the risk of cancer in PGB is much less than previously thought, and the incidence of porcelain gallbladder is more frequent with modern imaging techniques. The current trend is that cholecystectomy is not always indicated in asymptomatic porcelain gallbladder. However, the risk of gallbladder cancer, although low, prompts recommending cholecystectomy to

younger and otherwise healthy patients. Our opinion is this decision should be properly and adequately evaluated in countries where risk for GB cancer is high.

Pyogenic Liver Abscess

Pyogenic liver abscess may occur as result of cholecystohepatic fistula or ascending cholangitis. The most common cause remains biliary tract disease, although the majority of patients with liver abscess were those with no detectable cause (Seeto and Rockey 1996). The average age has been increasing with mean age 55–60 years (Holzman et al. 2004).

Diagnostic Studies for Biliary Disease (See Table 9)

US Abdomen (See Fig. 3)

US remains the initial test of choice in patients suspected to have acute cholecystitis (Yarmish et al. 2014). US had a sensitivity of 88% (95% CI: 74%, 100%) and a specificity of 80% (95% CI: 62%, 98%) in detecting cholecystitis. It has a 95% specificity and sensitivity in detecting stones > 1.5 mm in diameter. The limitation is that US has limited sensitivity (reported as 63%) in the evaluation for choledocholithiasis.

Table 9 Diagnostic modalities for gallstone disease

Imaging studies	Advantages	Limitations
US abdomen	Easy availability	Limited for choledocholithiasis and small stones
	Good sensitivity (81%) & specificity (83%) in acute cholecystitis	
	Detects gall stones more than 1.4 mm	
	Non-invasive	
	Low cost	
HIDA scan	Highest sensitivity (96%) and specificity (90%) in acute cholecystitis	Radiation exposure
		Prolonged study time
		Limited availability
CT abdomen	Easy availability	Radiation exposure
	Useful in emergencies	
	Sensitivity in acute cholecystitis 94% and specificity 59%	
	CBD stones sensitivity 87% specificity 96%	
	Evaluation of malignant lesions	
MRCP	No radiation exposure Sensitive to detect CBD stones	Contraindicated with pacemakers and aneurysm clips Claustrophobia
EUS	Detects microlithiasis	Limited availability
	High sensitivity 100% specificity 95% for CBD stones	Invasive
ERCP	Detects microlithiasis	Invasive procedure
	Can evaluate CBD stones and offer therapeutic intervention	Complications like pancreatitis and perforation

Data from Jordy J. S. Kiewiet et al. (2012), EASL (EASL 2016), and Oppenheimer and Rubens (2019)

Abdominal US findings seen in ACC are distended gallbladder, thickened gallbladder wall, pericholecystic fluid, gallstones, and a positive radiologic Murphy's sign (Ralls et al. 1985).

Cholescintigraphy (HIDA) Scan (See Figs. 4 and 5)

Cholescinitigraphy is useful in triaging patients with equivocal US findings of acute cholecystitis (Oppenheimer and Rubens 2019). It is done using radionuclides like technetium-labeled iminodiacetic acid (hepatobiliary iminodiacetic acid scan) to assess the gallbladder. It has the best sensitivity (97%; 95% confidence interval (CI): 96%, 98%) and specificity (90%; 95% CI: 86%, 95%) in acute cholecystitis. The test is losing its value due to prolonged scan time, radiation exposure, and availability. The lack of uptake of radioactive tracer is suggestive of acute cholecystitis. Delayed appearance may occur in nonfunctioning gallbladder and non-visualization in liver failure.

Computerized Tomography Scan

Computerized tomography scans of the abdomen are used widely in the evaluation of abdominal pain in an older adult because of inadequacy of history and non-classic presentations and the high possibility of surgical emergencies. CT is sensitive to evaluate biliary dilatation and useful in evaluation of the pancreas when malignancy is suspected. EUS and MRCP are superior in evaluation of biliary stones and the indications for CT are limited in uncomplicated acute cholecystitis, but needed. CT is useful in assessing for complications such as the identification of gas formation and perforation and to stratify patients who may

Fig. 3 US showing
gallstones

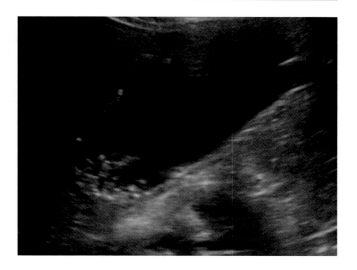

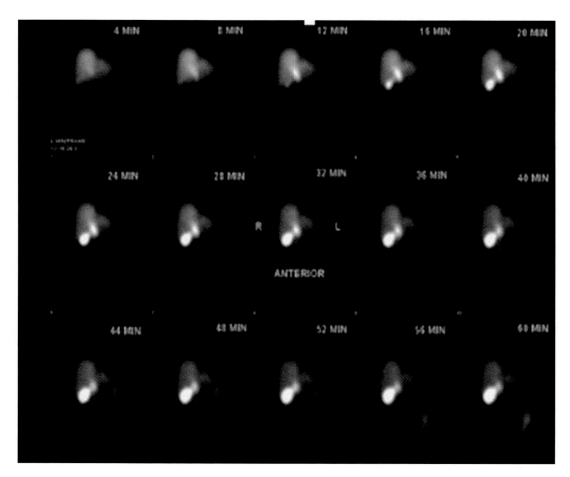

Fig. 4 Normal HIDA scan (The gallbladder is visualized seen with increased uptake)

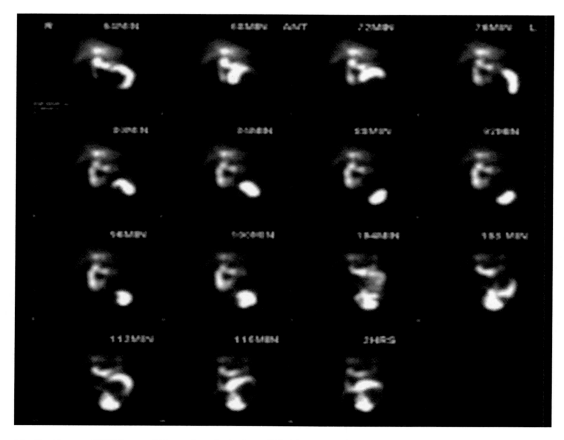

Fig. 5 Abnormal HIDA scan failure of uptake in the gallbladder so not visualized

need open cholecystectomy and identify any alternate diagnosis (Oppenheimer and Rubens 2019).

Magnetic Resonance Cholangiopancreatogram

MRCP is superior to CT and ultrasound in detecting gallstones in bile ducts (Grand et al. 2004). Stones as small as 2 mm can be seen, with excellent sensitivity (81–100% and specificity (85–99%). It can help in preoperative screening prior to cholecystectomy. MRCP is non-invasive and suitable in patients with altered gut anatomy. MRCP has limitations in viewing stones in pancreatic duct, artifacts, and claustrophobia and contraindicated in patients with pacemakers and aneurysm clips. There is no clear

evidence that EUS is superior to MRCP in the investigation of biliary stones (Giljaca et al. 2015).

Endoscopic Retrograde Cholangiopancreatogram

ERCP had been the gold standard for CBD stones but has risk of severe complications like pancreatitis, cholangitis, perforation, and hemorrhage and should be reserved for patients with proven stones or high likelihood of stones needing intervention. EUS or MRCP are nearly as accurate as ERCP. ERCP is indicated within 24 h in the presence of cholangitis (Boender et al. 1995; Acosta et al. 2006).

Endoscopic Ultrasound

Endoscopic ultrasound is helpful in detecting microlithiasis and small stones. It has a positive predictive value of 99% and a negative predictive value of 98% and is superior to other modalities in imaging the biliary system due to proximity (Endoscopic Ultrasound for Biliary Disease). It is a useful tool and can be helpful prior to ERCP in patients with low or intermediate probability of stones. It can be done in patients when MRCP is contraindicated.

Management of Gallstones and Complications

Asymptomatic Gallstones

The general recommendation is not to do cholecystectomy in asymptomatic patients, and this dictum applies to the older adult. Some patients with asymptomatic gallstones may be at increased risk of gallbladder cancer because of large stones (larger than 3 cm), patchy, or incomplete calcification of gallbladder wall (PGB). The risk for cancer is also high in Native Americans and in parts of Northern India. Prophylactic cholecystectomy may be considered based on life expectancy and comorbid conditions.

Management of Acute Calculous Cholecystitis (See Table 10)

Acute calculous cholecystitis (ACC) is the most common complication of gallstone disease, and the incidence is expected to increase. According to the Tokyo guidelines 2018, a definite diagnosis of ACC can be made on the basis of physical examination, early blood tests, and imaging findings that are characteristic of the diagnosis. (Local sign of inflammation (Murphy's sign or RUQ pain, mass, or tenderness) and one systemic sign of inflammation (fever, increased C-reactive protein level, increased white blood cell count) and imaging findings.) Age-related changes of pain perception, biliary physiology, and stress response can make the diagnosis more complicated in older adults. A combination of symptoms, signs, and laboratory tests helps in a more accurate diagnosis of ACC in the elderly as in other patients. As the majority of randomized controlled trials exclude older people, evidence from younger patients is extrapolated to the elderly, not ideal in developing guidelines. The Tokyo 2018 guidelines were not specific for geriatric patients, but the 2017 WSES and SICG guidelines on ACC addressed this in the elderly population; defining elderly as age 65 years and above (Pisano et al. 2019). A higher WBC count was reported in the elderly, and this unexpected result was explained as due to the more severe cholecystitis. Abdominal US is the preferred initial imaging for older patients suspected to have acute cholecystitis due to lower costs, better availability, lack of invasiveness, and good accuracy for stones. HIDA scan has the highest sensitivity and specificity but is limited by availability, long procedure time and exposure to radiation. Management

Table 10 Diagnosis of acute cholecystitis, CBD stone, and ascending cholangitis

	Acute cholecystitis	Acute cholangitis	CBD stones
Symptoms	Biliary pain	Abdominal pain fever jaundice	Biliary pain
	Nausea vomiting		
Physical findings	Murphy's sign	Fever, jaundice	Jaundice
		RUQ tenderness	
		Charcot's triad	
Lab findings	Leucocytosis	Leucocytosis	Elevated bilirubin & alkaline phosphatase
	Elevated CRP	Elevated CRP	
	Mild elevation of liver biochemistry	Elevated bilirubin and alkaline phosphatase	
Diagnostic tests	US abdomen	ERCP	EUS/MRCP/ ERCP
	HIDA scan		

recommendations were based on severity of cholecystitis – severe, moderate, or mild and comorbidities in both the guidelines. Acute cholecystitis should be treated with appropriate antibiotics. Empiric antibiotic therapy should be guided by bacteria most frequently isolated, antibiotic resistance and the severity of infection. Older institutionalized patients are at risk for MDR infections. For patients of advanced age preferred antibiotics are imipenem-cilastatin, meropenem, doripenem, piperacillin tazobactam, or ceftazidime/cefepime with metronidazole.

Uncomplicated Acute Cholecystitis in a Good Surgical Candidate

In patients with mild cholecystitis who present early antibiotics may not have much role other than prophylaxis prior to surgery when source control is achieved by cholecystectomy (Loozen et al. 2017). ASGE guidelines based on a meta-analysis of randomized controlled trials concluded that although antibiotics are not required in low-risk patients undergoing laparoscopic cholecystectomy (Level I, Grade A), antibiotics may reduce the incidence of wound infection in high risk patients (age > 60 years, diabetes, acute colic within 30 days of operation, jaundice, acute cholecystitis, or cholangitis) (Table 11) (Level I, Grade B). Among papers suggesting that antibiotic prophylaxis is helpful is a recent randomized study finding fewer wound infections in patients on ampicillin sulbactam versus cefuroxime particularly in enterococcal infections in high risk patients undergoing elective cholecystectomy. If

Table 11 High risk acute cholecystitis patient requiring antibiotics

Risk factors
Age > 60 years
Diabetes mellitus
Acute colic within 30 days of operation
Jaundice
Acute cholecystitis
Cholangitis

given, they should be limited to a single preoperative dose given within one hour of skin incision and re-dosed if the procedure is more than 4 h long (Dervisoglou et al. 2006).

Laparoscopic cholecystectomy (LC) is the standard of care in most patients with symptomatic gallstones and is a safe procedure in the older adult although outcomes may not be as good as younger patients (Nielsen et al. 2014). Parmar et al. used a large population-based cohort to describe the trajectory of care specifically in older patients presenting with an initial episode of symptomatic cholelithiasis who did not undergo elective cholecystectomy. The authors developed the PREOP-Gallstones model, a nomogram that reliably predicted patients with an over 40% 2-year risk of developing gallstone-related complications (approximately 10% of the cohort) and an additional 50% of patients with less than 10% 2-year risk. Older age, white race, male sex, initial visit to the emergency room department, and a diagnosis of complicated gallstone disease (gallstone pancreatitis, common bile duct stones, and acute cholecystitis) at initial presentation need urgent surgery. The PREOP-Gallstones model enables clinicians to use readily identifiable patient characteristics to quantify an individualized risk score requiring emergent biliary care. Active treatment of coexisting diseases, appropriate selection of surgical procedures, improvements in perioperative therapy, and timely management of postoperative complications are key factors in enhancing therapeutic efficacy in elderly patients with biliary diseases (Zhang et al. 2017).

Despite the proven safety of laparoscopic cholecystectomy, older patients with gallstone disease are less likely to undergo cholecystectomy than younger patients (Riall et al. 2010). However the super-elderly patients (>90 years) have a mortality of 3.7% after laparoscopic cholecystectomy and 12% after open cholecystectomy according to Irojah et al. (2017). Unsurprisingly in their study, postop myocardial infarction, pneumonia, sepsis, SIRS, pre-operative delirium, history of cigarette smoking, and corticosteroid use were predictive of poor outcome and death. In symptomatic gallstone disease, cholecystectomy should be done as early as possible, if no major contraindications exist, preferably in the same admission (Thangavelu et al. 2018; Oppenheimer and Rubens 2019). Gurusamy et al. (2010) in a meta-analysis compared early laparoscopic cholecystectomy (ELC 1 week of onset of symptoms) with delayed laparoscopic cholecystectomy (DLC at least 6 week after symptoms resolve) in patients with ACC (Gurusamy et al. 2010). The results were similar with regard to bile duct injury and conversion rate, but the hospital stay was shorter by 4 days for early LC (Gomes et al. 2017; Gurusamy et al. 2013). Mortality rates in the elderly undergoing emergency cholecystectomy are reported to range from 6% to 22% (Uecker et al. 2001; Glenn 1981; Harness et al. 1986). The conversion rate to open cholecystectomy is 7–32% in older patients. Patients with mild cholecystitis should have early surgery, within 7 days.

The role of medical therapy with ursodeoxycholic acid (UDCA) with or without extracorporeal shock wave lithotripsy is limited due to low rates of cure, ineffectiveness in preventing complications and high recurrence rates (O'Donnell and Heaton 1988; Carrilho-Ribeiro et al. 2006). Arguably UDCA can be considered in patients with non-calcified stones less than 1.5 mm and if the patient does not want surgery, although the benefit is disputed (Venneman et al. 2006). However, there is an indication for UDCA therapy in patients after bariatric surgery who have gallstones prior to surgery or are at high risk (Magouliotis et al. 2017).

Management of Complicated Gallbladder Disease in the Elderly

Supportive treatment like IV fluids and antibiotics are advisable. Antibiotic therapy should be instituted taking into consideration severity, hospitalized status, and cultures. Multi-specialty input including infectious disease may be needed in severely ill patients.

Gallbladder disease is the most common cause of acute abdominal pain in older patients and accounts for a third of abdominal operations in

patients older than 65 years (Hendrickson and Naparst 2003; Riall et al. 2015; Bugliosi et al. 1990; Ansaloni et al. 2016). Age is an independent risk factor for mortality related to surgery, and older age is a negative predictor for undergoing cholecystectomy (Bergman et al. 2011). The 2017 WSES guidelines on ACC considered the relationship between old age and surgery (Ansaloni et al. 2016).

Laparoscopic cholecystectomy (LC) is the standard approach of treatment for symptomatic gallstone disease with few relative or absolute contraindications, but elderly patients with gallstone complications are less likely to undergo surgery (Maple et al. 2010; Williams et al. 2008). Laparoscopic approach should always be attempted at first except in the case of absolute anesthetic contraindications and septic shock in older patients with acute cholecystitis (see Table 12).

Most geriatric patients today undergo laparoscopic cholecystectomy without increased morbidity or mortality even though obesity and other comorbid conditions would affect the outcome. LC was shown to be safe and feasible in octogenarians (De la Serna et al. 2019). However, another study based on a large number of adults aged 60 or older, age was associated negatively with complications. Older age however is not a major factor in conversion of LC to open surgery. The rate of complications between older and younger patients is not different (Nassar and Richter 2019). The mortality for the super-elderly (90 year and older) after laparoscopic or open

Table 12 Contraindications for laparoscopic cholecystectomy

ASGE guidelines – contraindications for LC include but are not limited to
Generalized peritonitis
Septic shock from cholangitis
Severe acute pancreatitis
Untreated coagulopathy
Lack of surgeon expertise
Previous abdominal operations which prevent safe abdominal access or progression of the procedure
Advanced cirrhosis with failure of hepatic function
Gallbladder cancer

cholecystectomy is 3.7% and 12%, respectively, significantly higher than the mortality in the general population of 0.3% to 3.8% (Irojah et al. 2017; Ingraham et al. 2010). Other factors increasing the risk further were reported to be Hispanic race, emergent procedures, open surgical approaches, poor preoperative functional status, postoperative myocardial infarction, delirium, and septic shock (Irojah et al. 2017).

Management of gallbladder disease varies according to complications and comorbidities. A reliable prognostic score in assessing frailty that can guide the management in ACC is necessary but can consider using ASA APACHE II Charlson Comorbidity Index (CCI) or P-POSUM score (Portsmouth Physiological and Operative Severity Score for the enUmeration of Mortality.) POSUM score is useful in assessing mortality and morbidity in elderly patients undergoing laparoscopic cholecystectomy (Tambyraja et al. 2005). POSUM score accurately predicts morbidity in emergency surgery in nonagenarians (Imaoka et al. 2017). CCI is a method to categorize a patient's comorbidities based on the International Classification of Diseases (ICD) codes used in regulatory data such as hospital summary data. There is agreement that the decision is based on comorbid conditions and risk stratification criteria like American Society of Anesthesiology (ASA) criteria. The above perceptions are to be critically reviewed with other options. Older individuals do better with elective surgery, so it is necessary to weigh the decision regarding surgery with great care. Patients on chronic anticoagulation on bridging heparin therapy had more bleeding in several studies and caution is needed in these patients (Ercan et al. 2010).

The Tokyo 2013 guidelines recommended surgery within 72 h and in the 2018 update early cholecystectomy was still advised in low risk patients beyond 72 h (Yokoe et al. 2018). Tokyo Guidelines 2018 are summarized as follows (see Fig. 6).

The ASA score or Charlson Comorbidity Index (CCI) can be used to stratify patients with high risk. Patients with moderate cholecystitis should have surgery early if the patient can withstand surgery, but if the patient is high risk for surgery, conservative treatment and biliary drainage should be considered. In patients with severe cholecystitis, after the patient has been resuscitated, with favorable organ system failure factors and negative predictive factors, early surgery can be considered in specialist centers.

Cholecystectomy should be performed as early as possible as it has less complications and shorter hospital stay but can be done within 10 days of onset of symptoms. There are no specific studies evaluating early versus delayed laparoscopic cholecystectomy for elderly patients. Conversion to open surgery may be predicted by fever, leucocytosis, elevated serum bilirubin, and extensive upper abdominal surgery. Laparoscopic or open subtotal cholecystectomy can be considered as an alternative for older patients with advanced inflammation, gangrenous gallbladder, and if gallbladder anatomy makes it difficult and main bile duct injuries are likely.

In individuals who may not withstand surgery, including the elderly, conservative treatment including early biliary drainage should be performed and surgery should be done once factors are favorable. Studies looking at the need for cholecystectomy after percutaneous cholecystostomy in high-risk patients are scant.

The role of cholecystostomy as a bridging therapy until cholecystectomy or as definitive treatment in elderly patients is uncertain due to lack of studies in the age group, but in high risk patients, a number of options are available like emergency ultrasonographic percutaneous cholecystostomy and interval laparoscopic cholecystectomy (Fleming et al. 2019; Radosa et al. 2019; Park et al. 2019). Endoscopic techniques are an alternate in older patients who are acutely ill and are at high risk for surgery (discussed in another chapter) (Mori et al. 2018; Siddiqui et al. 2019). Endoscopic US-guided gallbladder drainage is an emerging alternative as it provides highly effective drainage without the need for a percutaneous catheter via either a trans-ampullary or a transmural approach (Balmadrid 2018). Endoscopic gallbladder drainage is reported to have a high success rate with an acceptable rate of adverse events and can be considered in non-surgical patients to avoid long term percutaneous catheter (Adler 2019). Percutaneous transhepatic

Fig. 6 Adaptation of Tokyo guidelines 2018 for treatment of cholecystitis (Ref Management of acute cholecystitis Tokyo guidelines 2018)

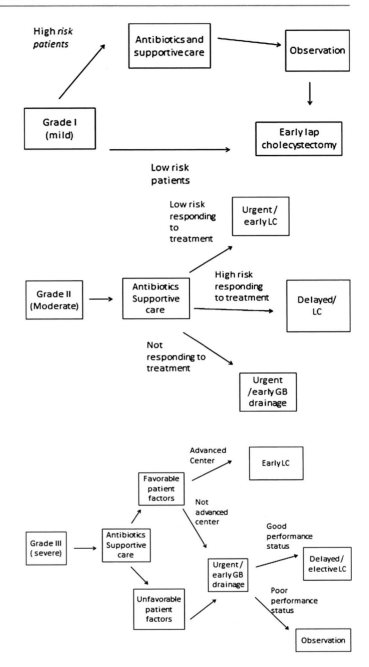

gallbladder aspiration though not a recommended standard procedure, is a simple and easy decompression method with a low complication rate (Itoi et al. 2017; Komatsu et al. 2016). It may also be reasonable to wait in high risk patients as about 30% of patients may not have recurrent biliary colic.

CBD Stones

The presence of biliary stones in patients with symptomatic gallbladder disease is about 10–20%, but in the absence of abnormal liver biochemical tests and CBD dilatation, risk of choledocholithiasis may be as low as 5% (Collins

Table 13 ASGE risk stratification and management

Probability for CBD stone	Predictors for choledocholithiasis	Recommended strategy
High	CBD stone on imagingor Clinical ascending cholangitis or Total bilirubin>4 mg/dl and dilated CBD stone on imaging	Proceed to ERCP
Intermediate	Abnormal liver biochemical tests or age > 55 years or Dilated CBD on imaging	EUS MRCP laparoscopic IOC or intraoperative US
Low	No predictors present	Cholecystectomy with/without IOC or intraoperative US

et al. 2004; Nebiker et al. 2009). The management of CBD stones is endoscopic or by surgery or by a combined approach. The general principles in the management of CBD stones were recently revised (Williams et al. 2017; Buxbaum et al. 2019). The ASGE 2019 guidelines should be used in older patients to risk stratify for CBD stones to reduce unnecessary ERCP (Buxbaum et al. 2019) (see Table 13). Direct ERCP was advised only in patients with confirmed CBD stones on abdominal ultrasound or high risk of choledocholithiasis (total bilirubin > 4 mg/dl, dilated bile duct and cholangitis) to allow immediate clearance of the duct. There was no conclusive superior outcome with ERCP done preoperatively, intraoperatively, or postoperatively. In patients undergoing cholecystectomy, timing of ERCP is advised based on available surgical and endoscopic expertise.

The British Society of Gastroenterology recommends laparoscopic bile duct exploration in patients undergoing cholecystectomy to reduce the number of interventions needed for biliary stones, as there was no difference in mortality or morbidity compared to perioperative ERCP. Laparoscopic biliary duct exploration was comparable to ERCP and associated with shorter hospital stay (Williams et al. 2017; Dasari et al. 2013). ERCP and intraoperative cholangiography (IOC) have showed excellent and comparable results (Dasari et al. 2013). Intraoperative cholangiogram is limited by its availability but is an option where available in patients with intermediate to high probability of gallstones

and where diagnosis has not been confirmed by other modalities. CBD stone removal with ERCP is associated with high efficiency (about 90%) and only a negligible rate of adverse events of about 5% including ERCP pancreatitis, bleeding, perforation, and death (less than 1%). ERCP leads to complications (pancreatitis, cholangitis, duodenal perforations, hemorrhage, contrast media allergy) in 1% to 2% of patients which increases to 10% in case of sphincterotomy (Sousa et al. 2019; Cotton et al. 2009). Endoscopic sphincterotomy (ES) followed by large balloon dilation over ES alone was advised in patients with large or difficult to remove bile duct stones. Intraductal therapy with electrohydraulic or laser lithotripsy was suggested for large intrahepatic and extrahepatic bile ducts stones that cannot be removed by conventional methods (Watson et al. 2018). Stent maintenance with exchange or removal is essential to reduce the risk for adverse events in patients who have stents placed.

MRCP, EUS, intraoperative cholangiography, or laparoscopic US can be done in older patients with moderate risk for choledocholithiasis depending on local availability and expertise.

Evaluation with tests including intraoperative cholangiogram was not felt to be necessary in the EASL 2016 guidelines in patients at low risk for CBD stones as small stones would pass spontaneously, while ASGE guidelines recommend cholecystectomy with or without IOC or intraoperative US in these patients (EASL 2016).

Primary CBD stones can occur in patients with risk factors for gallstones. CBD stones may recur in patients treated with ERCP+ES without cholecystectomy. Risk is high in patients with periampullary type A diverticulum and dilated CBD (Nzenza et al. 2018).

Acute Cholangitis

Acute cholangitis is a serious complication associated with significant morbidity and mortality especially in the geriatric population (Sugiyama and Atomi 1997). Presence of RUQ pain with fever and jaundice is highly suggestive of cholangitis. Abdominal US may show CBD dilatation but is less sensitive than EUS or MRCP. Treatment includes IV fluids and antibiotics alone in mild cholangitis and biliary drainage procedure usually ERCP+ES in moderate and severe cholangitis or if there is failure to improve in mild cholangitis (Lai et al. 1992). Antibiotic treatment should be guided by local microbial susceptibility patterns. ERCP +ES are procedures of choice in management of ascending cholangitis and has the additional benefit of obtaining bile cultures which are a reliable mechanism to evaluate ascending cholangitis and check sensitivity of organisms (Chandra et al. 2019).

In the Tokyo guidelines 2018, recommendations include treating mild community acquired infection with ampicillin sulbactam (unless local resistance is more than 20%), second- or third-generation cephalosporins, and quinolones with metronidazole. In patients with severe community-acquired infections or hospital acquired infections piperacillin tazobactam, third- or fourth-generation cephalosporins +/- metronidazole, and broad-spectrum carbapenems were recommended (Gomi et al. 2018; Pisano et al. 2019). High rate of multi-drug-resistant bacteria and polymicrobial culture is seen in patients who have had previous biliary stenting, especially those patients with multiple prior interventions (Schneider et al. 2014). Additional details on antimicrobial therapy in biliary infections are provided in another chapter.

In patients with septic shock or deterioration despite antibiotic therapy biliary decompression needs to be done urgently after adequate resuscitation, within 24 h of presentation although evidence on optimal timing is not clear. Early ERCP is associated with reduced hospital stay, while in patients who had ERCP after 72 h, increased vasopressor requirement was seen. If ERCP is not feasible then percutaneous drainage or surgical intervention may be required. Endoscopic therapy was seen to be superior to surgical treatment in patients needing biliary decompression for cholangitis due to gallstones, especially in the old, with lesser mortality and morbidity (Leese et al. 1986).

Among older patients including those with serious comorbidities early ERCP+ES followed by laparoscopic cholecystectomy is associated with a significant and clinically important reduction in complications compared to sphincterotomy alone. Patient's family members as well as physicians are often reluctant to proceed with cholecystectomy in elderly patients with cholangitis. Cholecystectomy followed by endoscopic intervention does not appear to increase surgical complications (Elmunzer et al. 2017; Tohda et al. 2016). Older age does not influence incidence or severity of post ERCP pancreatitis (Katsinelos et al. 2018).

Biliary pancreatitis has been discussed in another chapter. Urgent ERCP was not recommended in patients with gallstone pancreatitis without cholangitis or biliary obstruction; this was a strong recommendation with low quality of evidence in the recent ASGE guidelines. Same admission cholecystectomy was advised in mild gallstone pancreatitis.

DVT Prophylaxis

The American College of Chest Physicians (ACCP) guidelines for deep vein thrombosis (DVT) prophylaxis utilizing the venous thromboembolism (VTE) risk stratification systems were endorsed by the SAGES guidelines committee although they are not specifically directed at laparoscopic surgery patients (Gould et al. 2012; Richardson et al. 2017). There was a statistically significant reduction in VTE risk in laparoscopic procedures as seen in a study comparing the incidence of VTE following laparoscopic versus open surgery in 138,595 patients (Vedovati et al. 2014). Based on a meta-analysis on laparoscopic cholecystectomy patients routine use of VTE chemoprophylaxis showed no significant benefit and suggested its use only in higher risk patients based on risk stratification (Rondelli et al. 2013). Risk of bleeding should be considered when evaluating for chemoprophylaxis postoperatively. Although the optimal agent, dosing, duration, and timing of pharmacologic prophylaxis was not determined in the SAGES guidelines, ACCP guidelines recommend heparin and mechanical prophylaxis with elastic stockings or intermittent pneumatic compression in high-risk patients.

Acute Acalculous Cholecystitis

See Table 14.

Acute acalculous cholecystitis (AAC) is acute cholecystitis in the absence of gallstones, a rare but lethal condition, with a mortality rate of 30% (Kalliafas et al. 1998). A high index of suspicion is needed as it has no typical presentation, so diagnosis can be challenging and is a serious problem as can progress rapidly with a high prevalence of gangrene and perforation. It is usually seen in patients hospitalized for serious illnesses like trauma and burns but is not limited to critical illness. It can occur after gastrointestinal surgery and in the postoperative period is a devastating condition. It is seen more often in males (80%), especially elderly (Ryu et al. 2003).

Diagnosis of AAC can be made with use of US or CT abdomen accurately (Crichlow et al. 2012). US features for AAC are GB wall thickness of

Table 14 Risk factors for AAC

Risk factors
Burns
Trauma
Prolonged parenteral nutrition
Uncontrolled diabetes
Congestive heart failure
Vascular disease
Acquired immune deficiency syndrome
Drugs like hormonal agents and thiazides

more than 3.5 mm, subseroral edema or pericholecystic fluid, distention of more than 5 cm (without associated ascites or hypoalbuminemia) intramural gas and mucosal sloughing (Barie and Eachempati 2010).

E. coli and other gram-negative enteric bacteria are most frequently isolated. HIV-infected patients may have CMV, Cryptosporidium, *Mycobacterium* TB, MAI, or fungal infection as the agent (Elwood 2008). Bile stasis is implicated in its pathogenesis. Bile compounds like lysophosphatidyl choline and β glucuronidase may have a role, leading to inflammation of the gallbladder wall (Neiderhiser 1986; Kouroumalis et al. 1983). Infection with bacteria is a secondary event. Increasing rates of AAC is attributed to obesity and fat in the gallbladder wall.

Traditionally cholecystectomy has usually been the treatment but percutaneous cholecystostomy with antibiotics is emerging as an alternative (Glenn and Becker 1982; Horn et al. 2015). Percutaneous cholecystostomy is adequate in 85–90% of patients (Park et al. 2019; Akhan et al. 2002).

Cholecystectomy may be performed after the resolution of cholecystitis and optimization of associated medical illnesses to prevent recurrent cholecystitis.

Functional Gallbladder Disorder

Functional disorders of the gallbladder include acalculous biliary pain or biliary dyskinesia or dysmotility and Sphincter of Oddi dysfunction (SOD). Functional gallbladder disorder is biliary pain which is not due to structural disease. A previous classification (Milwaukee) defined type 1 as biliary type pain associated with abnormal liver/pancreatic chemistries in association with biliary or pancreatic changes. Type 2 refers to either abnormal liver or pancreatic chemistries, with either biliary or pancreatic ductal dilatation. Type 3 was based only on symptoms. Rome IV has eliminated type 3 (Geenen et al. 1989). According to the Rome IV criteria, Sphincter of Oddi disorders are now classified as functional biliary sphincter disorder and functional pancreatic sphincter disorder (Cotton et al. 2016).

According to the Rome IV criteria, biliary pain is defined as pain in the epigastrium or RUQ that meets the following criteria:

Builds up to a steady level and lasts at least 30 min
Occurs at different intervals
Is severe enough to interrupt daily activities or lead to an emergency department visit
Is not significantly related to bowel movements (< 20%) or relieved by postural change or acid suppression

It is more common in women and young to middle age. Pathophysiology is poorly understood, but dysmotility and crystal formation have been suggested. These patients should be evaluated with liver enzymes, pancreatic enzymes, and abdominal ultrasound. Cholecystokinin cholescintigraphy may be used to measure gallbladder ejection fraction. Normal GB EF is 35%. A low gallbladder EF is supportive of diagnosis. There is insufficient evidence on the role of cholecystectomy in patients with normal EF. In a recent study looked at the utility of scintigraphic studies in evaluation of chronic GB disease by reviewing 366 hepatobiliary scintigraphic studies the authors noted that the findings like small bowel delayed transit, GB filling time, and reversal of normal GB and small bowel filling sequence on HB scanning are not associated with GB EF. GB EF according to the authors should continue to be used as a diagnostic tool for chronic gallbladder disease (Christensen et al. 2018).

Chronic pain after laparoscopic cholecystectomy is not as common as with open cholecystectomy and appears to be associated with the intensity of acute postoperative pain (Bisgaard et al. 2005; Ahmed et al. 2008). This is a difficult issue for the patient and physician, and there is not much literature on its prevalence. Usually no clear etiology is found.

Biliary Strictures

Biliary strictures may be benign or malignant (Kapoor et al. 2018). Causes of benign biliary strictures include iatrogenic causes like biliary or hepatic surgery, chronic pancreatitis, parasites, and primary sclerosing cholangitis (Ferreira et al. 2016). Patients may present with abnormal liver biochemistry or obstructive jaundice. Differentiation whether stricture is benign or malignant maybe difficult especially in older people. The diagnosis of biliary lesions and strictures, and differentiating benign from malignant is important in the precise diagnosis of inflammatory activity and in management (Rey et al. 2014). The accurate assessment of bile duct stenosis may require MRCP, ERCP, EUS, and or spyglass technique of cholangioscopy. Brush cytology is the preferred investigation method for strictures. Cholangioscopy allows direct visualization, therapeutic maneuvers of the biliary ductal system and opportunity for obtaining sample for cytology (Ayoub et al. 2018). Cholangioscopy-guided biopsy appears to have the potential to overcome the problems associated with inadequate tissue sampling.

Key Points

The burden of gallstone disease is impressive because of its high frequency, relationship to advancing age, and the rising cost of care.

- Over 700,000 cholecystectomies are performed in the United States annually.
- With increasing obesity and aging populations, there is rising incidence and severity of gallstone disease.
- Gallstones are formed in the gallbladder or bile ducts, of cholesterol or bile pigments. Most gallstones are cholesterol stones.
- The risk of gallstones at age 80 years is near 50%.
- Asymptomatic in most people; about 20% develop symptoms, necessitating cholecystectomy in 1–2% yearly.
- Abdominal ultrasound is the preferred initial imaging technique in suspected acute cholecystitis, because of low cost, easy availability, non-invasive nature and high accuracy for gallbladder stones.
- Ultrasound abdomen has low sensitivity in detecting microlithiasis (50%).

- The combination of sonographic Murphy sign, gallbladder wall thickening > 3 mm, pericholecystic fluid are major criteria for diagnosis of acute cholecystitis. Biliary dilation and gallbladder hydrops are minor criteria.
- Hepatobiliary iminodiacetic acid scan (HIDA scan) has the highest sensitivity and specificity for acute cholecystitis, but the long time required to perform the test and exposure to ionizing radiation limit its use.
- Acute cholecystitis is an inflammatory process at the beginning.
- The use of antibiotics may be restricted to those likely to develop sepsis.
- Laparoscopic cholecystectomy for acute cholecystitis is safe and feasible and has a low complication rate in the older adult.

Key Points 2

- The incidence of choledocholithiasis in patients with cholelithiasis is 5–20%, of which 5% are asymptomatic.
- Charcot's triad had low sensitivity but high specificity.
- The complication of CBD stones are acute cholangitis acute pancreatitis and biliary cirrhosis.
- Sensitivity of abdominal US in detection of CBD stones is only 65–70%; however specificity is 90%.
- Endoscopic US has a sensitivity of 90% and a higher specificity.
- CT scan has variable accuracy for choledocholithiasis but lower than MRCP and EUS.
- ERCP should only be performed for therapeutic purposes and not as a diagnostic test.
- Ascending cholangitis should be treated with early biliary drainage.

References

Acalovschi M, Buzas C, Radu C, Grigorescu M. Hepatitis C virus infection is a risk factor for gallstone disease: a prospective hospital-based study of patients with chronic viral C hepatitis. J Viral Hepat. 2009;16(12):860–6.

Acosta JM, Katkhouda N, Debian KA, Groshen SG, Tsao-Wei DD, Berne TV. Early ductal decompression versus conservative management for gallstone pancreatitis with ampullary obstruction: a prospective randomized clinical trial. Ann Surg. 2006;243(1):33–40.

Adler DG. Endoscopic gallbladder drainage. Endosc. 2019;114(5):700–2.

Aerts R, Penninckx F. The burden of gallstone disease in Europe. Aliment Pharmacol Ther. 2003;18(s3):49–53.

Ahlberg J. Serum lipid levels and hyperlipoproteinaemia in gallstone patients. Acta Chir Scand. 1979;145(6):373–7.

Ahmed BH, Ahmed A, Tan D, Awad ZT, Al-Aali AY, Kilkenny J 3rd, et al. Post-laparoscopic cholecystectomy pain: effects of intraperitoneal local anesthetics on pain control – a randomized prospective double-blinded placebo-controlled trial. Am Surg. 2008;74(3):201–9.

Akhan O, Akıncı D, Özmen MN. Percutaneous cholecystostomy. Eur J Radiol. 2002;43(3):229–36.

Alemi F, Seiser N, Ayloo S. Gallstone disease: cholecystitis, Mirizzi syndrome, Bouveret syndrome, gallstone ileus. Surg Clin North Am. 2019;99(2):231–44.

Alvaro D, Angelico M, Gandin C, Ginanni Corradini S, Capocaccia L. Physico-chemical factors predisposing to pigment gallstone formation in liver cirrhosis. J Hepatol. 1990;10(2):228–34.

Amaral JF, Thompson WR. Gallbladder disease in the morbidly obese. Am J Surg. 1985;149(4):551–7.

Angelico M, Gandin C, Canuzzi P, Bertasi S, Cantafora A, De Santis A, et al. Gallstones in cystic fibrosis: a critical reappraisal. Hepatology (Baltimore, Md). 1991;14(5):768–75.

Angelin B. Effect of thiazide treatment on biliary lipid composition in healthy volunteers. Eur J Clin Pharmacol. 1989;37(1):95–6.

Ansaloni L, Pisano M, Coccolini F, Peitzmann AB, Fingerhut A, Catena F, et al. WSES guidelines on acute calculous cholecystitis. World J Emerg Surg. 2016;11(1):25.

Apstein MD, Dalecki-Chipperfield K. Spinal cord injury is a risk factor for gallstone disease. Gastroenterology. 1987;92(4):966–8.

Ata N, Kucukazman M, Yavuz B, Bulus H, Dal K, Ertugrul DT, et al. The metabolic syndrome is associated with complicated gallstone disease. Can J Gastroenterol = J Can de Gastroenterol. 2011;25(5):274–6.

Attasaranya S, Fogel EL, Lehman GA. Choledocholithiasis, ascending cholangitis, and gallstone pancreatitis. Med Clin North Am. 2008;92(4):925–60, x.

Ayoub F, Yang D, Draganov PV. Cholangioscopy in the digital era. Transl Gastroenterol Hepatol. 2018;3:82.

Balmadrid B. Recent advances in management of acalculous cholecystitis. F1000Research. 2018;7:1660.

Banim PJ, Luben RN, Wareham NJ, Sharp SJ, Khaw KT, Hart AR. Physical activity reduces the risk of symptomatic gallstones: a prospective cohort study. Eur J Gastroenterol Hepatol. 2010;22(8):983–8.

Barbara L, Sama C, Morselli Labate AM, Taroni F, Rusticali AG, Festi D, et al. A population study on the prevalence of gallstone disease: the Sirmione study. Hepatology (Baltimore, Md). 1987;7(5):913–7.

Barie PS, Eachempati SR. Acute Acalculous cholecystitis. Gastroenterol Clin. 2010;39(2):343–57.

Bateson MC. Gallstones and cholecystectomy in modern Britain. Postgrad Med J. 2000;76(901):700–3.

Beltran MA, Csendes A, KSJWJoS C. The relationship of Mirizzi syndrome and cholecystoenteric fistula: validation of a modified classification. World J Surg. 2008;32(10):2237–43.

Bennett GL, Balthazar EJ. Ultrasound and CT evaluation of emergent gallbladder pathology. Radiol Clin. 2003;41(6):1203–16.

Bergman S, Sourial N, Vedel I, Hanna WC, Fraser SA, Newman D, et al. Gallstone disease in the elderly: are older patients managed differently? Surg Endosc. 2011;25(1):55–61.

Bisgaard T, Rosenberg J, Kehlet H. From acute to chronic pain after laparoscopic cholecystectomy: a prospective follow-up analysis. Scand J Gastroenterol. 2005;40(11):1358–64.

Boender J, Nix GA, de Ridder MA, Dees J, Schutte HE, van Buuren HR, et al. Endoscopic sphincterotomy and biliary drainage in patients with cholangitis due to common bile duct stones. Am J Gastroenterol. 1995;90(2):233–8.

Bonatsos G, Birbas K, Toutouzas K, Durakis N. Laparoscopic cholecystectomy in adults with sickle cell disease. Surg Endosc. 2001;15(8):816–9.

Brink MA, Slors JF, Keulemans YC, Mok KS, De Waart DR, Carey MC, et al. Enterohepatic cycling of bilirubin: a putative mechanism for pigment gallstone formation in ileal Crohn's disease. Gastroenterology. 1999;116(6):1420–7.

Bugliosi TF, Meloy TD, Vukov LF. Acute abdominal pain in the elderly. Ann Emerg Med. 1990;19(12):1383–6.

Buxbaum JL, Abbas Fehmi SM, Sultan S, Fishman DS, Qumseya BJ, Cortessis VK, et al. ASGE guideline on the role of endoscopy in the evaluation and management of choledocholithiasis. Gastrointest Endosc. 2019;89(6):1075–105.

Carey MC, Cahalane MJ. Whither biliary sludge? Gastroenterology. 1988;95(2):508–23.

Carrilho-Ribeiro L, Pinto-Correia A, Velosa J, Carneiro De Moura M. A ten-year prospective study on gallbladder stone recurrence after successful extracorporeal shockwave lithotripsy. Scand J Gastroenterol. 2006;41(3):338–42.

Chandra S, Klair JS, Soota K, Livorsi DJ, Johlin FC. Endoscopic retrograde Cholangio-Pancreatography-obtained bile culture can guide antibiotic therapy in acute cholangitis. Dig Dis. 2019;37(2):155–60.

Chang Y, Sung E, Ryu S, Park Y-W, Jang YM, Park M. Insulin resistance is associated with gallstones even in non-obese, non-diabetic Korean men. J Korean Med Sci. 2008;23(4):644–50.

Chapman BA, Wilson IR, Frampton CM, Chisholm RJ, Stewart NR, Eagar GM, et al. Prevalence of gallbladder disease in diabetes mellitus. Dig Dis Sci. 1996;41(11):2222–8.

Chen W, Mo JJ, Lin L, Li CQ, Zhang JF. Diagnostic value of magnetic resonance cholangiopancreatography in choledocholithiasis. World J Gastroenterol. 2015;21(11):3351–60.

Christensen CT, Peacock JG, Vroman PJ, Banks KP. Scintigraphic findings beyond ejection fraction on hepatobiliary scintigraphy: are they correlated with chronic gallbladder disease? Clin Nucl Med. 2018;43(10):721–7.

Clemente G, Tringali A, De Rose AM, Panettieri E, Murazio M, Nuzzo G, et al. Mirizzi syndrome: diagnosis and Management of a Challenging Biliary Disease %J Canadian journal of gastroenterology and. Hepatology. 2018;2018:6.

Collins C, Maguire D, Ireland A, Fitzgerald E, O'Sullivan GC. A prospective study of common bile duct calculi in patients undergoing laparoscopic cholecystectomy: natural history of choledocholithiasis revisited. Ann Surg. 2004;239(1):28–33.

Comess LJ, Bennett PH, Burch TA. Clinical gallbladder disease in pima Indians. N Engl J Med. 1967;277(17):894–8.

Conte D, Fraquelli M, Fornari F, Lodi L, Bodini P, Buscarini L. Close relation between cirrhosis and gallstones: cross-sectional and longitudinal survey. Arch Intern Med. 1999;159(1):49–52.

Cotton PB, Garrow DA, Gallagher J, Romagnuolo J. Risk factors for complications after ERCP: a multivariate analysis of 11,497 procedures over 12 years. Gastrointest Endosc. 2009;70(1):80–8.

Cotton PB, Elta GH, Carter CR, Pasricha PJ, Corazziari ES. Gallbladder and sphincter of Oddi disorders. Gastroenterology. 2016;150(6):1420–9.e2.

Crespi M, Montecamozzo G, Foschi D. Diagnosis and treatment of biliary fistulas in the laparoscopic era. Gastroenterol Res Pract. 2016;2016:6293538.

Crichlow L, Walcott-Sapp S, Major J, Jaffe B, Bellows CF. Acute acalculous cholecystitis after gastrointestinal surgery. Am Surg. 2012;78(2):220–4.

Csendes A, Diaz JC, Burdiles P, Maluenda F, Nava O. Mirizzi syndrome and cholecystobiliary fistula: a unifying classification. Br J Surg. 1989;76(11):1139–43.

Dasari BVM, Tan CJ, Gurusamy KS, Martin DJ, Kirk G, McKie L, et al. Surgical versus endoscopic treatment of bile duct stones. Cochrane Database Syst Rev. 2013;9:CD003327.

De la Serna S, Ruano A, Perez-Jimenez A, Rojo M, Avellana R, Garcia-Botella A, et al. Safety and feasibility of cholecystectomy in octogenarians. Analysis of a single center series of 316 patients. HPB (Oxford). 2019;21(11):1570–6.

Dervisoglou A, Tsiodras S, Kanellakopoulou K, Pinis S, Galanakis N, Pierakakis S, et al. The value of chemoprophylaxis against Enterococcus species in elective cholecystectomy: a randomized study of cefuroxime vs ampicillin-sulbactam. Arch Surg (Chicago, Ill: 1960). 2006;141(12):1162–7.

Dowling RH. Review: pathogenesis of gallstones. Aliment Pharmacol Ther. 2000;14(Suppl 2):39–47.

EASL. Clinical practice guidelines on the prevention, diagnosis and treatment of gallstones. J Hepatol. 2016;65(1):146–81.

Elmunzer BJ, Noureldin M, Morgan KA, Adams DB, Cote GA, Waljee AK. The impact of cholecystectomy after endoscopic Sphincterotomy for complicated gallstone disease. Am J Gastroenterol. 2017;112(10):1596–602.

Elwood DR. Cholecystitis. Surg Clin North Am. 2008;88(6):1241–52, viii.

Ercan M, Bostanci EB, Ozer I, Ulas M, Ozogul YB, Teke Z, et al. Postoperative hemorrhagic complications after elective laparoscopic cholecystectomy in patients receiving long-term anticoagulant therapy. Langenbeck's Arch Surg. 2010;395(3):247–53.

Erlinger S. Gallstones in obesity and weight loss. Eur J Gastroenterol Hepatol. 2000;12(12):1347–52.

Everhart JE. Contributions of obesity and weight loss to gallstone disease. Ann Intern Med. 1993; 119(10):1029–35.

Everhart JE, Ruhl CE. Burden of digestive diseases in the United States part III: liver, biliary tract, and pancreas. Gastroenterology. 2009a;136(4):1134–44.

Everhart JE, Ruhl CE. Burden of digestive diseases in the United States part I: overall and upper gastrointestinal diseases. Gastroenterology. 2009b;136(2):376–86.

Everhart JE, Khare M, Hill M, Maurer KR. Prevalence and ethnic differences in gallbladder disease in the United States. Gastroenterology. 1999;117(3):632–9.

Ferreira R, Loureiro R, Nunes N, Santos AA, Maio R, Cravo M, et al. Role of endoscopic retrograde cholangiopancreatography in the management of benign biliary strictures: what's new? World of J Gastrointest Endosc. 2016;8(4):220–31.

Festi D, Dormi A, Capodicasa S, Staniscia T, Attili AF, Loria P, et al. Incidence of gallstone disease in Italy: results from a multicenter, population-based Italian study (the MICOL project). World J Gastroenterol. 2008;14(34):5282–9.

Fleming CA, Ismail M, Kavanagh RG, Heneghan HM, Prichard RS, Geoghegan J, et al. Clinical and survival outcomes using percutaneous cholecystostomy tube alone or subsequent interval cholecystectomy to treat acute cholecystitis. J Gastrointest Surg. 2019;21(2):302–11.

Geenen JE, Hogan WJ, Dodds WJ, Toouli J, Venu RP. The efficacy of endoscopic sphincterotomy after cholecystectomy in patients with sphincter-of-Oddi dysfunction. N Engl J Med. 1989;320(2):82–7.

Gibney EJ. Asymptomatic gallstones. Br J Surg. 1990;77(4):368–72.

Giljaca V, Gurusamy KS, Takwoingi Y, Higgie D, Poropat G, Stimac D, et al. Endoscopic ultrasound versus magnetic resonance cholangiopancreatography for common bile duct stones. Cochrane Database Syst Rev. 2015;2:Cd011549.

Gill KS, Chapman AH, Weston MJ. The changing face of emphysematous cholecystitis. Br J Radiol. 1997;70(838):986–91.

Glenn F. Surgical management of acute cholecystitis in patients 65 years of age and older. Ann Surg. 1981;193(1):56–9.

Glenn F, Becker CG. Acute acalculous cholecystitis. An increasing entity. Ann Surg. 1982;195(2):131–6.

Gomes CA, Junior CS, Di Saverio S, Sartelli M, Kelly MD, Gomes CC, et al. Acute calculus cholecystitis: review

of current best practices. World J Gastrointest Surg. 2017;9(5):118–26.

Gomi H, Solomkin JS, Takada T, Strasberg SM, Pitt HA, Yoshida M, et al. TG13 antimicrobial therapy for acute cholangitis and cholecystitis. J Hepatobiliary Pancreat Sci. 2013;20(1):60–70.

Gomi H, Solomkin JS, Schlossberg D, Okamoto K, Takada T, Strasberg SM, et al. Tokyo guidelines 2018: antimicrobial therapy for acute cholangitis and cholecystitis. J Hepatobiliary Pancreat Sci. 2018;25(1): 3–16.

Gould MK, Garcia DA, Wren SM, Karanicolas PJ, Arcelus JI, Heit JA, et al. Prevention of VTE in nonorthopedic surgical patients: antithrombotic therapy and prevention of thrombosis, 9th ed: American college of chest physicians evidence-based clinical practice guidelines. Chest. 2012;141(2 Suppl):e227S–e77S.

Gouveia C, Loureiro R, Ferreira R, Oliveira Ferreira A, Santos AA, Santos MPC, et al. Performance of the Choledocholithiasis diagnostic score in patients with acute cholecystitis. GE Port J Gastroenterol. 2018;25(1):24–9.

Grand D, Horton KM, Fishman EK. CT of the gallbladder: spectrum of disease. AJR Am J Roentgenol. 2004;183(1):163–70.

Guglielmi FW, Boggio-Bertinet D, Federico A, Forte GB, Guglielmi A, Loguercio C, et al. Total parenteral nutrition-related gastroenterological complications. Dig Liver Dis. 2006;38(9):623–42.

Gurusamy KS, Davidson BR. Gallstones. BMJ. 2014;348: g2669.

Gurusamy K, Samraj K, Gluud C, Wilson E, Davidson BR. Meta-analysis of randomized controlled trials on the safety and effectiveness of early versus delayed laparoscopic cholecystectomy for acute cholecystitis. Br J Surg. 2010;97(2):141–50.

Gurusamy KS, Davidson C, Gluud C, Davidson BR. Early versus delayed laparoscopic cholecystectomy for people with acute cholecystitis. Cochrane Database Syst Rev. 2013;6:Cd005440.

Haley K. Congenital hemolytic anemia. Med Clin North Am. 2017;101(2):361–74.

Harness JK, Strodel WE, Talsma SE. Symptomatic biliary tract disease in the elderly patient. Am Surg. 1986;52(8):442–5.

Hemminki K, Hemminki O, Forsti A, Sundquist K, Sundquist J, Li X. Familial risks for gallstones in the population of Sweden. BMJ Open Gastroenterol. 2017;4(1):e000188.

Hendrickson M, Naparst TR. Abdominal surgical emergencies in the elderly. Emerg Med Clin North Am. 2003;21(4):937–69.

Holzman RS, Oram V, Rahimian J, Wilson T. Pyogenic liver abscess: recent trends in etiology and mortality. Clin Infect Dis. 2004;39(11):1654–9.

Horn T, Christensen SD, Kirkegård J, Larsen LP, Knudsen AR, Mortensen FV. Percutaneous cholecystostomy is an effective treatment option for acute calculous cholecystitis: a 10-year experience. HPB. 2015;17(4):326–31.

Hu KC, Chu CH, Wang HY, Chang WH, Lin SC, Liu CC, et al. How does aging affect presentation and Management of Biliary Stones? J Am Geriatr Soc. 2016;64(11):2330–5.

Imaoka Y, Itamoto T, Nakahara H, Oishi K, Matsugu Y, Urushihara T. Physiological and operative severity score for the enUmeration of mortality and morbidity and modified physiological and operative severity score for the enUmeration of mortality and morbidity for the mortality prediction among nonagenarians undergoing emergency surgery. J Surg Res. 2017;210:198–203.

Ingraham AM, Cohen ME, Ko CY, Hall BL. A current profile and assessment of North American cholecystectomy: results from the American college of surgeons national surgical quality improvement program. J Am Coll Surg. 2010;211(2):176–86.

Irojah B, Bell T, Grim R, Martin J, Ahuja V. Are they too old for surgery? safety of cholecystectomy in superelderly patients (≥ age 90). Perm J. 2017;21:16–013.

Itoi T, Takada T, Hwang TL, Endo I, Akazawa K, Miura F, et al. Percutaneous and endoscopic gallbladder drainage for acute cholecystitis: international multicenter comparative study using propensity score-matched analysis. J Hepatobiliary Pancreat Sci. 2017;24(6):362–8.

Jansen S, Stodolski M, Zirngibl H, Godde D, Ambe PC. Advanced gallbladder inflammation is a risk factor for gallbladder perforation in patients with acute cholecystitis. World J Emerg Surg. 2018;13:9.

Johnston DE, Kaplan MM. Pathogenesis and Treatment of Gallstones. N Engl J Med. 1993;328(6):412–21.

Kalliafas S, Ziegler DW, Flancbaum L, Choban PS. Acute acalculous cholecystitis: incidence, risk factors, diagnosis, and outcome. Am Surg. 1998;64(5):471–5.

Kao LS, Kuhr CS, Flum DR. Should cholecystectomy be performed for asymptomatic cholelithiasis in transplant patients? J Am Coll Surg. 2003;197(2):302–12.

Kapoor BS, Mauri G, Lorenz JM. Management of Biliary Strictures: state-of-the-art review. Radiology. 2018;289(3):590–603.

Katsinelos P, Lazaraki G, Chatzimavroudis G, Terzoudis S, Gatopoulou A, Xanthis A, et al. The impact of age on the incidence and severity of post-endoscopic retrograde cholangiopancreatography pancreatitis. Ann Gastroenterol. 2018;31(1):96–101.

Khan ZS, Livingston EH, Huerta S. Reassessing the need for prophylactic surgery in patients with porcelain gallbladder: case series and systematic review of the literature. Arch Surg (Chicago, Ill: 1960). 2011;146(10):1143–7.

Kiewiet JJ, Leeuwenburgh MM, Bipat S, Bossuyt PM, Stoker J, Boermeester MA. A systematic review and meta-analysis of diagnostic performance of imaging in acute cholecystitis. Radiology. 2012;264(3):708–20.

Kimura Y, Takada T, Kawarada Y, Nimura Y, Hirata K, Sekimoto M, et al. Definitions, pathophysiology, and epidemiology of acute cholangitis and cholecystitis: Tokyo guidelines. J Hepato-Biliary-Pancreat Surg. 2007;14(1):15–26.

Kiriyama S, Kozaka K, Takada T, Strasberg SM, Pitt HA, Gabata T, et al. Tokyo guidelines 2018: diagnostic criteria and severity grading of acute cholangitis (with videos). J Hepatobiliary Pancreat Sci. 2018;25(1):17–30.

Knab LM, Boller AM, Mahvi DM. Cholecystitis. Surg Clin North Am. 2014;94(2):455–70.

Komatsu S, Tsuchida S, Tsukamoto T, Wakahara T, Ashitani H, Ueno N, et al. Current role of percutaneous transhepatic gallbladder aspiration: from palliative to curative management for acute cholecystitis. J Hepatobiliary Pancreat Sci. 2016;23(11):708–14.

Kouroumalis E, Hopwood D, Ross PE, Milne G, Bouchier IA. Gallbladder epithelial acid hydrolases in human cholecystitis. J Pathol. 1983;139(2):179–91.

Krawczyk M, Miquel JF, Stokes CS, Zuniga S, Hampe J, Mittal B, et al. Genetics of biliary lithiasis from an ethnic perspective. Clin Res Hepatol Gastroenterol. 2013;37(2):119–25.

Lai EC, Mok FP, Tan ES, Lo CM, Fan ST, You KT, et al. Endoscopic biliary drainage for severe acute cholangitis. N Engl J Med. 1992;326(24):1582–6.

Lam CM, Murray FE, Cuschieri A. Increased cholecystectomy rate after the introduction of laparoscopic cholecystectomy in Scotland. Gut. 1996;38(2):282–4.

Lee SP, Maher K, Nicholls JF. Origin and fate of biliary sludge. Gastroenterology. 1988;94(1):170–6.

Lee YS, Kang BK, Hwang IK, Kim J, Hwang JH. Longterm outcomes of symptomatic gallbladder sludge. J Clin Gastroenterol. 2015;49(7):594–8.

Leese T, Neoptolemos JP, Baker AR, Carr-Locke DL. Management of acute cholangitis and the impact of endoscopic sphincterotomy. Br J Surg. 1986;73(12):988–92.

Liang TJ, Liu SI, Chen YC, Chang PM, Huang WC, Chang HT, et al. Analysis of gallstone disease after gastric cancer surgery. Gastric Cancer: Off J Int Gastric Cancer Assoc and Jpn Gastric Cancer Assoc. 2017;20(5):895–903.

Loozen CS, Kortram K, Kornmann VN, van Ramshorst B, Vlaminckx B, Knibbe CA, et al. Randomized clinical trial of extended versus single-dose perioperative antibiotic prophylaxis for acute calculous cholecystitis. Br J Surg. 2017;104(2):e151–e7.

Lopez AJ, O'Keefe P, Morrissey M, Pickleman J. Ceftriaxone-induced Cholelithiasis. Ann Intern Med. 1991;115(9):712–4.

Loria P, Lonardo A, Lombardini S, Carulli L, Verrone A, Ganazzi D, et al. Gallstone disease in non-alcoholic fatty liver: prevalence and associated factors. J Gastroenterol Hepatol. 2005;20(8):1176–84.

Maclure KM, Hayes KC, Colditz GA, Stampfer MJ, Speizer FE, Willett WC. Weight, diet, and the risk of symptomatic gallstones in middle-aged women. N Engl J Med. 1989;321(9):563–9.

Magalhaes J, Rosa B, Cotter J. Endoscopic retrograde cholangiopancreatography for suspected choledocholithiasis: from guidelines to clinical practice. World J Gastrointest Endosc. 2015;7(2):128–34.

Magouliotis DE, Tasiopoulou VS, Svokos AA, Svokos KA, Chatedaki C, Sioka E, et al. Ursodeoxycholic acid in the prevention of gallstone formation after bariatric surgery: an updated systematic review and meta-analysis. Obes Surg. 2017;27(11):3021–30.

Maki T. Pathogenesis of calcium bilirubinate gallstone: role of *E. coli*, beta-glucuronidase and coagulation by inorganic ions, polyelectrolytes and agitation. Ann Surg. 1966;164(1):90–100.

Maple JT, Ben-Menachem T, Anderson MA, Appalaneni V, Banerjee S, Cash BD, et al. The role of endoscopy in the evaluation of suspected choledocholithiasis. Gastrointest Endosc. 2010;71(1):1–9.

Maringhini A, Ciambra M, Baccelliere P, Raimondo M, Orlando A, Tine F, et al. Biliary sludge and gallstones in pregnancy: incidence, risk factors, and natural history. Ann Intern Med. 1993;119(2):116–20.

McSherry CK, Ferstenberg H, Calhoun WF, Lahman E, Virshup M. The natural history of diagnosed gallstone disease in symptomatic and asymptomatic patients. Ann Surg. 1985;202(1):59–63.

Melmer A, Sturm W, Kuhnert B, Engl-Prosch J, Ress C, Tschoner A, et al. Incidence of gallstone formation and cholecystectomy 10 years after bariatric surgery. Obes Surg. 2015;25(7):1171–6.

Moore SW. Intramural formation of gallstones. Arch Surg. 1937;34(3):410–23.

Morfin E, Ponka JL, Brush BE. Gangrenous cholecystitis. Arch Surg (Chicago, Ill: 1960). 1968;96(4):567–73.

Mori Y, Itoi T, Baron TH, Takada T, Strasberg SM, Pitt HA, et al. Tokyo guidelines 2018: management strategies for gallbladder drainage in patients with acute cholecystitis (with videos). J Hepatobiliary Pancreat Sci. 2018;25(1):87–95.

Morris BS, Balpande PR, Morani AC, Chaudhary RK, Maheshwari M, Raut AA. The CT appearances of gallbladder perforation. Br J Radiol. 2007;80(959):898–901.

Nassar Y, Richter S. Management of complicated gallstones in the elderly: comparing surgical and non-surgical treatment options. Gastroenterol Rep. 2019;7(3):205–11.

Nebiker CA, Baierlein SA, Beck S, von Flue M, Ackermann C, Peterli R. Is routine MR cholangiopancreatography (MRCP) justified prior to cholecystectomy? Langenbeck's Arch Surg. 2009;394(6):1005–10.

Neiderhiser DH. Acute acalculous cholecystitis induced by lysophosphatidylcholine. Am J Pathol. 1986;124(3):559–63.

Nenner RP, Imperato PJ, Rosenberg C, Ronberg E. Increased cholecystectomy rates among Medicare patients after the introduction of laparoscopic cholecystectomy. J Community Health. 1994;19(6):409–15.

Nervi F, Miquel JF, Alvarez M, Ferreccio C, García-Zattera MJ, González R, et al. Gallbladder disease is associated with insulin resistance in a high risk Hispanic population. J Hepatol. 2006;45(2):299–305.

Nesland JM. Chronic cholecystitis. Ultrastruct Pathol. 2004;28(3):121.

Nielsen LB, Harboe KM, Bardram L. Cholecystectomy for the elderly: no hesitation for otherwise healthy patients. Surg Endosc. 2014;28(1):171–7.

Nomura H, Kashiwagi S, Hayashi J, Kajiyama W, Ikematsu H, Noguchi A, et al. Prevalence of gallstone disease in a general population of Okinawa, Japan. Am J Epidemiol. 1988;128(3):598–605.

Nzenza TC, Al-Habbal Y, Guerra GR, Manolas S, Yong T, McQuillan T. Recurrent common bile duct stones as a late complication of endoscopic sphincterotomy. BMC Gastroenterol. 2018;18(1):39.

O'Donnell LD, Heaton KW. Recurrence and re-recurrence of gall stones after medical dissolution: a longterm follow up. Gut. 1988;29(5):655–8.

Oppenheimer DC, Rubens DJ. Sonography of acute cholecystitis and its mimics. Radiol Clin. 2019;57(3):535–48.

Overby DW, Apelgren KN, Richardson W, Fanelli R. SAGES guidelines for the clinical application of laparoscopic biliary tract surgery. Surg Endosc. 2010;24(10):2368–86.

Park JK, Yang JI, Wi JW, Park JK, Lee KH, Lee KT, et al. Long-term outcome and recurrence factors after percutaneous cholecystostomy as a definitive treatment for acute cholecystitis. J Gastroenterol Hepatol. 2019;34(4):784–90.

Peery AF, Crockett SD, Murphy CC, Lund JL, Dellon ES, Williams JL, et al. Burden and cost of gastrointestinal, liver, and pancreatic diseases in the United States: update 2018. Gastroenterology. 2019;156(1):254–72. e11.

Petitti DB, Friedman GD, Klatsky AL. Association of a history of gallbladder disease with a reduced concentration of high-density-lipoprotein cholesterol. N Engl J Med. 1981;304(23):1396–8.

Pisano M, Ceresoli M, Cimbanassi S, Gurusamy K, Coccolini F, Borzellino G, et al. 2017 WSES and SICG guidelines on acute calcolous cholecystitis in elderly population. World J Emerg Surg. 2019;14(1):10.

Pitt HA, Lewinski MA, Muller EL, Porter-Fink V, DenBesten L. Ileal resection-induced gallstones: altered bilirubin or cholesterol metabolism? Surgery. 1984;96(2):154–62.

Portincasa P, Di Ciaula A, de Bari O, Garruti G, Palmieri VO, Wang DQ. Management of gallstones and its related complications. Expert Rev Gastroenterol Hepatol. 2016;10(1):93–112.

Radosa C, Schaab F, Hofmockel T, Kuhn JP, Hoffmann RT. Percutaneous biliary and gallbladder interventions. Radiologe. 2019;59(4):342–7.

Ralls PW, Colletti PM, Lapin SA, Chandrasoma P, Boswell WD Jr, Ngo C, et al. Real-time sonography in suspected acute cholecystitis. Prospective evaluation of primary and secondary signs. Radiology. 1985;155(3):767–71.

Reuken PA, Torres D, Baier M, Loffler B, Lubbert C, Lippmann N, et al. Risk factors for multi-drug resistant pathogens and failure of empiric first-line therapy in acute cholangitis. PLoS One. 2017;12(1):e0169900.

Rey JW, Hansen T, Dumcke S, Tresch A, Kramer K, Galle PR, et al. Efficacy of SpyGlass(TM)-directed biopsy compared to brush cytology in obtaining adequate tissue for diagnosis in patients with biliary strictures. World of J Gastrointest Endosc. 2014;6(4):137–43.

Riall TS, Zhang D, Townsend CM Jr, Kuo YF, Goodwin JS. Failure to perform cholecystectomy for acute cholecystitis in elderly patients is associated with increased morbidity, mortality, and cost. J Am Coll Surg. 2010;210(5):668–77–9.

Riall TS, Adhikari D, Parmar AD, Linder SK, Dimou FM, Crowell W, et al. The risk paradox: use of elective cholecystectomy in older patients is independent of their risk of developing complications. J Am Coll Surg. 2015;220(4):682–90.

Richardson WS, Hamad GG, Stefanidis D. SAGES VTE prophylaxis for laparoscopic surgery guidelines: an update. Surg Endosc. 2017;31(2):501–3.

Rondelli F, Manina G, Agnelli G, Becattini C. Venous thromboembolism after laparoscopic cholecystectomy: clinical burden and prevention. Surg Endosc. 2013;27(6):1860–4.

Roslyn JJ, Pitt HA, Mann LL, Ament ME, DenBesten L. Gallbladder disease in patients on long-term parenteral nutrition. Gastroenterology. 1983;84(1):148–54.

Roslyn JJ, Thompson JE Jr, Darvin H, DenBesten L. Risk factors for gallbladder perforation. Am J Gastroenterol. 1987;82(7):636–40.

Rosseland AR, Glomsaker TB. Asymptomatic common bile duct stones. Eur J Gastroenterol Hepatol. 2000;12(11):1171–3.

Ruhl CE, Everhart JE. Association of diabetes, serum insulin, and C-peptide with gallbladder disease. Hepatology (Baltimore, Md). 2000;31(2):299–303.

Ryu JK, Ryu KH, Kim KH. Clinical features of acute acalculous cholecystitis. J Clin Gastroenterol. 2003;36(2):166–9.

Sampliner RE, Bennett PH, Comess LJ, Rose FA, Burch TA. Gallbladder disease in pima Indians. N Engl J Med. 1970;283(25):1358–64.

Sarin SK, Negi VS, Dewan R, Sasan S, Saraya A. High familial prevalence of gallstones in the first-degree relatives of gallstone patients. Hepatology (Baltimore, Md). 1995;22(1):138–41.

Schneider J, De Waha P, Hapfelmeier A, Feihl S, Rommler F, Schlag C, et al. Risk factors for increased antimicrobial resistance: a retrospective analysis of 309 acute cholangitis episodes. J Antimicrob Chemother. 2014;69(2):519–25.

Schnelldorfer T. Porcelain gallbladder: a benign process or concern for malignancy? J Gastrointest Surg. 2013;17(6):1161–8.

Seeto RK, Rockey DC. Pyogenic liver abscess. Changes in etiology, management, and outcome. Medicine. 1996;75(2):99–113.

Shaffer E. Epidemiology and risk factors for gallstone disease: has the paradigm changed in the 21st century? Curr Gastroenterol Rep. 2005;7(2):132–40.

Shaffer EA. Gallstone disease: epidemiology of gallbladder stone disease. Best Pract Res Clin Gastroenterol. 2006;20(6):981–96.

Shoda J, Tanaka N, Osuga T. Hepatolithiasis – epidemiology and pathogenesis update. Front Biosci. 2003;8:e398–409.

Siddiqui A, Kunda R, Tyberg A, Arain MA, Noor A, Mumtaz T, et al. Three-way comparative study of endoscopic ultrasound-guided transmural gallbladder drainage using lumen-apposing metal stents versus endoscopic transpapillary drainage versus

percutaneous cholecystostomy for gallbladder drainage in high-risk surgical patients with acute cholecystitis: clinical outcomes and success in an international. Multicenter Study Surg Endosc. 2019;33(4):1260–1270. https://doi.org/10.1007/s00464-018-6406-7

Singh V, Trikha B, Nain C, Singh K, Bose S. Epidemiology of gallstone disease in Chandigarh: a community-based study. Eur J Gastroenterol Hepatol. 2001;16(5):560–3.

Somjen GJ, Gilat T. Contribution of vesicular and micellar carriers to cholesterol transport in human bile. J Lipid Res. 1985;26(6):699–704.

Sousa M, Pinho R, Proença L, Rodrigues J, Silva J, Gomes C, et al. ASGE high-risk criteria for choledocholithiasis – are they applicable in cholecystectomized patients? Dig Liver Dis. 2019;51(1):75–8.

Spes CH, Angermann CE, Beyer RW, Schreiner J, Lehnert P, Kemkes BM, et al. Increased incidence of cholelithiasis in heart transplant recipients receiving cyclosporine therapy. J Heart Transplant. 1990;9(4):404–7.

Stampfer MJ, Maclure KM, Colditz GA, Manson JE, Willett WC. Risk of symptomatic gallstones in women with severe obesity. Am J Clin Nutr. 1992;55(3):652–8.

Stephen AE, Berger DL. Carcinoma in the porcelain gallbladder: a relationship revisited. Surgery. 2001;129(6):699–703.

Stinton LM, Shaffer EA. Epidemiology of gallbladder disease: cholelithiasis and cancer. Gut and Liver. 2012;6(2):172–87.

Suarez AL, LaBarre NT, Cotton PB, Payne KM, Cote GA, Elmunzer BJ. An assessment of existing risk stratification guidelines for the evaluation of patients with suspected choledocholithiasis. Surg Endosc. 2016;30(10):4613–8.

Sugiyama M, Atomi Y. Treatment of acute cholangitis due to choledocholithiasis in elderly and younger patients. Arch Surg (Chicago, Ill: 1960). 1997;132(10):1129–33.

Tambyraja AL, Kumar S, Nixon SJ. POSSUM scoring for laparoscopic cholecystectomy in the elderly. ANZ J Surg. 2005;75(7):550–2.

Tanaka A, Takada T, Kawarada Y, Nimura Y, Yoshida M, Miura F, et al. Antimicrobial therapy for acute cholangitis: Tokyo guidelines. J Hepato-Biliary-Pancreat Surg. 2007;14(1):59–67.

Tazuma S. Gallstone disease: epidemiology, pathogenesis, and classification of biliary stones (common bile duct and intrahepatic). Best Pract Res Clin Gastroenterol. 2006;20(6):1075–83.

Thakrar R, Thomson S, Monib S, Pakdemirli E. Calcified gallbladder cancer: is it preventable? J Surg Case Rep. 2019;2019(3):rjz069.

Thangavelu A, Rosenbaum S, Thangavelu D. Timing of cholecystectomy in acute cholecystitis. J Emerg Med. 2018;54(6):892–7.

Tohda G, Ohtani M, Dochin M. Efficacy and safety of emergency endoscopic retrograde cholangiopancreatography for acute cholangitis in the elderly. World J Gastroenterol. 2016;22(37):8382–8.

Trendle MC, Moertel CG, Kvols LK. Incidence and morbidity of cholelithiasis in patients receiving chronic octreotide for metastatic carcinoid and malignant islet cell tumors. Cancer. 1997;79(4):830–4.

Trotman BW. Pigment gallstone disease. Gastroenterol Clin N Am. 1991;20(1):111–26.

Trowbridge RL, Rutkowski NK, Shojania KG. Does this patient have acute cholecystitis? JAMA. 2003;289(1):80–6.

Tsai CJ, Leitzmann MF, Willett WC, Giovannucci EL. Dietary carbohydrates and glycaemic load and the incidence of symptomatic gall stone disease in men. Gut. 2005;54(6):823–8.

Uecker J, Adams M, Skipper K, Dunn E. Cholecystitis in the octogenarian: is laparoscopic cholecystectomy the best approach? Am Surg. 2001;67(7):637–40.

Upala S, Sanguankeo A, Jaruvongvanich V. Gallstone disease and the risk of cardiovascular disease: a systematic review and meta-analysis of observational studies. Scand J Surg. 2017;106(1):21–7.

Van Erpecum KJ, Van Berge Henegouwen GP, Stoelwinder B, Stolk MFJ, Eggink WF, Govaert WHA. Cholesterol and pigment gallstone disease: comparison of the reliability of three bile tests for differentiation between the two stone types. Scand J Gastroenterol. 1988;23(8):948–54.

Vedovati MC, Becattini C, Rondelli F, Boncompagni M, Camporese G, Balzarotti R, et al. A randomized study on 1-week versus 4-week prophylaxis for venous thromboembolism after laparoscopic surgery for colorectal cancer. Ann Surg. 2014;259(4):665–9.

Venneman NG, van Erpecum KJ. Pathogenesis of gallstones. Gastroenterol Clin N Am. 2010;39(2):171–83, vii.

Venneman NG, Besselink MG, Keulemans YC, Vanberge-Henegouwen GP, Boermeester MA, Broeders IA, et al. Ursodeoxycholic acid exerts no beneficial effect in patients with symptomatic gallstones awaiting cholecystectomy. Hepatology (Baltimore, Md). 2006;43(6):1276–83.

Wang DQ, Afdhal NH. Genetic analysis of cholesterol gallstone formation: searching for Lith (gallstone) genes. Curr Gastroenterol Rep. 2004;6(2):140–50.

Wang HH, Portincasa P, Afdhal NH, Wang DQ. Lith genes and genetic analysis of cholesterol gallstone formation. Gastroenterol Clin N Am. 2010;39(2):185–207, vii–viii.

Wang HH, Li T, Portincasa P, Ford DA, Neuschwander-Tetri BA, Tso P, et al. New insights into the role of Lith genes in the formation of cholesterol-supersaturated bile. Liver Res. 2017;1(1):42–53.

Wang TY, Portincasa P, Liu M, Tso P, Wang DQ. Mouse models of gallstone disease. Curr Opin Gastroenterol. 2018;34(2):59–70.

Watson RR, Parsi MA, Aslanian HR, Goodman AJ, Lichtenstein DR, Melson J, et al. Biliary and pancreatic lithotripsy devices. VideoGIE. 2018;3(11):329–38.

Whorwell PJ, Hawkins R, Dewbury K, Wright RJDD. Ultrasound survey of gallstones and other hepatobiliary disorders in patients with Crohn's disease. Dig Dis Sci. 1984;29(10):930–3.

Williams EJ, Green J, Beckingham I, Parks R, Martin D, Lombard M. Guidelines on the management of common bile duct stones (CBDS). Gut. 2008;57(7):1004–21.

Williams E, Beckingham I, El Sayed G, Gurusamy K, Sturgess R, Webster G, et al. Updated guideline on the management of common bile duct stones (CBDS). Gut. 2017;66(5):765–82.

Yarmish GM, Smith MP, Rosen MP, Baker ME, Blake MA, Cash BD, et al. ACR appropriateness criteria right upper quadrant pain. J Am Coll Radiol. 2014;11(3):316–22.

Yokoe M, Hata J, Takada T, Strasberg SM, Asbun HJ, Wakabayashi G, et al. Tokyo guidelines 2018: diagnostic criteria and severity grading of acute cholecystitis (with videos). J Hepatobiliary Pancreat Sci. 2018;25(1):41–54.

Zaliekas J, Munson JL. Complications of gallstones: the Mirizzi syndrome, gallstone ileus, gallstone pancreatitis, complications of "lost" gallstones. Surg Clin North Am. 2008;88(6):1345–68, x.

Zhang ZM, Liu Z, Liu LM, Zhang C, Yu HW, Wan BJ, et al. Therapeutic experience of 289 elderly patients with biliary diseases. World J Gastroenterol. 2017;23(13):2424–34.

Zheng Y, Xu M, Heianza Y, Ma W, Wang T, Sun D, et al. Gallstone disease and increased risk of mortality: two large prospective studies in US men and women. J Gastroenterol Hepatol. 2018;33(11):1925–31.

Biliary Neoplasms

63

C. S. Pitchumoni and Nishal Ravindran

Contents

Abstract

Gallbladder polyps are mostly benign but may progress to cancer. In older age, single polyps and large and sessile polyps are more likely to undergo malignant transformation.

Adenomyomatosis is a benign hyperplastic lesion due to the excessive proliferation of the surface epithelium, which invaginates into the muscularis.

Gallbladder cancer is extremely rare in the USA and many Western countries. The incidence is high in certain ethnic groups such as Native Americans and Mexican Americans and some geographic areas including Chile, Bolivia, and Northern parts of India. Other risk factors include older age, history of chronic cholecystitis, the larger size of stones, gallbladder polyps, and certain types of porcelain gallbladder disease with patchy calcification of the wall of the gallbladder. Typhoid carrier state is an association in some countries.

Gallbladder cancer has a poor prognosis as it is usually detected late because symptoms are non-specific and cancer spreads early. The prognosis is good when the disease is incidentally detected in routine cholecystectomy.

C. S. Pitchumoni (✉)
Department of Medicine, Robert Wood Johnson School of Medicine, Rutgers University, New Brunswick, NJ, USA

Department of Medicine, New York Medical College, Valhalla, NY, USA

Division of Gastroenterology, Hepatology and Clinical Nutrition, Saint Peters University Hospital, New Brunswick, NJ, USA
e-mail: pitchumoni@hotmail.com

N. Ravindran
Robert Wood Johnson School of Medicine, Rutgers University, New Brunswick, NJ, USA

Saint Peters University Hospital, New Brunswick, NJ, USA
e-mail: nishal.c@gmail.com

© Springer Nature Switzerland AG 2021
C. S. Pitchumoni, T. S. Dharmarajan (eds.), *Geriatric Gastroenterology*,
https://doi.org/10.1007/978-3-030-30192-7_105

Keywords

Gallbladder polyps · Cholesterolosis ·
Adenomyomatosis · Adenomas ·
Inflammatory polyps · Porcelain gallbladder ·
Typhoid carrier state · Malignant polyps ·
Gallbladder cancer · Cholangiocarcinoma

Introduction

Biliary neoplasms may be benign or malignant, with the vast majority being benign polyps found incidentally. Both benign and malignant lesions are seen more often in women and increase with age. Biliary malignancies are rare in most parts of the Western world but are seen more often in certain parts of the world, such as in the Andes region of Chile and Bolivia, Eastern Europe, East Asia, and Northern parts of India as well as in certain populations like Native Americans (Malhotra et al. 2017; Hundal and Shaffer 2014). There has been a rise in incidentally detected malignancy in cholecystectomy specimens with the increase in laparoscopic cholecystectomy. Biliary malignancies can arise in the bile ducts or gallbladder and are divided, based on location, into intra- or extrahepatic, gallbladder malignancies, and ampullary lesions. They have different genetics, risk factors, and clinical presentation (Benavides et al. 2015). Gallbladder cancer is the commonest biliary malignancy. Estimates for cancer of the gallbladder and large bile ducts in the USA for 2019 by the American Cancer Society are about 12,360 new cases, 5,810 in men and 6,550 in women, and about 3,960 deaths from these cancers. About four in ten of these will be gallbladder cancers. Only 25% of patients with gallbladder cancer are detected early enough for curative surgery with a 5-year survival rate of 16%.

Gallbladder Polyps

Polyps in the gallbladder (GB) are mucosal projections into the lumen. Gallbladder polyps are formed as a result of a heterogeneous group of changes in the GB that result in the formation of cholesterol polyps, inflammatory polyps, adenomas, lipomas, and leiomyomas. Adherent

sludge or gallstones may give the appearance of polyps on imaging. Interestingly one study found a high number of gallstones in patients thought to have polyps initially (Kratzer et al. 2008). While nearly 5% of all adults have gallbladder polyps, the majority (95%) are pseudopolyps with no neoplastic potential. Polyps due to cholesterolosis are the commonest (60% of gallbladder polyps), while adenomyomas are 25%, inflammatory are 10%, and adenomas are less than 5% (Hundal and Shaffer 2014; McCain et al. 2018; Christensen and Ishak 1970). No consistent risk factors have been identified for polyps in most studies except presence of gallbladder polyps in familial polyposis syndrome-like Peutz-Jeghers and Gardener's syndrome and hepatitis B in the Chinese (Lin et al. 2008; Wada et al. 1987; Komorowski et al. 1986). In a recent meta-analysis from East Asia (China, Korea, and Japan), Yamin et al. identified additional risk factors for gallbladder polyps. According to the authors, the additional risk factors are male gender, higher BMI, higher waist circumference, higher LDL, low HDL, and higher diastolic BP and HBsAg in this population (Yamin et al. 2019). There is a trend toward an increase in gallbladder polyps with age, mostly in 40–59 years old with a drop in the above 65 age group (Heitz et al. 2019).

Gallbladder polyps are usually found incidentally on abdominal ultrasound (US) examination. The prevalence of gallbladder polyps based on abdominal US studies ranges from 0.3% to 26%. A follow-up study in a random population observed that nearly 80% of polyps did not significantly change in size (Moriguchi et al. 1996). GB polyps may disappear in a large number of patients (Heitz et al. 2019). The majority of polyps are hyperechoic on the abdominal US exam. Imaging findings like polyp size, shape, wide base, wall thickening, and coexistent gallstones aid in diagnosis (Mellnick et al. 2015). Histology is necessary to confirm the diagnosis through radiographic appearance may be suggestive. Age, risk factors for gallbladder cancer, and radiological appearance are useful in clinical decision-making.

In cholesterolosis, the lamina propria is infiltrated with lipid-laden macrophages and can be diffuse or form polyps. It is characterized by villous mucosal hyperplasia with excessive accumulation of cholesterol esters within epithelial macrophages (Owen and Bilhartz 2003). In the diffuse form of cholesterolosis, the bright red mucosa with interposed areas of yellow lipid gives a characteristic appearance, "strawberry gallbladder." Cholesterol polyps are pedunculated, are multiple, and are usually less than 10 mm in size (Owen and Bilhartz 2003; Gallahan and Conway 2010). They may be solitary in about 20%. They are generally benign and do not cause symptoms but rarely can cause acute pancreatitis, often attributed as idiopathic (Parrilla Paricio et al. 1990).

Adenomyomatosis is a benign hyperplastic lesion due to the excessive proliferation of the surface epithelium, which invaginates into the muscularis. Increased intraluminal pressure in the gallbladder from mechanical obstruction is thought to lead to cystic dilatation of the Rokitansky sinuses and results in hyperplasia of the muscularis. The incidence increases after 50 years of age (Golse et al. 2017). Adenomyomatosis may resemble more serious and emergent gallbladder disease in the US (Mariani and Hsue 2011). It is reported to have a twinkling or comet tail appearance in the US. Adenomyomatosis may be segmental, fundal, or diffuse. They are usually seen in the fundus, are solitary, and range in size from 10 to 20 mm (Gallahan and Conway 2010; Ram and Midha 1975). Segmental adenomyomatosis may coexist with gallbladder cancer (Ootani et al. 1992). Segmental adenomyomatosis has a high risk of gallbladder cancer in elderly patients (Nabatame et al. 2004). Asymptomatic adenomyomatosis is not an indication for surgery. In older adults especially those from the gallbladder cancer (GBC) belt with increased risk of GBC, cholecystectomy is justified when in doubt (Golse et al. 2017) (Fig. 1).

Inflammatory polyps resulting from chronic inflammation are typically less than 10 mm (Gallahan and Conway 2010). They are made up of granulation and fibrous tissue and are small sessile lesions.

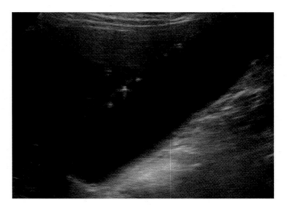

Fig. 1 The US showing adenomyomatosis

Adenomas are usually solitary, are pedunculated masses, and vary in size from 5 to 20 mm (Persley 2005). They may be papillary or non-papillary. They are often associated with gallstones. Although adenomas are neoplastic, they are mostly benign. The progression from adenoma to carcinoma has been reported but is not thought to be the predominant pathway (Albores-Saavedra et al. 2012).

There is an increased risk of malignant polyps noted with age above 50, history of primary sclerosing cholangitis, Northern Indian population, large polyps, and sessile polyps (McCain et al. 2018). Several studies have shown that large polyps (more than 10 mm) have increased the probability of adenomas and 50% may have carcinoma (Park et al. 2008). Gallbladder polyps were reported to be associated with colorectal adenomas in Taiwanese men (Liu et al. 2018).

Usually, polyps are asymptomatic, but there are reports of biliary colic, obstruction, cholecystitis, and hemobilia. The sonographic findings suggestive of a polyp on the abdominal US are immobility of the shadow with changes in patient position and lack of acoustic shadowing. Sonographic features suggestive of malignancy are solitary lesions, size above 1 cm, increased vascularity, sessile shape, rapid growth noted on serial studies, and invasion into the liver but are unreliable (Li et al. 2018). Although EUS is more accurate, there is no evidence to support its use as a more definitive diagnostic test but could be considered in centers that have availability. In a retrospective study of 2290 cholecystectomies, malignancy was seen only in 0.4%; risk factors identified were age more than 40 and polyp size more than 10 mm (Li et al. 2018).

Cholecystectomy is advised for gallbladder polyps with symptoms or if more than 10 mm or if 6–9 mm with risk factors. If the polyp is less than 6 mm or if 6–9 mm without risk factors, serial follow-up imaging is recommended in 6 months, 1 year, and yearly for 5 years (Wiles et al. 2017). A predictive model based on older age, single lesion, sessile polyp, and size showed statistical significance for neoplastic potential (probability of 7.4%) and could guide the decision for cholecystectomy (Yang et al. 2018). Open cholecystectomy is advisable if there is a high suspicion of malignancy, but laparoscopic cholecystectomy should be adequate in most patients (Gallahan and Conway 2010; Persley 2005).

Gallbladder Cancer

Gallbladder cancer is the most common malignancy of the biliary tract, representing 80–95% of biliary tract cancers worldwide. The prevalence of gallbladder cancer and mortality rates tends to increase with advancing age. In the USA, where GB cancer is not so common, data from 2016 reveals that age-adjusted incidence rates were 1.2/100,000 with 28% in 65–74 age group and 26% in 75–84 age group.

The highest mortality rate was in individuals over the age of 75 at 5.05/100,000, according to the SEER data (2013).

Risk factors are similar to gallstones like increasing age, female gender, ethnicity, family history, smoking, obesity, and diet and much less often attributed to gallstones, chronic inflammation, congenital abnormalities, and polyps (Malhotra et al. 2017; Randi et al. 2006). GBC is more often diagnosed in women, Hispanics, Native Alaskans, and Natives Americans. The highest incidence of GBC is seen in those above 65, with an average age of 72 years. Women have a risk of two to eight times that of men and are more common in older women (Kiran et al. 2007). The high incidence in women suggests that female sex hormones play a role in the pathogenesis. In a majority of patients with gallbladder cancer, Chen and Huminer found high levels of estrogen and its receptor (ER) in the gallbladder (Chen and Huminer 1991). Chronic infection with *Salmonella* Typhi is associated with an increased risk of gallbladder cancer, up to a 12-fold increase (Caygill et al. 1994; Nath et al. 1997). High incidence areas include parts of Andean regions of South America (Peru, Chile, Bolivia), Eastern Europe (Hungary, Poland), Northern India, Southern Pakistan, and Korea, with the highest rates in Korean males (Randi et al. 2006; Batra et al. 2005; Bhattacharjee and Nanda 2019; Barreto et al. 2018; Nagaraja and Eslick 2014).

The incidence of gallbladder cancer in North and Central India is very high. It is the most common gastrointestinal cancer in women there (Kapoor and McMichael 2003). Population-based data reveals that while the incidence of gallbladder cancer in Northern Indian cities is 5–7 per 100,000 women, it is low in Southern India, 0–0.7 per 100,000 women (Dhir and Mohandas 1999). The prevalence of gallbladder cancer is especially high along the banks of the Ganga, two to three times higher than other parts of India. The possibility of heavy metal poisoning in this area was studied by Shukla, who found high concentrations of cadmium and chromium in drinking water and gallbladder specimens (Shukla et al. 1998) (Fig. 2 and Table 1).

A genetic role is possible in gallbladder cancer but is not clear. The expression of p53 in gallbladder dysplasia suggests that the p53 mutation could be an early event in the evolution of some gallbladder cancers (Wee et al. 1994) (Fig. 3).

Larger stones (more than 3 cm) have a higher risk of malignancy (Diehl 1983). Porcelain gallbladder occurs in chronic cholecystitis with mural calcification of the gallbladder, and incomplete calcification of gallbladder is a risk factor (Gore et al. 2002; Patel et al. 2011). Traditional teaching is that porcelain gallbladder is strongly associated with gallbladder cancer with older reports quoting the prevalence of 12–61%. However, the risk is much lower than previously reported. It is prudent

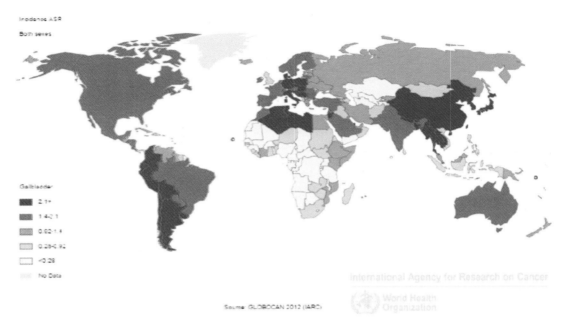

Fig. 2 Map showing the incidence of gallbladder cancer worldwide

Table 1 Gallbladder cancer rates worldwide in both sexes

Rank	Country	Age-standardized rate per 100,000
1	Bolivia	14.0
2	Chile	9.3
3	Thailand	7.4
4	South Korea	6.8
5	Nepal	6.7

Bolivia had the highest rate of gallbladder cancer in 2018, followed by Chile
Source: Bray F, Ferlay J, Soerjomataram I, Siegel RL, Torre LA, Jemal A. Global Cancer Statistics 2018

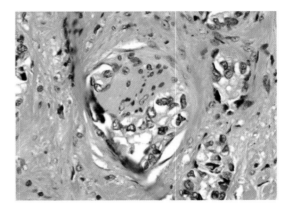

Fig. 3 Gallbladder cancer histopathology

to do prophylactic cholecystectomy in young, healthy, and symptomatic patients, but surveillance in those patients who are poor surgical candidates is a reasonable approach (DesJardins et al. 2018) (Table 2).

The presenting symptoms that occur in patients with GBC are similar to symptoms seen in a benign disease like biliary colic, right upper quadrant pain, or obstructive jaundice. In general, patients found to have obstructive jaundice are more likely to have metastatic disease and unresectable GBC. Other factors that influence survival are gastric outlet obstruction, nodal involvement and extension to adjacent organs, and higher cancer staging (Hickman and Contreras 2019; Mishra et al. 2017).

Gallbladder cancer has a poor prognosis as is usually detected late because symptoms are non-specific, and also the anatomy of the gallbladder leads to cancer spreading early (Chan et al. 2008). It is usually advanced when it causes symptoms. Only about one of five gallbladder

Table 2 Risk factors for gallbladder cancer

Risk factors		
Increasing age	Mean age at diagnosis is 65 years Incidence increases with age	Hickman and Contreras (2019)
Female gender	Female to male ratio of 2:1 Higher risk in females is independent of gallstone disease Risk increases after menopause Mortality rate higher in females	Wernberg and Lucarelli (2014)
Obesity	The relative risk of 1.66 Stronger association in women	Larsson and Wolk (2007)
Ethnicity/geography	Native Americans, Indian, Pakistani, Japanese, and Korean Eastern Europe, Andes region of South America	Hundal and Shaffer (2014)
Genetic predisposition	Genetic predisposition to lithogenic bile in certain ethnicities suggests a possible genetic link Familial risk in Swedish, Italian, and American reports relative risk range 2.1–13.9 for first-degree relatives	Wernberg and Lucarelli (2014)
Cholelithiasis	Gallstones in 70–88% of GBC patients but the incidence of gallbladder cancer 0.3–3.0% with gallstones Increased risk with larger gallstones Stones larger than 3 cm increases risk tenfold Increased number, weight, and volume of gallstones increase risk	Wernberg and Lucarelli (2014)
Porcelain gallbladder	12–60% incidence of gallbladder cancer with GB calcification in older literature Current consensus weak association 2–3% and only in patchy calcification	Hundal and Shaffer (2014)
Gallbladder polyps	Size >1 cm increases risk Especially those older than 50–60 years with polyps larger than 1 cm	Hundal and Shaffer (2014)
Choledochal cysts	Incidence of malignancy 11% Higher risk of cholangiocarcinoma	Sastry et al. (2015)
Anomalous junction of the pancreaticobiliary ductal system	Reflux of pancreatic secretions into the biliary tree Seen more in Asia especially Japanese Seen in 10% of patients with gallbladder cancer Seen more in younger women	Hundal and Shaffer (2014)
Typhoid carrier state	Chronic salmonellosis – a 12-fold increase	Koshiol et al. (2016)
Environmental risk factors	Exposure to industrial chemicals Cigarette smoking	Wernberg and Lucarelli (2014)

Data from Hickman and Contreras (2019), Kanthan et al. (2015), Koshiol et al. (2016), and Hundal and Shaffer (2014)

cancers is found in the early stages. Incidental identification of gallbladder cancer occurs in 0.2–3% of all cholecystectomies done for presumed benign disease. Only 30% of patients with gallbladder cancer are suspected of harboring a malignancy preoperatively, and such patients have a good prognosis after surgery (Kanthan et al. 2015). The increase in the number of laparoscopic cholecystectomies currently being performed is associated with an increase in the identification of incidental gallbladder cancer.

Adenocarcinomas are the most common gallbladder cancer (80%), and the fundus is the commonest site. Others are sarcoma, lymphoma, and carcinoid. There is no reliable tumor marker in the diagnosis of gallbladder cancer. The only two markers, carcinoembryonic antigen (CEA) and carbohydrate antigen 19-9, are most often elevated in advanced stages, have low specificity, and are useless for early diagnosis (Srivastava et al. 2013).

Genetics of GB cancer shows that the common genetic alterations are in the oncogenes, tumor suppressor genes, microsatellite instability, methylation of gene promoter areas, p53 mutation, and K-ras point mutations (Hundal and Shaffer 2014). The Oxford hepatobiliary 2015 consensus statement recommendations included high-quality cross-sectional imaging with CT or MRI and selective use of PET scan to clarify features of concerns before resection. Gallbladder cancer staging is done by the American Joint Committee on Cancer (AJCC) TNM system which is based on tumor size, lymph node involvement, and metastasis. The SEER database uses staging as localized (within the gallbladder), regional (spread outside to the gallbladder to nearby structures), and distant stage (metastases to other organs). The 5-year survival rate from 2008 to 2014 for localized GBC was 61%, with regional spread was 26%, and in the distant spread was 2%.

The alarming incidence of GBC in India has prompted investigators there to re-evaluate the need to consider prophylactic cholecystectomy in selected populations. The long-standing correlation of gallstones and GBC prompted Mohandas et al. to advise prophylactic cholecystectomy in young women from high-risk areas with asymptomatic gallstones based on prospective population-based data (Mohandas and Patil 2006). Although the chapter specifically mentions young women, the observation can be extended to the healthy elderly population with many years of life expectancy. Prophylactic cholecystectomy may not be acceptable in the Western world, where the incidence of GBC is very low in contrast to high prevalence areas. The risk-benefit ratio is dramatic in India, with 1 GBC prevented with 67 cholecystectomies (Mathur 2015).

For GBC diagnosed after cholecystectomy, tumors T1b and greater necessitate radical cholecystectomy. Radical cholecystectomy includes staging laparoscopy, hepatic resection, and locoregional lymph node clearance to achieve R0 resection (Cavallaro et al. 2014). Resection of the adjacent liver and lymph nodes is also advised in incidentally identified T2 or T3 disease in a cholecystectomy specimen unless contraindicated by advanced disease or poor performance status (Aloia et al. 2015). Although in patients with early cancer laparoscopic cholecystectomy has not been shown to have a worse prognosis than open cholecystectomy, it was recommended only in specialized centers (Zhao et al. 2018). Laparoscopic cholecystectomy does not affect survival in incidental GBC.

Patients with locally advanced disease (T3 or T4), hepatic-sided T2 tumors, node positivity, or R1 resection may benefit from adjuvant chemotherapy. Chemotherapy increases survival in unresectable disease (Hickman and Contreras 2019). Patients with advanced cancer may benefit from palliative endoscopic or percutaneous procedures to relieve the obstruction.

Details of current treatment of gallbladder cancer are available in "Update in GBC management" by Zaidi and Maithel (2018). Chemotherapy with targeted therapeutic agents may be available in the future for treatment of advanced gallbladder cancer with potential target genes at *ERBB2* amplification, mutations or amplification of the PI3-kinase family genes, *FGFR* mutations or fusions, and aberrations of the chromatin modulating genes (Jiao et al. 2013; Javle et al. 2013).

Cholangiocarcinoma

Cholangiocarcinoma arises from biliary epithelium in both the intrahepatic and extrahepatic biliary tree (de Groen et al. 1999). It is a rare malignancy but is the second most common hepatic malignancy after hepatocellular carcinoma, and the incidence is rising (Hsing et al. 2006).

Risk factors for cholangiocarcinoma are primary sclerosing cholangitis, choledochal cysts, inflammatory bowel disease, cirrhosis, congenital fibrosis, hepatolithiasis, and parasitic infections (*Opisthorchis*, *Clonorchis*) (Shin et al. 2010; Edil et al. 2008; Mabrut et al. 2013; Chapman et al. 2012). Parasitic infection of the biliary tract is the commonest risk factor worldwide for cholangiocarcinoma as the highest incidence of cholangiocarcinoma is seen in Southeast Asia (Blechacz 2017). In patients with primary

Fig. 4 Classification of cholangiocarcinoma

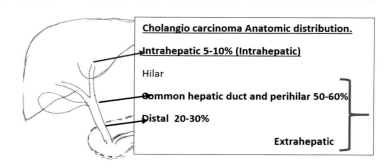

Table 3 Risk factors for cholangiocarcinoma

Risk factors		
Increasing age	74% of cases after 65 years	Tyson and El-Serag (2011)
Sex	Incidence higher in men than women range from 1.2 to 1.5:1	Tyson and El-Serag (2011)
Genetics	Acquired genetic mutations in some poorer prognosis	Razumilava and Gores (2014)
Ethnicity/race	Increased in Hispanic and Asian populations 2.8–3.3/100,000 Highest incidence rates in Southeast Asia and China Mortality rates highest in Native Americans, Native Alaskans, and Asians	Razumilava and Gores (2014)
Cirrhosis	Odds ratio 22.92 Viral hepatitis B and C not clear	Razumilava and Gores (2014)
Exposure to Thorotrast (radiographic contrast agent)	Thorotrast used until 1960s latency >16 years between exposure and malignancy	Tyson and El-Serag (2011)
Choledochal cysts	Risk 30 times higher Seen more in Asians	Tyson and El-Serag (2011)
Primary sclerosing cholangitis	Chronic inflammation and segmental stenosis of bile ducts Strong risk factor for (6–36%) cholangiocarcinoma (CC) Not more than 10% of all cases Risk 1% per year	Tyson and El-Serag (2011)
Inflammatory bowel disease	Difficult to define due to complex association	Tyson and El-Serag (2011)
Caroli's disease	Risk up to 30 times higher	Tyson and El-Serag (2011)
Hepatolithiasis	2–10% of patients develop CC	Tyson and El-Serag (2011)
Parasites	Liver flukes including *Opisthorchis viverrini*, *Opisthorchis/Clonorchis sinensis* Attributable risk 27% in men	Tyson and El-Serag (2011)

Data from Tyson and El-Serag (2011) and Blechacz (2017)

sclerosing cholangitis, about 50% of cholangiocarcinoma is diagnosed within 2 years. It is rarely diagnosed before 40 years; mean age at diagnosis is 50 years globally and 65 in Western nations (Rizvi and Gores 2013). In the USA, incidence rates are 2.1–3.3 per 100,000 population, while rates are as high as 113 per 100,000 population in Southeast Asia.

It is usually asymptomatic in the early stages but in the late stages may present with jaundice, abdominal pain, abdominal mass, ascites, and hepatomegaly. Malaise and weight loss may be the only features. Jaundice is more likely in perihilar or distal cholangiocarcinoma.

Depending on the relationship to second-degree bile duct, they are divided into intrahepatic and extrahepatic; extrahepatic may be perihilar or distal. Proximal to second-degree bile ducts, they are called intrahepatic, and between second-degree bile duct and cystic duct, they are perihilar, and between the cystic duct and ampulla of Vater, it is distal. Perihilar cholangiocarcinoma is further stratified depending on biliary and vascular involvement. Extrahepatic cholangiocarcinomas comprise about 90% of these cancers, and perihilar type is about 50%. Klatskin tumor is another term for hilar cholangiocarcinoma. Mixed hepatocellular cholangiocarcinoma is a distinct subtype.

Intrahepatic cholangiocarcinoma usually has non-specific symptoms, while extrahepatic presents with jaundice. CEA and CA 19-9 may be elevated. Most cholangiocarcinomas are adenocarcinomas (Fig. 4 and Table 3).

Endoscopic ultrasonography and endoscopic retrograde cholangiopancreatography are usually required for obtaining biopsy or cytology for diagnosis. TNM classification, according to the American Joint Committee on Cancer, is used for staging.

The most common method of tumor spread in intrahepatic cholangiocarcinoma is via portal vein invasion, similar to hepatocellular carcinoma. Surgical resection has the best outcome in intrahepatic cholangiocarcinoma if the tumors are potentially resectable, with a 5-year survival range of 22–45% (Endo et al. 2008). Liver transplantation does not appear to be an option in these patients due to poor survival rates based on several multicenter trials (Rosen et al. 2010). Transarterial chemoembolization and radiofrequency ablation are treatment options in inoperable intrahepatic cholangiocarcinoma (Kuhlmann and Blum 2013). Liver transplantation in combination with neoadjuvant chemotherapy has the best outcomes in perihilar cholangiocarcinoma with a 5-year survival rate approaching 68% (Gores et al. 2013). In advanced

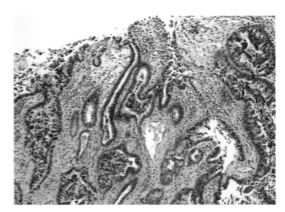

Fig. 5 Neuronal invasion by gallbladder cancer

disease single-agent chemotherapy with gemcitabine or combination with cisplatinum is used though evidence is limited (Boimel et al. 2018) (Fig. 5).

Key Points

- Most common biliary neoplasms are benign polyps.
- Cholesterol polyps are the commonest polyp (95%).
- Polyps more than 1 cm require cholecystectomy.
- High prevalence of gallbladder cancer in Native Americans and certain geographical areas like Northern India, Eastern Europe, and the Andes.
- Gallstones are commonly seen in patients with gallbladder cancer.
- Incomplete gallbladder calcification but not complete calcification is associated with gallbladder cancer.
- Gallbladder cancer has a poor prognosis unless detected incidentally.

References

Albores-Saavedra J, Chable-Montero F, Gonzalez-Romo MA, Ramirez Jaramillo M, Henson DE. Adenomas of the gallbladder. Morphologic features, expression of gastric and intestinal mucins, and incidence of high-grade dysplasia/carcinoma in situ and invasive carcinoma. Hum Pathol. 2012;43 (9):1506–13.

Aloia TA, Jarufe N, Javle M, Maithel SK, Roa JC, Adsay V, et al. Gallbladder cancer: expert consensus statement. HPB (Oxford). 2015;17(8):681–90.

Barreto SG, Dutt A, Sirohi B, Shrikhande SV. Gallbladder cancer: a journey of a thousand steps. Future Oncol. 2018;14(13):1299–306.

Batra Y, Pal S, Dutta U, Desai P, Garg PK, Makharia G, et al. Gallbladder cancer in India: a dismal picture. J Gastroenterol Hepatol. 2005;20(2):309–14.

Benavides M, Anton A, Gallego J, Gomez MA, Jimenez-Gordo A, La Casta A, et al. Biliary tract cancers: SEOM clinical guidelines. Clin Transl Oncol. 2015;17(12): 982–7.

Bhattacharjee P, Nanda D. Prospective observational study on cholelithiasis in patients with carcinoma gall bladder in a tertiary referral hospital of Eastern India. J Cancer Res Ther. 2019;15(1):153–6.

Blechacz B. Cholangiocarcinoma: current knowledge and new developments. Gut Liver. 2017;11(1):13–26.

Boimel PJ, Binder KR, Hong TS, Feng M, Ben-Josef E. Cholangiocarcinoma and gallbladder cases: an expert panel case-based discussion. Semin Radiat Oncol. 2018;28(4):351–61.

Cavallaro A, Piccolo G, Di Vita M, Zanghì A, Cardì F, Di Mattia P, et al. Managing the incidentally detected gallbladder cancer: algorithms and controversies. Int J Surg. 2014;12:S108–19.

Caygill CP, Hill MJ, Braddick M, Sharp JC. Cancer mortality in chronic typhoid and paratyphoid carriers. Lancet. 1994;343(8889):83–4.

Chan SY, Poon RT, Lo CM, Ng KK, Fan ST. Management of carcinoma of the gallbladder: a single-institution experience in 16 years. J Surg Oncol. 2008;97(2):156–64.

Chapman MH, Webster GJ, Bannoo S, Johnson GJ, Wittmann J, Pereira SP. Cholangiocarcinoma and dominant strictures in patients with primary sclerosing cholangitis: a 25-year single-centre experience. Eur J Gastroenterol Hepatol. 2012;24(9):1051–8.

Chen A, Huminer D. The role of estrogen receptors in the development of gallstones and gallbladder cancer. Med Hypotheses. 1991;36(3):259–60.

Christensen AH, Ishak KG. Benign tumors and pseudo-tumors of the gallbladder. Report of 180 cases. Arch Pathol. 1970;90(5):423–32.

de Groen PC, Gores GJ, LaRusso NF, Gunderson LL, Nagorney DM. Biliary tract cancers. N Engl J Med. 1999;341(18):1368–78.

DesJardins H, Duy L, Scheirey C, Schnelldorfer T. Porcelain gallbladder: is observation a safe option in select populations? J Am Coll Surg. 2018;226(6): 1064–9.

Dhir V, Mohandas KM. Epidemiology of digestive tract cancers in India IV. Gall bladder and pancreas. Indian J Gastroenterol. 1999;18(1):24–8.

Diehl AK. Gallstone size and the risk of gallbladder cancer. JAMA. 1983;250(17):2323–6.

Edil BH, Cameron JL, Reddy S, Lum Y, Lipsett PA, Nathan H, et al. Choledochal cyst disease in children and adults: a 30-year single-institution experience. J Am Coll Surg. 2008;206(5):1000–5; discussion 5–8.

Endo I, Gonen M, Yopp AC, Dalal KM, Zhou Q, Klimstra D, et al. Intrahepatic cholangiocarcinoma: rising frequency, improved survival, and determinants of outcome after resection. Ann Surg. 2008;248(1): 84–96.

Gallahan WC, Conway JD. Diagnosis and management of gallbladder polyps. Gastroenterol Clin. 2010;39(2): 359–67.

Golse N, Lewin M, Rode A, Sebagh M, Mabrut JY. Gallbladder adenomyomatosis: diagnosis and management. J Visc Surg. 2017;154(5):345–53.

Gore RM, Yaghmai V, Newmark GM, Berlin JW, Miller FH. Imaging benign and malignant disease of the gallbladder. Radiol Clin North Am. 2002;40(6): 1307–23, vi.

Gores GJ, Darwish Murad S, Heimbach JK, Rosen CB. Liver transplantation for perihilar cholangiocarcinoma. Dig Dis. 2013;31(1):126–9.

Heitz L, Kratzer W, Grater T, Schmidberger J. Gallbladder polyps – a follow-up study after 11 years. BMC Gastroenterol. 2019;19(1):42.

Hickman L, Contreras C. Gallbladder cancer: diagnosis, surgical management, and adjuvant therapies. Surg Clin North Am. 2019;99(2):337–55.

Hsing AW, McGlynn KA, Pfeiffer RM, Welzel TM, O'Brien TR. Impact of classification of hilar cholangio-carcinomas (Klatskin tumors) on the incidence of intra- and extrahepatic cholangiocarcinoma in the United States. J Natl Cancer Inst. 2006;98(12):873–5.

Hundal R, Shaffer EA. Gallbladder cancer: epidemiology and outcome. Clin Epidemiol. 2014;6:99–109.

Javle MM, Rashid A, Kar SP, Schalper K, Wang N, Peto M, et al. Identification of unique somatic mutations with functional relevance through genetic characterization of gallbladder cancer (GB ca). J Clin Oncol. 2013; 31(4_Suppl):214.

Jiao Y, Pawlik TM, Anders RA, Selaru FM, Streppel MM, Lucas DJ, et al. Exome sequencing identifies frequent inactivating mutations in BAP1, ARID1A and PBRM1 in intrahepatic cholangiocarcinomas. Nat Genet. 2013; 45(12):1470–3.

Kanthan R, Senger JL, Ahmed S, Kanthan SC. Gallbladder cancer in the 21st century. J Oncol. 2015;2015:967472.

Kapoor VK, McMichael AJ. Gallbladder cancer: an 'Indian' disease. Natl Med J India. 2003;16(4):209–13.

Kiran RP, Pokala N, Dudrick SJ. Incidence pattern and survival for gallbladder cancer over three decades – an analysis of 10301 patients. Ann Surg Oncol. 2007;14(2):827–32.

Komorowski RA, Tresp MG, Wilson SD. Pancreaticobiliary involvement in familial polyposis coli/Gardner's syndrome. Dis Colon Rectum. 1986; 29(1):55–8.

Koshiol J, Wozniak A, Cook P, Adaniel C, Acevedo J, Azocar L, et al. *Salmonella enterica* serovar Typhi and gallbladder cancer: a case-control study and meta-analysis. Cancer Med. 2016;5(11):3235–310.

Kratzer W, Haenle MM, Voegtle A, Mason RA, Akinli AS, Hirschbuehl K, et al. Ultrasonographically detected gallbladder polyps: a reason for concern? A seven-year follow-up study. BMC Gastroenterol. 2008;8:41.

Kuhlmann JB, Blum HE. Locoregional therapy for cholangiocarcinoma. Curr Opin Gastroenterol. 2013; 29(3):324–8.

Larsson SC, Wolk A. Obesity and the risk of gallbladder cancer: a meta-analysis. Br J Cancer. 2007;96(9):1457–61.

Li Y, Tejirian T, Collins JC. Gallbladder polyps: real or imagined? Am Surg. 2018;84(10):1670–4.

Lin WR, Lin DY, Tai DI, Hsieh SY, Lin CY, Sheen IS, et al. Prevalence of and risk factors for gallbladder polyps detected by ultrasonography among healthy Chinese: analysis of 34 669 cases. J Gastroenterol Hepatol. 2008;23(6):965–9.

Liu YL, Wu JS, Yang YC, Lu FH, Lee CT, Lin WJ, et al. Gallbladder stones and gallbladder polyps associated with increased risk of colorectal adenoma in men. J Gastroenterol Hepatol. 2018;33(4):800–6.

Mabrut JY, Kianmanesh R, Nuzzo G, Castaing D, Boudjema K, Letoublon C, et al. Surgical management of congenital intrahepatic bile duct dilatation, Caroli's disease and syndrome: long-term results of the French Association of Surgery Multicenter Study. Ann Surg. 2013;258(5):713–21; discussion 21.

Malhotra RK, Manoharan N, Shukla NK, Rath GK. Gallbladder cancer incidence in Delhi urban: a 25-year trend analysis. Indian J Cancer. 2017;54(4):673–7.

Mariani PJ, Hsue A. Adenomyomatosis of the gallbladder: the good omen comet. J Emerg Med. 2011;40(4):415–8.

Mathur AV. Need for prophylactic cholecystectomy in silent gall stones in North India. Indian J Surg Oncol. 2015;6(3):251–5.

McCain RS, Diamond A, Jones C, Coleman HG. Current practices and future prospects for the management of gallbladder polyps: a topical review. World J Gastroenterol. 2018;24(26):2844–52.

Mellnick VM, Menias CO, Sandrasegaran K, Hara AK, Kielar AZ, Brunt EM, et al. Polypoid lesions of the gallbladder: disease spectrum with pathologic correlation. Radiographics. 2015;35(2):387–99.

Mishra PK, Saluja SS, Prithiviraj N, Varshney V, Goel N, Patil N. Predictors of curative resection and long term survival of gallbladder cancer – a retrospective analysis. Am J Surg. 2017;214(2):278–86.

Mohandas KM, Patil PS. Cholecystectomy for asymptomatic gallstones can reduce gall bladder cancer mortality in northern Indian women. Indian J Gastroenterol. 2006;25(3):147–51.

Moriguchi H, Tazawa J, Hayashi Y, Takenawa H, Nakayama E, Marumo F, et al. Natural history of polypoid lesions in the gall bladder. Gut. 1996; 39(6):860–2.

Nabatame N, Shirai Y, Nishimura A, Yokoyama N, Wakai T, Hatakeyama K. High risk of gallbladder carcinoma in elderly patients with segmental adenomyomatosis of the gallbladder. J Exp Clin Cancer Res. 2004;23(4):593–8.

Nagaraja V, Eslick GD. Systematic review with meta-analysis: the relationship between chronic Salmonella typhi carrier status and gall-bladder cancer. Aliment Pharmacol Ther. 2014;39(8):745–50.

Nath G, Singh H, Shukla VK. Chronic typhoid carriage and carcinoma of the gallbladder. Eur J Cancer Prev. 1997;6(6):557–9.

Ootani T, Shirai Y, Tsukada K, Muto T. Relationship between gallbladder carcinoma and the segmental type of adenomyomatosis of the gallbladder. Cancer. 1992;69(11):2647–52.

Owen CC, Bilhartz LE. Gallbladder polyps, cholesterolosis, adenomyomatosis, and acute acalculous cholecystitis. Semin Gastrointest Dis. 2003;14(4): 178–88.

Park JK, Yoon YB, Kim YT, Ryu JK, Yoon WJ, Lee SH, et al. Management strategies for gallbladder polyps: is it possible to predict malignant gallbladder polyps? Gut Liver. 2008;2(2):88–94.

Parrilla Paricio P, Garcia Olmo D, Pellicer Franco E, Prieto Gonzalez A, Carrasco Gonzalez L, Bermejo Lopez J. Gallbladder cholesterolosis: an aetiological factor in acute pancreatitis of uncertain origin. Br J Surg. 1990;77(7):735–6.

Patel S, Roa JC, Tapia O, Dursun N, Bagci P, Basturk O, et al. Hyalinizing cholecystitis and associated carcinomas: clinicopathologic analysis of a distinctive variant of cholecystitis with porcelain-like features and accompanying diagnostically challenging carcinomas. Am J Surg Pathol. 2011;35(8):1104–13.

Persley KM. Gallbladder polyps. Curr Treat Options Gastroenterol. 2005;8(2):105–8.

Ram MD, Midha D. Adenomyomatosis of the gallbladder. Surgery. 1975;78(2):224–9.

Randi G, Franceschi S, La Vecchia C. Gallbladder cancer worldwide: geographical distribution and risk factors. Int J Cancer. 2006;118(7):1591–602.

Razumilava N, Gores GJ. Cholangiocarcinoma. Lancet. 2014;383(9935):2168–79.

Rizvi S, Gores GJ. Pathogenesis, diagnosis, and management of cholangiocarcinoma. Gastroenterology. 2013; 145(6):1215–29.

Rosen CB, Heimbach JK, Gores GJ. Liver transplantation for cholangiocarcinoma. Transpl Int. 2010;23(7):692–7.

Sastry AV, Abbadessa B, Wayne MG, Steele JG, Cooperman AM. What is the incidence of biliary carcinoma in choledochal cysts, when do they develop, and how should it affect management? World J Surg. 2015;39(2):487–92.

Shin HR, Oh JK, Lim MK, Shin A, Kong HJ, Jung KW, et al. Descriptive epidemiology of cholangiocarcinoma and clonorchiasis in Korea. J Korean Med Sci. 2010; 25(7):1011–6.

Shukla VK, Prakash A, Tripathi BD, Reddy DC, Singh S. Biliary heavy metal concentrations in carcinoma of the gall bladder: case-control study. BMJ. 1998; 317(7168):1288–9.

Srivastava K, Srivastava A, Mittal B. Potential biomarkers in gallbladder cancer: present status and future directions. Biomarkers. 2013;18(1):1–9.

Tyson GL, El-Serag HB. Risk factors for cholangiocarcinoma. Hepatology. 2011;54(1):173–84.

Wada K, Tanaka M, Yamaguchi K, Wada K. Carcinoma and polyps of the gallbladder associated with Peutz-Jeghers syndrome. Dig Dis Sci. 1987;32(8):943–6.

Wee A, Teh M, Raju GC. Clinical importance of p53 protein in gall bladder carcinoma and its precursor lesions. J Clin Pathol. 1994;47(5):453–6.

Wernberg JA, Lucarelli DD. Gallbladder cancer. Surg Clin North Am. 2014;94(2):343–60.

Wiles R, Thoeni RF, Barbu ST, Vashist YK, Rafaelsen SR, Dewhurst C, et al. Management and follow-up of gallbladder polyps: joint guidelines between the European Society of Gastrointestinal and Abdominal Radiology (ESGAR), European Association for Endoscopic Surgery and other Interventional Techniques (EAES), International Society of Digestive Surgery – European Federation (EFISDS) and European Society of Gastrointestinal Endoscopy (ESGE). Eur Radiol. 2017;27(9):3856–66.

Yamin Z, Xuesong B, Guibin Y, Liwei L, Fei L. Risk factors of gallbladder polyps formation in East Asian population: a meta-analysis and systematic review. Asian J Surg. 2019;43:52.

Yang JI, Lee JK, Ahn DG, Park JK, Lee KH, Lee KT, et al. Predictive model for neoplastic potential of gallbladder polyp. J Clin Gastroenterol. 2018;52(3):273–6.

Zaidi MY, Maithel SK. Updates on gallbladder cancer management. Curr Oncol Rep. 2018;20(2):21.

Zhao X, Li XY, Ji W. Laparoscopic versus open treatment of gallbladder cancer: a systematic review and meta-analysis. J Minim Access Surg. 2018;14(3):185–91.

Acute Pancreatitis

64

C. S. Pitchumoni

Contents

C. S. Pitchumoni (✉)
Department of Medicine, Robert Wood Johnson School of
Medicine, Rutgers University, New Brunswick, NJ, USA

Department of Medicine, New York Medical College,
Valhalla, NY, USA

Division of Gastroenterology, Hepatology and Clinical
Nutrition, Saint Peters University Hospital, New
Brunswick, NJ, USA
e-mail: pitchumoni@hotmail.com

© Springer Nature Switzerland AG 2021
C. S. Pitchumoni, T. S. Dharmarajan (eds.), *Geriatric Gastroenterology*,
https://doi.org/10.1007/978-3-030-30192-7_55

Abstract

Roughly one-third of patients with acute pancreatitis (AP) admitted to hospitals are reported to be over 65 years, and the number is expected to increase along with changes in the demographics. In younger patients, the diagnosis of AP is valid if the patient has a sudden onset of epigastric pain radiating to the back, associated with elevated serum levels of amylase or lipase more than three times of normal levels. In the older adults, the diagnosis may be difficult without an early CT scan of abdomen (considered unnecessary in younger adults) because a number of other abdominal emergencies that require prompt surgery, such as intestinal ischemia, perforated peptic ulcer, appendicitis, volvulus, and abdominal aortic aneurysm, may also be associated with elevations of serum levels of amylase and/or lipase .

Older age has been recognized as a marker of severity in all scoring systems of severity, such as Ranson's criteria, modified Glasgow, Imrie, BISAP, and the APACHE II score. The overall mortality is approximately 1–3% among all AP patients but reaches 20–30% in older adults. The etiological factors, while the same in younger adults, a biliary etiology, drug-induced, and a procedure-related AP and less often an early manifestation of an occult pancreatic cancer are to be emphasized. The Atlanta II classification of AP (2013) clarifies the terms acute pancreatic fluid collection, pseudocyst, sterile, and infected necrotizing and walled-off pancreatic necrosis.

Older patients with CBD stones, ascending cholangitis, and persistent biliary obstruction require prompt endoscopic therapy, which may be life-saving even in advanced age. In the care of older adults, aggressive fluid administration, recommended as early therapy in younger patients, is associated with risk of pulmonary edema. AP in the older adult is to be considered an indication for ICU care.

Keywords

Acute pancreatitis · Drug induced pancreatitis · Gallstones · Alcoholism · Hyperlipdemia · Trauma · Cholangitis. Contrast enhanced CT · MRCP · ERCP · Pseudocyst · Pleural effusion · Sterile necrosis · Infected necrosis · Walled off necrosis · Organ system failure · Atlanta criteria · Ranson criteria · BISAP · Criteria · SIRS criteria · Amylase · Lipase · Abdominal ultrasound · Antibiotics · Enteral nutrition · Parenteral nutrition · Intensive care

Introduction

Acute pancreatitis (AP) is an acute inflammatory disorder of the pancreas clinically characterized by sudden onset of epigastric pain radiating to the back associated with anorexia, nausea, and vomiting. Other features are low-grade fever, tachycardia, and in severe cases, shortness of breath and features of Systemic Inflammatory Response Syndrome (SIRS). AP is morphologically associated with varying degrees of

Table 1 Revised ATLANTA definitions of morphological features of acute pancreatitis

A. Two morphological types
Interstitial edematous (without recognizable tissue necrosis CECT criteria) and necrotizing
B. **Two peaks of severity. Early and late**
C. **Three degrees of severity**
Mild: No organ failure, no local complications (e.g., peripancreatic fluid collections, pancreatic necrosis, peripancreatic necrosis), no systemic complications, typically resolves in first week
Moderate: Transient organ failure (≤48 h), local complications. Exacerbation of comorbid disease
Severe: Persistent organ failure (>48 h), presence of findings of peripancreatic necrosis
Fluid collections
Edematous pancreatitis
I) Acute peripancreatic fluid collections (APFC). < 4 weeks, fluid only, not or only partially encapsulated. Often regress spontaneously
II) Pseudocyst. > 4 weeks, encapsulated, no necrotic material, may disappear without intervention. May cause abdominal pain, compress upon adjacent organs, grow progressively, and/or get infected I infected pseudocyst)
Edematous pancreatitis
Necrotizing pancreatitis
I) *Acute Necrotic Collections (ANC)*: a mixture of fluid and necrotic material, not or only partially encapsulated, <4 weeks lack of pancreatic parenchymal enhancement by IV contrast/presence of findings of peripancreatic necrosis. May get infected
II) *Walled-off necrosis (WON)*: encapsulated heterogenous collection of pancreatic and/or peripancreatic necrosis, after >4 weeks of onset. May get infected

Modified from Banks et al. (2013)

pancreatic inflammation from minimal edema to necrosis and fluid collections. The natural history of AP and its complications in the older adult are discussed in this chapter.

A clinically based classification system for AP was available since (Atlanta I) 1992 (Bradley 1993). The Atlanta classification was revised in 2012 and provided clear definitions to classify AP using easily identifiable clinical and radiologic criteria (Table 1). Also, greater emphasis was stressed on organ failure and severity was graded as mild, moderately severe, and severe acute pancreatitis. The two terms phlegmon and pancreatic abscess were deleted from the terminologies (Banks et al. 2013).

Epidemiology

Independent of the growing number of older adults, the incidence of AP and in particular severe AP (SAP) is increasing. Worldwide, the incidence of AP widely varies between 4.5 and 73.4 per hundred thousand population and is increasing (Peery et al. 2015; Yadav and Lowenfels 2006; Tenner et al. 2013; Crockett et al. 2018; Krishna et al. 2017; Gullo et al. 2002; Whitcomb 2006). Three major factors, the prevalence of obesity, the genetic predisposition for gallstones, and prevalence of alcoholism in the community significantly affect the etiology, epidemiology, and severity of AP (Yadav and Lowenfels 2006). The spectrum of severity varies from a brief self-limited course to a fulminant disease associated with multiple organ dysfunction syndrome (MODS) and death. In the United States, AP is the leading cause of hospitalization for any gastrointestinal disorder with >275,000 admissions per year, and the rate is increasing. The annual cost of care is an aggregate cost of >$2.6 billion per year (Krishna et al. 2017; Whitcomb 2006; Tinto et al. 2002).

The number of patients with AP admitted and readmitted to hospitals has also increased irrespective of age (Noel et al. 2016; Otsuki et al. 2013; Martin and Ulrich 1999). Roughly, one-third of patients admitted to US hospitals are reported to be >65 years, and the number is expected to increase along with changes in the demographics (Martin and Ulrich 1999; Yadav and Lowenfels 2006; Carvalho et al. 2018; Gullo et al. 2002; Gloor et al. 2002; Peery et al. 2015; Fagenholz et al. 2007). Routine evaluation of serum pancreatic enzymes and imaging studies, including ultrasound and or CT scans of the abdomen, certainly contribute to the increase in the number of cases diagnosed.

Older Age Increases the Severity of AP and Mortality (Kara et al. 2018; Forsmark et al. 2016; Ahn et al. 2010)

Older age has been recognized as a marker of severity in most severity scoring systems such as Ranson criteria, modified Glasgow, Imrie, BISAP, and the

APACHE II score (Wu et al. 2008). The overall mortality is approximately 1–3% among all AP patients but reaches 20–30% in older adults (Kesselman and Holt 1991; Xin et al. 2008; Gardner et al. 2008; van Dijk et al. 2017; Losurdo et al. 2016; Somasekar et al. 2011). Many older patients, even with moderately severe and SAP, require Intensive care unit (ICU) management given the presence of comorbid conditions. The risk of increased systemic inflammatory response syndrome (SIRS), local complications, and sepsis needs early monitoring and special attention (Frossard et al. 2008).

In managing AP in the older adult, the three major steps are (1) establish the diagnosis of AP excluding other causes of acute abdomen, (2) assess the severity of AP initially and through the clinical course, (3) establish the etiology for AP by biochemical and imaging studies, and (4) in biliary AP where emergency therapy is available, initiate appropriate and prompt management strategies including early therapeutic endoscopic interventions.

AP is morphologically defined as interstitial, edematous, and necrotizing pancreatitis (Figs. 1 and 2). In very mild cases, the pancreas may appear normal with no morphological changes even in contrast-enhanced CT scans (CECT). Necrotizing pancreatitis occurs in 5–10% of patients. The extent of necrosis may vary and involve the pancreatic parenchyma, the peripancreatic tissue, or both.

AP has two peaks of severity, an early peak occurring within a week of onset and a second peak after the second week. Organ system dysfunctions and mortality occur in both peaks, in the first peak with no morphological changes visible in imaging studies and in the second peak with evidence of pancreatic necrosis with or without infection. In the early peak of severity, death may occur even before the patient seeks medical attention (McKay et al. 1999) with no cause identifiable except in an autopsy examination.

The diagnosis of AP requires two out of the three items in the following diagnostic criteria. (1) A history of abdominal pain is consistent with AP (epigastric, sudden in onset, radiating to back), (2) serum level of amylase or lipase >3 times the upper limit of normal, and (3) the characteristic

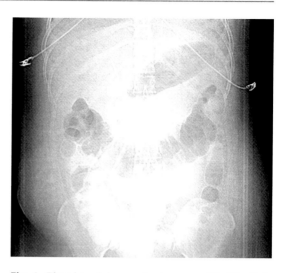

Fig. 1 Flat plate abdomen. Acute pancreatitis. The findings are not specific for acute pancreatitis. The dilatation of transverse colon and stomach indicate ileus. Once popular **colon cut-off sign** is as a result of gaseous distension of proximal colon associated with narrowing of the spleen, originally described in plain X-ray of abdomen has also been demonstrated in computed tomography of abdomen. A "sentinel loop" is a dilated segment of small intestine that indicates localized ileus from nearby inflammation

imaging findings in CT, MRI, or abdominal ultrasound. Serum levels of amylase and lipase are required only for diagnosing AP but not useful for assessment of severity. An initial abdominal plain x-ray may not be diagnostic (Fig. 1). On the other hand, an initial abdominal ultrasound is mandatory in all patients to identify the presence of gallstones, the size of the common bile duct, CBD stones, and other findings. Abdominal ultrasound is often not useful in imaging the pancreas since abdominal fat and gas in the intestine obscure the findings. According to guidelines in the younger population, an initial CT scan of the abdomen is not recommended to diagnose AP except in circumstances when other diagnostic considerations exist. Routine CT abdomen is considered overuse of the resources. However, in the older adult, the indications for a CT scan with or without IV contrast on admission are invariably indicated given the many other critical abdominal emergencies in the differential diagnosis, inadequate history, and many comorbid conditions confusing the picture. It is important to recognize that a number of conditions

Table 2 Conditions associated with elevation of serum amylase and/or lipase in the older adult

With abdominal pain	Without abdominal pain
Pancreatic causes	Malignancies of
Acute pancreatitis	Lung
Chronic pancreatitis (acute exacerbation)	Ovary
Trauma	Pancreas
Abdominal surgery	Colon
Intervention (ERCP)	Thymus
Nonpancreatic abdominal causes	Bone marrow
Mesenteric infarction	Breast
Intestinal obstruction	Tongue
Appendicitis	Esophagus
Systemic disorders (abdominal pain due to a nonpancreatic cause)	Stomach
Diabetic ketoacidosis	Small bowel
	Liver
	Other causes
	Renal failure
	Liver failure
	Shock
	ARDS
	Postburn
	Cardiac surgery
	Pneumonia
	Benign hyperlipasemia/ Hypermylasemia

other than AP cause elevation of amylase and lipase (see Table 2); in particular, a few other ICU-related disorders may also cause incidental elevations of pancreatic enzymes. In the latter category are diabetic ketoacidosis, liver disease, renal failure, severe burns, head injury/stroke, abdominal trauma (blunt or penetrating), abdominal surgery, shock, pulmonary disease (ARDS, lung cancer, pulmonary embolism, perforated peptic ulcer, post-transplant (cardiac, liver, renal, bone marrow)), ruptured abdominal aortic aneurysm, and post-cardiac surgery (Muniraj and Dang 2015).

There are three grades of severity of AP: mild, moderately severe (MSAP), and severe acute pancreatitis (SAP). Mild AP is defined as AP with no organ failure and no systemic complications. MSAP is associated with organ failure, but it resolves within 48 h (transient organ failure). In MSAP, local or systemic complications may be present but without persistent organ failure. In SAP, there is persistent single organ failure (>48 h) or multiple organ failure. SAP is associated with high morbidity and mortality as a result of pancreatic and extra-pancreatic necrosis, subsequent infection, and MODS. SAP accounts for around 20% of AP patients and is associated with a high mortality rate (Johnson and Abu-Hilal 2004; Mofidi et al. 2006).

Difficulties in Diagnosing AP in the Older Adult

Acute abdominal pain, a frequent presentation of elderly patients to any emergency department, poses a significant challenge for various reasons (Lyon and Clark 2006). The initial diagnosis of the acute abdomen made in the emergency department often needs to be revised based on changes in subsequent clinical assessments, imaging studies, and laboratory results (Laurell et al. 2006; Lyon and Clark 2006). The diagnosis of AP may be missed in some cases (underdiagnosis) due to lack of classic history, or over-diagnosed because of a large number of nonpancreatic causes for serum pancreatic enzymes elevation (see Table 2) (Yegneswaran and Pitchumoni 2010). The classic teaching is that evaluation of abdominal pain necessarily starts with a good history. However, in many older adults, in particular in the oldest old (>85 years), severe cognitive impairment may make it impossible. The patient may be disoriented, demented, depressed, or aphasic, and a complete history from the patient may be difficult. The health care provider or a proxy may be the source of history, which may not be accurate. A delay in recognition of abdominal pain is not unusual. Often the older patient's symptoms initially get ignored until the disease advances to a critical situation. In the absence of an accurate history, AP may be confused with several disorders that need emergency surgery. The differential diagnosis of sudden onset abdominal pain with or without elevation of serum pancreatic enzymes in the older adult is broad. A surgical diagnosis such as acute appendicitis, cholecystitis, intestinal ischemia, intestinal obstruction, volvulus, diverticulitis, or perforated peptic ulcer (related to increased use of NSAIDs for many chronic painful conditions) is more often in the picture compared to that in the younger adult. On the other hand, older adults often complain of vague abdominal pain of musculoskeletal origin when the diagnosis of AP is considered and serum pancreatic enzymes are appropriately evaluated. Mild to moderate elevations of pancreatic enzymes even twofold to threefold occur in many instances with any inflammatory process (Table 2). Persons with Type 2 diabetes have an increased incidence of AP (Girman et al. 2010). It has been noted that many patients with diabetes and with acidosis of any etiology including diabetic ketoacidosis (DKA) have elevated levels of serum amylase and lipase (Steinberg 2011). A few elderly patients with AP may present with organ failure of unknown origin, hyperglycemia, and hypothermia. There may be a total absence of abdominal pain in the setting of even SAP (Gullo et al. 1994; Gloor et al. 2002) or if the patient is already on therapy with NSAIDs or another narcotic analgesic.

Although small in number, it is reported that some patients may be brought to the emergency department in a state of shock, respiratory difficulties, or evidence of multiple organ system dysfunctions. AP is a multisystem disease (see Table 3) and one or more organ system dysfunction may be the presenting feature (Coelho et al. 2019; Szakács et al. 2018).

Early identification with interventions is crucial for AP irrespective of age. There is evidence that after the initial 48–72 h, the progression of the disease may be fully established, leading to multisystem organ failure. The diagnosis of AP should be included in older patients with unexplained organ system dysfunction because of the urgent need for effective treatment options to prevent disease progression. Despite the availability of multiple scoring systems and their use in the emergency departments, more than 15–20% of patients with AP will develop SAP and according to one study up to 40% of this subgroup will die as a result (Sarri et al. 2019). Physical examination findings are also often unimpressive or misleading. Many findings of concomitant disorders

Table 3 Complications of acute pancreatitis (AP)

Systemic complications
Pulmonary
Early arterial hypoxia
Atelectasis, pneumonia, pleural effusion, and mediastinal abscess
Acute respiratory distress syndrome
Cardiac: shock, pericardial effusion, EKG changes, arrhythmias, SIRS
Hematologic: disseminated intravascular coagulation, thrombotic thrombocytopenic purpura/hemolytic uremic syndrome
Gastrointestinal: gastrointestinal bleeding (portal-splenic vein thrombosis, colonic infarction)
Renal: azotemia, oliguria
Metabolic: hyperkalemia, hypocalcemia, hypophosphatemia, hyperglycemia, hypertriglyceridemia, acidosis, elevation of free fatty acids, hypoalbuminemia
Central nervous system: psychosis, pancreatic encephalopathy, Purtscher-like retinopathy
Peripheral: fat necrosis (skin and bones), arthritis
Rhabdomyolysis
Pancreatic/peripancreatic complications
Acute fluid collection
Necrosis, sterile and infected, walled off pancreatic necrosis (WOPN)
Pseudocyst
Infected pseudocyst
Local extrapancreatic complications
Involvement of contiguous organs (intraperitoneal hemorrhage, gastrointestinal bleeding, thrombosis of spleen vein, bowel infarction)
Obstructive jaundice
Colonic involvement (necrosis, stricture)
Abdominal compartment syndrome

divert the path to the correct diagnosis. It is also likely that older people may have had previous abdominal surgical procedures complicating the history and physical findings (Sandblom et al. 2008).

AP Based on Etiological Factors

The etiological factors for AP are tabulated (Tables 4 and 5). While the etiological factors are the same as in the young, the frequency of

Table 4 Etiologic factors for acute pancreatitis (AP) in the older adult

Common
Gallstones
Alcohol
Drugs
Hypertriglyceridemia
Rare
Hypercalcemia
Obstruction of the ampulla of Vater, pancreatic adenocarcinoma, IPMN
Post-ERCP
Genetic
Pancreas divism
Trauma to abdomen
Viral (CMV, EBV, Mumps, Coxsackie B)
Parasitic (Toxoplasma, Cryptosporidium, Ascaris, *Clonorchis sinensis*, *Fasciola hepatica*)
Bacterial (Legionella)
Shock/ischemia/reperfusion injury (ICU pancreatitis)
Vasculitis
Duodenal diverticula
Choledochocele
Metastasis from primary tumor (lung, breast)
Abdominal and cardiac Surgery
Organophosphate poisoning
Idiopathic
Organ transplantation
Scorpion bite (in Trinidad)

Table 5 Obscure causes for acute pancreatitis (AP)

Microlithiasis
Ampullary tumors
Mucinous tumors of the pancreas (IPMN)
Undiagnosed chronic pancreatitis (early stages)
Anomalies of the pancreatic duct
Hereditary pancreatitis (initial episodes)
Sphincter of Oddi dysfunction
Choledochocele (type III choledochal cyst)
Annular pancreas
Anomalous pancreato-biliary junction
Duodenal diverticulum
Autoimmune
Even after completion of all tests, 15% of AP cases, an etiology is not identifiable

cases due to different factors varies. In general, the etiology of AP does not influence the course.

Gallstones

Similar to the younger age groups, gallstone-induced AP is the most frequent. The prevalence of gallstones increases as age advances and is over 25–30% in those aged >50. At least half of all cases of AP are due to the passage of small stones, usually 5 mm or less in diameter (Fogel and Sherman 2014). Common bile duct (CBD) stones are seen more often in older adults than in the general populations. Overall, 5% of patients presenting with cholecystitis have coexisting CBD stones in contrast to 10–20% of the elderly (Siegel and Kasmin 1997). Nationwide increases in the incidence of gallstones and obesity (a well-known risk for gallstones and a marker of severe AP) are expected to increase the incidence and severity of AP.

There is a greater incidence of complications of AP, CBD stones, ascending cholangitis, portal vein thrombosis, a higher need for therapeutic procedures in the management of complications, and higher susceptibility to infections (Roulin et al. 2018). Given the frequency of CBD stones and the possibility of ascending cholangitis more often, there is an indication for MRCP, EUS, and therapeutic ERCP (Trust et al. 2011; Roulin et al. 2018). The pathogenesis of biliary pancreatitis is not completely understood. In 1901, Eugene Opie postulated that impairment of the pancreatic outflow due to obstruction of the pancreatic duct causes pancreatitis. Gallstones (and sludge) small enough to pass through the biliary tract, rather than the ones that remain asymptomatically in the gallbladder, confer risk for AP. The mechanisms of biliary pancreatitis are many and include a reflux of bile into the pancreatic duct – either through a common channel created by an impacted gallstone or through an incompetent sphincter, changes in intra-acinar cell calcium signaling, or injury to acinar cells by bile acids (Markus and Lerch 2016). Once a patient has developed AP, it is likely to recur if the gallbladder, the source of migrating bile duct stones, is not removed or their impaction at the duodenal papilla is not prevented (Markus and Lerch 2016). AP due to bile duct stones may rarely occur even years after cholecystectomy and one should not exclude a biliary cause because of previous cholecystectomy (Gloor et al. 2003).

The initial diagnosis of a biliary etiology for AP is made by the combination of history, physical examination findings, serum biochemical studies, and transabdominal ultrasound (stones in the gallbladder and main bile duct). Charcot's triad (jaundice associated with biliary colic, fever, and chills), indicates acute cholangitis. However, currently, a diagnosis of CBD stone or ascending cholangitis need not wait for Charcot's triad to develop.

The diagnosis of AP of biliary etiology is essentially by imaging studies but is complemented by the evaluation of liver chemistry. The elevated liver enzymes alanine aminotransferase [ALT] or aspartate aminotransferase [AST]) in the setting of AP suggest a biliary etiology (Tenner et al. 1994). The AST/ALT levels may be markedly elevated to thousands in acute biliary obstruction mimicking acute hepatitis. However, normal serum levels do not totally exclude a biliary etiology (Dholakia et al. 2004). Years ago, ERCP was a primary diagnostic tool in suspected biliary pancreatitis, but currently, there is little role for diagnostic ERCP. The availability of endoscopic ultrasound (EUS) of the biliary system and MRCP has changed the diagnostic algorithm (see ASGE guidelines). In addition to CBD stones, EUS identifies microlithiasis, pancreaticobiliary neoplasms, pancreas divisum, and often the most frequent occult causes for AP, sometimes classified as Idiopathic AP.

Once an initial etiology of biliary AP is established, the broad principles of management of biliary pancreatitis involve:

1. The treatment of mild biliary AP is conservative, followed by cholecystectomy in the same admission if there is no contraindication. Early cholecystectomy in the setting of gallstone pancreatitis (i.e., during the index admission) reduces the incidence of repeat biliary-related events, including pancreatitis, cholecystitis, and biliary colic (Hwang et al. 2013; Garber et al. 2018).

2. There is no indication for urgent ERCP in patients with mild pancreatitis without cholangitis (Kapetanos 2010). If cholecystectomy is contraindicated in patients because of comorbidities, ERCP and sphincterotomy should be considered before discharge. ERCP is not indicated in predicted severe biliary pancreatitis without cholangitis (Working Group IAP/APA Acute Pancreatitis Guidelines 2013).

3. Endoscopic therapy is indicated when there is evidence of CBD obstruction. A strong indication for early therapeutic intervention is when patients are suspected with CBD stones and with one of the following: ascending cholangitis (fever, jaundice, sepsis), persistent biliary obstruction (serum conjugated bilirubin of >5 mg/dL), and clinical deterioration (worsening pain, increasing white cell count, and worsening vital signs) (Kapetanos 2010; Takada et al. 2013). Endoscopic therapy may be palliative or in some cases curative even in advanced age. One can safely perform ERCP procedures for patients aged 85 years or older (Sugiyama and Atomi 2000; Obana et al. 2010).

4. Before performing ERCP, MRCP and/or EUS are useful in the diagnosis of biliary obstruction. MRCP is a noninvasive procedure for the detection of CBD stone, with 85–92% sensitivity and 93–97% specificity (Costi et al. 2014). However, it is not recommended in an unstable patient who cannot be monitored in the MRCP chamber (Romagnuolo et al. 2003).

5. Endoscopic ultrasound (EUS) is an excellent modality to detect CBD stones (Garrow et al. 2007). MRCP may not detect small stones lodged near the ampulla. EUS under IV sedation can be followed by ERCP and stone removal if indicated in the same sitting of IV sedation.

6. According to ASGE guideline, the predictor for a CBD stone is very strong when CBD stone is noted on transabdominal ultrasonography (US), the presence of clinical ascending cholangitis or when total serum bilirubin is >4 mg/dL. It is considered strong (dilated CBD > 6 mm on the US with gallbladder in situ and a total bilirubin level of 1.8–4.0 mg/dL) and moderate (abnormal liver biochemical test other than bilirubin, age more than 55 years, and clinical findings of biliary pancreatitis) (Maple et al. 2010; Kuzu et al. 2017;

Forsmark et al. 2007). Endoscopic therapy is needed as an emergency. The frequency of ERCP-related complications is almost the same in older as compared to younger individuals except for a lower rate of post-ERCP pancreatitis in the elderly group (Tohda et al. 2016; Greenberg et al. 2016).

Alcoholic Pancreatitis

Alcoholic pancreatitis is generally a disease of the younger generation more than in the elderly based on drinking habits. However, one cannot ignore alcoholism in the older adult with new-onset AP. Although descriptions vary, it is generally accepted that drinking >80 g of alcohol a day in men and lesser amounts in women for 5–10 years or more is a prerequisite for developing alcoholic AP. Alcoholism in the older population is a "silent epidemic" ignored by all (Barry and Blow 2016). The National Institute of Alcohol Abuse and Alcoholism found that about 40 % of adults ages 65 and older drink alcohol (Gunzerath et al. 2004; Rigler 2000; Hall et al. 2005). About 10–15% start drinking in older age as a result of the loss of a spouse, loneliness, a feeling of abandonment, depression, and many other factors. The sensitivity of MCV or GGT in detecting alcohol misuse is higher in older than in younger populations (Caputo et al. 2012). Older adults are more vulnerable to the physiological effects of alcohol than younger adults (Gargiulo et al. 2013). The risk of alcohol-associated disorders is higher since it is processed differently. Reduced activity of gastric and liver alcohol dehydrogenase (ADH) leads to the elevation of blood alcohol level by 20–50% (Lieber 2005). Comorbid conditions and a decrease in lean body mass result in a decrease in the aqueous volume of cells, which in turn increases the effective concentration of alcohol in the body (Ferreira and Weems 2008; Gargiulo et al. 2013). It is likely although not proven that the risk of alcohol-associated disorders is higher as reported in a Japanese study showing that a high consumption of alcohol over a short period as may happen in the older adult could be an independent risk factor for AP. The synergistic effect of cigarette smoking in increasing the risk is well recognized (Yadav et al. 2009; Burns 2000). Older smokers are less likely than younger smokers to attempt quitting (Masamune et al. 2013).

Post ERCP Pancreatitis (PEP)

Diagnostic ERCP has decreased substantially, but ERCP for therapeutic indications has increased irrespective of age. Older age is not a contraindication for ERCP and ERCP as a palliative care in biliary pancreatitis may be needed often in the older adult. Perhaps the indications for ERCP are more in the older adult. Choledocholithiasis, biliary and pancreatic cancer, and the postoperative management of adverse events following biliary surgery are all more prevalent in the old age (Day et al. 2014; Lukens et al. 2010). Since endoscopic treatment of pancreaticobiliary disorders is a preferred alternative to surgery in the frail elderly, more procedures are performed. PEP is a complication in up to 10% of cases requiring the procedure and carries significant morbidity and mortality (Sheiybani et al. 2018). AP is a reported complication in 35/1000 ERCPs, but the range varies widely from 16–157/1000 (Day et al. 2014). A prior history of PEP, female sex, normal CBD size, and normal bilirubin are factors that increase the risk. A systematic review in 2015 revealed that rectal NSAIDs significantly reduce the risk. Diclofenac is more effective than indomethacin (Sajid et al. 2015). A risk assessment for PEP is necessary before ERCP and prophylactic measure to prevent PEP are highly recommended.

Pancreatic Cancer

Pancreatic cancer is increasing in incidence in Western countries. AP, although is only a rare manifestation of pancreatic cancer, clinicians fail to recognize the association. Other overwhelming confounding factors such as the use of medications, history of alcohol use, or a coexistent incidental gallstone evade the diagnosis. The association of AP with pancreatic cancer is well documented, with a 20-fold increase in the risk of pancreatic cancer within the first 2 years after diagnosis of AP (Kirkegård et al. 2018). Patients admitted with AP in one study had an increased risk of pancreatic cancer compared with age- and sex-matched comparison subjects from the general (Kirkegård et al. 2018). Although relatively small when pancreatic cancer is diagnosed early, there is a survival benefit in cases presenting with AP (>25%) than with other causes (20%) (Mujica et al. 2000). Thus it is important to exclude pancreatic cancer in an elderly patient with AP (Mujica et al. 2000; Kimura et al. 2015; Köhler and Lankisch 1987; Morales-Oyarvide et al. 2015; Rigler 2000). Endoscopic ultrasound evaluation of the pancreas in AP a few weeks after the acute episode is to be recommended.

Drug-Induced AP (DIP)

The topic of DIP is riddled with many doubts, and the cause and effect of the association are rarely established. However, DIP is a real entity and cannot be dismissed. One should be vigilant to the possibility along with consideration of other causes such as biliary disease, alcoholism, hyperlipidemia, and pancreatic cancer.

According to WHO, 525 different drugs can induce AP as an adverse reaction, but a recent publication listed only 31 drugs to be associated with an established definite causality (Nitsche et al. 2010). Many individual case reports of DIP are probably incidental findings (Balani and Grendell 2008; Trivedi and Pitchumoni 2005; Tenner 2014; Nitsche et al. 2010).

The confounding issues are many. The elderly population is at higher risk for AP for a variety of reasons such as increased incidence of gallstones and hypertriglyceridemia. The incidence of AP in people with type 2 diabetes is higher than in those without diabetes. Although a definite cause and effect cannot be established, the following medications are frequently cited as to cause AP (Table 6). Many of these drugs are often used by older people. A few medications frequently used by older adults for the age-related diseases are emphasized below. Furosemide-induced AP is often mentioned, but its

incidence must be extremely low considering the high frequency of its use. Use of incretin-based drugs ((DPP-4 inhibitors [sitagliptin, vildagliptin, and saxagliptin] or GLP-1 analogs [exenatide, liraglutide]) alone or in combination with other anti-diabetic drugs are reported to cause AP. Some of these observations have overlooked the facts that there is an increased incidence of AP in diabetics unrelated to medications (Tenner 2014). Modest elevations of serum amylase levels in diabetics in particular with DKA is not unusual. Analysis of data from 14,611 patients with type 2 diabetes from 25 clinical trials in the sitagliptin database provided no compelling evidence of an increased risk of pancreatitis or pancreatic cancer (Lyon and Clark 2006). FDA concludes that "assertions concerning a causal relationship between incretin drugs are inconsistent with the scientific literature" and does not support exenatide-induced AP (Tenner 2014).

AP-induced by statins has been reported from hours to years after initiation of treatment. Drug-induced AP by HMG-CoA reductase inhibitors (statins) is a class effect. The exact incidence is likely to be extremely low. ACE inhibitors (benazepril, captopril, enalapril, lisinopril, quinapril, and ramipril) extensively used by older adults are also associated with drug-induced AP (Laurell et al. 2006). AP is commonly associated with both HIV and the use of HAART in HIV-positive patients. Many chemotherapeutic agents and hormonal agents can cause AP. There are several case reports of AP associated with medications used in the management of inflammatory bowel diseases (5-aminosalicylic acid (5-ASA), immunomodulators, 6-mercaptopurine, and azathioprinez) (Pitchumoni et al. 2010). The association of AP induced by azathioprine is strong.

Other drugs suspected are antibiotics (tetracyclines, macrolides, metronidazole, ampicillin, amoxicillin, and amphotericin), cimetidine, clozapine, corticosteroids, methyldopa, metronidazole, salicylates, and zalcitabine, acetaminophen, cyclosporine, cytarabine, erythromycin and roxithromycin, ketoprofen, metolazone, and octreotide. Opiates are used extensively for pain control, including in patients with AP, although AP is a rare adverse effect of opiates.

Table 6 Drug-induced pancreatitis in the older adult (Egan et al. 2014; Kaurich 2008)

Medications implicated in acute pancreatitis in the elderly
Cardiovascular agents
Antihypertensives
ACE-I (Benzapril, captopril, enalapril, forinopril, lisinopril, moexipril, quinapril, ramipril, transolapril)
Diuretics (thiazide diuretics, loop diuretics, ethacrynic acid, furosemide)
Calcium channel blockers
Cholesterol-lowering agents
HMG-CoA reductase inhibitors (fluvastatin, lovastatin, pravastatin, simvastatin, atorvastatin, rosuvastatin)
Fibrates (genfibrozil, fenofibrate)
Anti-platelets/thrombolytics
ASA, alteplase, anagrelide, dipyridamole, reteplase, streptokinase
Anti-arrhythmics
Smiodarone, mexiletine
Antibacterials
Tetracyclines (doxycycline, demeclocycline, minocycline)
Macrolides (azithromycin, clarithromycin)
Quinolones (clatrofloxacin, ciprofloxacin, levofloxacin, norfloxacin, trovafloxacin)
Others (atovaquone, metronidazole, secnidazole, ertapenem, nitrofurantoin, trimethoprim/sulfamethoxazole, quinpristin/dalfopristin)
TNF-a inhibitors
Etanercept, infliximab
Anti-inflammatory agents
NSAIDS (diclofenac, ibuprofen, ketorolac, meloxicam, sulindac, mefenamic acid, nabumetone, naproxen, indomethacin, piroxicam
COX-II inhibitors (celecoxib, rofecoxib)
Acetaminophen
Hypoglycemic agents
Incretin mimetics (exenatide, liraglutide)
Glitazones (troglitazone, rosiglitazone, pioglitazone)
GI agents
PPIs (omeprazole, pantroprazole, rabeprazole)
Antacids (cimetidine, ranitidine)
IBD medications
Aminosalicylates (balsalazide, mesalamine, olsalazine, sulfasalazine)
Others (azathioprine, mercaptopurine)
Hormones
Steroids (cortisone, dexamethasone, fludrocortisone, methylprednisolone, prednisone)
Others (somatropin, octretide)

(continued)

Table 6 (continued)

Antineoplastic drugs
L-asparaginase, 6-mercaptopurine, vincristine, vinblastine)
Immunemodulators
Cyclosporine, glatiramer, interferon b-1B, interferon g-1B, mycophenolate, sirolimus, tacrolimus, thalidomide, PegInterferon a-2B

Modified from Trivedi and Pitchumoni (2005)

Idiopathic AP

Idiopathic AP accounts for 20–40% of patients influenced by the diligence with which one would look for an etiological factor. Idiopathic AP by definition is AP with no identifiable etiological factor after a thorough evaluation with biochemical (including the exclusion of hypercalcemia, hyperlipidemia) and imaging studies (including MRI, CT scan abdomen with pancreatic protocol, exclusion of pancreas divisum and neoplasms). Genetic predisposition to pancreatitis is a topic of importance, but it is less likely in the elderly. Mutations of the trypsinogen PRSS1gene, SPINK1, and CFTR gene (cystic fibrosis) are known to have a high risk of developing pancreatitis. There is a possibility that many cases of idiopathic AP cases are erroneously attributed to one or more medications that the older adult is taking. Although obesity in itself is not a cause for AP, it is an association with gallstones and a risk for severe AP.

Physical Examination Findings

There is no specific or diagnostic finding that would strongly suggest AP but epigastric tenderness is a prominent sign that may not be reliably elicited if the patient is demented or not capable of verbalizing. Cholecystitis, perforated peptic ulcer, intestinal ischemia, and a few other conditions are also associated with epigastric tenderness. The finding of hypoactive bowel sounds is unreliable. Cullen and Grey- Turner signs (periumbilical and flank echymoses) are text book signs of curiosity, extremely rare, and are seldom useful in the diagnosis. When present in a patient with proven AP, the signs indicate severity. Many older persons may be on anticoagulants with a higher tendency for easy echymosis unrelated to AP.

Initial Laboratory Studies

The initial tests are a complete blood count, serum electrolytes, liver tests, and other tests that evaluate the severity as discussed below. Serum amylase levels rapidly increase first but decrease rapidly. This gradual decrease in serum amylase may delay early treatment in patients with a long interval between the onset of symptoms and admission to the hospital, often the case in elderly patients. The sensitivity of serum lipase ranges from 85% to 100%, and it is more specific than amylase and useful in patients who present after several days. The critically ill patient in an intensive care unit and patients with DKA may have false elevations of serum pancreatic enzymes (Muniraj and Dang 2015). C-reactive protein (CRP) is an acute phase reactant that usually rises after 36 h of pancreatic inflammation and peaks at 48 h. When distinguishing between mild and severe disease, CRP was shown to be the most useful biomarker if serum levels are greater than 150 mg/dl; CRP is especially useful in the elderly in whom the initial diagnosis can be a great challenge.

Severity Assessment

AP may be severe in nearly 20% of all cases of pancreatitis, but a larger percentage of patients in the older age group is logically expected to suffer a serious course. Severe AP causes significant morbidity and increased mortality due to numerous local and systemic complications, an intense inflammatory response that may progress to multiorgan failure and or pancreatic necrosis. In the geriatric population, AP is reported to be associated with a more severe course than the nongeriatric population with a longer duration of hospital stay (Kara et al. 2018) and a higher incidence of organ failure and mortality (Gardner et al. 2008). Age > 70 years is noted as an

independent risk factor for mortality in patients with SAP (Gardner et al. 2008; Carvalho et al. 2018). Not all studies agree; there is a considerable conflict about the effect of older age and outcomes in AP (Fan et al. 1988; Kim et al. 2012; Schütte and Malfertheiner 2008).

One large study concluded that despite multiple comorbidities and higher Charlson index in the elderly at admission, old age solely did not affect mortality or severity of acute biliary pancreatitis (Roulin et al. 2018). Since comorbidity is a common feature of old age, it is irrelevant to state that AP in the older adult is intrinsically not more serious, if not for the presence of concomitant diseases with advanced age.

The need to predict the severity of AP is because, in the first 24–48 h of the onset of symptoms, aggressive treatment may benefit the patient. A delay in transferring the patient to ICU is associated with poor prognosis. Unfortunately, on day one of AP, it may be difficult to differentiate a mild case of AP from a severe case with an increase in mortality (Brivet et al. 1999). Hence the predictors of severity of AP are important (Tables 7, 8, and 9). There are single markers of severity (Table 7) and multiple scoring systems. There is not one sure prognostic factor for mortality in patients with AP and only an association between several factors can lead to an accurate mortality prediction (Popa et al. 2016). Judgment based on findings, clinical as well as laboratory,

Table 7 Single markers of severity and comments

Obesity: BMI >30 is a poor prognostic marker
Ecchymosis (Cullen and Grey Turner signs); both signs are very rare
Admission hemoconcentration >44%: (lack of hemoconcentration denotes milder pancreatitis)
Failure to correct hemoconcentration to <44% within 24 h of hospitalization: suggests the need for early and adequate intravenous hydration
Serum creatinine >2 mg/dL on admission and failure to decline below 2 mg/dL with adequate fluid administration is a marker of volume depletion
Fasting blood glucose >125 mg/dL (in nondiabetics)
C-reactive protein >150 mg/L at 48 h after admission
Fall in serum calcium, albumin
CT scan of abdomen: not necessary in most, but is a good marker when used appropriately

Table 8 Scoring system for Bedside Index of Severity in Acute Pancreatitis (BISAP)

Score one point for each of the following criteria:
Blood urea nitrogen level > 8.9 mmol/L
Impaired mental status
Systemic inflammatory response syndrome is present
Age > 60 years
Pleural effusion on radiography
A score of more than three indicates an increased risk of death

Wu et al. (2008)

Table 9 Systemic inflammatory response syndrome (SIRS)

SIRS criteria
Temperature > 38 or < 36 °C
Respiratory rate >20 breaths/minute or $PaCO_2 < 32$ mmHg
Pulse >90 beats/minute
White blood cell count <4000 cells/mm^3 or 12,000 cells/mm^3 or >10% immature bands

Note: SIRS is defined as the presence of two or more SIRS criteria

should be the basis of an assessment of severity. Older age, comorbid conditions, multiorgan dysfunction syndrome, the extent of pancreatic necrosis, infection, and sepsis are the major determinants of mortality in AP (Buter et al. 2002; Khanna et al. 2013; Otsuki et al. 2013).

The severity prediction systems include, importantly, frequent clinical assessment, early and repeated biochemical markers, and a scoring system. Multiple scoring systems are available, and early assessment of severity using one or more of the above is necessary to triage the patient to a medical floor or the ICU. A recent multivariate analysis revealed that patients suffering from severe comorbidities commonly noted in older patients were about 4.5 times more likely to have a fatal episode of AP and about two times more likely to develop severe AP than those having no comorbidities. In the same study, the authors noted that aging and comorbidities influenced the development of local and systemic complications in a completely different manner. Charlson Comorbidity Index (CCI) covering preexisting chronic conditions is to be included in the prognostic assessment (Szakács et al. 2018; Quero et al. 2019; Carvalho et al. 2018).

The single markers of severity.

1. Obesity (BMI) (Khatua et al. 2017).
   Obesity is a risk factor for the development of local and systemic complications in AP, and also increases the mortality of this disease.
2. Hemoconcentration on admission is a reflection of fluid loss and hypovolemia that leads to microcirculatory compromise and a potential cause of pancreatic necrosis. Hemoconcentration with a hematocrit >44% on admission and failure to correct within 48 h are markers of severity. A normal or low hematocrit at admission and during the first 24 h has a negative predictive value in that it is generally associated with a milder clinical course. Overall, initial hematocrit evaluation is a simple and useful predictor of severe pancreatitis (Gan and Romagnuolo 2004).
3. Blood urea nitrogen. BUN, as a single marker of severity in AP is easy to perform and inexpensive.
4. Creatinine. Increased serum creatinine in the first 48 h of admission is strongly associated with the development of pancreatic necrosis.
5. Blood sugar level. An elevated blood sugar in a nondiabetic and hypoglycemia indicate severity.
6. C-reactive protein. As an acute phase, reactant CRP levels in serum help to predict severity. Levels of CRP >150 mg/L at 48 h denotes SAP (Lin et al. 2017; Wu et al. 2009). C reactive protein assay is a simple and inexpensive method (Neoptolemos et al. 2000). Elevated levels, however, are not specific to AP since many other causes of inflammation such as cholangitis and pneumonia also raise the levels.
7. Hypocalcemia occurs in severe AP the pathophysiology of the finding is not clear. The fall is mostly in the unionized form and hence tetany is a rare finding.
8. Hypoalbuminemia a day after admission indicates severity attributed to various causes including extravasation of protein rich

exudates in the retroperitoneal space, calcium trapping in the peripancreatic tissues (soap formation) and muscles. The role of calcitonin and other hormones release is speculated.

9. Pleural effusion. Often considered a marker of pancreatitis in the past, is indeed a sign of severity.
10. Plain X-ray abdomen in severe AP shows ileus but is not a reliable sign of severity (see Fig. 1).

Many other less-often used single markers are trypsinogen activation peptide, carboxypeptidase B activation peptide, procalcitonin, interleukins polymorphonuclear elastase, and coagulation parameters. Serum levels of IL-6 and procalcitonin have the highest sensitivity for prediction of severity (Mofidi et al. 2009).

Modalities of assessment of the severity of AP are Ranson and Glasgow Criteria, but both require 48 h for accurate assessment of mortality and cannot be used beyond 48 h after admission to the hospital (Mounzer et al. 2012; Harshit Kumar and Singh Griwan 2018). The APACHE II scoring system takes into account 12 variables which include, (Bradley 1993) body temperature (Banks et al. 2013), mean arterial pressure (mm Hg) (Peery et al. 2015), Heart rate (HR) (Yadav and Lowenfels 2006), respiratory rate (R.R/mt) (Tenner et al. 2013), Oxygenation (mm Hg) (Crockett et al. 2018), pH (Krishna et al. 2017), Na (mmol/l) (Gullo et al. 2002), K (mmol/l) (Whitcomb 2006), creatinine (mg/100 ml) (Tinto et al. 2002), hematocrit (Noel et al. 2016), total leucocyte count, and the (Otsuki et al. 2013) Glasgow coma score. The scoring system can be used on admission as well as to reassess the severity and disease progression. By adding obesity to the scoring system, APACHEO was introduced to include the added prognostic marker. APACHE II has not been developed specifically for AP but has been proven to be an early and reliable tool. APACHE II measures the physiological response to injury and inflammation-driven stress designed to predict prolonged intensive care unit treatment and mortality and is not specific for AP. Other limitations of the APACHE II system are the requirement for multiple parameters. Older age is given a high negative score to start with. Age over 65 to 74 is given 5 points and over 75 carries 6 points.

Bedside index of severity in acute pancreatitis (BISAP) is a newer scoring system that needs to be carefully interpreted in the elderly with AP (see Table 8 for BISAP score (Wu et al. 2008)). In a recent study a BISAP score at a cut-off of >3 had a moderate sensitivity and a high specificity for predicting mortality and severe AP. In comparison, at a cut-off of <2, the sensitivity increased whereas the specificity decreased for both outcomes (Gao et al. 2015). BISAP score is a reliable and accurate means for predicting the severity of AP in the early phase and younger patients. BISAP score is higher in older patients and patients with altered mental status (Khanna et al. 2013). Impaired mental status (the "I" of BISAP) is a subjective assessment that is often positive in the older adult as a result of preexisting conditions or a state of delirium in the older adult as a result of an acute illness (Table 8) (Wu et al. 2008).

SIRS is the clinical manifestation of the inflammatory process. The markers of SIRS occur in a variety of infectious and noninfectious conditions. The markers of SIRS are tabulated (Table 9). The measurement of SIRS during the first day of hospitalization provides important information in assessing severity (Singh et al. 2009). Sequential Organ Failure Assessment (SOFA) Score. SOFA is composed of six parameters that can be measured daily. They involve the following organ systems; Pulmonary (PaO2/FIO2), hematologic (platelet count), gastrointestinal (serum bilirubin), cardiovascular (hypotension), neurologic (Glasgow coma scale) and renal (creatinine or urine output). Each organ is graded from 0 to 4 (most abnormal), and one may get a daily score of 0 to 24. The SOFA score provides potentially valuable prognostic information on in-hospital survival (Jones et al. 2009).

Ranson criteria originally established in 1974 and revised in 1979 is nearly obsolete currently.

Imaging Studies

A chest x-ray to exclude pleural effusion is indicated on admission and subsequently if clinically indicated. Pleural effusion is a marker of severity. Pleural effusion has been reported in 4–20% of patients with AP. Pleural effusion is associated with SAP and poor outcome.

CT scan abdomen. Given the difficulties in obtaining an accurate history of abdominal pain in many or some older adults, particularly in those with dementia or taking NSAIDs or other analgesics for preexisting chronic diseases, the classic history of AP pain may not be available. Elderly patients may seek medical attention not for pain but with altered mental status, or in a delayed stage of AP. Physical examination findings may be misleading. Various imaging studies are necessary early during the initial evaluation; some of the tests may be considered unwanted in the young according to well-accepted practice guidelines. Early imaging studies may be unavoidable.

Abdominal ultrasound is routinely performed to evaluate a biliary etiology in all patients. Because of the overlying bowel gas, it makes it difficult to study the pancreas. Abdominal US is to evaluate the presence or absence of gallstones, CBD size, stones, distension of gallbladder, and other findings of cholecystitis. Several incidental age-related findings may mislead the diagnosis. The normal diameter of the common bile duct can be up to 10 mm. There is a high probability of seeing incidental gallstones.

In the management of AP in the large majority of younger patients, CT abdomen on admission is not indicated. The radiological manifestations may be absent or only mild. In most inpatient hospital settings, attempt to do a CT, or any other special radiological procedure, often delays the initiation of treatment. Early CT scan with IV contrast in a dehydrated patient poses a high risk for kidney injury in an older patient.

Despite arguments against an early CT scan of the abdomen in a younger patient in the management of elderly patients with acute abdominal pain, a liberal attitude is essential. Unlike in the young, the differential diagnosis of abdominal pain is wider, and exclusion of a surgical condition mimicking AP is crucial. Ischemic bowel disease, a perforated viscus, intestinal obstruction, and acalculous cholecystitis are conditions that require prompt surgical intervention while AP needs only nonsurgical management with scrutiny. Whether the initial CT abdomen is to be a contrast-enhanced one or not is to be decided based on the clinical condition of the patient. A noncontrast CT scan of the abdomen performed in the Emergency Department is very valuable in excluding a surgical disease (Payor et al. 2015). A history of abdominal pain and findings on physical examination may be unreliable or confusing; other conditions in the differential diagnosis may be associated with elevation of serum amylase and or lipase. A contrast-enhanced computed tomography (CECT) performed on initial evaluation cannot be used to reliably determine the morphological changes that would appear later.

A CT study, when done properly, will help to assess the severity. Imaging studies, in particular, computed tomography severity index of Balthazar, has a good correlation with the development of complications and mortality in patients with AP (Balthazar 2002). Imaging studies do not identify the risk of organ system dysfunction, in particular, in the first week of the disease when morphological changes are not present or only minimal.

CECT helps in the staging of the inflammatory process and early detection of possible complications of the inflamed pancreas, including pancreatic necrosis. A CECT performed in the first several days of onset of AP helps determine whether AP is localized or diffuse enlargement of the pancreas with normal homogenous enhancement suggestive of edematous pancreatitis. Other findings include fat stranding and acute peripancreatic fluid collections (APFC). In less than 5% of cases of acute pancreatitis, CECT helps to identify pancreatic necrosis by areas of the pancreas with lack of parenchymal enhancement (necrosis) (Thoeni 2012). Weeks later on in the clinical course, APFC may disappear, form a pseudocyst, or infrequently get infected. Similarly, necrotized areas may get walled off (Walled off necrosis, WON). The area of necrosis and WON may be sterile or less often infected.

Magnetic resonance imaging (MRI) is indicated when a CBD stone is suspected. It is also a good alternative to CT for detecting parenchymal necrosis. The limitations include: technical difficulties, obesity, pacemaker, claustrophobia, difficult implementation in critically ill patients, and gadolinium toxicity (in patients with renal insufficiency) (Abou Rached et al. 2014). MRCP findings help to decide the need for ERCP and stone extraction in biliary AP.

Patients with AP may also be evaluated with a magnetic resonance image (MRI); however, implanted cardiac devices, such as cardiac pacemakers, preclude the use of MRI in the elderly. Ultrasonography does not have an important role in the diagnosis or staging of acute pancreatitis but may be useful in the determination of common bile duct stones or dilatation of the bile duct or stones within the gallbladder.

Many professional organizations have published guidelines for the management of acute pancreatitis (Crockett et al. 2018; Koutroumpakis et al. 2017; van Dijk et al. 2017).

General Management of AP

The broad principles of initial management of AP irrespective of age are largely supportive therapy with IV fluids, nutritional support, and appropriate pain control with parenteral analgesics. One should adhere to recent guidelines in the management of AP in all healthy elderly, but based on age-related comorbid conditions one should use clinical judgment and modify the management in providing the best care without causing any iatrogenic complications.

An important aspect of care is that more frequent monitoring is needed because the initial diagnosis may have to be changed based on newer developments, rapid deterioration in the patient's clinical condition, signs of fluid overload, and the need for additional consultations from specialists in pain management, pulmonologists, and surgeons. Frequent monitoring of vital signs, including oxygen saturation, is needed. Appropriate respiratory support is to be given. Various cardiovascular manifestations may occur (Table 10) (Yegneswaran et al. 2011). Hypoxia may occur due to various causes. Pleural effusions, atelectasis, and acute respiratory distress syndrome (ARDS) are important pulmonary complications. As early as possible using one of the prognostic criteria complemented by using the single markers of prognosis, a clinical judgment about the potential severity is to be assessed and the decision has to be made regarding the need for ICU care

Table 10 Cardiac manifestations of (AP)

Hemodynamic changes
Tachycardia
Low total peripheral resistance
Increased cardiac index
Hypovolemia
Decreased left ventricular stroke volume
Myocardial depression
Cardiac regional wall motion abnormalities
Impaired diastolic function
Decreased peak blood flow velocity
Electrocardiographic changes
Ventricular fibrillation
Bradycardia
Atrial flutter
Atrial fibrillation
Supraventricular premature contractions, ventricular ectopic arrhythmias
QRS prolongation
QT prolongation
Shortened PQ interval
Left bundle branch block
Right bundle branch block
Left anterior hemi-block
Nonspecific changes in repolarization
Decreased T-wave voltage
T-wave changes
ST-segment depression
ST-segment elevation
Pericardial changes
Pericardial effusion
Chylous pericardial effusion with tamponade
Fibrinous constrictive pericarditis

Modified from Yegneswaran et al. 2011

(van Dijk et al. 2017). IV hydration is to be carefully adjusted to the needs of avoiding overhydration and development of pulmonary edema and or abdominal compartment syndrome. Other items to be frequently assessed are the development of hypo or hyperglycemia, rapid change in hemoglobin levels (hemoconcentration indicating inadequate hydration and compromise of microcirculation in the pancreas, fall in hemoglobin indicative of internal bleeding (often retroperitoneal) and hypokalemia) are to be assessed frequently for early diagnosis and appropriate management.

Pain Management

The Pain in AP is Quite Variable in Severity. Older adults are less sensitive to pain, and this increased threshold to pain may lead to delays in the diagnosis and result in poor prognosis (Pergolizzi et al. 2008). The increased prevalence of dementia and communication disorders adds another dimension of challenges in pain control in the elderly (Cavalieri 2002). The management of pain in the older adult, in particular in ones with frailty, is complicated by the added risks posed by changes in pharmacokinetics and pharmacodynamics, polypharmacy, and drug-disease interactions. Clinical studies evaluating the efficacy of analgesics often exclude older people, in particular, frail patients. Therefore, the true efficacy and side-effect profiles in these population groups are largely unknown (Veal and Peterson 2015). On the other hand, adequate control of pain is necessary as in any other patient.

Adequate control of pain in the older adult without causing side effects such as confusion, delirium, and instability is a delicate balance. Opioids are effective but need individual dose titration. The appropriate analgesic should be chosen based on safety and tolerability considerations. The half-life of the active drug and metabolites is increased with age and in those with renal dysfunction; the dosage has to be appropriately decreased. Opioid analgesics could be safely administered with an excellent benefit (Schorn et al. 2015). There is no evidence for a long-standing belief that they cause sphincter of Oddi spasm (Lee and Cundiff 1998) or any difference in the risk of complications or clinically serious adverse events between opioids and other analgesia options (Chau et al. 2008). There are many opioids (buprenorphine, fentanyl, hydromorphone, methadone, morphine, and oxycodone) available and the superiority of one over another is not established. Respiratory depression is a major side effect in those with underlying pulmonary pathology such as COPD or when receiving concomitant central nervous system (CNS) drugs associated with hypoventilation (Pergolizzi et al. 2008). Tramadol, a narcotic analgesic, is an atypical opioid with opioid and non-opioid activity. The adverse effects of opioids are nausea, dizziness, headache, hypotension, and seizures. On the one hand, the elderly are often untreated or undertreated for pain; on the other hand, the incidence of serious side effects increases with the patient's age. Compared with other analgesics, opioids may decrease the need for supplementary analgesics. There is no increased risk of complications of AP with the use of opioid analgesics (Basurto Ona et al. 2013). In the older adult, there is potential for more side effects or treatment failures (Linnebur et al. 2005). Debilitated patients or those with COPD are at higher risk for hypoxia if over sedated.

Given age-related pharmacokinetic and pharmacodynamic changes, opioids should be started at a lower dose, about 25–50% of the dose given to younger patients (Chau et al. 2008; Clark 2002). In assessing the relief of pain, one should be aware of the following. In demented patients, there may be an impaired perception of pain, ability to report pain, ability to recall pain sensation for evaluating relief, and the ability to communicate about relief (Chau et al. 2008; AGS Panel on Persistent Pain in Older Persons 2002). Thus, the potential for unrelieved and unrecognized pain is greater among those who cannot reliably evaluate and verbally express their discomfort. Fentanyl (intravenous) may be used for pain relief in AP. However, one should titrate fentanyl cautiously. There is lower fentanyl clearance in older patients explained by lower plasma albumin, decreased hepatic blood flow, or decreased renal function (Kuip et al. 2017). There may be a need for consulting a pain specialist in selected patients with COPD and with severe and prolonged pain from AP and those on sedatives and hypnotics for coexisting conditions.

Fluid Administration in Older Adults

The recommendations about IV fluid therapy in the management of dehydration in the elderly, the best type of fluid to use for fluid resuscitation, optimal volume, and rate of delivery are not uniform. The National Institute for Health and Care Excellence (NICE) published guidance in 2014. The aim of NICE guideline helps the clinicians understand the physiological principles that underscore fluid prescribing pathophysiological changes that affect fluid balance in disease states indications for IV fluid therapy, reasons for the choice of the various fluids available and principles of assessing fluid balance (Sansom and Duggleby 2014). A variety of crystalloids, artificial colloids, and human albumin solutions are available for resuscitation.

AP is associated with increased microvascular permeability, leading to significant volume loss and causing decreased perfusion to the lungs, kidneys, and other vital organs (Mayer et al. 2000). Therefore, the single most important treatment is vigorous fluid resuscitation with crystalloids to maintain hemodynamic stability and to avoid or to minimize the degree of ischemia and reperfusion injury. The delicate balance in providing rapid and adequate hydration and the risk of pulmonary edema in the older adult with or without cardiac failure and/or renal disease is an art and science best performed by the intensivists (Zhao et al. 2013). Fluid requirements need to be frequently assessed and reassessed and the rate adjusted (Trikudanathan et al. 2012). However, the amount of fluid getting sequestrated in the retroperitoneal space in AP is not easily assessed. Monitoring of the central venous pressure in AP is not perfect, yet helps in the accuracy of the fluid replacement concerning cardiac reserve. Several recent studies suggest that Ringer lactate is superior to normal saline in AP. Ringer lactate has anti-inflammatory effects and is associated with decreased odds of persistent SIRS, which is a marker of severity in AP patients (De-Madaria et al. 2018; Iqbal et al. 2018; Wu et al. 2011). Ringer lactate is less likely to induce acidosis which in itself may cause acinar cell injury. In clinical practice, it is not the wrong choice of fluid administration that worsens the outcome. Faster rate of hydration early in the course of severe AP diminishes in-hospital stay (Gardner et al. 2009). Often it is the inadequate hydration in the first 24 h that influences the prognosis. The total volume of IV hydration at 48 h after the onset of AP appears to have little effect or impact on the outcome (Tenner et al. 2013). The difficulties in delicately balancing adequate hydration versus the risk of precipitating pulmonary edema in an older adult itself is a reason to treat the patient initially in an ICU setting.

Nutritional Care

The metabolic state of severe AP resembles that of severe sepsis, burns, or major trauma. There is increased protein catabolism, an inability of exogenous glucose to inhibit gluconeogenesis, increased energy expenditure, increased insulin resistance, and increased dependence on fatty acid oxidation to provide energy substrates. Energy needs vary and change according to the severity and stage of AP, comorbid conditions, and specific complications (sterile or infected pancreatic necrosis) occurring during the clinical course of AP (Gianotti et al. 2009).

The standard of care of patients with suspected AP is keeping the patient on IV fluids with no oral feedings (nothing by mouth -NPO) for 2–3 days. The long-held notion is that we are offering "rest to the pancreas" avoiding stimulation by food. Initially, almost all patients with AP will have worsening of abdominal pain with oral intake of solid or liquid foods. There are other potential benefits for the initial "NPO" status, more so in older adults. In many cases, the diagnosis may not be clear in the emergency room. There is a possibility of a change in the diagnosis and that the patient may even require emergency surgery or endoscopy. Keeping the patient NPO will avoid any delay in the needed procedure. Other benefits for the initial short duration NPO include keeping the stomach empty to reduce vomiting and aspiration. However, with regard to the "NPO status," many questions remain unanswered and are left to clinical judgment. The prolonged need for NPO, the duration of NPO, and the risks of NPO in an older adult are unanswered questions. It has become clear that the order "NPO" is frequently overused in hospitals with no regard to the age of the patient. Prolonged NPO subjects an already elderly frail patient to malnutrition in the hospital. There is no clinical or laboratory evidence that the inflamed pancreas requires prolonged NPO in the management. However, in the absence of pain, there is no evidence that inappropriate early feeding converts mild pancreatitis to a severe one or promote complications.

Traditional practices of placing patients nil per os (NPO) or on a clear liquid diet (CLD) for prolonged periods delay adequate nutritional support and often is without any scientific basis (Franklin et al. 2011; Giner et al. 1996). There is increasing evidence that prolonged bowel rest is associated with intestinal mucosal atrophy and increased infectious complications as a result of bacterial translocation from the gut. Early oral feedings will result in better patient satisfaction, a shorter hospital stay (LOS), decreased infectious complications, decreased morbidity, and decreased mortality (Tenner et al. 2013). Recent studies, although not specifically in older patients, have shown that early oral feeding in mild AP is safe (Eckerwall et al. 2007).

The optimal energy intake in critically ill patients in severe AP is debatable, but undernutrition is not helpful (Preiser et al. 2015). In the older patient in a critically ill state with higher nutritional requirements malnutrition, in particular, protein deficiency will become an added insult and will require prolong recovery. After a period of NPO, it is a tradition to initiate feedings gingerly with clear liquids first, followed by full liquids but low in fat, to a soft diet, and full diet as a step up approach. The scientific need for such a cautious approach is unclear but is not harmful. The value of clear vs. more nutritious liquid feeds is also not well studied. Interestingly a low-fat solid diet is safe compared with clear liquids, providing more calories (Jacobson et al. 2007). Oral feeding with a soft diet is safe compared with clear liquids, and it shortens the hospital stay (Tenner et al. 2013; Sathiaraj et al. 2008; Moraes et al. 2010). In summary, early feeding with a nutritious liquid diet is preferred to prolonged NPO, to maintain nutrition, to avoid hospital related malnutrition in the older adult, to avoid septic complications, and to reduce the length of stay.

The indication for nutritional support by enteral or parenteral nutritional support in AP is an actual or anticipated inadequate oral intake for 5–7 days (Gianotti et al. 2009). If the older adult is malnourished initially, this period may be shorter. The ASPEN guidelines recommend against routine use of nutritional support in patients with mild or moderately severe AP and emphasize the need for professional help in evaluating the nutritional needs of the patient with severe AP (Meier et al. 2006). The hospitalized older adult is highly susceptible to malnutrition, with the incidence of malnutrition in the group ranging from 12% to 50% (Wallace 1999). Many recent studies have evaluated the need for maintaining the gut barrier, decreasing translocation of bacteria, and infection of the necrotic area of the pancreas (Feng et al. 2017). The ACG guidelines recommend nasojejunal or nasogastric enteral feeding in severe AP (Gupta et al. 2003). In providing enteral nutrition, continuous infusion is preferred over cyclic or bolus administration (Tenner et al. 2013). Nasogastric feeding is currently preferred to nasojejunal approach. The benefit of supplementation of enteral formulas with prebiotics and probiotics are not proven and thus cannot be routinely recommended (Spanier et al. 2011; Gou et al. 2014). There is no firm evidence for immune-enhancing formulas or "immunonutrition" in severe acute pancreatitis (Zou et al. 2010; Pan et al. 2017; Feng et al. 2017).

Intravenous nutrition (TPN) may be needed in a small number of patients who develop severe pain on oral or enteral feedings or cannot tolerate total parenteral nutrition (Zou et al. 2010). There are several reasons for the above. Recurrence of pain on EN, vomiting, severe diarrhea, prolonged ileus, complex pancreatic fistulae, and abdominal compartment syndrome are some of the reasons for considering PPN or TPN. TPN is labor intensive and associated with many complications. Line sepsis and fungal sepsis are serious and potentially fatal. Peripheral parenteral nutrition can be the preferred option if the anticipated period of nutritional support is less than 14 days. PPN needs less special expertise, no need for a central line, and lower morbidity than TPN. The increased calorie requirements are as in severe sepsis (Zou et al. 2010). A frequent question is on lipid infusions. Lipids are an efficient source of calories. The use of intravenous lipids in AP is safe if hypertriglyceridemia is avoided. Obviously, in cases of hypertriglyceridemic pancreatitis, it is prudent to avoid lipid emulsions. Hyperglycemia, hypoglycemia, and electrolyte imbalances are other complications associated with TPN.

Pharmacological Agents

Many pharmacological interventions are tried in a small number of patients without any definite benefit. In a Cochrane meta-analysis, 78 studies that included a total of 7366 participants, the treatments assessed included antioxidants, aprotinin, atropine, calcitonin, cimetidine, EDTA (ethylenediaminetetraacetic acid), gabexate, glucagon, iniprol, lexipafant, NSAIDs (non-steroidal anti-inflammatory drugs), octreotide, oxyphenonium, probiotics, activated protein C, somatostatin, somatostatin plus omeprazole, somatostatin plus ulinastatin, thymosin, and ulinastatin; the benefit of anyone of the above was questionable (Moggia et al. 2017). The utility of antibiotics is discussed below.

Antibiotics

Most guidelines advise against prophylactic antibiotics in the management of AP initially. In mild AP, there is no indication for prophylactic antibiotic therapy. The consensus of many recent studies is that there is no benefit in prophylactic antibiotic therapy in the large majority of even severe cases in reducing important outcome measures such as persistent single organ failure, or multiple organ failure, or multiple organ dysfunction of unclear duration, or single organ dysfunction of unclear duration and length of stay (Crockett et al. 2018; Barrie et al. 2018). The use of antibiotics in pancreatic necrosis must be restricted to patients with documented infection that usually occurs after the third week (Rasslan et al. 2017). Most used antibiotics are those with good penetration in the pancreatic tissue, such as carbapenems, quinolones, and metronidazole.

Prophylactic antibiotics are justifiable if there is more than 50% necrosis, detection of inflammatory markers (indication for a high risk of secondary infection (Pezzilli et al. 2015; Mourad et al. 2017). Older age alone is not an indication for antibiotic therapy because of the high risk for opportunistic infections (*C. diificle*, MRSA, Fungal sepsis if on TPN) (Mowbray et al. 2018). Fungal infection is a serious complication with a higher risk of mortality (Reuken et al. 2018).

Emergent ERCP in AP

Obstruction of common bile duct with stones or any other cause increases intraductal pressure and predisposes to cholangitis. The clinical findings are known as "Charcot triad" (fever, abdominal pain, and jaundice). According to Tokyo criteria in diagnosing cholangitis, the clinical features are a history of bile duct disease, fever, chills, jaundice, and right upper quadrant abdominal pain, laboratory findings as signs of inflammatory response (increasing leukocyte count, elevated CRP), abnormal liver function tests (increased ALT, AST, ALP, and GGT), and dilated bile ducts (Buyukasik et al. 2013). Many of the features may be absent or subtle in older adults. A high index of suspicion is needed to suspect cholangitis, which is an indication for urgent ERCP and therapeutic intervention. MRCP examination before ERCP is complimentary. Delayed and failed ERCP is associated with prolonged hospital stays and increased costs of hospitalization. The timing of ERCP is crucial. When a therapeutic ERCP is delayed, it can be associated with poor outcome and death. Even in advanced age, ERCP is an effective and safe procedure when indicated and performed by experienced endoscopists (Yıldırım et al. 2017; Iida et al. 2018).

Early ERCP in most patients with predicted mild and severe acute biliary pancreatitis without cholangitis is an unnecessary invasive procedure associated with unwanted complications. The delicate balance in choosing the procedure at the right time and when indicated is a careful judgment call.

Surgery in Acute Pancreatitis

The indications for surgery in AP are limited. Cholecystectomy in biliary pancreatitis and surgery for complications of AP are the two major divisions. Therapeutic endoscopy and/or interventional radiology are currently valuable options. These procedures have either reduced the need or replaced or helped to delay open surgery (Banks et al. 2013; Navadgi et al. 2015).

Complications and Their Management

Complications may be systemic or related to the pancreas and peripancreatic area. The systemic complications are tabulated (Tables 3 and 10) (Yegneswaran et al. 2011).

Acute pancreatic fluid collections (APFC). (Figs. 2, 3, 4, 5, and 6a, b).

There are two types of fluid collections in AP with different clinical courses and management options. Acute Pancreatic Fluid Collections (APFC) without nonliquefied components may

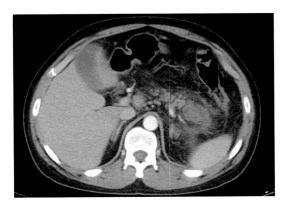

Fig. 3 There is inflammatory stranding surrounding the distal pancreatic body and the pancreatic tail, consistent with acute pancreatitis. There is an approximately 3.3 cm region of the pancreatic tail which demonstrates hypo-enhancement, consistent with necrosis. No gas or drainable fluid collection is present

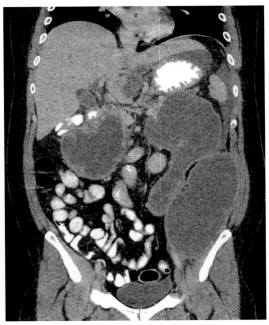

Fig. 4 Acute pancreatic fluid collections (APFC). Fluid collections in *interstitial edematous pancreatitis*. APFC occurs in the first 4 weeks and they are nonencapsulated peripancreatic fluid collections. *Pseudocysts* are encapsulated and develop after 4 weeks

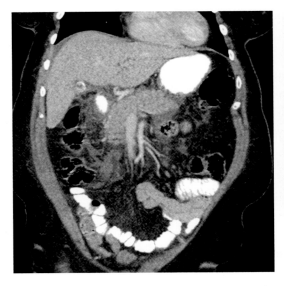

Fig. 2 Peripancreatic inflammatory change tracking in the retroperitoneum, most compatible with acute pancreatitis. Perihepatic ascites. Cholelithiasis, with prominence of the common bile duct. Sigmoid diverticulosis without diverticulitis

develop in edematous pancreatitis within the first 4 weeks of onset. There is a clear distinction between fluid and nonliquified fluid collections. In APFC there is no necrosis of the pancreas. In the first week of AP, a radiological distinction between APFC and ANC may even be difficult in certain cases. APFC in the large majority of cases get reabsorbed and disappear and do not need any treatment. It is important not to needle the fluid for diagnostic or therapeutic purposes and introduce infection. Only infected APF, which is rare, needs

drainage. When APFC has not resolved as in approximately 10% of the cases, it acquires a well-defined capsule and becomes a pseudocyst. Pancreatic pseudocyst has no necrotic material (Fig. 7).

All pseudocysts are not symptomatic, and they do not need any specific treatment. Approximately 60% of pseudocysts resolve spontaneously. A pseudocyst may be painful, may enlarge on follow up, may compress upon the adjacent viscera (gastric antrum or duodenum or biliary system, rarely transverse colon), and may get infected. Irrespective of the size of the cyst or duration of the cyst intervention is indicated in the above situations. Complications of pseudocyst include enlargement, infection, compression of adjacent viscera such as gastric antrum, duodenum, transverse colon, and or biliary system, rupture, pancreatic ascites, pleural effusion, aneurysm formation in neighboring blood vessels, and rarely herniation into the thoracic cavity. In 25% of cases, a pseudocyst may communicate with the pancreatic duct.

The management of pseudocyst is endoscopic, radiologic, or rarely surgical (Yip and Teoh 2017; Teoh et al. 2015, 2018). The decision is mostly based on the availability of experts locally for these procedures, but surgical drainage is not currently popular. Most prefer the EUS-guided approach for pseudocyst drainage (Varadarajulu et al. 2013).

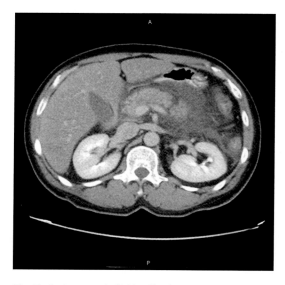

Fig. 5 Peripancreatic fluid collection

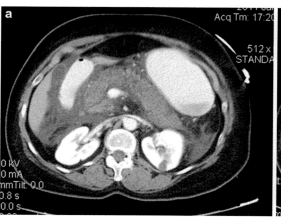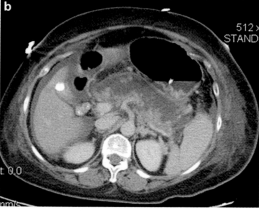

Fig. 6 (a) CT abdomen on day 1 of AP. (b) Same patient CT abdomen day 9. An initial CT scan may be misleadingly less severe since the radiological changes are late to appear. The early peak of severity is not associated with morphological changes

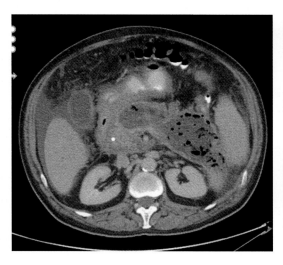

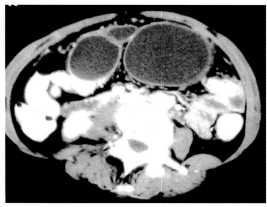

Fig. 9 Walled off pancreatic necrosis (WON). WON may be sterile or get infected

Fig. 7 Pseudocysts of the pancreas. The fluid collection is homogenous without any necrotic material within

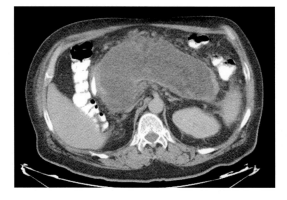

Fig. 8 Infected pancreatic necrosis with gas bubbles in the pancreas. The figure is characteristic but often not seen. A fine needle aspiration and gram staining may be needed when the image is not pathognomonic

Pancreatic necrosis (Figs. 8 and 9). The incidence of necrotizing AP is approximately 20% of patients with AP, with an associated mortality rate of 15%. Secondary infection of pancreatic necrosis develops in approximately 30% of patients with pancreatic necrosis. The natural history of ANCs is as follows. ANCs may be sterile or get infected. Necrotizing collections may resolve. Presence of infection can be diagnosed with CT scan of the pancreas (air bubbles showing the presence of gas within the collection is diagnostic), fine needle aspiration of the necrotic material, the presence of a positive culture, and gram staining. The ANCs may mature and develop liquefaction necrosis and gets encapsulated when the collection is called Walled off necrosis. ANCs may get reabsorbed or develop into walled-off necrosis (WON) (Ahmed et al. 2016). The severity of AP is associated with the extent of pancreatic or peripancreatic tissue necrosis, and the presence or absence of infection. Infected pancreatic necrosis is associated with a high rate of mortality. When it is combined with organ failure, the mortality is higher. It is difficult to predict infection. A pancreatitis activity scoring system (PASS) showed a strong association between PASS score and clinical outcomes (Buxbaum et al. 2018).

Acute necrotizing collections (ANC) from acute necrotizing pancreatitis can affect the pancreatic parenchyma only, peripancreatic tissues only or most commonly both the pancreatic parenchyma and the peripancreatic tissues (Ahmed et al. 2016). Infected pancreatic necrosis is a serious disease associated with a high mortality rate. However, the evolving management of IPN by early drainage and delayed surgery helps to lower mortality rates and improve outcomes (Donald et al. 2012).

Asymptomatic pancreatic and extra-pancreatic necrosis does not require intervention regardless of size, location, and extension. They are likely to resolve spontaneously, even if infected (Freeman et al. 2012).

The management of infected pancreatic necrosis years ago was early, open necrosectomy, which was associated with significant mortality. Infected acute necrotic collections may occasionally require early intervention, but because early open surgery is associated with high morbidity and mortality, it should be avoided whenever possible. Instead, radiologic or endoscopic drainage should be used before surgery to treat the infection and to postpone or obviate the need for surgical debridement (Freeman et al. 2012). The mortality of infected necrosis was falsely believed to be almost 100% in patients with infected pancreatic necrosis if not surgically treated promptly (Tenner et al. 2013). The step-up approach in the management of necrotizing pancreatitis is nicely summarized as a "3D" concept "delay, drain and debride" (Besselink 2011).

Asymptomatic walled-off necrosis (WON) does not require intervention regardless of the size and extension of the collection; it may eventually resolve spontaneously, even in rare cases of infected necrosis; and symptomatic WON generally requires intervention late in the course (i.e., after 4 weeks) if there is intractable pain, visceral obstruction (e.g., the stomach or bile duct), or infection (Puli et al. 2014).

Abdominal compartment syndrome (ACS) and intraabdominal hypertension (IAH). Both are complications of AP. Some patients with IAP develop ACS. ACS is characterized by the elevated intraabdominal pressure of >20 mmHg (with or without an abdominal perfusion pressure < 60 mmHg) with organ failure (Kirkpatrick et al. 2013; Marcos-Neira et al. 2017). ACS is probably secondary to either the severity of AP and or overhydration. In ACS, the increased pressure in a confined anatomical space adversely affects circulation and threatens the perfusion of tissues therein. A similar complication is IAH, characterized by repeated pathological elevation of intraabdominal pressure increase of 12 mm Hg or more. IAP and ACS imply severity and predict high mortality. The incidence of IAP and ACS is quite variable and probably not determined by age. IAH leads to a reduction of chest wall compliance

and hypoperfusion of the gastrointestinal tract contributing to the pathogenesis of organ dysfunction (Radenkovic et al. 2016). The reduction of peripheral blood CD4+ T lymphocytes is associated with ACS in SAP and may act as a potential predictor of ACS in SAP (Liu et al. 2015).

The frequency of ACS in SAP may be rising due to more aggressive fluid resuscitation that is recommended in the management of AP. Therefore a delicate balance exists between adequate hydration and aggressive overhydration precipitating ACS.

The diagnosis of ACS requires a high index of clinical suspicion combined with an increased IAP, measured by urinary bladder pressure (UBP) measurement. First line therapy is a conservative treatment to decrease IAP and to restore organ dysfunction. All patients with bladder pressure of >20 mmHg benefit from decompression methods, abdominal percutaneous decompression drainage, or decompressive laparotomy.

Many older adults with moderately severe and severe AP require ICU care. A well-staffed ICU provides a capacity for proper respiratory and cardiovascular care and life support that is typically unavailable elsewhere in the hospital. Patients with organ system dysfunction need ICU care irrespective of age. There are no rigid criteria for ICU admission. In general, not specifically for AP, patients aged 85 years and older are less likely to be admitted into the ICU compared to those between 65 and 84 years. This attitude will not help the sick AP patient who primarily requires adequate hydration and supportive care.

Key Points

- Acute pancreatitis (AP) is an acute inflammatory disorder of the pancreas clinically characterized by sudden onset of epigastric pain radiating to the back associated with anorexia, nausea, and vomiting.
- The Atlanta II classification in 2012 provided clear definitions to classify AP using easily identifiable clinical and radiologic criteria.

- AP morphologically is defined as interstitial edematous and necrotizing pancreatitis.
- Two peaks of severity (early and late) and three degrees of severity (mild, moderately severe, and severe) are recognized. The two terms: phlegmon and pancreatic abscess have been deleted from the terminologies. The new terms include necrotizing pancreatitis (sterile or infected, walled off necrosis (WON)) and infected pseudocyst.
- Complications include organ system dysfunction early or late in the course.
- Older age increases the severity of AP and mortality.
- In managing AP in the older adult, the three major steps are: (1) establish the diagnosis of AP excluding other causes of acute abdomen in the older adult, (2) assess the severity of AP initially and in an ongoing manner, and (3) establish the etiology for AP by biochemical and imaging studies.
- In biliary AP where emergency therapy is available, initiate appropriate and prompt management strategies including early therapeutic endoscopic interventions.
- The diagnosis of AP in the older adult can be missed in some cases (underdiagnosis) due to lack of classic history or overdiagnosed because of a large number of nonpancreatic causes for serum pancreatic enzymes elevation.
- Biliary diseases and alcoholism are the most frequent etiological factors.
- According to WHO, 525 different drugs can induce AP as an adverse reaction.
- Older patients suffering from severe comorbidities are about 4.5 times more likely to have a fatal episode of AP and about two times more likely to develop severe AP than those having no comorbidities.
- The increased prevalence of dementia and communication disorders adds a new dimension of challenges in pain control in the elderly.
- Traditional practices of placing patients nil per os (NPO) or on a clear liquid diet (CLD) for prolonged periods delay adequate nutritional support and often is without any scientific basis.
- Biliary pancreatitis with evidence of CBD obstruction needs therapeutic ERCP. Even in advanced age, ERCP is an effective and safe procedure when indicated and performed by experienced endoscopists.
- Necrotizing pancreatitis, sterile or even infected, does not need emergency surgery. Infected pancreatic necrosis needs early drainage and delayed surgery.

References

Abou Rached A, Basile M, El Masri H. Gastric leaks post sleeve gastrectomy: review of its prevention and management. World J Gastroenterol [Internet]. 2014 [cited 2019 Jun 21];20(38):13904–10. Available from: http://www.ncbi.nlm.nih.gov/pubmed/25320526

AGS Panel on Persistent Pain in Older Persons. The management of persistent pain in older persons. J Am Geriatr Soc [Internet]. 2002 [cited 2018 Dec 24];50 (6 Suppl):S205–24. Available from: http://www.ncbi.nlm.nih.gov/pubmed/12067390

Ahmed A, Gibreel W, Sarr MG. Recognition and importance of new definitions of peripancreatic fluid collections in managing patients with acute pancreatitis. Dig Surg [Internet]. 2016 [cited 2018 Dec 24];33 (4):259–66. Available from: https://www.karger.com/Article/FullText/445005

Ahn JR, Lee SH, Kim JE, Cha BH, Hwang J-H, Ryu JK, et al. The etiology, severity, and clinical outcome of acute pancreatitis in the elderly. HPB [Internet]. 2010;12:305. Available from: http://www.embase.com/search/results?subaction=viewrecord&from=export&id=L70458889%5Cn. https://doi.org/10.1111/j.1477-2574.2010.00165.x. http://sfx.library.uu.nl/utrecht?sid=EMBASE&issn=1365182X&id=doi:10.1111%2Fj.1477-2574.2010.00165.x&atitle=The+etio

Balani AR, Grendell JH. Drug-induced pancreatitis. Drug Saf [Internet]. 2008 [cited 2018 Dec 24];31(10):823–37. Available from: http://www.ncbi.nlm.nih.gov/pubmed/18759507

Balthazar EJ. Acute pancreatitis: assessment of severity with clinical and CT evaluation. Radiology [Internet]. 2002 [cited 2018 Dec 24];223(3):603–13. Available from: http://pubs.rsna.org/doi/10.1148/radiol.2233010680

Banks PA, Bollen TL, Dervenis C, Gooszen HG, Johnson CD, Sarr MG, et al. Classification of acute pancreatitis—2012: revision of the Atlanta classification and definitions by international consensus. Gut [Internet]. 2013 [cited 2018 Dec 24];62(1):102–11. Available from: http://www.ncbi.nlm.nih.gov/pubmed/23100216

Barrie J, Jamdar S, Smith N, McPherson SJ, Siriwardena AK, O'Reilly DA. Mis-use of antibiotics in acute pancreatitis: insights from the United Kingdom's national confidential enquiry into patient outcome and death (NCEPOD) survey of acute pancreatitis. Pancreatology [Internet]. 2018 [cited 2019 Jun 22];18(7):721–6. Available from: https://www.sciencedirect.com/science/article/abs/pii/S142439031830591X?via%3Dihub

Barry KL, Blow FC. Drinking over the lifespan: focus on older adults. Alcohol Res [Internet]. 2016 [cited 2018 Dec 24];38(1):115–20. Available from: http://www.ncbi.nlm.nih.gov/pubmed/27159818

Basurto Ona X, Rigau Comas D, Urrútia G. Opioids for acute pancreatitis pain. Cochrane Database Syst Rev [Internet]. 2013 [cited 2019 Jun 21];(7). Available from: http://doi.wiley.com/10.1002/14651858.CD009179.pub2

Besselink MGH. The "step-up approach" to infected necrotizing pancreatitis: delay, drain, debride. Dig Liver Dis [Internet]. 2011 [cited 2018 Dec 24];43(6):421–2. Available from: https://linkinghub.elsevier.com/retrieve/pii/S1590865811001253

Bradley EL. A clinically based classification system for acute pancreatitis. Arch Surg [Internet]. 1993 [cited 2019 Jun 21];128(5):586. Available from: http://archsurg.jamanetwork.com/article.aspx?doi=10.1001/archsurg.1993.01420170122019

Brivet FG, Emilie D, Galanaud P. Pro- and anti-inflammatory cytokines during acute severe pancreatitis: an early and sustained response, although unpredictable of death. Parisian Study Group on Acute Pancreatitis. Crit Care Med [Internet]. 1999 [cited 2018 Dec 24];27(4):749–55. Available from: http://www.ncbi.nlm.nih.gov/pubmed/10321665

Burns DM. Cigarette smoking among the elderly: disease consequences and the benefits of cessation. Am J Health Promot [Internet]. 2000 [cited 2018 Dec 24];14(6):357–61. Available from: http://journals.sagepub.com/doi/10.4278/0890-1171-14.6.357

Buter A, Imrie CW, Carter CR, Evans S, McKay CJ. Dynamic nature of early organ dysfunction determines outcome in acute pancreatitis. Br J Surg [Internet]. 2002 [cited 2019 Jun 21];89(3):298–302. Available from: http://www.ncbi.nlm.nih.gov/pubmed/11872053

Buxbaum J, Quezada M, Chong B, Gupta N, Yu CY, Lane C, et al. The pancreatitis activity scoring system predicts clinical outcomes in acute pancreatitis: findings from a prospective cohort study. Am J Gastroenterol [Internet]. 2018 [cited 2018 Dec 24];113(5):755–64. Available from: http://www.ncbi.nlm.nih.gov/pubmed/29545634

Buyukasik K, Toros AB, Bektas H, Ari A, Deniz MM. Diagnostic and therapeutic value of ERCP in acute cholangitis. ISRN Gastroenterol [Internet]. 2013 [cited 2019 Jun 22];2013:191729. Available from: http://www.ncbi.nlm.nih.gov/pubmed/23997958

Caputo F, Vignoli T, Leggio L, Addolorato G, Zoli G, Bernardi M. Alcohol use disorders in the elderly: a brief overview from epidemiology to treatment options. Exp Gerontol [Internet]. 2012 [cited 2018 Dec 24];47(6):411–6. Available from: https://linkinghub.elsevier.com/retrieve/pii/S0531556512000745

Carvalho JR, Fernandes SR, Santos P, Moura CM, Antunes T, Velosa J. Acute pancreatitis in the elderly: a cause for increased concern? Eur J Gastroenterol Hepatol. 2018;30(3):337–41.

Cavalieri TA. Pain management in the elderly. J Am Osteopath Assoc [Internet]. 2002 [cited 2018 Dec 24];102(9):481–5.

Available from: http://www.ncbi.nlm.nih.gov/pubmed/12361180

Chau DL, Walker V, Pai L, Cho LM. Opiates and elderly: use and side effects. Clin Interv Aging [Internet]. 2008 [cited 2018 Dec 24];3(2):273–8. Available from: http://www.ncbi.nlm.nih.gov/pubmed/18686750

Clark JD. Chronic pain prevalence and analgesic prescribing in a general medical population. J Pain Symptom Manage [Internet]. 2002 [cited 2018 Dec 24];23(2):131–7. Available from: http://www.ncbi.nlm.nih.gov/pubmed/11844633

Coelho AMM, Machado MCC, Sampietre SN, da Silva FP, Cunha JEM, D'Albuquerque LAC. Local and systemic effects of aging on acute pancreatitis. Pancreatology [Internet]. 2019 [cited 2019 Jun 22]. Available from: http://www.ncbi.nlm.nih.gov/pubmed/31204259

Costi R, Gnocchi A, Di Mario F, Sarli L. Diagnosis and management of choledocholithiasis in the golden age of imaging, endoscopy and laparoscopy. World J Gastroenterol [Internet]. 2014 [cited 2018 Dec 24];20(37):13382–401. Available from: http://www.wjgnet.com/1007-9327/full/v20/i37/13382.htm

Crockett SD, Wani S, Gardner TB, Falck-Ytter Y, Barkun AN, American Gastroenterological Association Institute Clinical Guidelines Committee S, et al. American gastroenterological association institute guideline on initial management of acute pancreatitis. Gastroenterology [Internet]. 2018 [cited 2018 Dec 24];154(4):1096–101. Available from: https://linkinghub.elsevier.com/retrieve/pii/S0016508518300763

Day LW, Lin L, Somsouk M. Adverse events in older patients undergoing ERCP: a systematic review and meta-analysis. Endosc Int open [Internet]. 2014 [cited 2018 Dec 24];2(1):E28–36. Available from: http://www.thieme-connect.de/DOI/DOI?10.1055/s-0034-1365281

De-Madaria E, Herrera-Marante I, González-Camacho V, Bonjoch L, Quesada-Vázquez N, Almenta-Saavedra I, et al. Fluid resuscitation with lactated Ringer's solution vs normal saline in acute pancreatitis: a triple-blind, randomized, controlled trial. United Eur Gastroenterol J [Internet]. 2018 [cited 2018 Dec 24];6(1):63–72. Available from: http://journals.sagepub.com/doi/10.1177/2050640617707864

Dholakia K, Pitchumoni CS, Agarwal N. How often are liver function tests normal in acute biliary pancreatitis? J Clin Gastroenterol [Internet]. 2004 [cited 2018 Dec 24];38(1):81–3. Available from: http://www.ncbi.nlm.nih.gov/pubmed/14679333

Donald G, Donahue T, Reber HA, Hines OJ. The evolving management of infected pancreatic necrosis. Am Surg [Internet]. 2012 [cited 2018 Dec 24];78(10):1151–5. Available from: http://www.ncbi.nlm.nih.gov/pubmed/23025961

Eckerwall GE, Tingstedt BBA, Bergenzaun PE, Andersson RG. Immediate oral feeding in patients with mild acute pancreatitis is safe and may accelerate recovery–a randomized clinical study. Clin Nutr [Internet]. 2007 [cited 2018 Dec 24];26(6):758–63. Available from: http://linkinghub.elsevier.com/retrieve/pii/S0261561407000714

Egan AG, Blind E, Dunder K, de Graeff PA, Hummer BT, Bourcier T, et al. Pancreatic safety of incretin-based drugs–FDA and EMA assessment. N Engl J Med [Internet]. 2014 [cited 2018 Dec 24];370(9):794–7. Available from: http://www.nejm.org/doi/10.1056/NEJMp1314078

Fagenholz PJ, Del Castillo CF, Harris NS, Pelletier AJ, Camargo CA. Increasing United States hospital admissions for acute pancreatitis, 1988–2003. Ann Epidemiology. 2007;17(7):491–7

Fan ST, Choi TK, Lai CS, Wong J. Influence of age on the mortality from acute pancreatitis. Br J Surg [Internet]. 1988 [cited 2018 Dec 24];75(5):463–6. Available from: http://www.ncbi.nlm.nih.gov/pubmed/3390679

Feng P, He C, Liao G, Chen Y. Early enteral nutrition versus delayed enteral nutrition in acute pancreatitis. Medicine (Baltimore) [Internet]. 2017 [cited 2018 Dec 24];96(46):e8648. Available from: http://www.ncbi.nlm.nih.gov/pubmed/29145291

Ferreira MP, Weems MKS. Alcohol consumption by aging adults in the United States: health benefits and detriments. J Am Diet Assoc [Internet]. 2008 [cited 2018 Dec 24];108(10):1668–76. Available from: http://linkinghub.com/retrieve/pii/S0002822308014089

Fogel EL, Sherman S. ERCP for gallstone pancreatitis. N Engl J Med. 2014;370(2):150–7

Forsmark CE, Baillie J, AGA Institute Clinical Practice and Economics Committee, AGA Institute Governing Board. AGA Institute technical review on acute pancreatitis. Gastroenterol [Internet]. 2007 [cited 2019 Jun 22];132(5):2022–44. Available from: http://www.ncbi.nlm.nih.gov/pubmed/17484894

Forsmark CE, Swaroop Vege S, Wilcox CM. Acute pancreatitis. N Engl J Med [Internet]. 2016;375(20):1972–81. Available from: http://www.nejm.org/doi/10.1056/NEJMra1505202

Franklin GA, McClave SA, Hurt RT, Lowen CC, Stout AE, Stogner LL, et al. Physician-delivered malnutrition: why do patients receive nothing by mouth or a clear liquid diet in a university hospital setting? JPEN J Parenter Enteral Nutr [Internet]. 2011 [cited 2018 Dec 24];35(3):337–42. Available from: http://doi.wiley.com/10.1177/0148607110374060

Freeman ML, Werner J, van Santvoort HC, Baron TH, Besselink MG, Windsor JA, et al. Interventions for necrotizing pancreatitis: summary of a multidisciplinary consensus conference. Pancreas [Internet]. 2012 [cited 2018 Dec 24];41(8):1176–94. Available from: http://content.wkhealth.com/linkback/openurl?sid=WKPTLP:landingpage&an=00006676-201211000-00004

Frossard J-L, Steer ML, Pastor CM. Acute pancreatitis. Lancet (London, England) [Internet]. 2008 [cited 2018 Dec 24];371(9607):143–52. Available from: http://www.ncbi.nlm.nih.gov/pubmed/18191686

Gan SI, Romagnuolo J. Admission hematocrit: a simple, useful and early predictor of severe pancreatitis. Dig Dis Sci [Internet]. 2004 [cited 2018 Dec 24];49(11–12):1946–52. Available from: http://www.ncbi.nlm.nih.gov/pubmed/15628731

Gao W, Yang HX, Ma CE. The value of BISAP score for predicting mortality and severity in acute pancreatitis: a systematic review and meta-analysis. PLoS One [Internet]. 2015 [cited 2019 Jun 21];10(6). Available from: https://journals.plos.org/plosone/article/file?id=10.1371/journal.pone.0130412&type=printable

Garber A, Frakes C, Arora Z, Chahal P. Mechanisms and management of acute pancreatitis. Gastroenterol Res Pract [Internet]. 2018 [cited 2018 Dec 24];2018. Available from: https://www.hindawi.com/journals/grp/2018/6218798/

Gardner TB, Vege SS, Chari ST, Pearson RK, Clain JE, Topazian MD, et al. The effect of age on hospital outcomes in severe acute pancreatitis. Pancreatol [Internet]. 2008;8(3):265–70. Available from: http://ovidsp.ovid.com/ovidweb.cgi?T=JS&PAGE=reference&D=med5&NEWS=N&AN=18497539

Gardner TB, Vege SS, Chari ST, Petersen BT, Topazian MD, Clain JE, et al. Faster rate of initial fluid resuscitation in severe acute pancreatitis diminishes in-hospital mortality. Pancreatol [Internet]. 2009 [cited 2018 Dec 24];9(6):770–6. Available from: https://linkinghub.elsevier.com/retrieve/pii/S1424390309801154

Gargiulo G, Testa G, Cacciatore F, Mazzella F, Galizia G, Della-Morte D, et al. Moderate alcohol consumption predicts long-term mortality in elderly subjects with chronic heart failure. J Nutr Health Aging [Internet]. 2013 [cited 2019 Jun 22];17(5):480–5. Available from: http://link.springer.com/10.1007/s12603-012-0430-4

Garrow D, Miller S, Sinha D, Conway J, Hoffman BJ, Hawes RH, et al. Endoscopic ultrasound: a meta-analysis of test performance in suspected biliary obstruction. Clin Gastroenterol Hepatol [Internet]. 2007 [cited 2018 Dec 24];5(5):616–23. Available from: http://linkinghub.elsevier.com/retrieve/pii/S1542356507002212

Gianotti L, Meier R, Lobo DN, Bassi C, Dejong CHC, Ockenga J, et al. ESPEN guidelines on parenteral nutrition: pancreas. Clin Nutr [Internet]. 2009 [cited 2018 Dec 24];28(4):428–35. Available from: https://linkinghub.elsevier.com/retrieve/pii/S026156140900082X

Giner M, Laviano A, Meguid MM, Gleason JR. In 1995 a correlation between malnutrition and poor outcome in critically ill patients still exists. Nutrition [Internet]. 1996 [cited 2018 Dec 24];12(1):23–9. Available from: http://www.ncbi.nlm.nih.gov/pubmed/8838832

Girman CJ, Kou TD, Cai B, Alexander CM, O'Neill EA, Williams-Herman DE, et al. Patients with type 2 diabetes mellitus have higher risk for acute pancreatitis compared with those without diabetes. Diabetes Obes Metab [Internet]. 2010 [cited 2018 Dec 24];12(9):766–71. Available from: http://doi.wiley.com/10.1111/j.1463-1326.2010.01231.x

Gloor B, Ahmed Z, Uhl W, Buchler MW. Pancreatic disease in the elderly. Best Pract Res Clin Gastroenterol. 2002;16(1):159–70.

Gloor B, Stahel PF, Müller CA, Worni M, Büchler MW, Uhl W. Incidence and management of biliary pancreatitis in cholecystectomized patients. Results of a 7-year study. J Gastrointest Surg [Internet]. 2003 [cited 2018 Dec 24];7(3):372–7. Available from: http://www.ncbi.nlm.nih.gov/pubmed/12654562

Gou S, Yang Z, Liu T, Wu H, Wang C. Use of probiotics in the treatment of severe acute pancreatitis: a systematic review and meta-analysis of randomized controlled trials. Crit Care [Internet]. 2014 [cited 2018 Dec 24];18(2): R57. Available from: http://ccforum.biomedcentral. com/articles/10.1186/cc13809

Greenberg JA, Hsu J, Bawazeer M, Marshall J, Friedrich JO, Nathens A, et al. Clinical practice guideline: management of acute pancreatitis. Can J Surg. 2016;59:128–40.

Gullo L, Sipahi HM, Pezzilli R. Pancreatitis in the elderly. J Clin Gastroenterol. 1994;19(1):64–8.

Gullo L, Migliori M, Oláh A, Farkas G, Levy P, Arvanitakis C, et al. Acute pancreatitis in five European countries: etiology and mortality. Pancreas [Internet]. 2002 [cited 2018 Dec 24];24(3):223–7. Available from: http://www.ncbi.nlm.nih.gov/pubmed/11893928

Gunzerath L, Faden V, Zakhari S, Warren K. National Institute on Alcohol Abuse and Alcoholism report on moderate drinking. Alcohol Clin Exp Res [Internet]. 2004 [cited 2018 Dec 24];28(6):829–47. Available from: http://www.ncbi.nlm.nih.gov/pubmed/15201626

Gupta R, Patel K, Calder PC, Yaqoob P, Primrose JN, Johnson CD. A randomised clinical trial to assess the effect of total enteral and total parenteral nutritional support on metabolic, inflammatory and oxidative markers in patients with predicted severe acute pancreatitis (APACHE II > or =6). Pancreatol [Internet]. 2003 [cited 2018 Dec 24];3(5):406–13. Available from: http://linkinghub.elsevier.com/retrieve/pii/ S1424390303800352

Hall KE, Proctor DD, Fisher L, Rose S. American gastroenterological association future trends committee report: effects of aging of the population on gastroenterology practice, education, and research. Gastroenterol [Internet]. 2005 [cited 2018 Dec 24];129(4):1305–38. Available from: http://www.ncbi.nlm.nih.gov/pubmed/16230084

Harshit Kumar A, Singh Griwan M. A comparison of APACHE II, BISAP, Ranson's score and modified CTSI in predicting the severity of acute pancreatitis based on the 2012 revised Atlanta Classification. Gastroenterol Rep [Internet]. 2018 [cited 2019 Jun 21];6(2):127–31. Available from: https://academic. oup.com/gastro/article/6/2/127/4055926

Hwang SS, Li BH, Haigh PI. Gallstone pancreatitis without cholecystectomy. JAMA Surg [Internet]. 2013 [cited 2018 Dec 24];148(9):867–72. Available from: http://archsurg.jamanetwork.com/article.aspx?doi=10. 1001/jamasurg.2013.3033

Iida T, Kaneto H, Wagatsuma K, Sasaki H, Naganawa Y, Nakagaki S, et al. Efficacy and safety of endoscopic procedures for common bile duct stones in patients aged 85 years or older: a retrospective study. PLoS One [Internet]. 2018 [cited 2019 Jun 22];13(1): e0190665. Available from: http://www.ncbi.nlm.nih. gov/pubmed/29298346

Iqbal U, Anwar H, Scribani M. Ringer's lactate versus normal saline in acute pancreatitis: a systematic review and meta-analysis. J Dig Dis [Internet]. 2018 [cited 2018 Dec 24];19(6):335–41. Available from: http:// doi.wiley.com/10.1111/1751-2980.12606

Jacobson BC, Vander Vliet MB, Hughes MD, Maurer R, McManus K, Banks PA. A prospective, randomized trial of clear liquids versus low-fat solid diet as the initial meal in mild acute pancreatitis. Clin Gastroenterol Hepatol [Internet]. 2007 [cited 2018 Dec 24];5(8):946–51; quiz 886. Available from: http://linkinghub.elsevier.com/ retrieve/pii/S1542356507004533

Johnson CD, Abu-Hilal M. Persistent organ failure during the first week as a marker of fatal outcome in acute pancreatitis. Gut. 2004;

Jones AE, Trzeciak S, Kline JA. The sequential organ failure assessment score for predicting outcome in patients with severe sepsis and evidence of hypoperfusion at the time of emergency department presentation. Crit Care Med [Internet]. 2009 [cited 2018 Dec 24];37(5):1649–54. Available from: https://insights. ovid.com/crossref?an=00003246-200905000-00015

Kapetanos DJ. ERCP in acute biliary pancreatitis. World J Gastrointest Endosc [Internet]. 2010 [cited 2018 Dec 24];2(1):25–8. Available from: http://www.wjgnet. com/1948-5190/full/v2/i1/25.htm

Kara B, Olmez S, Yalcın MS, Tas A, Ozturk NA, Sarıtaş B. Update on the effect of age on acute pancreatitis morbidity: a retrospective, single-center study. Prz Gastroenterol [Internet]. 2018 [cited 2018 Dec 24];13(3):223–7. Available from: https://www.termedia. pl/doi/10.5114/pg.2018.75677

Kaurich T. Drug-induced acute pancreatitis. Proc (Bayl Univ Med Cent) [Internet]. 2008 [cited 2018 Dec 24];21(1):77–81. Available from: http://www.ncbi. nlm.nih.gov/pubmed/18209761

Kesselman MS, Holt PR. Acute pancreatitis in the elderly. J Am Geriatr Soc [Internet]. 1991 [cited 2018 Dec 24];39(10):1043. Available from: http://doi.wiley. com/10.1111/j.1532-5415.1991.tb04055.x

Khanna AK, Meher S, Prakash S, Tiwary SK, Singh U, Srivastava A, et al. Comparison of Ranson, Glasgow, MOSS, SIRS, BISAP, APACHE-II, CTSI Scores, IL-6, CRP, and Procalcitonin in Predicting Severity, Organ Failure, Pancreatic Necrosis, and Mortality in Acute Pancreatitis. HPB Surg [Internet]. 2013 [cited 2019 Jun 21];2013:367581. Available from: http://www. ncbi.nlm.nih.gov/pubmed/24204087

Khatua B, El-Kurdi B, Singh VP. Obesity and pancreatitis. Curr Opin Gastroenterol [Internet]. 2017 [cited 2018 Dec 24];33(5):374–382. Available from: http://insights. ovid.com/crossref?an=00001574-201709000-00010

Kim JE, Hwang JH, Lee SH, Cha BH, Park YS, Kim JW, et al. The clinical outcome of elderly patients with acute pancreatitis is not different in spite of the different etiologies and severity. Arch Gerontol Geriatr. 2012;54(1):256–60.

Kimura Y, Kikuyama M, Kodama Y. Acute pancreatitis as a possible indicator of pancreatic cancer: the importance of mass detection. Intern Med [Internet]. 2015 [cited 2018 Dec 24];54(17):2109–14. Available from: https:// www.jstage.jst.go.jp/article/internalmedicine/54/17/54_ 54.4068/_article

Kirkegård J, Cronin-Fenton D, Heide-Jørgensen U, Mortensen FV. Acute pancreatitis and pancreatic cancer risk: a nationwide matched-cohort study in Denmark. Gastroenterol [Internet]. 2018 [cited 2018 Dec 24];154(6):1729–36. Available from: https://linkinghub.elsevier.com/retrieve/pii/S0016508518302002

Kirkpatrick AW, Roberts DJ, De Waele J, Jaeschke R, Malbrain MLNG, De Keulenaer B, et al. Intra-abdominal hypertension and the abdominal compartment syndrome: updated consensus definitions and clinical practice guidelines from the world society of the abdominal compartment syndrome. Intensive Care Med [Internet]. 2013 [cited 2018 Dec 24];39(7):1190–206. Available from: http://link.springer.com/10.1007/s00134-013-2906-z

Köhler H, Lankisch PG. Acute pancreatitis and hyperamylasaemia in pancreatic carcinoma. Pancreas [Internet]. 1987 [cited 2018 Dec 24];2(1):117–9. Available from: http://www.ncbi.nlm.nih.gov/pubmed/2437571

Koutroumpakis E, Slivka A, Furlan A, Dasyam AK, Dudekula A, Greer JB, et al. Management and outcomes of acute pancreatitis patients over the last decade: a US tertiary-center experience. Pancreatol [Internet]. 2017 [cited 2018 Dec 24];17(1):32–40. Available from: http://www.ncbi.nlm.nih.gov/pubmed/28341116

Krishna SG, Kamboj AK, Hart PA, Hinton A, Conwell DL. The changing epidemiology of acute pancreatitis hospitalizations. Pancreas [Internet]. 2017 [cited 2018 Dec 24];46(4):482–8. Available from: http://www.ncbi.nlm.nih.gov/pubmed/28196021

Kuip EJM, Zandvliet ML, Koolen SLW, Mathijssen RHJ, van der Rijt CCD. A review of factors explaining variability in fentanyl pharmacokinetics; focus on implications for cancer patients. Br J Clin Pharmacol [Internet]. 2017 [cited 2018 Dec 24];83(2):294–313. Available from: http://doi.wiley.com/10.1111/bcp.13129

Kuzu UB, Ödemiş B, Dişibeyaz S, Parlak E, Öztaş E, Saygılı F, et al. Management of suspected common bile duct stone: diagnostic yield of current guidelines. HPB [Internet]. 2017 [cited 2019 Jun 22];19(2):126–32. Available from: https://www.sciencedirect.com/science/article/pii/S1365182X16319724

Laurell H, Hansson L-E, Gunnarsson U. Acute abdominal pain among elderly patients. Gerontology [Internet]. 2006 [cited 2018 Dec 24];52(6):339–44. Available from: https://www.karger.com/Article/FullText/94982

Lee F, Cundiff D. Meperidine vs morphine in pancreatitis and cholecystitis. Arch Intern Med [Internet]. 1998 [cited 2018 Dec 24];158(21):2399. Available from: http://www.ncbi.nlm.nih.gov/pubmed/9827794

Lieber CS. Metabolism of alcohol. Clin Liver Dis [Internet]. 2005 [cited 2018 Dec 24];9(1):1–35. Available from: http://www.ncbi.nlm.nih.gov/pubmed/15763227

Lin S, Hong W, Basharat Z, Wang Q, Pan J, Zhou M. Blood urea nitrogen as a predictor of severe acute pancreatitis based on the revised Atlanta criteria: timing of measurement and cutoff points. Can J Gastroenterol Hepatol [Internet]. 2017 [cited 2019 Jun 21];2017:9592831. Available from: http://www.ncbi.nlm.nih.gov/pubmed/28487848

Linnebur SA, O'Connell MB, Wessell AM, McCord AD, Kennedy DH, DeMaagd G, et al. Pharmacy practice, research, education, and advocacy for older adults. Pharmacother [Internet]. 2005 [cited 2019 Jun 21];25(10):1396–430. Available from: http://doi.wiley.com/10.1592/phco.2005.25.10.1396

Liu Y, Wang L, Cai Z, Zhao P, Peng C, Zhao L, et al. The decrease of peripheral blood CD4+ T cells indicates abdominal compartment syndrome in severe acute pancreatitis. Strnad P, editor. PLoS One [Internet]. 2015 [cited 2018 Dec 24];10(8):e0135768. Available from: https://dx.plos.org/10.1371/journal.pone.0135768

Losurdo G, Iannone A, Principi M, Barone M, Ranaldo N, Ierardi E, et al. Acute pancreatitis in elderly patients: a retrospective evaluation at hospital admission. Eur J Intern Med [Internet]. 2016 [cited 2018 Dec 24];30:88–93. Available from: https://linkinghub.elsevier.com/retrieve/pii/S0953620516000121

Lukens FJ, Howell DA, Upender S, Sheth SG, Jafri S-MR. ERCP in the very elderly: outcomes among patients older than eighty. Dig Dis Sci [Internet]. 2010 [cited 2018 Dec 24];55(3):847–51. Available from: http://www.ncbi.nlm.nih.gov/pubmed/19337836

Lyon C, Clark DC. Diagnosis of acute abdominal pain in older patients. Am Fam Physician [Internet]. 2006 [cited 2018 Dec 24];74(9):1537–44. Available from: http://www.ncbi.nlm.nih.gov/pubmed/17111893

Maple JT, Ben-Menachem T, Anderson MA, Appalaneni V, Banerjee S, Cash BD, et al. The role of endoscopy in the evaluation of suspected choledocholithiasis. Gastrointest Endosc [Internet]. 2010 [cited 2018 Dec 24];71(1):1–9. Available from: http://www.ncbi.nlm.nih.gov/pubmed/20105473

Marcos-Neira P, Zubia-Olaskoaga F, López-Cuenca S, Bordejé-Laguna L, Epidemiology of acute pancreatitis in intensive care medicine study group. Relationship between intra-abdominal hypertension, outcome and the revised Atlanta and determinant-based classifications in acute pancreatitis. BJS Open [Internet]. 2017 [cited 2018 Dec 24];1(6):175–81. Available from: http://doi.wiley.com/10.1002/bjs5.29

Markus M, Lerch AA. Gallstone-related pathogenesis of acute pancreatitis. Pancreapedia Exocrine Pancreas Knowl Base [Internet]. 2016 [cited 2018 Dec 24]; Available from: https://www.pancreapedia.org/reviews/gallstone-related-pathogenesis-of-acute-pancreatitis

Martin SP, Ulrich CD. Pancreatic disease in the elderly. Clin Geriatr Med [Internet]. 1999;15(3):579–605. Available from: http://www.ncbi.nlm.nih.gov/pubmed/10393743

Masamune A, Kume K, Shimosegawa T. Sex and age differences in alcoholic pancreatitis in Japan: a multicenter nationwide survey. Pancreas [Internet]. 2013 [cited 2018 Dec 24];42(4):578–83. Available from: http://insights.ovid.com/crossref?an=00006676-201305000-00003

Mayer J, Rau B, Gansauge F, Beger HG. Inflammatory mediators in human acute pancreatitis: clinical and pathophysiological implications. Gut [Internet]. 2000 [cited 2018 Dec 24];47(4):546–52. Available from: http://www.ncbi.nlm.nih.gov/pubmed/10986216

McKay CJ, Evans S, Sinclair M, Carter CR, Imrie CW. High early mortality rate from acute pancreatitis in Scotland, 1984–1995. Br J Surg [Internet]. 1999 [cited 2018 Dec 24];86(10):1302–5. Available from: http://www.blackwell-synergy.com/links/doi/10.1046/j.1365-2168.1999.01246.x

Meier R, Ockenga J, Pertkiewicz M, Pap A, Milinic N, Macfie J, et al. ESPEN guidelines on enteral nutrition: pancreas. Clin Nutr [Internet]. 2006 [cited 2018 Dec 24];25(2):275–84. Available from: http://linkinghub.elsevier.com/retrieve/pii/S0261561406000392

Mofidi R, Duff MD, Wigmore SJ, Madhavan KK, Garden OJ, Parks RW. Association between early systemic inflammatory response, severity of multiorgan dysfunction and death in acute pancreatitis. Br J Surg [Internet]. 2006 [cited 2019 Jun 21];93(6):738–44. Available from: http://doi.wiley.com/10.1002/bjs.5290

Mofidi R, Suttie SA, Patil P V, Ogston S, Parks RW. The value of procalcitonin at predicting the severity of acute pancreatitis and development of infected pancreatic necrosis: systematic review. Surgery [Internet]. 2009 [cited 2018 Dec 24];146(1):72–81. Available from: https://linkinghub.elsevier.com/retrieve/pii/S0039606009001561

Moggia E, Koti R, Belgaumkar AP, Fazio F, Pereira SP, Davidson BR, et al. Pharmacological interventions for acute pancreatitis. Cochrane database Syst Rev [Internet]. 2017 [cited 2019 Jun 22];4(4):CD011384. Available from: http://www.ncbi.nlm.nih.gov/pubmed/28431202

Moraes JMM, Felga GEG, Chebli LA, Franco MB, Gomes CA, Gaburri PD, et al. A full solid diet as the initial meal in mild acute pancreatitis is safe and result in a shorter length of hospitalization: results from a prospective, randomized, controlled, double-blind clinical trial. J Clin Gastroenterol [Internet]. 2010 [cited 2018 Dec 24]; 44(7):517–22. Available from: http://content.wkhealth.com/linkback/openurl?sid=WKPTLP:landingpage&an=00004836-900000000-99447

Morales-Oyarvide V, Mino-Kenudson M, Ferrone CR, Gonzalez-Gonzalez LA, Warshaw AL, Lillemoe KD, et al. Acute pancreatitis in intraductal papillary mucinous neoplasms: a common predictor of malignant intestinal subtype. Surgery [Internet]. 2015 [cited 2018 Dec 24];158(5):1219–25. Available from: https://linkinghub.elsevier.com/retrieve/pii/S003960601500358X

Mounzer R, Langmead CJ, Wu BU, Evans AC, Bishehsari F, Muddana V, et al. Comparison of existing clinical scoring systems to predict persistent organ failure in patients with acute pancreatitis. Gastroenterol [Internet]. 2012 [cited 2019 Jun 21];142(7):1476–82. Available from: http://www.ncbi.nlm.nih.gov/pubmed/22425589

Mourad MM, Evans R, Kalidindi V, Navaratnam R, Dvorkin L, Bramhall SR. Prophylactic antibiotics in acute pancreatitis: endless debate. Ann R Coll Surg Engl [Internet]. 2017 [cited 2018 Dec 24];99(2):107–12. Available from: http://publishing.rcseng.ac.uk/doi/10.1308/rcsann.2016.0355

Mowbray NG, Ben-Ismaeil B, Hammoda M, Shingler G, Al-Sarireh B. The microbiology of infected pancreatic necrosis. Hepatobiliary Pancreat Dis Int [Internet]. 2018 [cited 2018 Dec 24];17(5):456–60. Available from: https://linkinghub.elsevier.com/retrieve/pii/S1499387218301887

Mujica VR, Barkin JS, Go VL. Acute pancreatitis secondary to pancreatic carcinoma. Study Group Participants. Pancreas [Internet]. 2000 [cited 2018 Dec 24];21(4):329–32. Available from: http://www.ncbi.nlm.nih.gov/pubmed/11075985

Muniraj T, Dang S, Pitchumoni CS. PANCREATITIS OR NOT?–Elevated lipase and amylase in ICU patients. J Crit Care [Internet]. 2015 [cited 2018 Dec 24];30(6):1370–5. Available from: https://linkinghub.elsevier.com/retrieve/pii/S0883944115004554

Navadgi S, Pandanaboyana S, Windsor JA. Surgery for acute pancreatitis. Indian J Surg [Internet]. 2015 [cited 2019 Jun 22];77(5):446–52. Available from: http://www.ncbi.nlm.nih.gov/pubmed/26722210

Neoptolemos JP, Kemppainen EA, Mayer JM, Fitzpatrick JM, Raraty MG, Slavin J, et al. Early prediction of severity in acute pancreatitis by urinary trypsinogen activation peptide: a multicentre study. Lancet (London, England) [Internet]. 2000 [cited 2018 Dec 24];355(9219):1955–60. Available from: http://www.ncbi.nlm.nih.gov/pubmed/10859041

Nitsche CJ, Jamieson N, Lerch MM, Mayerle J V. Drug induced pancreatitis. Best Pract Res Clin Gastroenterol [Internet]. 2010 [cited 2018 Dec 24];24(2):143–55. Available from: http://www.ncbi.nlm.nih.gov/pubmed/20227028

Noel P, Patel K, Durgampudi C, Trivedi RN, de Oliveira C, Crowell MD, et al. Peripancreatic fat necrosis worsens acute pancreatitis independent of pancreatic necrosis via unsaturated fatty acids increased in human pancreatic necrosis collections. Gut [Internet]. 2016 [cited 2018 Aug 29];65(1):100–11. Available from: http://www.ncbi.nlm.nih.gov/pubmed/25500204

Obana T, Fujita N, Noda Y, Kobayashi G, Ito K, Horaguchi J, et al. Efficacy and safety of therapeutic ERCP for the elderly with choledocholithiasis: comparison with younger patients. Intern Med [Internet]. 2010 [cited 2018 Dec 24];49(18):1935–41. Available from: http://www.ncbi.nlm.nih.gov/pubmed/20847495

Otsuki M, Takeda K, Matsuno S, Kihara Y, Koizumi M, Hirota M, et al. Criteria for the diagnosis and severity stratification of acute pancreatitis. World J Gastroenterol [Internet]. 2013 [cited 2018 Dec 24];19 (35):5798–805. Available from: http://www.wjgnet.com/1007-9327/full/v19/i35/5798.htm

Pan L-L, Li J, Shamoon M, Bhatia M, Sun J. Recent advances on nutrition in treatment of acute pancreatitis. Front Immunol [Internet]. 2017 [cited 2018 Dec 24];8:762. Available from: http://journal.frontiersin.org/article/10.3389/fimmu.2017.00762/full

Payor A, Jois P, Wilson J, Kedar R, Nallamshetty L, Grubb S, et al. Efficacy of noncontrast computed tomography of the abdomen and pelvis for evaluating nontraumatic acute abdominal pain in the emergency department. J Emerg Med [Internet]. 2015 [cited 2018 Dec 24];49 (6):886–92. Available from: https://linkinghub.elsevier.com/retrieve/pii/S0736467915006848

Peery AF, Crockett SD, Barritt AS, Dellon ES, Eluri S, Gangarosa LM, et al. Burden of gastrointestinal, liver, and pancreatic diseases in the United States.

Gastroenterology [Internet]. 2015 [cited 2018 Dec 24];149(7):1731–41.e3. Available from: http://www.ncbi.nlm.nih.gov/pubmed/26327134

Pergolizzi J, Böger RH, Budd K, Dahan A, Erdine S, Hans G, et al. Opioids and the management of chronic severe pain in the elderly: consensus statement of an International Expert Panel with focus on the six clinically most often used World Health Organization Step III opioids (buprenorphine, fentanyl, hydromorphone, methadone, morphine, oxycodone). Pain Pract [Internet]. 2008 [cited 2018 Dec 24];8(4):287–313. Available from: http://doi.wiley.com/10.1111/j.1533-2500.2008.00204.x

Pezzilli R, Zerbi A, Campra D, Capurso G, Golfieri R, Arcidiacono PG, et al. Consensus guidelines on severe acute pancreatitis. Dig Liver Dis. 2015;47(7):532–43.

Pitchumoni CS, Rubin A, Das K. Pancreatitis in inflammatory bowel diseases. J Clin Gastroenterol [Internet]. 2010 [cited 2018 Dec 24];44(4):246–53. Available from: https://insights.ovid.com/crossref?an=00004836-201004000-00009

Popa CC, Badiu DC, Rusu OC, Grigorean VT, Neagu SI, Strugaru CR. Mortality prognostic factors in acute pancreatitis. J Med Life. 2016;9(4):413–8.

Preiser J-C, van Zanten ARH, Berger MM, Biolo G, Casaer MP, Doig GS, et al. Metabolic and nutritional support of critically ill patients: consensus and controversies. Crit Care [Internet]. 2015 [cited 2019 Jun 21];19(1):35. Available from: http://www.ncbi.nlm.nih.gov/pubmed/25886997

Puli SR, Graumlich JF, Pamulaparthy SR, Kalva N. Endoscopic transmural necrosectomy for walled-off pancreatic necrosis: a systematic review and meta-analysis. Can J Gastroenterol Hepatol [Internet]. 2014 [cited 2018 Dec 24];28(1):50–3. Available from: http://www.ncbi.nlm.nih.gov/pubmed/24212912

Quero G, Covino M, Fiorillo C, Rosa F, Menghi R, Simeoni B, et al. Acute pancreatitis in elderly patients: a single-center retrospective evaluation of clinical outcomes. Scand J Gastroenterol [Internet]. 2019 [cited 2019 Jun 21];54(4):492–8. Available from: http://www.ncbi.nlm.nih.gov/pubmed/30905212

Radenkovic D V., Johnson CD, Milic N, Gregoric P, Ivancevic N, Bezmarevic M, et al. Interventional treatment of abdominal compartment syndrome during severe acute pancreatitis: current status and historical perspective. Gastroenterol Res Pract [Internet]. 2016 [cited 2019 Jun 22];2016:5251806. Available from: http://www.ncbi.nlm.nih.gov/pubmed/26839539

Rasslan R, Novo FdaCF, Bitran A, Utiyama EM, Rasslan S. Management of infected pancreatic necrosis: state of the art. Rev Col Bras Cir [Internet]. 2017 [cited 2018 Dec 24];44(5):521–9. Available from: http://www.scielo.br/scielo.php?script=sci_arttext&pid=S0100-69912017000500521&lng=en&tlng=en

Reuken PA, Albig H, Rödel J, Hocke M, Will U, Stallmach A, et al. Fungal infections in patients with infected pancreatic necrosis and pseudocysts: risk factors and outcome. Pancreas [Internet]. 2018 [cited 2019

Jun 22];47(1):92–8. Available from: http://www.ncbi.nlm.nih.gov/pubmed/29215543

Rigler SK. Alcoholism in the elderly. Am Fam Physician [Internet]. 2000 [cited 2018 Dec 24];61(6):1710–6, 1883–4, 1887–8 passim. Available from: http://www.ncbi.nlm.nih.gov/pubmed/10750878

Romagnuolo J, Bardou M, Rahme E, Joseph L, Reinhold C, Barkun AN. Magnetic resonance cholangiopancreatography: a meta-analysis of test performance in suspected biliary disease. Ann Intern Med [Internet]. 2003 [cited 2018 Dec 24];139(7):547–57. Available from: http://www.ncbi.nlm.nih.gov/pubmed/14530225

Roulin D, Girardet R, Duran R, Hajdu S, Denys A, Halkic N, et al. Outcome of elderly patients after acute biliary pancreatitis. Biosci Trends. 2018;12(1):54–9.

Sajid MS, Khawaja AH, Sayegh M, Singh KK, Philipose Z. Systematic review and meta-analysis on the prophylactic role of non-steroidal anti-inflammatory drugs to prevent post-endoscopic retrograde cholangiopancreatography pancreatitis. World J Gastrointest Endosc [Internet]. 2015 [cited 2018 Dec 24];7(19):1341–9. Available from: http://www.wjgnet.com/1948-5190/full/v7/i19/1341.htm

Sandblom G, Bergman T, Rasmussen I. Acute pancreatitis in patients 70 years of age or older [Internet]. Clinical Medicine: Geriatrics. 2008 [cited 2019 Jun 22]. Available from: https://pdfs.semanticscholar.org/9c19/d72a25247e8e1f2906673203f126e636e841.pdf

Sansom LT, Duggleby L. Intravenous fluid prescribing: improving prescribing practices and documentation in line with NICE CG174 guidance. BMJ Qual Improv reports [Internet]. 2014 [cited 2019 Jun 21];3(1). Available from: http://www.ncbi.nlm.nih.gov/pubmed/26734287

Sarri G, Guo Y, Iheanacho I, Puelles J. Moderately severe and severe acute pancreatitis: a systematic review of the outcomes in the USA and European Union-5. BMJ open Gastroenterol [Internet]. 2019 [cited 2019 Jun 22];6(1):e000248. Available from: http://www.ncbi.nlm.nih.gov/pubmed/30899535

Sathiaraj E, Murthy S, Mansard MJ, Rao G V, Mahukar S, Reddy DN. Clinical trial: oral feeding with a soft diet compared with clear liquid diet as initial meal in mild acute pancreatitis. Aliment Pharmacol Ther [Internet]. 2008 [cited 2018 Dec 24];28(6):777–81. Available from: http://www.ncbi.nlm.nih.gov/pubmed/19145732

Schorn S, Ceyhan GO, Tieftrunk E, Friess H, Demir IE. Pain management in acute pancreatitis. 2015 [cited 2019 Jun 21]; Available from: https://www.pancreapedia.org/sites/default/files/DOI V2. Pain management in acute pancreatitis 5–22-15_0.pdf.

Schütte K, Malfertheiner P. Markers for predicting severity and progression of acute pancreatitis. Best Pract Res Clin Gastroenterol [Internet]. 2008 [cited 2018 Dec 24];22(1):75–90. Available from: http://linkinghub.elsevier.com/retrieve/pii/S1521691807001199

Sheiybani G, Brydon P, Toolan M, Linehan J, Farrant M, Colleypriest B. Does rectal diclofenac reduce post-ERCP pancreatitis? A district general hospital experience. Frontline Gastroenterol [Internet]. 2018 [cited 2018 Dec 24];9(1):73–7. Available from:

http://fg.bmj.com/lookup/doi/10.1136/flgastro-2017-100832

Siegel JH, Kasmin FE. Biliary tract diseases in the elderly: management and outcomes. Gut [Internet]. 1997 [cited 2018 Dec 24];41(4):433–5. Available from: http://www.ncbi.nlm.nih.gov/pubmed/9391238

Singh VK, Wu BU, Bollen TL, Repas K, Maurer R, Mortele KJ, et al. Early systemic inflammatory response syndrome is associated with severe acute pancreatitis. Clin Gastroenterol Hepatol [Internet]. 2009 [cited 2018 Dec 24];7(11):1247–51. Available from: https://linkinghub.elsevier.com/retrieve/pii/S1542356509007745

Somasekar K, Foulkes R, Morris-Stiff G, Hassn A. Acute pancreatitis in the elderly - can we perform better? Surgeon. 2011;9(6):305–8.

Spanier BWM, Bruno MJ, Mathus-Vliegen EMH. Enteral nutrition and acute pancreatitis: a review. Gastroenterol Res Pract [Internet]. 2011 [cited 2019 Jun 22];2011. Available from: http://www.ncbi.nlm.nih.gov/pubmed/20811543

Steinberg WM. Comment: acute pancreatitis associated with liraglutide. Ann Pharmacother [Internet]. 2011 [cited 2018 Dec 24];45(9):1169. Available from: http://journals.sagepub.com/doi/10.1345/aph.1P714a

Sugiyama M, Atomi Y. Endoscopic sphincterotomy for bile duct stones in patients 90 years of age and older. Gastrointest Endosc [Internet]. 2000 [cited 2018 Dec 24];52(2):187–91. Available from: http://www.ncbi.nlm.nih.gov/pubmed/10922089

Szakács Z, Gede N, Pécsi D, Izbéki F, Papp M, Kovács G, et al. Aging and comorbidities in acute pancreatitis II.: a cohort-analysis of 1203 prospectively collected cases. Front Physiol [Internet]. 2018 [cited 2019 Jun 21];9:1776. Available from: http://www.ncbi.nlm.nih.gov/pubmed/31001148

Takada T, Strasberg SM, Solomkin JS, Pitt HA, Gomi H, Yoshida M, et al. TG13: updated Tokyo guidelines for the management of acute cholangitis and cholecystitis. J Hepatobiliary Pancreat Sci [Internet]. 2013 [cited 2018 Dec 24];20(1):1–7. Available from: http://www.ncbi.nlm.nih.gov/pubmed/23307006

Tenner S. Drug induced acute pancreatitis: does it exist? World J Gastroenterol [Internet]. 2014 [cited 2019 Jun 21];20(44):16529–34. Available from: http://www.ncbi.nlm.nih.gov/pubmed/25469020

Tenner S, Dubner H, Steinberg W. Predicting gallstone pancreatitis with laboratory parameters: a meta-analysis. Am J Gastroenterol [Internet]. 1994 [cited 2018 Dec 24];89(10):1863–6. Available from: http://www.ncbi.nlm.nih.gov/pubmed/7942684

Tenner S, Baillie J, DeWitt J, Vege SS, American College of Gastroenterology. American college of gastroenterology guideline: management of acute pancreatitis. Am J Gastroenterol [Internet]. 2013 [cited 2018 Sep 5];108(9):1400–15. Available from: http://www.ncbi.nlm.nih.gov/pubmed/23896955

Teoh AYB, Ho LKY, Dhir VK, Jin ZD, Kida M, Seo DW, et al. A multi-institutional survey on the practice of endoscopic ultrasound (EUS) guided pseudocyst drainage in the Asian EUS group. Endosc Int open [Internet]. 2015 [cited 2018 Dec 24];3(2):E130–3. Available from: http://www.thieme-connect.de/DOI/DOI?10.1055/s-0034-1390890

Teoh AYB, Dhir V, Kida M, Yasuda I, Dong Jin Z, Wan Seo D, et al. Consensus guidelines on the optimal management in interventional EUS procedures: results from the Asian EUS group RAND/UCLA expert panel. Gut [Internet]. 2018 [cited 2019 Jun 22];67:1209–28. Available from: http://gut.bmj.com/

Thoeni RF. The revised atlanta classification of acute pancreatitis: its importance for the radiologist and its effect on treatment. Radiology [Internet]. 2012;262(3):751–64. Available from: http://pubs.rsna.org/doi/10.1148/radiol.11110947

Tinto A, Lloyd DAJ, Kang J-Y, Majeed A, Ellis C, Williamson RCN, et al. Acute and chronic pancreatitis – diseases on the rise: a study of hospital admissions in England 1989/90–1999/2000. Aliment Pharmacol Ther [Internet]. 2002 [cited 2018 Dec 24];16(12):2097–105. Available from: http://www.ncbi.nlm.nih.gov/pubmed/12452943

Tohda G, Ohtani M, Dochin M. Efficacy and safety of emergency endoscopic retrograde cholangiopancreatography for acute cholangitis in the elderly. World J Gastroenterol [Internet]. 2016 [cited 2018 Dec 24];22(37):8382–8. Available from: http://www.wjgnet.com/1007-9327/full/v22/i37/8382.htm

Trikudanathan G, Navaneethan U, Vege SS. Current controversies in fluid resuscitation in acute pancreatitis: a systematic review. Pancreas [Internet]. 2012 [cited 2018 Dec 24];41(6):827–34. Available from: http://content.wkhealth.com/linkback/openurl?sid=WKPTLP:landingpage&an=00006676-201208000-00001

Trivedi CD, Pitchumoni CS. Drug-induced pancreatitis: an update. J Clin Gastroenterol [Internet]. 2005 [cited 2018 Dec 24];39(8):709–16. Available from: http://www.ncbi.nlm.nih.gov/pubmed/16082282

Trust MD, Sheffield KM, Boyd CA, Benarroch-Gampel J, Zhang D, Townsend CM, et al. Gallstone pancreatitis in older patients: are we operating enough? Surgery [Internet]. 2011 [cited 2018 Dec 24];150(3):515–25. Available from: https://linkinghub.elsevier.com/retrieve/pii/S0039606011004284

van Dijk SM, Hallensleben NDL, van Santvoort HC, Fockens P, van Goor H, Bruno MJ, et al. Acute pancreatitis: recent advances through randomised trials. Gut [Internet]. 2017 [cited 2018 May 16];66(11):2024–32. Available from: http://gut.bmj.com/lookup/doi/10.1136/gutjnl-2016-313595

Varadarajulu S, Bang JY, Sutton BS, Trevino JM, Christein JD, Wilcox CM. Equal efficacy of endoscopic and surgical cystogastrostomy for pancreatic pseudocyst drainage in a randomized trial. Gastroenterol [Internet]. 2013 [cited 2018 Dec 24];145(3):583–90.e1. Available from: https://linkinghub.elsevier.com/retrieve/pii/S0016508513008445

Veal FC, Peterson GM. Pain in the frail or elderly patient: does tapentadol have a role? Drugs Aging [Internet].

2015 [cited 2018 Dec 24];32(6):419–26. Available from: http://link.springer.com/10.1007/s40266-015-0268-7

Wallace JI. Malnutrition and enteral/parenteral alimentation. In: Hazzard W, Blass J, Ettinger WJ, Halter J, Ouslander J, editors. Principles of geriatric medicine and gerontology. 4th ed. New York: McGraw-Hill; 1999. p. 1455–69.

Whitcomb DC. Clinical practice. Acute pancreatitis. N Engl J Med [Internet]. 2006;354(20):2142–50. Available from: http://www.ncbi.nlm.nih.gov/pubmed/16707751

Working Group IAP/APA Acute Pancreatitis Guidelines. IAP/APA evidence-based guidelines for the management of acute pancreatitis Working Group IAP/APA Acute Pancreatitis Guidelines. Pancreat. 2013;13:e1–15.

Wu BU, Johannes RS, Sun X, Tabak Y, Conwell DL, Banks PA. The early prediction of mortality in acute pancreatitis: a large population-based study. Gut [Internet]. 2008 [cited 2018 Dec 24];57(12):1698–703. Available from: http://gut.bmj.com/cgi/doi/10.1136/gut.2008.152702

Wu BU, Johannes RS, Sun X, Conwell DL, Banks PA. Early changes in blood urea nitrogen predict mortality in acute pancreatitis. Gastroenterology [Internet]. 2009 [cited 2019 Jun 21];137(1):129–35. Available from: http://www.ncbi.nlm.nih.gov/pubmed/19344722

Wu BU, Hwang JQ, Gardner TH, Repas K, Delee R, Yu S, et al. Lactated ringer's solution reduces systemic inflammation compared with saline in patients with acute pancreatitis. Clin Gastroenterol Hepatol [Internet]. 2011 [cited 2018 Dec 24];9(8):710–7.e1. Available from: http://www.ncbi.nlm.nih.gov/pubmed/21645639

Xin M-J, Chen H, Luo B, Sun J-B. Severe acute pancreatitis in the elderly: etiology and clinical characteristics. World J Gastroenterol [Internet]. 2008;14(16):2517–21. Available from: http://www.pubmedcentral.nih.gov/articlerender.fcgi?artid=2708362&tool=pmcentrez&rendertype=abstract

Yadav D, Lowenfels AB. Trends in the epidemiology of the first attack of acute pancreatitis. Pancreas [Internet]. 2006 [cited 2018 Dec 24];33(4):323–30. Available from: http://www.ncbi.nlm.nih.gov/pubmed/17079934

Yadav D, Hawes RH, Brand RE, Anderson MA, Money ME, Banks PA, et al. Alcohol consumption, cigarette smoking, and the risk of recurrent acute and chronic pancreatitis. Arch Intern Med [Internet]. 2009 [cited 2018 Dec 24];169(11):1035–45. Available from: http://www.ncbi.nlm.nih.gov/pubmed/19506173

Yegneswaran B, Pitchumoni CS. When should serum amylase and lipase levels be repeated in a patient with acute pancreatitis?|Cleveland Clinic Journal of Medicine. Cleve Clin J Med [Internet]. 2010;77(4):230–1. Available from: https://www.mdedge.com/ccjm/article/95282/gastroenterology/when-should-serum-amylase-and-lipase-levels-be-repeated-patient

Yegneswaran B, Kostis JB, Pitchumoni CS. Cardiovascular manifestations of acute pancreatitis. J Crit Care [Internet]. 2011 [cited 2019 Jun 22];26(2):225.e11–225.e18. Available from: https://www.sciencedirect.com/science/article/abs/pii/S0883944110002959?via%3Dihub

Yıldırım AE, Öztürk ZA, Konduk BT, Balkan A, Edizer B, Gulsen MT, et al. The safety and efficacy of ERCP in octogenarians: a comparison of two geriatric age cohorts. Acta Gastroenterol Belg [Internet]. 2017 [cited 2018 Dec 24];80(2):263–70. Available from: http://www.ncbi.nlm.nih.gov/pubmed/29560692

Yip HC, Teoh AYB. Endoscopic management of peripancreatic fluid collections. Gut Liver [Internet]. 2017 [cited 2018 Dec 24];11(5):604–11. Available from: http://www.gutnliver.org/journal/view.html?doi=10.5009/gnl16178

Zhao G, Zhang J-G, Wu H-S, Tao J, Qin Q, Deng S-C, et al. Effects of different resuscitation fluid on severe acute pancreatitis. World J Gastroenterol [Internet]. 2013 [cited 2018 Dec 24];19(13):2044–52. Available from: http://www.wjgnet.com/1007-9327/full/v19/i13/2044.htm

Zou X-P, Chen M, Wei W, Cao J, Chen L, Tian M. Effects of enteral immunonutrition on the maintenance of gut barrier function and immune function in pigs with severe acute pancreatitis. JPEN J Parenter Enteral Nutr [Internet]. 2010 [cited 2018 Dec 24];34(5):554–66. Available from: http://doi.wiley.com/10.1177/0148607110362691

Chronic Pancreatitis

65

Sonmoon Mohapatra, Gaurav Aggarwal, and Suresh T. Chari

Contents

Conflicts of Interest/Disclosures: None

S. Mohapatra (✉)
Division of Gastroenterology and Hepatology, Saint
Peter's University Hospital – Rutgers Robert Wood
Johnson School of Medicine, New Brunswick, NJ, USA

G. Aggarwal
GA Bellevue Medical Center, Bellevue, WA, USA

Division of Epidemiology, Mayo Clinic, Rochester, MN,
USA

S. T. Chari
Department of Gastroenterology, Hepatology and
Nutrition, Division of Internal Medicine, The University of
Texas MD Anderson Cancer Center, Houston, TX, USA
e-mail: stchari@mdanderson.org

© Springer Nature Switzerland AG 2021
C. S. Pitchumoni, T. S. Dharmarajan (eds.), *Geriatric Gastroenterology*,
https://doi.org/10.1007/978-3-030-30192-7_56

Abstract

Chronic pancreatitis refers to progressive chronic inflammation and fibrosis along with impaired exocrine and endocrine pancreatic function, eventually leading to endocrine and exocrine failure. In the USA, pancreatitis is not an uncommon diagnosis in an ambulatory care setting in subjects over 65 years of age. While alcohol is the most common cause of chronic pancreatitis in the general population, most cases of chronic pancreatitis in the older adult are idiopathic. Other causes in the geriatric population include those related to obstruction (e.g., ampullary malignancy or pancreatic cancer). Most older adults with idiopathic chronic pancreatitis do not have pain and instead present with exocrine and endocrine insufficiency. No single test is adequately sensitive for the diagnosis of chronic pancreatitis. The diagnosis is based on clinical presentation with stool testing and radiologic imaging. Exocrine function testing and endoscopic evaluation for diagnosis are typically used when the imaging is inconclusive. Therapy targets the prevention of ongoing damage to the pancreas, alleviation of symptoms, and treating complications. Exclusion of malignancy, pancreatic enzyme replacement, and treatment of diabetes along with the cessation of tobacco and alcohol use are mainstays of therapy. Surgical and endoscopic interventions are reserved for those who do not respond to conservative therapy and for complications.

Keywords

Chronic pancreatitis · Alcoholic pancreatitis · Pancreatic pseudocyst · Amylase · Lipase · Autoimmune pancreatitis · Pancreatic cancer · Steatorrhea · Diabetes · Smoking · Exocrine insufficiency · Amylase · Lipase · Elastase · Fecal fat · Endoscopic ultrasound · Steroids · Chronic abdominal pain · ERCP · Pseudoaneurysm · Gastric varices · Splenic vein thrombosis · Pancreatic fistula · Pancreatic ascites

Introduction

Chronic pancreatitis is characterized by progressive chronic inflammation and fibrosis of the pancreas resulting in impaired exocrine and endocrine function (Aggarwal and Chari 2012). In true acute pancreatitis, there is restitution of the gland to structural and functional normalcy after an acute attack, characterized by acute abdominal pain, elevated serum amylase/lipase, and morphological changes on imaging. In chronic pancreatitis, patients often experience attacks of clinically acute pancreatitis, but in contrast to true acute pancreatitis, there is progressive structural and functional damage to the pancreas despite clinical recovery from the attacks. Despite the differences in the two entities, a subset of patients with (recurrent) acute pancreatitis will progress to chronic pancreatitis (Dimagno and Dimagno 2010).

Epidemiology

The incidence rate of clinical chronic pancreatitis has increased significantly from 2.94/100,000 during 1977–1986 to 4.35/100,000 person years during 1997–2006 ($P < 0.05$) because of an increase in the incidence of alcoholic chronic pancreatitis. (Yadav et al. 2011) In the USA, pancreatitis was listed among the top three principal diagnoses with a 291,915 annual number of admissions in 2014 (Peery et al. 2019). Although the peak age for diagnosis of alcohol-related chronic pancreatitis is the 45–54 age group, the age of diagnosing nonalcoholic chronic pancreatitis is most common in the 65–74 age group (Yadav et al. 2011). A survey in Japan revealed the prevalence of chronic pancreatitis in men between 65 and 69 years of age to be 115 per 100,000 population and in women aged 75–79 years to be 39.6 per 100,000 population (Lin et al. 2000). A prospective survey in France yielded a crude prevalence rate of 26 per 100,000 population and estimated that about 20% of chronic pancreatitis cases occurred in the over 65 year age group (Levy et al. 2006). The most common causes of death in chronic pancreatitis include malignancies (23%) and cardiovascular causes (21%). (Yadav et al. 2011).

Effects of Aging on the Pancreas

The effect of aging on the pancreas has been well described (Ross and Forsmark 2001). They involve not only pancreatic parenchyma but also functional, pathological, and ductal changes as described below.

Functional Changes

Studies of changes on exocrine pancreatic function with aging yield conflicting data. Early studies showed a 10–30% reduction in the volume, bicarbonate, and lipase in pancreatic juice in the older adults (Ross and Forsmark 2001). In contrast, there was no difference in secretin-stimulated pancreatic secretion between 25 older subjects and 30 young controls (Gullo et al. 1983). These contradictory data may be due to differences in methodology and inadvertent inclusion of patients with asymptomatic pancreatic disease. In a population-based German study of nearly 1000 healthy individuals with normal serum lipase and amylase, there was a significant 30% reduction in secretin-stimulated output in those

>80 years (Bulow et al. 2014). An age-related decrease in the secretory flow of pancreatic juice in the main pancreatic duct has been demonstrated noninvasively by cine-dynamic MRCP using spatially selective inversion recovery pulse (Torigoe et al. 2014). A decrease in fecal elastase-1 (level <200 lg g^1) was observed in 21.7% of subjects who were >60 years with no history of gastrointestinal disease, gastrointestinal surgery, or diabetes mellitus (Herzig et al. 2011). In contrast, another study on fecal elastase-1 has shown no functional impairment in those over 90 years old (Gullo et al. 2009). Regardless, even if there was some age-related decline (10–30%), this would not be clinically relevant since >90% of the pancreas has to be damaged to cause clinically evident exocrine insufficiency (Dimagno et al. 1973).

Pathological Changes

In contrast to the effects of age on function, marked changes in pancreatic structure occur with aging. Autopsy series reveal duct proliferation, lobular degeneration, and fatty infiltration (Pitchumoni et al. 1984; Shimizu et al. 1989; Ross and Forsmark 2001). Severe pancreatic steatosis was demonstrated in 15% of those 60- to 69-year-olds compared to no severe pancreatic steatosis in subjects below 40 years (Olsen 1978). There is a marginal decline in volume densities of islets and loss of both β- and non-β-cells with aging (Matsuda 2018). Mild focal or segmental ductal ectasia of the main or branched pancreatic ducts can also be seen. Main pancreatic ductal dilation greater than 4 mm in diameter has been reported in 16% of patients at autopsy (Stamm 1984). Pancreatic lithiasis ranges from being absent in those <70 years to being present in 16% of patients >90 years (Nagai and Ohtsubo 1984). Pancreatic lithiasis was found in the peripheral ducts upstream from sites of squamous metaplasia, in asymptomatic persons, not associated with alcoholism or hypercalcemia (Nagai and Ohtsubo 1984). Extensive parenchymal atrophy and fibrosis were also seen in areas upstream from the stones.

Morphological Changes

A significant negative correlation was reported between age and pancreatic size based on ultrasound (US) in 1000 males and females aged between 18 and 65 years (Niederau et al. 1983). In a large CT-based study on the pancreatic volume in humans from birth to age 100 years, the reported volumes of the pancreas increased linearly with age during childhood and adolescence, reached a plateau at age 20–60 years, and declined thereafter (Saisho et al. 2007). Postmortem pancreatography performed by physicians trained in Endoscopic Retrograde Cholangio-Pancreatography (ERCP) found ductal changes similar to those seen in chronic pancreatitis in 81% of older adults (Schmitz-Moormann et al. 1985; Gloor et al. 2002). However, histopathology in the same cases confirmed the findings to be age-related and not due to chronic pancreatitis (Schmitz-Moormann et al. 1985). Compared to subjects <50 years, the ductal diameter of those >90 years old increased significantly from 3.3 to 5.3 mm 2.3 to 3.7 mm, and 1.6 to 2.6 mm in the head, body, and tail of the pancreas, respectively (Hastier et al. 1998). The suggested ERCP criteria for diagnosing of chronic pancreatitis in older adults are summarized in Table 1 (Jones et al. 1989; Gloor et al. 2002). Age-related pancreatic changes are also seen on endoscopic ultrasonography (EUS). In a prospective study of 120 patients without pancreatic disease, 39% of patients >60 years had at least one EUS abnormality of chronic pancreatitis (Rajan et al. 2005). In this study, the presence of >3 EUS abnormalities, ductal or parenchymal stones, ductal narrowing, or dilation were more likely to represent disease than age-related changes (Rajan et al. 2005). Thus, caution should be exercised when interpreting ERCP and EUS findings in the geriatric patient.

Table 1 ERCP criteria for diagnosis of chronic pancreatitis in the elderly. (*Adapted from* Jones et al. 1989, Gloor et al. 2002)

Ductal obstruction and stricture
Gross irregularity of the main pancreatic duct
Presence of large cavities (>5 mm) (due to pre-stenotic ductal dilation)

Risk Factors

Idiopathic Chronic Pancreatitis

Most of the cases of chronic pancreatitis identified in the older subjects are due to "late-onset" idiopathic disease, described initially as "senile" chronic pancreatitis by Amman et al. and characterized by the age of onset of 56 years, absence of pain, and early development of structural (diffuse calcifications) and functional (exocrine and endocrine) abnormalities (Ammann and Sulser 1976; Layer et al. 1994). This is in contrast to "early-onset" idiopathic disease with a mean age of onset of 20 years, presence of pain, and long delay to the development of pancreatic abnormalities (Ammann et al. 1987; Layer et al. 1994).

Obstructive Pancreatitis

Obstruction of the main pancreatic duct (e.g., by an ampullary malignancy or cancer in the pancreatic head) can be an important cause in the elderly patient with new-onset chronic pancreatitis (Gloor et al. 2002; Cavallini and Frulloni 2009). This form of chronic pancreatitis differs from other varieties in the absence of calcifications and higher prevalence of a dilated pancreatic duct (Cavallini and Frulloni 2009).

Alcoholic Chronic Pancreatitis

In the general population, alcohol is the most common cause of chronic pancreatitis, accounting for 70–80% cases; however in patients with onset of pancreatitis after the age of 65, alcohol is an exceedingly uncommon cause (Yang et al. 2008). The risk increases with increasing dose (>4 drinks/day) and duration (>10 years) of alcohol consumption (Yadav et al. 2007). While alcohol appears to play an essential role in the development of chronic pancreatitis, only 5–15% of alcoholics develop the disease, suggesting a role for cofactors such as genetics, tobacco, etc. (Yadav et al. 2007).

Tobacco

While smoking is an independent risk factor for chronic pancreatitis, the damage to the pancreas is often compounded by ongoing alcohol use (Andriulli et al. 2010). After adjusting for alcohol use, the pooled risk estimate for chronic pancreatitis was 2.5 (95% CI 1.3–4.6) for current smokers when compared with never smokers (Andriulli et al. 2010). Also, the association between smoking and chronic pancreatitis was dose dependent, with a pooled risk estimate of 3.3 (95% CI 1.4–7.9) for people smoking one or more packs per day, compared with 2.4 (95% CI 0.9–6.6) for those smoking less than one pack per day and 1.4 (95% CI 1.1–1.9) for former smokers (Andriulli et al. 2010). The detrimental effects of smoking seem synergistic with alcohol use in patients with chronic pancreatitis (Yadav et al. 2009).

Recurrent Acute Pancreatitis

Approximately one out of every five patients with acute alcoholic pancreatitis will progress to chronic pancreatitis (Yadav 2011).

Other Causes

- *Hereditary pancreatitis:* Hereditary pancreatitis is an uncommon cause of chronic pancreatitis and is rare in the older adults (Rebours et al. 2009). While mutations in the cationic trypsinogen gene (PRSS1) are most commonly associated with chronic pancreatitis, mutated cystic fibrosis gene (CFTR) and trypsin inhibitor (SPINK1) genes are being increasingly identified in patients with idiopathic chronic pancreatitis (Etemad and Whitcomb 2001; Bishop et al. 2005).
- *Autoimmune pancreatitis:* Autoimmune pancreatitis (AIP) is a rare autoimmune disorder that is subclassified into two types, based on distinct pathological and clinical profiles (Sah et al. 2010). Type 1 or lymphoplasmacytic sclerosing pancreatitis is characterized by infiltration of the pancreas by IgG4-positive plasma cells and typically affects older men. Over 80% of patients with type 1 AIP are males, with >80% over age 50 (Sah et al. 2010). Type 1 disease is also associated with a higher relapse rate as well as extra-pancreatic involvement. In contrast, type 2 or idiopathic duct-centric pancreatitis is characterized by a granulocytic epithelial lesion (GEL) with minimal IgG4-positive cells and affects younger patients (affecting males and females equally). This entity is discussed in detail in a separate chapter.
- *Tropical pancreatitis:* Although the life expectancy of patients with tropical pancreatitis has considerably improved, it is not yet a geriatric problem. The entity is common in southern India, and is characterized by onset at young age, severe malnutrition, diabetes mellitus, and pancreatic calculi.

In summary, the etiology of chronic pancreatitis may be attributed to a complex interplay of environmental and genetic factors. The former include alcohol, tobacco, and occupational chemicals (volatile hydrocarbons) (Braganza et al. 2011) while the genetic factors include mutations in trypsin-controlling or cystic fibrosis genes (Whitcomb 2004).

Clinical Presentation

Abdominal pain, an uncommon symptom in late-onset idiopathic chronic pancreatitis, is often a major complaint in alcoholic chronic pancreatitis (Layer et al. 1994; Gloor et al. 2002). The typical pain is epigastric, post-prandial, radiates to the back, and is relieved by sitting up or leaning forward. However, the severity and character of pain are highly variable in chronic pancreatitis, with some patients having severe daily pain (continuous pattern) while others have fleeting discomfort (intermittent pattern). The continuous and intermittent pain patterns do not seem to be the result of distinctly different pathophysiological entities (Kempeneers et al. 2020). The subjectively reported character of the pain often does not correlate with morphologic changes or disease duration, indicating a complex mechanism of pain in chronic pancreatitis (Wilcox et al. 2015; Kempeneers et al. 2020). Earlier theories focused on a mechanical cause of pain related to pancreatic ductal or parenchymal hypertension (White and Bourde 1970). An inflammatory mass in the head of the pancreas is reported in nearly one-third of patients with chronic pain (Frey and Reber 2005; Roch et al. 2014). Other factors such as activation of intrapancreatic nociceptors, hypertrophy, and inflammation of intrapancreatic nerves and abnormal pain processing in the central nervous system have been suggested (Drewes et al. 2008). The pancreatic nociceptive afferent injury over time leads to peripheral sensitization, central sensitization, or both, characterized by neuronal hyperresponsiveness, which results in a continuous state of pain independent of peripheral nociceptive input (Olesen et al. 2010). The persistence of pain despite complete removal of the noxious stimulus (e.g., total pancreatectomy) supports this central sensitization hypothesis.

Pancreatic exocrine insufficiency is often the presenting symptom in patients with late-onset idiopathic chronic pancreatitis (Layer et al. 1994). While protein and carbohydrate malabsorption might occur in advanced pancreatic insufficiency, they are generally less pronounced than fat malabsorption due to compensatory secretions from intact salivary amylase and brush border peptidases in most patients. Most patients with exocrine insufficiency present with greasy, foul-smelling stools (steatorrhea). Patients might also present with weight loss, malnutrition, fat-soluble vitamin deficiencies (Vitamin A, D, E, and K), and vitamin B12 deficiency (due to noncleavage of R-factor from vitamin B12, dependent on pancreatic function). Malnutrition is common in patients with chronic pancreatitis. Anorexia secondary to abdominal pain, pancreatic enzyme insufficiency, alcohol abuse, and diabetes mellitus may contribute to malnutrition in chronic pancreatitis.

Endocrine pancreatic insufficiency (type 3c diabetes, also known as pancreatogenic diabetes) eventually develops in most patients due to progressive beta-cell loss (American Diabetes 2013). The patients with type 3c diabetes are at a higher risk of hypoglycemia because of concomitant loss of counter-regulatory hormones such as glucagon and pancreatic polypeptide (Hart et al. 2016). The risk of developing type 3c diabetes increases with increasing age, duration of disease, surgical intervention (especially distal pancreatectomy), smoking, and the presence of pancreatic calcifications.

Patients with chronic pancreatitis are at significantly higher risk (relative risk 13.3, 95% CI 6.1–28.9) of pancreatic adenocarcinoma, although this risk is greatest for early-onset disease and in patients with hereditary and tropical pancreatitis (Raimondi et al. 2010). Some other common complications in patients with long-standing chronic pancreatitis include pseudocysts, common bile duct stricture; duodenal stenosis; pleural effusion; splenic vein thrombosis with the formation of gastric varices; portal vein thrombosis; pseudoaneurysm affecting the splenic, hepatic, gastroduodenal, and pancreaticoduodenal arteries; and pancreatic ascites.

Diagnosis

No single diagnostic test is adequately sensitive or specific for chronic pancreatitis in all patients. Age-related structural changes in the older adult may make the diagnosis even more difficult. A suggested diagnostic algorithm for chronic pancreatitis is outlined in Fig. 1.

Tests of Function

- *Amylase and lipase levels*: Amylase and lipase levels are generally normal and are not useful in the diagnosis of chronic pancreatitis.
- *Stool fat quantitation*: A 72-hour fecal fat quantitation is useful in patients with steatorrhea. Patients with pancreatic insufficiency typically excrete >10–14 grams of fat. Since exocrine pancreatic insufficiency develops only when <10% secretory capacity remains, this test is not useful in the diagnosis of early disease (Dimagno et al. 1973). Further, the test is cumbersome in older adults.

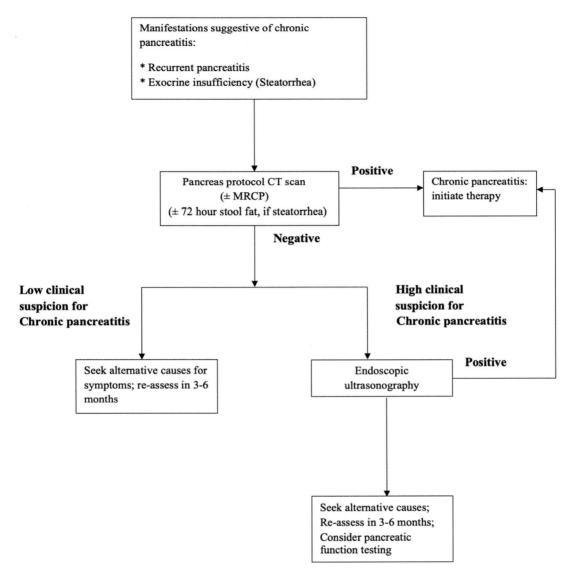

Fig. 1 Diagnostic algorithm for suspected chronic pancreatitis. *(Adapted from* Etemad and Whitcomb 2001*)*

- *Stool elastase and chymotrypsin:* These tests are a measure of the secretion of elastase and chymotrypsin by the pancreas on random stool samples (Keim et al. 2003). However, they provide yield only in the presence of steatorrhea, obviating their utility in the diagnosis of early disease (Lankisch 2004).
- *Hormonal stimulation tests:* They measure pancreatic secretory capacity by collecting pancreatic fluid following stimulation with a

secretagogue (e.g., secretin). Hormonal stimulation tests are considered the most sensitive tests (70–90%) for chronic pancreatitis (Chowdhury and Forsmark 2003). Secretin stimulation test can be combined with EUS during which pancreatic fluid is collected by duodenal aspirate endoscopically after secretin stimulation, allowing for a functional assessment of the pancreas in the same setting. However, this technique is not widely used. Also, while they detect early disease, there is a risk of complications from invasive endoscopic procedures (Dominguez-Munoz 2011).

Tests of Structure

- *Plain radiography:* Diffuse calculi in the pancreatic duct are very specific for chronic pancreatitis and often seen in elderly smokers with late-onset idiopathic disease (Imoto and Dimagno 2000) (Fig. 2).
- *Ultrasonography (USG):* Trans-abdominal ultrasound has limited utility in evaluation of the pancreas due to interference by bowel gas and body fat (Ikeda et al. 1994).
- *Computed tomography (CT):* CT has the advantage of adequate imaging regardless of body habitus, but carries risk of radiation exposure. However, the higher sensitivity (80–90%) and specificity (85%) for diagnosis of chronic pancreatitis justify its widespread use (Choueiri et al. 2010).
- *Magnetic Resonance Cholangio-Pancreatography (MRCP):* MRCP is increasingly becoming the preferred test in the diagnosis of chronic pancreatitis since it can detect ductal abnormalities with a similar frequency to ERCP and avoids the risks associated with ERCP (Fig. 3) (Calvo et al. 2002; Sandrasegaran et al. 2010). The presence of typical imaging findings

for chronic pancreatitis with MRCP is often sufficient for diagnosis, although a normal MRCP cannot exclude mild forms of the disease. Intravenous administration of secretin during MRCP increases sensitivity to diagnose ductal changes in chronic pancreatitis (Lohr et al. 2018).

- *Endoscopic Retrograde Cholangio-Pancreatography (ERCP)*: ERCP has the highest sensitivity (70–90%) and specificity (80–100%) for the diagnosis of chronic pancreatitis but carries a risk of complications (Calvo et al. 2002). As discussed earlier, ERCP findings of chronic pancreatitis in the older adults (Fig. 4) can be confounded by age-related changes in the normal pancreas (Forsmark and Toskes 1995; Gleeson and Topazian 2007). The guidelines by the American Society for Gastrointestinal Endoscopy (ASGE) in 2006 recommended reserving the use of ERCP for patients in whom diagnosis is inconclusive despite pancreatic function testing CT/MRI or EUS (Adler et al. 2006).
- *Endoscopic ultrasound (EUS):* EUS criteria for diagnosis of chronic pancreatitis include ductal abnormalities (dilation, irregularity, calcification, etc.) and parenchymal abnormalities (cysts, hyperechoic foci, lobularity, etc.) (Fig. 5 **a–c**) (Gleeson and Topazian 2007; Varadarajulu et al. 2007). Pancreatic changes on EUS can be seen in the absence of any symptoms of pancreatic disease. Besides aging, alcohol, smoking, diabetes,

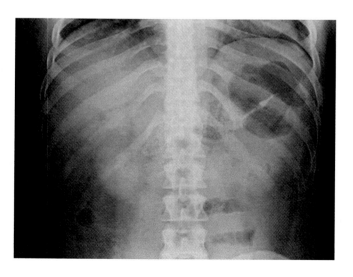

Fig. 2 Abdominal plain film in a patient with chronic pancreatitis with diffuse calcifications in the pancreas. *(Adapted from Aggarwal and Chari 2012)*

Fig. 3 MRI/MRCP showing dilated, irregular pancreatic duct with a filling defect secondary to intra-ductal calculus in a 72-year-old female

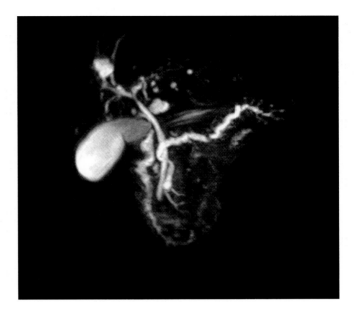

Fig. 4 Endoscopic Retrograde Cholangio-Pancreatography showing classic changes of chronic pancreatitis in an elderly patient, grossly irregular and dilated main pancreatic duct, dilated side branches, filling defects, and stone in the main pancreatic duct. *(Adapted from* Aggarwal and Chari 2012*)*

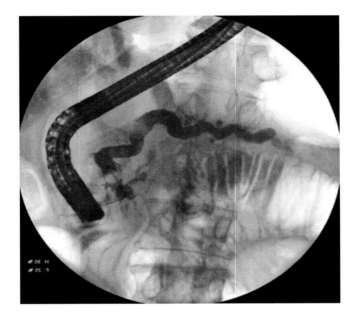

and acute pancreatitis can all cause EUS abnormalities in the absence of chronic pancreatitis (Yusoff and Sahai 2004; Rajan et al. 2005). EUS diagnosis, therefore, should always be interpreted in the appropriate clinical context and is rarely diagnostic of chronic pancreatitis in isolation.

As chronic pancreatitis is a complex disease, EUS-based criteria for diagnosis have differed widely. A consensus study has established major and minor EUS-based criteria for chronic pancreatitis in the "Rosemont Classification" (Catalano et al. 2009). Further, EUS may be complemented by digital imaging analysis and functional testing;

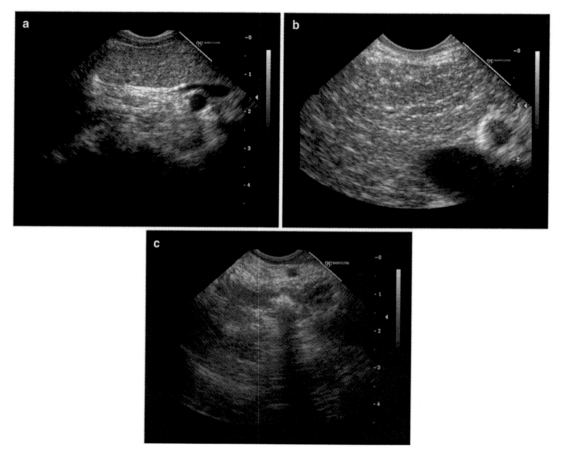

Fig. 5 EUS findings in chronic pancreatitis. *(Courtesy: Dr. Michael J. Levy, Mayo Clinic, Rochester, MN, Adapted from Aggarwal and Chari 2012)*

(a) Normal pancreas
(b) Hyperechoic foci
(c) Dilated main pancreatic duct, intra-ductal calculus

EUS may also be used for celiac plexus blockade and ductal access techniques (Stevens 2011).

Treatment

Therapy for chronic pancreatitis is centered around the management of symptoms. Complications and approach to management are listed in Table 2.

Abdominal Pain

Lifestyle modifications including abstinence from alcohol and cessation of smoking are associated with a reduction in pain (Strum 1995). Supplemental antioxidants (selenium, Vitamin A, Vitamin C, and Vitamin E) have a modest effect on reducing pain (Bhardwaj et al. 2009). However, most patients require some form of analgesia for pain control. When prescribing analgesics in the elderly, the strategy is to begin with non-narcotic analgesics followed by low-potency opioids (e.g., tramadol) and finally higher-potency narcotics. The goal is to reduce pain to a manageable level and not complete alleviation. Since chronic pain can lead to depression which in turn exacerbates pain, there is a role for adjunct therapy such as antidepressants. The role of oral pancreatic enzyme therapy to reduce pain is doubtful and is markedly limited to patients with small duct disease, women, and those with idiopathic chronic pancreatitis (Slaff et al. 1984). Patients with

Table 2 Complications of chronic pancreatitis (Lowenfels et al. 1993; Balachandra and Siriwardena 2005; Morgan and Adams 2007; Habashi and Draganov 2009)

Complication	Cause	Presentation	Diagnosis	Treatment
Pseudocyst	Ductal disruption	Abdominal pain Bleeding Bowel/Biliary obstruction Ascites (from disruption)	Imaging with USG, CT, MRI, and EUS	No treatment, if asymptomatic Drainage, if symptomatic, enlarging, or complicated
Biliary/ Duodenal obstruction	Inflammation or fibrosis in the head leading to compression	Jaundice nausea, vomiting, abdominal pain	CT MRCP EGD	Surgical bypass or endoscopic stenting
Pancreatic fistulae and ascites	Ductal disruption, pseudocyst rupture	Abdominal pain Ascites	High amylase on paracentesis	TPN, NPO, octreotide Endoscopic stenting Surgery
Splenic vein thrombosis	Contiguous inflammation	Gastrointestinal bleeding from gastric varices	EGD USG with doppler CT	No treatment if asymptomatic Endoscopic glue for bleeding Splenectomy is curative
Pseudoaneurysm	Enzymatic digestion of arterial wall	Bleeding	Urgent EGD CT Angiography	Angiographic embolization Surgery, if embolization fails
Pancreatic cancer	Highest risk in active smokers	No specific symptoms Abdominal pain, weight loss, jaundice	CA19–9 CT EUS	Surgery, if resectable

worsening abdominal pain require evaluation for complications such as pseudocysts, cancer, stricture, etc.

Endoscopic Therapy

In patients with large duct disease and evidence of pancreatic ductal obstruction (strictures or stones), endoscopic therapy with a pancreatic sphincterotomy with or without pancreatic stenting might be useful (Tringali et al. 2008). Endoscopic therapy may be performed when there are 3 or fewer small (<1 cm) stones located in the head or body of the pancreas (Dumonceau et al. 2019). Large stones usually require extracorporeal shockwave lithotripsy before endoscopic removal. However, this procedure is not approved by the Food and Drug Administration for pancreatic stones and requires urologist assistance at US centers. The use of straight polyethylene pancreatic stents (8.5–10 Fr) is generally recommended for managing main pancreatic duct strictures

(Dominguez-Munoz et al. 2018). Stent exchange can be performed either "on-demand" (preferred strategy) or at regular intervals (e.g., every 3 months) in patients with recurrence of abdominal pain or main pancreatic duct dilatation.

Since the celiac plexus transmits nociceptive impulses from the pancreas to the spinal cord, blocking these signals (percutaneously, endoscopically, or surgically) can help treat pain in chronic pancreatitis. While EUS guided celiac plexus block (injecting steroids) is safer and more cost-effective than CT-guided techniques, the pain relief is temporary (Gress et al. 2001). A study of 90 patients showed pain relief in 55% at 4 weeks but by 24 weeks only 10% reported sustained benefit (Gress et al. 1999). EUS-guided celiac plexus block might be useful in the older adults since pain relief was more evident in those over age 45 years in the previously mentioned study (Gress et al. 1999). However, most recent evidence supporting the efficacy of endoscopic celiac plexus block remains weak and this approach is not recommended for patients with painful chronic pancreatitis in the absence of a concomitant pancreatic malignancy (Stevens et al. 2012; Dumonceau 2013).

Surgery

Surgical intervention with ductal drainage or pancreatic resection is reserved for medically refractory disease, suspected malignancy, and complications such as pseudocysts (Buchler and Warshaw 2008). Compared with an endoscopy-first approach, early surgery is more effective in managing painful chronic pancreatitis as per a recent randomized clinical trial (Issa et al. 2020).

In drainage procedures, a dilated pancreatic duct is cut and anastomosed to the bowel (most commonly jejunum). The pancreatic duct should be dilated to 6 mm or more for the long-term patency of the pancreatico-jejunostomy anastomosis. The most frequently performed drainage procedures are the modified Puestow procedure (lateral pancreatico-jejunostomy) and the Frey procedure, which in addition to a pancreatico-jejunostomy includes coring of the pancreatic head. Both of these procedures are relatively safe (mortality <1%) and effective for managing pain in chronic pancreatitis. However, in patients with persistent inflammation of the pancreatic head without upstream ductal dilatation, pancreaticoduo-denectomy (Whipple) or a duodenum-preserving head resection (Beger) can be done. Distal pancreatectomy should be reserved for patients with disease limited to the pancreatic tail region and is rarely performed to manage pain in chronic pancreatitis. The long-term outcomes of total pancreatectomy with auto-islet transplantation have shown a mixed response (Beyer et al. 2020). Regardless, the procedure is not practical in the older adults especially when associated with multiple comorbid conditions.

Steatorrhea

The mainstay of treatment for pancreatic steatorrhea is pancreatic enzyme supplementation. Lipase (30,000–50,000 IU) spread over each meal is generally adequate (Chowdhury and Forsmark 2003). A smaller amount is required with snacks. If a nonenteric coated formulation is selected, concomitant acid suppression (e.g., proton pump inhibitor or H2 blocker) is necessary. In addition, fat-soluble vitamins should be replaced in patients with steatorrhea. In patients who do not respond, dietary restriction of fat to less than 20 grams per day may help relief of steatorrhea, but prevents weight gain. Bacterial overgrowth may complicate steatorrhea and require treatment. Medium chain triglycerides (MCTs), which do not need lipase for absorption, are rarely required to treat pancreatic steatorrhea (Chowdhury and Forsmark 2003).

Diabetes Mellitus

Type 3c diabetes secondary to chronic pancreatitis is usually insulin requiring. Patients with type 3c diabetes are often difficult to manage with potential life-threatening acute complications such as hypoglycemia and ketoacidosis. Up to 25% of these patients have "brittle diabetes" because of rapid swings in glucose levels. Therapy with metformin can be considered if the hyperglycemia is mild and concomitant insulin resistant is suspected or present. Sulfonylureas, thiazolidines, alpha-glycosidase inhibitors, incretin-based therapies, and sodium glucose cotransporter-2 should not be used because of the risk of hypoglycemia and prominent side effects.

Nutritional Deficiencies

Small, frequent, and high-calorie meals should be recommended for patients with malnutrition. For patients who are undernourished and cannot meet their nutritional requirements despite dietary intervention, oral nutritional supplementations may be helpful. Enteral feeding is indicated in patients with malnutrition who do not respond to oral nutritional support. Parenteral nutrition is required in patients with severe malnutrition, gastric outlet obstruction from duodenal stenosis, or complex fistulizing disease when enteral feeding is not possible.

Screening for fat-soluble vitamin deficiency (A, D, E, and K), zinc, and magnesium should be performed in all patients with chronic pancreatitis. Patients with chronic pancreatitis are at high risk of developing osteoporosis and osteopenia, thus regular assessment of bone density by dual-energy X-ray absorptiometry, along with regular measurement of serum 25(OH)-vitamin D, should be considered.

Key Points

- While alcohol is the most common cause of chronic pancreatitis in the general population, alcoholic pancreatitis rarely has its onset over age 60 years. Late-onset idiopathic pancreatitis is a possibility to be considered.
- Pancreatic cancer can mimic chronic pancreatitis in the older adults.
- Older patients often present with exocrine insufficiency without significant abdominal pain.
- Age-related changes in pancreatic structure can resemble the changes of chronic pancreatitis.
- Diffuse pancreatic calcifications on abdominal radiographs are specific for chronic pancreatitis but are generally seen in late stages of the disease. In early chronic pancreatitis, CT and MRI may be normal.
- EUS findings of chronic pancreatitis may be confounded by changes due to aging, alcohol, and smoking.
- Patients with chronic pancreatitis are at increased risk of pancreatic cancer

References

Adler DG, Lichtenstein D, Baron TH, Davila R, Egan JV, Gan SL, Qureshi WA, Rajan E, Shen B, Zuckerman MJ, Lee KK, Vanguilder T, Fanelli RD. The role of endoscopy in patients with chronic pancreatitis. Gastrointest Endosc. 2006;63:933–7.

Aggarwal G, Chari ST. Chronic pancreatitis. In: Pitchumoni CS, Dharmarajan TS, editors. Geriatric gastroenterology. New York: Springer; 2012.

American Diabetes A. Diagnosis and classification of diabetes mellitus. Diabetes Care. 2013;36(Suppl 1):S67–74.

Ammann R, Sulser H. "Senile" chronic pancreatitis; a new nosologic entity? Studies in 38 cases. Indications of a vascular origin and relationship to the primarily painless chronic pancreatitis. Schweiz Med Wochenschr. 1976;106:429–37.

Ammann RW, Buehler H, Muench R, Freiburghaus AW, Siegenthaler W. Differences in the natural history of idiopathic (nonalcoholic) and alcoholic chronic pancreatitis. A comparative long-term study of 287 patients. Pancreas. 1987;2:368–77.

Andriulli A, Botteri E, Almasio PL, Vantini I, Uomo G, Maisonneuve P, Ad Hoc Committee of the Italian Association for the Study of the Pancreas. Smoking as a cofactor for causation of chronic pancreatitis: a meta-analysis. Pancreas. 2010;39:1205–10.

Balachandra S, Siriwardena AK. Systematic appraisal of the management of the major vascular complications of pancreatitis. Am J Surg. 2005;190:489–95.

Beyer G, Habtezion A, Werner J, Lerch MM, Mayerle J. Chronic pancreatitis. Lancet. 2020;396:499–512.

Bhardwaj P, Garg PK, Maulik SK, Saraya A, Tandon RK, Acharya SK. A randomized controlled trial of antioxidant supplementation for pain relief in patients with chronic pancreatitis. Gastroenterology. 2009;136:149–159 e2.

Bishop MD, Freedman SD, Zielenski J, Ahmed N, Dupuis A, Martin S, Ellis L, Shea J, Hopper I, Corey M, Kortan P, Haber G, Ross C, Tzountzouris J, Steele L, Ray PN, Tsui LC, Durie PR. The cystic fibrosis transmembrane conductance regulator gene and ion channel function in patients with idiopathic pancreatitis. Hum Genet. 2005;118:372–81.

Braganza JM, Lee SH, Mccloy RF, Mcmahon MJ. Chronic pancreatitis. Lancet. 2011;377:1184–97.

Buchler MW, Warshaw AL. Resection versus drainage in treatment of chronic pancreatitis. Gastroenterology. 2008;134:1605–7.

Bulow R, Simon P, Thiel R, Thamm P, Messner P, Lerch MM, Mayerle J, Volzke H, Hosten N, Kuhn JP. Anatomic variants of the pancreatic duct and their clinical relevance: an MR-guided study in the general population. Eur Radiol. 2014;24:3142–9.

Calvo MM, Bujanda L, Calderon A, Heras I, Cabriada JL, Bernal A, Orive V, Astigarraga E. Comparison between magnetic resonance cholangiopancreatography and ERCP for evaluation of the pancreatic duct. Am J Gastroenterol. 2002;97:347–53.

Catalano MF, Sahai A, Levy M, Romagnuolo J, Wiersema M, Brugge W, Freeman M, Yamao K, Canto M, Hernandez LV. EUS-based criteria for the diagnosis of chronic pancreatitis: the Rosemont classification. Gastrointest Endosc. 2009;69:1251–61.

Cavallini G, Frulloni L. Pathophysiology of chronic pancreatitis. In: Balthazar EJ, Megibow AJ, Pozzi Mucelli R, editors. Imaging of the pancreas: Springer; 2009.

Choueiri NE, Balci NC, Alkaade S, Burton FR. Advanced imaging of chronic pancreatitis. Curr Gastroenterol Rep. 2010;12:114–20.

Chowdhury RS, Forsmark CE. Review article: pancreatic function testing. Aliment Pharmacol Ther. 2003;17:733–50.

Dimagno MJ, Dimagno EP. Chronic pancreatitis. Curr Opin Gastroenterol. 2010;26:490–8.

Dimagno EP, Go VL, Summerskill WH. Relations between pancreatic enzyme outputs and malabsorption in severe pancreatic insufficiency. N Engl J Med. 1973;288:813–5.

Dominguez-Munoz JE. Pancreatic exocrine insufficiency: diagnosis and treatment. J Gastroenterol Hepatol. 2011;26(Suppl 2):12–6.

Dominguez-Munoz JE, Drewes AM, Lindkvist B, Ewald N, Czako L, Rosendahl J, Lohr JM, HaPanEU/UEG Working Group. Recommendations from the United European Gastroenterology evidence-based guidelines for the diagnosis and therapy of chronic pancreatitis. Pancreatology. 2018;18:847–54.

Drewes AM, Krarup AL, Detlefsen S, Malmstrom ML, Dimcevski G, Funch-Jensen P. Pain in chronic pancreatitis: the role of neuropathic pain mechanisms. Gut. 2008;57:1616–27.

Dumonceau JM. Endoscopic therapy for chronic pancreatitis. Gastrointest Endosc Clin N Am. 2013;23:821–32.

Dumonceau JM, Delhaye M, Tringali A, Arvanitakis M, Sanchez-Yague A, Vaysse T, Aithal GP, Anderloni A, Bruno M, Cantu P, Deviere J, Dominguez-Munoz JE, Lekkerkerker S, Poley JW, Ramchandani M, Reddy N, Van Hooft JE. Endoscopic treatment of chronic pancreatitis: European Society of Gastrointestinal Endoscopy (ESGE) guideline – updated August 2018. Endoscopy. 2019;51:179–93.

Etemad B, Whitcomb DC. Chronic pancreatitis: diagnosis, classification, and new genetic developments. Gastroenterology. 2001;120:682–707.

Forsmark CE, Toskes PP. What does an abnormal pancreatogram mean? Gastrointest Endosc Clin N Am. 1995;5:105–23.

Frey CF, Reber HA. Local resection of the head of the pancreas with pancreaticojejunostomy. J Gastrointest Surg. 2005;9:863–8.

Gleeson FC, Topazian M. Endoscopic retrograde cholangiopancreatography and endoscopic ultrasound for diagnosis of chronic pancreatitis. Curr Gastroenterol Rep. 2007;9:123–9.

Gloor B, Ahmed Z, Uhl W, Buchler MW. Pancreatic disease in the elderly. Best Pract Res Clin Gastroenterol. 2002;16:159–70.

Gress F, Schmitt C, Sherman S, Ikenberry S, Lehman G. A prospective randomized comparison of endoscopic ultrasound- and computed tomography-guided celiac plexus block for managing chronic pancreatitis pain. Am J Gastroenterol. 1999;94:900–5.

Gress F, Schmitt C, Sherman S, Ciaccia D, Ikenberry S, Lehman G. Endoscopic ultrasound-guided celiac plexus block for managing abdominal pain associated with chronic pancreatitis: a prospective single center experience. Am J Gastroenterol. 2001;96:409–16.

Gullo L, Priori P, Daniele C, Ventrucci M, Gasbarrini G, Labo G. Exocrine pancreatic function in the elderly. Gerontology. 1983;29:407–11.

Gullo L, Simoni P, Migliori M, Lucrezio L, Bassi M, Frau F, Costa PL, Nestico V. A study of pancreatic function among subjects over ninety years of age. Pancreatology. 2009;9:240–4.

Habashi S, Draganov PV. Pancreatic pseudocyst. World J Gastroenterol. 2009;15:38–47.

Hart PA, Bellin MD, Andersen DK, Bradley D, Cruz-Monserrate Z, Forsmark CE, Goodarzi MO, Habtezion A, Korc M, Kudva YC, Pandol SJ, Yadav D, Chari ST, Consortium for the Study of Chronic Pancreatitis, Diabetes, and Pancreatic Cancer (CPDPC). Type 3c (pancreatogenic) diabetes mellitus secondary to chronic pancreatitis and pancreatic cancer. Lancet Gastroenterol Hepatol. 2016;1:226–37.

Hastier P, Buckley MJ, Dumas R, Kuhdorf H, Staccini P, Demarquay JF, Caroli-Bosc FX, Delmont JP. A study of the effect of age on pancreatic duct morphology. Gastrointest Endosc. 1998;48:53–7.

Herzig KH, Purhonen AK, Rasanen KM, Idziak J, Juvonen P, Phillps R, Walkowiak J. Fecal pancreatic elastase-1 levels in older individuals without known gastrointestinal diseases or diabetes mellitus. BMC Geriatr. 2011;11:4.

Ikeda M, Sato T, Morozumi A, Fujino MA, Yoda Y, Ochiai M, Kobayashi K. Morphologic changes in the pancreas detected by screening ultrasonography in a mass survey, with special reference to main duct dilatation, cyst formation, and calcification. Pancreas. 1994;9:508–12.

Imoto M, Dimagno EP. Cigarette smoking increases the risk of pancreatic calcification in late-onset but not early-onset idiopathic chronic pancreatitis. Pancreas. 2000;21:115–9.

Issa Y, Kempeneers MA, Bruno MJ, Fockens P, Poley JW, Ahmed Ali U, Bollen TL, Busch OR, Dejong CH, Van Duijvendijk P, Van Dullemen HM, Van Eijck CH, Van Goor H, Hadithi M, Haveman JW, Keulemans Y, Nieuwenhuijs VB, Poen AC, Rauws EA, Tan AC, Thijs W, Timmer R, Witteman BJ, Besselink MG, Van Hooft JE, Van Santvoort HC, Dijkgraaf MG, Boermeester MA, Dutch Pancreatitis Study G. Effect of early surgery vs endoscopy-first approach on pain in patients with chronic pancreatitis: the ESCAPE randomized clinical trial. JAMA. 2020;323:237–47.

Jones SN, Mcneil NI, Lees WR. The interpretation of retrograde pancreatography in the elderly. Clin Radiol. 1989;40:393–6.

Keim V, Teich N, Moessner J. Clinical value of a new fecal elastase test for detection of chronic pancreatitis. Clin Lab. 2003;49:209–15.

Kempeneers MA, Issa Y, Verdonk RC, Bruno M, Fockens P, Van Goor H, Alofs E, Bollen TL, Bouwense S, Van Dalen A, Van Dieren S, Van Dullemen HM, Van Geenen EJ, Hoge C, Van Hooft JE, Kager LM, Keulemans Y, Nooijen LE, Poley JW, Seerden TCJ, Tan A, Thijs W, Timmer R, Vleggaar F, Witteman B, Ahmed Ali U, Besselink MG, Boermeester MA, Van Santvoort HC, Dutch Pancreatitis Study, Group. Pain patterns in chronic pancreatitis: a nationwide longitudinal cohort study. Gut. 2020; Epub ahead of print. https://doi.org/10.1136/gutjnl-2020-322117.

Lankisch PG. Now that fecal elastase is available in the United States, should clinicians start using it? Curr Gastroenterol Rep. 2004;6:126–31.

Layer P, Yamamoto H, Kalthoff L, Clain JE, Bakken LJ, Dimagno EP. The different courses of early- and late-onset idiopathic and alcoholic chronic pancreatitis. Gastroenterology. 1994;107:1481–7.

Levy P, Barthet M, Mollard BR, Amouretti M, Marion-Audibert AM, Dyard F. Estimation of the prevalence and incidence of chronic pancreatitis and its complications. Gastroenterol Clin Biol. 2006;30:838–44.

Lin Y, Tamakoshi A, Matsuno S, Takeda K, Hayakawa T, Kitagawa M, Naruse S, Kawamura T, Wakai K, Aoki R, Kojima M, Ohno Y. Nationwide epidemiological survey of chronic pancreatitis in Japan. J Gastroenterol. 2000;35:136–41.

Lohr JM, Panic N, Vujasinovic M, Verbeke CS. The ageing pancreas: a systematic review of the evidence and analysis of the consequences. J Intern Med. 2018;283:446–60.

Lowenfels AB, Maisonneuve P, Cavallini G, Ammann RW, Lankisch PG, Andersen JR, Dimagno EP, Andren-Sandberg A, Domellof L. Pancreatitis and the risk of pancreatic cancer. International Pancreatitis Study Group. N Engl J Med. 1993;328:1433–7.

Matsuda Y. Age-related pathological changes in the pancreas. Front Biosci (Elite Ed). 2018;10:137–42.

Morgan KA, Adams DB. Management of internal and external pancreatic fistulas. Surg Clin North Am. 2007;87:1503–13, x.

Nagai H, Ohtsubo K. Pancreatic lithiasis in the aged. Its clinicopathology and pathogenesis. Gastroenterology. 1984;86:331–8.

Niederau C, Sonnenberg A, Muller JE, Erckenbrecht JF, Scholten T, Fritsch WP. Sonographic measurements of the normal liver, spleen, pancreas, and portal vein. Radiology. 1983;149:537–40.

Olesen SS, Frokjaer JB, Lelic D, Valeriani M, Drewes AM. Pain-associated adaptive cortical reorganisation in chronic pancreatitis. Pancreatology. 2010;10: 742–51.

Olsen TS. Lipomatosis of the pancreas in autopsy material and its relation to age and overweight. Acta Pathol Microbiol Scand A. 1978;86A:367–73.

Peery AF, Crockett SD, Murphy CC, Lund JL, Dellon ES, Williams JL, Jensen ET, Shaheen NJ, Barritt AS, Lieber SR, Kochar B, Barnes EL, Fan YC, Pate V, Galanko J, Baron TH, Sandler RS. Burden and cost of gastrointestinal, liver, and pancreatic diseases in the United States: update 2018. Gastroenterology. 2019;156:254–272 e11.

Pitchumoni CS, Glasser M, Saran RM, Panchacharam P, Thelmo W. Pancreatic fibrosis in chronic alcoholics and nonalcoholics without clinical pancreatitis. Am J Gastroenterol. 1984;79:382–8.

Raimondi S, Lowenfels AB, Morselli-Labate AM, Maisonneuve P, Pezzilli R. Pancreatic cancer in chronic pancreatitis; aetiology, incidence, and early detection. Best Pract Res Clin Gastroenterol. 2010;24:349–58.

Rajan E, Clain JE, Levy MJ, Norton ID, Wang KK, Wiersema MJ, Vazquez-Sequeiros E, Nelson BJ, Jondal ML, Kendall RK, Harmsen WS, Zinsmeister AR. Age-related changes in the pancreas identified by EUS: a prospective evaluation. Gastrointest Endosc. 2005;61:401–6.

Rebours V, Boutron-Ruault MC, Schnee M, Ferec C, Le Marechal C, Hentic O, Maire F, Hammel P, Ruszniewski P, Levy P. The natural history of hereditary pancreatitis: a national series. Gut. 2009;58:97–103.

Roch A, Teyssedou J, Mutter D, Marescaux J, Pessaux P. Chronic pancreatitis: a surgical disease? Role of the Frey procedure. World J Gastrointest Surg. 2014;6:129–35.

Ross SO, Forsmark CE. Pancreatic and biliary disorders in the elderly. Gastroenterol Clin North Am. 2001;30: 531–45, x.

Sah RP, Chari ST, Pannala R, Sugumar A, Clain JE, Levy MJ, Pearson RK, Smyrk TC, Petersen BT, Topazian MD, Takahashi N, Farnell MB, Vege SS. Differences in clinical profile and relapse rate of type 1 versus type 2 autoimmune pancreatitis. Gastroenterology. 2010;139: 140–8; quiz e12-3.

Saisho Y, Butler AE, Meier JJ, Monchamp T, Allen-Auerbach M, Rizza RA, Butler PC. Pancreas volumes in humans from birth to age one hundred taking into account sex, obesity, and presence of type-2 diabetes. Clin Anat. 2007;20:933–42.

Sandrasegaran K, Lin C, Akisik FM, Tann M. State-of-the-art pancreatic MRI. AJR Am J Roentgenol. 2010;195: 42–53.

Schmitz-Moormann P, Himmelmann GW, Brandes JW, Folsch UR, Lorenz-Meyer H, Malchow H, Soehendra LN, Wienbeck M. Comparative radiological and morphological study of human pancreas. Pancreatitis like changes in postmortem ductograms and their morphological pattern. Possible implication for ERCP. Gut. 1985;26:406–14.

Shimizu M, Hayashi T, Saitoh Y, Itoh H. Interstitial fibrosis in the pancreas. Am J Clin Pathol. 1989;91:531–4.

Slaff J, Jacobson D, Tillman CR, Curington C, Toskes P. Protease-specific suppression of pancreatic exocrine secretion. Gastroenterology. 1984;87:44–52.

Stamm BH. Incidence and diagnostic significance of minor pathologic changes in the adult pancreas at autopsy: a systematic study of 112 autopsies in patients without known pancreatic disease. Hum Pathol. 1984;15:677–83.

Stevens T. Update on the role of endoscopic ultrasound in chronic pancreatitis. Curr Gastroenterol Rep. 2011;13: 117–22.

Stevens T, Costanzo A, Lopez R, Kapural L, Parsi MA, Vargo JJ. Adding triamcinolone to endoscopic ultrasound-guided celiac plexus blockade does not reduce pain in patients with chronic pancreatitis. Clin Gastroenterol Hepatol. 2012;10:186–91, 191 e1.

Strum WB. Abstinence in alcoholic chronic pancreatitis. Effect on pain and outcome. J Clin Gastroenterol. 1995;20:37–41.

Torigoe T, Ito K, Yamamoto A, Kanki A, Yasokawa K, Tamada T, Yoshida K. Age-related change of the secretory flow of pancreatic juice in the main pancreatic duct: evaluation with cine-dynamic MRCP using spatially selective inversion recovery pulse. AJR Am J Roentgenol. 2014;202:1022–6.

Tringali A, Boskoski I, Costamagna G. The role of endoscopy in the therapy of chronic pancreatitis. Best Pract Res Clin Gastroenterol. 2008;22:145–65.

Varadarajulu S, Eltoum I, Tamhane A, Eloubeidi MA. Histopathologic correlates of noncalcific chronic pancreatitis by EUS: a prospective tissue characterization study. Gastrointest Endosc. 2007;66:501–9.

Whitcomb DC. Value of genetic testing in the management of pancreatitis. Gut. 2004;53:1710–7.

White TT, Bourde J. A new observation on human intraductal pancreatic pressure. Surg Gynecol Obstet. 1970;130:275–8.

Wilcox CM, Yadav D, Ye T, Gardner TB, Gelrud A, Sandhu BS, Lewis MD, Al-Kaade S, Cote GA, Forsmark CE, Guda NM, Conwell DL, Banks PA, Muniraj T, Romagnuolo J, Brand RE, Slivka A, Sherman S, Wisniewski SR, Whitcomb DC, Anderson MA. Chronic pancreatitis pain pattern and severity are independent of abdominal imaging findings. Clin Gastroenterol Hepatol. 2015;13:552–60; quiz e28-9.

Yadav D. Recent advances in the epidemiology of alcoholic pancreatitis. Curr Gastroenterol Rep. 2011;13: 157–65.

Yadav D, Papachristou GI, Whitcomb DC. Alcohol-associated pancreatitis. Gastroenterol Clin N Am. 2007;36:219–38, vii.

Yadav D, Hawes RH, Brand RE, Anderson MA, Money ME, Banks PA, Bishop MD, Baillie J, Sherman S, Disario J, Burton FR, Gardner TB, Amann ST, Gelrud A, Lawrence C, Elinoff B, Greer JB, O'connell M, Barmada MM, Slivka A, Whitcomb DC, North American Pancreatic Study Group. Alcohol consumption, cigarette smoking, and the risk of recurrent acute and chronic pancreatitis. Arch Intern Med. 2009;169:1035–45.

Yadav D, Timmons L, Benson JT, Dierkhising RA, Chari ST. Incidence, prevalence, and survival of chronic pancreatitis: a population-based study. Am J Gastroenterol. 2011;106:2192–9.

Yang AL, Vadhavkar S, Singh G, Omary MB. Epidemiology of alcohol-related liver and pancreatic disease in the United States. Arch Intern Med. 2008;168:649–56.

Yusoff IF, Sahai AV. A prospective, quantitative assessment of the effect of ethanol and other variables on the endosonographic appearance of the pancreas. Clin Gastroenterol Hepatol. 2004;2:405–9.

Autoimmune Pancreatitis

66

Sajan Nagpal

Contents

Abstract

Autoimmune pancreatitis (AIP) is an umbrella term for two forms of autoimmune chronic pancreatitides that share certain features but are distinct with regards to others. Lymphoplasmacytic sclerosing pancreatitis (LPSP), often also called Type 1 AIP, is the pancreatic manifestation of immunoglobulin 4-related disease (IgG4-RD), a multisystemic fibroinflammatory process which typically affects males in the geriatric age group and is characterized by a relapsing course, a brisk

S. Nagpal (✉)
University of Chicago, Chicago, IL, USA
e-mail: snagpal@medicine.bsd.uchicago.edu

© Springer Nature Switzerland AG 2021
C. S. Pitchumoni, T. S. Dharmarajan (eds.), *Geriatric Gastroenterology*,
https://doi.org/10.1007/978-3-030-30192-7_115

response to steroid treatment, and a high likelihood of requirement of long-term immunosuppression or Rituximab in certain cases. The other subtype of AIP, referred to as Type II AIP or idiopathic duct centric pancreatitis (IDCP), usually affects young adults, and males and females equally. While IDCP tends to be very steroid responsive as well, the likelihood of relapse is low. LPSP and IDCP also have very distinct histological characteristics. The precise antigen responsive for AIP remains unknown and is a subject of ongoing investigation. This chapter explores these two subtypes of AIP in further detail, with a focus on the geriatric population.

Keywords

Autoimmune pancreatitis (AIP) · Etiology of autoimmune pancreatitis · Subtypes of AIP · Diagnosis of AIP · Lymphoplasmacytic sclerosing pancreatitis · Idiopathic duct centric pancreatitis · IgG4-related disease · IgG4 antibody

Introduction

In 1961, Sarles et al. reported a case of a patient with pancreatitis associated with increased immunoglobulin levels (Sarles et al. 1961). Soon after two reports of patients with concurrent pancreatitis along with retroperitoneal fibrosis and Reidel thyroiditis, respectively, were published in 1963 (Bartholomew et al. 1963). These patients were diagnosed after surgery done for suspected pancreatic malignancy presenting with obstructive jaundice. However, biopsies were not consistent with cancer and instead showed eosinophilia and inflammatory fibrosis. Comings et al. reported another similar patient with retroperitoneal and mediastinal fibrosis, sclerosing cholangitis, and orbital pseudotumor. They proposed that these apparently distinct clinical manifestations may actually be due to a single underlying inflammatory process (Comings et al. 1967). Numerous cases of patients with suspected primary sclerosing cholangitis (PSC) with coexisting pancreatic involvement or other autoimmune disorders such as Sjogren syndrome, systemic lupus erythematosus (SLE), and inflammatory bowel disease in various combinations were reported then and over the next two to three decades (Axon et al. 1979; Ball et al. 1950; Borum et al. 1993; Epstein et al. 1982; Gurian and Keeffe 1982; Laszik et al. 1988; Lindstrom et al. 1991; Lysy and Goldin 1992; Seyrig et al. 1985; Sjogren et al. 1979; Smith and Loe 1965; Sood et al. 1995; Waldram et al. 1975). Interestingly, a number of these patients had complete gross and histological resolution with steroids. In 1991, Kawaguchi et al. coined the term lymphoplasmacytic sclerosing pancreatitis (LPSP), based on their histological findings from a case they described as "a variant of primary sclerosing cholangitis extensively involving pancreas" (Kawaguchi et al. 1991). Just a little over 2 years later, Chari et al. described that certain subsets of chronic pancreatitis seemed to be associated with autoimmune diseases, proposing that they be classified separately as "chronic autoimmune pancreatitis" (Chari and Singer 1994). Yoshida et al. demonstrated a brisk response to steroids in a case of chronic pancreatitis with elevated gammaglobulin levels and established the concept of autoimmune pancreatitis (AIP) (Yoshida et al. 1995). It was not until 2001 that patients with AIP were found to have elevated IgG4 antibodies – findings which were reported in a landmark study by Hamano (Hamano et al. 2001). Subsequently, Kamisawa et al. concluded that AIP is a multisystemic immunoglobulin G4 (IgG4)-related disease (IgG4-RD) by describing similar histologic findings from anatomically distinct sites, e.g., bile ducts (now known as IgG4-associated cholangitis or IAC), salivary glands (chronic sclerosing sialadenitis), kidney (tubulointerstitial nephritis), and retroperitoneal fibrosis. The histologic changes described by them were characterized by infiltration of tissues with IgG4-positive plasma cells along with storiform fibrosis and obliterative phlebitis (Kamisawa et al. 2003a, b; Kamisawa and Okamoto 2006). This systemic form of AIP characterized by involvement of multiple organs, association with elevated IgG4 levels in most patients, and histological findings of LPSP is now known as Type 1 AIP.

Meanwhile, investigators from Europe described a group of patients with "nonalcoholic duct destructive chronic pancreatitis." These patients appeared to have features very distinct from alcoholic chronic pancreatitis. Some of these features overlapped with LPSP, such as lymphoplasmacytic infiltration and fibrosis, but others were characteristically different such as the presence of a duct-centric neutrophilic infiltrate along with duct destruction. The authors described this form of pancreatitis as a "chronic duct destructive pancreatitis." Only 4 out of the 12 patients initially reported had a clear association with any extrapancreatic autoimmune diseases (Ectors et al. 1997). A later series of patients from Mayo Clinic, Rochester, described 35 patients with idiopathic chronic pancreatitis who had periductal lymphoplasmacytic infiltration on histology. While 22 of these patients appeared to have the features described for LPSP above, the remaining 13 were younger, had a nearly equal male–female distribution of cases, and had a very unique histological feature – the presence of a neutrophilic infiltrate associated with duct destruction and obliteration (Notohara et al. 2003), very similar to the subset described in Europe (Ectors et al. 1997; Zamboni et al. 2004). This form of pancreatitis was termed idiopathic duct-centric pancreatitis (IDCP). The neutrophilic lesion described was termed granulocyte epithelial lesion (GEL) and is now recognized as the histologic hallmark of IDCP (Kloppel et al. 2010). With time, IDCP was even better defined and ultimately became established as a type of autoimmune pancreatitis (Type 2 AIP). The defining characteristics of Type 2 AIP included a younger age at presentation, lack of extrapancreatic involvement, absence of association with elevated IgG4 elevation, and particularly its association with inflammatory bowel disease (Sah et al. 2010). In 2011, the International Consensus Diagnostic Criteria (ICDC) for AIP were established and aimed to have consistency in the description and terminology of AIP. The ICDC criteria also aimed to define formal criteria for the diagnosis of type 1 and type 2 AIP (Shimosegawa et al. 2011).

To avoid confusion between the two subtypes of AIP, we will refer to Type 1 AIP as LPSP and Type 2 AIP as IDCP in subsequent sections of this chapter. The term AIP will be used as an umbrella term to define any characteristics that overlap between LPSP and IDCP. Moreover, since LPSP is a disease that typically presents much more commonly in the geriatric population than IDCP, we will attempt to focus more on LPSP in subsequent sections of this chapter.

Lymphoplasmacytic Sclerosing Pancreatitis (LPSP)

The most common clinical presentation of LPSP is obstructive jaundice. LPSP tends to be relatively painless and if patients are requiring narcotics for pain control, this may suggest an alternative diagnosis such as pancreatic cancer. LPSP usually manifests in the seventh to eighth decade of life and affects males almost three times more commonly as females. Other presentations can include the presence of diffuse or focal pancreatic enlargement, a pancreatic mass on imaging similar to malignancy, pancreatic ductal strictures, and very rarely as acute pancreatitis (Sah et al. 2010; Sandanayake et al. 2009). Involvement of other organs outside the pancreas is often seen with LPSP, with the biliary system the most commonly involved extrapancreatic site, in up to 80% patients with LPSP. The involvement of the biliary system is often referred to as Ig4-associated cholangitis (Ghazale et al. 2008; Sandanayake et al. 2009). LPSP can also affect a number of other organs in the body. LPSP can manifest as an orbital pseudotumor (referred to as IgG4-associated pseudolymphoma), IgG4-related plasmacytic exocrinopathy of the salivary gland, pulmonary interstitial fibrosis and nodules, mediastinal or retroperitoneal fibrosis, and tubulointerstitial nephritis (Hamano et al. 2002; Kaji et al. 2012; Stone et al. 2012; Zhang and Smyrk 2010).

Although involvement of multiple organs is supportive of a diagnosis of LPSP (especially when accompanied by similar histological findings at involved sites), the absence of involvement of more than one organ does not rule out LPSP. In fact, ~50% of patients with LPSP have isolated pancreatic involvement (Sah et al. 2010). Finally, while both LPSP and pancreatic cancer usually present in a geriatric population and can present as a pancreatic mass, the diagnosis of one is not mutually exclusive of the other, i.e., LPSP may coexist with underlying pancreatic adenocarcinoma. Therefore, steroids should only be initiated after malignancy has been reliably ruled out.

Diagnosis

The modified HISORt (*h*istology, *i*maging, *s*erology, *o*ther organ involvement, and *r*esponse to *t*herapy) criteria can be used for the diagnosis of AIP. A schematic of these criteria and how they can be used for diagnosis of AIP is shown below in Fig. 1 (Chari et al. 2006, 2009).

Histology

Characteristic histological features include lymphoplasmacytic infiltration surrounding the duct (Fig. 2a, b), storiform fibrosis (Fig. 2c), obliterative phlebitis (Fig. 2d), and IgG4+ cell infiltration (>10/hpf) (Fig. 2e). IgG4+ cell infiltration is not seen in patients with IDCP. Patients with IDCP may have GEL (granulocyte epithelial lesion) showing neutrophilic infiltration with duct epithelial destruction (Fig. 2f).

Because exclusion of malignancy is of paramount importance, obtaining pancreatic tissue is critical to definitively distinguish AIP from pancreatic cancer. While fine needle aspiration (FNA) usually suffices for the diagnosis of adenocarcinoma, the diagnosis of AIP can be difficult and often requires a larger sample than can be provided by FNA. Endoscopic ultrasound (EUS) guided trucut biopsy has been proposed as a means to overcome this difficulty and allows for a larger tissue sample with preserved architecture to be collected (Levy et al. 2005). The use of trucut biopsy is also endorsed by the ICDC (Shimosegawa et al. 2011). However, when needles for EUS-trucut biopsy sampling are not commercially available, the use of 22G and 19G needles has been reported (Kanno et al. 2016; Iwashita et al. 2012). Besides definitive histology, no other feature is pathognomonic for AIP.

Patients with LPSP have characteristic histologic features comprising of lymphoplasmacytic infiltration, usually in a single file between thick, swirling collagen fibers (storiform fibrosis), along with obliterative phlebitis (Kawaguchi et al. 1991) (Fig. 2). The presence of positive immunostaining for IgG4 in plasma cell infiltrates (>10 cells/high power field) provides support for LPSP (Deshpande et al. 2012). Lymphoid follicles may be seen at the periphery of the interlobular pancreatic ducts and in adipose tissue. Fat necrosis and pseudocyst formation and calcification are not observed (Sah et al. 2010; Zhang et al. 2007; Park et al. 2009; Zamboni et al. 2004). Similar histological changes can be appreciated on biopsies from extrapancreatic sites (Wallace et al. 2014; Plaza et al. 2011; Ohno et al. 2014; Inoue et al. 2012; Baer et al. 2013; Himi et al. 2012; Watanabe et al. 2013; Dahlgren et al. 2010; Zen et al. 2004, 2012; Nishi et al. 2011; Inokuchi et al. 2014).

Imaging

Imaging findings can include a diffuse enlargement of the pancreas with peripheral rim-like hypoenhancement, diffuse enlargement without peripheral hypoenhancement, or a pancreatic mass.

An abnormal abdominal CT or magnetic resonance imaging (MRI) is usually the initial test that first prompts further workup in many cases of AIP as diffuse pancreatic swelling or a pancreatic mass many be seen, which often raises suspicion for pancreatic cancer as well. As AIP (LPSP and IDCP) are overall rare as compared to pancreatic cancer, the diagnosis of AIP should be considered once a thorough workup for underlying pancreatic cancer is negative. If diffuse enlargement of the pancreas (also referred to as sausage-shaped pancreas) with delayed enhancement on CT suggests is seen, this is in fact a Level 1 diagnostic criterion for diagnosis of AIP (Suzuki et al. 2010; Huggett et al. 2014; Shimosegawa et al. 2011; Takahashi et al. 2009). While a low-attenuating rim-like capsule may be seen in only about 30–40% patients with AIP, it is very specific AIP (Takahashi et al. 2009). MRI often shows diffuse hypointensity on T1-weighted images, and slight hyperintensity on T2-weighted images, in

A	B	C

• Histology: Diagnostic histology on resection specimen or pancreatic core biopsy
 	
  • LPSP, OR
  • >10 IgG4 cells/hpf
  +2/3 out of:
    •Periductal lymphoplasmacytic infiltrate
    •Obliterative phlebitis
    •Storiform Fibrosis
 	
  • IDCP, OR
  • GEL with minimal IgG4 positive cells.
	• Imaging: Diffusely enlarged gland with featureless borders and delayed enhancement with/without capsule-like rim AND any one of the following:
	
	  • Elevated IgG4
	
	  • Other organ involvement*
	
	  • Storiform fibrosis with lymphoplasmacytic infiltration (but not meeting all criteria in A)
		• Response to steroids** (resolution/marked improvement in pancreatic/extrapancreatic manifestations in patients meeting criteria for steroid use:
		  • Groups A or B
		  • Patients without typical imaging features¶ and negative cancer workup who have
		    • One highly suggestive feature for AIP#, OR
		    • Two supportive features of AIP&

Fig. 1 Diagnosis of autoimmune pancreatitis. Patients meeting criteria as listed in any of the boxes A, B, and C can be diagnosed as having AIP. **The authors strongly discourage using a trial of steroids in the absence of collateral evidence and definitive histology, solely to distinguish between AIP and PDAC. *Typical histology in affected organ OR typical radiologic features + positive IgG4 immunostain in affected organ OR radiologic evidence of hilar/intrahepatic biliary strictures, renal involvement, retroperitoneal fibrosis, parotid/lacrimal gland enlargement, positive IgG4 immunostaining in other organs (gallbladder, ampulla), and inflammatory bowel disease (seen in 30% patients with IDCP; Only 6% with LPSP so not considered other organ involvement for LPSP). ¶Focally enlarged gland without features highly suggestive of cancer (low density mass, pancreatic ductal dilatation/cutoff, upstream pancreatic atrophy or liver lesions suggestive of, or biopsy proven metastases). #Serum IgG4 >2× upper limit of normal or definitive other organ involvement and supportive features of AIP: less than twofold elevation of IgG4, clinical/radiologic, evidence of other organ involvement (radiologic evidence of hilar/intrahepatic biliary strictures, renal involvement, retroperitoneal fibrosis, parotid/lacrimal gland enlargement, positive IgG4 immunostaining in other organs, inflammatory bowel disease, and compatible histology) as listed in box B. *LPSP* lymphoplasmacytic sclerosing pancreatitis, *IDCP* idiopathic duct centric pancreatitis, *GEL* granulocyte epithelial lesion, *AIP* autoimmune pancreatitis, *hpf* high-power field (Adapted with permission from Nagpal et al. 2018)

addition to heterogeneously diminished enhancement during the early phase and delayed enhancement during the late phase of contrast enhancement (Sahani et al. 2004; Yang et al. 2006). Pancreatic imaging findings in AIP are shown in Fig. 3. Positron emission tomography (PET) scans are not required for diagnosis. If a PET scan ends up getting performed due to suspected underlying pancreatic cancer, it may show diffuse or focal fluorine-18 fluorodeoxyglucose (FDG) uptake in the inflamed areas of the pancreas, which resolves with steroid treatment. Therefore, a single PET scan may not allow for a distinction to be made between pancreatic cancer and AIP (Nakamoto et al. 2000).

MRCP and endoscopic retrograde cholangiopancreatography (ERCP) may reveal diffuse narrowing of the pancreatic duct with long (greater than one-third of the pancreatic duct) or multifocal strictures, with lack of upstream dilatation and side branches originating from a strictured segment (Sugumar et al. 2011). However, it should be noted that ERCP alone is not a reliable modality to diagnose AIP. ERCP is also not reliably able to distinguish IAC, which is the most common extrapancreatic manifestation of AIP, from primary sclerosing cholangitis or cholangiocarcinoma (Kalaitzakis et al. 2011).

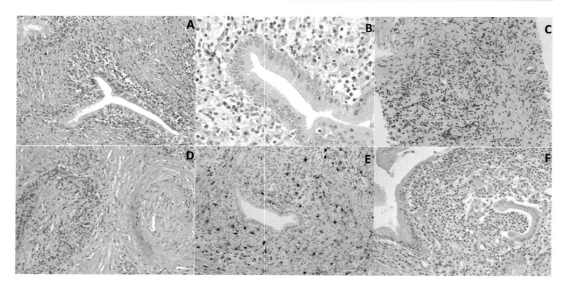

Fig. 2 Characteristic features of LPSP and IDCP. Histological features of LPSP (**a–e**) and IDCP (**f**). (**a**) Low power and (**b**) high power view of lymphoplasmacytic infiltration surrounding the duct, (**c**) storiform fibrosis, (**d**) obliterative phlebitis, (**e**) IgG4 infiltration (>10/hpf) and (**f**) GEL (granulocyte epithelial lesion) showing neutrophilic infiltration with duct epithelial destruction (Adapted with permission from Nagpal et al. 2018)

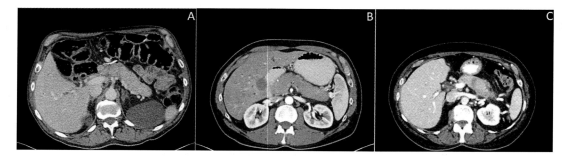

Fig. 3 Pancreatic imaging findings of AIP. (**a**) Diffuse enlargement of the pancreas with peripheral rim-like hypoenhancement; (**b**) diffuse enlargement without peripheral hypoenhancement; and (**c**) mass-like presentation (Adapted with permission from Nagpal et al. 2018)

Serology

The serologic criteria required for diagnosis involve measurement of IgG4 levels. Elevated levels of IgG4 (>2× the upper limit of normal) are a "Level 1" criterion for the diagnosis of LPSP according to our diagnostic algorithm and are seen in about two-third of patients with LPSP (Chari et al. 2006; Shimosegawa et al. 2011). Using a higher threshold of IgG4 levels (i.e., >2× the normal IgG4) leads to a lower sensitivity in differentiating LPSP from pancreatic cancer but increases the specificity to 99% (Ghazale et al. 2007). A diagnosis of LPSP can be made even when the levels of IgG4 are elevated less than twofold. As demonstrated in Fig. 1, this requires the presence of other features as well (such as other certain imaging features, other organ involvement, histologic features that meet some but not all criteria for diagnosis, etc.). Elevation in serum IgG4 levels is not specific to LPSP and up to 10% of patients with pancreatic cancer may have elevated serum IgG4 values, out of which 1% may even have elevation >2× the upper limit of normal (Ghazale et al. 2007).

Other Organ Involvement

Other organs are involved in individuals with LPSP. Extrapancreatic involvement is most commonly seen in the biliary system (IAC), but can also be seen in other areas of the body such as eyes (orbital pseudolymphoma), salivary glands, lungs and mediastinum (interstitial lung disease and mediastinal fibrosis), kidneys and retroperitoneum, and even prostate gland. Examples of extrapancreatic involvement are shown in Fig. 4.

Response to Therapy

Even though the risk of relapse in patients with LPSP is high, whenever a recurrence occurs, each episode is highly responsive to treatment (e.g., with steroids). In fact, response to treatment for the initial and subsequent episodes is one of the diagnostic criteria within the HiSORt criteria for diagnosis of AIP. An example of response to treatment is shown in Fig. 5.

Other Criteria for Diagnosis

Various criteria for diagnosis of AIP have been proposed from societies and institutions around the world. These include the Japanese Pancreatic Society, HISORt, Korean, Asian, Mannheim, and Italian criteria (Chari et al. 2009; Kamisawa et al. 2008; Kwon et al. 2007; Okazaki et al. 2006; Pearson et al. 2003; Schneider and Lohr 2009; Shimosegawa et al. 2011). After a review of these criteria, the ICDC (International Consensus Diagnostic Criteria) were developed. However, in their current form, ICDC suggests the use of endoscopic retrograde pancreatography (ERP) for ductal imaging, which is not routinely performed to diagnose AIP in the West (Shimosegawa et al. 2011), and may also be associated with a higher risk of complications than noninvasive imaging. As noninvasive imaging modalities such as computed tomography (CT) and magnetic resonance cholangiopancreatography (MRCP) are more commonly used in the West for diagnosing AIP, we suggest using those for pancreatic ductal imaging as reasonable alternatives to ERP when using the ICDC criteria in the Western setting.

Other Laboratory Findings

Patients with LPSP most commonly present with a cholestatic pattern of liver enzyme elevation, i.e., elevated alkaline phosphatase and/or bilirubin levels. Other antibodies that have been reported to be associated with autoimmune pancreatitis but are not a part of the diagnostic criteria include antibodies to carbonic anhydrase, Lactoferrin, antimitochondrial antibodies (AMA), antismooth muscle antibodies (ASMA), and antithyroglobulin (Kino-Ohsaki et al. 1996; Kim et al. 2004; Yoshida et al. 1995; Deshpande et al. 2005; Uchida et al. 2000). Antibodies against a peptide homologous to an amino acid sequence of plasminogen-binding protein (PBP) of Helicobacter pylori was reported to be positive in patients with AIP but was also found to be positive in 5% patients with pancreatic cancer (Frulloni et al. 2009). A more recent study identified antibodies to laminin 511-E8, a truncated laminin 511, an extracellular matrix protein in patients with AIP (Shiokawa et al. 2018).

Treatment and Long-Term Outcomes

While steroids have been traditionally considered the mainstay of initial treatment, there is also emerging evidence on the use of other immunomodulators and Rituximab. Most patients with LPSP have remarkable initial improvement with the use of Prednisone, both biochemically (based on liver biochemistries) as well as on imaging. A high dose of prednisone at 40 mg/day for 4 weeks is recommended, although some have suggested that a lower dose (20 mg/day) may be used (Buijs et al. 2014). After 4 weeks, response can be assessed with clinical evaluation, radiology, and serology (IgG4 levels) (Ghazale et al. 2008). If there is clinical, serologic, and radiologic improvement at 4 weeks, the dose of prednisone can start to be tapered by 5 mg/week. A lower dose (30 mg/day) can be the initial dose for

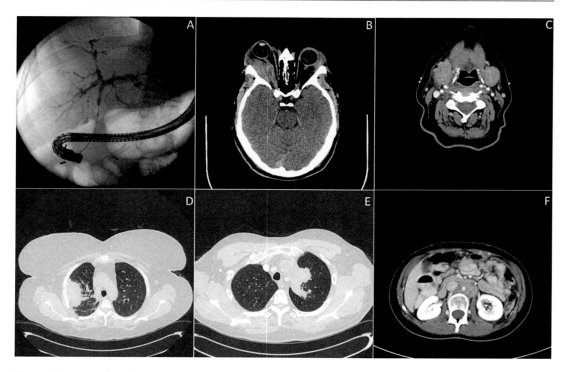

Fig. 4 Other organ involvement in LPSP. (**a**) Cholangiogram revealing extensive biliary stricturing from IgG4-associated cholangitis; (**b**) orbital pseudolymphoma; (**c**) submandibular gland involvement; (**d**) interstitial lung disease; (**e**) mediastinal involvement, and (**f**) retroperitoneal involvement (Adapted with permission from Nagpal et al. 2018)

patients with diabetes. A thorough evaluation for underlying malignancy is recommended in all cases. Only in a very select group of patients a therapeutic trial of steroids may be undertaken for 2 weeks with reassessment at the end of the trial period after ensuring there is no malignancy (Moon et al. 2008). Recent data suggests that Rituximab can also be used for as an induction agent for remission as a first-line agent if steroids are absolutely contraindicated (Hart et al. 2013b). Rituximab may also be considered as first-line treatment for patients at a high risk of relapse, such as those with proximal biliary involvement, younger age, and high alkaline phosphatase levels at initial presentation (Majumder et al. 2018). There is no data from randomized clinical trials for patients with AIP assessing or comparing the efficacy of steroids or other therapies for the induction of remission in these patients.

There is a high likelihood of relapses in patients with LPSP, despite the brisk response to steroids seen upon initial treatment. Relapses can be seen in up to 60% of patients and can happen even during the steroid taper and in many cases within the first 3 years of treatment (Hart et al. 2013a; Zamboni et al. 2004; Kamisawa et al. 2009; Huggett et al. 2014; Ryu et al. 2008). In a previous study from Mayo Clinic, Rochester, relapse rates of 25%, 44%, and 59% were seen at 1, 2, and 3 years, respectively (Sah et al. 2010). Relapses are managed with another course of steroids or Rituximab. As the likelihood of relapsing disease is very high in patients with LPSP, it is advised that consideration be given to an immunosuppressive regimen for maintenance early in the course of the treatment. In fact, immunosuppression can be considered at the first episode of LPSP as the likelihood of relapse is high. Recent studies have identified patients at a high risk of relapsing disease (those with intrahepatic and suprapancreatic portion of the common bile duct, those with diffuse pancreatic enlargement, younger age, higher IgG4-responder index

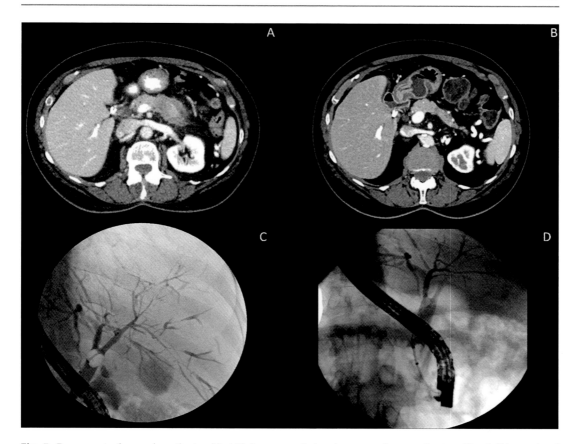

Fig. 5 Response to therapy in patients with AIP. Images (a) and (b) show a computed tomography (CT) scan of a patient with LPSP and images (c) and (d) show the cholangiogram of a patient with IgG4-associated cholangitis (IAC) demonstrating response to treatment (Adapted with permission from Nagpal et al. 2018)

(IgG4-RI) score after induction therapy, and elevated serum alkaline phosphatase levels either at baseline or after RTX induction) (Majumder et al. 2018). These patients may especially be considered for immunosuppression at the first episode of LPSP. While in the West steroids are not given for prolonged periods and alternative immunosuppressive agents such as azathioprine and mycophenolate are preferred, studies from Japan suggest the use of a prolonged taper followed by a low dose of steroids (2.5–10 mg/day) for 1–3 years and sometimes even indefinitely (Kamisawa et al. 2010). We recommend azathioprine (2 mg/kg daily) or mycophenolate mofetil (750 mg twice daily) also appear to be effective in maintaining remission and allow for a steroid-free regimen to be used for these patients (REF). Alternatively, Rituximab is an agent that can be used to maintain remission (Hart et al. 2013b).

Idiopathic Duct-Centric Pancreatitis (IDCP)

Clinical Presentation

Demographic characteristics of the typical patient with IDCP are different from those with LPSP. IDCP is not commonly seen among the geriatric population and mostly afflicts a younger age group, with a mean age at presentation usually between 40 and 50 years. Additionally, IDCP has no predilection towards a particular sex and affects males and females equally. Patients with IDCP tend to present mostly with recurrent acute pancreatitis (up to 50% of these patients present with that history). It should be mentioned here that IgG4 is very commonly checked in patients with acute pancreatitis in hospitals around the world, but since IgG4 levels can be falsely elevated during an episode of acute pancreatitis and are not good markers of IDCP (which can present with acute pancreatitis), checking IgG4 levels for acute pancreatitis is not advised. Other presentations of IDCP may include painless obstructive jaundice, pancreatic ductal stricture, or a focal pancreatic mass. As opposed to LPSP, IDCP is a disease of the pancreas alone and extrapancreatic involvement is characteristically absent. However, it can be associated with independent autoimmune processes elsewhere in the body, most characteristically concurrent IBD (predominantly ulcerative colitis) as compared to LPSP (Sah et al. 2010). In fact, a diagnosis of IBD is a supportive diagnostic criterion in a patient suspected to have IDCP (Shimosegawa et al. 2011).

Laboratory Findings

There is no specific laboratory-based test for IDCP, therefore its diagnosis can be challenging. Therefore, histopathology remains the cornerstone of diagnosis. Other laboratory tests may reveal a cholestatic pattern of liver enzyme elevation as seen in LPSP as well. As opposed to LPSP, only about 25% of patients with IDCP have elevated IgG4 levels which is why IgG4 levels are not good markers for IDCP (Kamisawa et al. 2011).

Histopathology

On histology, intense lymphoplasmacytic infiltration and inflammation are seen in patients with IDCP. These are more marked in the periductal regions as compared to the acini (Kloppel et al. 2010; Notohara et al. 2003; Zamboni et al. 2004; Zhang and Smyrk 2010). The ductal epithelium may be infiltrated by neutrophils. This lesion has been referred to as a GEL (granulocyte epithelial lesion), and is diagnostic of IDCP (Notohara et al. 2003; Zamboni et al. 2004) (Fig. 2). Staining for IgG4+ cells may reveal scattered positive cells but in much lower numbers as typically seen in LPSP.

Similar to LPSP, an EUS-guided trucut biopsy is important as it can provide a better yield of tissue as compared to fine needle aspiration (Levy et al. 2011).

Imaging and Endoscopy

Endoscopic findings from ERCP and imaging findings on CT and MRCP can be similar to IDCP in patients with IDCP.

Treatment

IDCP is treated similar to a first episode of LPSP using steroids. Any symptoms and inflammation associated with IDCP respond rapidly to corticosteroid therapy. We recommend starting prednisone at an initial dose of 40 mg/day for 4 weeks followed by reassessment using clinical evaluation, radiology, and measurement of liver biochemistries. Once response is documented, the dose of steroids can begin to be tapered at 5 mg/week for the next 8 weeks. The likelihood of relapses is much lower in IDCP than LPSP (<10%). Therefore, long-term immunomodulator therapy (e.g., azathioprine) is not recommended as risks of long-term immunosuppression outweigh any benefits. In rare cases that do end up having a relapse, the subsequent episode can be treated similarly.

Complications of AIP

A delay in diagnosis and treatment can have significant consequences for patients with AIP and lead to preventable complications. Pancreatic atrophy can be seen in up to 25% of patients and this may manifest as impairment of glucose tolerance or even frank diabetes mellitus or exocrine pancreatic insufficiency. If untreated, patients with extrapancreatic involvement (e.g., IAC) may have a rapid progression to secondary biliary cirrhosis. In a previous study from Mayo Clinic on patients with IAC, 4 out 53 patients developed portal hypertension due to rapid progression to

Table 1 Features of Lymphoplasmacytic sclerosing pancreatitis (LPSP; Type 1 AIP) and Idiopathic duct-centric pancreatitis (IDCP; Type 2 AIP). *LPSP* lymphoplasmacytic sclerosing pancreatitis, *IDCP* idiopathic duct centric pancreatitis, *hpf* high-power field

Feature	LPSP	IDCP
Clinical		
Age at presentation/diagnosis	Decade 7	Decade 5
Sex (M:F ratio)	3:1	1:1
> 2× elevation of IgG4 levels	~2/3rd	~1/4th
Association with inflammatory bowel disease	Weak	Strong (10–20%)
Imaging	Similar imaging features in both	
Histology		
Lymphoplasmacytic infiltration	Yes	Yes
Periductal inflammation	Yes	Yes
Storiform fibrosis	Prominent	Less prominent
Obliterative phlebitis	Characteristic	Rare
Granulocyte epithelial lesion (GEL)	Absent	Characteristic
IgG4 staining	Abundant; >10/hpf	Rare; <10/hpf
Treatment		
Response to steroids	~100%	~100%
Relapse	Up to 60%	<10%

secondary biliary cirrhosis. Three out of these were treatment-naive and the fourth patient was a non-responder to treatment (Ghazale et al. 2008). The relationship of AIP to the development of pancreatic malignancy has remained elusive, but overall it does not appear to be the case (Majumder et al. 2017). On the other hand, AIP has been suggested to be a paraneoplastic phenomenon by some, as a high incidence of extrapancreatic cancers was reported within the first year of diagnosis of AIP (Shiokawa et al. 2013). Other reports have also suggested this association but more data is required to definitively establish this phenomenon (Schneider et al. 2017) (Table 1).

Key Points

- The term AIP comprises two distinct forms of steroid response chronic pancreatitis, LPSP and IDCP.
- LPSP is a disease of the geriatric population and predominantly affects males more than females.
- Both LPSP and IDCP are clinically and histopathologically distinct but are characterized by a brisk initial response to steroids.
- LPSP has a relapsing-remitting course and often requires the use of maintenance immunomodulation.
- On the other hand, IDCP tends not to relapse after initial treatment.
- Subsequent episodes of IDCP are also very responsive to steroids.
- IgG4 levels can fluctuate with steroid use and may even go up after initiation of steroids, and should not be used as the sole indicator of response to treatment.
- As pancreatic cancer is much more common than AIP, malignancy should be ruled out before considering an empiric trial of steroids with short-term imaging in a select group of patients.
- Timely treatment of AIP can prevent complications such as pancreatic atrophy which can further lead to exocrine and endocrine pancreatic insufficiency.
- In patients with extrapancreatic involvement (IAC), delayed treatment can lead to rapid development of secondary biliary cirrhosis.

References

Axon AT, Ashton MG, Lintott DJ. Chronic pancreatitis and inflammatory bowel disease. Clin Radiol. 1979;30: 179–82.

Baer AN, Gourin CG, Westra WH, Cox DP, Greenspan JS, Daniels TE. Rare diagnosis of IgG4-related systemic disease by lip biopsy in an international Sjogren syndrome registry. Oral Surg Oral Med Oral Pathol Oral Radiol. 2013;115:e34–9.

Ball WP, Baggenstoss AH, Bargen JA. Pancreatic lesions associated with chronic ulcerative colitis. Arch Pathol. 1950;50:347–58.

Bartholomew LG, Cain JC, Woolner LB, Utz DC, Ferris DO. Sclerosing cholangitis: its possible association with Riedel's struma and fibrous retroperitonitis. Report of two cases. N Engl J Med. 1963;269:8–12.

Borum M, Steinberg W, Steer M, Freedman S, White P. Chronic pancreatitis: a complication of systemic lupus erythematosus. Gastroenterology. 1993;104:613–5.

Buijs J, van Heerde MJ, Rauws EA, de Buy Wenniger LJ, Hansen BE, Biermann K, Verheij J, Vleggaar FP, Brink MA, Beuers UH, Kuipers EJ, Bruno MJ, van Buuren HR. Comparable efficacy of low- versus high-dose induction corticosteroid treatment in autoimmune pancreatitis. Pancreas. 2014;43:261–7.

Chari ST, Singer MV. The problem of classification and staging of chronic pancreatitis. Proposals based on current knowledge of its natural history. Scand J Gastroenterol. 1994;29:949–60.

Chari ST, Smyrk TC, Levy MJ, Topazian MD, Takahashi N, Zhang L, Clain JE, Pearson RK, Petersen BT, Vege SS, Farnell MB. Diagnosis of autoimmune pancreatitis: the Mayo Clinic experience. Clin Gastroenterol Hepatol. 2006;4:1010–6; quiz 934.

Chari ST, Takahashi N, Levy MJ, Smyrk TC, Clain JE, Pearson RK, Petersen BT, Topazian MA, Vege SS. A diagnostic strategy to distinguish autoimmune pancreatitis from pancreatic cancer. Clin Gastroenterol Hepatol. 2009;7:1097–103.

Comings DE, Skubi KB, van Eyes J, Motulsky AG. Familial multifocal fibrosclerosis. Findings suggesting that retroperitoneal fibrosis, mediastinal fibrosis, sclerosing cholangitis, Riedel's thyroiditis, and pseudotumor of the orbit may be different manifestations of a single disease. Ann Intern Med. 1967;66:884–92.

Dahlgren M, Khosroshahi A, Nielsen GP, Deshpande V, Stone JH. Riedel's thyroiditis and multifocal fibrosclerosis are part of the IgG4-related systemic disease spectrum. Arthritis Care Res. 2010;62:1312–8.

Deshpande V, Mino-Kenudson M, Brugge W, Lauwers GY. Autoimmune pancreatitis: more than just a pancreatic disease? A contemporary review of its pathology. Arch Pathol Lab Med. 2005;129:1148–54.

Deshpande V, Zen Y, Chan JK, Yi EE, Sato Y, Yoshino T, Kloppel G, Heathcote JG, Khosroshahi A, Ferry JA, Aalberse RC, Bloch DB, Brugge WR, Bateman AC, Carruthers MN, Chari ST, Cheuk W, Cornell LD, Fernandez-Del Castillo C, Forcione DG, Hamilos DL, Kamisawa T, Kasashima S, Kawa S, Kawano M, Lauwers GY, Masaki Y, Nakanuma Y, Notohara K, Okazaki K, Ryu JK, Saeki T, Sahani DV, Smyrk TC, Stone JR, Takahira M, Webster GJ, Yamamoto M, Zamboni G, Umehara H, Stone JH. Consensus statement on the pathology of IgG4-related disease. Mod Pathol. 2012;25:1181–92.

Ectors N, Maillet B, Aerts R, Geboes K, Donner A, Borchard F, Lankisch P, Stolte M, Luttges J, Kremer B, Kloppel G. Non-alcoholic duct destructive chronic pancreatitis. Gut. 1997;41:263–8.

Epstein O, Chapman RW, Lake-Bakaar G, Foo AY, Rosalki SB, Sherlock S. The pancreas in primary biliary cirrhosis and primary sclerosing cholangitis. Gastroenterology. 1982;83:1177–82.

Frulloni L, Lunardi C, Simone R, Dolcino M, Scattolini C, Falconi M, Benini L, Vantini I, Corrocher R, Puccetti A. Identification of a novel antibody associated with autoimmune pancreatitis. N Engl J Med. 2009;361:2135–42.

Ghazale A, Chari ST, Smyrk TC, Levy MJ, Topazian MD, Takahashi N, Clain JE, Pearson RK, Pelaez-Luna M, Petersen BT, Vege SS, Farnell MB. Value of serum IgG4 in the diagnosis of autoimmune pancreatitis and in distinguishing it from pancreatic cancer. Am J Gastroenterol. 2007;102:1646–53.

Ghazale A, Chari ST, Zhang L, Smyrk TC, Takahashi N, Levy MJ, Topazian MD, Clain JE, Pearson RK, Petersen BT, Vege SS, Lindor K, Farnell MB. Immunoglobulin G4-associated cholangitis: clinical profile and response to therapy. Gastroenterology. 2008;134:706–15.

Gurian LE, Keeffe EB. Pancreatic insufficiency associated with ulcerative colitis and pericholangitis. Gastroenterology. 1982;82:581–5.

Hamano H, Kawa S, Horiuchi A, Unno H, Furuya N, Akamatsu T, Fukushima M, Nikaido T, Nakayama K, Usuda N, Kiyosawa K. High serum IgG4 concentrations in patients with sclerosing pancreatitis. N Engl J Med. 2001;344:732–8.

Hamano H, Kawa S, Ochi Y, Unno H, Shiba N, Wajiki M, Nakazawa K, Shimojo H, Kiyosawa K. Hydronephrosis associated with retroperitoneal fibrosis and sclerosing pancreatitis. Lancet. 2002;359:1403–4.

Hart PA, Kamisawa T, Brugge WR, Chung JB, Culver EL, Czako L, Frulloni L, Go VL, Gress TM, Kim MH, Kawa S, Lee KT, Lerch MM, Liao WC, Lohr M, Okazaki K, Ryu JK, Schleinitz N, Shimizu K, Shimosegawa T, Soetikno R, Webster G, Yadav D, Zen Y, Chari ST. Long-term outcomes of autoimmune pancreatitis: a multicentre, international analysis. Gut. 2013a;62:1771–6.

Hart PA, Topazian MD, Witzig TE, Clain JE, Gleeson FC, Klebig RR, Levy MJ, Pearson RK, Petersen BT, Smyrk TC, Sugumar A, Takahashi N, Vege SS, Chari ST. Treatment of relapsing autoimmune pancreatitis with immunomodulators and rituximab: the Mayo Clinic experience. Gut. 2013b;62:1607–15.

Himi T, Takano K, Yamamoto M, Naishiro Y, Takahashi H. A novel concept of Mikulicz's disease as IgG4-related disease. Auris Nasus Larynx. 2012;39:9–17.

Huggett MT, Culver EL, Kumar M, Hurst JM, Rodriguez-Justo M, Chapman MH, Johnson GJ, Pereira SP, Chapman RW, Webster GJM, Barnes E. Type 1 autoimmune pancreatitis and IgG4-related sclerosing cholangitis is associated with extrapancreatic organ failure, malignancy, and mortality in a prospective UK cohort. Am J Gastroenterol. 2014;109:1675–83.

Inokuchi G, Hayakawa M, Kishimoto T, Makino Y, Iwase H. A suspected case of coronary periarteritis due to IgG4-related disease as a cause of ischemic heart disease. Forensic Sci Med Pathol. 2014;10:103–8.

Inoue D, Zen Y, Sato Y, Abo H, Demachi H, Uchiyama A, Gabata T, Matsui O. IgG4-related perineural disease. Int J Rheumatol. 2012;2012:401890.

Iwashita T, Yasuda I, Doi S, Ando N, Nakashima M, Adachi S, Hirose Y, Mukai T, Iwata K, Tomita E, Itoi T, Moriwaki H. Use of samples from endoscopic ultrasound-guided 19-gauge fine-needle aspiration in diagnosis of autoimmune pancreatitis. Clin Gastroenterol Hepatol. 2012;10:316–22.

Kaji R, Takedatsu H, Okabe Y, Ishida Y, Sugiyama G, Yonemoto K, Mitsuyama K, Tsuruta O, Sata M. Serum immunoglobulin G4 associated with number and distribution of extrapancreatic lesions in type 1 autoimmune pancreatitis patients. J Gastroenterol Hepatol. 2012;27:268–72.

Kalaitzakis E, Levy M, Kamisawa T, Johnson GJ, Baron TH, Topazian MD, Takahashi N, Kanno A, Okazaki K, Egawa N, Uchida K, Sheikh K, Amin Z, Shimosegawa T, Sandanayake NS, Church NI, Chapman MH, Pereira SP, Chari S, Webster GJ. Endoscopic retrograde cholangiography does not reliably distinguish IgG4-associated cholangitis from primary sclerosing cholangitis or cholangiocarcinoma. Clin Gastroenterol Hepatol. 2011;9:800–803.e2.

Kamisawa T, Okamoto A. Autoimmune pancreatitis: proposal of IgG4-related sclerosing disease. J Gastroenterol. 2006;41:613–25.

Kamisawa T, Egawa N, Nakajima H. Autoimmune pancreatitis is a systemic autoimmune disease. Am J Gastroenterol. 2003a;98:2811–2.

Kamisawa T, Funata N, Hayashi Y, Eishi Y, Koike M, Tsuruta K, Okamoto A, Egawa N, Nakajima H. A new clinicopathological entity of IgG4-related autoimmune disease. J Gastroenterol. 2003b;38:982–4.

Kamisawa T, Okazaki K, Kawa S. Diagnostic criteria for autoimmune pancreatitis in Japan. World J Gastroenterol. 2008;14:4992–4.

Kamisawa T, Shimosegawa T, Okazaki K, Nishino T, Watanabe H, Kanno A, Okumura F, Nishikawa T, Kobayashi K, Ichiya T, Takatori H, Yamakita K, Kubota K, Hamano H, Okamura K, Hirano K, Ito T, Ko SB, Omata M. Standard steroid treatment for autoimmune pancreatitis. Gut. 2009;58:1504–7.

Kamisawa T, Okazaki K, Kawa S, Shimosegawa T, Tanaka M. Japanese consensus guidelines for management of autoimmune pancreatitis: III. Treatment and prognosis of AIP. J Gastroenterol. 2010;45:471–7.

Kamisawa T, Chari ST, Giday SA, Kim MH, Chung JB, Lee KT, Werner J, Bergmann F, Lerch MM, Mayerle J, Pickartz T, Lohr M, Schneider A, Frulloni L, Webster GJ, Reddy DN, Liao WC, Wang HP, Okazaki K, Shimosegawa T, Kloeppel G, Go VL. Clinical profile of autoimmune pancreatitis and its histological subtypes: an international multicenter survey. Pancreas. 2011;40:809–14.

Kanno A, Masamune A, Fujishima F, Iwashita T, Kodama Y, Katanuma A, Ohara H, Kitano M, Inoue H, Itoi T, Mizuno N, Miyakawa H, Mikata R, Irisawa A, Sato S, Notohara K, Shimosegawa T. Diagnosis of autoimmune pancreatitis by EUS-guided FNA using a 22-gauge needle: a prospective multicenter study. Gastrointest Endosc. 2016;84:797–804.e1.

Kawaguchi K, Koike M, Tsuruta K, Okamoto A, Tabata I, Fujita N. Lymphoplasmacytic sclerosing pancreatitis with cholangitis: a variant of primary sclerosing cholangitis extensively involving pancreas. Hum Pathol. 1991;22:387–95.

Kim KP, Kim MH, Song MH, Lee SS, Seo DW, Lee SK. Autoimmune chronic pancreatitis. Am J Gastroenterol. 2004;99:1605–16.

Kino-Ohsaki J, Nishimori I, Morita M, Okazaki K, Yamamoto Y, Onishi S, Hollingsworth MA. Serum antibodies to carbonic anhydrase I and II in patients with idiopathic chronic pancreatitis and Sjogren's syndrome. Gastroenterology. 1996;110:1579–86.

Kloppel G, Detlefsen S, Chari ST, Longnecker DS, Zamboni G. Autoimmune pancreatitis: the clinicopathological characteristics of the subtype with granulocytic epithelial lesions. J Gastroenterol. 2010;45:787–93.

Kwon S, Kim MH, Choi EK. The diagnostic criteria for autoimmune chronic pancreatitis: it is time to make a consensus. Pancreas. 2007;34:279–86.

Laszik GZ, Pap A, Farkas G. A case of primary sclerosing cholangitis mimicking chronic pancreatitis. Int J Pancreatol. 1988;3:503–8.

Levy MJ, Reddy RP, Wiersema MJ, Smyrk TC, Clain JE, Harewood GC, Pearson RK, Rajan E, Topazian MD, Yusuf TE, Chari ST, Petersen BT. EUS-guided trucut biopsy in establishing autoimmune pancreatitis as the cause of obstructive jaundice. Gastrointest Endosc. 2005;61:467–72.

Levy MJ, Smyrk TC, Takahashi N, Zhang L, Chari ST. Idiopathic duct-centric pancreatitis: disease description and endoscopic ultrasonography-guided trucut biopsy diagnosis. Pancreatology. 2011;11:76–80.

Lindstrom E, Lindstrom F, von Schenck H, Ihse I. Pancreatic ductal morphology and function in primary Sjogren's syndrome. Int J Pancreatol. 1991;8:141–9.

Lysy J, Goldin E. Pancreatitis in ulcerative colitis. J Clin Gastroenterol. 1992;15:336–9.

Majumder S, Takahashi N, Chari ST. Autoimmune pancreatitis. Dig Dis Sci. 2017;62:1762–9.

Majumder S, Mohapatra S, Lennon RJ, Piovezani Ramos G, Postier N, Gleeson F, Levy MJ, Pearson RK, Petersen BT, Vege SS, Chari ST, Topazian M, Witzig TE. Rituximab maintenance therapy reduces rate of relapse of pancreaticobiliary immunoglobulin G4-related disease. Clin Gastroenterol Hepatol. 2018;16 (12):1947–53.

Moon SH, Kim MH, Park DH, Hwang CY, Park SJ, Lee SS, Seo DW, Lee SK. Is a 2-week steroid trial after initial negative investigation for malignancy useful in differentiating autoimmune pancreatitis from pancreatic cancer? A prospective outcome study. Gut. 2008;57:1704–12.

Nagpal SJ, Sharma A, Chari ST. Autoimmune pancreatitis. Am J Gastroenterol. 2018;113(9):1301. PMID: 29910463. https://doi.org/10.1038/s41395-018-0146-0. https://pubmed.ncbi.nlm.nih.gov/29910463/.

Nakamoto Y, Saga T, Ishimori T, Higashi T, Mamede M, Okazaki K, Imamura M, Sakahara H, Konishi J. FDG-

PET of autoimmune-related pancreatitis: preliminary results. Eur J Nucl Med. 2000;27:1835–8.

Nishi S, Imai N, Yoshida K, Ito Y, Saeki T. Clinicopathological findings of immunoglobulin G4-related kidney disease. Clin Exp Nephrol. 2011;15:810–9.

Notohara K, Burgart LJ, Yadav D, Chari S, Smyrk TC. Idiopathic chronic pancreatitis with periductal lymphoplasmacytic infiltration: clinicopathologic features of 35 cases. Am J Surg Pathol. 2003;27:1119–27.

Ohno K, Sato Y, Ohshima K, Takata K, Ando M, Abd Al-Kader L, Iwaki N, Takeuchi M, Orita Y, Yoshino T. IgG4-related disease involving the sclera. Mod Rheumatol. 2014;24:195–8.

Okazaki K, Kawa S, Kamisawa T, Naruse S, Tanaka S, Nishimori I, OharA H, Ito T, Kiriyama S, Inui K, Shimosegawa T, Koizumi M, SUDA K, Shiratori K, Yamaguchi K, Yamaguchi T, Sugiyama M, Otsuki M. Clinical diagnostic criteria of autoimmune pancreatitis: revised proposal. J Gastroenterol. 2006;41:626–31.

Park DH, Kim MH, Chari ST. Recent advances in autoimmune pancreatitis. Gut. 2009;58:1680–9.

Pearson RK, Longnecker DS, Chari ST, Smyrk TC, Okazaki K, Frulloni L, Cavallini G. Controversies in clinical pancreatology: autoimmune pancreatitis: does it exist? Pancreas. 2003;27:1–13.

Plaza JA, Garrity JA, Dogan A, Ananthamurthy A, Witzig TE, Salomao DR. Orbital inflammation with IgG4-positive plasma cells: manifestation of IgG4 systemic disease. Arch Ophthalmol. 2011;129:421–8.

Ryu JK, Chung JB, Park SW, Lee JK, Lee KT, Lee WJ, Moon JH, Cho KB, Kang DW, Hwang JH, Yoo KS, Yoo BM, Lee DH, Kim HK, Moon YS, Lee J, Lee HS, Choi HS, Lee SK, Kim YT, Kim CD, Kim SJ, Hahm JS, Yoon YB. Review of 67 patients with autoimmune pancreatitis in Korea: a multicenter nationwide study. Pancreas. 2008;37:377–85.

Sah RP, Chari ST, Pannala R, Sugumar A, Clain JE, Levy MJ, Pearson RK, Smyrk TC, Petersen BT, Topazian MD, Takahashi N, Farnell MB, Vege SS. Differences in clinical profile and relapse rate of type 1 versus type 2 autoimmune pancreatitis. Gastroenterology. 2010;139:140–8; quiz e12–3.

Sahani DV, Kalva SP, Farrell J, Maher MM, Saini S, Mueller PR, Lauwers GY, Fernandez CD, Warshaw AL, Simeone JF. Autoimmune pancreatitis: imaging features. Radiology. 2004;233:345–52.

Sandanayake NS, Church NI, Chapman MH, Johnson GJ, Dhar DK, Amin Z, Deheragoda MG, Novelli M, Winstanley A, Rodriguez-Justo M, Hatfield AR, Pereira SP, Webster GJ. Presentation and management of post-treatment relapse in autoimmune pancreatitis/immunoglobulin G4-associated cholangitis. Clin Gastroenterol Hepatol. 2009;7:1089–96.

Sarles H, Sarles JC, Muratore R, Guien C. Chronic inflammatory sclerosis of the pancreas – an autonomous pancreatic disease? Am J Dig Dis. 1961;6:688–98.

Schneider A, Lohr JM. Autoimmune pancreatitis. Internist. 2009;50:318–30.

Schneider A, Hirth M, Munch M, Weiss C, Lohr JM, Ebert MP, Pfutzer RH. Risk of cancer in patients with autoimmune pancreatitis: a single-center experience from Germany. Digestion. 2017;95:172–80.

Seyrig JA, Jian R, Modigliani R, Golfain D, Florent C, Messing B, Bitoun A. Idiopathic pancreatitis associated with inflammatory bowel disease. Dig Dis Sci. 1985;30:1121–6.

Shimosegawa T, Chari ST, Frulloni L, Kamisawa T, Kawa S, Mino-Kenudson M, Kim MH, Kloppel G, Lerch MM, Lohr M, Notohara K, Okazaki K, Schneider A, Zhang L. International consensus diagnostic criteria for autoimmune pancreatitis: guidelines of the International Association of Pancreatology. Pancreas. 2011;40:352–8.

Shiokawa M, Kodama Y, Yoshimura K, Kawanami C, Mimura J, Yamashita Y, Asada M, Kikuyama M, Okabe Y, Inokuma T, Ohana M, Kokuryu H, Takeda K, Tsuji Y, Minami R, Sakuma Y, Kuriyama K, Ota Y, TANABE W, Maruno T, Kurita A, Sawai Y, Uza N, Watanabe T, Haga H, Chiba T. Risk of cancer in patients with autoimmune pancreatitis. Am J Gastroenterol. 2013;108:610–7.

Shiokawa M, Kodama Y, Sekiguchi K, Kuwada T, Tomono T, Kuriyama K, Yamazaki H, Morita T, Marui S, Sogabe Y, Kakiuchi N, Matsumori T, Mima A, Nishikawa Y, Ueda T, Tsuda M, Yamauchi Y, Sakuma Y, Maruno T, Uza N, Tsuruyama T, Mimori T, Seno H, Chiba T. Laminin 511 is a target antigen in autoimmune pancreatitis. Sci Transl Med. 2018;10:eaaq0997.

Sjogren I, Wengle B, Korsgren M. Primary sclerosing cholangitis associated with fibrosis of the submandibular glands and the pancreas. Acta Med Scand. 1979;205:139–41.

Smith MP, Loe RH. Sclerosing cholangitis; review of recent case reports and associated diseases and four new cases. Am J Surg. 1965;110:239–46.

Sood S, Fossard DP, Shorrock K. Chronic sclerosing pancreatitis in Sjogren's syndrome: a case report. Pancreas. 1995;10:419–21.

Stone JH, Khosroshahi A, Deshpande V, Chan JK, Heathcote JG, Aalberse R, Azumi A, Bloch DB, Brugge WR, Carruthers MN, Cheuk W, Cornell L, Castillo CF, Ferry JA, Forcione D, Kloppel G, Hamilos DL, Kamisawa T, Kasashima S, Kawa S, Kawano M, Masaki Y, Notohara K, Okazaki K, Ryu JK, Saeki T, Sahani D, Sato Y, Smyrk T, Stone JR, Takahira M, Umehara H, Webster G, Yamamoto M, Yi E, Yoshino T, Zamboni G, Zen Y, Chari S. Recommendations for the nomenclature of IgG4-related disease and its individual organ system manifestations. Arthritis Rheum. 2012;64:3061–7.

Sugumar A, Levy MJ, Kamisawa T, Webster GJ, Kim MH, Enders F, Amin Z, Baron TH, Chapman MH, Church NI, Clain JE, Egawa N, Johnson GJ, Okazaki K, Pearson RK, Pereira SP, Petersen BT, READ S, Sah RP, Sandanayake NS, Takahashi N, Topazian MD, Uchida K, Vege SS, Chari ST. Endoscopic retrograde pancreatography criteria to diagnose autoimmune pancreatitis: an international multicentre study. Gut. 2011;60:666–70.

Suzuki K, Itoh S, Nagasaka T, Ogawa H, Ota T, Naganawa S. CT findings in autoimmune pancreatitis: assessment using multiphase contrast-enhanced multisection CT. Clin Radiol. 2010;65:735–43.

Takahashi N, Fletcher JG, Hough DM, Fidler JL, Kawashima A, Mandrekar JN, Chari ST. Autoimmune pancreatitis: differentiation from pancreatic carcinoma and normal pancreas on the basis of enhancement characteristics at dual-phase CT. AJR Am J Roentgenol. 2009;193:479–84.

Uchida K, Okazaki K, Konishi Y, Ohana M, Takakuwa H, Hajiro K, Chiba T. Clinical analysis of autoimmune-related pancreatitis. Am J Gastroenterol. 2000;95:2788–94.

Waldram R, Kopelman H, Tsantoulas D, Williams R. Chronic pancreatitis, sclerosing cholangitis, and sicca complex in two siblings. Lancet. 1975;1:550–2.

Wallace ZS, Deshpande V, Stone JH. Ophthalmic manifestations of IgG4-related disease: single-center experience and literature review. Semin Arthritis Rheum. 2014;43:806–17.

Watanabe T, Maruyama M, Ito T, Fujinaga Y, Ozaki Y, Maruyama M, Kodama R, Muraki T, Hamano H, Arakura N, Kadoya M, Suzuki S, Komatsu M, Shimojo H, Notohara K, Uchida M, Kawa S. Clinical features of a new disease concept, IgG4-related thyroiditis. Scand J Rheumatol. 2013;42:325–30.

Yang DH, Kim KW, Kim TK, Park SH, Kim SH, Kim MH, Lee SK, Kim AY, Kim PN, HA HK, Lee MG.

Autoimmune pancreatitis: radiologic findings in 20 patients. Abdom Imaging. 2006;31:94–102.

Yoshida K, Toki F, Takeuchi T, Watanabe S, Shiratori K, Hayashi N. Chronic pancreatitis caused by an autoimmune abnormality. Proposal of the concept of autoimmune pancreatitis. Dig Dis Sci. 1995;40:1561–8.

Zamboni G, Luttges J, Capelli P, Frulloni L, Cavallini G, Pederzoli P, Leins A, Longnecker D, Kloppel G. Histopathological features of diagnostic and clinical relevance in autoimmune pancreatitis: a study on 53 resection specimens and 9 biopsy specimens. Virchows Arch. 2004;445:552–63.

Zen Y, Harada K, Sasaki M, Sato Y, Tsuneyama K, Haratake J, Kurumaya H, Katayanagi K, Masuda S, Niwa H, Morimoto H, Miwa A, Uchiyama A, Portmann BC, Nakanuma Y. IgG4-related sclerosing cholangitis with and without hepatic inflammatory pseudotumor, and sclerosing pancreatitis-associated sclerosing cholangitis: do they belong to a spectrum of sclerosing pancreatitis? Am J Surg Pathol. 2004;28:1193–203.

Zen Y, Kasashima S, Inoue D. Retroperitoneal and aortic manifestations of immunoglobulin G4-related disease. Semin Diagn Pathol. 2012;29:212–8.

Zhang L, Smyrk TC. Autoimmune pancreatitis and IgG4-related systemic diseases. Int J Clin Exp Pathol. 2010;3:491–504.

Zhang L, Notohara K, Levy MJ, Chari ST, Smyrk TC. IgG4-positive plasma cell infiltration in the diagnosis of autoimmune pancreatitis. Mod Pathol. 2007;20:23–8.